Fundamentals of X-ray Imaging

Dibya Prakash • Rahul Pratap Kotian

Fundamentals of X-ray Imaging

Basic Principles, Quality Control, Clinical Applications, and Safety

Springer

Dibya Prakash
Advanced Centre for Treatment,
Research and Education in Cancer
(ACTREC)
Tata Memorial Centre, Department of
Atomic Energy
Kharghar, Navi Mumbai, Maharashtra,
India

Rahul Pratap Kotian
Customer Lifetime Success Manager
(MRI) - META
Philips Middle East & Turkey & Africa
Dubai, United Arab Emirates

ISBN 978-981-96-7327-8 ISBN 978-981-96-7328-5 (eBook)
https://doi.org/10.1007/978-981-96-7328-5

This Springer imprint is published by the registered company Springer Nature Singapore Pte Ltd.
The registered company address is: 152 Beach Road, #21-01/04 Gateway East, Singapore 189721, Singapore

Preface

This textbook is conceptualized as a single, comprehensive reference that meticulously covers all X-ray imaging modalities, catering to a wide spectrum of readers, from diploma students to doctoral candidates in radiology and nuclear medicine, as well as educators, medical physicists, clinicians, and other healthcare professionals. The book presents underlying physics, operational principles, quality control measures, and safety protocols in a manner that is both accessible and thorough. The use of clear and simple language ensures that complex concepts are easily understandable meeting the diverse needs of its audience. The authors have endeavored to address questions that commonly arise in the minds of students and practitioners. To nurture curiosity and critical thinking, the manuscript is, in many places, written in a question-and-answer format, encouraging readers to actively engage with the content and stimulate their own thought process. In each section, the historical aspect of a particular discovery has been discussed in detail to further inspire the thought process behind that discovery and encourage new achievements. The chapters have been crafted so that readers feel they are reading a storybook or novel, allowing them to enjoy the journey of learning science in a more engaging and immersive manner.

The textbook is organized into 12 chapters, starting with foundational concepts and advancing to specialized topics such as X-ray imaging, CT, mammography, fluoroscopy, dental radiography, and hybrid imaging. It serves as a practical reference for professionals, covering routine tasks like X-ray quality control, radiation safety, and patient care. It also addresses the planning and design of radiology departments, with a focus on global standards, safety, and pediatric considerations. Each chapter includes multiple-choice, short-answer, and long-answer questions to support students' exam preparation and reinforce learning.

Chapter 1 provides a thorough foundation in basic radiation science, which is essential for understanding the more advanced concepts discussed in subsequent chapters. Divided into seven sections, it begins with an atomic structure, starting from the evolution of atomic theory and introducing fundamental concepts essential for understanding the nature of matter. The chapter then digs into the principles of electricity and magnetism, explaining how these forces are interconnected and their significance in radiation science. Following this, the book explains radiation quantities and units, providing a clear understanding of how radiation is measured and quantified. The interaction of radiation with matter is another area covered, detailing the various ways in which radiation behaves when it encounters different materials. The fifth section explains the historical evolution of X-rays, its production, X-ray spectrum, hard and soft X-rays, clinical applications of X-rays and its hazards. The sixth section talks about production of radionuclides, highlighting the processes involved and their significance in medical and scientific applications. Finally, the chapter addresses the concept of radioactivity, discussing its discovery, the different modes of radioactive decay, and its applications.

Chapter 2 begins with an overview of X-ray technology, goes in detail about the historical development of X-ray tubes from Wilhelm Conrad Roentgen's groundbreaking discovery to the rapid advancements that integrated X-ray technology into medical practice. Significant milestones in X-ray tube technology are highlighted, including the evolution from early Crookes tubes to modern innovations like the multi-source X-ray tube and advancements in cathode technology for spectral CT. The basic principles of X-ray tube operation are thoroughly explained, followed by a detailed examination of the different types of X-ray tubes, such as stationary and rotating anode tubes, as well as specialized tubes for various medical applications. The components used in X-ray production are explored in depth, providing insights into the construction and functionality of key parts like the cathode, anode, tube housing, and heat dissipation systems. The chapter then explains manufacturing process of X-ray tubes, ensuring a comprehensive understanding of how these critical devices are produced, tested, and maintained. The chapter also discusses routine quality control measures, safety protocols, and the common causes of X-ray tube failures, along with practical recommendations to maximize tube life. Advancements in X-ray tube technology are highlighted, showcasing innovations that have enhanced performance, power, and safety.

Chapter 3 explains digital radiography systems, focusing on their principles of operation, clinical applications, and the importance of quality control. The chapter is divided into two main sections: computed radiography (CR) and digital radiography (DR). The first section begins with an introduction to computed radiography, tracing its historical development and the factors that should be considered when planning a CR installation. It then explores the working principles of CR, highlighting its benefits and the key instrumentation involved. The chapter also covers the dynamic range of CR, its clinical applications, and the advantages it offers over traditional radiography systems. The discussion on CR concludes with an examination of common image artifacts and the quality control measures necessary to ensure optimal performance, including an overview of top CR manufacturers. The second section shifts focus to digital radiography systems, offering a comprehensive overview of their history, classification, and the major components of a DR imaging system. The chapter explains the technology behind DR flat panel detectors (FPDs), distinguishing between direct and indirect detector technologies. It also explores the advantages of FPDs, the role of charged-coupled devices (CCDs), and the classification of various detector types. The working principles of both indirect and direct flat panel detectors are thoroughly examined, along with a detailed discussion on CCD and Thin Film Transistor (TFT) detectors. The clinical applications of DR are highlighted, showcasing how this advanced technology is utilized in medical imaging. The chapter also addresses common artifacts associated with flat panel detectors, offering insights into their types, causes, and methods for mitigation. Quality control in DR is emphasized, with practical guidance on the tools and equipment needed to implement QC tests effectively. The chapter concludes with a look at recent technological advancements in digital radiography, ensuring readers are up-to-date with the latest innovations in the field.

Chapter 4 focuses on mammography, detailing the essential physics, principles of operation, quality control, and safety protocols integral to this imaging technique. It begins with an introduction and historical overview, tracing the evolution of mammography and its technological advancements. Understanding breast anatomy is also emphasized, laying the foundation for accurate imaging. The chapter then explores the key components of mammography equipment, including the anode heel effect, tube housing, filters, compression devices, and digital mammography technology. Special attention is given to digital breast tomosynthesis (DBT), discussing its principles, advantages, and limitations. Quality control in mammography is thoroughly covered, from the history of QC practices to specific tests for both 2D and DBT imaging. The chapter outlines essential QC procedures, including the evaluation of image quality, AEC performance, and spatial resolution, ensuring high standards are maintained in mammography.

Chapter 5 explores the essential aspects of fluoroscopy, focusing on its physics, operational principles, and the critical quality control measures necessary for effective imaging. It begins with an overview of the evolution of fluoroscopic imaging, tracing its development from early techniques to modern advancements, and includes some lesser-known historical insights. Key topics include the special demands of fluoroscopic imaging and its mechanism of action. The chapter also delves into fluoroscopy instrumentation, highlighting the role of image intensifiers and radiation protection devices in ensuring patient safety. The clinical applications of fluoroscopy are discussed, along with the principles of digital fluoroscopy and the working mechanisms of various flat panel detectors. Radiation dose considerations and protection measures are emphasized to ensure safe practice. The chapter also covers room design for fluoroscopy, ensuring optimal setup for effective imaging. It addresses the importance of image quality control, technological advancements in the field, and common image-related artifacts. Quality assurance (QA) and quality control (QC) practices are also outlined to maintain high standards in fluoroscopic imaging.

Chapter 6 provides a comprehensive exploration of computed tomography (CT) with a focus on its physics, operational principles, quality control, and safety. It begins with a historical overview of CT, tracing its evolution from the earliest scanners to the cutting-edge technologies used today. The chapter covers the different generations of CT scanners, including the latest innovations such as dual-source CT and photon-counting CT, explaining their principles, benefits, and clinical applications. Key concepts such as Hounsfield Units, the Beer-Lambert Law, and the technological components of CT scanners—gantries, X-ray tubes, and data acquisition systems—are thoroughly discussed. The chapter also delves into CT image reconstruction methods, including Fourier transform and iterative reconstruction techniques. It provides a detailed analysis of the various types of artifacts that can occur in CT images, both 2D and 3D, and offers practical guidance on their prevention and correction. Quality control procedures for CT are emphasized, with a focus on the importance of regular testing, calibration, and dosimetry to ensure accurate and safe imaging. The chapter also addresses the clinical applications of CT across a wide range of medical fields, including cardiac imaging, oncology, and guided biopsies. Additionally, it covers CT room design and safety considerations, with an emphasis on dose reduction techniques and adherence to regulatory guidelines.

Chapter 7 introduces hybrid imaging technologies, providing an in-depth exploration of their physics, operational principles, and quality control requirements. The chapter begins with an introduction to hybrid imaging, explaining the rationale behind combining different imaging modalities and highlighting the limitations of standalone modalities such as PET, SPECT, CT, and MR imaging. It discusses the advantages of hybrid imaging systems, such as improved diagnostic accuracy and enhanced clinical applications. It provides a detailed explanation on positron emission tomography (PET) and single photon emission computed tomography (SPECT) technology, covering its historical development, fundamental principles, and clinical applications, including their significance in diagnosing and managing various diseases. A detailed procedural explanation of quality control is provided with full of images and techniques so that physicist/technologist understand the logic of QC procedure and perform it on ground. The chapter also discuss the technical challenges, advantages, and clinical applications of these hybrid systems.

Chapter 8 explains the field of dental radiography, focusing on its physics, operational principles, quality control, and safety. It begins with an overview of the history of dental radiography, tracing its evolution from the earliest X-rays to the modern digital techniques used today. The chapter covers the different types of dental radiographic techniques, including intraoral and extraoral imaging, and discusses the advantages and limitations of each. The technical components of dental radiography, such as X-ray tubes, film holders, and digital sensors, are thoroughly explained. The chapter also addresses the principles of panoramic radiography, cephalometric analysis, and cone-beam computed tomography (CBCT) in dental imaging. Quality control procedures for dental radiography are emphasized, with a focus on the importance of regular testing, calibration, and adherence to radiation protection guidelines to ensure accurate and safe imaging. The chapter also covers the clinical applications of dental radiography, including its use in diagnosis, treatment planning, and monitoring of dental and maxillofacial conditions.

Chapter 9 addresses the critical aspects of radiology department planning, offering a comprehensive guide to the design, construction, and operation of radiology facilities. It begins with an introduction to the key considerations in site planning, including the selection of a suitable location, the layout of the department, and the importance of ensuring adequate space for both current operations and future expansion. The chapter covers the regulatory requirements for radiology department design, including building codes, radiation shielding, and environmental considerations. The principles of radiation protection are thoroughly explained, with guidance on how to incorporate these principles into the design of the department. The chapter also addresses the specific needs of different types of radiology facilities, including outpatient clinics, hospitals, and specialized imaging centers. The importance of workflow optimization is emphasized, with practical advice on how to design a department that supports efficient patient flow, staff productivity, and high standards of patient care. The chapter also covers the selection and installation of radiology equipment, including considerations for electrical, mechanical, and IT infrastructure.

Chapter 10 is a practical guide on radiation safety to radiological professionals for the safety of patients as well as practitioners. It provides an in-depth explanation of radiation protection principles, dose terminology, and best practices for ensuring safe and effective operation. The chapter begins with an introduction to the basic principles of radiation protection, including the ALARA (As Low As Reasonably Achievable) principle; the concepts of justification, optimization, and dose limits; and the importance of understanding the risks associated with radiation exposure. The chapter then covers the various types of radiation protection devices, including lead aprons, thyroid shields, and protective barriers, and discusses their proper use and maintenance. A special attention is given on how to handle female patients, and as female radiation workers, what precautions are supposed to be followed. A number of questions have been answered which can arise in the mind of radiation worker related to pregnancy and foetal protection. The importance of dose reduction techniques is emphasized, with practical guidance on how to minimize patient and staff exposure during imaging procedures. The chapter also addresses the regulatory requirements for radiation safety, including the roles and responsibilities of radiation safety officers, the importance of maintaining accurate records, and the procedures for reporting radiation incidents.

Chapter 11 focuses on field of pediatric radiology, exploring the unique challenges and considerations associated with imaging children. The chapter begins with an introduction to the anatomical and physiological differences between children and adults, highlighting how these differences impact the selection and performance of imaging procedures. The chapter covers the various types of imaging techniques used in pediatric radiology, including X-ray, ultrasound, CT, MRI, and nuclear medicine, and discusses the advantages and limitations of each. The importance of radiation protection in pediatric imaging is emphasized, with practical guidance on how to minimize radiation exposure while still obtaining high-quality diagnostic images. The chapter also addresses the specific challenges associated with imaging infants and young children, including the need for sedation, the importance of effective communication with both the child and their parents, and the role of child life specialists in supporting the imaging process.

Chapter 12 concludes the textbook by focusing on the critical role of nursing care in radiology, highlighting the importance of patient care, infection control, and emergency protocols in the imaging environment. The chapter begins with an introduction to the role of the radiology nurse, outlining their responsibilities in patient preparation, procedure assistance, and post-procedure care. The chapter covers the principles of patient care in radiology, including the importance of communication, patient education, and the management of anxiety and pain. The chapter also addresses the specific infection control challenges associated with radiology procedures, providing guidance on how to prevent the transmission of infectious agents in the imaging environment. The importance of emergency protocols is emphasized, with practical advice on how to respond to medical emergencies that may occur during imaging procedures, including the management of contrast media reactions, the handling of radiopharmaceuticals, and the provision of basic life support.

We have strived hard to provide valuable content to the radiological and nuclear medicine community, and hope our efforts will serve as a helpful resource. It is our sincere hope that this work benefits and supports the broader field of radiology.

Kharghar, Navi Mumbai, Maharashtra, India Dibya Prakash
Dubai, United Arab Emirates Rahul Pratap Kotian

Acknowledgments

Writing this book has been a journey of discovery, perseverance, and growth. It would not have been possible without the unwavering support and love of those closest to me.

First and foremost, I wish to express my deepest gratitude to my wife, Mausam Singh. Her constant encouragement, patience, and understanding have been the bedrock of my efforts. Her unwavering belief in me has been a source of strength and inspiration throughout this project.

To my beloved sons, Shwetank and Saanidhya, thank you for your boundless love and joy. You have motivated me to strive for excellence, and I hope this work reflects the values of dedication and hard work that I wish to pass on to you.

In loving memory of my mother, Late Ramavati Singh, whose nurturing love, strength, and wisdom continue to guide me daily. Her sacrifices and principles have been the foundation of my life and career. I am forever indebted to my father, Indrajeet Singh, whose wisdom and guidance have shaped me into the person I am today. My deepest gratitude also goes to my elder brother, Dr. Shashi Prakash, for his invaluable intellectual guidance and encouragement. To my younger brother, Mani Prakash, thank you for your unwavering support and for always being there whenever needed. Your belief in me has been a source of great comfort.

I extend my heartfelt thanks to Dr. Rahul Kotian, my esteemed co-author. Despite facing significant health and personal challenges, his dedication and support were instrumental in completing this book.

I also wish to acknowledge Sonveer for his exceptional skill in figure drawing, which has greatly enhanced the quality and clarity of this book. Your work has brought my ideas to life, and I am sincerely grateful.

To all those mentioned and others whose names may not appear here but who have contributed in various ways, I offer my heartfelt thanks. This book is as much a product of your support as it is of my own efforts.

Dibya Prakash

I want to express my deepest gratitude to my wife, Disha Kotian, for her unwavering support and encouragement throughout the journey of writing this book.

Her belief in me never wavered, even in moments when I doubted myself. She was my constant source of inspiration, providing me with the strength and motivation to keep going. This book would not have been possible without her patience, love, and understanding. For all the late nights, the endless conversations, and her steadfast presence by my side, I am forever grateful. This book is as much hers as it is mine.

I would like to extend my deepest appreciation to my co-author, Dibya Prakash, whose collaboration and dedication made this book possible. Working together has been an incredible experience, and your insights, creativity, and commitment have enriched this project beyond measure. Your expertise and hard work have been invaluable, and I am grateful for the many hours of discussion, revision, and mutual support that went into crafting this book. Thank you for being a true partner in this endeavor.

I would like to express my sincere gratitude to my friends, Sharath S., Assistant Professor at Manipal College of Health Professions, Manipal Academy of Higher Education, and Adithya G. Rao, Assistant Professor in Medical Imaging at Yenepoya University whose steadfast support and encouragement were instrumental in bringing this book to life. Thank you for being my sounding boards, cheerleaders, and sources of motivation throughout this journey. Your belief in me, whether through thoughtful advice, constructive feedback, or simply being there when I needed it most, has meant the world to me. I am incredibly fortunate to have friends like you, and this book reflects the unwavering support you've shown me.

Last but not the least, I want to extend my heartfelt thanks to my family for their unwavering support and encouragement throughout the writing of this book. To my sibling Dr. Sneha, your patience, understanding, and love have been my greatest source of strength. You've been there for me through every step of this journey, offering kind words, thoughtful advice, and, most importantly, your belief in me. This book is a testament to the love and support you've always given me, and I am forever grateful.

Dr. Rahul Pratap Kotian

Contents

Principle of Radiation Science: Basic Physics, the Interaction of Radiation with Matter, and Radiation Production

1

Learning Objectives

Introduction
- Why is radiation classified as an electromagnetic wave?

Section A: Atom and Its Structure
- Historical discovery of the atom
  - Ancient Indian philosophy.
  - Greek philosophy.
  - Sixteenth century onward.
  - Dalton's atomic theory.
  - Atomic nomenclature and symbols.
  - IUPAC and standardized naming.
  - Table of elements with atomic numbers 1 to 118: Etymology, discovery, and discoverer information.
- **Atomic Models**
  - Thomson's atomic model.
  - Rutherford's atomic model.
  - Bohr's atomic model.
  - The discovery of the neutron.
  - Modern atomic model.
  - Size of atom vs size of the nucleus.
  - Quantum numbers.
  - Pauli's exclusion principle.
  - The Aufbau principle.
  - Hund's rule.
- **Terms Related to Atomic Theory**
  - Atomic number.
  - Atomic mass.
  - Nuclear notations.
  - Isotopes.
  - Isomers.
  - Isotones.
  - Isobars.
  - Binding energy.
  - Nuclear stability.

Section B: Fundamental Concepts of Electricity and Magnetism
- Electricity.
- Unit of electricity.
- Coulomb's law and Lorentz force.
- Concept of mAs used in X-ray machines.
- Concept of voltage.
- Electric power.
- Magnetism.
- An electric field is always associated with the magnetic field.
- Electromagnetic radiation and electromagnetic spectrum.

Section C: Radiation Quantities and Units
- Exposure, "X".
- Exposure rate, "X^0".
- Dose and absorbed dose "D".
- Dose rate.
- Equivalent dose.
- Effective dose.
- Kerma, "K" (kinetic energy released in material).

Section D: Interaction of Radiation with Matter
- Charged particle interaction.
- Photon interaction with the medium.
  - Photoelectric effect.
  - Compton scattering.
  - Pair production.
  - Rayleigh scattering.
  - Auger effect.
  - Photodisintegration.
- Interaction of neutron with matter.

Section E: Production of X-rays
- Historical background.
- Interaction of electron with the target.
- The process of production of X-rays.
- X-ray spectrum.
- X-ray properties and energy ranges —Soft and hard X-rays.
- Some of the common uses of soft X-rays include:
- Other uses of hard X-rays apart from medical imaging.
- Clinical X-ray applications, hazards, and significance in diagnostic radiography.
- Hazards from the X-rays.
- Significance of X-rays in diagnostic radiography.

Section F: Production of Radionuclides
- Reactor-based.
- Cyclotron-based.
- Generator-based.

Section G: Radioactivity
- Discovery of radioactivity.
- Unit of radioactivity.
- Radioactive decay equation and half-life.
- Modes of radioactive decay.

D. Prakash, R. P. Kotian, *Fundamentals of X-ray Imaging*,
https://doi.org/10.1007/978-981-96-7328-5_1

1.1 Introduction

Radiation is a form of energy that originates from a source and propagates through space. It exists in two main forms: electromagnetic radiation and particle radiation. Electromagnetic radiation travels at the speed of light and exhibits both wavelike and particle-like properties. It consists of oscillating electric and magnetic fields that are perpendicular to each other and to the direction of propagation, forming what is known as an "electromagnetic wave." In contrast, particle radiation consists of subatomic particles, such as alpha and beta particles, which move at speeds lower than that of light, depending on their energy.

We are constantly exposed to radiation from our surroundings, including the air we breathe, the food we consume, the water we drink, and even the homes we live in. Everything around us contains some level of radiation; even our bodies naturally harbor radioactive elements such as potassium-40, carbon-14, and radium-226, which circulate in our blood and are present in our bones [1, 2]. The sun, the primary energy source for our planet, emits radiation that sustains life. Since radiation is an inescapable part of our environment, the best approach is to understand it and its effects.

Radiation is a broad term, and it is classified based on its interaction with matter, primarily as ionizing and non-ionizing radiation. Ionizing radiation has enough energy to remove electrons from atoms, creating charged particles (ions). Examples include X-rays, gamma rays, and particle radiation such as alpha, beta, and neutron radiation. In contrast, non-ionizing radiation has lower energy and cannot ionize atoms, though it can transfer energy in the form of excitation. Examples include radio waves, microwaves, visible light, ultraviolet (UV, noting that high-energy UV, such as ultravoilet C (UVC), can cause ionization in specific cases), and infrared radiation.

> ? Why does radiation called as electromagnetic wave despite there is no electric charge or magnetism in it and how they carry momentum despite there is no mass?

Electromagnetic radiation, despite having no electric charge or magnetism in the classical sense, is still called an electromagnetic wave because it consists of oscillating electric and magnetic fields that propagate through space. These fields are inherently linked; according to Maxwell's equations, a changing electric field generates a magnetic field, and a changing magnetic field generates an electric field. This continuous interaction allows electromagnetic waves to travel even through a vacuum without requiring a medium. The most common example of electromagnetic radiation in daily life is sunlight, which consists of energy packets called photons. These photons do not have mass or charge but still possess both energy and momentum, exhibiting both wavelike and particle-like behavior.

The energy of a photon is given by $E = h\nu$, where h (Planck's constant) is $6.62607015 \times 10^{-34}$ $m^2 \cdot kg/s$ and ν is the frequency of the radiation. Alternatively, since the speed of light in a vacuum, c (approximately 3×10^8 m/s), is related to the wavelength λ and frequency by $c = \lambda\nu$, we can also express the energy as:

$$E = \frac{hc}{\lambda}$$

Despite being massless, photons carry momentum, which seems counterintuitive in classical physics where momentum is defined as the product of mass and velocity. However, in quantum mechanics, the momentum of a photon is determined by its energy and wavelength. The momentum of a photon is given by.

$$p = \frac{E}{c}$$

$$\text{Substituting } E = h\nu, \text{ we get:}$$

$$p = \frac{h}{\lambda}$$

This relationship shows that the momentum of a photon is directly proportional to its frequency and inversely proportional to its wavelength. This fundamental concept has been experimentally confirmed through the photoelectric effect and Compton scattering, reinforcing the idea that photons, though massless, do indeed carry momentum.

To visualize electromagnetic radiation, consider thermal imaging. In movies and scientific videos, we often see infrared thermal images of the human body. These images reveal that we constantly emit infrared radiation (Figs. 1.1 and 1.2), which is a type of electromagnetic wave. Although invisible to the naked eye, infrared waves can be detected using thermal cameras, allowing us to see the heat emitted by objects. Now, looking at a larger scale, the Sun also emits electromagnetic waves, which reach us in the form of sunlight.

A close-up image of the Sun's surface (Fig. 1.3) illustrates the broad spectrum of elec-

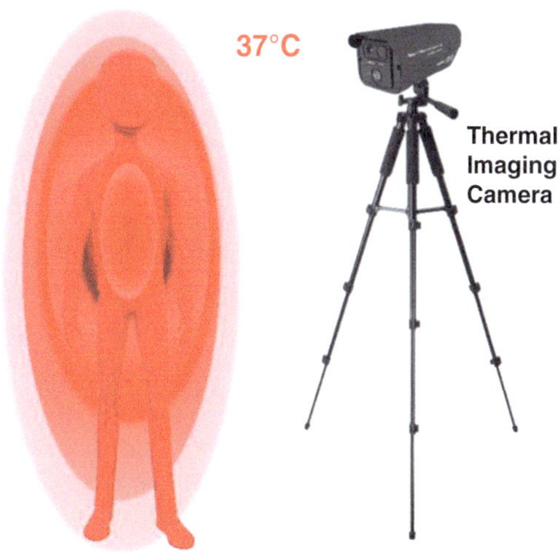

Fig. 1.1 Thermal radiation from the human body and detection by a special thermal imaging camera

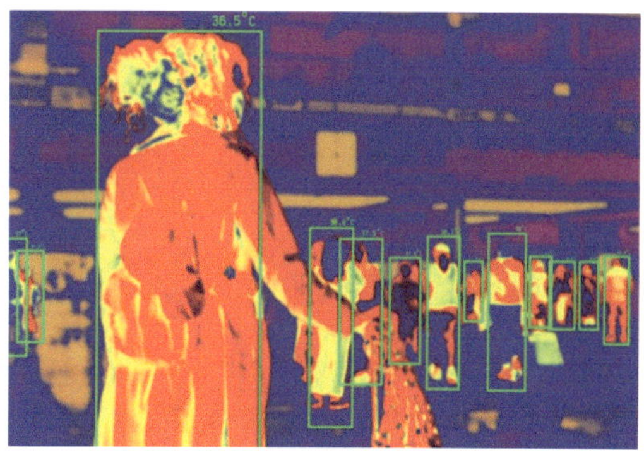

Fig. 1.2 Thermal image of the human. (Image courtesy: Designed by Freepik)

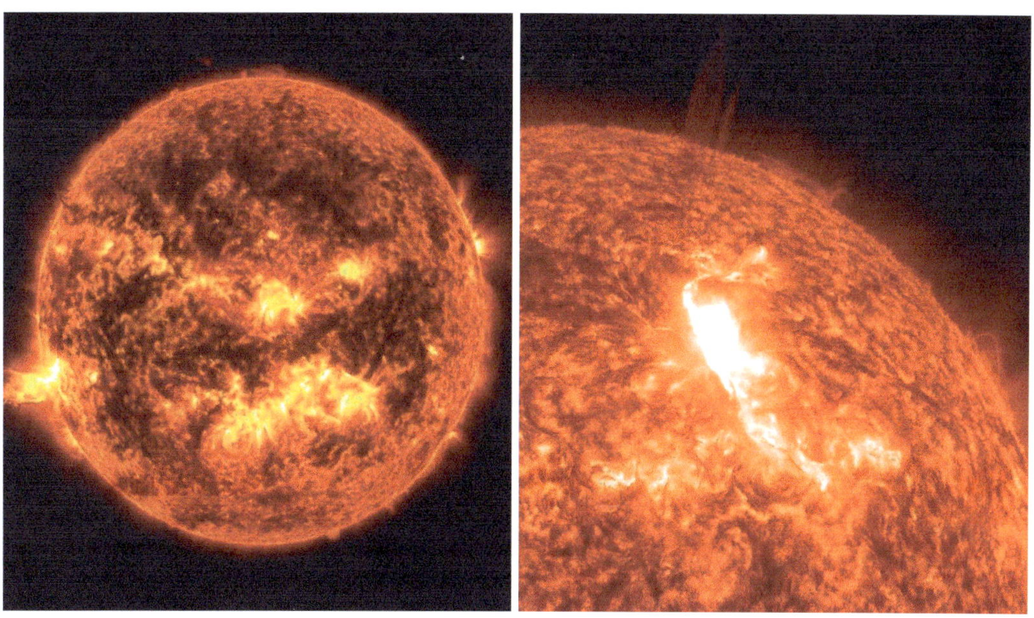

Fig. 1.3 Close-up images of the sun. (Image courtesy NASA)

tromagnetic radiation it produces, including visible light, ultraviolet (UV) radiation, and infrared (IR) radiation. The Sun's surface temperature, around 5500 °C (9,932 F), determines the range of wavelengths it emits. The core temperature, much higher at approximately 15 million degrees Celsius (27 million degrees Fahrenheit), results in nuclear fusion reactions that generate an even broader range of radiation.

Everything in the universe, from our bodies to the Sun, is composed of atoms. Atoms contain charged particles such as electrons and protons, and any charged particle is always associated with an electric field. When a charged particle accelerates, it generates a changing magnetic field, as explained by Maxwell's theory. A key principle of electromagnetism states that a changing electric field creates a magnetic field, and a changing magnetic field, in turn, induces an electric field. If a charged particle is accelerated, it disturbs the surrounding electric and magnetic fields, producing electromagnetic waves that propagate through space at the speed of light. This interdependence of electric and magnetic fields is the essence of electromagnetic radiation (Fig. 1.4). The generated waves continue to spread through space due to this mutual disturbance process, forming self-sustaining electromagnetic waves.

Electromagnetic waves are ubiquitous, as they are generated whenever charged particles move, accelerate, or change direction. Within atoms, electrons are bound in discrete energy levels, and any excitation or disturbance can lead to electromagnetic wave generation. When an atom vibrates, it causes its electron cloud to oscillate, similar to how a stretched rubber band vibrates when disturbed. This results in continuous electromagnetic wave emission, which becomes more energetic as the object's temperature increases. For example, the human body, with a temperature of about 37 °C, constantly emits infrared radiation. While this radiation is invisible to the naked eye, thermal cameras (Fig. 1.2) can detect and visualize it.

Depending on how a particle accelerates, electromagnetic waves can vary in energy. These waves are classified into different categories based on their frequency, forming the electromagnetic spectrum. Visible light, which we perceive as different colors in a rainbow, is only a small fraction of the spectrum. Beyond visible light, there exist many other types of electromagnetic waves, such as infrared, ultraviolet, radio waves, X-rays, and gamma rays. The vast majority of these radiations are invisible to us, but technological advancements allow us to detect and utilize them for various applications. Examples

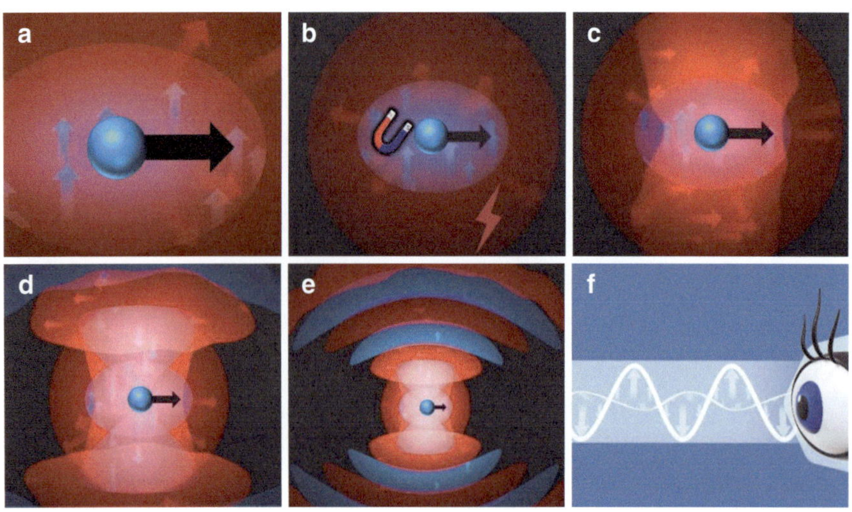

Fig. 1.4 Formation of electromagnetic waves: (**a**) movement of a charged particle, (**b**) formation of the electric and magnetic field, (**c–e**) propagation of electromagnetic waves, (**f**) the EM waves seen by us

include medical imaging, microwave ovens, telecommunications systems, and space telescopes.

In addition to movement-induced radiation, electromagnetic waves can also be generated by atomic disturbances such as excitation and ionization. When an electron absorbs energy, it moves to a higher energy state within an atom. This process is called excitation. When the electron returns to its ground state, it releases the excess energy as electromagnetic radiation. The frequency of this radiation depends on the energy gap between the excited and ground states, resulting in emissions ranging from infrared to ultraviolet light. Ionization, on the other hand, occurs when an atom loses one or more electrons, forming an ion. This process can generate high-energy electromagnetic radiation, such as X-rays or gamma rays, depending on the energy involved.

Both excitation and ionization occur naturally in many environments. In the upper atmosphere, solar radiation causes these processes, leading to the emission of various types of electromagnetic radiation. In controlled laboratory settings, excitation and ionization are utilized in plasma devices, laser technologies, and medical applications such as radiation therapy and spectroscopy. The ability to manipulate electromagnetic radiation has led to groundbreaking advancements in science and technology, from communication systems to advanced medical treatments.

To understand the above concept in detail, we must understand the atomic structure and other related concepts given below.

1.2 Section A: The Evolution of Atomic Theory: Historical Discoveries, Models, and Terminologies

As discussed in the previous section, an atom comprises a cloud of electrons and a nucleus at the center, where electrons revolve around the nucleus, containing protons and neutrons. Now if we think with a common understanding, *electrons are negatively charged whereas nucleus is positively charged, technically they should attract each other and combine, and the atom should collapse, whereas in reality, the atoms do exist, how?* Also, *since atoms exist and electrons rotate around the nucleus, any idea what would be the speed of these electrons?* Let us find the answer to these questions before proceeding to the historical development of atomic structure.

As per Bohr's atomic model (discussed later), the electrons rotate move in fixed energy states in a fixed energy state at a speed proportional to the distance from the nucleus, and the electrons in higher energy levels have higher speeds. With an approximation and calculation using the Bohr radii formula, the electrons may have a speed of 10^5 m/s to 10^7 m/s. The quantum theory (discussed later) says the speed of an electron cannot be determined with complete accuracy, and there will always be some level of uncertainty.

Electrons do not fall into the nucleus primarily due to their quantum mechanical wavelike behavior, which creates stable, quantized energy levels or "orbitals" around the nucleus. Electron-electron repulsion contributes to stability in multi-electron atoms.

The repulsive forces between electrons are typically between electrons in different orbitals or energy levels rather than within the same orbital. This is because the same wave function describes electrons within the same orbit and therefore share the same spatial probability distribution around the nucleus, so they do not experience significant repulsion from one another. For K-shell electrons, the repulsive force between electrons is weaker than the attractive force of the nucleus, and the electrons are stabilized in their minimum energy state by the wavelike behavior of electrons. This balance of forces prevents the K-shell electrons from falling into the nucleus.

The wavelike behavior of electrons creates standing wave patterns in which the electron wave interferes constructively with itself, leading to stable energy states. The energy levels of these states are quantized, meaning they can only take on specific discrete values. When an electron absorbs energy, it can move to a higher energy level but cannot occupy a position between the energy levels. When electrons return to lower energy level, they emit energy through light or other electromagnetic radiation.

In summary, electrons do not fall into the nucleus primarily due to their quantum mechanical wavelike behavior, which creates stable, quantized energy levels or orbitals. Electron-electron repulsion contributes to stability in multi-electron atoms.

The above concept is to understand it from the current understanding of science and possibly at the advanced level. Let us understand from the beginning and start with the basics.

1.2.1 Historical Discovery of the Atom

1.2.1.1 Ancient Indian Philosophy

The fundamental particle of matter has been researched and explained for ages. The written evidence is found in Maharshi Kanada's "Vaisheshika Darshanam," written between the sixth and second centuries BCE (Before Common Era) [3]. The concept may be even older than that as in ancient Indian philosophy, the concepts were taught from generation to generation in the form of shruti (शुरुति) and smriti (स्मृति), that is, listening and remembering and least in the form of writing with a thought process if things are written, the reader will have their interpretation, and the originality of the concept may be lost. This may be why, despite being such an advanced science, most things could not be carried forward to the forthcoming generation, as Indian civilization was continuously exposed to various invaders for thousands of years. The concept of "listening, remembering, and transferring the knowledge to the next generation by verbal communication" may not work in the modern days, and today we think that whatever is published in journals and can be proven is the only truth. Though oral traditions continue to be an important way of passing down knowledge in many cultures worldwide, modern technology has made it possible to record and preserve these traditions for future generations.

Maharshi Kanada (कणाद) explained the smallest particle of matter with "Darshan" or "Philosophy," considering life as a whole in its entirety. There were "six" philosophies in ancient India, viz., "Sankhya" (संख्या) means "numbers" by Sage Kapila, "Yoga" (योग) by Sage Patanjali, "Nyaya" (न्याय) or "justice" by Gautam Muni, "Vaisheshika" (वैशेषिका) derived from "Vishesh" or "Special" by sage Kanada, "Mimamsa" (मीमांसा) means "profound thought" or "consideration" by sage Jaimini, and "Vedanta" (वेदान्त) means the "conclusion of Vedas"' by Maharshi Ved Vyas and as said "Vaisheshika Darshanam" was one of them.

Maharshi Kanada (कणाद) was known for his philosophy on kana (कण), a Sanskrit word for the fundamental particle of matter. He was also known as Ulūka, Kashyapa, Kaṇabhaksha, and Kaṇabhuj and was an ancient Indian natural scientist and philosopher. He founded the "Vaisheshika School of Indian Philosophy," representing the earliest Indian physics [3]. According to him, every element of creation is composed of atoms (paramanu), which combine to form molecules (Anu). They are eternal, and the empirical material world comprises their numerous combinations [4]. Although in sutras, he mentioned the word "anu" and not the word (Fig. 1.5).

"paramanu," all other scholars of his school talk of "paramanu" as the most fundamental particle of matter [5]. Kanada enumerates real entities irrespective of whether they can be perceived through the sense organs, but they are conceivable by the observer's mind. He explained nine dravyas (द्रव्य) or matter which constitute everything existing in the universe. These nine dravyas are earth, water, fire, air, akasa, time, space, atma, and mind (slok 1.1.5) [5]. These nine dravyas have specific attributes related to them with an understanding of their interaction with the rest of the world [5].

1.2.1.2 Greek Philosophy

Around the same era, ancient Greek Philosophers Leucippus and his famous disciple "Democritus" suggested about 430 BCE that "if we keep on dividing matter, at one stage, it will come when particles obtained cannot be further divided" [6]. Democritus called these indivisible particles atoms [a (not) + temon (cut)]. Democritus thought atoms were uniform, hard, solid, incompressible, and unbroken, traveling endlessly across empty space until coming to a stop and varied qualities of matter depending on atomic

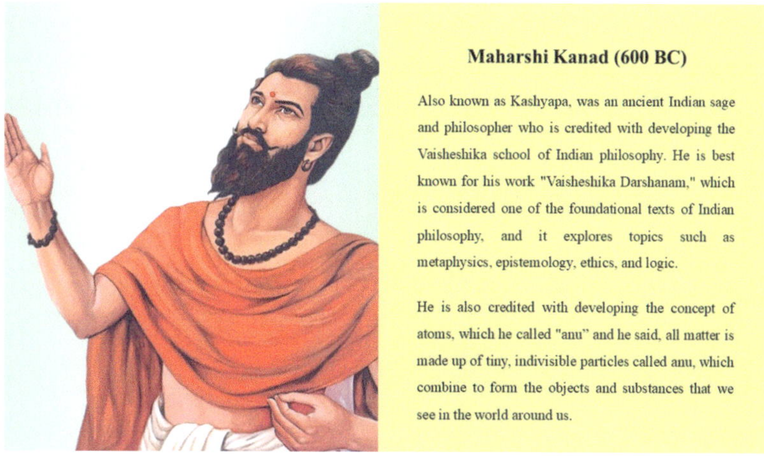
Maharshi Kanad (600 BC)
Also known as Kashyapa, was an ancient Indian sage and philosopher who is credited with developing the Vaisheshika school of Indian philosophy. He is best known for his work "Vaisheshika Darshanam," which is considered one of the foundational texts of Indian philosophy, and it explores topics such as metaphysics, epistemology, ethics, and logic.
He is also credited with developing the concept of atoms, which he called "anu" and he said, all matter is made up of tiny, indivisible particles called anu, which combine to form the objects and substances that we see in the world around us.

Fig. 1.5 Maharshi Kanada, who explained the smallest particle of matter with "Darshan" or "Philosophy" and called it "Anu." (Image Courtesy: Kiddle Encyclopedia, CC BY-SA 4.0)

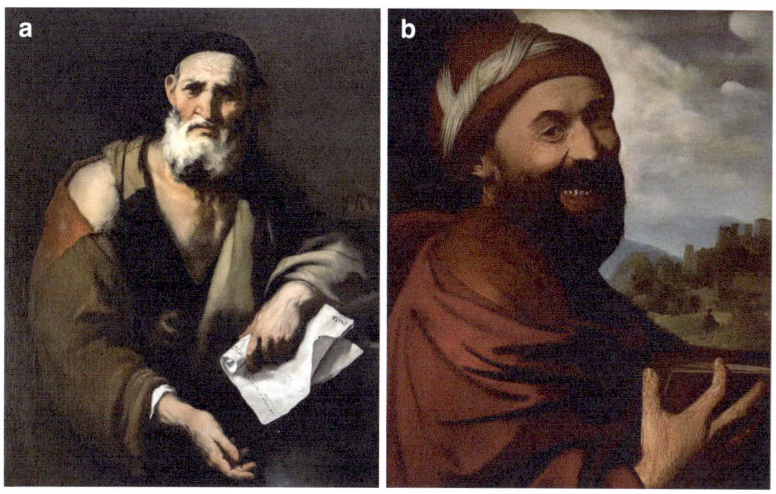
a
b

Fig. 1.6 Ancient Greek Philosophers. (**a**). Leucippus and his disciple. (Image courtesy, Didier Descouens, CC BY-SA 4.0, https://commons.wikimedia.org/w/index.php?curid=89994561). (**b**). "Democritus" (Image courtesy: Dosso and Battista Dossi, World History Encyclopedia, published under Wikipedia license)

size and form variations [6]. All this was based on philosophical assumptions, and no experimental work to validate this could be done until the eighteenth century (Fig. 1.6).

Aristotle (384–322 BCE), who was an ancient Greek philosopher and scientist and was a student of the philosopher Plato, opposed this theory and believed that substances on Earth are made up of five elements as earth, fire, water, air, and ether (worlds of the outer celestial spheres) instead of atoms. As most people adopted his philosophy, Democritus' hypothesis of "substances of Earth is composed of tiny particles known as atoms" was ignored for approximately 2000 years. Finally, Aristotle's theory was disproven, and the modern understanding of the atom does not reflect his ideas (Fig. 1.7).

1.2.1.3 Sixteenth Century Onward

Atomism theme was running through science from the late sixteenth century onward [7]. Anglo-Irish chemist Robert Boyle published his paper in 1662 on gaseous behaviors and expressed his law as an equation $P_1V_1 = P_2V_2$, describing pressure and volume as constant for an ideal gas. From his air-pressure experiments, Boyle commented, "all matter is composed of solid particles which are arranged into molecules to give its different properties." Sir Isaac Newton, in 1704, in his book *Opticks* stated a typical eighteenth-century view of the atom, similar to that of Democritus and Boyle.

In the late eighteenth century, chemists started to understand how chemicals interact with each

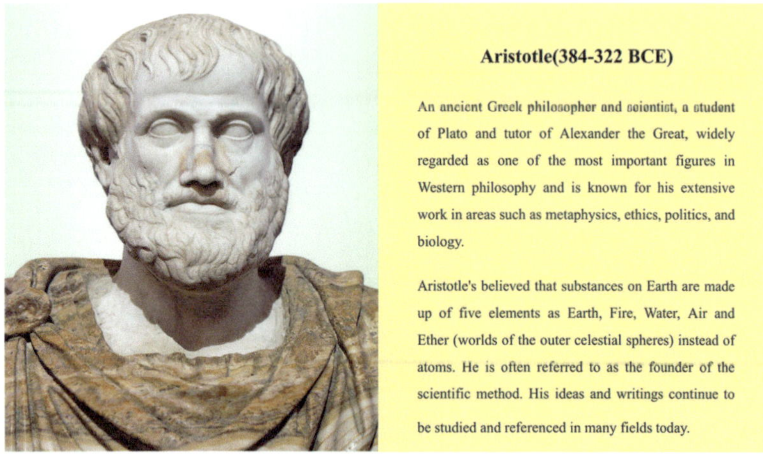
Aristotle(384-322 BCE)
An ancient Greek philosopher and scientist, a student of Plato and tutor of Alexander the Great, widely regarded as one of the most important figures in Western philosophy and is known for his extensive work in areas such as metaphysics, ethics, politics, and biology.
Aristotle's believed that substances on Earth are made up of five elements as Earth, Fire, Water, Air and Ether (worlds of the outer celestial spheres) instead of atoms. He is often referred to as the founder of the scientific method. His ideas and writings continue to be studied and referenced in many fields today.

Fig. 1.7 An ancient Greek philosopher and scientist, Aristotle. (Image Courtesy: Jastrow, CC BY-SA 4.0)

other. Two important laws of chemical combination laid the foundation of chemical sciences and were the trigger for the modern understanding of atomic structure. In 1789, Antoine Lavoisier's published "the law of conservation of mass," which stated that "in chemical reactions, mass can neither be created nor destroyed" [8]. Whereas French chemist Joseph-Louis Proust presented his "law of constant proportions" in 1794 [9]. As per his law, chemical compounds are made up of elements with a fixed ratio by mass.

However, these two laws were just philosophies, and contemporary scientists were looking to provide justifications for these rules. The British chemist John Dalton provided the basic theory of matter and believed that it was presented in 1802–1803 during his lectures at Manchester but was first published in 1805 [7]. He picked the term "atom" from Greek, adopted the matter's divisibility concept, and asserted the tiniest particles of a substance are called atoms. Both the laws, that is, the **law of constant proportions** as well as the **law of conservation of mass,** were explained in Dalton's atomic hypothesis. He presented the first table of relative atomic weights (Table 1.1). These values were based on hydrogen = 1; however, except this, no other element or compound could hold its values with time (Fig. 1.8).

Table 1.1 First Table of relative weights of ultimate particles of gaseous and other bodies by John Dalton, published in 1805 [10]. Table extract from "Biodiversity Heritage Library" published under CC-BY-NC 3.0

Name of the element	Relative atomic weight
Hydrogen	1
Azote (currently known as nitrogen)	4.2
Carbone	4.3
Ammonia	5.2
Oxygen	5.5
Water	6.5
Phosphorus	7.2
Phosphuretted hydrogen	8.2
Nitrous gas	9.3
Ether	9.6
Gaseous oxide of carbon	9.8
Nitrous oxide	13.7
Sulfur	14.4
Nitric acid	15.2
Sulphurated hydrogen	15.4
Carbonic acid	15.3
Alcohol	15.1
Sulfurous acid	19.9
Sulfuric acid	25.4
Carburetted hydrogen from the stag. Water	6.3
Olefiant gas	5.3

1.2.1.4 Dalton's Atomic Theory

Dalton's atomic model was an important step in the development of modern chemistry and provided a framework for understanding the behavior of matter at the atomic level. However, the model had some limitations, as it did not clearly explain how atoms were connected or interacted with other atoms. The five main propositions of his theory are as follows:

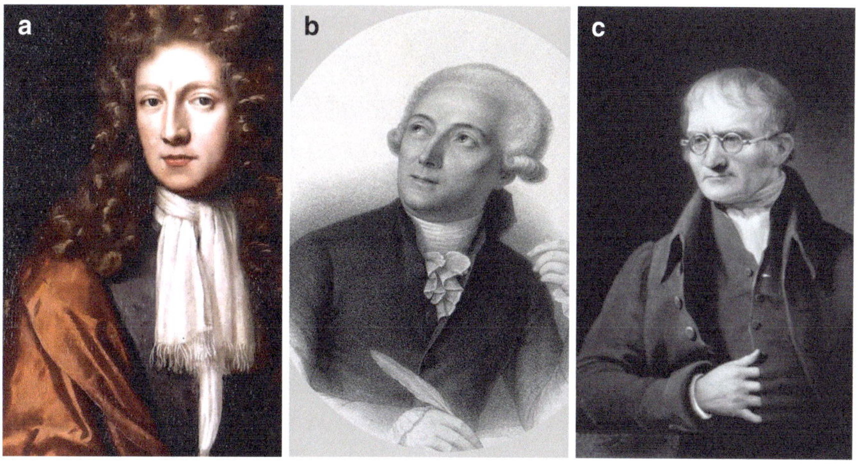

Fig. 1.8 (**a**). Robert Boyle, Image courtesy: Wellcome Library, London. (**b**). Antoine Lavoisier. Image courtesy: Wellcome Library, London (**c**). John Dalton, Image courtesy: the United States Library of Congress. (All images published under Creative Commons Attribution only license CC BY 4.0)

1. All matter is composed of extremely small and definite particles called atoms.
2. Atoms are indivisible, neither can be created nor destroyed.
3. Atoms of certain elements are identical in size, mass, and other properties, whereas atoms of different elements differ.
4. Chemical compounds can be created by combining atoms of various elements in simple whole-number ratios.
5. Atoms can be combined, separated, or rearranged during chemical processes.

Though this theory was largely accepted, however with continuous advancement in the field, we know that

(a) Atoms can be further subdivided.
(b) All atoms of a particular element are not identical in mass.
(c) Using artificial methods such as nuclear fission or fusion, atoms can be created or destroyed by changing into other atoms.

1.2.1.5 Atomic Nomenclature and Symbols

The late eighteenth century is considered the foundation for modern chemistry. Many new elements and compounds were discovered and named; however, there naming pattern was chaotic and mainly based on the discoverer's name. Louis-Bernard Guyton de Morveau (1737–1816) is considered instrumental in establishing the modern "system" of chemical nomenclature and raised the need through his paper in 1782 [11]. He collaborated with Antoine-Laurent Lavoisier (1743–1794), the father of modern chemistry, along with two more authors Claude-Louis Berthollet and Antoine de Fourcroy, to formulate a system of chemical nomenclature through the book *Method of Chemical Nomenclature* published in 1787. In this book, vitriolic acid became sulfuric acid along with the coining of many other modern names [12].

John Dalton is known for the "invention of atomic symbols" and introduced it in 1803, though his symbols were not frequently used in literature and were thought to be challenging to write and print (Fig. 1.9) [7]. In 1814, a Swedish chemist, Jöns Jacob Berzelius, published an easy method of expressing elements and suggested, "The chemical signs ought to be letters." His method of naming elements was.

"the chemical sign is to be the initial letter of the Latin name. If many have the same initial letter, the first two letters of the word shall be employed, and if the first two letters are the same, the letter followed by the first consonant which they do not have common shall be employed."

The examples based on his suggestion are H = hydrogen, He = Helium (though it was discovered in 1868), C = carbonicum, Co = cobaltium (cobalt), Cu = cuprum (copper), phosphorus

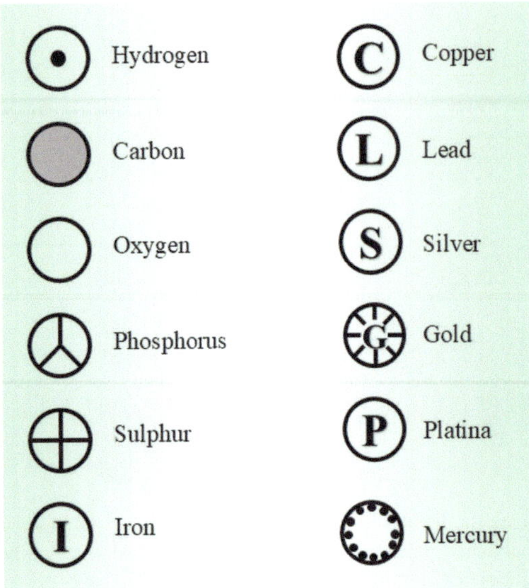

Fig. 1.9 John Dalton's atomic symbols

(P), lead (plumbum, Pb), plutonium (Pu), palladium (Pd), iron (ferrum, Fe), copper (cuprum, Cu), tin (stannum, Sn), silver (Argentum, Ag), gold (aurum, Au), antimony (stibium, Sb), oxygen (O), osmium (Os), etc.

1.2.1.6 IUPAC and Standardized Naming

The International Union of Pure and Applied Chemistry (IUPAC) is an international organization that aims to advance the chemical sciences and contribute to the application of chemistry in the service of humankind. Approves the name of new elements. The naming process is standardized, and that includes verification of the discovery. Once verification is over, the discoverer(s) proposes the name, and the proposed name passes through several steps of review before approval. If the IUPAC rejects the proposed name, the discovering group is given another opportunity to suggest a different name. Once IUPAC approves the name, it becomes the official name of the element. As per IUPAC 2002 rule [13] and subsequent amendment in 2016 [14], the new elements can be named on the following criteria:

- A mythological concept or character that may include an astronomical object.
- A mineral or similar substance.
- A place or geographical region.
- A property of the element.
- A scientist.

The name of new elements to end with "ium" for elements of 1–16 group of the periodic table, "-ine" for the elements of group 17 and "-on" for the elements of group 18 to maintain historical and chemical consistency [14]. Also, the new names in English should allow translation into other major languages [14]. Now there are 118 elements in the periodic table (Fig. 1.10); the last naming of elements was done in the UPAC 2016 press release [15]. The interactive electronic version of the periodic table of elements and their isotopes was introduced by IUPAC in August 2016 and can be viewed at www.isotopesmatter.com.

The atomic weights of the seventh row or period 7 in the periodic table are typically written in brackets because they are uncertain. This is because these elements are all either radioactive or have very short half-lives, making it difficult to measure their atomic weights accurately. In addition, some of these elements may have different isotopes with varying atomic weights, further complicating determining their exact atomic weights. Therefore, the values in brackets indicate an estimate or a range of possible values for the atomic weight of each element.

The elements such as iron, copper, silver, tin, antimony, gold, mercury, arsenic, zinc, and lead have been known since ancient times [16]. Many elements, such as hydrogen, lithium, sodium, potassium, boron, carbon, nitrogen, phosphorus, etc., were found in the late seventeenth and early eighteenth century. However, no formal naming system existed until 1786, and the discoverer kept names of substances that were sometimes founded upon loose analogies or false theoretical views [17].

The suffix "-gen" in the names of elements such as oxygen, nitrogen, and hydrogen comes from the Greek word "gennao," which means "to produce" or "to create." The scientist observed that many compounds could be formed by combining certain elements, and they used the suffix "-gen" to indicate that these elements were essential in creating these compounds. Oxygen was named by Antoine Lavoisier in 1777, who recognized that it was a necessary component of many

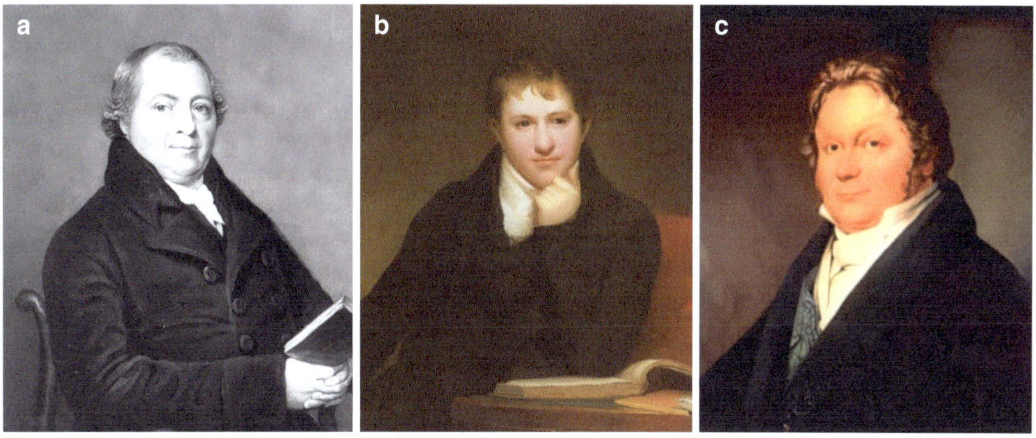

Fig. 1.10 (**a**). Martin Heinrich Klaproth, image courtesy: welcomelibrary.org. (**b**). Humphry Davy, image courtesy: Dr. Manuel, (**c**). Jons Jacob Berzelius, image courtesy: National Portrait Gallery. All images are published under a creative commons license

compounds, and he named it "oxygen" from the Greek words "oxys," meaning "acid," and "gennao," meaning "to produce," since he believed it was an essential component of all acids.

Similarly, nitrogen was discovered by the Scottish chemist Daniel Rutherford in 1772 and named by Jean-Antoine Chaptal in 1790 after the Greek words "nitron," meaning "native soda," and "gennao," meaning "to produce," due to its presence in saltpeter (also known as potassium nitrate (KNO_3), used in gunpowder and fertilizers. Hydrogen was named by the French chemist Antoine Lavoisier in 1783, though it was discovered in 1766 by Henry Cavendish. He named it "hydrogen" from the Greek words "hydro," meaning water, and "gennao," meaning "to produce," since he observed that hydrogen was produced when water was split into its parts by electrolysis. The name "hydrogen" reflects that hydrogen is a component of water, a compound made up of hydrogen and oxygen atoms.

Martin Heinrich Klaproth is credited with being one of the first chemists to propose using the "-ium" suffix for naming newly discovered elements. Klaproth believed that using a standardized suffix for element names would help to bring order and clarity to the rapidly growing field of chemistry, which was seeing an influx of new elements being discovered and isolated at an unprecedented rate during his time.

Klaproth's idea of using the "-ium" suffix was based on the Latin word "ium," which is a neuter noun ending (does not have a gender) often used in scientific nomenclature. By appending this suffix to the end of an element's name, Klaproth believed it would indicate that the substance was a new, distinct element. Other chemists of the time, including Humphry Davy (1778–1829) and Jöns Jacob Berzelius (1779–1848), also adopted this naming convention and helped to establish it as a standard practice in the field. Humphry Davy named his discoveries including potassium, sodium, calcium, and magnesium and proposed scientific community in his discovery of sodium and potassium in 1807, which was accepted widely and still used today [18].

Today, the "-ium" suffix is still common in naming elements, although there are some exceptions to the rule. For example, some elements that were discovered before Klaproth's time, such as gold (Au) and iron (Fe), do not have the "-ium" suffix in their names. Other elements, such as helium (He), neon (Ne), and argon (Ar), were given names that do not follow the "-ium" convention because they were discovered before the idea of using a standardized suffix for element names had become widespread.

Table 1.2 gives information about all the elements discovered to date as per their atomic number and lets readers know their atomic symbol, the origin of the name with its meaning, the inventor's name, and the year in which they were discovered.

Table 1.2 Table of elements with atomic numbers 1 to 118: Etymology, Discovery, and Discoverer Information. Significant portion of this table is extracted from reference [19]

Atomic number	Element name	Atomic symbol	Name derived from	Invented by	Year
1	Hydrogen	H	The Greek word "hydro" = water and "gennao" = to produce, as it forms water when burned.	English physicist Henry Cavendish in 1766 and named by Antoine Lavoisier in 1783.	1766
2	Helium	He	The Greek word "helios" for "sun" as it was discovered during spectroscopy of a solar eclipse	French astronomer Pierre-Jules-Cesar Janssen	1868
3	Lithium	Li	The Latin word "lithos" for "stone" as lithium was thought to exist only in minerals during that time	Swedish mineralogist Johan August Arfivedson	1818
4	Beryllium	Be	The Greek word "berryllos" is for "Beryl," the gemstone in which it was found	French chemist and pharmacist Nicholas-Louis Vauquelin	1797
5	Boron	B	The Arabic word "buraq" is for "white"	Known for thousands of years, but isolated independently in the impure state by French chemists Louis-Joseph Gay-Lussac and Louis-Jacques Thenard in Paris and pure state in London by English chemist, Humphry Davy	1808
6	Carbon	C	The Latin word "carbo" means "charcoal"	Though known for prehistoric times in the form of charcoal and soot, the English chemist Smithson Tennant has shown that diamond is pure carbon	1797
7	Nitrogen	N	The Greek word "nitron" means "saltpeter", and "gennao = to produce" because of its presence in saltpeter i.e. potassium nitrate (KNO_3)	Scottish physician and chemist Daniel Rutherford in 1772 and named by Jean-Antoine Chaptal in 1790.	1772
8	Oxygen	O	The Greek word "oxys" = acid and "gennao" = to produce. The French chemist Antoine Lavoisier initially thought that oxygen is an acid producer because burning phosphorus with sulfur and dissolving that in water produces acid	In 1771, the Swedish pharmacist and chemist Carl-Wilhelm Scheele and in 1774, the English clergyman and scientist Joseph Priestly separately discovered oxygen. Since Priestly published first and Scheele's "Chemical Treatise on Air and Fire" was not published until 1777, Priestley is credited for the discovery. Named by Antoine Lavoisier in 1777.	1774
9	Fluorine	F	The Latin word "fluere" means "flow or flux." Fluorspar or CaF_2 was used as a flux in metallurgy since it has a low melting point	Discovered in hydrofluoric acid (HF) by Swedish pharmacist and chemist Carl-Wilhelm Scheele	1771

(continued)

Table 1.2 (continued)

Atomic number	Element name	Atomic symbol	Name derived from	Invented by	Year
10	Neon	Ne	The Greek word "neos" means "new." discovered from its bright red spectral lines	Scottish chemist William Ramsay and English chemist Morris William travers	1898
11	Sodium	Na	Symbol Na derives from the Latin word "natron" means "soda" in English, and hence the element name "Natrium" in Latin or "sodium" in English	English chemist Humphry Davy	1807
12	Magnesium	Mg	Derived from the word "Magnesia," a district in the northeastern region of Greece called Thessalia	In 1755, Scottish chemist distinguished magnesia alba (a magnesium compound) from other substances, but in 1808, the English chemist Humphry Davy isolated impure magnesium metal. He suggested to name "magnium," but later on, it was named magnesium.	1755
13	Aluminum	Al	The Latin word "alum" and alumen for "stringent" since the early romans called "alum"' for any substance with a stringent taste	Known since the prehistoric era. In 1825, impure aluminum was isolated by the Danish physicist Hans Christian Oersted. The pure metal was isolated in 1827 by German scientist Friedrich Wöhler.	1825
14	Silicon	Si	The Latin words "silex" and "silicis" for "flint" are very hard gray stones that can produce sparks and are also used in cigarette lighters. The early name was "silicium," considering it as metal. When found this to be incorrect, the name changed to silicon	Swedish chemist Jons Jacob Berzelius	1823
15	Phosphorus	P	The name derives from the Greek word "phosphorous" means "bringing light," since white phosphorus oxidizes spontaneously in air and glows in the dark. Phosphorus was the ancient name in Greek for Planet Venus, which appears before sunrise	German merchant Hennig Brand	1669

(continued)

Table 1.2 (continued)

Atomic number	Element name	Atomic symbol	Name derived from	Invented by	Year
16	Sulfur	S	The Latin word "sulfurium" means "to burn." sulfur was known as brenne stone or combustible stone from which brimstone is derived. Brimstone is commonly found on the brims (rims) of volcanoes, a flammable mineral. The American name "sulfur" was preferred over the English name "Sulphur" as many languages have a spelling using an "f."	Known from prehistoric times, but proved element by French chemists Louis-Joseph Gay-Lussac and Louis-Jacques Thenard	1809
17	Chlorine	Cl	The Greek word "chlooros" for "pale green" or "greenish-yellow" color of the element	Discovered by the Swedish pharmacist and chemist Carl-Wilhelm Scheele in 1774, but English chemist Humphry Davy proved it as an element and named it chlorine in 1810	1774
18	Argon	Ar	The Greek word "Argos" for "lazy or inactive" as it did not combine with other elements	Scottish chemist William Ramsay and English physicist Robert John Strutt (Lord Rayleigh)	1895
19	Potassium	K	English word "potash or pot ashes" as it is found in caustic potash (KOH). The chemical symbol K derives from the Latin word "kalium" via the Arabic "qali" for alkali	British chemist Humphry Davy	1807
20	Calcium	Ca	The Latin word "calx" for "lime" (CaO) or "limestone" ($CaCO_3$) in which it was found	British chemist Humphry Davy with help from Swedish chemist Jons Jacob Berzelius and physician MM afPontin prepared calcium amalgam	1808
21	Scandium	Sc	Latin word "Scandia" for "Scandinavia," where the mineral was found	Swedish chemist Lars-Fredrik Nilson from an ytterbium sample	1879
22	Titanium	Ti	The Latin word "titans" who were the mythological "first sons of the earth"	Initial discovery by English clergyman William Gregor in the mineral ilmenite in 1791 but in 1795, German chemist Martin Heinrich Klaproth rediscovered it and called it titanium	1791
23	Vanadium	V	Because of its multicolored compound, the name is derived from the Scandinavian goddess of love and beauty "Freyja Vanadis"	Swedish physician and chemist Nils-Gabriel Sefstrom	1830
24	Chromium	Cr	Greek chroma for "color," as it has many colored compounds	French chemist and pharmacist Nicolas-Louis Vauquelin	1797

(continued)

Table 1.2 (continued)

Atomic number	Element name	Atomic symbol	Name derived from	Invented by	Year
25	Manganese	Mn	The Latin word "magnes" is for "magnet" since pyrolusite (MnO_2) has magnetic properties	Swedish pharmacist and chemist Carl-Wilhelm Scheele	1774
26	Iron	Fe	Anglo-Saxon "iron" of unknown origin. The symbol "Fe" is taken from the Latin word "ferrum" for "firmness."	The element is known since prehistoric times, but evidence of use by man has been found since 5000–3000 BCE.	Not known
27	Cobalt	Co	The Greek word "kobalos" means "mine." the name derives from the German word "kobold" means "evil spirits." this was superstitiously thought to cause trouble for miners. The minerals contained arsenic, injured their health and metallic ores, and did not yield metals when treated with the normal methods	Swedish chemist Georg Brandt	1735
28	Nickel	Ni	The German word "nickel" for "deceptive little spirit," as miners called "mineral niccolite" (NiAs) by the name "kupfernickel," that is, a false copper since it resembled copper ores in appearance, but copper was not found in the ore	Swedish metallurgist Axel-Fredrik Cronstedt	1751
29	Copper	Cu	Latin Cuprum for "Cyprus," the island of Cyprus where the romans first obtained copper. The symbol also comes from the Latin "cuprum"	Evidence shows man has been using this metal for over 10,000 years. However, the exact discovery is not known	Not known
30	Zinc	Zn	The German word "zink" is of unknown origin	Used since prehistoric times, where its compounds were used for healing wounds and eye sores and for making brass	Recognized as metal in early 1374
31	Gallium	Ga	The Latin word "Gallia" means "France" as the French chemist discovered it	French chemist Paul-Emile Lecoq de Boisbaudan	1875
32	Germanium	Ge	The Latin word "Germania" is for "Germany"	German chemist, Clemens-Alexander Winkler	1886
33	Arsenic	As	The Latin word "Arsenicum" and the Greek "arsenikos" for the arsenic ore "yellow orpiment (an ancient dye stuff)" and sounds similar to the Greek word "arsenikon" for "male or potent," possibly referring to its poisonous properties	Known since prehistoric times for its poisonous sulfides. The German scientist and philosopher Albert von Bollstadt is thought to have obtained arsenic around 1250, but this is uncertain	Considered to be in 1250

(continued)

Table 1.2 (continued)

Atomic number	Element name	Atomic symbol	Name derived from	Invented by	Year
34	Selenium	Se	The Greek word "Selene" who was the Greek goddess of the moon	Swedish chemist Jons Jacob Berzelius	1817
35	Bromine	Br	The Greek word "bromos" is for "stench or bad odor"	First prepared by German chemist Carl Lowig in 1825 but the first public announcement by French chemist and pharmacist Antoine-Jerome Balard in 1826; therefore, Balard is credited for the discovery	1826
36	Krypton	Kr	The Greek word "Kryptos" for "concealed or hidden"	Scottish chemist William Ramsay and English chemist Morris William travers	1898
37	Rubidium	Rb	The Latin "rubidus" is for "deepest red" because two "deep red spectral lines" are observed in its spectrum	German chemist Robert Wilhelm Bunsen and physicist Gustav-Robert Kirchoff	1861
38	Strontium	Sr	The name derived from Strontian, "a town in Scotland"	Scottish chemist and physician Thomas Charles Hope	1792
39	Yttrium	Yt	The name derived from the "Swedish village of Ytterby," where the mineral gadolinite was found	Finnish chemist Johan Gadolin	1794
40	Zirconium	Zr	The Arabic word "zargun" for "gold-like"	Discovered in zirconia (North Carolina, United States) by the German chemist Martin-Heinrich Klaproth	1789
41	Niobium	Nb	Greek mythological character "Niobe," a daughter of Tantalus	British chemist and manufacturer Charles Hatchett	1801
42	Molybdenum	Mo	The Greek word "molybdos" means "lead." in ancient days term lead was used for any black mineral which gives a mark on paper	Swedish pharmacist and chemist Carl Wilhelm Scheele	1778
43	Technetium	Tc	The Greek word "technetos" means "artificial" because it was the first element produced by artificial means	Claims of discovery started in 1828, but the first synthesized was done by Italian physicists C. Perrier and Emilio Segre in 1937	1937
44	Ruthenium	Ru	The Latin word "Ruthenia" is the "old name of Russia"	Russian chemist Gottfried Wilhelm Osann	1828
45	Rhodium	Rh	The Greek word "rhodon" means "rose" because of the rose color of its dilute solutions of salts	English chemist and physicist William Hyde Wollaston	1803
46	Palladium	Pd	The name is derived from the word "Pallas," based on the second largest asteroid of the solar system, discovered 1 year before, that is, in 1802	English chemist and physicist William Hyde Wollaston	1803

(continued)

Table 1.2 (continued)

Atomic number	Element name	Atomic symbol	Name derived from	Invented by	Year
47	Silver	Ag	Old English "seolfor," of Germanic origin, is related to the Dutch word "zilver" and German "Silber," but the origin of these words is unknown. The chemical symbol, Ag, is derived from the Latin word "Argentum" and Sanskrit "argunas" for "bright"	The element was known since prehistoric times, but evidence of use since 5000–3000 BCE	Not known
48	Cadmium	Cd	The Greek word "kadmeia" means "calamine or zinc carbonate," which was found as an impurity	German physician Friedrich Stromeyer	1817
49	Indium	In	The name is derived from the word "Indigo" for the "indigo-blue" line in its spark spectrum. The word "indigo" comes from the Latin word "indicum" which means "Indian," as the dye was originally exported to Europe from India [20]	German physicist Ferdinand Reich and German metallurgist Hieronymus Theodor Richter	1863
50	Tin	Sn	The origin of the "tin" word is unknown. The symbol "Sn" is based on the Latin word "stannum" for alloys containing lead	The element is known since prehistoric times but is believed to be first used in 3500 BCE in the "Ur" city of southern Mesopotamia (now Iraq) [21]	Not known
51	Antimony	Sb	Greek word "anti + monos" for "not alone or not one" as it was found along many compounds. The symbol "Sb" is taken from the original name, stibium, derived from the Greek word "stibi" means "mark," as it was used for blackening eyebrows and eyelashes	The element is known since prehistoric times, and evidence of use has existed since 3100 BCE [22]	Not known
52	Tellurium	Te	The Latin word "Tellus," who was the "Roman goddess of the earth"	Roumanian mine director Franz Joseph Miiller von Reichenstein	1782
53	Iodine	I	The Greek word "ioeides" for "violet colored" because of its violet vapors	French chemist Bernard Courtois	1811
54	Xenon	Xe	The Greek word "xenos" is for "the stranger"	Scottish chemist William Ramsay along with English chemist Morris William travers	1898
55	Caesium	Cs	The Latin word "caesius" means "sky blue color," as it was the color of the caesium line in the spectroscope	German scientist Robert Wilhelm Bunsen with compatriot physicist Gustav Robert Kirchhoff	1860
56	Barium	Ba	The Greek word "barys" for "heavy" since it was found in the heavy mineral spar (BaS04).	Swedish pharmacist and chemist Carl Wilhelm Scheele	1774

(continued)

Table 1.2 (continued)

Atomic number	Element name	Atomic symbol	Name derived from	Invented by	Year
57	Lanthanum	La	The Greek word "lanthanein" means "to be hidden or to escape notice" as it hid in cerium ore and was difficult to separate	Swedish surgeon and chemist Carl-Gustav Mosander	1839
58	Cerium	Ce	The name derives from the planetoid "Ceres," the Roman goddess of agriculture discovered in 1801	Swedish chemists Jöns Jacob Berzelius and Wilhelm Hisinger and during the same time working independently by German chemist Martin Klaproth	1803
59	Praseodym ium	Pr	Initially named "praseodidymium" and was later shortened to praseodymium. The Greek word "prasios" means "green" and "didymos" for "twin" because of the pale green salts it forms	Austrian chemist Carl Auer von Welsbach	1885
60	Neodymium	Nd	Initially "neodidymium" but later shortened to "neodymium." Greek word "neos" for "new" and "didymos" for "twin"	Swedish surgeon and chemist Carl Gustav Mosander	1841
61	Promethium	Pm	The name derives from the Greek Mythological character "Prometheus," who stole fire from god and gave it to the humanity	American scientists J.A. Marinsky, L.E. Glendenin and Charles D. Coryell	1945, but published in 1947 [23]
62	Samarium	Sm	The name derived from the mineral "Samarskite," which was found and named for "Colonel von Samarski" a Russian mine official	Swiss chemist Marc Delafontaine	1878
63	Europium	Eu	The name derives from the continent of "Europe"	French chemist Eugene-Anatole Demarcay in Paris	1896
64	Gadolinium	Gd	The name derived from the mineral "gadolinite," in which it was found, and was named after Finnish rare earth chemist "Johan Gadolin"	Swiss chemist Jean-Charles Galissard de Marignac in Switzerland. He also suggested the possibility of isotopes and the packing fraction of nuclei	1886
65	Terbium	Tb	The name derived from the name of the village in Sweden called "Ytterby," where its source "Ytterbite" was first found	Swedish surgeon and chemist Carl-Gustav Mosander in Sweden	1843
66	Dysprosium	Dy	The Greek word "dysprositos" means "hard to get at," as it is difficult to separate from the holmium mineral in which it was found	French scientist Paul-Emile Lecoq de Boisbaudron in Paris	1886

(continued)

Table 1.2 (continued)

Atomic number	Element name	Atomic symbol	Name derived from	Invented by	Year
67	Holmium	Ho	The Latin word "holmia" is for "Stockholm"	Swiss chemist J. L. Soret in Sweden	1878
68	Erbium	Er	The name derived from the Swedish town of "Ytterby," where the mineral "gadolinite" (in which it was found) was first mined	Swedish surgeon and chemist Carl-Gustav Mosander in Sweden	1843
69	Thulium	Tm	The name derived from the word "Thule," the earliest name of the northernmost part of the civilized world—"Scandinavia (Norway, Sweden, and Iceland)"	Swedish chemist Per Theodor Cleve in Sweden	1879
70	Ytterbium	Yb	The name derived from the "Swedish village of Ytterby," where the ore ytterbite (the source of ytterbium) was originally found	Swiss chemist Jean-Charles Galissard de Marignac in Switzerland	1878
71	Lutetium	Lu	The name is derived from the word "Lutetia," an ancient Latin name for "Paris"s	French chemist George Urbain in Paris	1907
72	Hafnium	Hf	A Latin name "hafnia" for "Copenhagen"	George Charles de Hevesy and Dirk Coster in Denmark	1923
73	Tantalum	Ta	The name is derived from the word "Tantalos," a Greek mythological character. This name was selected because of its insolubility in acids	Swedish chemist and mineralogist Anders-Gustav Ekeberg	1802
74	Tungsten	W	Swedish word "tungsten" for "heavy stone." symbol W is derived from the German word "wolfram," which was found with tin and interfered with smelting. It was said the "tin" was eaten up like a wolf eats up the sheep	Swedish pharmacist and chemist Carl-Wilhelm Scheele	1781
75	Rhenium	Re	The Latin word "rhenus" is "the Rhine river in Germany"	German scientists Walter Noddack, Ida Tacke and Otto Berg	1925
76	Osmium	Os	The Greek word "osme" for "smell" because of the sharp odor of the volatile oxide	English chemist Smithson Tennant	1803
77	Iridium	Ir	The Latin word "iris," the Greek goddess of rainbows as the element's salt solution, has various colors	English chemist Smithson Tennant	1803
78	Platinum	Pt	The Spanish word "Platina" for "little silver" as platinum was considered an unwanted impurity in silver	Spanish mathematician Don Antonio de Ulloa in Peru, South America	1735

(continued)

Table 1.2 (continued)

Atomic number	Element name	Atomic symbol	Name derived from	Invented by	Year
79	Gold	Au	The name derived from the Sanskrit word "jval" means shine, the Teutonic (indo-European speakers of Germanic languages) word "gulth" for shining metal and the Anglo-Saxon gold of unknown origin. The symbol "Au" has a Latin origin from the word "aurum" for the goddess of dawn	It is known since prehistoric times and is highly valued. Discovery dates back to 5000 BCE	Not known
80	Mercury	Hg	The Mercury originates from the Roman god "Mercury," who was considered "the nimble messenger of the gods." the symbol, Hg, is derived from the Greek word "hydragyrium" for "liquid silver" or "quick silver"	Known from prehistoric times. Thirty thousand years ago, paleolithic painters decorated caves in Spain and France [24]	Not known
81	Thallium	Tl	The Greek word "thallos" is for "green shoot or twig" because its spectrum has a bright green line	English physicist and chemist William Crookes	1861
82	Lead	Pb	The symbol Pb is derived from the Latin word "plumbum" for "lead"	The element was known from prehistoric times. But found used in the Middle East at about 7000 BCE [25]	Not known
83	Bismuth	Bi	The German word "Weisse masse" for "white mass" comes from the color of its oxides. The ancients could not distinguish bismuth from lead	The French chemist Claude-Francois Geoffioy (the younger) showed that bismuth was distinct from lead	1753
84	Polonium	Po	The name derived from the country name "Poland," the native country of Marie Curie	Pierre and Marie curie	1898
85	Astatine	At	The Greek word "astatos" means "unstable" since it is an unstable element	American physicists Dale R. Corson, Kenneth R. MacKenzie, and Emilio Segrè at the University of California, USA	1940
86	Radon	Rn	The name indicates its origin from "radium," and radon is a decay product of radium	German chemist Friedrich Ernst Dorn	1900
87	Francium	Fr	The name derives from the country "France"	French physicist Marguerite Perey in Paris	1939
88	Radium	Ra	Latin word "radius" for "beam or ray" because of its tremendous ray-emitting power	French physicist Pierre Curie and French chemist Marie Sklodowska Curie	1898

(continued)

Table 1.2 (continued)

Atomic number	Element name	Atomic symbol	Name derived from	Invented by	Year
89	Actinium	Ac	The Greek word "aktis or akinis" means "beam or ray" since it is a powerful source of alpha radiation in equilibrium and its daughter products	French chemist Andre-Louis Debierne	1899
90	Thorium	Th	The name derives from the Greek mythological name "Thor," the "Scandinavian god of thunder"	Swedish chemist Jons Jacob Berzelius	1828
91	Protactinium	Pa	The Greek word "protos" means "first," and the suffix "actinium" because it was found to be the parent of actinium	German chemists Kasimir Fajans and O. H. Gohring	1913
92	Uranium	U	The name derived from the planet "Uranus," which in Roman mythology was "Father Heaven." Uranus was discovered in 1781	German chemist Martin-Heinrich Klaproth	1789
93	Neptunium	Np	The name is derived from the planet "Neptune" which, per Roman mythology, is "god of the sea." Neptunium was named so since it is the next outermost planet in the solar system after planet Uranus. And this is the next element in the periodic table after uranium	Edwin M. McMillan and Philip H. Abelson	1940
94	Plutonium	Pu	The name is derived from the planet "Pluto," (the Roman mythological god). Pluto was named the next planet in the solar system after planet Neptune and Plutonium is the next element in the periodic table after neptunium	American scientists Glenn T. Seaborg, Edwin M. McMillan, Joseph W. Kennedy and Arthur C. Wahl	1940
95	Americium	Am	The name derived from the country name "America," where it was first synthesized	American scientists under the leadership of Glenn T. Seaborg at the University of California	1944
96	Curium	Cm	The name derived from "Pierre and Marie Curie"	American chemist Glenn T. Seaborg at the University of California lab in Berkeley, California	1944
97	Berkelium	Bk	The name is derived from Berkeley, the town in California where the element was first synthesized	American scientists under the leadership of Glenn T. Seaborg at the University of California	1949

(continued)

Table 1.2 (continued)

Atomic number	Element name	Atomic symbol	Name derived from	Invented by	Year
98	Californium	Cf	The name is derived from the state and the university of California in the United States, where the element was first synthesized	American scientists under the leadership of Glenn T. Seaborg at the University of California	1950
99	Einsteinium	Es	The name derived from the name of scientist "Albert Einstein," the German physicist who proposed the famous theory of relativity	A group of scientists from the Argonne National Laboratory, Illinois, the Los Alamos scientific laboratory, New Mexico and the University of California lab, Berkeley	1952
100	Fermium	Fm	The name derived from the Italian physicist "Enrico Fermi," who built the first nuclear reactor	A group of scientists from the Argonne National Laboratory, Illinois, the Los Alamos Scientific Laboratory, New Mexico, and the University of California lab, Berkeley	1952
101	Mendelevium	Md	The name was derived from the Russian chemist "Dimitrii Mendeleev," who gave the periodic table of elements	American scientists under the leadership of Glenn T. Seaborg at the University of California	1958
102	Nobelium	No	The name derived from the scientist name "Alfred Nobel," who is the discoverer of dynamite and founder of the Nobel prizes	A group of Russian scientists from the Joint Institute for Nuclear Research (JNIR) lab in Dubna, Russia, under the leadership of Georgi Flerov	1966
103	Lawrencium	Lr	The name is derived from the American physicist, "Ernest O. Lawrence," who developed the cyclotron	A group of scientists in collaboration with the University of California laboratory, Berkeley, under Albert Ghiorso and the joint Institute for Nuclear Reactions (JINR) lab, Russia, under the leadership of Georgi N. Flerov	1971
104	Rutherfordium	Rf	The name was derived from the English physicist "Ernest Rutherford," a Nobel laurette for developing the theory of radioactive transformations	A group of scientists, in collaboration with the University of California laboratory, Berkeley, under Albert Ghiorso and the joint Institute for Nuclear Reactions (JINR) lab in Russia, under the leadership of Georgi N. Flerov	1964
105	Dubnium	Db	The name is derived from "Dubna," in Russia, where the Russian research center "Joint Institute for Nuclear Research (JINR)" is situated	A group of scientists, in collaboration with the University of California laboratory, Berkeley, under Albert Ghiorso and the joint Institute for Nuclear Reactions (JINR) lab in Russia, under the leadership of Georgi N. Flerov	1970

(continued)

Table 1.2 (continued)

Atomic number	Element name	Atomic symbol	Name derived from	Invented by	Year
106	Seaborgium	Sg	The name derived from the American chemist "Glenn Theodore Seaborg," who was instrumental in synthesizing several transuranium elements	American scientist group of California University, Berkeley, under the leadership of Albert Ghiorso	1974
107	Bohrium	Bh	The name derives from the Danish physicist "Niels Bohr," who gave the theory of the electronic structure of the atom	A group of scientists in Germany at the Center for Heavy-Ion Research, under German scientists Peter Armbruster and Gunther Munzenberg	1981
108	Hassium	Hs	The name derived from the Latin word "Hassia" for the German state of "Hesse"; the former capital was Darmstadt	A group of German Physicist at the Center for Heavy-Ion Research Lab at Darmstadt, Germany	1984
109	Meitnerium	Mt	The name derived from the Austrian physicist "Lise Meitner," who co-discovered the element protactinium	A group of German Physicist at the Center for Heavy-Ion Research, Gesellschaft fir Schwerionenforschung (GSI) Lab at Darmstadt, Germany	1982
110	Darmstadtium	Ds	The name derived from the place name "Darmstadt," Germany, where the element was first produced	A multi-national team of experts at the Center for Heavy-Ion Research, Gesellschaft fir Schwerionenforschung (GSI) Lab at Darmstadt, Germany. The teams comprised scientists from the GSI lab, scientists from the Joint Institute for Nuclear Research (JINR), Dubna, Russia, scientists from the Comenius University, Bratislava, Slovakia, and the scientist from the University of Jyvaskyla, Finland	1994
111	Roentgenium	Rg	The name derived from scientist "Wilhelm Conrad Röntgen," the discoverer of X-rays	A multinational team of experts at the Center for Heavy-Ion Research, Gesellschaft fir Schwerionenforschung (GSI) Lab at Darmstadt, Germany. The teams comprised scientists from the GSI lab, scientists from the Joint Institute for Nuclear Research (JINR), Dubna, Russia, scientists from the Comenius University, Bratislava, Slovakia, and the scientist from the University of Jyvaskyla, Finland	1994

(continued)

Table 1.2 (continued)

Atomic number	Element name	Atomic symbol	Name derived from	Invented by	Year
112	Copernicium	Cn	The name derived from the influential sixteenth-century astronomer "Nicolaus Copernicus"	A multinational team of experts at the Center for Heavy-Ion Research, Gesellschaft fir Schwerionenforschung (GSI) Lab at Darmstadt, Germany. The teams comprised scientists from the GSI lab, the Joint Institute for Nuclear Research, Dubna, Russia, scientists from the Comenius University, Bratislava, Slovakia and the scientist from the University of Jyvaskyla, Finland	1996
113	Nihonium	Nh	The name is derived from the word "Nihon" which is one way to say the country's name in Japanese	Team of Japanese scientists at Riken in Wakō, Japan	2004
114	Flerovium	Fl	The name is derived from Russian physicist "Georgy Flerov" known for the discovery of spontaneous fission	A multinational team of experts working at the Joint Institute for Nuclear Research (JINR), Dubna, Russia. The team comprised scientists from JINR and the Lawrence Livermore Laboratory in Livermore, California, USA	1998
115	Moscovium	Mc	Named after the name of the place "Moscow" where the element was discovered	A joint team of Russian and American scientists at JINR, that is, Joint Institute for Nuclear Research (JINR), in Dubna, Russia	2003
116	Livermorium	Lv	The name was selected to honor the scientists' contributions in Livermore to heavy and superheavy element research	A group of Russian scientists from the Joint Institute for Nuclear Research, Dubna, Russia and American scientists from the Lawrence Livermore Laboratory, California, USA	2000
117	Tennessine	Ts	The name derived from the US state of "Tennessee" where the element was discovered	A team from the Joint Institute for Nuclear Research (JINR) in Dubna, Russia, the Lawrence Livermore National Laboratory in California, USA, and Oak Ridge National Laboratory in Tennessee, USA	2010
118	Oganesson	Og	Named after Russian nuclear physicist "Yuri Oganessian," a leader of the Russian American team which created most of the elements with atomic numbers >110 [26]	The team consists of scientists from the Joint Institute for Nuclear Research at Dubna, Russia and Lawrence Livermore National Laboratory, California	2002

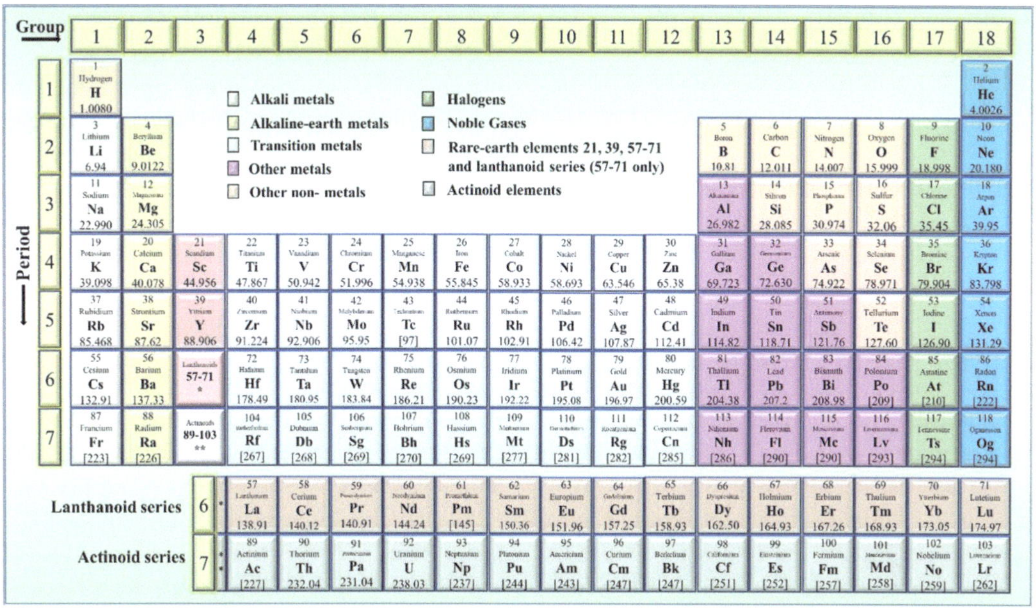

Fig. 1.11 The periodic table

1.2.2 Atomic Models

1.2.2.1 Thomson's Atomic Model

Dalton assumed atoms are indivisible and further components such as negatively charged electrons (−) and positively charged protons (+) were not considered then. In an experiment with cathode ray tubes, Sir Joseph John Thomson (1856–1940), a British physicist and Nobel Laureate, discovered the first subatomic particle called "electrons." In the paper "Cathode Rays, 1897" [27], he displayed that all atoms contain very small negatively charged subatomic particles or electrons, as in positively charged plum pudding, and the negatively charged electrons are embedded within it (Fig. 1.12). He called those tiny negatively charged particles "corpuscles." The term "electron" was first proposed by the Irish physicist George Johnstone Stoney in 1891; it was adopted widely in the early 1900s. Before that, electrons were often referred to as "corpuscles," a term used since the seventeenth century to describe small, discrete particles of matter. The "electron" discovery and its properties were a breakthrough in the development of modern physics.

Sir J.J. Thomson presented his atomic theory model in a series of papers published in 1904 and 1906, later called the "plum pudding" model. His model can be summarized as follows:

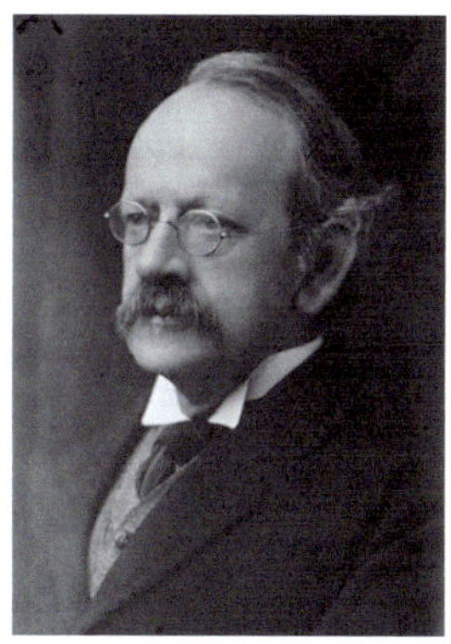

Fig. 1.12 Sir JJ Thomson. Image published under creative commons license

1. Atoms have a spherical shape and are composed of a uniform, positively charged material with negatively charged electrons embedded in them.
2. The negatively charged electrons were evenly distributed throughout the positively charged material, like raisins in a pudding.
3. The total charge of the atom is assumed to be neutral, where the total negative charge of the

electrons is balanced out with the total positive charge of the material.
4. The electrons have a much smaller mass than atoms.

Limitations of the Thomson Atomic Model

This model has several major limitations that other scientists later discovered. Some of the key defects of the model include:

1. *Lack of a nuclear structure*: As per the model, "Positive charge of the atom is distributed uniformly throughout the atom," whereas it is concentrated in a small, positively charged nucleus, as later experiments showed.
2. *Failure to explain atomic spectra*: The model could not explain the complex emission and absorption spectra patterns observed in atomic spectra.
3. *Inability to explain the stability of atoms*: The model could not explain why atoms are stable and did not simply collapse under the influence of the force of attraction between the negatively charged electrons and the positively charged sphere.
4. *Ignorance about the existence of isotopes*: The model was developed before the existence of isotopes was discovered, and it assumed all atoms of a given element had the same mass.

These defects in the "plum pudding model" of the atom led to the development of more refined models, such as the Rutherford atomic model and the Bohr atomic model, which better explained the behavior and properties of atoms (Fig. 1.13).

1.2.2.2 Rutherford's Atomic Model

A New Zealand physicist, Ernest Rutherford (1871–1937), is considered the father of nuclear physics and credited with discovering the "nucleus" and "protons." In a series of papers titled "The Scattering of α and β Particles by Matter and the Structure of the Atom" and later on its Part II and Part III, all published in 1911 (March, April, and June), he found that some of the alpha particles were deflected at large angles, indicating that they were encountering a very small, dense, positively charged object in the center of the atom. Rutherford proposed that this object was the atomic nucleus.

In 1919, he discovered protons published in a paper titled "The Artificial Disintegration of Light Elements." In this paper, he described experiments in which he bombarded nitrogen gas with alpha particles and observed the emission of a new type of radiation. He concluded that this radiation was composed of positively charged particles, which he named protons.

He proposed his atomic model in several papers, but the most famous is "The Structure of the Atom," published in 1911. His model can be summarized as follows (Fig. 1.14):

1. Atoms have small, dense, positively charged "nuclei" at their center, surrounded by negatively charged electrons that orbit the nucleus.
2. The nucleus is comparatively very small compared to the entire atom, containing most of the mass.

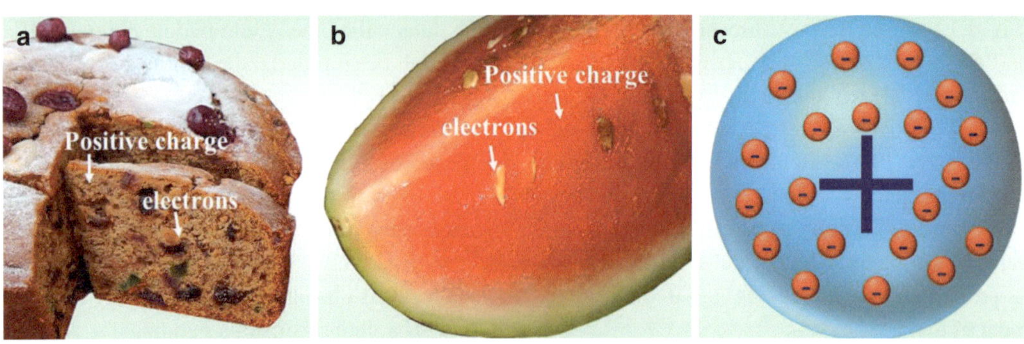

Fig. 1.13 Thomson atomic model: (**a**) plum cake showing the arrangement of electrons and positively charged mass, (**b**) watermelon shows an arrangement of electrons and positive charge in an atom, (**c**) Graphical representation of Thomson model

3. The protons inside an atom are all gathered at the center (nucleus) of the atom, with the electrons orbiting around, as the fruit of a peach is formed around the stone in the center.

This model is also called the "nuclear model" and the "planetary model." The nuclear model is named as it was the first model to describe the nucleus, and the planetary model is because it proposes that electrons orbit the nucleus of an atom like the way planets orbit the Sun in our solar system. However, planetary model names are less common (Fig. 1.15).

Limitations of the Rutherford Model

Rutherford's model was a significant breakthrough in the understanding of the atomic structure, but it had some drawbacks, including:

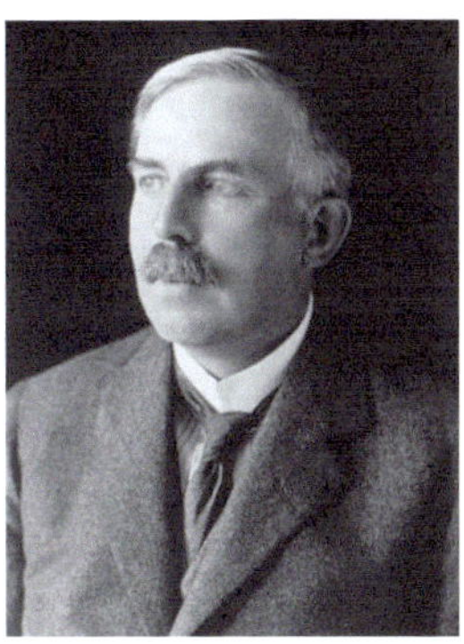

Fig. 1.14 Sir Ernest Rutherford. Image published under creative commons license

1. *Unable to explain the distribution of electrons*: The Rutherford model predicted that the size of the nucleus was much smaller than the size of the atom, which was confirmed by the experiments. However, the model did not explain the distribution of the electrons around the nucleus.
2. *Stability of the atom*: According to this model, electrons revolve around the nucleus in circular orbits. However, according to classical electromagnetism, charged particles moving in a circular path emit energy in the form of electromagnetic radiation. Thus, the electrons in the Rutherford model would lose energy and spiral into the nucleus, making the atom unstable.
3. *Absence of atomic spectra*: The Rutherford model did not explain the characteristic atomic spectra observed experimentally. The model suggested that the electrons could occupy any orbit around the nucleus, leading to a continuous radiation spectrum. However, experimental observations showed that atoms emit radiation at specific wavelengths, indicating that electrons occupy only specific energy levels.
4. *Does not account for other subatomic particles*: The Rutherford model did not consider the existence of subatomic particles such as neutrons (discovered later), work laid the groundwork for linking the number of protons in the nucleus to its atomic number and the chemical properties of the element.

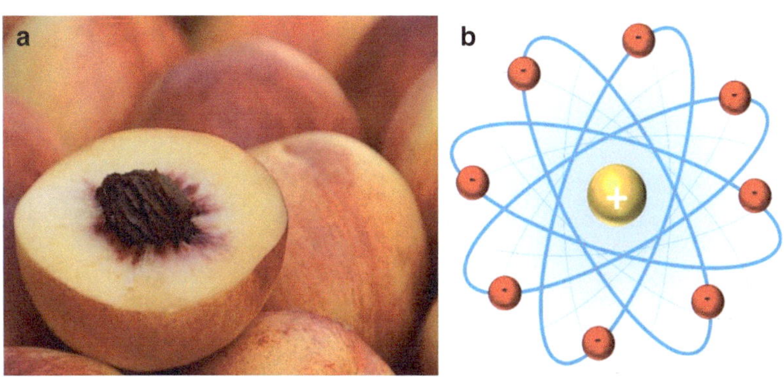

Fig. 1.15 Rutherford atomic model: (**a**) peach fruit showing positive charge at the center, (**b**) graphical representation of Rutherford's atomic model

Overall, the Rutherford model was a significant step forward in understanding the atomic structure, but it had some limitations that the Bohr model and quantum mechanics later addressed.

1.2.2.3 Bohr's Atomic Model

In 1900, the German physicist Max Planck hypothesized "quantum theory" in 1900. It was based on his experimental observations of black-body radiation, which is the radiation emitted by a heated object. According to his hypothesis, "electromagnetic radiation, such as light, could only be emitted or absorbed in discrete packets of energy, called "quanta." (Fig. 1.16)

Niels Bohr was examining the movement of electrons, and based on Planck's quantum theory and Rutherford's atomic model, he proposed his atomic theory with the help of the line spectrum of hydrogen atoms in 1913.

His postulates can be summarized as follows:

1. Electrons orbit the nucleus in circular paths, or orbits, at fixed energy levels.
2. The energy levels or "shells" are quantized, meaning they can only take on certain values.
3. These shells are called principal quantum numbers and can be denoted by letters K, L, M, N, O,... or by positive integer numbers such as "n" = 1, 2, 3, ... They represent lower to higher energy levels. The higher the number, the higher the energy state.

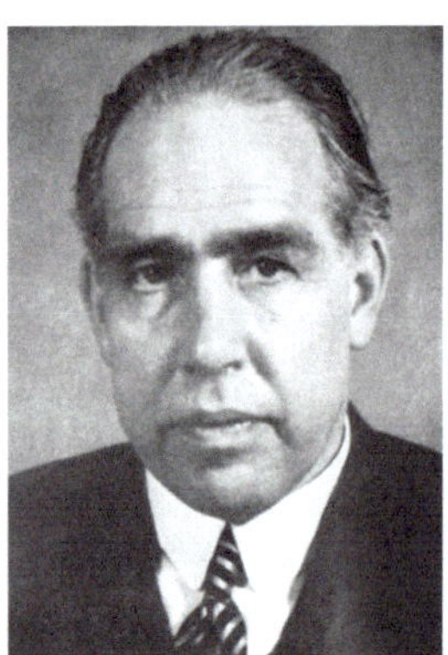

Fig. 1.16 Niel Bohr (1885–1962). Image published under creative commons license

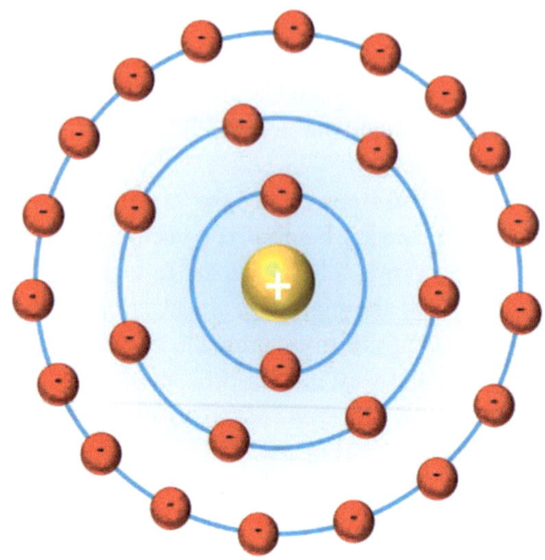

Fig. 1.17 Bohr atomic model

4. When electrons move from a higher energy level to a lower energy level, they emit photons of light with a specific wavelength (Fig. 1.17).

Shortcomings of Bohr's Atomic Model

Bohr's atomic model was a significant step forward in understanding the atomic structure and laid the foundations for developing quantum mechanics. However, it was eventually replaced by more sophisticated models that provided a better description of the behavior of the atoms. Some of the drawbacks of his postulates are as follows:

1. *Limited to hydrogen atom*: Bohr's model was designed specifically for the hydrogen atom, which is the simplest atom with only one electron. It failed to explain the electronic structure of other, more complex atoms.
2. *Non-explanation of nuclear structure*: Bohr's model focused on electron energy levels and did not address the nuclear structure, including protons (discovered in 1919) and neutrons (discovered in 1932).
3. *Absence of electron movement details*: Bohr's model did not explain the path that electrons follow around the nucleus, only the allowed energy levels. This implied that electrons

move in circular orbits around the nucleus, which is an oversimplification.

4. *Unable to sync with advancements such as Heisenberg's uncertainty principle*: As per Heisenberg's uncertainty principle (1927), "it is not possible to measure position and momentum of an electron simultaneously with absolute certainty." There was no such description in Bohr model.

Despite these limitations, Bohr's atomic model significantly contributed to the field of atomic theory and played an important role in developing modern atomic theory. Figure 1.18 gives a comparative image of all four models discussed so far.

1.2.2.4 The Discovery of the Neutron

After the discovery of the nucleus and protons, the atom's existence was still questionable as to how all positive charges could be in one place, and still, the atom exists. In May 1932, Sir James Chadwick (1891–1974), a British physicist, discovered "neutrons" and published his discovery in the journal *Nature* titled "The Existence of a Neutron" [28]. Although Ernest Rutherford (the discoverer of the nucleus and protons) did not directly participate in the discovery of the neutron, he was a mentor and the head of the department at Cavendish Laboratory in Cambridge, where Sir James Chadwick was working.

Chadwick bombarded alpha particles at a sample of beryllium metal, which caused the release of neutral particles that had never been observed before. These neutral particles were identified as neutrons, and Chadwick was able to measure their mass and other properties. This landmark discovery revolutionized the field of nuclear physics and helped to explain certain properties of atomic nuclei, such as their stability, the presence of isotopes, the development of nuclear power, and nuclear weapons. Sir James Chadwick was awarded the Nobel Prize in Physics in 1935 for this discovery (Fig. 1.19).

The neutron has no charge, and its mass is about 1.67493×10^{-27} kg which is slightly less than the sum of a proton (1.67262×10^{-27} kg) and an electron ($9.10938356 \times 10^{-31}$ kg) plus binding energy. Chadwick mentioned that the mass of a neutron is a little less than the sum of the mass of a proton and an electron and concluded neutron is a complex particle consisting of a proton and an electron in close combination with some binding energy [28], later on with the discovery of artificial radioactivity by F. Joliot and I. Curie in 1934 and further subsequent research demonstrated

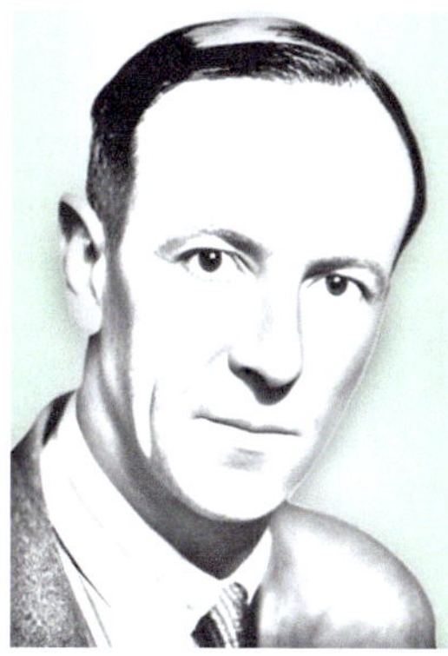

Fig. 1.19 James Chadwick, who is credited with discovering the neutron. Image courtesy: Los Alamos National Laboratory. Published under Creative Commons CC0 License

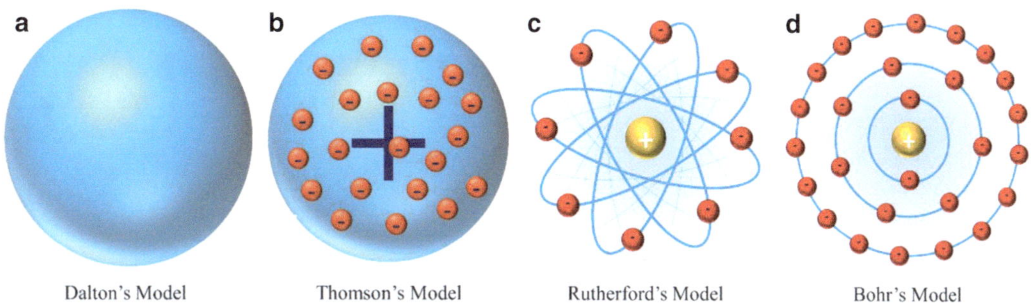

Fig. 1.18 Classical physics atomic model: (**a**) Dalton's model, (**b**) Thomson's model, (**c**). Rutherford's model, (**d**) Bohr's model

neutron is another subatomic particle and the same was accepted by James Chadwick too.

1.2.2.5 Modern Atomic Model

The modern atomic theory is a scientific model that describes the nature and behavior of atoms, which are the basic building blocks of matter. The pioneers of this theory are Lois de Broglie, Heisenberg, and Schrödinger. One of the key concepts in the modern atomic theory is the wave-particle duality of matter, which states that particles such as electrons can exhibit wavelike and particle-like properties. This is known as the wave-particle duality, a fundamental principle of quantum mechanics. French physicist Louis de Broglie gave this principle in his doctoral thesis in 1924 [29]. Quantum mechanics predicts that the position and momentum of particles such as electrons cannot be known simultaneously with certainty. This principle was proposed by Werner Heisenberg in 1927 [30] and called the Heisenberg uncertainty principle.

According to this theory,

- Atoms are composed of a central nucleus containing positively charged "protons" and neutral subatomic particle "neutrons," surrounded by negatively charged "electrons" that orbit the nucleus in specific energy levels or shells.
- Atoms are electrically neutral, meaning they have equal protons and electrons.
- Number of protons in the nucleus is known as its atomic number, which determines the element to which the atom belongs. For example, atoms having eight protons are oxygen atoms, while those with one proton are hydrogen atoms.
- The electrons in an atom revolve in different energy levels, or shells, located at varying distances from the nucleus and not between them. The lowest energy level, the ground state, is closest to the nucleus and holds two electrons. Each energy shell can hold up to $2n^2$ electrons, where $n = 1, 2, 3, 4, \ldots$, that is, the energy shell can hold up to 2, 8, 18, 32, ... electrons in each subsequent orbital.
- These energy levels are described by quantum numbers, which are four numbers that describe the energy, angular momentum, magnetic moment, and spin of an electron.
- The behavior of electrons within an atom describes how particles behave on a very small scale.
- When an electron absorbs energy, it can move to a higher energy level or orbital, but it will eventually release that energy and return to its original energy level.
- Atoms can combine to form molecules through chemical bonding. They can share, gain, lose, or transfer electrons to form new chemical bonds. These interactions between atoms give rise to the properties of matter, such as its density, melting point, and reactivity.

In modern atomic theory, the concept of the orbit is replaced by the concept of orbitals, which better reflects the probabilistic nature of electron behavior. To understand, orbits are specific paths followed by electrons in the Bohr model, whereas orbitals are the regions of space where electrons are likely to be found in the quantum mechanical description. A demonstrative quantum mechanical atom model is shown in Figs. 1.20 and 1.21.

1.2.2.6 Size of Atom vs Size of the Nucleus

The size of the atom is on the order of nanometers (10^{-9} m), whereas the size of an atom's nucleus is on the order of femtometers (10^{-15} m), and the difference between an atom and its nucleus is about 10^6 (one million) times. For an approximation and simplification to understand with real-world examples, the following analo-

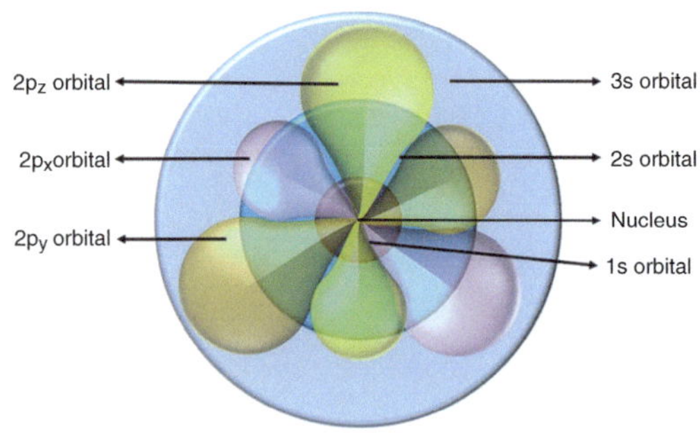

Fig. 1.21 Quantum mechanical model of the relatively small atom with a maximum of 14 electrons

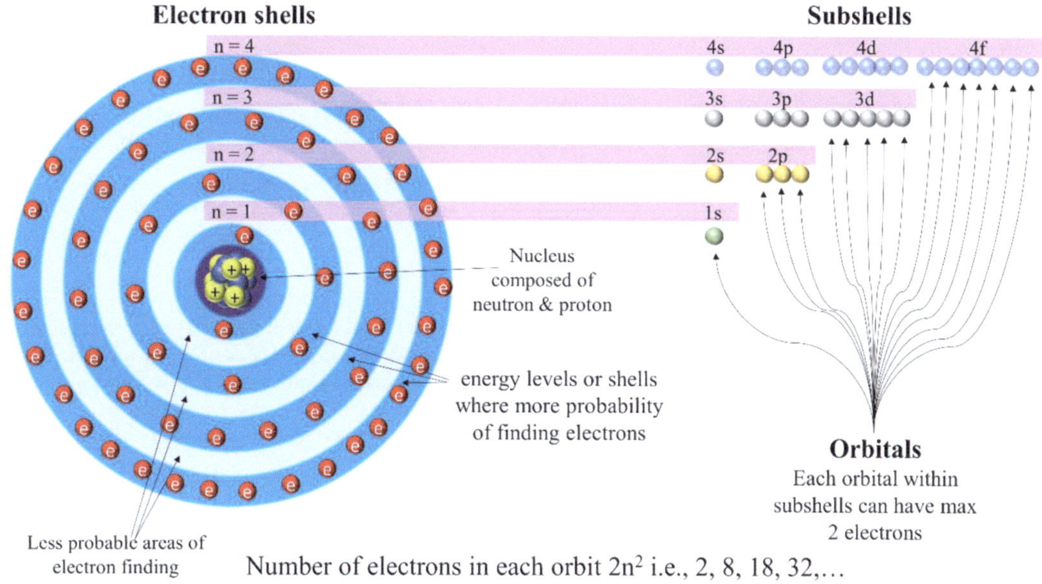

Fig. 1.20 Atomic structure as per modern atomic theory. S-subshell contains one orbital, p-subshell contains three orbitals, d-subshell contains five orbitals, and f-subshell contains seven orbitals, each can hold maximum 2 electrons in each of their orbitals

gies can be used to understand the differences between the two.

Imagine a tiny grain of sand placed at the center of a football field. Here, the grain of sand represents the atom's nucleus, while the football field represents the electron cloud. The electron cloud would extend far beyond the football field's boundaries, illustrating the electron cloud's vast size compared to the nucleus.

Again, it is important to note that this analogy is imperfect and only meant to provide a general understanding of size differences. The electron cloud does not have a well-defined boundary like the walls of a stadium, and the nature of electron behavior is inherently probabilistic according to quantum mechanics.

1.2.2.7 Quantum Numbers

Quantum numbers are a set of values used to describe various properties and characteristics of particles in quantum mechanics. They provide information about the allowed energy levels, spatial distribution, and other attributes of particles, such as electrons in atoms. The four quantum numbers, which describe the quantum state of an electron in an atom are (Table 1.3):

Principal quantum number (n): This number describes the electron's energy level and distance from the nucleus. It can take on integer values from 1 to n, where n can go up to infinity.

Azimuthal quantum number or angular momentum quantum number (l): This number describes the shape of the orbital (s, p, d, f) and its angular momentum. It can take on integer values ranging from 0 to n-1. The rule for the shape of the orbital follows the following rules:

- For l = 0, the orbital is an s (sharp) orbital with a spherical shape.
- For l = 1, the orbital is a p (principal) orbital with a dumbbell shape with two lobes on the x, y, and z axes called p_x, p_y, and p_z orbitals.
- For l = 2, the orbital is a d (diffuse) orbital, which has a more complex shape with four lobes and a doughnut-shaped region between them. There are five types of d orbitals, commonly called d subshells. They are *dxy*, *dyz*, *dzx*, *dx²-y²*, *dz²*. Each d orbital has a different shape and orientation

Table 1.3 Quantum numbers

Name of quantum number	Symbol	Representation	Can take values	Example of values
Principal	N	Electron's energy level and its distance from the nucleus	1 to n	Positive integers (1, 2, 3, ...theoretically to infinity)
Azimuthal	L	Describes the shape of the orbital (s, p, d, f) and its angular momentum	0 to n-1	0, 1, 2, ...
Magnetic	m_l	Orbital's orientation in space	–l to +l	The magnetic quantum number (m_l) ranges from –l to +l, including zero (e.g., –1, 0, +1 for l = 1), and defines the orbital's orientation in space, such as the p_x, p_y, and p_z orbitals along the x-, y-, and z-axes for l = 1, influencing electron interactions in chemical bonds.
Spin	m_s	Describes the electron's intrinsic spin	$+\frac{1}{2}, -\frac{1}{2}$	Represents as "spin-up" or "spin-down"

in space, contributing to the overall electron density distribution in the d subshell.

- For l = 3, the orbital is an f (fundamental) orbital, with an even more complex shape with eight lobes and multiple nodes. There are seven f orbitals with different shapes and orientations, contributing to the overall electron density distribution in complex ways. They are named as $fx(x^2 - 3y^2)$ or $fxz^2, fy(3x^2 - y^2)$ or $fyz^2, fx(5z^2 - r^2), fy(5z^2 - r^2), fz(5z^2 - 3r^2), fz(x^2 - y^2), fxyz$.

Therefore, an electron with an azimuthal quantum number of 4 (l = 3) is in an f orbital with a very complex shape starting from one lobe to eight lobes and multiple nodes. The exact shape and orientation of the orbital can be determined by combining the azimuthal quantum number with the other three quantum numbers. Figure 1.22 shows the indicative three-dimensional structure of s, p, d, and f orbitals; however, it is important to note that the shape of these orbitals represents the electron density distribution and should not be interpreted as a physical object in space. The shapes are derived from mathematical calculations and visually represent the probability of finding an electron at different locations within the orbital.

The angular momentum quantum number (l), often called the azimuthal quantum number, describes the orbital's angular momentum magnitude in the quantum mechanical description of atomic orbitals.

The magnetic quantum number (m_l) describes the orbital's orientation in space. It can take on integer values ranging from –l to +l. For l = 1, it defines the p_x, p_y, and p_z orbitals along the x-, y-, and z-axes. Positive m_l values correspond to a positive z-component of angular momentum (L_z), negative values to a negative L_z, and $m_l = 0$ to no z-component, influencing orbital alignment in bonding.

Spin quantum number (s): This quantum number describes the electron's intrinsic spin. It can take on a value of +1/2 or – 1/2 representing a particle's two possible spin orientations. These orientations are often called "spin-up" and "spin-down," respectively. They are conventionally denoted as ↑ (spin-up) and ↓ (spin-down).

These four quantum numbers (Fig. 1.23) uniquely identify each electron in an atom and define its quantum state. These quantum numbers can be considered as if they exactly define the address of an electron and represent its street number, building number, floor number, and flat number.

1.2.2.8 Pauli's Exclusion Principle

In 1925, Austrian physicist Wolfgang Pauli proposed another fundamental principle of quantum

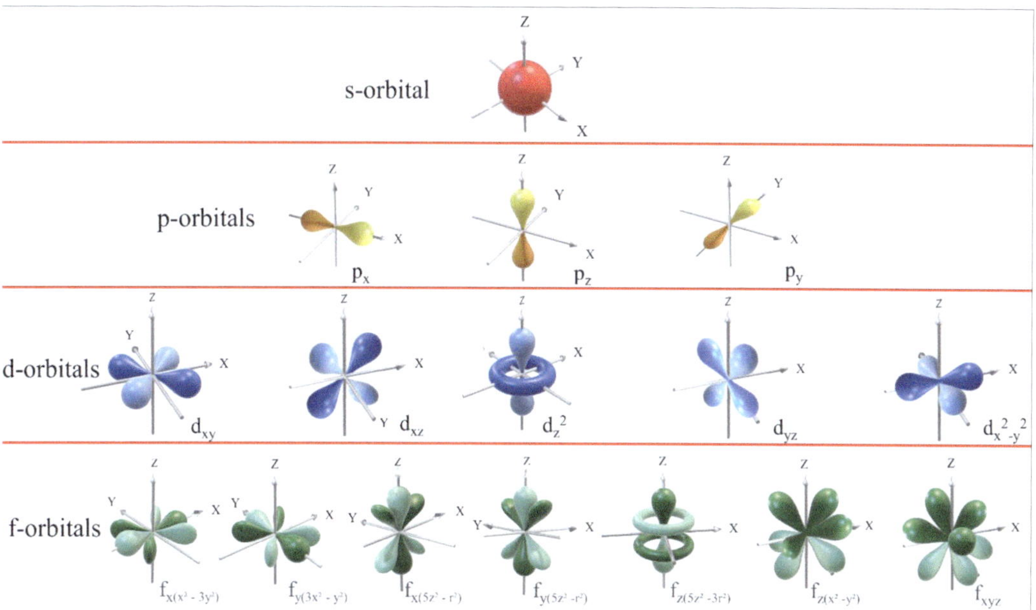

Fig. 1.22 Indicative three-dimensional structure of s, p, d, and f orbitals

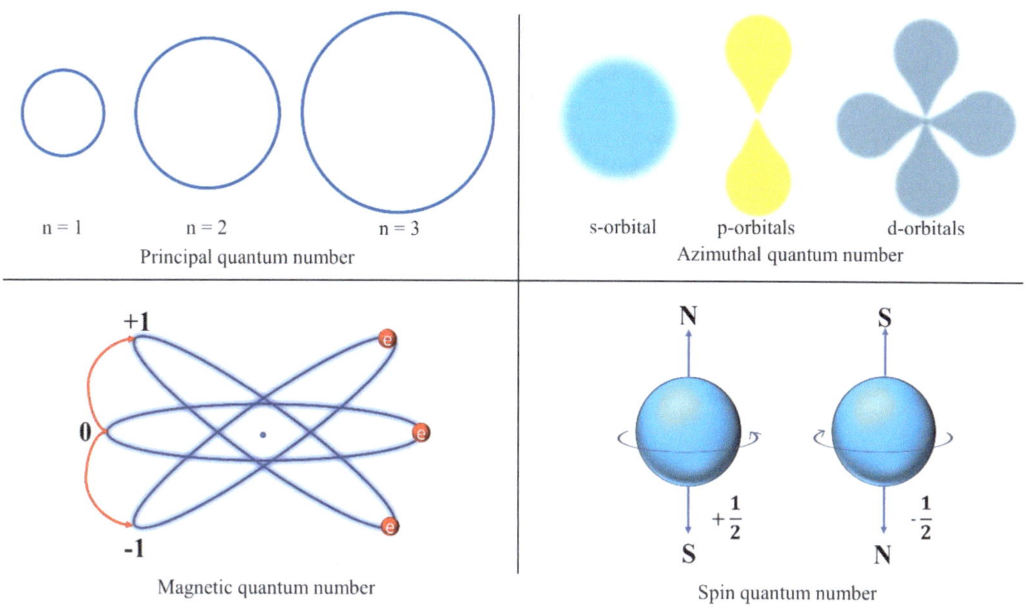

Fig. 1.23 All quantum numbers

mechanics called "Pauli's exclusion principle." This principle states, "No two electrons in an atom can have the same quantum numbers." In other words, no two electrons in an atom can occupy the same energy level, with the same values of the principal quantum number (n), azimuthal quantum number (l), magnetic quantum number (m), and spin quantum number (s).

The exclusion principle has important implications for the electronic structure of atoms and the behavior of electrons in materials. It helps to explain why certain electron configurations are more stable than others and why certain elements have unique chemical and physical properties.

For example, the exclusion principle explains why the first energy level ($n = 1$) can hold only two electrons (one with $s = +1/2$ and one with $s = -1/2$), the second energy level ($n = 2$) can hold up to eight electrons, that is, two in the s orbital and six in the p orbital, and so on. The exclusion principle also underlies the periodicity of the periodic table and the trends in the chemical and physical properties of the elements (Fig. 1.24).

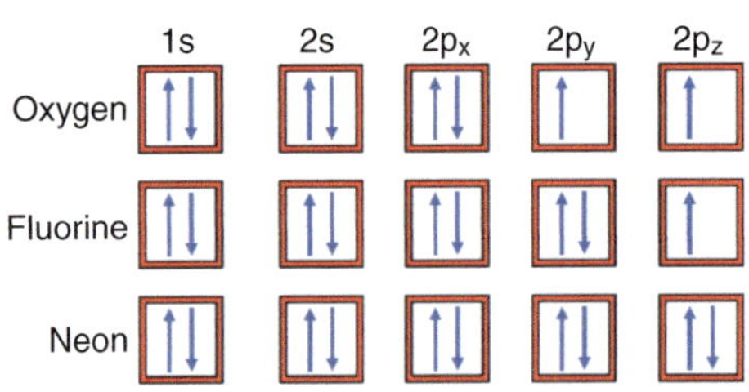

Fig. 1.24 Pauli's exclusion principle examples

1.2.2.9 The Aufbau Principle

The Aufbau principle was first proposed by Niels Bohr in 1921 as part of his work on the electron configuration of atoms. It was later refined and formalized by Erwin Madelung in 1936 through the (n + ℓ) rule, building on earlier contributions from German physicist Arnold Sommerfeld's (1868–1951), whose work on quantum numbers in 1916 provided the theoretical framework for orbital classification [31]. This principle is also sometimes called the building-up principle (in German, Aufbau means building up). It states that the lowest energy orbitals are filled first. In other words, electrons will occupy the lowest energy orbital available before moving on to higher energy orbitals. The Aufbau principle is fundamental to quantum mechanics and is essential for understanding the electronic structure of atoms and molecules.

Arnold Sommerfeld was consistently nominated for Nobel Prize on 84 occasions (the maximum number for any person) from 1917 to 1951 but never received the award [32]. However, his many students, including Wolfgang Pauli and Werner Heisenberg, received Nobel prizes. He gave the concept of azimuthal and magnetic quantum numbers along with many other notable scientific works. He also gave a modified version of Bohr's atomic model in 1916 which was called as Bohr–Sommerfeld atomic model [33] (Fig. 1.25).

1.2.2.10 Hund's Rule

German physicist Friedrich Hund (1896–1997) proposed the principle of filling up atomic orbitals in an atom in 1927. It states that when elec-

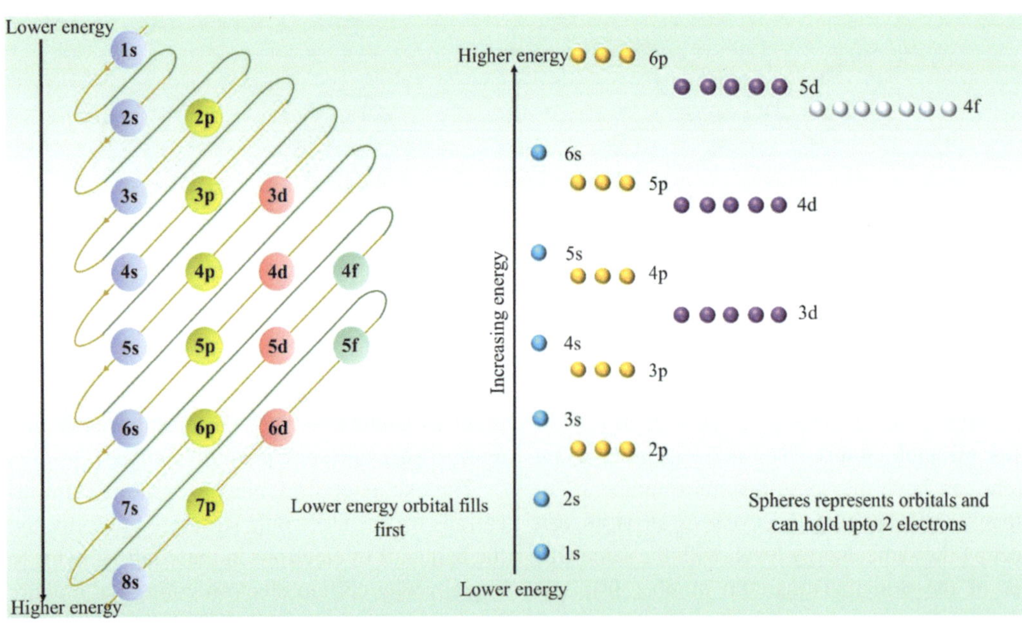

Fig. 1.25 Afbau principle or building-up principle given by Arnold Sommerfeld

trons occupy orbitals with the same energy, they fill each orbital singly before pairing up.

In other words, if an atom has multiple orbitals with the same energy level, for example, p_x, p_y, p_z, each will be filled first by a single electron and then occupied by the second electron. This is known as "maximizing spin" and results in all of the electrons in the atom having unpaired spins.

Hund's rule helps to explain the behavior of atoms and the properties of materials, particularly in terms of their magnetism and conductivity (Fig. 1.26).

In summary, the modern atomic theory is a fundamental framework for understanding the behavior of matter at the atomic and molecular levels. It describes the structure of atoms, the behavior of electrons within atoms as well as in chemical reactions, the interactions between atoms that give rise to the properties of matter and other areas of science, such as materials science and nanotechnology. The modern atomic theory also provides a framework for understanding the periodic table of elements, which arranges elements according to their electron configurations and chemical properties. The periodic table is divided into 18 groups and 7 periods, with elements in the same group having similar chemical properties because of their similar electron configurations (Fig. 1.11). By understanding the behavior of atoms and molecules at the atomic and molecular levels, scientists can design new materials and develop new technologies with specific properties and functions.

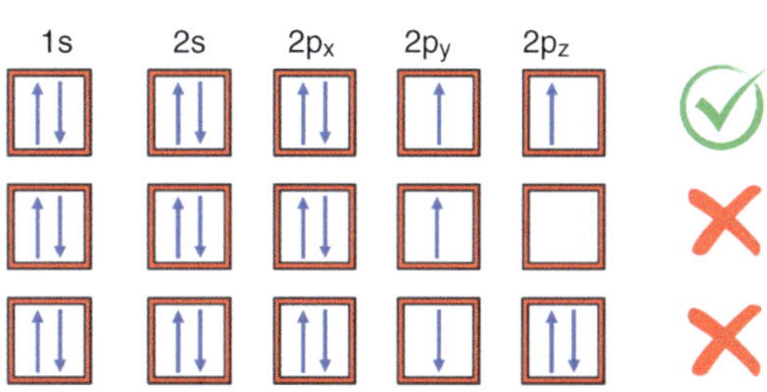

Fig. 1.26 Hund's rule. Electrons fill subshells singly before forming pairs, and each electron in a single orbital has the same spin

1.2.3 Terms Related to Atomic Theory

1.2.3.1 Atomic Number

The atomic number is a fundamental property of an element defined as the number of protons in the nucleus of an atom. It is denoted by the symbol "Z" and is used to identify the element (Fig. 1.27). Each element has a unique atomic number, determining its chemical properties and position in the periodic table. The atomic number also provides information about the atom's isotopes, that is, atoms of the same element having different numbers of neutrons in their nuclei.

The number of protons in nucleus is balanced by equal number of negatively charged electrons which occupy in different energy shells or energy levels. The number of electrons and protons remains equal in an electrically neutral atom.

1.2.3.2 Atomic Mass

Atomic mass is the mass of an individual atom of an element, expressed in atomic mass units (amu). It is denoted by the symbol "A" and determined by adding the mass of total protons and total neutrons. In periodic table, the atomic mass is typically reported beneath the element's symbol (Fig. 1.27), and it is a proportionate average of each isotope that exists in nature for that particular element. Isotopes are the atoms of the

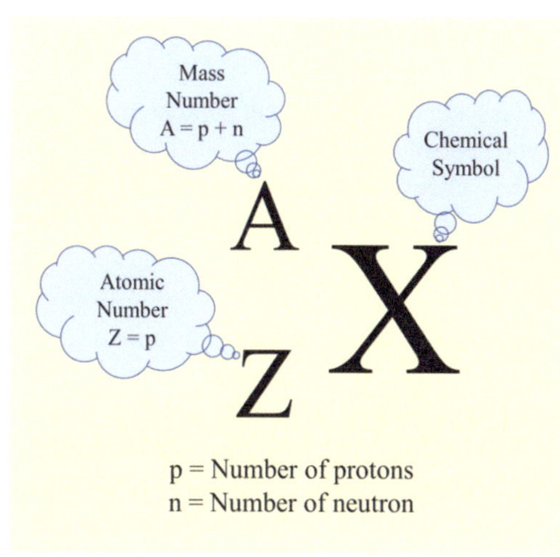

Fig. 1.27 Atomic Notations

same element with the same number of protons but a different number of neutrons. Since isotopes can have different atomic masses, taking an average gives a more accurate representation of the typical mass of that atom.

The unit of atomic mass, that is, the atomic mass unit (amu), is defined as one-twelfth of the mass of neutral atom of carbon-12.

$$1\ \text{amu} = 1.66054 \times 10^{-27}\ \text{kg} \tag{1.1}$$

> ? Why is the mass of electrons not considered when calculating the mass of an atom?

In calculation of atomic mass of an element, typically, only the masses of the protons and neutrons are considered, not the electrons. This is because the mass of an electron is considerably smaller than the mass of a proton or neutron. Mass of an electron is approximately 1/1836th of the mass of a proton or neutron. Since electrons occupy the space outside the atomic nucleus, their mass does not significantly contribute to the total mass of an atom, and hence they are not taken into account.

1.2.3.3 Nuclear Notations

Nuclear notation or nuclear symbol, also known as atomic notation, is a way to represent the structure of an atom using symbols and numbers. It provides information about an atom's number of protons, neutrons, and electrons.

The atomic notation consists of three parts:

- Atomic number (Z): the number of protons (p).
- Mass number (A): total number of protons and neutrons (p + n).
- The chemical symbol of the element. Examples of nuclear notations are ${}^{16}_{8}O$, ${}^{184}_{74}W$, ${}^{204}_{82}Pb$, ${}^{99m}_{43}Tc$.

Sometimes, atomic notation also includes the charge of the atom. An atom is neutral when it has an equal number of protons and electrons but can become charged by gaining or losing electrons. A positive charge indicates the loss of electrons, and a negative charge indicates the gain. The positive or negative charge is written as a superscript on the right side of the nuclear symbol. For example, a carbon atom with a positive charge would be represented as ${}^{12}C^{2+}$.

1.2.3.4 Isotopes

The atoms of the same element with an equal number of protons in their nuclei but different numbers of neutrons are called as isotopes. The identity of a particular element is not changed; however, their atomic masses remain different as they have different numbers of neutrons in their nucleus.

Isotopes are denoted by their element name followed by their atomic mass number. For example, iodine-127 and iodine-131, nitrogen-13 and nitrogen-14. Iodine-127 has 53 protons and 84 neutrons in its nucleus, whereas iodine-131 has 53 protons and 88 neutrons. Nitrogen-13 has 7 protons and 6 neutrons, whereas nitrogen-14 has 7 protons and 7 neutrons.

Some isotopes of elements are stable; however, some can be radioactive. For example, I-127 is stable, whereas I-131 is radioactive; similarly, nitrogen-14 is stable, and nitrogen-13 is radioactive.

The presence and abundance of different isotopes of an element can be determined through various analytical techniques, including mass spectrometry, which separates and measures the mass-to-charge ratios of ions based on their atomic masses. The isotopic composition of an element can provide valuable information about its origin, formation, and history.

1.2.3.5 Isomers

Different types of isomers, such as structural isomers, stereoisomers, conformational isomers, and nuclear isomers, have different structural arrangements in chemistry. But here, we will discuss nuclear isomers only, as they are relevant in medical imaging. The isomers in nuclear physics are defined as any of two or more nuclides of the same element that consist of the same number of protons as well as the same number of neutrons but differ in energy state and the manner of radioactive decay and exist for a measurable duration of time.

The measurable duration of time can have a lower limit of several picoseconds (10^{-12} seconds); however, in general, half-life of >1 nanosecond (10^{-9} seconds) or greater is considered as isomers [34, 35]. The isomers can have their half-life in several years as well.

Nuclear isomers can be formed through various processes, including nuclear reactions, beta decay, and gamma decay. They can also be artificially created in nuclear reactors, accelerators, or radioactive generators.

One example of a nuclear isomer is metastable technetium-99 m (half-life: 6.0066 h), used in medical imaging. This isotope has a half-life of about 6 h and emits gamma rays, which can be detected and used to produce an image inside the body. The following isomers have been considered as potential candidates: ^{58m}Co (8.853 h), ^{60m}Co (10.467 min), ^{103m}Rh (56.114 min), ^{117m}Sn (116.2 min), ^{125m}Te (57.40 days), ^{189m}Os (5.81 h), ^{193m}Ir (10.53 days), ^{193m}Pt (4.33 days), ^{195m}Pt (4.010 days), and ^{197m}Hg (23.82 h) [35]. Nuclear isomers can have important technological and scientific applications due to their unique properties and long half-lives (Table 1.4).

1.2.3.6 Isotones

Isotones are atoms of different elements with the same number of neutrons in their nuclei but different numbers of protons. Since the number of protons in an atom's nucleus determines its atomic number and thus its identity as a particular element, isotones are different elements with the same neutron number.

Table 1.4 Atoms, their composition, and related terms

Atom, their composition, and related terms
The atom is the basic unit of any element. It retains the chemical and physical properties of the element.
It is mostly empty space with its mass concentrated in the central nucleus and contains nucleons (**protons** and **neutrons**).
Protons are positively charged, and neutrons have zero charge. Atoms are electrically neutral (number of protons = number of electrons).
Atomic mass (**A**) = number of protons + neutrons.
Atomic number (**Z**) = number of protons.
Short-range forces hold nucleons together. The neutrons in the nucleus help reduce the repulsive forces of the positively charged protons as they "space" them out.
When there are less than 25 protons in a nucleus, there are the same number of neutrons. As nuclei get heavier (Z > 25), the relative number of neutrons needs to increase to counteract the increased electrostatic repulsive forces [36].

For example, carbon-14, nitrogen-15, and oxygen-16 are isotones with the same number of neutrons (eight) but different protons (six, seven, and eight). Similarly, chlorine-37, potassium-39, and calcium-40 are also isotones, all having the same number of neutrons (20) but different protons (17, 19, and 20, respectively).

Isotones have similar nuclear properties, such as nuclear spin, magnetic moment, and nuclear energy levels. This similarity can be attributed to the fact that the neutrons in isotones contribute more significantly to nuclear properties than protons.

1.2.3.7 Isobars

The different chemical elements with the same atomic mass but different atomic numbers are called as isobars. This means that isobars have the same number of nucleons (protons and neutrons) in their nuclei but a different number of protons.

For example, carbon-14 and nitrogen-14 are isobars with an atomic mass 14, but carbon-14 has 6 protons, and nitrogen-14 has 7 protons. Similarly, potassium-40 and calcium-40 are isobars, with an atomic mass of 40, but potassium-40 has 19 protons, and calcium-40 has 20 protons.

Due to the differences in atomic numbers and electron configurations, isobars have different chemical and physical properties. However, they can have similar nuclear properties, such as the same half-life or nuclear decay modes. This makes them useful in nuclear physics and applications such as radiotherapy.

1.2.3.8 Binding Energy

The amount of energy, required to break the nucleus of an atom into its constituent, that is, protons and neutrons, is called binding energy. The neutrons and protons are combinedly called nucleons. The binding energy per nucleon is important, as it indicates a nucleus's stability and can be used to predict the energy released in nuclear reactions. Nuclear forces operate over short distances but are very powerful. It overcomes the electromagnetic repulsion forces between the positively charged protons in the nucleus and holds the nucleus together.

When proton and neutron form a nucleus, some of their mass is converted into energy. According to Einstein's famous mass-energy equivalence eq. ($E = mc^2$), this energy is equivalent to the binding energy of the nucleus, and it is responsible for holding the nucleus together. The higher binding energy per nucleon gives more stable nucleus.

1.2.3.9 Nuclear Stability

Nuclear stability refers to the ability of an atomic nucleus to maintain its structural integrity and resist decay. Nuclear stability is generally determined by the balance between the forces that hold the nucleus together, such as the strong nuclear force, and the electrostatic repulsion forces between protons that pull it apart. The stability of a nucleus is measured by its binding energy per nucleon, which is the amount of energy required to separate the nucleons in a nucleus. Generally, nuclei with higher binding energies per nucleon are more stable than those with lower binding energies.

Nuclei with unequal numbers of neutrons and protons tend to be unstable. Neutron-rich nuclei tend to undergo beta-minus decay, also known as beta decay. In this, the neutron in the nucleus decays into a proton, an electron, and antineutrino. The electron (β^-) and antineutrino ($\bar{\nu}$) are emitted from the nucleus, and the proton remains in the nucleus. The atomic number of the nucleus is changed since a neutron has been converted into a proton, and it typically moves the nucleus toward a more stable configuration.

The proton-rich nuclei tend to undergo beta-plus decay, also known as positron emission. In this decay, the proton decays into a neutron, a positron, and a neutrino. The positron (β^+) and neutrino (ν) are emitted from the nucleus, and the neutron remains in the nucleus. The atomic number of the nucleus is changed since a proton has been converted into a neutron, and it typically moves the nucleus toward a more stable configuration.

1.3 Section B: Fundamental Concepts of Electricity and Magnetism

In the first and second sections, we understood radiation, the structure of atoms and radioactive decay, and other concepts of atomic physics. Our main aim is to understand X-rays, their physics, and equipment based on X-rays. Since an X-ray machine needs electricity to produce X-rays, we must also understand electricity. Electricity is always associated with magnetism and vice versa; therefore, understanding magnetism becomes essential. Understanding electricity and magnetism becomes important since X-rays are also called electromagnetic radiation. While operating X-ray machines, we encounter terms such as mAs and kVp. These are abbreviations of "milliampere-second" and "kilovolt peak." In a later section, "Production of X-rays," we will also learn how the current is converted into X-rays. mAs and kVp are associated with electric current or electricity.

1.3.1 Electricity

The flow of electrons or ions through a conductor medium is called "electricity." In a typical electrical circuit, electrons flow from the negative terminal to the positive terminal of a voltage source (such as a battery), while conventional current is defined as flowing from positive to negative. This flow of electrons generates a current that can be used to power electrical devices.

A single person did not discover electricity; its discovery and development were gradual. However, many scientists and inventors significantly contributed to our understanding and use of electricity. One of the earliest known discoveries related to electricity was made by the ancient Greeks, who observed that rubbing amber against fur would cause the amber to become charged and attract small objects. This phenomenon was later named "electricity" after the Greek word for amber, "Elektron." Amber has been a fossilized tree resin used for decorative and medicinal purposes for thousands of years. It is typically yellow, orange, or brown and can be found in many areas of the world (Fig. 1.28).

In the eighteenth century, scientists such as Benjamin Franklin (1706–1790) and Italian physicist Alessandro Volta (1745–1827) made important electricity-related discoveries. Franklin is best known for his kite experiment, in which he demonstrated the electrical nature of lightning and explored the polarity of electric charge (positive and negative), while Volta is credited with inventing the first battery in 1800, which paved the way for the development of modern electronics.

Later in the nineteenth century, scientists such as British scientist Michael Faraday (1791–1867) and Scottish physicist James Clerk Maxwell (1831–1879) made significant contributions to the field of electromagnetism, a field where which relationship between electricity and magnetism is studied. Faraday discovered electromagnetic induction, the principle behind the operation of generators and transformers, while Maxwell developed a set of equations that unified the fields of electricity and magnetism.

1.3.2 Unit of Electricity

The unit of electricity is Ampere, denoted by "A" as recommended by the International System of Units (SI); however, the abbreviation of ampere "Amp" is also used. The ampere is named on French physicist André-Marie Ampère (1775–1836), who is known for his contributions in the field of electromagnetism. *The ampere is the electric current corresponding to a flow of one coulomb of charge per sec-*

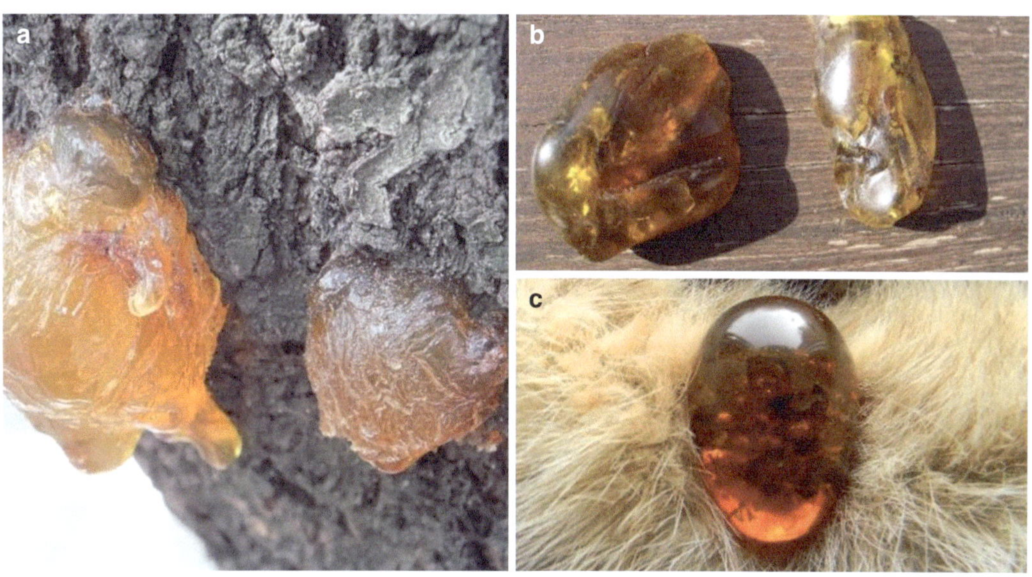

Fig. 1.28 Amber images: (**a**) Tree trunk with resin, (**b**) amber, (**c**) amber with fur. Image courtesy: Pixabay.com

ond through a conductor. The formula for electric current is:

$$I = \frac{Q}{t} \tag{1.2}$$

where I is the electric current, Q is the electric charge, and t is the time the current flows.

The electric charge "Q" is measured in "coulomb," and 1 coulomb of electric charge equals total charges of approximately 6.24×10^{18} electrons.

1 coulomb of charge is equal to 6.24×10^{18} electrons. How did this figure arrive?

The value of 6.24×10^{18} electrons per coulomb is derived from the fundamental physical constant known as the elementary charge or the charge of an electron, meaning it is a value that has been measured experimentally and is considered a fixed value. The charge of an electron is a fundamental constant of nature, represented by the symbol "e," and has a value of approximately -1.602×10^{-19} coulombs, where the negative sign indicates that the electron has a negative charge.

$$\because 1\,\text{electron} = 1.602 \times 10^{-19}\,\text{C}$$

$$\therefore 1\,\text{coulomb} = \frac{1}{1.602 \times 10^{-19}}\,\text{electrons}$$

$$\therefore 1\,\text{coulomb} = 6.24 \times 10^{18}\,\text{electrons}$$

One coulomb of electrical charge is the amount of charge that flows in a conductor when a current of one ampere flows in one second.

Now if we see coulomb and ampere, both are interdependent, related by the equation I = Q/t, where 1 ampere corresponds to 1 coulomb of charge flowing per second. To understand this, let us see the International System of Units (SI) definition of "Ampere."

"The ampere is that constant current which, if maintained in two straight parallel conductors of the infinite length of negligible circular cross section, and placed 1 meter apart in vacuum, would produce between these conductors a force equal to 2×10^{-7} newtons per meter of length" [37]. The coulomb, on the other hand, is defined as the SI unit of electric charge. It is defined as the amount of electric charge that flows through a cross section of a conductor in per second when a current of one ampere flows through the conductor.

As can be seen, the definition of the ampere involves the force between two conductors carrying a certain current, which is related to the magnetic field created by the current. Meanwhile, the definition of the coulomb involves the flow of electric charge, which is related to the current passing through a conductor. Therefore, electric charge is not typically used as a force, as it is a property of a particle or object rather than a force that can be applied to another object. The force in electric circuits is typically associated with electric current, which is the flow of electric charge through a conductor.

1.3.3 Coulomb's Law and Lorentz Force

The force between two charged particles or objects is described by Coulomb's law, which states that "the force between two point charges is directly proportional to the product of the individual charges and inversely proportional to the square of the distance between them." This force is an electric force, and it can be attractive or repulsive force depending on the sign of the charges. The mathematical expression of Coulomb's law is as follows:

$$F = \frac{k.q1.q2}{r^2} \tag{1.3}$$

where F is the electrostatic force between two point charges, q_1 and q_2 are charges, r is the distance between the charges, and k is Coulomb's constant, a proportionality constant that depends on the medium between the charges.

In electric circuits, charges primarily experience an electric force due to the electric field that drives the current. When these charges or a current-carrying conductor move through a magnetic field, they also experience a magnetic force. This magnetic component of the Lorentz force acts perpendicular to both the magnetic field and the direction of current flow. The Lorentz force finds practical applications in devices such as cyclotrons and other particle accelerators. The application of this force is in cyclotrons and other particle accelerators (Fig. 1.29).

Overall, the ampere is an important unit of measurement in electricity and plays a key role in the design and operation of electrical systems and devices.

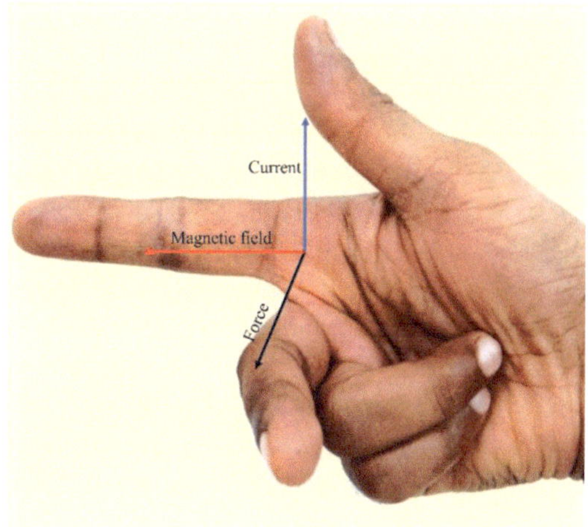

Fig. 1.29 Right-hand rule—Lorentz's force

> ? Is there any way to visualize the units such as ampere and coulomb as we do it for meter, kilogram and second?

Units such as meter, kilogram, and second can be easily visualized because they correspond to physical quantities that are directly observable and tangible. However, units like ampere and coulomb, used to measure electrical quantities, are not as easily visualized in the same way.

The Ampere (A) is unit of electric current, and represents the flow of electric charge. It can be defined as the amount of charge passing through a given point in a conductor per unit time. While we cannot directly see or visualize electric current, we can use analogies to help understand it. One common analogy is to think of electric current as the water flow in a pipe. The current is analogous to the water flow rate, and the ampere represents the quantity of electric charge flowing per unit of time.

Coulomb (C) is the unit of electric charge and defined as the amount of charge transported by a current of one ampere in 1 s. Visualizing the coulomb directly is challenging because it is an abstract unit representing a specific charge quantity. However, we can consider it a measure of the total charge carried by a certain number of electrons. For example, one coulomb is approximately equal to the charge of 6.24×10^{18} electrons.

> ? What are the differences in electricity, electric current and charge?

When we refer to "electricity" in a more general sense, it can refer to both static and flowing electric charge, but we typically use the term "electric current" when we specifically refer to the flow of electric charge. Static electricity involves the build-up of electric charge on an object that is not in motion, and there is no flow of electric charge between the charged objects. An example is rubbing a balloon against hair, the balloon and hair both become charged, but there is no electric charge flows between them, and therefore no electric current.

A coulomb is an important unit in electricity used to measure an electrical system's charge. For example, the capacity of a battery is measured in coulombs, as is the amount of charge that a capacitor can hold. The coulomb is also used in calculations of electric force, such as the force between two charged particles, which is proportional to the product of their charges in coulombs. Electric charge is the property of matter that describes how much electricity is present in a particle, like an electron or proton. Just like we use grams to measure the weight of an object, we use coulombs to measure the amount of electric charge in an object.

One coulomb of charge is a lot of charges! It is equal to the charge that passes through a wire in 1 s when a current of one ampere flows. One ampere measures how many electrons flow through the wire each second.

Generally, household items are designed to operate on standard electrical outlets, which supply an alternating current (AC) voltage of around 120 or 230 volts RMS (root mean square) at a frequency of 60 Hz. The current that flows through these devices is typically measured in amperes (A), the unit of electric current.

1.3.4 Concept of mAs Used in X-Ray Machines

We are familiar with mobile phone battery capacities, measured in milliampere-hours (mAh), for example, 2000 mAh and 5000 mAh. The mAh stands for milliampere-hour and theoretically delivers a current of, for example, 2000 mAh (or 2 amperes) for 1 h before running out of charge. But again, the battery life depends on various factors, such as the device's power consumption, usage patterns, and battery health. *In practical terms, a battery's capacity is determined by its current product and the time it can sustain that current.*

But the concepts of mAh in batteries and mAs in X-ray tubes differ.

In radiology, the mAs stand for milliampere-second, a unit that measures the product of the X-ray tube current (in milliamperes) and exposure time (in seconds), which determines the number of electrons emitted and thus correlates with the amount of X-ray radiation produced by an X-ray tube. It represents the product of the tube current (measured in milliamperes) and the exposure time (measured in seconds). For instance, an X-ray tube operated at 100 mA for 0.1 s would produce an exposure of 10 mAs.

Higher mAs values result in more X-rays, which can provide better image quality and increase the patient's radiation exposure. It is used to control the amount of radiation exposure to a patient during an X-ray procedure. Therefore, radiographers use a combination of mAs and other factors, such as kVp (kilovoltage peak) and filtration, to optimize image quality while minimizing radiation exposure.

An X-ray machine passes an electrical current through a cathode filament, which heats up and emits electrons. These electrons are then accelerated toward the anode target, which produces X-rays. The amount of X-rays produced is directly proportional to the current flowing through the filament and the duration of exposure, that is, the mAs value is directly proportional to the amount of X-rays produced, and increasing the mAs value will increase the number of X-rays that pass through the patient's body and reach the detector. This increased number of X-rays will create a brighter image with more contrast, making it easier to see details in the image.

Conversely, decreasing the mAs value will result in a darker image with less contrast and details. However, reducing the mAs value can be useful in some situations to minimize the radiation dose to the patient while still obtaining a diagnostic image. Therefore, using the appropriate mAs setting for each imaging scenario is important to balance image quality and radiation safety.

> ? Compare the number of electrons flowing in 300 mAs versus 500 mAs.

The number of electrons flowing through an X-ray tube depends on the current (measured in milliamperes) and exposure time (measured in seconds) used in the X-ray machine, collectively expressed as mAs. To calculate the number of electrons, the X-ray tube takes into account the current and exposure time.

The following formula for calculating the number of electrons in an X-ray tube is used:

$$\text{Number of electrons} = \frac{mAs \times 10^{-3}}{1.602 \times 10^{-19}}$$

Where mAs are the milliampere-seconds.

Using the mAs value of 300, the calculation would be:

$$\text{Number of electrons} = \frac{300 \times 10^{-3}}{1.602 \times 10^{-19}}$$

$$\therefore \text{Number of electrons} \approx 1.872 \times 10^{18} \text{ electrons}$$

Therefore, the number of electrons in an X-ray tube required to deliver 300 mAs is approximately 1.872×10^{18} electrons.

Assuming the same conditions, the number of electrons flowing in an X-ray tube for 500 mAs would be:

$$\text{Number of electrons} = \frac{500 \times 10^{-3}}{1.602 \times 10^{-19}}$$

We get

$$\text{Number of electrons} \approx 3.120 \times 10^{18} \text{ electrons}$$

Therefore, the number of electrons flowing in an X-ray tube for 500 mAs is higher than for 300 mAs.

1.3.5 Concept of Voltage

Voltage, also known as electric potential difference, measures the electrical energy per unit of charge in a circuit. It is the force that drives electrical current through a conductor or circuit. Voltage is measured in units of volts (V) and represented by the symbol "V." A voltage of one volt is defined as the amount of electrical potential difference required to drive a current of one ampere (A) through a resistance of one ohm (Ω) in a circuit. In practical terms, voltage can be considered the pressure that moves electrical current through a circuit. Just as water flows from high pressure area to a low pressure area, electrical current flows from an area of high voltage to an area of low voltage.

Various sources, such as batteries, generators, and power supplies, can produce voltage. The amount of voltage produced by a source depends on the properties of the source, such as its design, materials, and operating conditions. In electrical circuits, voltage controls current flow through different components, such as resistors, capacitors, and inductors. Adjusting the voltage in a circuit makes it possible to control the behavior of these components and produce the desired electrical output.

In radiology, the voltage measures the electrical potential difference between the cathode and anode of the tube. When voltage is applied to the X-ray tube, it accelerates the electrons emitted by the cathode toward the anode, causing them to collide with the atoms of the anode material and produce X-rays.

The voltage applied to the X-ray tube is typically measured in kilovolts (kV) and is referred to as the tube voltage, tube potential, or X-ray generator voltage. The voltage can be adjusted using a control panel on the X-ray machine to produce X-rays of different energy levels. Higher voltage settings result in X-rays with higher energy levels, which can penetrate deeper into the body for imaging dense tissue. However, higher-energy X-rays also carry a greater risk of radiation exposure and must be used with care.

- *kVp*

The term kVp is used more often in radiology, and it stands for kilovoltage peak and describes the peak voltage applied to an X-ray tube. It is a primary factor affecting the quality (photon energy) of X-rays produced during a radiographic examination.

The kVp controls the energy of the X-ray photons produced by the tube. Higher kVp values result in higher-energy photons, which can penetrate deeper into the body and produce less contrast in the X-ray image. Conversely, lower kVp values produce lower-energy photons that are absorbed more easily by the body, resulting in more contrast in the image.

In practice, the kVp is set based on the type of examination being performed and the body part being imaged. For example, high kVp values are typically used for examinations of dense body parts, such as the chest, while lower kVp values may be used for examinations of less dense body parts, such as the extremities.

It is worth noting that the kVp setting is only one factor affecting the quality of X-rays produced during a radiographic examination. Other factors include the mAs (milliampere-seconds), which control the overall quantity of X-rays produced, and the filtration, which removes low-energy photons from the X-ray beam to reduce patient radiation exposure.

The term "peak voltage" is used in X-ray machines because the voltage applied to the X-ray tube varies over time (often from rectified alternating current) and rises to a maximum value during each cycle. The maximum value is referred to as the peak voltage (kVp), and it determines the maximum energy of the X-ray photons produced.

In contrast, in household electrical systems, the supply is also alternating current, but the quoted value (e.g., 120 V in the US, 230 V in many countries) is the root-mean-square (RMS) voltage, not the peak voltage. The RMS value is used because it reflects the equivalent heating or power-delivery capability of the AC voltage. Therefore, "voltage" is typically used to describe the electrical potential difference between two points in the circuit.

Additionally, the voltage used in household electrical systems is typically much lower than the peak voltage used in X-ray machines. The voltage supplied to a typical household outlet may be 120 volts, while the kVp used in diagnostic X-ray imaging can range from around 40 kVp to over 150 kVp, depending on the imaging modality and the patient's anatomy.

In summary, the use of the term "peak voltage" in X-ray machines reflects the fact that the voltage applied to the X-ray tube is time-varying and that its peak value determines the maximum photon energy, whereas the term "voltage" used in household electrical systems generally refers to the RMS value of the alternating voltage.

? Why is peak voltage term used in X-rays, whereas in households uses only voltage?

1.3.6 Electric Power

It is the rate at which electrical energy is transferred or converted from one form to another. It is expressed in units of watts (W), equivalent to joules per second (J/s), and represents the amount of energy transferred per unit of time. The formula for calculating power is:

$$\text{Power}(\text{P}) = \frac{Energy(E)}{Time(t)} \quad (1.4)$$

In an electrical circuit, power can also be calculated using the following formula:

$$\text{Power} = \text{Voltage} \times \text{Current} \quad (1.5)$$

Where voltage is the electrical potential difference across the circuit, and current is the rate of flow of electric charge through the circuit.

Based on Eq. (1.14), if a circuit delivers 10 joules of energy in 1 s, the power delivered by the circuit is 10 watts. Similarly, if a circuit delivers 100 joules of energy in 10 s, the power is also 10 watts.

The power delivered to the X-ray tube is typically measured in units of kilowatts (kW) or megawatts (MW) and is dependent on the tube current (mA) and the applied voltage (kVp). X-ray tubes used for medical diagnostic imaging typically operate at much lower power levels, typically on a few kilowatts (kW) or less. This is because the imaging requirements for medical X-rays do not typically require the high energies or intensities used in industrial or research applications and because the low power levels help to minimize the radiation dose to the patient. However, due to the required high-power levels, X-ray tubes used for industrial or research applications, such as nondestructive testing or high-energy physics experiments, may be measured in megawatts (MW).

1.3.7 Magnetism

Magnetism is a fundamental aspect of the electromagnetic force, one of the four fundamental force of nature responsible for many phenomena we observe in the physical world. At its core, magnetism is caused by the movement of electric charges, specifically electrons, within a material (Fig. 1.30).

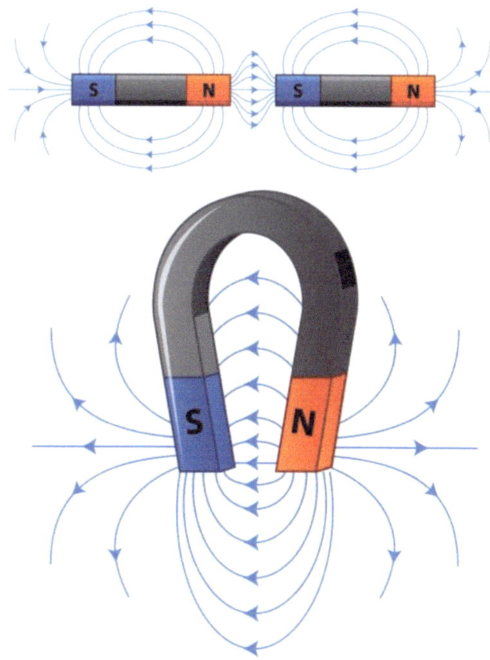

Fig. 1.30 Magnetism. (Image by brgfx on Freepik)

When electrons move through a material, they create a magnetic field. In most materials, these magnetic fields are randomly oriented and cancel each other out, resulting in no net magnetism. However, in certain materials called ferromagnets, the magnetic moments of the electrons align with each other, creating a net magnetic field that can be observed on a larger scale.

Magnetism has many practical applications, such as electric motors, generators, and magnetic storage devices like hard drives. Magnets, such as magnetic resonance imaging (MRI) machines, are also used in medical imaging. Magnetic fields have many properties, including polarity (north and south), strength, and direction.

The unit of magnetic field strength is teslas (T), and the direction of the field is defined as the direction that a north-seeking compass needle points in the field. Magnetic fields can interact with other magnetic fields, electric fields, and moving charges. This interaction allows magnets to attract or repel each other and can be used to generate electrical currents through a process called electromagnetic induction.

1.3.8 An Electric Field Is Always Associated with the Magnetic Field

Electric and magnetic fields are always associated in situations where charges are moving or fields are changing, as described by the theory of electromagnetism.

Electromagnetism studies the relationship between electric charges and electric and magnetic fields. Whenever an electric charge is present, it creates an electric field that exerts a force on other electric charges. Similarly, when an electric charge is in motion, it creates a magnetic field which exerts a force on other moving charges (Fig. 1.31).

The electric and magnetic fields relationship is so intimate that they are often described as two sides of the same coin. Specifically, a changing

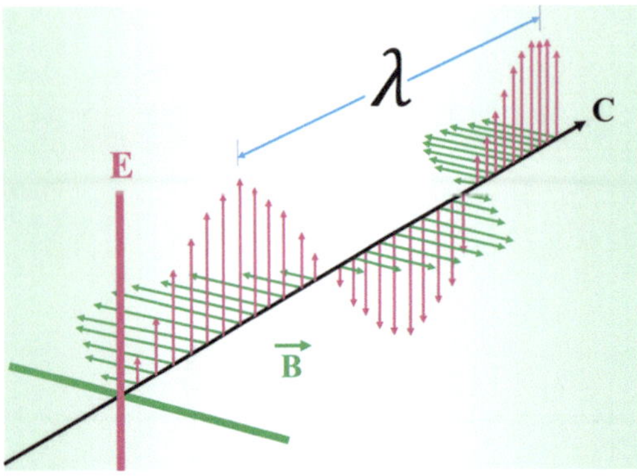

Fig. 1.31 Electromagnetism. If *C* represents energy density, *E* represents electric field strength, and *B* represents magnetic field strength, then according to the Poynting theorem, the energy flux (S) is given by the Poynting vector $S = E \times H$, and the energy density (u) is given by $u = (\varepsilon_0 E^2 + B^2/\mu_0)/2$. Electromagnetic energy is the cross product of electric field intensity and magnetic field intensity, making it inherently directional

electric field creates a magnetic field, and vice versa a changing magnetic field creates an electric field. This process is called electromagnetic induction and is the basis for many important technologies, including generators, transformers, and electric motors.

Moreover, the interplay between electric and magnetic fields is also responsible for the propagation of electromagnetic waves, such as light, radio waves, and X-rays. In all these cases, the electric and magnetic fields oscillate together, perpendicular to each other and to the direction of wave propagation.

1.3.9 Electromagnetic Radiation and Electromagnetic Spectrum

1.3.9.1 Electromagnetic Radiation

Electromagnetic radiation is energy propagated through space in the form of oscillating electric and magnetic fields. These fields can be generated by the acceleration of charged particles.

When charged particles are accelerated, they create disturbances in the surrounding electric and magnetic fields, propagating outward as electromagnetic waves. These waves are characterized by their frequency, wavelength, and amplitude and can travel through a vacuum at the speed of light.

Photons, on the other hand, are quanta of energy associated with electromagnetic waves. They are not themselves charged particles and thus do not have an electric charge (in the classical sense; they have an intrinsic quantum spin but no rest mass or net charge). Instead, they are best understood as discrete packets of energy emitted or absorbed when electrons transition between energy states.

> ? Photons do not have electrons, but still, they are electromagnetic radiation; how?

While photons are not particles in the classical sense, they are often described as particles because they exhibit some properties of particles, such as momentum, energy, and the ability to interact with matter discretely.

The relationship between photons and electromagnetic radiation is established through wave-particle duality. This principle holds that particles like photons can exhibit wavelike and particle-like behavior, depending on the experimental conditions. Photons can be considered both wavelike disturbances in the electric and magnetic fields and particles that carry discrete amounts of energy.

Therefore, while photons do not have an electric charge in the classical sense, they are still considered electromagnetic radiation because they are intimately connected with the electric and magnetic fields and are the quanta of these fields. The interaction of photons with matter allows us to detect and measure electromagnetic radiation and is the basis for many important technologies, such as X-ray imaging, solar cells, and lasers.

> **?** Calculate the momentum of 100 keV photons.

The photon momentum can be calculated using the photon momentum–wavelength relation:

$$p = \frac{h}{\lambda} \tag{1.6}$$

where p is the photon's momentum, h is Planck's constant, and λ is the photon's wavelength.

First, we need to calculate the photon's wavelength to calculate the momentum. Let us first convert the photon's energy from keV to joules since Planck's constant is typically given in joule-seconds.

$$\because 1\,\text{keV} = 1.602 \times 10^{-16}\,\text{joules}$$

$$\therefore 100\,\text{keV} = 1.602 \times 10^{-14}\,\text{joules}.$$

Next, we can use the formula for the energy of a photon:

$$E = h\nu \tag{1.7}$$

E is the photon's energy, h is Planck's constant, and ν is the frequency. On rearranging this formula to solve for the frequency:

$$\nu = \frac{E}{h}$$

Substituting in the energy of the 100 keV photons and Planck's constant, we get:

$$\nu = \frac{1.602 \times 10^{-14}\,J}{6.626 \times 10^{-34}\,J.\text{sec}}$$

$$\nu = 2.41 \times 10^{19}\,\text{Hz} \;\{1/\text{s} = \text{Hertz}(\text{Hz}), \text{unit of frequency}\}$$

∴ the wavelength of 100 keV photon

$$\lambda = \frac{c}{\nu} = \frac{299{,}792{,}458\,\text{m/s}}{2.41 \times 10^{19}\,\text{Hz}} = 1.24 \times 10^{-11}\,\text{m}$$

c is the speed of light and equivalent to 299,792,458 m/s, and ν is the frequency of the photon. Now since we have the wavelength of the 100 keV photons, using the formula (Eq. 1.16) to calculate its momentum:

$$p = \frac{h}{\lambda}$$

$$p = \frac{6.626 \times 10^{-34}\,J.\text{sec}}{1.24 \times 10^{-11}\,m}$$

$$p = 5.34 \times 10^{-23}\,Kg.m/s \left(\text{Joule} = \frac{Kg.m^2}{s^2}\right)$$

Therefore, the momentum of a 100 keV photon is approximately 5.34×10^{-23} kg m/s.

1.3.9.2 Electromagnetic Spectrum

The electromagnetic spectrum describes a range of all types of electromagnetic radiation, which are waves of energy that travel through space at the speed of light. These waves have different wavelengths and frequencies and are classified according to their properties. Depending on the wavelength and frequency of radiation, they are classified as follows:

1.3.9.2.1 Radio Waves

Radio waves have the longest wavelengths and lowest frequencies of all types of electromagnetic radiation. They are typically used for communication, such as radio and television broadcasting, cell phone communication, and navigation systems like GPS. They are also used for scientific research in radio astronomy, which studies celestial objects and phenomena by observing their radio waves. They typically have wavelengths between 1 mm and 100 km, corresponding to frequencies ranging from 300 GHz to 3 kHz (Fig. 1.32).

1.3.9.2.2 Microwaves

Microwaves have shorter wavelengths and higher frequencies than radio waves. They are used in everyday applications, such as cooking, commu-

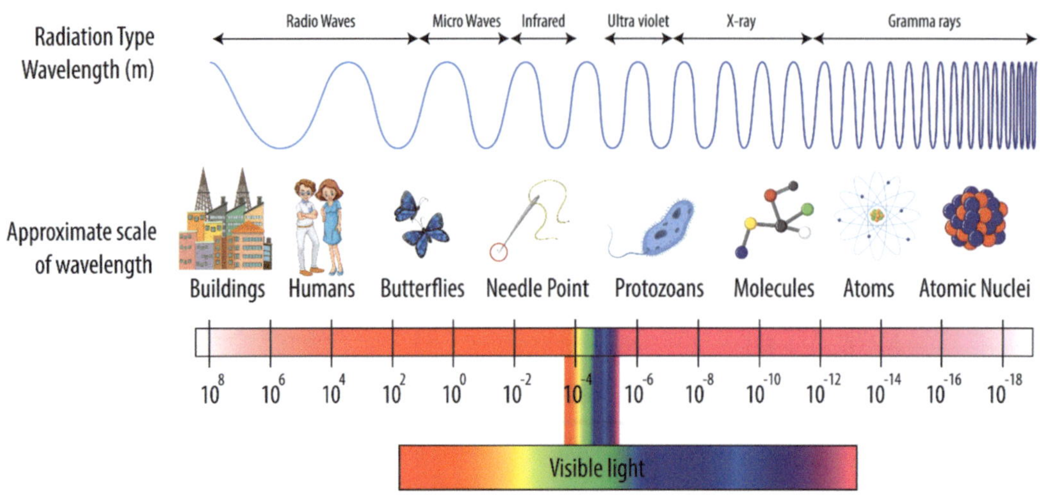

Fig. 1.32 Wavelength and frequency range of electromagnetic radiation. Image by brgfx on Freepik

nication, and radar systems. In cooking, the water molecules in the food to vibrate and generate heat microwaves heat food by causing the water molecules in the food to vibrate and generate heat. In communication, microwaves are used for satellite communication, cell phone networks, and wireless Internet. In radar systems, microwaves detect objects and measure their distance and speed.

1.3.9.2.3 Infrared Radiation

Infrared radiation has shorter wavelengths and higher frequencies than microwaves. All warm objects emit it and can be detected by infrared cameras. Infrared radiation is used in many applications, such as thermal imaging for medical diagnosis, industrial inspection, and surveillance. It is also used in heating systems, such as infrared heaters, which heat objects directly rather than heating the air around them.

1.3.9.2.4 Visible Light

Visible light has wavelengths in the range of approximately 380–750 nanometers, which the human eye can detect, producing the sensation of color. It ranges from violet, which has the shortest wavelength, to red, which has the longest wavelength. Each light color has a different wavelength and frequency, determining its properties. Visible light is used in many applications, such as photography, lighting, and optical microscopy and certain medical imaging techniques (Table 1.5).

Table 1.5 Range of wavelengths and frequency for different types of electromagnetic radiation

Type of radiation	Wavelength range	Frequency range
Radio waves	>1 mm	<300 GHz
Microwaves	1 mm–30 cm	300 GHz–1 GHz (some definitions extend to 300 MHz)
Infrared radiation	750 nm–1 mm	400 THz–300 GHz
Visible light	~380–750 nm	790 THz–400 THz
Ultraviolet radiation	10 nm–400 nm	30 PHz–790 THz
X-rays	0.01 nm–10 nm	30 EHz–30 PHz (overlaps with gamma rays at high end)
Gamma rays	<0.01 nm	>30 EHz

mm = millimeter (10^{-3} m), m = meter, nm = nanometer (10^{-9} m), MHz = Mega Hertz (10^{6} Hertz), GHz = Giga Hertz (10^{9} Hertz), THz = Tera Hertz (10^{12} Hertz), PHz = Peta Hertz (10^{15} Hertz), EHz = Exa Hertz (10^{18} Hz).

1.3.9.2.5 Ultraviolet Radiation

Ultraviolet radiation has shorter wavelengths and higher frequencies than visible light. It is responsible for causing sunburns and can damage the DNA in cells, which can lead to skin cancer. Ultraviolet radiation is also used in tanning beds, sterilization devices, and scientific research.

1.3.9.2.6 X-Rays

X-rays have shorter wavelengths and higher frequencies than ultraviolet radiation. They are used in medical imaging to create images of the body's internal structures, as well as in scientific research and industrial inspection. X-rays are highly energetic and can penetrate many dense materials, such as bone and to some extent metal, but can also cause damage to living cells if exposure is not carefully controlled.

1.3.9.2.7 ϒ-Rays

Gamma rays are a type of electromagnetic radiation with the highest frequency and shortest wavelength in the electromagnetic spectrum. They are generated by the most energetic processes in the universe, such as nuclear explosions, supernovae, and the annihilation of matter with antimatter. Gamma rays can also be produced artificially in particle accelerators or through the radioactive decay of certain isotopes. Gamma rays are highly energetic and can penetrate most materials, including thick layers of lead and concrete. They can cause significant damage to living tissues and are thus used in radiation therapy to destroy cancer cells. In addition, gamma rays are also used in various industrial and scientific applications, such as detecting defects in metal components, sterilizing medical equipment, and the study of the properties of matter at the atomic and subatomic levels.

In summary, the electromagnetic spectrum includes a wide range of radiation with different wavelengths and frequencies, each with unique properties and applications.

? What is the difference between gamma and x-rays?

Gamma and X-rays are both forms of electromagnetic radiation, but they differ in origin and energy levels. Nuclear processes, such as radioactive decay, nuclear fusion or fission, and particle annihilation, produce gamma rays. They have the highest energy and the shortest wavelength in the electromagnetic spectrum, with typical energies ranging from hundreds of keV (kiloelectron volts) to many MeV (megaelectron volts).

On the other hand, X-rays are typically generated by the interaction of fast-moving electrons with matter, such as the electron beams in X-ray tubes or the synchrotron radiation emitted by charged particles traveling at near-light speeds. They have a lower energy and longer wavelength than gamma rays, with typical energies ranging from a few keV to a few hundred keV.

Because of their higher energy and shorter wavelength, gamma rays are more penetrating than X-rays and can pass through thicker materials, such as concrete and lead. This property makes them useful in various applications, such as radiation therapy and detecting defects in materials. On the other hand, X-rays are used in various applications, including medical imaging, airport security, and materials analysis.

Gamma rays and X-rays are both forms of electromagnetic radiation with different energies and origins. Nuclear processes typically produce gamma rays, and a range of gammas have higher energy and shorter wavelength and are more penetrating than X-rays, while X-rays are typically generated by the interaction of fast-moving electrons with matter and have lower energy and longer wavelength than gamma rays.

1.4 Section C: Radiation Quantities and Units

1.4.1 Exposure, "X"

Exposure is the amount of radiation an individual receives from a particular source. It can occur through various routes, such as inhalation, ingestion, or direct radiation exposure. The exposure is proportional to the number of ionizations created in a given air volume, which is affected by the radiation's intensity and exposure time.

It is defined as the amount of X- or ϒ-rays radiation which produces ionization of 1 electrostatic unit (1 esu) of either positive or negative charge per cubic centimeter of dry air at standard temperature and pressure (STP) (i.e., 0 °C of temperature and one atmospheric pressure).

$$\text{Exposure}\left(\text{X}\right)=\frac{dQ}{dm} \quad (1.8)$$

where dQ is the total charge of ions of a single sign produced (either positive or negative) in the air by ionizing radiation, and dm is the mass of air irradiated.

The SI (the International System of Units) exposure unit is expressed in coulombs per kilogram (C/kg). However, the unit of exposure in use is Roentgen, "R," and

$$1\text{R}=2.58\times10^{-4}\,\text{C}\,\text{Kg}^{-1}\left(\text{air}\right)$$

Except at very high energies, the exposure defined above is the ionization equivalent of the air kerma, and by definition, exposure is a quantity restricted to photons and air as the medium.

1.4.2 Exposure rate, "X^0"

Exposure per unit of time is called exposure rate and is represented as X^0.

$$\text{Exposure rate}\left(X^{0}\right)=\frac{\text{Exposure}}{\text{time}}=\frac{X}{t} \quad (1.9)$$

SI unit of exposure rate is $\frac{C}{Kg.t}$ or $\frac{Ampere}{Kg}$

∵ 1 ampere = $\frac{Coulomb}{time.}$

However, in common use, exposure rate is measured in Roentgen/hour (R/h) or milli roentgen/h (mR/h). The exposure rate can also be measured in microsieverts per hour (μSv/h). A microsievert is a unit of radiation dose equivalent that considers both the energy deposited by ionizing radiation in a material and the biological effect of the radiation on human tissue. For gamma and X-ray radiation, in air;

$$1\ \text{R}/\text{h}\approx 8770\ \mu Sv/\text{h}$$
$$\&1\ \mu Sv/\text{h}=0.114\ \text{mR}/\text{h}$$

However, for other types of radiation, such as alpha and beta particles, the conversion factor is different and can vary depending on the energy of the radiation and the material that the radiation is passing through.

1.4.3 Dose and Absorbed Dose "D"

The dose is a broader term that refers to the amount of energy deposited in a material or tissue by radiation and can be subdivided into three related but distinct terms: absorbed dose, equivalent dose, and effective dose. However, as per International Commission on Radiation Units and Measurements (ICRU), the dose is absorbed dose only, but it is used as a generic term also [38]. Terms such as emergency dose, collective absorbed dose, median lethal dose, permissible dose, threshold dose, dose tolerance etc., may also be broadly generalized as "dose"' terms. The absorbed dose specifically refers to the amount of energy deposited in a specific material or tissue per unit mass.

The absorbed dose is the energy deposited per unit mass on any specific material. This energy can be related to any ionizing radiation, such as gamma rays, X-rays, or alpha particles, and it can be absorbed by any type of matter, such as air, water, or human tissue.

It is denoted as D. The equation for absorbed dose:

$$D=\frac{\text{d}E}{\text{d}m} \quad (1.10)$$

Unit: Système International (SI) unit is joule/kilogram (J/kg), and the special unit is gray. The traditional unit is erg/gram (erg/gm) or rad (acronym of "radiation absorbed dose").

Gy = 1 joule/kg 1 rad = 100 ergs/gm

∵ 1 joule = 10^7 ergs and 1 kg = 1000 gm

1Gy = 100 rad or, 1 cGy = 1 rad

The quantities rad, gray, and sievert are collective nouns such as staff, team, army, etc., and should not be spoken as rads, sieverts, etc. However, this is seen in books and papers.

The absorbed dose is a fundamental concept in radiation dosimetry, which studies how radiation affects living organisms and how to measure and control radiation exposure. It quantifies the amount of energy absorbed by a material or organism due to exposure to ionizing radiation.

1.4.4 Dose Rate

Absorbed dose per unit time is called dose rate and is denoted as $\dot{D}$.

$$\dot{D} = \frac{D}{t} \quad (1.11)$$

The unit is gray/time, that is, gray/h or gray/s.

Short half-lives imply high dose rates and, conversely, long half-lives. The absorbed dose rate may affect the biological response of tissues to irradiation.

1.4.5 Equivalent Dose

The equivalent dose accounts for the different types of radiation and their different biological effectiveness in causing radiation damage. An equivalent dose is calculated by multiplying the absorbed dose by a radiation weighting factor, which reflects the relative biological effectiveness of the type of radiation being considered. It is represented as "H_T" and

$$H_T = \sum \text{Absorbed dose} \times w_R \quad (1.12)$$

Where w_R is called the radiation weighting factor, different for different types of radiation (Table 1.6) and is a dimensionless quantity. The SI unit of the equivalent dose is sievert (Sv). The term "rem" (roentgen equivalent to men) was also used for an equivalent dose.

$$1\,\text{Sv} = 100\,\text{Rem}$$

1.4.6 Effective Dose

Different organs have different radiosensitivity, and therefore, they receive different doses. The effective dose accounts for different organ sensitivity along with different types of radiation.

Table 1.6 Radiation weighing factors for various ionizing radiation. Copyright Springer Nature Singapore [39]. Reprinted with permission

Ionizing radiation	ICRP 103 recommendations
Photons, electrons, positrons, and β-particles	1
Alpha	20
Protons and charged pions	(In ICRP 60, it was 5)
Neutron	A continuous function of neutron energy varies between 2.5 and 20.7
Auger electrons (in nuclear medicine, emitters such as ^{99m}Tc, ^{123}I, ^{125}I, and ^{201}Tl)	Varies from 1 to 20 on a case-to-case basis, for example, 1 when ^{125}I is localized in the cytoplasm, 4 in the nucleus, and 7–9 when bound to DNA. It can be up to 20 depending on the proportion of DNA-bound emitters (MIRD pamphlet 21)

Table 1.7 Tissue weighting factors as per ICRP 103. Copyright ICRP. Reprinted with permission

Tissue	w_T	No. of tissues	Summation
Red bone marrow, colon, lung, stomach, breast, and remainder tissue[a]	0.12 each	06	0.72
Gonads	0.08	01	0.08
Urinary bladder, esophagus, liver, thyroid	0.04 each	04	0.16
Bone surface, brain, salivary glands, skin	0.01	04	0.04
Total	1.00		

[a]Remainder tissues include adrenals, extra-thoracic region, gall bladder, heart, kidneys, lymphatic system, muscles, oral mucosa, pancreas, prostate, small intestine, spleen, thymus, and uterus/cervix

Effective dose is calculated by multiplying the absorbed dose (in gray or Gy), radiation weighting factor (dimensionless) and tissue weighting factor (dimensionless). It is represented as "E" and

$$E = \sum \text{Absorbed dose} \times w_R \times w_T \quad (1.13)$$

where w_R is tissue weighting factor and w_T is a tissue weighting factor that differs for different organs (Table 1.7). The SI unit of effective dose is sievert (Sv). w_T is also a dimensionless quantity.

1.4.7 Kerma, "K" (Kinetic Energy Released in Material)

Kerma or Kinetic Energy Released in Material is the sum of the initial kinetic energies of all the charged particles liberated by the radiation per unit mass of the material.

The SI unit of kerma is gray, and 1 Gy = 1 J kg^{-1} (joules per kilogram)

When the reference material is air, the quantity is termed as "air kerma." The concept of kerma was originally defined as "Kinetic Energy Released per unit Mass" by ICRU (The International Commission on Radiation Units and Measurements) in the 1960s, but the definition was revised to "Kinetic Energy Released in Material" in ICRU Report 33 published in 1980 to more accurately reflect the nature of the energy transfer that occurs when ionizing radiation interacts with matter (Table 1.8).

? Is there any difference between the equivalent dose and dose equivalent?

Equivalent dose and dose equivalent are two different terms; however, many people use them interchangeably mistakenly. "Equivalent dose" is a dosimetric quantity used in radiation protection, whereas "dose equivalent" is an operational quantity. Operational quantities are those which are used to monitor and control radiation exposure in a particular situation, such as personal monitoring or area monitoring, whereas radiation protection quantities are used to assess the risk of radiation-induced health effects, typically based on standardized models for a reference person.

The dose equivalent is a measured quantity for external radiation used to estimate the effective dose, whereas the equivalent dose is an intermediate quantity in calculating the effective dose. The equivalent dose is represented as H_T, whereas the "dose equivalent" is represented as H.

Generally, the International Commission on Radiological Protection (ICRP) provides recommendations on radiation protection quantities (publication 1977, 1990, 2007) and International Commission on Radiological Units and Measurements (ICRU) provides reports on operational quantities (1985, 1988, 1993, 2020). However, joint reports are also published, and ICRU report 95 in 2020 [42] is recent, but a separate recommendation by ICRP has also been published in publication 147 [40]. ICRU report 95 (2020) and ICRP publication 147 (2021) discuss refinements to radiation protection quantities, but the term "equivalent dose" remains in use and is not discontinued, though its application is clarified in these reports. The ICRP considers that the absorbed dose is more appropriate instead of using an equivalent dose to set limits to prevent tissue

Table 1.8 Quantities and their units

Quantity	Old unit	SI unit	Relationship between units
Radioactivity	Ci (curie)	Bq (becquerel)	1 Bq = 2.7×10^{-11} Ci 1 ci = 3.7×10^{10} Bq
Exposure	R (roentgen)	C/kg (coulombs per kg)	1 R = 2.58×10^{-4} C/kg
Exposure rate	R/h	C/kg.t or ampere/kg	1 R/h = 10 μSv/h 1 μSv/h = 0.1 mR/h
Absorbed dose	rad	Gy (gray)	1 gray = 100 rads
Equivalent dose	rem	Sv (sievert)	1 Sv = 100 rems
Effective dose	rem	Sv (sievert)	1 Sv = 100 rems

reactions. This change will draw a clear distinction between limits applying to tissue reactions, set in absorbed dose (Gy), and those applying to probabilistic effects, set in effective dose (Sv).

The International Commission on Radiological Protection (ICRP) has used radiation protection quantities such as absorbed, equivalent, and effective doses. The term effective dose was introduced in the ICRP 60, 1990 [41] to use a single quantity for the control of occupational and public exposures and later extended its application to include exposures for all ages and in utero exposures [42]–[44]. In addition, it is widely used in medical applications for which the primary requirement is for estimates of detriment, mainly from cancer, to understand the implications of different diagnostic modalities [40].

Measuring the absorbed dose is possible using dosimeters, but measuring the equivalent dose and effective dose requires knowledge of the type and energy of the radiation, the tissues or organs exposed, and the sensitivity of those tissues or organs to radiation, which are difficult to measure directly. Therefore, these quantities are typically calculated using mathematical models based on measurements of the absorbed dose and other factors related to radiation exposure.

On the other hand, operational quantities are practical and measurable quantities used in radiation protection to monitor and control radiation exposure. They are defined based on the types of detectors or measurement instruments commonly used in radiation protection and are related to the absorbed dose in a particular material or tissue.

Though the term "dose equivalent" is also not used directly and is named as personal dose equivalent and ambient dose equivalent. The personal dose equivalent is measured at different depths, Hp(d), for assessment of whole-body exposure and skin and lens of the eye doses. Hp(10) is representative of whole-body exposure, and the dosimeter is worn at a depth of 10 mm on a position of the body. For dose assessment to the skin and the extremities, the personal dose equivalent, Hp(0.07), with a depth of 0.07 mm, is recommended as an operational quantity. These terms are defined as the product of fluence or air kerma and conversion coefficients based on conversion coefficients provided in ICRP Publication 116 (Table 1.9), which relate operational quantities to effective dose for various particles and energies.

Table 1.9 Operation dose quantities for the area and individual monitoring

Operational dose quantities	Dose equivalent
For area monitoring	Ambient dose equivalent H*(10) Directional dose equivalent H (0.07, Ω)
Operational dose quantities for individual monitoring	Personal dose equivalent, H_p (10) Personal dose equivalent, H_p (0.07)

1.5 Section D: Interaction of Radiation with Matter

Various forms of radiation, including photons, electrons, positrons, neutrons, protons, pions, muons, or helium ions, interact with the medium through which they pass. Based on these interactions, they are detected and used in various radiation applications, including medical imaging. These radiations can be divided into particulate and non-particulate or electromagnetic radiation. Both behave differently with the medium and therefore are described separately.

While interacting with matter, particulate radiation transfers its energy and causes excitation and ionization of the atoms. In another type of interaction, due to coulombic forces of the positively charged nucleus, the velocity of incident electrons is decelerated, and in response, bremsstrahlung radiation is produced. Non-particulate radiation, specifically photons, interacts with matter through processes such as the photoelectric effect, Compton scattering, and pair production, depending on the photon's energy. The photoelectric effect and Compton scattering are particularly relevant for medical imaging.

1.5.1 Charged Particle Interaction

The charged particles collide with electrons in orbit and the nuclei of the atoms in the medium and cause these particles to lose energy

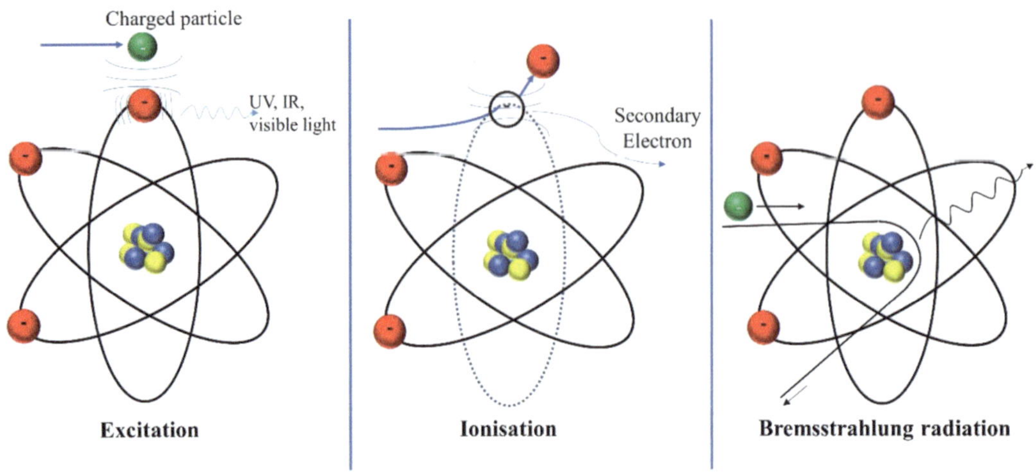

Fig. 1.33 Charged particle interaction with matter

(Fig. 1.33). Along the path of a charged particle in the medium, the following interaction may occur:

1.5.1.1 Excitation

The charged particle can transfer energy to atoms or molecules in the medium, causing them to become excited (move to a higher energy state) without ionizing.

1.5.1.2 Ionization

The charged particle can transfer energy to atoms or molecules in the medium, causing them to ionize (lose or gain electrons) and become charged particles, forming ions.

1.5.1.3 Radiative Energy Loss

The charged particle can emit radiation (such as photons) as it passes through the medium, losing energy due to interaction with the electric and magnetic fields of the medium. The energy loss can result in bremsstrahlung radiation, synchrotron radiation, or transition radiation.

1.5.1.4 Bremsstrahlung Radiation

It is a special case of radiative energy loss caused by the deceleration of a charged particle. When a charged particle, for example, an electron, passes through a medium, it can be deflected by the nuclei of the atoms in the medium, causing it to change direction and lose kinetic energy. This loss of kinetic energy is equivalent to decelerating the charged particle.

As the charged particle decelerates, it emits electromagnetic radiation in the form of photons. This is because the changing velocity of the charged particle produces an oscillating electric field, which in turn generates an oscillating magnetic field. Combining these two fields produces electromagnetic radiation, which is emitted as photons.

This process is known as bremsstrahlung radiation, a German term meaning "braking radiation." The term reflects that the emission of photons is due to the deceleration of the charged particle as it passes through the medium.

Bremsstrahlung radiation is an important phenomenon in various fields, including medical imaging, nuclear physics, and materials science. It can be used, for example, in X-ray imaging to produce images of the internal structure of objects or in particle accelerators to generate high-energy photons for research purposes.

1.5.1.5 Scattering

The charged particle can be deflected from its path as it passes through the medium due to collisions with atoms or molecules.

1.5.1.6 Nuclear Interactions

If the charged particle has sufficient energy, it can interact with atomic nuclei in the medium, causing nuclear reactions.

The nature and extent of these interactions depend on the energy and type of the charged particle, as well as the properties of the medium (such as its density, composition, and temperature). These interactions are important in various applications, from particle physics experiments to medical imaging and radiation therapy.

1.5.2 Photon Interaction with the Medium

Photon interaction with matter refers to how photons, packets of electromagnetic energy, interact with atoms or molecules in a material medium. The nature of this interaction depends on many factors, including the energy of the photon, the composition of the medium, and the properties of the atoms or molecules in the medium. The following are the major interactions:

1.5.2.1 Photoelectric Effect

This occurs when a photon is absorbed by an atom, causing an electron to be ejected from atom. The ejected electron is known as a photoelectron, and its energy is equal to the energy of the absorbed photon minus the electron's binding energy to the atom. The energy of photoelectron, mathematically expressed as:

$$E_e = h\nu - E_B \tag{1.14}$$

where E_e is the energy of the photoelectron, h is Planck's constant, ν is the frequency of the incident photon, and E_b is the electron's binding energy.

The probability of the photoelectric effect occurring depends on the photon's energy and the absorbing material's properties. Materials with higher atomic numbers and densities are more likely to undergo photoelectric interactions, and the probability decreases with increasing photon energy.

Properties of Photoelectric Effect

- The photoelectric effect only occurs when the incident photon's energy exceeds the electron's binding energy in the atom.
- The energy of the incident photon is completely transferred to the ejected electron and the atom.
- The energy of the emitted electron equals the energy of the absorbed photon minus the electron's binding energy to the atom.
- The probability of the photoelectric effect occurring depends on the properties of the absorbing material, including its atomic number and density.
- The cross section of the photoelectric effect is proportional to the number of electrons available for interaction and the probability of the photon being absorbed.
- The threshold energy required for the photoelectric effect depends on the absorbing material's atomic number and electron configuration.
- The absorption edge, corresponding to the threshold energy for photoelectric absorption, depends on the absorbing material's atomic number and electron configuration.
- The photoelectric effect has important applications in X-ray imaging, radiation therapy, and X-ray spectroscopy.

1.5.2.2 Compton Scattering

This occurs when a photon collides with an electron in the material and transfers part of its energy to the electron, causing it to recoil. The scattered photon has less energy and a longer wavelength than the original. Suppose the energy of the incident photon is hν, the energy of the scattered photon is E_{sc}, and the energy of recoil electron E_{re} then, the energy of scattered photons:

$$E_{sc} = \frac{h\nu}{\left[1 + \left(\frac{h\nu}{0.511}\right)(1 - cos\theta)\right]} \tag{1.15}$$

The energy of recoil electron:

$$E_{re} = h\nu - E_{sc} \tag{1.16}$$

where h is Planck's constant, ν is the frequency of the incident photon, 0.511 MeV is the electron's rest mass, θ is the scattering angle, and cosθ is the cosine of the scattering angle.

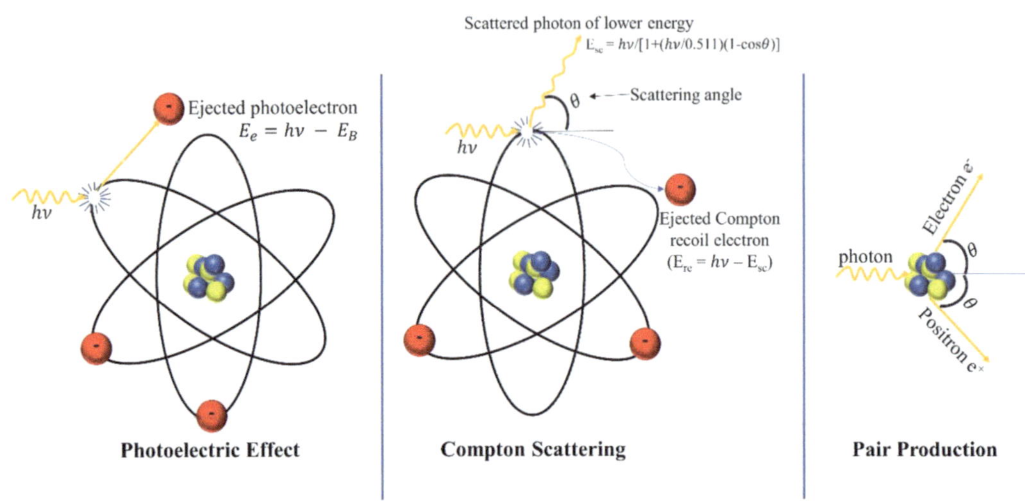

Fig. 1.34 Interaction of photons with matter

The energy of the scattered photon and recoil electron depends on the scattering angle and the initial energy of the incident photon. The probability of Compton scattering is dominant at intermediate photon energies (approximately 0.1 to 10 MeV) and is nearly independent of the material's atomic number (Fig. 1.34).

Properties of Compton Effects

- The Compton effect is a form of scattering of photons by loosely bound or free electrons.
- The scattered photon energy is lower than the incident photon.
- The energy transfer from the photon to the electron is maximum when the photon scatters at 180 degrees.
- The probability of Compton scattering is nearly independent of the atomic number of the scattering material.
- Compton scattering is an important process in X-ray and gamma ray imaging and spectroscopy.

1.5.2.3 Pair Production

Pair production is a process in which a photon is converted into an electron–positron pair in the presence of a nucleus or an electron. Pair production occurs when the photon has energy greater than the rest mass energy of the electron–positron pair, which is 1.022 MeV. When a high-energy photon interacts with a nucleus, it can produce an electron–positron pair through the following reaction:

$$h\nu + Z \rightarrow e^+ + e^- + Z \tag{1.17}$$

Properties of Pair Production

- Pair production occurs only when the photon has energy greater than 1.022 MeV.
- Pair production can occur in the presence of a nucleus or an electron. When a photon interacts with an electron, it can produce an electron–positron pair in a process called triplet production, with the original electron recoiling.
- The probability of pair production increases with the photon energy and the atomic number of the target material.
- Pair production is an important process in medical physics, where high-energy photons are used for radiation therapy. When a high-energy photon interacts with a patient's body tissue, it can produce electron–positron pairs, which can deposit energy and damage the DNA of cancer cells.
- Pair production is also an important process in astrophysics, where high-energy photons from outer space can produce electron–positron pairs when they interact with the interstellar medium. This can lead to the creation of gamma ray bursts and other energetic phenomena.

1.5.2.4 Rayleigh Scattering

This occurs when a photon interacts with the entire atom and causes it to vibrate, reradiating the photon, with the same energy as the original photon. Rayleigh scattering occurs most frequently at low photon energies, and the probability decreases with increasing photon energy. It is named after Lord Rayleigh (1842–1919), who first described the phenomenon in 1871.

Rayleigh scattering is responsible for the blue color of the sky, which is caused by the scattering of sunlight by atmospheric gases, such as nitrogen and oxygen. The other important applications of Rayleigh scattering are in astronomy, radar and communication systems, nanoparticle characterization, remote sensing, and other applications in science and technology.

1.5.2.5 Auger Effect

It occurs when a photoelectron is ejected from an atom, leaving behind an inner-shell vacancy. Another electron from a higher shell can fill this vacancy, releasing energy as an Auger electron.

1.5.2.6 Photodisintegration

This occurs when a high-energy photon interacts with an atom's nucleus, causing it to break apart into smaller nuclei or particles.

Understanding the different forms of photon interactions with matter is important in many applications, including medical imaging, radiation therapy, and materials science. Different materials are better suited for different types of interactions, and optimizing these interactions can help improve the sensitivity and specificity of imaging techniques and the effectiveness of radiation therapy.

1.5.3 Interaction of Neutron with Matter

When a neutron interacts with matter, several possible outcomes depend on the neutron's energy and the material's nature. Some of the common interactions of neutrons with matter are:

1.5.3.1 Elastic Scattering

It occurs when a neutron collides with an atomic nucleus in the material and transfers part of its energy to the nucleus, causing it to recoil. The neutron may change direction and lose some of its energy.

1.5.3.2 Inelastic Scattering

This occurs when a neutron collides with an atomic nucleus and transfers a significant amount of energy to the nucleus, causing it to become excited, to a higher energy state.

1.5.3.3 Absorption

This occurs when a neutron is captured by the nucleus of an atom in the material, forming a heavier isotope. The absorbed neutron may also cause the nucleus to become excited, emitting gamma rays.

1.5.3.4 Fission

This occurs when a neutron is absorbed by a heavy nucleus, causing it to become unstable and break apart into two or more smaller nuclei, with the release of a large amount of energy and often additional neutrons.

The probability of each of these interactions depends on the neutron's energy and the material's properties, such as its composition and density. The interaction of neutrons with matter is important in various fields, including nuclear engineering, materials science, and medical physics.

1.6 Section E: Production of X-Rays

1.6.1 Historical Background

In the late nineteenth century, Wilhelm Conrad Roentgen (1845–1923) discovered X-rays on November 8, 1895 [45]. Though he did not mention a specific date of discovery in his original paper on X-rays, it is generally accepted that Roentgen made his discovery on November 8, 1895, based on his own recollections, personal diary, and other historical evidence. Roentgen

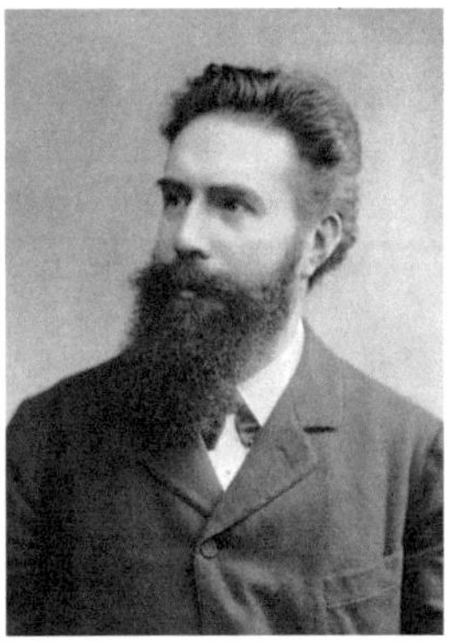

Fig. 1.35 Wilhelm C. Roentgen. (Image courtesy: Deutsches Röntgen-Museum. Published with permission)

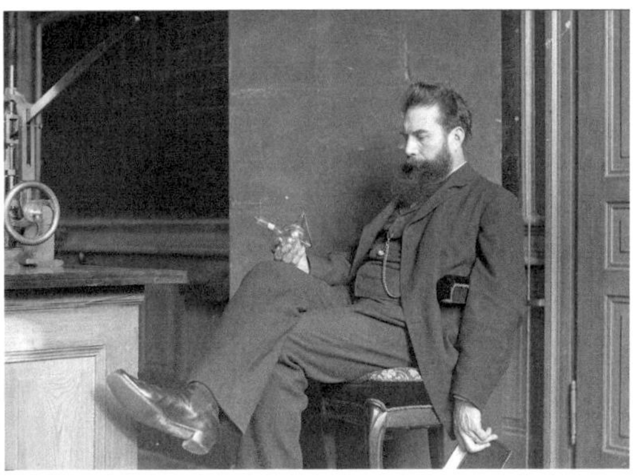

Fig. 1.36 WC Roentgen with early gas (ion) X-ray tube. (Image courtesy: Deutsches Röntgen-Museum, printed with permission)

was a German physicist experimenting with cathode ray tubes, a common apparatus in the study of electricity at the time. He noticed that when the tubes were energized with high-voltage electricity, they emitted a new type of invisible ray that could penetrate many substances, including the human body (Figs. 1.35 and 1.36).

Roentgen's discovery caused a sensation in the scientific community, and within months, X-rays were being used for medical purposes, particularly in diagnosing bone fractures and other internal injuries. X-ray machines were rapidly developed and deployed in hospitals and clinics worldwide. The technology quickly spread, and within a year, X-ray machines were being used in hospitals and clinics worldwide. In 1901, Roentgen was awarded the Nobel Prize in Physics for discovering X-rays [46].

The early X-ray machines were relatively simple: a cathode ray tube that produced X-rays when energized with high-voltage electricity and a photographic plate that captured the X-ray image. The X-ray machine required a high-voltage power source and an operator who could adjust the settings to manipulate the intensity and duration of the X-ray exposure.

As X-ray technology advanced, so did the machines themselves. New designs and features were added, such as the rotating anode X-ray tube, which allowed for higher-intensity X-ray beams, and the use of lead shielding to protect patients and operators from excessive radiation exposure.

However, the widespread use of X-rays also led to the concerns about potentially harmful effects of radiation exposure. Many early X-ray technicians and patients suffered from radiation burns and other health problems due to excessive exposure to X-rays. This led to the development of radiation protection measures and regulations, including the use of lead aprons, collimators, and dosimeters to measure radiation exposure.

Despite these concerns, X-ray technology continued to advance, and new applications were found for X-rays in fields such as dentistry, veterinary medicine, and industrial testing. Today, X-rays are still widely used for medical imaging, and new technologies such as digital X-rays and computed tomography (CT) have further expanded the capabilities of this powerful diagnostic tool.

1.6.2 Interaction of Electron with the Target

The production of X-rays in an X-ray machine involves the interaction of high-energy electrons with a metal target. When a high-energy electron is directed toward a metal target, it is decelerated by the electric field of the atomic nucleus in the target material, and the energy lost by the electron is emitted as an X-ray photon. This process is known as bremsstrahlung radiation or braking radiation. The photon's energy is equal to the dif-

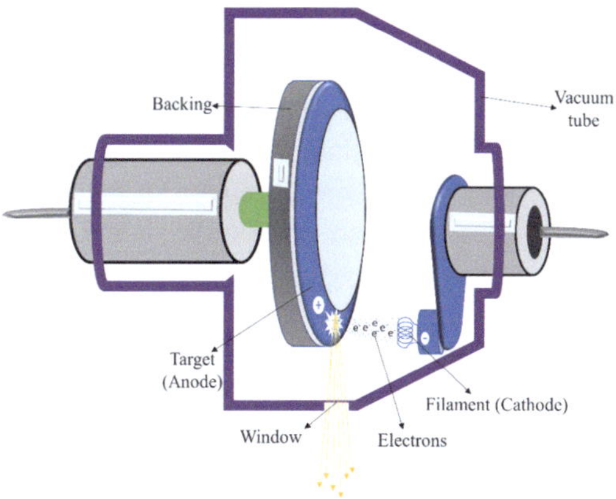

Fig. 1.37 Cross-sectional diagram of the X-ray tube

ference between the electron's initial and final kinetic energy (Fig. 1.37).

There are two main types of interactions between the incident electrons and the target atoms: elastic and inelastic. In elastic scattering, the incident electron interacts with an atomic electron, causing it to be deflected from its path. The electron little to no energy and retains its initial kinetic energy. In inelastic scattering, the incident electron collides with an atomic electron, transferring enough energy to eject it from the atom. This is known as ionization.

The interaction between the electrons and the target material can be further broken down into two main processes: bremsstrahlung and characteristic radiation. Most X-rays produced in an X-ray machine are bremsstrahlung radiation, which occurs when the electric field of the target atom decelerates the incident electron. The resulting X-ray photon has a continuous energy spectrum, ranging from zero to the maximum energy of the incident electron. The maximum energy of the X-ray photon is equal to the energy of the incident electron, while the minimum energy is typically near zero due to the continuous nature of the bremsstrahlung spectrum (Fig. 1.37).

In addition to bremsstrahlung radiation, X-rays can also be produced through a process known as characteristic radiation. This occurs when an incident electron collides with an inner-shell electron in the target material, causing it to be ejected from the atom. When an outer-shell electron fills the resulting vacancy, it emits an X-ray photon with characteristic energy specific to the target material.

1.6.3 The Process of Production of X-Rays

The process of production of X-rays can be broken down into several steps:

1.6.3.1 Generation of Electrons

Electrons are produced by a cathode, a heated filament or a wire that emits electrons when heated. The electrons are then accelerated toward the anode by an electric field.

1.6.3.2 Interaction with the Target

When the high-energy electrons collide with the target material (usually a metal such as tungsten or molybdenum), they transfer some of their kinetic energy to the target atoms. This can cause the atoms to ionize or excite, which releases energy in the form of X-rays. Tungsten and molybdenum are commonly used as target materials in X-ray tubes because of their high melting points and ability to produce X-rays efficiently. Tungsten has atomic number ($Z = 74$) and is an efficient producer of high-energy X-rays. Molybdenum ($Z = 42$) has a lower melting point than tungsten (tungsten has 3422 °C whereas molybdenum has 2623 °C), which can make it more suitable for applications requiring lower-energy X-rays, such as mammography. The choice of material depends on the specific application and desired X-ray energy range.

Tungsten (W) is commonly used as a target material in high-energy X-ray tubes, such as those used in CT scanners and other diagnostic imaging applications that require high penetrating power. On the other hand, molybdenum is commonly used as a target material in mammography X-ray tubes requiring lower energies, as a lower atomic number allows it to produce lower energy range X-rays. However, it should be noted that other factors can also influence the choice of target material, such as cost, availability, and the specific requirements of the imaging system.

1.6.3.3 Production of X-rays

The X-rays produced by the interaction between the electrons and the target material are then emitted in all directions from the target. Some X-rays pass through the patient's body and are detected by a detector on the other side, creating an image of the internal structures.

Overall, the interaction of high-energy electrons with a metal target is a complex process that involves elastic and inelastic scattering, ionization, and the emission of bremsstrahlung and characteristic X-rays. These processes are carefully controlled in an X-ray machine to produce the desired X-ray energy spectrum and optimize image quality.

1.6.4 X-Ray Spectrum

The X-ray spectrum produced by an X-ray tube comprises two fundamental components: bremsstrahlung radiation and characteristic X-rays. These components arise from distinct interactions between high-energy electrons and the atoms of the target material in the X-ray tube.

1.6.4.1 Bremsstrahlung Radiation

Bremsstrahlung, or "braking radiation," is the primary mechanism for X-ray production in an X-ray tube. It occurs when high-energy electrons, accelerated by a large potential difference (typically between 20,000 and 150,000 volts) between the cathode and the anode, collide with the target material, usually tungsten due to its high atomic number and high melting point and thermal stability. As these electrons approach the positively charged nuclei of the target atoms, they are decelerated by the nuclear electric field. This deceleration causes the electrons to lose kinetic energy, which is emitted as X-ray photons. The energy of these emitted photons varies depending on how close the electrons come to the nucleus during their deceleration: the closer the encounter, the greater the energy loss and, consequently, the higher the energy of the emitted X-ray photon.

The resulting bremsstrahlung radiation forms a continuous spectrum because deceleration can occur over a wide range of distances and intensities. On an X-ray spectrum graph, this continuous spectrum is represented by a smooth curve that starts from zero and increases to a peak before gradually declining. The maximum energy of the X-rays in this spectrum corresponds to the peak voltage applied across the X-ray tube, known as the tube potential.

1.6.4.2 Characteristic X-Rays

In addition to bremsstrahlung radiation, X-ray tubes also produce characteristic X-rays, which result from specific interactions between the incident electrons and the inner-shell electrons of the target atoms. When the high-energy electrons strike the target, they can eject inner-shell electrons (such as those in the K or L shells) from the atoms, creating vacancies. Electrons from higher energy levels (outer shells) then transition down to fill these vacancies, and the energy difference between these levels is emitted as X-ray photons. These photons have discrete energies that are characteristic of the target material's atomic structure.

For example, in a tungsten target, an electron transition from the L shell (with a binding energy of about 10.2 (L_3), 11.5 (L_2), 12.1 (L_1) keV) to a K shell vacancy (binding energy of about 69.525 keV) produces a characteristic X-ray with an energy of approximately 59.3 keV ($K\alpha_1$, $L_3 \rightarrow K$) or 58.0 keV ($K\alpha_2$, $L_2 \rightarrow K$). These discrete energy emissions appear as sharp peaks on the X-ray spectrum graph and are specific to the element used in the target. The binding energy of the K shell in a tungsten target is approximately 69.525 keV, and the binding energy of the L shell is about 10.2 – 12.1 keV. Therefore, the energy of the K_α X-ray photon is approximately 59.3 keV ($K\alpha_1$) (69.5 keV–10.2 keV) or 58.0 keV ($K\alpha_2$) (69.5 keV–11.5 keV). This peak is typically the most intense and prominent in the characteristic X-ray spectrum of tungsten.

The second peak, known as the K_β peak, arises from the transition of an electron from the M shell (third energy level) to the K shell. The binding energy of the M shell in tungsten is approximately 1.78 – 2.8 keV. Consequently, the energy of the K_β X-ray photon is about 67.7 keV

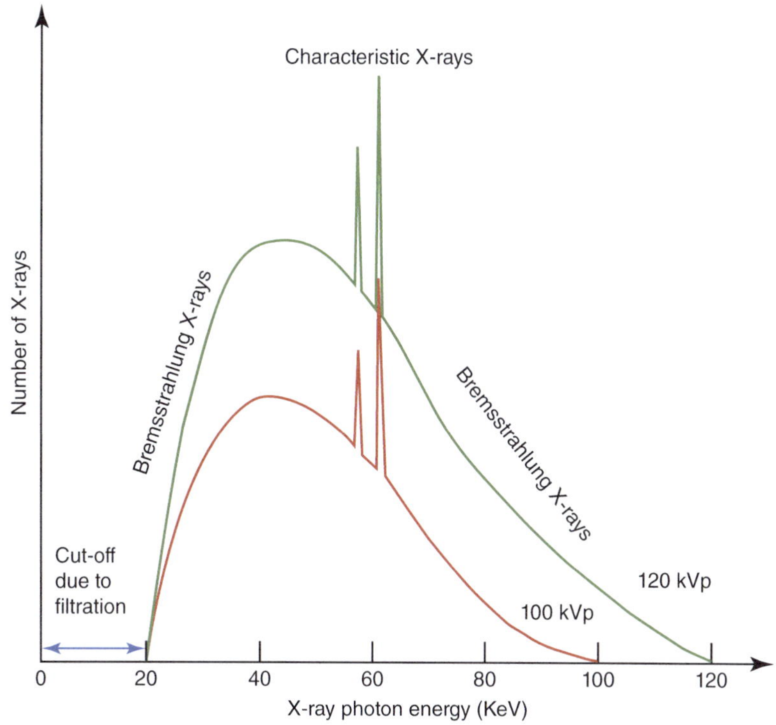

Fig. 1.38 Schematic representation of X-ray spectrum graph

(69.5 keV–1.8 keV). The K_β peak is generally less intense than the Kα peak.

1.6.4.3 Combined X-Ray Spectrum

The X-ray spectrum from an X-ray tube thus comprises both the continuous bremsstrahlung spectrum and the discrete characteristic peaks. The continuous spectrum covers a broad range of energies, while the characteristic spectrum is superimposed on this continuum with distinct peaks corresponding to the target material's specific energy transitions.

Adjusting the voltage applied to the X-ray tube affects both the continuous and characteristic components of the spectrum. Higher tube voltages increase the maximum energy of the bremsstrahlung spectrum and can enhance the intensity of characteristic peaks. Additionally, filtration can be used to remove lower-energy X-rays from the spectrum, optimizing it for specific imaging purposes by reducing patient dose and improving image quality.

Figure 1.38 illustrates a combined X-ray spectrum, showing both the continuous bremsstrahlung spectrum and the discrete characteristic peaks. It demonstrates how the X-ray spectrum changes with different tube voltages (100 kVp and 120 kVp) and highlights the cutoff due to filtration, which removes low-energy X-rays to enhance the quality of the imaging. The peaks at around 57.4 keV and 66.7–67.7 keV correspond to the K_α and K_β characteristic X-rays of tungsten, respectively. These peaks are superimposed on the continuous bremsstrahlung spectrum, adding specific energy lines to the overall X-ray output of the tube (Fig. 1.38).

1.6.5 X-Ray Properties and Classification Based on Energy Ranges

1.6.5.1 Properties of X-Rays

X-rays have several properties that make them useful in medical imaging and other applications:

- **Penetrating power**: X-rays can penetrate through materials which are opaque to visible light, such as skin, muscle, and bone. The pen-

etration depends on the X-rays energy and the material's density and thickness.
- **Ionizing ability**: X-rays have enough energy to ionize atoms, which means they can remove electrons from atoms and create charged particles. This property is used in radiation therapy to kill cancer cells and in radiography to produce images of the inside of the body.

Absorption and scattering: X-rays are absorbed or scattered by materials with high atomic numbers, such as bone and metal. This property is used to produce contrast in X-ray images, where the X-rays that pass through the body and are detected by a sensor or film are attenuated differently depending on the tissue density and composition.

1.6.5.2 Classification Based on Energy Ranges

Based on their energy ranges, X-rays are categorized into two main types: soft X-rays and hard X-rays.

Soft X-rays

Soft X-rays are characterized by their lower energy levels and longer wavelengths, typically ranging from about 0.1 to 5 keV (kiloelectron volts). This range of X-rays is more readily absorbed by matter, which limits their penetration power. Due to their lower energy, soft X-rays are commonly used in applications such as radiography for imaging soft tissues. They are also employed in some scientific research. It is important to note that there is some variation in the energy ranges defined for soft X-rays; some references suggest that X-rays from 100 eV (electronvolts) to less than 5 keV fall into this category, while others extend this range up to 10 keV [47] [49] [50] [51, 52]. In X-ray mammography, X-rays with energies ranging from 15 keV to 30 keV are used. Although these are often referred to as soft X-rays, the term "low-energy X-rays" is more accurate, given that mammography uses relatively low-energy X-rays compared to other diagnostic techniques like conventional X-rays and computed tomography (CT) scans.

Some of the common uses of soft X-rays include:

- ***Imaging and microscopy***: Soft X-rays can be used for high-resolution imaging and microscopy of biological samples, materials, and surfaces. This can provide detailed information about the samples' structure, composition, and properties.
- ***Spectroscopy***: Soft X-rays can be used for X-ray absorption spectroscopy (XAS) and X-ray emission spectroscopy (XES), which can provide detailed information about materials' electronic and chemical properties.
- ***Material science***: Soft X-rays can be used for surface analysis, thin film characterization, and other applications in materials science.
- ***Synchrotron radiation***: Soft X-rays can be produced by synchrotron radiation sources, which are powerful research tools for various experiments and studies in physics, chemistry, and biology.

Hard X-rays

Hard X-rays, on the other hand, have higher energy levels and shorter wavelengths, generally ranging from 5 keV to 100 keV or more. This high energy allows hard X-rays to penetrate matter more deeply, making them suitable for applications requiring high-resolution imaging and detailed structural analysis. They are extensively used in industrial inspections, crystallography, and advanced medical imaging techniques. The distinction between hard and soft X-rays is not strictly well-defined, with hard X-rays typically being those with energies of 5 keV or more [47, 48]. This classification helps in choosing the appropriate type of X-ray based on the specific requirements of penetration depth and imaging resolution. Hard X-rays have a wide range of applications in science, technology, and industry apart from medical imaging. Some of the common uses of hard X-rays:

- ***Materials science***: Hard X-rays can be used for studying the structure and properties of materials, including crystallography, small-angle scattering, and imaging of defects and cracks in metals and alloys.

- ***Nondestructive testing***: Hard X-rays can be used for the nondestructive testing of materials and components in the industry, including the inspection of welds, castings, and aerospace components.
- ***Security and defense***: Hard X-rays can be used for security and defense applications, including scanning for weapons and explosives and imaging hidden objects.
- ***High-energy physics***: Hard X-rays are used in high-energy physics experiments to probe the properties of subatomic particles.
- ***Astronomy***: Hard X-rays study high-energy phenomena such as black holes, neutron stars, and supernovae.
- ***Environmental science***: Hard X-rays can be used for studying the structure and properties of soils, sediments, and rocks and for environmental monitoring and analysis.

X-rays have unique properties that make them valuable in medical imaging and other applications. The energy range of the X-rays produced can be controlled by adjusting the voltage and current applied to the X-ray tube and the target material used. Soft X-rays have lower energies and are primarily absorbed by soft tissue, while hard X-rays have higher energies and can penetrate denser materials.

1.6.6 Clinical X-Ray Applications, Hazards, and Significance in Diagnostic Radiography

1.6.6.1 Clinical Applications

X-rays play a crucial role in various clinical applications in diagnostic radiography, providing essential information for diagnosing and treating a wide range of medical conditions:

- **Radiography:** X-rays are extensively used to visualize the internal structures of the human body, allowing for the detection of abnormalities and diseases. Radiography is employed to examine bones, teeth, and soft tissues, and is instrumental in diagnosing conditions such as pneumonia, lung cancer, and heart disease.
- **Computed tomography (CT):** CT scans combine X-rays with advanced computer technology to produce detailed cross-sectional images of the body. This technique is highly valuable in patient care, offering insights for diagnosing and managing conditions such as cancer, cardiovascular disease, and stroke.
- **Fluoroscopy:** This technique utilizes X-rays to create real-time images of the body, enabling continuous monitoring during procedures. Fluoroscopy is commonly used to guide surgical interventions and to examine the digestive system.
- **Mammography:** X-rays are utilized in mammography to detect breast cancer at an early stage, when it is most treatable. The low-energy X-rays used in mammography are specifically designed to produce high-quality images with minimal radiation exposure, enhancing the accuracy of breast cancer detection.
- **Dental imaging:** In dental clinics, X-rays are used to capture images of teeth and jaws, aiding in the diagnosis and treatment of dental issues such as cavities, abscesses, and impacted teeth. This imaging technique is crucial for effective dental care.
- **Angiography:** X-rays are employed in angiography to visualize blood vessels throughout the body. This application is essential for diagnosing and treating vascular conditions such as heart disease, stroke, and peripheral artery disease.
- **Radiation therapy:** In the field of oncology, high-energy X-rays are used in radiation therapy to target and destroy cancer cells. This treatment requires meticulous planning and monitoring to ensure precise delivery of radiation to the cancerous tissues while minimizing damage to healthy surrounding tissues.
- **Interventional radiology:** X-rays are used in various interventional radiology procedures, such as catheter placements and biopsies. These procedures often require real-time imaging to guide the instruments accurately and ensure optimal outcomes.

- **Nuclear medicine:** While not exclusively X-ray based, nuclear medicine sometimes utilizes X-ray imaging in conjunction with radioactive tracers to diagnose and monitor conditions, such as bone scans or PET (positron emission tomography) scans.
- **Pediatric imaging:** X-ray techniques are adapted for pediatric patients to ensure appropriate radiation doses and to address specific diagnostic needs in children, who are more sensitive to radiation.
- **Forensic medicine:** X-rays are used in forensic medicine to examine human remains, often aiding in the identification of deceased individuals or in determining the cause of injury or death.
- **Preoperative and postoperative imaging:** X-rays are commonly used before and after surgeries to assess the condition of the surgical site, verify the placement of implants or devices, and monitor the healing process.

Each of these applications underscores the versatility and importance of X-rays in modern medicine, contributing significantly to diagnostic accuracy and effective patient care.

1.6.6.2 Hazards from the X-Rays

X-rays, due to their ionizing nature, present several hazards that can affect both patients and healthcare workers. Ionizing radiation can remove tightly bound electrons from atoms, leading to the ionization of atoms and molecules within the body. This ionization can cause various types of tissue damage and increase the risk of long-term health effects. Understanding these hazards and implementing effective safety measures is crucial.

- **Radiation exposure:** X-ray exposure, even at low doses, can potentially cause tissue damage and increase the risk of cancer over time. The risk is proportional to the dose and frequency of exposure. For instance, patients undergoing multiple X-ray examinations or radiation therapies may accumulate a significant dose of radiation, which can have cumulative effects. Healthcare professionals employ various strategies, such as dose optimization and regular monitoring, to manage and minimize these risks.
- **Skin burns:** High doses of X-rays can result in skin burns, especially if there is prolonged exposure or inadequate shielding. These burns can vary from mild erythema to severe skin damage, depending on the dose. It is essential to use appropriate protective measures and monitor the dose closely during procedures involving high radiation.
- **Reproductive damage:** Exposure to X-rays can lead to damage to the reproductive organs, affecting fertility and potentially causing genetic abnormalities in offspring. This risk is particularly significant for patients of childbearing age. Techniques such as lead shielding and careful planning of exposure are employed to protect reproductive organs during diagnostic and therapeutic procedures.
- **Radiation sickness:** Radiation sickness is a condition resulting from exposure to high doses of radiation and can manifest as nausea, vomiting, fatigue, and in severe cases, more serious health effects. While this is more common in cases of accidental high-dose exposure or certain therapeutic procedures, it highlights the importance of adhering to safety protocols to avoid excessive exposure.
- **Increased risk of cancer:** Long-term or high-dose exposure to X-rays increases the risk of cancer, particularly in tissues that are more sensitive to radiation, such as the breast, thyroid, and bone marrow. This risk underscores the necessity of using X-rays judiciously and employing strategies to minimize radiation exposure, such as utilizing alternative imaging modalities when appropriate and implementing regular dose tracking.
- **Cumulative radiation effects:** Cumulative radiation exposure can have long-term health implications, particularly for patients who undergo frequent imaging or radiation treatments. Chronic exposure may increase the risk of various health conditions, including cancer. Monitoring cumulative dose levels and evaluating the risk–benefit ratio of

repeated imaging are important practices to manage this risk.

- **Radiation-induced genetic mutations:** Exposure to X-rays can induce genetic mutations, which may not only affect the exposed individual but also have potential implications for future generations. This is particularly concerning for reproductive cells and developing embryos. Efforts to minimize radiation exposure and protect sensitive populations are critical in mitigating these risks.
- **Potential effects on health workers:** Healthcare workers are also at risk from occupational exposure to X-rays. Chronic exposure can lead to health issues such as an increased risk of cancer, skin problems, and reproductive issues. Protective measures, including the use of lead aprons, shields, and regular health screenings, are essential to protect those who work with X-ray equipment.
- **Mitigation strategies:** To address these hazards, healthcare professionals follow rigorous safety guidelines, including using the lowest radiation dose necessary for diagnostic purposes, applying shielding to protect sensitive areas, and using advanced imaging technologies that reduce radiation levels. Additionally, patient and staff education on radiation safety and the importance of reporting pregnancy or potential pregnancy are vital components of minimizing risk. The careful balancing of diagnostic and therapeutic benefits with potential risks ensures that X-rays continue to be a valuable tool in medical practice while safeguarding health and safety.

To minimize these hazards, healthcare professionals follow strict guidelines for X-ray use, including using the lowest possible dose of radiation necessary to produce a diagnostic image. Patients are also advised to inform their healthcare provider if they are pregnant or could be pregnant, as the developing fetus is particularly sensitive to radiation. Overall, the benefits of X-rays in medical diagnosis and treatment must be carefully weighed against the potential risks.

1.6.7 Significance of X-Rays in Diagnostic Radiography

X-rays are an essential component of diagnostic radiography, offering the capability to penetrate the human body and produce detailed images of internal structures. This imaging modality is invaluable for identifying and diagnosing a wide array of medical conditions. Here are some of the key applications and significance of X-rays in diagnostic radiography:

- **Detection of fractures and bone injuries:** X-rays are highly effective in detecting fractures and bone injuries due to their ability to penetrate bone tissue and produce clear, detailed images of the skeletal system. This capability allows for precise identification of fractures, dislocations, and other bone-related injuries, facilitating timely and appropriate treatment. X-ray imaging is often the first step in assessing bone trauma and guiding subsequent medical interventions.
- **Identification of tumors and abnormalities:** X-rays are instrumental in identifying tumors, masses, and other abnormalities within the body. They are particularly useful for detecting anomalies in vital organs such as the lungs, breast, and digestive tract. For instance, chest X-rays can reveal the presence of lung tumors, while mammograms are essential for early breast cancer detection. This diagnostic capability aids in early disease detection and monitoring, improving patient outcomes through timely intervention.
- **Evaluation of lung function:** X-ray imaging plays a crucial role in evaluating lung function by producing images of the lungs and airways. It is used to diagnose and assess conditions such as pneumonia, emphysema, and lung cancer. By visualizing the structure and condition of the lungs, X-rays help healthcare professionals understand the extent of lung disease and guide appropriate treatment strategies.

- **Diagnosis of dental problems:** In dental practice, X-rays are commonly used to diagnose a range of dental issues, including cavities, impacted teeth, and jaw disorders. Dental X-rays provide detailed images of the teeth, roots, and surrounding bone structure, enabling dentists to detect problems that may not be visible during a routine examination. This diagnostic tool is crucial for planning effective treatment and ensuring optimal oral health.
- **Monitoring of medical treatments:** X-rays are also valuable for monitoring the progress of various medical treatments, including radiation therapy. By producing images of the affected area, X-rays allow healthcare professionals to assess the effectiveness of treatment, track changes in the condition being treated, and make necessary adjustments to the therapeutic approach.
- **Preoperative and postoperative imaging:** Before and after surgical procedures, X-ray imaging is used to evaluate the condition of the surgical site. This includes assessing the placement of implants or devices, monitoring healing, and detecting any complications that may arise. Accurate imaging before and after surgery ensures that the procedure's outcomes are as expected and helps in managing postoperative care.
- **Assessment of cardiovascular health:** X-rays, particularly through techniques like angiography, are employed to assess cardiovascular health. They provide images of the blood vessels and heart structures, aiding in the diagnosis and treatment of cardiovascular conditions such as coronary artery disease, aneurysms, and vascular blockages.
- **Screening and preventive health:** In addition to diagnostic uses, X-rays are also employed in screening programs for early detection of diseases, such as lung cancer and breast cancer. Screening X-rays help identify asymptomatic conditions in their early stages, enabling preventive measures and improving long-term health outcomes.

X-rays are an indispensable tool in diagnostic radiography, offering a noninvasive, effective means of visualizing internal structures and diagnosing medical conditions. Their ability to provide detailed images quickly and accurately supports healthcare professionals in delivering timely and effective care, ultimately enhancing patient outcomes and advancing medical practice.

1.7 Section F: Production of Radionuclides

There are three main methods for producing radionuclides: (A) reactor-based, (B) accelerator-based (cyclotron), and (C) generator-based.

1.7.1 Reactor-Based

Reactor-based radionuclide generation involves using nuclear reactors to produce radionuclides using nuclear reactions. The process involves the bombardment of stable nuclei with neutrons, which results in the formation of radionuclides. Reactors are typically used to produce large quantities of radionuclides, which can be used for various purposes such as medical imaging, radiation therapy, and research (Fig. 1.39).

The process of radionuclide generation in a reactor involves the following steps:

1.7.1.1 Neutron Activation

In this step, a stable target nucleus is bombarded with neutrons, forming a radioactive nucleus. The nucleus absorbs the neutron, which then becomes unstable and undergoes a nuclear transformation to produce a radioactive isotope. The radionuclides used more commonly in gamma camera studies or SPECT (single photon emission computed tomography) studies are produced in a reactor. Molybdenum-99 (Mo-99) is a radioactive isotope widely used for medical imaging to generate technetium-99 m (Tc-99 m), a reactor-produced radionuclide. One of the most common methods for producing Mo-99 is the (n, ϒ) reaction, which involves irradiating a target material with neutrons in a nuclear reactor.

$$^{98}\mathrm{Mo} + \mathrm{n} \rightarrow {}^{99}\mathrm{Mo}^{*} \rightarrow {}^{99\mathrm{m}}\mathrm{Tc} + \gamma$$

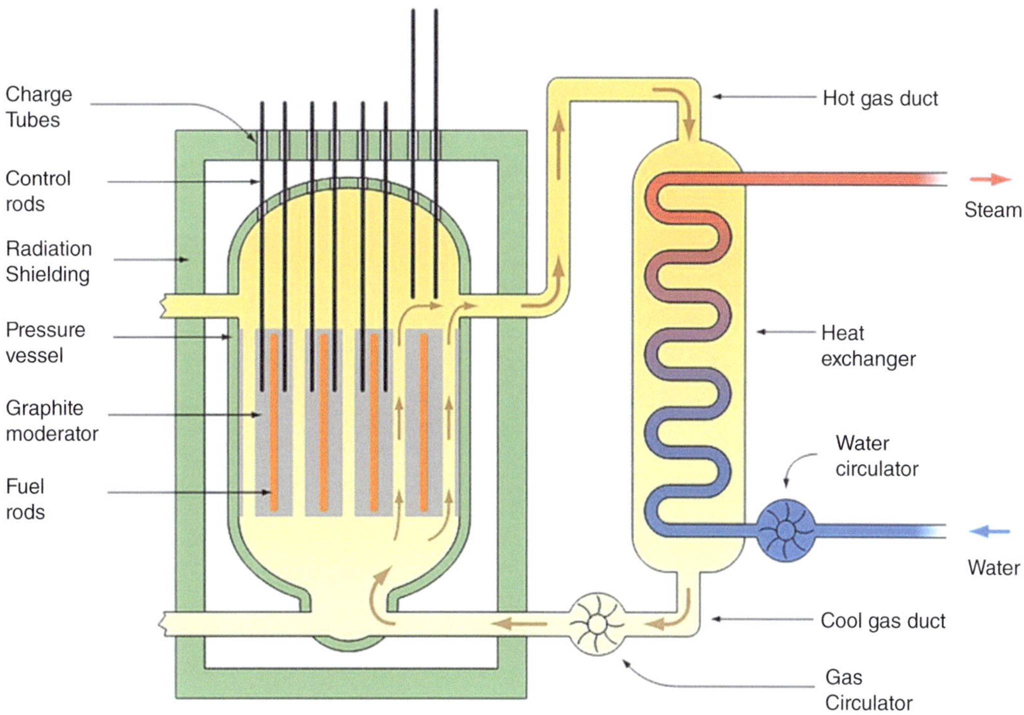

Fig. 1.39 Reactor working principles. (Image courtesy: Creative Commons, Attribution 2.5 Generic (CC BY 2.5))

In this reaction, a small fraction of the target nuclei are converted to the product radionuclide, resulting in a low specific activity product that is chemically identical to the target and difficult to separate. The fission of uranium is another process employed in reactors. This reaction is used to make a high-specific activity product, which is presently employed to make ^{99}Mo/^{99m}Tc generators (column type).

$$^{235}U + n \rightarrow {}^{99}Mo + \text{fission products} + 2-3\,\text{neutrons} + \textit{energy}$$

The amount of the radionuclide compared to the total quantity of the stable isotope is known as a *specific activity*. Fission occurs when a nucleus splits, releasing energy and neutrons. Other radionuclides useful in nuclear medicine are created in the reactor and are mentioned further down.

1.7.1.2 Decay and Isolation

Once the radionuclide is produced, it undergoes radioactive decay, which can result in the emission of gamma rays, beta particles, or alpha particles. The radionuclide must be isolated from the reactor environment to prevent contamination and exposure to personnel.

1.7.1.3 Processing and Purification

The radionuclide is processed and purified to remove impurities or unwanted isotopes. This can involve chemical separation techniques such as ion exchange, precipitation, or chromatography.

1.7.1.4 Packaging and Delivery

The purified radionuclide is packaged and delivered to end-users for their intended application. This can involve transporting the radionuclide to medical facilities for imaging or therapy or to research laboratories for further experimentation.

Using nuclear reactors for radionuclide generation offers several advantages over other methods, such as cyclotrons or accelerators. Reactors can produce large quantities of radionuclides in a relatively short time, and the process can be automated for efficient and consistent production. Additionally, reactors can produce a

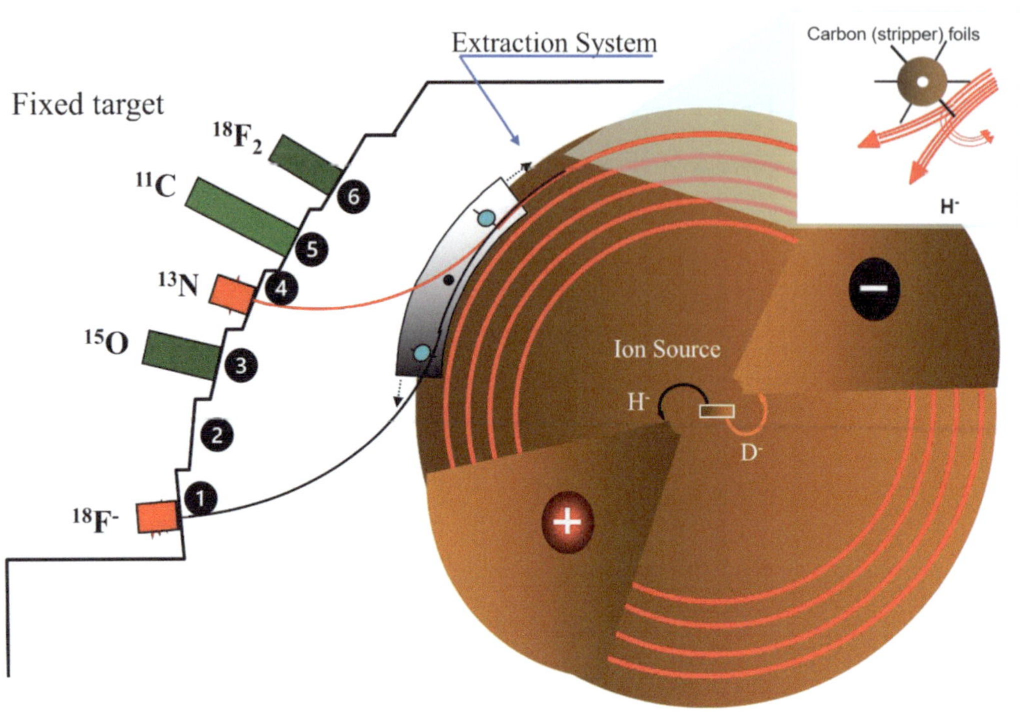

Fig. 1.40 Cyclotron principles

wider range of radionuclides than cyclotrons or accelerators, making them suitable for broader applications.

However, reactor-based radionuclide generation also presents some risks and challenges. The handling and processing radioactive materials require strict safety measures to prevent exposure to personnel and the environment. Additionally, the disposal of radioactive waste must be carefully managed to prevent contamination of the surrounding area. Proper management and regulation of reactor facilities are necessary to ensure radionuclides' safe and effective products for medical, research, and industrial applications.

1.7.2 Cyclotron-Based

Cyclotron-based radionuclide generation involves using a cyclotron particle accelerator to produce short-lived radioisotopes through nuclear reactions. The process involves accelerating charged particles, usually protons, to high energies and directing them toward a target material (Fig. 1.40). When the accelerated particle collides with the target nucleus, it can cause various nuclear reactions, producing the desired radionuclide.

One common method of cyclotron-based radionuclide production is through the proton bombardment of stable target nuclei, such as natural or enriched stable isotopes. The reaction may involve proton capture, proton emission, or nuclear spallation, producing short-lived radioisotopes.

Another method involves using a cyclotron to produce neutrons through proton-induced nuclear reactions. These neutrons can then be used to induce nuclear reactions in target materials, resulting in the production of various radionuclides.

Cyclotron-based radionuclide production is widely used in nuclear medicine to produce various positron-emitting radionuclides, such as fluorine-18, carbon-11, nitrogen-13, and oxygen-15. These radionuclides are used in PET imaging, a noninvasive medical imaging technique that allows the visualization and quantification of biological processes in vivo.

1.7.3 Generator-Based

Generator-based radionuclide production produces radionuclides that involve using a parent radionuclide to produce a daughter radionuclide through radioactive decay. The parent radionuclide is typically a long-lived isotope that can be easily obtained in large quantities, while the daughter radionuclide is typically short-lived and used for medical imaging or therapy.

The generator is typically a column filled with solid support material, such as alumina, silica gel, or ion exchange resin, coated or impregnated with the parent radionuclide. The coating or impregnation process allows the parent radionuclide to adhere to the surface of the solid support material, which increases the surface area available for the elution of the daughter radionuclide.

During the elution process, a suitable solvent is passed through the column, which selectively removes the daughter radionuclide from the solid support material. The elution process may be carried out using various solvents depending on the specific generator and the daughter radionuclide to be produced. Once the daughter radionuclide has been eluted from the generator, it can be used for medical imaging or therapy. The elution can be repeated after a certain time depending upon generator to generator. Here are some examples:

1.7.3.1 Technetium-99 m Generator

Nuclear medicine's most commonly used radionuclide generator. It is used for diagnostic imaging procedures such as renal scans, bone scans, myocardial perfusion imaging, and many others. The parent isotope is molybdenum-99, which decays to technetium-99 m, the daughter isotope. The generator usually comprises an alumina column containing the parent isotope, which is eluted with a saline solution to obtain the daughter isotope.

1.7.3.2 Gallium-68 Generator

This generator is used for positron emission tomography (PET) imaging. The parent isotope is germanium-68, which decays to gallium-68, the daughter isotope. The generator usually comprises a column containing the parent isotope bound to a resin, which is eluted gallium-68 generator: This generator is used in positron emission tomography (PET) imaging. The parent isotope is germanium-68, which decays to gallium-68, the daughter isotope. The generator usually comprises a column containing the parent isotope bound to a resin, which is eluted with a hydrochloric acid solution to obtain the daughter isotope.

1.7.3.3 Strontium-82/Rubidium-82 Generator

This generator is used for cardiac PET imaging. The parent isotope is strontium-82, which decays to rubidium-82, the daughter isotope. The generator usually comprises a column containing the parent isotope bound to a resin, which is eluted with a saline solution to obtain the daughter isotope.

1.7.3.4 Actinium-225/Bismuth-213 Generator

This generator is used for targeted alpha therapy (TAT) for cancer treatment. The parent isotope is actinium-225, which decays to bismuth-213, the daughter isotope. The generator usually comprises a column containing the parent isotope bound to a resin, which is eluted with an acid solution to obtain the daughter isotope (Fig. 1.41).

Generator-based radionuclide production is a highly efficient and cost-effective method of producing short-lived radionuclides for medical applications. It allows for the continuous production of the daughter radionuclide without the need for costly and time-consuming nuclear reactions (Fig. 1.42).

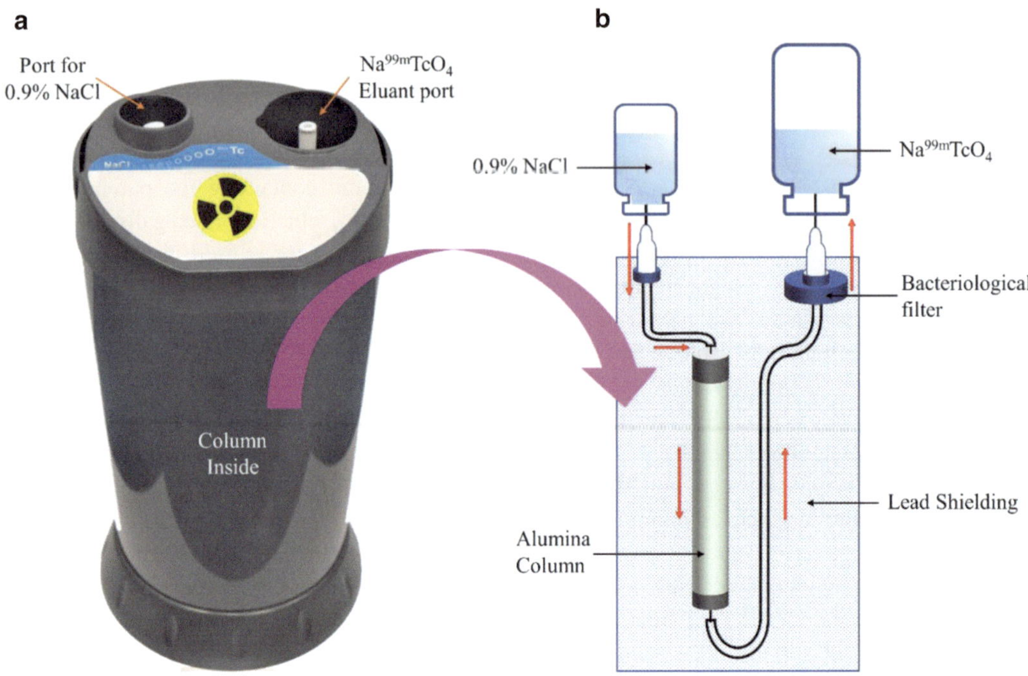

Fig. 1.41 (**a**) A typical dry technetium generator, (**b**) Cross-sectional diagram of technetium generator

Fig. 1.42 Decay and growth pattern of ^{99}Mo-^{99m}Tc generator

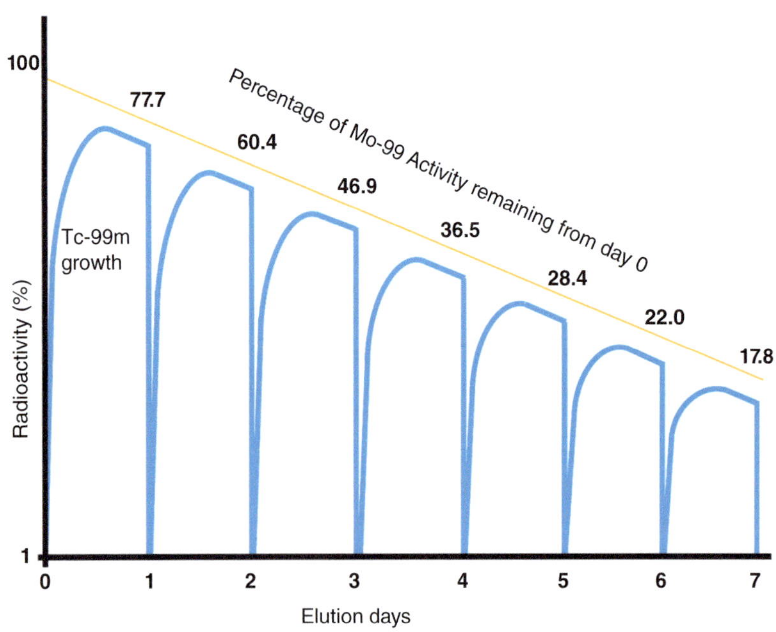

1.8 Section G: Radioactivity

Radioactivity refers to the process by which unstable atomic nuclei undergo spontaneous decay, releasing energy in the form of radiation. This radiation can be alpha particles, beta particles, gamma rays, positron decay, internal conversion, and isomeric transition.

1.8.1 Discovery of Radioactivity

French physicist Henri Becquerel (1852–1908) discovered Radioactivity in 1896 [53]. Becquerel was investigating the properties of a mineral called uranium when he observed that a photographic plate placed near the mineral became fogged, even though it had not been exposed to any visible light. He hypothesized that the uranium mineral emitted radiation that could penetrate solid objects and affect photographic plates.

Becquerel's discovery led to further investigations by other scientists, including Marie Curie (1867–1934) and her husband, Pierre Curie (1859–1906). The Curies identified two new elements, polonium and radium, that were highly radioactive, and they conducted extensive research on the properties of these and other radioactive substances. Their work led to the development of the field of nuclear physics and the understanding of the structure of the atom. Becquerel, Marie Curie, and Pierre Curie were awarded the Nobel Prize in Physics in 1903 for research on Radioactivity. For the discovery of elements such as radium and polonium, Marie Curie was awarded the Nobel Prize in Chemistry too in 1911.

1.8.2 Unit of Radioactivity

As per the International System of Units (SI), the unit of radioactivity is becquerel (Bq), named after the French physicist Henri Becquerel who discovered radioactivity in 1896. One Becquerel is defined as one radioactive decay event per second.

However, another commonly used unit of radioactivity is the Curie (Ci), named after the pioneering researchers Marie and Pierre Curie. One Curie is equal to 3.7×10^{10} radioactive decays per second or disintegrations per second (dps), which is equivalent to the activity of one gram of radium-226.

? Does temperature has any affect on radioactivity?

Radioactivity, or the spontaneous decay of atomic nuclei, cannot be directly controlled or stopped. The rate of radioactive decay is determined solely by the nuclear properties of the radioactive substance and is not affected by factors such as temperature, pressure, or chemical reactions. Also, there is no way to predict with certainty when a specific unstable nucleus will decay. Radioactive decay is a probabilistic process, and only mathematically average decay rates can be ascertained.

1.8.3 Radioactive Decay Equation and Half-Life

Let us suppose a radioactive sample contains N radioactive atoms; if ΔN atoms undergo radioactive decay in Δt time, the average decay rate for that sample is directly proportional to the initial number of atoms present and is given by

$$\frac{N}{t} \propto N \tag{1.18}$$

Or

$$\frac{N}{t} = -\lambda N \tag{1.19}$$

Where λ is called the decay constant, the negative symbol denotes the reduction in numbers or N decreasing with time. The decay constant is the characteristic property of each radionuclide and is defined as the fraction of atoms that undergo radioactive decay per unit time.

The unit of decay constant is per unit time or $(\text{time})^{-1}$ or $s - {}^{1}$. If the decay constant is $0.05\ s - {}^{1}$, 5% of atoms undergo radioactive decay in 1 s.

From Eq. (1.2)

$$\frac{N}{t} = -\lambda N$$

$$\text{Or,} \frac{N}{N} = -\lambda \quad t$$

$$\text{Or,} \frac{dN}{N} = -\lambda \, dt$$

On integration,

$$\int \frac{dN}{N} = -\lambda \int dt$$

$$\log_e N = -\lambda t + C \quad (1.20)$$

If the initial number of nuclei is N_0 and $N = N_0$ when $t = 0$, then Eq. (1.20) becomes

$$\log_e N_0 = C$$

Putting the value of C in Eq. (1.20)

$$\log_e N = -\lambda t + \log_e N_0$$

$$\log_e N - \log_e N_0 = -\lambda t$$

$$\log_e \frac{N}{N_0} = -\lambda t$$

$$\frac{N}{N_0} = e^{-\lambda t}$$

$$N = N_0 \, e^{-\lambda t} \quad (1.21)$$

Equation (1.4) is called the radioactive decay equation. It can also be represented as

$$A = A_0 \, e^{-\lambda t} \quad (1.22)$$

where A_0 is initial activity, A is the remaining activity after time t, and λ is the decay constant. $e^{-\lambda t}$ is called the "decay factor." The decay factor refers to the fraction of the radioactive substance remaining after time t. When the decay factor is 0.5, half of the radioactive material is decayed. The time any radioactive material takes to become half (50%) of its original is called the *half-life*. Considering initial activity, that is, A_0 = 1 and after T time, it becomes A = ½, putting the value in Eq. (1.4)

$$\frac{1}{2} = 1.e^{-\lambda T_{1/2}}$$

$$2 = e^{\lambda T_{1/2}}$$

$$\text{Or, In } 2 = \lambda T_{1/2}$$

$$\text{Or,} T_{1/2} = \frac{\ln 2}{\lambda}$$

$$\text{Or,} T_{1/2} = \frac{0.693}{\lambda} \quad (1.23)$$

$T_{1/2}$, is called the half-life, and it is a characteristic property of each radioactive substance and can range from fractions of a second to billions of years, depending on the type of nucleus (Fig. 1.43).

1.8.4 Modes of Radioactive Decay

1.8.4.1 Alpha Decay

Alpha decay is a type of radioactive decay in which an atomic nucleus emits an alpha particle consisting of two protons and two neutrons (essentially a helium-4 nucleus), thereby reducing the atomic number by two and the mass number by four. This process transforms the remaining nucleus into a different, more stable one. Standard notations for alpha decay are

$$^{A}_{Z}X \xrightarrow{\alpha} {}^{A-4}_{Z-2}Y \quad (1.24)$$

Alpha decay is commonly observed in heavy, unstable isotopes of uranium, thorium, and radium. An example of alpha decay is

$$^{238}_{92}U \xrightarrow{\alpha\left(^{4}_{2}He\right)} {}^{234}_{90}Th$$

An alpha particle has a limited range and can be stopped by a few centimeters of air or a sheet of paper. However, their dose delivery in a shorter range is very high. Actinium-225 and thorium-227 have been used for the treatment of metastatic castration-resistant-prostate cancer (mCRPC), acute myeloid leukemia (AML), neuroendocrine tumors (NETs), and glioma therapy.

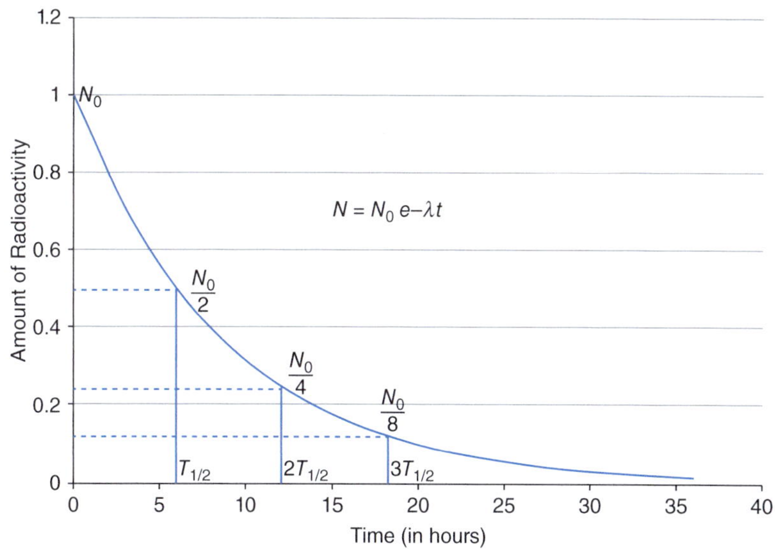

Fig. 1.43 Time-activity curve of ^{99m}Tc

1.8.4.2 Beta Decay

In beta decay or beta minus (β^-) decay, a neutron in the nucleus of an atom changes into a proton, an electron and antineutrino. The electron and antineutrino come out of the nucleus, and the proton changes the atomic number, and so is the element. The following equation can represent this:

$$n \rightarrow p + e^- + \bar{v} \tag{1.25}$$

Here, "n" represents a neutron, "p" represents a proton, "e^-" represents an electron, and "$\bar{v}$" represents an antineutrino. The electron emitted in the decay is called a beta particle, and it shares the excess energy of the nucleus with antineutrino. In nuclear notations, beta decay can be represented as

$$^{A}_{Z}X \xrightarrow{\beta} {}^{A}_{Z+1}Y \tag{1.26}$$

As a result of beta-negative decay, the atomic number of the nucleus increases by one since a neutron has been converted into a proton. However, the mass number of the nucleus remains the same since the total number of protons and neutrons has not changed. An example of beta decay is:

$$^{14}_{6}C \xrightarrow{\beta} {}^{14}_{7}N + \bar{v}$$

The beta particle has a greater range than alpha particles and can penetrate through a few millimeters of aluminum or other materials.

1.8.4.3 Gamma Decay

Gamma decay, also known as gamma emission or gamma rays, is a type of radioactive decay in which an unstable atomic nucleus releases high-energy gamma radiation. Gamma rays are high-energy photons emitted by the nucleus, and they have the greatest range of the three types of radiation.

During gamma decay, the nucleus emits a gamma ray, a type of electromagnetic radiation with a very short wavelength and high frequency. Gamma rays have neither mass nor charge and are highly penetrating, meaning they can pass through most materials, including dense materials like lead and concrete. Though by adjusting the thickness of lead and concrete, they can be absorbed within this and unjustified exposures to the human can be minimized (Table 1.10).

Gamma decay does not change the atomic or mass number of the nucleus since it only involves energy emission in gamma radiation. Thus, the resulting nucleus is a different energy state of the same atom. The amount of energy released during gamma decay depends on difference in energy between the initial and final states of the nucleus. Gamma rays can have energies ranging from a few kiloelectronvolts (keV) to several megaelectronvolts (MeV) (Fig. 1.44).

In many cases, gamma decay does occur in conjunction with other types of radioactive decay,

Table 1.10 Various modes of radioactive decay

Type of Decay	Notation	Generic Equation	Graphical representation
Alpha decay (α)	${}^4_2He$	${}^A_ZX \rightarrow {}^{A-4}_{Z-2}Y + {}^4_2He$	
Beta decay (β^-)	${}^0_{-1}\beta$	${}^A_ZX \rightarrow {}_{Z+1}^{A}Y + {}^0_{-1}\beta$	
Gamma emission (γ)	${}^0_0\gamma$	${}^A_ZX^* \rightarrow {}^A_ZX + {}^0_0\gamma$	
Positron emission (β^+)	${}^0_{+1}\beta$	${}^A_ZX \rightarrow {}_{Z-1}^{A}Y + {}^0_{+1}\beta$	
Electron capture (EC)	X-rays	${}^A_ZX + {}^0_{-1}e \rightarrow {}_{Z-1}^{A}Y + X\ rays$	
Neutron decay (n)	${}^1_0n$	${}^{A+B+C}_{Z_1+Z_2}X \rightarrow {}^A_{Z_1}Y' + {}^B_{Z_2}Y'' + C{}^1_0n$	

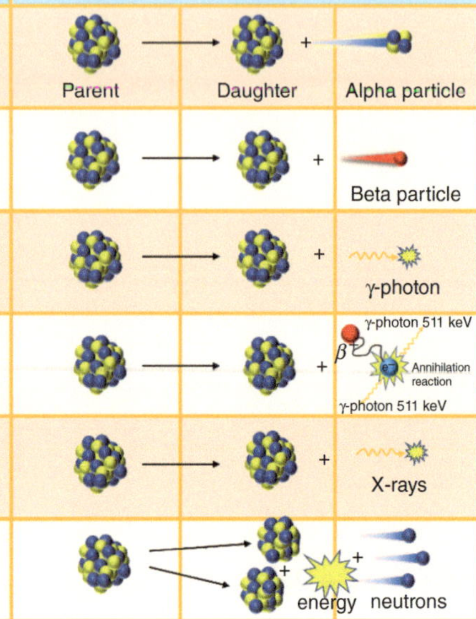

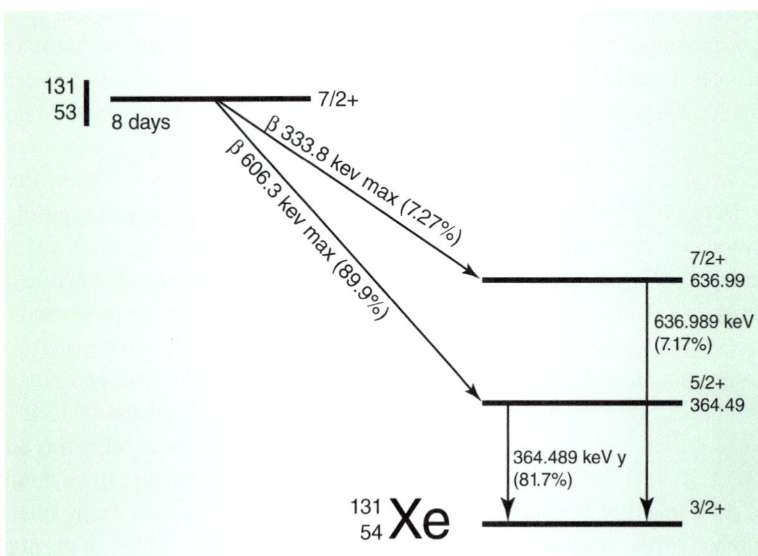

Fig. 1.44 I-131 decay scheme

such as alpha or beta decay. When a nucleus undergoes alpha or beta decay, it often leaves the daughter nucleus excited, releasing gamma radiation to return to a lower energy state. The nuclear notations accompanied with β^- are shown below:

$$ {}^A_ZX \xrightarrow{\beta} {}_{Z+1}^{A}Y^* \xrightarrow{\gamma} {}_{Z+1}^{A}Y \quad (1.27)$$

Example

$$ {}^{131}_{53}I \xrightarrow{\beta} {}^{131}_{54}Xe^* \xrightarrow{\gamma} {}^{131}_{54}Xe $$

Gamma decay is an important process in many areas of science and technology, including nuclear physics, medical imaging, and radiation therapy. In nuclear physics, gamma

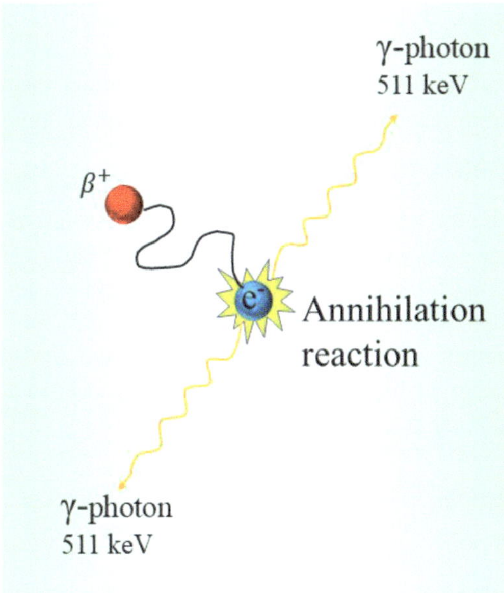

Fig. 1.45 Annihilation reaction between a positron (β^+) and an electron (e^-)

decay is used to study the properties of atomic nuclei and their interactions with other particles. In medical imaging, gamma rays are extensively used in positron emission tomography (PET) and single-photon emission computed tomography (SPECT) imaging. In radiation therapy, using sources like cobalt-60 or linear accelerators in external beam radiation therapy (EBRT), gamma rays kill cancer cells by damaging their DNA.

1.8.4.4 Positron Decay

Positron decay occurs when a nucleus has excess protons, resulting in unstable nuclei. The nucleus can stabilize itself by emitting a positron by converting one of its protons into a neutron and a positive electron called "positron." This process reduces the atomic number of the nucleus by one while leaving the mass number unchanged (Fig. 1.45). The following equation represents the decay:

$$ {}_{Z}^{A}X \xrightarrow{\beta+} {}_{Z-1}^{A}Y + \nu \tag{1.28}$$

Example

$$ {}_{9}^{18}F \xrightarrow{\beta+} {}_{8}^{18}O + \nu $$

When a positron is emitted from a nucleus, it interacts with an electron in the surrounding matter, resulting in their annihilation and producing two gamma rays of 511 kiloelectron volt (keV).

Positron decay is common in certain isotopes, including carbon-11, nitrogen-13, oxygen-15, fluorine-18, and rubidium-82. These isotopes are often used in medical imaging techniques such as PET (positron emission tomography).

1.8.4.5 Electron Capture

In electron caption (EC) decay, the nucleus captures an orbital electron and combines with a proton to form a neutron. This process looks like an "inverse β^- decay," and a neutrino carries away the transition energy. The vacancy created in the inner shells of the electron further triggers the production of characteristic X-rays and Auger electrons, same as above. The nuclear notation for electron capture is as follows:

$$ p^{+} + e^{-} = n + \nu + \text{energy} \tag{1.29}$$

This can be represented as

$$ {}_{Z}^{A}X \xrightarrow{EC} {}_{Z-1}^{A}Y $$

Generally, inner shells such as K or L shell orbital electrons are captured, denoted as EC(K) or EC(L).

1.8.4.6 Neutron Decay

Neutrons are uncharged particles and, therefore, cannot be stopped by electric or magnetic fields, as with charged particles such as alpha and beta particles. Neutron emission is a type of nuclear decay in which an unstable atomic nucleus spontaneously emits a neutron. This process can occur in isotopes with too many neutrons, causing the nucleus to become unstable and decay into a more stable configuration. The following equation can represent neutron emission:

$$ {}_{Z}^{A}X \xrightarrow{n} {}_{Z}^{A-1}X \tag{1.30}$$

Neutron emissions can also occur due to nuclear reactions, for those that take place in nuclear fission or nuclear fusion. In nuclear fission, a heavy nucleus is split into two lighter nuclei, releasing one or more neutrons. These neutrons can cause additional fission reactions, leading to a chain reaction that releases large amounts of energy. The nuclear fission reaction with neutron decay can be represented as follows:

$$^{A+B+C}_{Z_1+Z_2}X \rightarrow {}^{A}_{Z_1}Y' + {}^{B}_{Z_2}Y'' + \mathrm{C}\,{}^{1}_{0}n \quad (1.31)$$

An example can be

$$^{235}_{92}U \rightarrow {}^{140}_{54}Xe + {}^{94}_{38}Sr + {}^{1}_{0}n$$

In nuclear fusion, two lighter nuclei are combined to form a heavier nucleus, releasing energy. Neutrons are often used to initiate nuclear fusion reactions, as they can penetrate the positively charged nuclei and trigger the fusion process.

$$^{2}_{1}H + {}^{3}_{1}H \rightarrow {}^{4}_{2}He + {}^{1}_{0}n$$

Neutron emission is important in many areas of science and technology, including nuclear physics, nuclear engineering, and medical imaging. In particular, neutron radiation can be used in cancer treatment to destroy cancer cells, and neutron imaging can be used to study the structure and the properties of materials at the atomic level.

The most effective way to stop neutrons is through neutron moderation, which involves slowing down the neutrons to a speed where atomic nuclei can capture them in a material. There are two main ways that neutron moderation can be achieved:

Using a moderator material: Certain materials, such as water, heavy water (deuterium oxide), graphite, and beryllium, are effective at slowing down neutrons through collisions with the atoms in the material. By placing a neutron source near a moderator material, the neutrons can be slowed down and eventually captured by the nuclei in the moderator.

Using a neutron absorber material: Some materials, such as boron-10, cadmium, or gadolinium, have a high probability of capturing neutrons. By surrounding a neutron source with a layer of neutron absorber material, the neutrons can be absorbed and stopped, preventing them from reaching other materials or sensitive areas (Fig. 1.46).

It is important to note that the effectiveness of neutron moderation and absorption depends on the energy of the neutrons and the thickness and density of the materials used for shielding. For very high-energy neutrons, such as those produced in nuclear reactions, thicker and denser materials like concrete or lead may be needed to stop them effectively.

1.8.4.7 Characteristic X-Rays, Auger Electrons, and Conversion Electrons

When an unstable nucleus transfers its energy to an orbital electron, as if γ ray is "internally absorbed" within the atom and the orbital electron overcomes its binding energy to eject out from the nucleus, this electron is called a conversion electron. This can happen with any unstable nuclei but is commonly seen with metastable nuclei, for example, in the case of 99mTc, but other medically important radionuclides that emit conversion electrons are ^{111}In, ^{67}Ga, ^{125}I, ^{153}Sm. These conversion electrons generally originate from lower orbitals such as K, L, or M (Fig. 1.47).

Shells and the energy excess to the binding energy are imparted to them as kinetic energy. This results in the vacancy of an electron in a lower orbit, which is subsequently filled by an outer shell electron. The difference in binding energies between outer and inner shells is released, resulting in characteristic X-rays. In a second condition, the difference in binding energy generated from the higher to the lower orbit can be transferred to some other orbital electron, which can be ejected. This process is called the Auger effect, and the released electron is called the Auger electron.

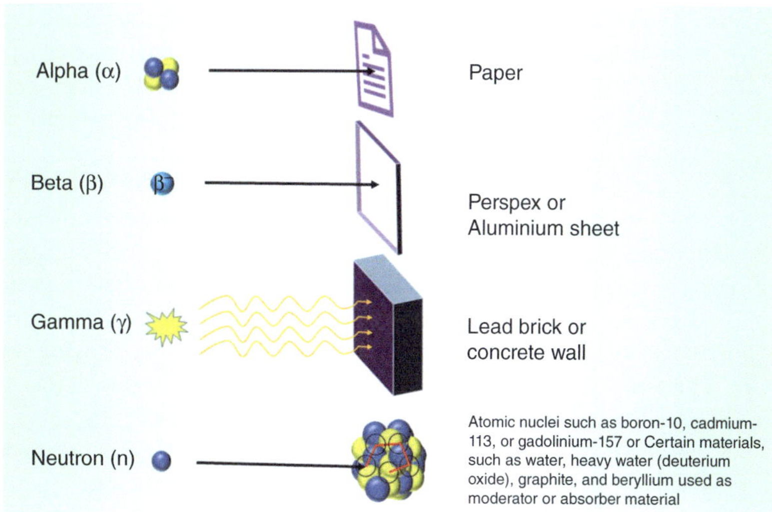

Fig. 1.46 Radiation shielding

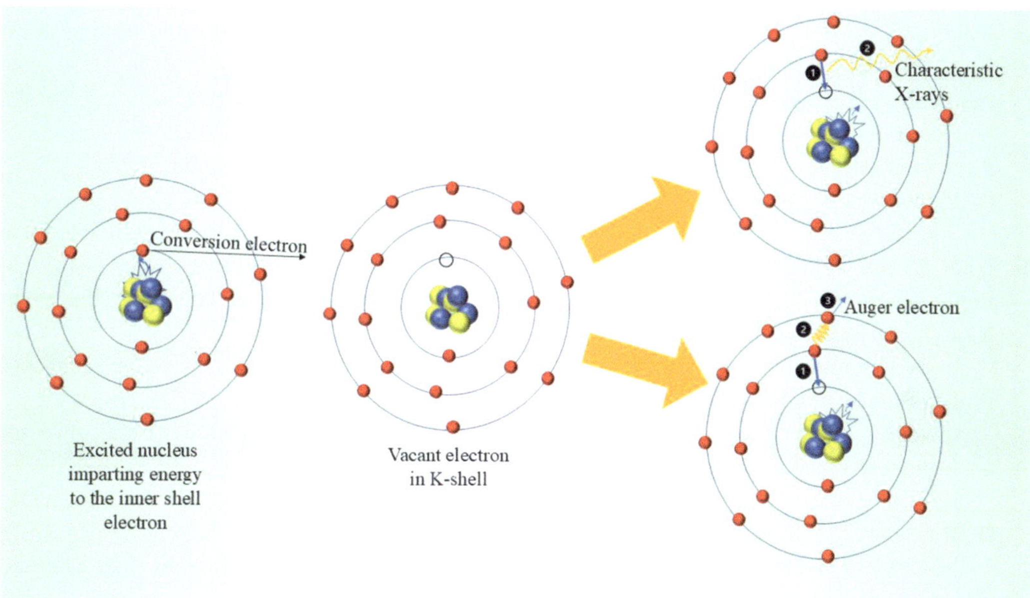

Fig. 1.47 Internal conversion (IC): Formation of characteristics X-ray and Auger electrons

Exercise

Multiple-Choice Questions (MCQs)

1. Which of the following types of radiation is classified as ionizing radiation?
   A. Radio waves
   B. Microwaves
   C. X-rays
   D. Infrared radiation
2. What determines the energy of an electromagnetic wave?
   A. Its amplitude
   B. Its frequency
   C. Its speed
   D. Its direction
3. What does the term "electromagnetic wave" refer to in the context of radiation?
   A. A wave that only contains an electric field

   B. A wave that travels through a vacuum and includes both electric and magnetic fields
   C. A wave that can only be detected by specialized instruments
   D. A wave with energy only in the visible light spectrum
4. According to Bohr's atomic model, why do electrons not fall into the nucleus?
   A. Because of the electron's wavelike behavior creating standing wave patterns
   B. Due to the constant energy absorption by electrons
   C. Because the nucleus repels electrons
   D. Due to the gravitational force between electrons and the nucleus
5. Which philosopher is known for introducing the concept of "atoms" as indivisible particles in ancient Greece?
   A. Aristotle
   B. Leucippus
   C. Pythagoras
   D. Socrates
6. What is the main limitation of Dalton's atomic theory?
   A. It did not account for the chemical reactions of atoms
   B. It assumed atoms could not be further divided
   C. It proposed that all atoms are identical in size and mass
   D. It incorrectly described the wavelike behavior of electrons
7. Which of the following is NOT a criterion for naming new elements according to IUPAC rules?
   A. A mythological concept or character
   B. A scientist's name
   C. A random combination of letters
   D. A property of the element
8. Who is credited with establishing the modern system of chemical nomenclature in the late eighteenth century?
   A. Antoine-Laurent Lavoisier
   B. Jöns Jacob Berzelius
   C. Louis-Bernard Guyton de Morveau
   D. John Dalton
9. What key feature distinguishes Rutherford's atomic model from Thomson's atomic model?
   A. The presence of electron shells
   B. The existence of a small, dense nucleus
   C. The concept of quantized energy levels
   D. The distribution of electrons in a uniform positive charge
10. According to Bohr's atomic model, how do electrons emit photons of light?
   A. By moving from a lower to a higher energy level
   B. By absorbing energy and moving to a higher energy level
   C. By moving from a higher to a lower energy level
   D. By colliding with other electrons
11. Which quantum number describes the shape of an orbital?
   A. Principal quantum number
   B. Azimuthal quantum number
   C. Magnetic quantum number
   D. Spin quantum number
12. What does Pauli's exclusion principle state about electrons in an atom?
   A. No two electrons can have the same energy level
   B. No two electrons can have the same spin quantum number
   C. No two electrons can have the same set of quantum numbers
   D. No two electrons can occupy the same orbital
13. What is the main limitation of Bohr's atomic model?
   A. It does not account for the stability of atoms
   B. It does not explain the existence of neutrons
   C. It only applies to hydrogen atoms
   D. It cannot explain the emission spectra of atoms
14. Which of the following correctly describes the atomic number of an element?
   A. The number of neutrons in the nucleus
   B. The number of protons in the nucleus
   C. The sum of protons and neutrons in the nucleus

D. The total number of electrons in an atom
15. How is atomic mass calculated?
A. By adding the number of protons and electrons
B. By taking the average of the number of neutrons
C. By summing the masses of protons and neutrons
D. By subtracting the number of protons from the mass number
16. What information does the atomic notation $^{16}_{8}O$ provide?
A. The number of protons and neutrons in the oxygen atom
B. The number of neutrons and electrons in the oxygen atom
C. The atomic number and mass number of the oxygen atom
D. The charge and mass number of the oxygen atom
17. Which term describes atoms of the same element that have different numbers of neutrons?
A. Isotones
B. Isobars
C. Isotopes
D. Isomers
18. Which of the following is true about isobars?
A. They have the same number of protons but different numbers of neutrons
B. They have different atomic masses but the same number of protons
C. They have the same number of nucleons but different numbers of protons
D. They are isotopes of the same element
19. Who is credited with inventing the first battery, which paved the way for modern electronics?
A. Michael Faraday
B. Alessandro Volta
C. James Clerk Maxwell
D. Benjamin Franklin
20. Which unit measures the amount of electric charge passing through a conductor in one second?
A. Volt
B. Coulomb
C. Ampere
D. Ohm
21. What does the term "mAs" stand for in radiology?
A. Milliampere-seconds
B. Milliampere-strategy
C. Microampere-seconds
D. Megaampere-seconds
22. According to Coulomb's law, the force between two point charges is directly proportional to
A. The distance between the charges
B. The sum of the charges
C. The product of the charges
D. The square root of the product of the charges
23. Which scientist discovered electromagnetic induction, which is crucial for the operation of generators and transformers?
A. Alessandro Volta
B. Michael Faraday
C. James Clerk Maxwell
D. Isaac Newton
24. What is the SI unit of exposure?
A. Roentgen (R)
B. Gray (Gy)
C. Coulombs per kilogram (C/kg)
D. Sievert (Sv)
25. Which equation represents the exposure rate?
A. $D = \frac{dE}{dm}$
B. $E = \frac{dQ}{dm}$
C. $X^0 = \frac{X}{t}$
D. $H_t = Absorbed\ dose \times w_R$
26. How is the equivalent dose calculated?
A. Absorbed dose × tissue weighting factor
B. Absorbed dose × radiation weighting factor
C. Absorbed dose × dose rate
D. Exposure rate × time
27. What does the term "kerma" stand for?
A. Kinetic Energy Released in Material
B. Kinetic Energy Received in Material

C. Kinetic Energy Required in Material
D. Kinetic Energy Ratio in Material

28. Which quantity is used to measure the impact of different types of radiation on biological tissues?
A. Absorbed dose
B. Effective dose
C. Exposure
D. Dose rate

29. What is the primary mechanism by which bremsstrahlung radiation is produced?
A. Interaction with atomic nuclei causing ionization
B. Acceleration of charged particles in a magnetic field
C. Deceleration of a charged particle when it interacts with the nucleus of an atom
D. Absorption of a photon by an atom causing electron ejection

30. In the photoelectric effect, which of the following statements is correct?
A. The probability of the photoelectric effect increases with increasing photon energy
B. The energy of the emitted photoelectron is equal to the photon energy plus the electron's binding energy
C. The photoelectric effect is more likely to occur in materials with higher atomic numbers
D. The photoelectric effect results in the emission of a positron

31. Who discovered X-rays and when?
A. Marie Curie, December 12, 1898
B. Wilhelm Conrad Roentgen, November 8, 1895
C. Albert Einstein, September 15, 1905
D. Thomas Edison, July 4, 1897

32. Which of the following materials is commonly used as a target in high-energy X-ray tubes?
A. Lead
B. Gold
C. Tungsten
D. Aluminum

33. What type of X-ray radiation is produced when an incident electron interacts with an inner-shell electron in the target material?
A. Bremsstrahlung radiation
B. Characteristic radiation
C. Scattering radiation
D. Reflection radiation

34. In X-ray imaging, which type of X-rays is characterized by lower energy levels and longer wavelengths?
A. Hard X-rays
B. Soft X-rays
C. Gamma rays
D. Alpha particles

35. Which of the following is NOT a clinical application of X-rays?
A. Radiography
B. Fluoroscopy
C. Magnetic resonance imaging (MRI)
D. Computed tomography (CT)

36. What is the primary advantage of reactor-based radionuclide production over cyclotron-based methods?
A. Reactor-based methods are more suited for producing short-lived radionuclides
B. Reactor-based methods can produce a wider range of radionuclides and in larger quantities
C. Reactor-based methods are more cost-effective than cyclotron-based methods
D. Reactor-based methods do not require any safety measures

37. Which of the following reactions describes the production of technetium-99m (Tc-99m) from molybdenum-99 (Mo-99)?
A. $^{98}\text{Mo} + \text{n} \rightarrow {}^{99}\text{Mo}* \rightarrow {}^{99m}\text{Tc} + \gamma$
B. $^{99}\text{Mo} + \text{n} \rightarrow {}^{99m}\text{Tc}+\gamma$
C. $^{99}\text{Mo} \rightarrow {}^{99m}\text{Tc} + \gamma$
D. $^{99}\text{Mo} + \text{n} \rightarrow {}^{99}\text{Tc} + \gamma$

38. Which of the following is a common radionuclide produced using a cyclotron?
A. Technetium-99m
B. Gallium-68
C. Strontium-82
D. Actinium-225

39. In generator-based radionuclide production, what is the role of the parent radionuclide?
A. To be directly used for medical imaging
B. To produce a short-lived daughter radionuclide through radioactive decay
C. To undergo chemical separation techniques

   D. To be used in the cyclotron-based production of other radionuclides
40. Which method is used to produce technetium-99m for medical imaging?
   A. Neutron activation in a reactor
   B. Proton bombardment in a cyclotron
   C. Generator-based elution
   D. Fission of uranium in a reactor
41. Who discovered radioactivity?
   A. Marie Curie
   B. Henri Becquerel
   C. Pierre Curie
   D. Ernest Rutherford
42. Which unit is equivalent to 3.7×10^{10} decays per second?
   A. Curie (Ci)
   B. Becquerel (Bq)
   C. Gray (Gy)
   D. Sievert (Sv)
43. Which type of radioactive decay involves the emission of an alpha particle?
   A. Beta decay
   B. Gamma decay
   C. Alpha decay
   D. Positron decay
44. What is the characteristic property of a radioactive substance that is determined by the decay constant?
   A. Half-life
   B. Atomic number
   C. Mass number
   D. Energy level
45. Which type of decay results in the emission of a positron?
   A. Alpha decay
   B. Beta minus decay
   C. Beta plus decay
   D. Gamma decay
46. Who were the scientists awarded the Nobel Prize in physics in 1903 for their research on radioactivity?
   A. Henri Becquerel and Pierre Curie
   B. Marie Curie and Pierre Curie
   C. Henri Becquerel, Marie Curie, and Pierre Curie
   D. Henri Becquerel and Marie Curie
47. What is the primary difference between alpha decay and beta decay?
   A. Alpha decay involves the emission of high-energy photons, while beta decay involves the emission of electrons
   B. Alpha decay reduces both the atomic number and mass number, while beta decay only changes the atomic number
   C. Beta decay emits a neutron, while alpha decay emits a proton
   D. Alpha decay occurs in lighter isotopes, while beta decay occurs in heavier isotopes
48. Which unit of radioactivity is defined as one radioactive decay event per second?
   A. Curie (Ci)
   B. Gray (Gy)
   C. Becquerel (Bq)
   D. Sievert (Sv)
49. In which radioactive decay process does the nucleus emit a positron?
   A. Alpha decay
   B. Beta minus decay
   C. Beta plus decay (positron emission)
   D. Gamma decay
50. What is the relationship between the decay constant (λ) and the half-life ($T_{1}/_{2}$) of a radioactive substance?
   A. $T_{1}/_{2} = \lambda * 0.693$
   B. $T_{1}/_{2} = 0.693/\lambda$
   C. $\lambda = 0.693/T_{1}/_{2}$
   D. $T_{1}/_{2} = \lambda/0.693$

Short Questions

1. Explain the role of photons in electromagnetic radiation.
2. Describe how the temperature of an object influences the type of electromagnetic radiation it emits.
3. Explain the significance of Maharshi Kanada's concept of "paramanu" in ancient Indian philosophy.
4. Discuss the main contributions of Antoine Lavoisier to the understanding of atomic structure and chemical reactions.
5. Explain how the discovery of the neutron contributed to the understanding of atomic structure.

6. Describe the main differences between classical and modern atomic models in terms of electron behavior and energy levels.
7. Why is the mass of electrons typically not considered in the calculation of atomic mass?
8. Explain the role of neutrons in maintaining nuclear stability.
9. Explain the relationship between voltage and electric current in a circuit.
10. Describe how the concept of mAs is used to adjust the amount of X-ray exposure in radiology.
11. Define the term "absorbed dose" and its unit in the International System of Units (SI).
12. Explain the difference between "dose equivalent" and "equivalent dose."
13. Describe the process and significance of Compton scattering in radiation physics.
14. Explain the difference between elastic scattering and inelastic scattering of neutrons with matter.
15. Explain the difference between bremsstrahlung and characteristic radiation in X-ray production.
16. Describe the role of X-rays in mammography and why low-energy X-rays are used in this technique.
17. Describe the process of neutron activation in reactor-based radionuclide production.
18. Explain the significance of specific activity in the context of radionuclide production.
19. Explain why the rate of radioactive decay is unaffected by temperature.
20. Describe the role of gamma decay in medical imaging techniques.

Long Question

1. Discuss the relationship between electric and magnetic fields in the formation of electromagnetic waves. Include how the acceleration of a charged particle contributes to the generation and propagation of these waves.
2. Analyze the historical development of atomic theory from ancient Greek philosophy through Dalton's atomic theory, highlighting the key contributions of various scientists and philosophers. Explain how these theories laid the groundwork for modern atomic theory and its impact on chemistry.
3. Discuss the evolution of atomic models from Thomson to Bohr, highlighting the key contributions and limitations of each model. How did these models pave the way for the development of the modern atomic theory?
4. Discuss the concept of binding energy and its significance in understanding nuclear stability. Include how binding energy per nucleon is related to the stability of a nucleus and describe the process by which mass is converted into energy according to Einstein's mass-energy equivalence equation.
5. Discuss the historical development of electricity from ancient discoveries to modern understanding, including key contributions from scientists such as Benjamin Franklin, Alessandro Volta, Michael Faraday, and James Clerk Maxwell. Explain how these contributions have led to the development of technologies like X-ray machines.
6. Describe the process of calculating the effective dose in radiation protection. Include in your answer the roles of absorbed dose, radiation weighting factor, and tissue weighting factor. Discuss how this approach helps in assessing the impact of radiation on different organs and tissues.
7. Discuss the various interactions of photons with matter, including the photoelectric effect, Compton scattering, pair production, and Rayleigh scattering. Highlight the conditions under which each interaction is most likely to occur and their applications in fields such as medical imaging and radiation therapy.
8. Discuss the evolution of X-ray technology from its early use to modern applications. Include details on the advancements in X-ray machines, the development of radiation protection measures, and the significance of X-rays in various medical and industrial fields.
9. Discuss the advantages and challenges associated with reactor-based radionuclide production, and compare it with cyclotron-based

and generator-based methods in terms of efficiency, safety, and application.

10. Discuss the process of neutron emission in the context of nuclear fission and fusion. How does neutron emission influence these reactions, and what are some of its applications in science and technology?

Answers to MCQs

1. C. X-rays.
2. B. Its frequency.
3. B. A wave that travels through a vacuum and includes both electric and magnetic fields.
4. A. Because of the electron's wavelike behavior creating standing wave patterns.
5. B. Leucippus.
6. B. It assumed atoms could not be further divided.
7. C. A random combination of letters.
8. C. Louis-Bernard Guyton de Morveau.
9. B. The existence of a small, dense nucleus.
10. C. By moving from a higher to a lower energy level.
11. B. Azimuthal quantum number.
12. C. No two electrons can have the same set of quantum numbers.
13. C. It only applies to hydrogen atoms.
14. B. The number of protons in the nucleus.
15. C. By summing the masses of protons and neutrons.
16. C. The atomic number and mass number of the oxygen atom.
17. C. Isotopes.
18. C. They have the same number of nucleons but different numbers of protons.
19. B. Alessandro Volta.
20. C. Ampere.
21. A. Milliampere-seconds.
22. C. The product of the charges.
23. B. Michael Faraday.
24. C. Coulombs per kilogram (C/kg).
25. C. $X^0 = \frac{X}{t}$.
26. B. Absorbed dose ×\times× radiation weighting factor.
27. A. Kinetic Energy Released in Material.
28. B. Effective dose.
29. C. Deceleration of a charged particle when it interacts with the nucleus of an atom.
30. C. The photoelectric effect is more likely to occur in materials with higher atomic numbers.
31. B. Wilhelm Conrad Roentgen, November 8, 1895.
32. C. Tungsten.
33. B. Characteristic radiation.
34. B. Soft X-rays.
35. C. Magnetic Resonance Imaging (MRI).
36. B. Reactor-based methods can produce a wider range of radionuclides and in larger quantities.
37. A. 98Mo + n → 99Mo∗ → 99mTc + γ.
38. B. Gallium-68.
39. B. To produce a short-lived daughter radionuclide through radioactive decay.
40. C. Generator-based elution.
41. B. Henri Becquerel.
42. A. Curie (Ci).
43. C. Alpha decay.
44. A. Half-life.
45. C. Beta plus decay.
46. C. Henri Becquerel, Marie Curie, and Pierre Curie.
47. B. Alpha decay reduces both the atomic number and mass number, while beta decay only changes the atomic number.
48. C. Becquerel (Bq).
49. C. Beta plus decay (positron emission).
50. B. $T_{1/2} = 0.693/\lambda$.

References

1. Radiation in Everyday Life | IAEA. https://www.iaea.org/Publications/Factsheets/English/radlife. Accessed 22 Feb 2023.
2. U. Nations Scientific Committee on the Effects of Atomic Radiation, "Sources and effects of ionizing radiation United Nations Scientific Committee on the Effects of Atomic Radiation UNSCEAR 2000 Report to the General Assembly, with Scientific Annexes Volume I: Sources United Nations."
3. Kaṇāda (philosopher) – Wikipedia. https://en.wikipedia.org/wiki/Ka%E1%B9%87%C4%81da_(philosopher). Accessed 04 Mar 2023.

4. The Vaisesika sutras of Kanada. Translated by Nandalal Sinha : Kanada : Free Download, Borrow, and Streaming : Internet Archive. https://archive.org/details/thevaiasesikasut00kanauoft/page/16/mode/2up?view=theater. Accessed 04 Mar 2023.
5. Narayan R. Space, Time and Anu in Vaisheshika.
6. Atom – Development of atomic theory | Britannica. https://www.britannica.com/science/atom/Development-of-atomic-theory. Accessed 05 Mar 2023.
7. Constable EC. John Dalton—the man and the myth. Dalton Trans. 2022;51(3):768–76. https://doi.org/10.1039/d1dt04135e.
8. The Conservation of Mass | Learn Science at Scitable. https://www.nature.com/scitable/knowledge/library/the-conservation-of-mass-17395478/. Accessed 10 Mar 2023.
9. Law of definite proportions | Definition, Discovery, & Facts | Britannica. https://www.britannica.com/science/law-of-definite-proportions. Accessed 10 Mar 2023.
10. M. L. and P. Society., Memoirs of the literary and philosophical society of Manchester, vol. ser.2:v.1 (1805). Manchester: The Society, 1805. Accessed: 10 Mar 2023. [Online]. Available: https://www.biodiversitylibrary.org/item/20167
11. Guyton de Morveau LB. Ann. Chim. Phys, J. Phys. 1782;19(310)
12. Chemical element – The Earth's mantle | Britannica. https://www.britannica.com/science/chemical-element/The-Earths-mantle Accessed 16 Mar 2023.
13. Koppenol WH. International union of pure and applied chemistry inorganic chemistry division commission on nomenclature of inorganic chemistry* Naming of new elements (IUPAC Recommendations 2002) Naming of new elements (IUPAC Recommendations 2002).
14. Koppenol WH, Corish J, García-Martínez J, Meija J, Reedijk J. How to name new chemical elements (IUPAC Recommendations 2016). Pure Appl Chem. 2016;88(4):401–5. https://doi.org/10.1515/pac-2015-0802.
15. Karol PJ, Barber RC, Sherrill BM, Vardaci E, Yamazaki T. Discovery of the elements with atomic numbers Z = 113, 115 and 117 (IUPAC technical report). Pure Appl Chem. 2016;88(1–2):139–53. https://doi.org/10.1515/pac-2015-0502.
16. Antoine Lavoisier, Douglas McKie (Introduction), Robert Kerr – Elements of Chemistry-Dover Publications (1984).
17. Elements of Chemical Philosphy Davy. 1812.
18. Transactions. [Online]. Available: https://royalsocietypublishing.org/
19. Holden NE. History of the origin of the chemical elements and their discoverers.
20. Indigo – Wikipedia. https://en.wikipedia.org/wiki/Indigo. Accessed 19 Mar 2023.
21. History of Tin | Home | Website | Makin Metal Powders (UK). http://www.makin-metals.com/history-of-tin/. Accessed 19 Mar 2023.
22. Antimony – Wikipedia. https://en.wikipedia.org/wiki/Antimony. Accessed 21 Mar 2023.
23. Marinsky JA, Glendenin LE, Coryell CD. The chemical identification of radioisotopes of neodymium and of element 61. J Am Chem Soc. 1947;69(11):2781–5. https://doi.org/10.1021/JA01203A059/ASSET/JA01203A059.FP.PNG_V03.
24. Mercury – Element information, properties and uses | Periodic Table. https://www.rsc.org/periodic-table/element/80/mercury. Accessed 20 Mar 2023.
25. Lead – Wikipedia. https://en.wikipedia.org/wiki/Lead. Accessed 20 Mar 2023.
26. Oganesson – American Chemical Society. https://www.acs.org/molecule-of-the-week/archive/o/oganesson.html. Accessed 20 Mar 2023.
27. thomson, 1897.
28. Chadwick J. Existence of a neutron. The Nature, 1932. https://royalsocietypublishing.org/doi/pdf/10.1098/rspa.1932.0112. Accessed 06 Apr 2023.
29. de Broglie L. Research on the theory of quanta. Minkowski Institute Press; 2021.
30. Heisenberg, W. (1927) The physical content of quantum kinematics and mechanics. In Wheeler, J.A. and Zurek, W.H., Eds., Quantum theory and measurement, Princeton University Press, Princeton, 62–84. [Originally Published Z. Phys., 1927, 43(3–4), 172–198]. – References – Scientific Research Publishing. https://www.scirp.org/(S(351jmbntvnsjt1aadkposzje))/reference/ReferencesPapers.aspx?ReferenceID=1935091. Accessed 07 Apr 2023.
31. MPRL | Research and Pedagogy | Sommerfeld's Atombau und Spektrallinien. https://www.mprl-series.mpg.de/studies/2/7/index.html. Accessed 08 Apr 2023.
32. Nomination archive – NobelPrize.org. https://www.nobelprize.org/nomination/archive/show_people.php?id=8661. Accessed 08 Apr 2023.
33. Sci-Hub. The Bohr–sommerfeld theory. Niels Bohr and the Quantum Atom, 140–181. https://doi.org/10.1093/acprof:oso/9780199654987.003.0004. https://sci-hub.se/https://doi.org/10.1093/acprof:oso/9780199654987.003.0004 Accessed 08 Apr 2023.
34. Sci-Hub. Atlas of nuclear isomers. Nucl Data Sheets, 128, 1–130 | https://doi.org/10.1016/j.nds.2015.08.001." https://sci-hub.se/https://doi.org/10.1016/j.nds.2015.08.001. Accessed 11 Apr 2023.
35. Garg S, Maheshwari B, Singh B, Sun Y, Goel A, Jain AK. Atlas of nuclear isomers. 2nd ed.
36. Lilley JS. Nuclear physics_ principles and applications. Wiley; 2001.
37. Ampere. The IUPAC compendium of chemical terminology. Research Triangle Park: International Union of Pure and Applied Chemistry (IUPAC); 2021. https://doi.org/10.1351/goldbook.A00300.
38. Trubey DK. Neutron physics division use of icru-defined quantities and units in shielding oak ridge national laboratory, 1968.
39. Tandon P, Prakash D, Kheruka SC, Bhat NN. Nuclear medicine internal dose assessment. In: Radiation safety guide for nuclear medicine professionals. Singapore: Springer Nature Singapore; 2022. p. 281–97. https://doi.org/10.1007/978-981-19-4518-2_19.

40. Harrison JD, et al. ICRP publication 147: use of dose quantities in radiological protection. Ann ICRP. 2021;50(1):9–82. https://doi.org/10.1177/01466453209 11864/FORMAT/EPUB.
41. Clarke RH et al.. Annals of the ICRP published on behalf of the international commission on radiological protection members of the main commission of the ICRP.
42. Annual Report of the International Commission on Radiological Protection. 2001.
43. Annual Report of the International Commission on Radiological Protection. 2003.
44. Clement CH. Annals of the ICRP compendium of dose coefficients based on ICRP Publication 60. ICRP Publica. 2013;123(4)
45. Sci -Hub | On a new kind of rays. Science, 3(59), 227–231 | https://doi.org/10.1126/science.3.59.227. https://sci-hub.se/10.1126/science.3.59.227 Accessed 03 May 2023.
46. A. M. K, The history of radiology.
47. Hard X-Rays. https://hesperia.gsfc.nasa.gov/sftheory/xray.htm Accessed 08 May 2023.
48. Attwood DT. Soft x-rays and extreme ultraviolet radiation : principles and applications. Cambridge University Press; 2000.
49. Tillman C. Development and characterisation of a laser-based hard X-ray source. 1996.
50. Woicik JC Editor. Springer series in surface sciences 59 Hard X-ray Photoelectron Spectroscopy (HAXPES). [Online]. Available: http://www.springer.com/series/409
51. Science with Soft X-Rays.
52. Rez P. Coherent and incoherent imaging of biological specimens with electrons and X-rays. Ultramicroscopy. 2021;231:113301. https://doi.org/10.1016/j.ultramic.2021.113301.
53. Badash L. Citation. Phys Today. 1996;49:21. https://doi.org/10.1063/1.881485.

Standard X-Ray Tubes: Basic Principles, Types of X-Ray Tubes, and Routine Quality Control

2

Learning Objectives

Overview of X-ray Technology and Tubes **Historical Development of X-Ray Tubes** Wilhelm Conrad Röntgen's discovery journey Rapid advancement in X-ray technology and swift integration into the medical practice **Major Milestones in X-Ray Tubes** Crookes tubes and early X-ray production challenges 1913: Thermionic cathodes—a milestone in X-ray tube technology 1918: Goetze's line focus 1925: The Philips Metalix tube 1926: J.E. Lilienfeld's pioneering work in vacuum tube amplification 1929: The introduction of rotating anode tubes 1959: High-speed tubes—the Super Rotalix (SRO) tubes by Philips 1973: The Super Rotalix Metal (SRM) X-ray tube by Philips 1979: The Super Rotalix Ceramic (SRC) X-ray tube 1987: Enhanced heat transfer rotating anode X-ray tubes with interleaved fins by Varian Medical Systems Inc. 1989: Maximus Rotalix Ceramic (MRC) 1996: Rotating anode cooled by high thermal conductivity fluid by Varian Medical Systems Inc 2003: Rotating frame X-ray tubes by Siemens 2005: The GE breakthrough: largest commercial anode 2007: Philips' innovation: the iMRC® tube for enhanced power density CT tube 2018: GE's breakthrough in cathode innovation for spectral CT 2020: Multisource X-ray tube to reduce imaging duration in digital breast tomosynthesis 2023: Line-focus X-ray tube for microbeam radiotherapy with very high dose rates	**Components Used in X-Ray Production** **X-Ray Tube Insert Assembly** Cathode assembly Filament Focusing cup Anode assembly Anode target and focal spot Anode angle and line focus principle The heel effect Crazing of the anode surface Anode disk and stem Bearing and lubrication Heat dissipation system Tube envelope Glass envelope Metal-ceramic envelope **Tube envelope/tube frame** Materials used Glass Ceramics Use of metal in X-ray tube envelopes X-ray tube housing assembly Lead shielding High-tension voltage cable sockets Stator electromagnetic coils Components and construction Beam collimation X-ray radiation port and window Radiation control timer circuit Bellows in X-ray tubes Heat exchanger parts **X-Ray Tube Housing Assembly** Lead shielding High-tension voltage cable sockets Stator electromagnetic coils Beam pre-collimation

(continued)

D. Prakash, R. P. Kotian, *Fundamentals of X-ray Imaging*,
https://doi.org/10.1007/978-981-96-7328-5_2

2.1 Overview of X-Ray Technology and Tubes

X-rays have become essential tools across various scientific fields, from physics to astronomy, biology, and chemistry, enabling us to uncover previously hidden phenomena. They aid in understanding the intricate structures of atoms and genes and exploring the mysteries surrounding black holes in our galaxy. The development of X-ray technology, including the types of X-ray tubes required, has greatly impacted medical diagnostics, radiotherapy, industrial radiography, and X-ray crystallography. X-ray technology plays a crucial role in medical diagnostics, providing invaluable insights into the internal structures of the human body. Central to this technology is the X-ray tube, which generates the X-ray beams used in medical imaging. It is essential to grasp the fundamental principles, various types, and routine quality-control procedures associated with standard X-ray tubes to ensure optimal performance and patient safety in diagnostic radiography (Table 2.1).

The fundamental principle underlying X-ray tube operation involves converting electrical energy into X-ray radiation. When a high voltage is applied across the tube, it establishes a potential difference that propels electrons from the cathode (negative electrode) to the anode (positive electrode). As electrons strike the anode target, they lose energy, emitting X-ray photons. This process's efficiency and the characteristics of the resulting X-rays depend on factors such as tube voltage, tube current, and the material composition of the anode.

X-ray tubes are engineered to operate across a broad spectrum of voltages and currents to accommodate diverse medical imaging modalities and therapeutic applications. For instance, lower tube voltages (20–50 kV) are typically employed in mammography to capture high-

Table 2.1 Applications of X-ray technology

Health care	Industrial usage
1. **Diagnostics** (a) General radiography (b) Computed tomography (c) Fluoroscopy (d) Mammography (e) Cath-lab angiography (f) Mobile C-arm (g) Portable and mobile X-ray (h) Dual-energy X-ray absorptiometry (DEXA) (i) Intraoral dental X-rays (j) Extraoral dental X-rays, such as panorama type and cone-beam computed tomography (CBCT) 2. **Therapeutics** (a) **Radiotherapy (photon-based)**—Superficial and deep radiotherapy units, for example, external beam radiation therapy (precisely targeting the tumor with high-energy X-rays, while minimizing exposure to surrounding healthy tissue) and brachytherapy (radioactive sources emitting gamma rays, and in some cases beta particles, are placed directly inside or near the tumor to deliver radiation internally) (b) **Interventional radiotherapy**—Uses precise imaging to deliver high doses of radiation directly to the tumor, minimizing damage to surrounding healthy tissue	1. **Food and agro**—Quality control, contaminant detection, foreign material detection, seed inspection, and poultry product screening 2. **Veterinary**—Diagnosing fractures, detecting foreign objects, and assessing internal health issues in animals 3. **Automotive**—Inspecting welds, detecting defects, and examining the internal structures of components like engines and tyres 4. **Aerospace**—Nondestructive testing of materials, inspecting welds, and analyzing the integrity of critical components like turbine blades and aircraft structures 5. **Electronics**—Quality control, inspecting solder joints, and analyzing the internal structure of electronic components such as integrated circuits and circuit boards 6. **Metallurgy**—Nondestructive testing, examining internal structures, detecting defects, and analyzing material composition in metal alloys and components 7. **Military and defense**—Nondestructive testing of weapons and equipment, inspecting munitions, and analyzing structural integrity 8. **Nanotechnology**—Imaging and analyzing nanostructures, characterizing materials at the nanoscale, and studying nanomaterial properties and behaviors 9. **Pharmaceuticals**—Quality control, analyzing crystal structures of drugs, and studying drug formulations and interactions at the molecular level 10. **Forensics**—Examining skeletal remains, identifying foreign objects within the body, and analyzing evidence in criminal investigations 11. **Security**—Screening baggage and cargo to detect concealed weapons, explosives, and other contraband items

contrast images of soft tissues, while higher voltages (70–150 kV) are commonly utilized in computed tomography (CT) scans to penetrate denser tissues and produce detailed cross-sectional images. In interventional radiology and fluoroscopy, the dynamic adjustment of tube current and voltage enables real-time imaging with optimal quality and minimal patient exposure. The market for X-ray tubes is highly competitive, with several leading companies dominating the industry and the key players include Varex Imaging (formerly part of Varian Medical Systems), GE, Canon Electron (formerly Toshiba Electron Tubes & Devices), Siemens, Dunlee, IAE, Comet Technologies, Hangzhou Wandong, Oxford Instruments, Kailong Medical, Sandt, Gulmay, and Keyway Electron [1].

The operational parameters and photon energy ranges for X-ray tubes used in various medical modalities are summarized in the table below. These ranges cover most typical clinical scenarios for each modality, although actual values may vary based on equipment, clinical protocols, and patient-specific factors (Table 2.2).

X-ray technology has revolutionized medical practice by offering noninvasive diagnostic methods and precise treatment options for various conditions. Ongoing innovations in X-ray tube design and materials enhance medical imaging systems' capabilities, improving diagnostic accuracy and patient outcomes. A thorough understanding of X-ray tube operational parameters and physical principles is essential for healthcare professionals and technologists to utilize these devices effectively and safely in clinical settings.

Table 2.2 Operational parameters and photon energy ranges for X-ray tubes used in different modalities[a]

Modality	Tube voltage (kV)	Tube current (mA)	Energy per patient (kWs)	Photon energy range (keV/MeV)
Mammography	20–45	20–200	2.5–90	20–45 keV
General radiography/mobile/surgical/dental panoramic	40–125	10–800	0.2–8.5	40–125 keV
Interventional cardiac and vascular X-rays	60–125	100–1000	120–900	60–125 keV
Computed tomography	70–150	10–800	55–1750	70–150 keV
Fluoroscopy	50–150	0.5–5	Varies widely	50–150 keV
Bone densitometry (DXA)	50–100	0.1–2	0.1–0.5	50–100 keV
Dental intraoral X-rays	60–70	4–10	0.1–0.5	60–70 keV
Radiation therapy for superficial tissues (X-ray)	100–400	10–50	Variable (kWs)	100–400 keV
Radiation therapy for deep-seated tumors (X-ray)	4–25 MV (megavolts)	100–400	Variable (kWs)	upto 25 MeV

[a] The values mentioned in the table are representative estimates. The actual range used in a specific diagnostic procedure/treatment may vary depending on clinical requirements, equipment specifications, and patient-specific factors.

In addition to their medical applications, X-rays have found widespread use across scientific and professional disciplines due to their penetrating power and ability to interact with matter. As the primary generators of these essential X-ray beams, X-ray tubes play a pivotal role in various fields, including industrial testing, security screening, and materials analysis.

2.2 Historical Development of X-Ray Tubes

The ancient Egyptians made remarkable advances in many fields, but the scientific study of electricity, including the concept of high voltage, developed much later, with significant contributions in the eighteenth and nineteenth centuries [2, 3]. The modern history of artificial X-ray generation traces back to pioneering experiments conducted from the seventeenth to the mid-nineteenth century [4]. In 1644, Evangelista Torricelli conducted an experiment involving a glass tube filled with mercury, demonstrating the creation of a vacuum when inverted over a dish. Otto von Guericke's attempts to separate large evacuated "Magdeburg hemispheres" in 1654 furthered the understanding of vacuum physics [5]. In 1705, Francis Hauksbee, the elder, observed light flashes in partially evacuated glass tubes using an electrostatic high-voltage generator, contributing to early investigations into electrical phenomena [5].

Around 1785, William Morgan observed a greenish glow near the surface of a glass container when applying high voltage after admitting a small quantity of air into it, which hinted at the phenomenon of gas discharge [6]. By the mid-nineteenth century, advancements in technology allowed for the provision of high voltage and power, paving the way for significant developments in the generation of artificial X-rays [4].

Scientists such as Julius Plücker and Johann Wilhelm Hittorf began generating cathode rays in the 1860s, later identified as free electrons by J. J. Thomson in 1897 [5]. Sir William Crookes and Philipp Lenard conducted further experiments, deflecting these charge carriers by magnetic fields and sending them through thin metal sheets into free air [4]. These innovative experiments inadvertently generated artificial X-rays of decent intensity as side effects since at least the late 1850s, laying the groundwork for subsequent discoveries in X-ray technology [4]. RF Mould [4] summarized the work done on electric discharge in a table from 1650 to 1879 (see Table 2.3 and Fig. 2.1).

Before 1895, the precursor to the X-ray tube originated from cathode ray tubes developed by scientists like Crookes, Hittorf, and other physicists of the nineteenth century who were studying

Table 2.3 Milestones in the development of vacuum tubes [4]

Year	Scientist	Description
1650	Otto von Guericke	Conducted the first vacuum experiment and created the first air pump. He used glass globes in his experiments to study electricity
1740	Abbe Nollet	Experimented with electricity and discovered that the length of an electric spark changes with the pressure of the gas
1834	W. Snow Harris	Studied electric discharges in tubes with improved methods, observing dark spaces around electrodes
1838	Michael Faraday	Developed better glass tubes for electric discharge studies and invented a pump for removing air from them
1838	Heinrich Geissler	Conducted experiments with modified glass tubes and improved vacuum conditions
1860	Kelvin, Rhumkorff, and others	Studied electric discharge phenomena, leading to the development of better equipment
1860	Gassiot	Used a large battery to demonstrate that vacuum tubes emit light under certain conditions
1865	Hermann Sprengel	Invented a pump capable of creating very low air pressure in tubes
1869	Johann Hittorf	Conducted experiments using specialized tubes named after him
1879	William Crookes	Presented his research on vacuum tubes at a scientific meeting in 1879
1895	Wilhelm Conrad Röntgen	Discovered X-rays, paving the way for their application in vacuum tube.
1896	O. L. Barringer, E. Hardie, E. P. Porter	Produced the first intentional X-ray picture in the United States, demonstrating practical applications of vacuum tube technology

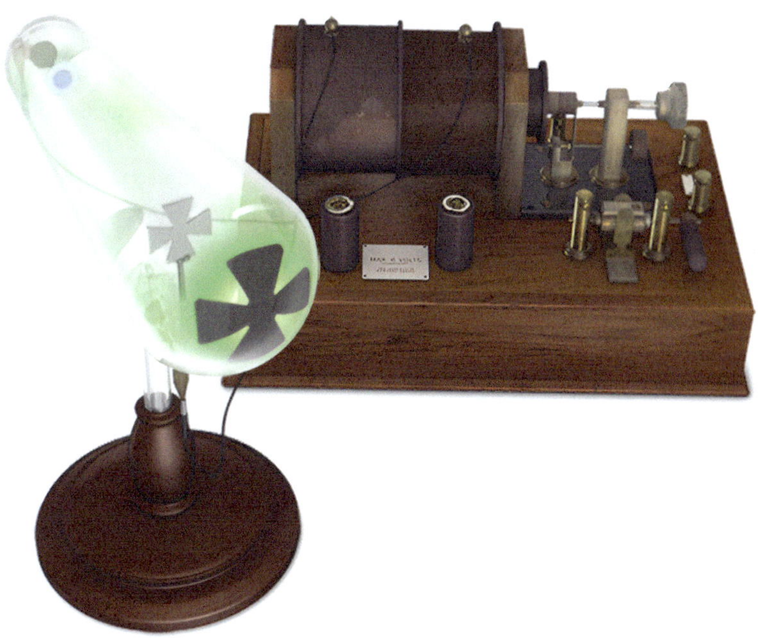

Fig. 2.1 Crookes tube (1870)—invented by Sir William Crookes, it led to the discovery of the electron and X-ray machines. (Image courtesy: National Magnet Academy and Florida State University. Printed with permission)

electric discharges through gases. The first published illustration of tube variants in 1896 suggests that the discharge tubes typically had a cylindrical shape and had a wide array of designs available at that time (Fig. 2.2). This diagram was initially featured in the French journal *La Nature* and later reproduced in *Nature* on January 23, 1897. The early tubes were often referred to as *Geissler tubes* [4]. Philips [7], the first British hospital physicist, reviewed tubes of that time

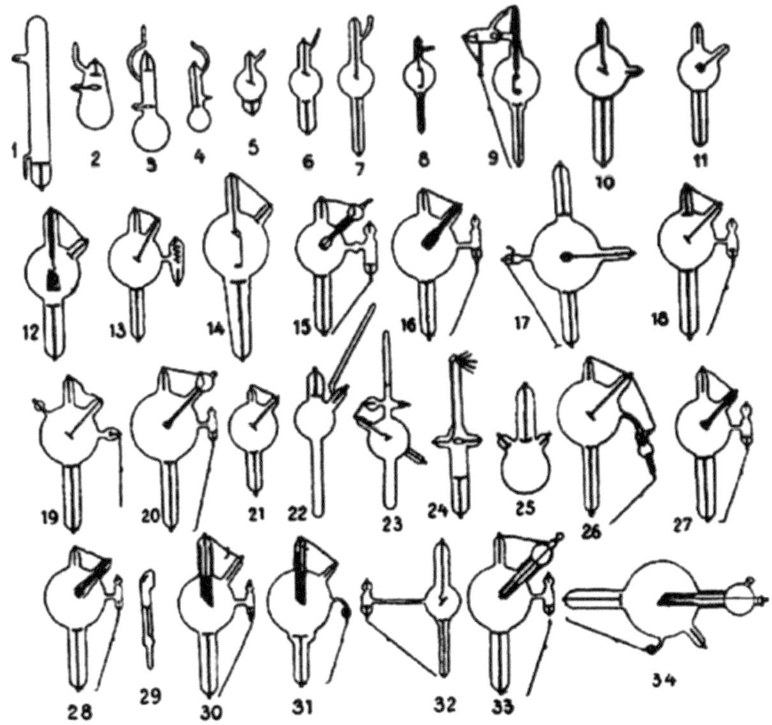

Fig. 2.2 C.H.F. Mueller's catalog of X-ray tubes, around 1898. (Image Courtesy: Rolf Behling [8]. Printed with permission)

and concluded with the remark, "Truly the 'electric egg' has been well hatched!" reflecting on the 60 years of progress in electric discharge research. In these tubes, the cathode disk is supported by a small rod, typically made of platinum, while the disk material itself would have been aluminum or an aluminum alloy. To ensure an airtight seal through the glass wall, a metal with the same coefficient of expansion as the glass had to be used. Platinum was often employed, with the tube glass around the rod often reinforced by lead glass. The anode of these early tubes was usually an aluminum stick placed in a small lateral glass pipe stub [4].

2.2.1 Wilhelm Conrad Röntgen's Discovery Journey

Wilhelm Conrad Röntgen's discovery of X-rays on the evening of November 8, 1895, marked a significant turning point in scientific history. While experimenting with cathode rays in a partially evacuated glass tube, Röntgen noticed an unusual fluorescence on the tube's glass wall when operated with high voltage and gas pressure. This fluorescence persisted even when he attempted to block it with various materials, leading Röntgen to suspect the presence of an unknown form of radiation. His meticulous observations revealed that this radiation, which he termed "X-rays," could penetrate solid objects and create shadows on a nearby screen coated with a fluorescent material.

Röntgen's initial experiments took place in his laboratory in Würzburg, Germany, where he worked diligently to understand the properties of X-rays. He observed that X-rays emerged from the region of the glass tube exhibiting the strongest fluorescence, where cathode rays interacted with the glass. By manipulating the voltage and gas pressure in the tube, Röntgen could control the intensity and direction of the emitted X-rays. Through systematic experimentation, he determined that X-rays exhibited characteristics distinct from both cathode rays and ultraviolet light, leading to their classification as a new form of electromagnetic radiation (Fig. 2.3).

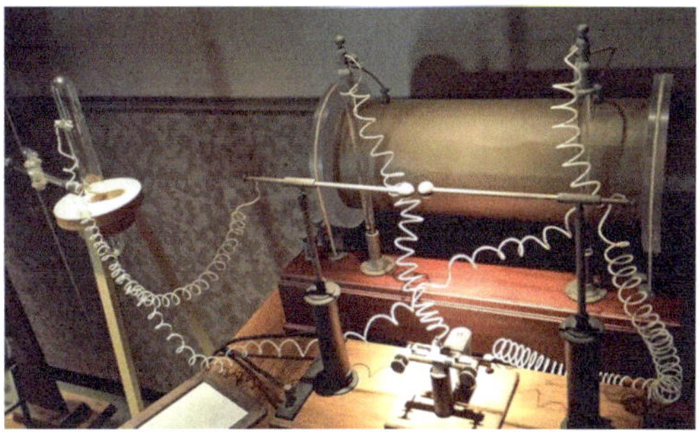

Fig. 2.3 Replica of W.C. Röntgen's first experiment. It shows an actively pumped simple Crookes tube and a "large" Ruehmkorff inductor. Röntgen discovered X-rays at dawn on Friday, November 8, 1895. (Image copyright: Rolf Behling, republished with permission [8])

Many academicians/researchers think the discovery of X-rays by Röntgen was a casual affair and mistakenly perceive his work as a typical end-of-the-week Friday afternoon fluke [9]. However, this discovery resulted from Röntgen's meticulous planning and dedication to his experiments. On November 8, 1895, he was experimenting to confirm Philipp Lenard's findings on cathode rays using specialized equipment in his laboratory in Würzburg, Germany. Working late into the night in his dimly lit laboratory, Röntgen's keen observational skills proved instrumental, aided by the darkness of a rainy late fall evening. After experimenting alone for hours, Röntgen was struck by the peculiar glow of barium platinocyanide on a cardboard screen [4]. As he experimented with the screen, his hand came in between the tube and the fluoroscopic screen, and he witnessed the bones of his hand and documented the observation [10]. This unexpected discovery led him to investigate the cathode rays and ultraviolet light further. Nearly a fortnight following his discovery, he captured the X-ray image of his wife Anna Bertha's hand [10].

Röntgen's meticulous experimentation involved varying voltage and vacuum levels to extreme extents, and through trial and error, he optimized detection methods and identified key characteristics of the newly discovered X-rays despite the challenges of working with primitive equipment. In 1896, Röntgen acknowledged that he struggled to fully understand the essence of the novel "X-rays," which were subsequently termed "Röntgenstrahlen" and "Röntgen rays" [9].

He did not apply for a patent for his discovery and devoted it to mankind, which revolutionized the field of medicine, saving countless lives and earned him the prestigious Nobel Prize in Physics in 1901.

2.2.2 Rapid Advancement in X-Ray Technology and Swift Integration into the Medical Practice

Following Röntgen's groundbreaking discovery of X-rays, there was a rapid advancement in technology and widespread knowledge about this invisible form of light. Just weeks after Röntgen's revelation in January 1896, news of X-rays spread swiftly worldwide, sparking curiosity and experimentation. Within a year, over a thousand articles were published, reflecting the profound impact of this discovery on global scientific discourse.

In the United States, three students—O. L. Barringer, E. Hardie, and E. P. Porter—persuaded a janitor to grant them access to the laboratory at Davidson College, North Carolina, on the night of January 12, 1896. After 3 h of tinkering with the available equipment, they successfully captured their first deliberate X-ray image on the American continent. Barringer later confessed, "We kept our achievement and adventure confidential, and it wasn't until later that we recognized we were not only breaking the rules but also making history for the college" [11].

Similarly, diagnostic X-rays were swiftly put to use in medical settings. On February 3, 1896, a diagnostic X-ray of a broken wrist was taken at Dartmouth College in New Hampshire, with claims of an earlier image taken at Yale University just days prior. Inspired by newspaper reports, chief surgeon Hermann Kümmell of the New General Hospital in Hamburg-Eppendorf, Germany, wasted no time acquiring an X-ray apparatus for clinical use, initiating the integration of X-ray technology into medical practice.

The commercial production of X-ray tubes also saw rapid development. C.H.F. Müller, a glass blower based in Hamburg, Germany, quickly pivoted to producing X-ray tubes in response to growing demand. Within weeks, Müller's company had manufactured and delivered X-ray tubes to medical facilities, laying the foundation for the mass production of this essential component of X-ray equipment.

Despite early challenges such as tube implosions, overheating, and air leakage, manufacturers endeavored to improve X-ray tube technology, striving for greater reliability and image quality. X-ray applications expanded beyond medicine to include skin therapy and industrial inspections, driving innovation and spurring a surge in patent filings related to X-ray technology.

The period following Röntgen's discovery witnessed a flurry of activities as scientists, engineers, and entrepreneurs worked tirelessly to harness the potential of X-rays for various applications, laying the groundwork for modern medical imaging and industrial testing techniques. N.A. Dyson [12] divides the historical perspective on the development of X-ray physics, broadly dividing it into three key periods:

1. *Discovery (1895–1922)*
   - This period marked the dawn of X-ray physics, encompassing the initial discovery by Wilhelm Röntgen in 1895 and extending to elucidate the Compton effect in 1923.
   - During this time, fundamental X-ray phenomena were unveiled and investigated, laying the groundwork for future advancements.
2. *Consolidation (1922–1945)*
   - This period focused on the in-depth study of X-ray spectroscopy and the development of sophisticated instruments for such analysis.
   - X-ray crystallography flourished as a scientific discipline, with significant progress in theoretically interpreting atomic energy levels.
   - X-ray tube technology also witnessed significant advancements as researchers pursued methods to achieve higher voltages and energy.
3. *Revival and new discoveries (1945–present)*
   - This period witnessed a resurgence in X-ray physics, fueled by the availability of new tools and isotopes resulting from advancements in nuclear research.
   - Muonic X-rays were discovered, and the field expanded into previously unforeseen areas like solar and stellar physics.
   - New phenomena emerged, including intense soft X-ray beams from electron synchrotrons and the "isotope effect" in X-ray emission.

Extensive research explored the production of X-rays through bombardment with protons and heavy ions, finding applications in elemental analysis across various materials. This field has significantly revitalized as a dynamic field of fundamental importance. With its ever-evolving nature, it will continue attracting the interest of physicists and researchers for years to come.

2.3 Major Milestones in X-Ray Tubes

2.3.1 Crookes Tubes and Early X-Ray Production Challenges

Crookes tubes, developed by physicist William Crookes in the late nineteenth century, were early experimental discharge tubes used to investigate cathode rays, later identified as streams of electrons. These tubes, consisting of a partially evacuated glass vessel with metal electrodes sealed inside, played a crucial role in Wilhelm Conrad Röntgen's discovery of X-rays in 1895.

Despite their significance, Crookes tubes faced several technical challenges that hampered clinical workflow and image quality. One major issue was the difficulty in liberating electrons from the electrode. Electrons were generated through discharge ionization of residual gas within the tube, causing a sharp increase in tube current as the voltage rose. Ideally, a higher voltage should have corresponded to a lower current to maximize the anode's cooling capacity. However, higher currents at lower voltages were needed for X-ray transparency and tissue contrast, complicating the process. This gap between desired outcomes and technical feasibility persisted until W. D. Coolidge and J. E. Lilienfeld introduced improvements in 1913, 18 years after Röntgen's discovery.

In the early days, additional "anticathodes" were also used to enhance electron current density by reducing negative space charge, thereby improving electron trajectory and focus on the target. However, gas pressure within the tubes was unstable due to contamination of built-in components. Heating of the anode and glass wall increased pressure, reducing the electrons' free path length and resulting in softer X-rays. High electric fields caused ions to be implanted into the glass wall and negatively charged electrodes, irreversibly burying them. Internal coating of the glass with target material helped remove residual gas by binding it, leading to self-cleaning of vacuum-tight tubes.

Handling ion X-ray tubes in those days required expertise in physics, electrical technology, and medical knowledge. Radiographers needed to be proficient in adjusting parameters such as high voltage while observing gas discharge characteristics in the tube to ensure acceptable image quality. Risks of electrical shock, tube implosion, and radiation burns necessitated caution during operation (Fig. 2.4).

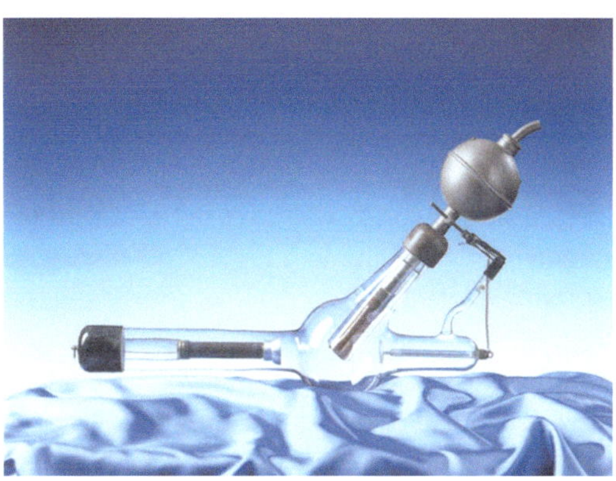

Fig. 2.4 An ion tube featuring a water-cooled target, produced by C.H.F. Müller in Hamburg around 1910. (Image Copyright: Springer Nature [13]. Reprinted with permission)

2.3.2 1913: Thermionic Cathodes—A Milestone in X-Ray Tube Technology

In 1913, American engineer and physicist William D. Coolidge introduced the concept of hot cathode X-ray tubes, a groundbreaking innovation that revolutionized X-ray technology. Coolidge earned his undergraduate degree in electrical engineering from the Massachusetts Institute of Technology (MIT) in 1896 and his doctorate in physics from the University of Leipzig in 1899. Coolidge joined the General Electric (GE) Research Laboratory in 1905, and his work at GE was pivotal in advancing X-ray technology and other areas of applied physics. By 1930, he led the GE Research Laboratory, and his legacy lives on through the Coolidge tube, still widely used today. And retired from GE in 1940 but remained active in the scientific community until his death on February 3, 1975, at age 101 [10] (Fig. 2.5).

Rontgen utilized a Crookes tube filled with gas, leading to inconsistent X-ray output; however, Coolidge developed a cathode vacuum tube that emitted stable X-rays [14]. Subsequently, he introduced a tungsten alloy for both the cathode and the anode, establishing tungsten as the standard material for X-ray tubes [14]. Unlike the Crookes tube, the Coolidge tube, known as the hot cathode tube, operated with a superior vacuum (around 10^{-4} pascal). Electrons were now produced by "thermionic emission," where a

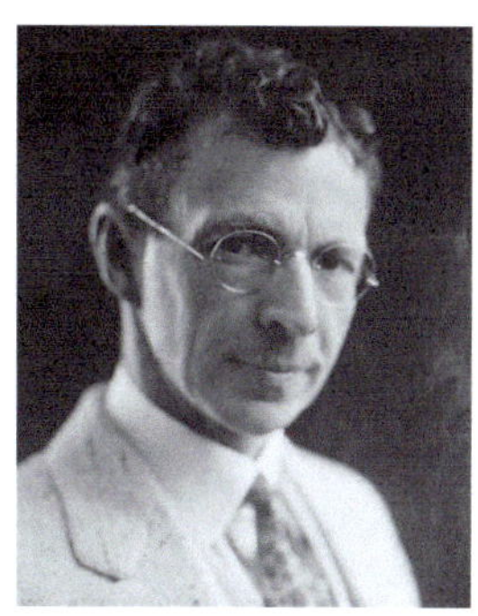

Fig. 2.5 William D. Coolidge (October 23, 1873—February 3, 1975). (Image Courtesy: Wikipaedia, published under Creative Commons license)

tungsten filament, heated by electricity, acted as the cathode (electron emitter). A high-voltage difference between the cathode and the anode accelerated these electrons toward the anode, generating X-rays.

These tubes were called the "second-generation" hot cathode X-ray tube and featured a spherical tempered borosilicate (pyrex) structure with high vacuum, two cylindrical arms serving as cathode and anode, and a tungsten anode embedded in copper. The anode's shape varies between circular, square, or rectangular, with thickness and size ranging from 2 to 10 mm and 10 to 20 mm, respectively, and an anode angle typically around 7 to 20 degrees [15]. A tungsten filament acts as the cathode, with a molybdenum focusing cup coated in nickel to streamline emitted electrons. Upon heating, the cathode filament emits electrons via thermionic emission, which are then accelerated and strike the anode, producing bremsstrahlung and characteristic X-rays with an output power ranging from 0.1 to 100 kW, depending on the application.

While serving as the prototype for modern X-ray tubes, it faces technical limitations, including slow temporal response time, high-power consumption of the thermionic cathode, and potential filament failure due to high temperatures, leading to reduced tube lifespan (Figs. 2.6, 2.7 and Table 2.4).

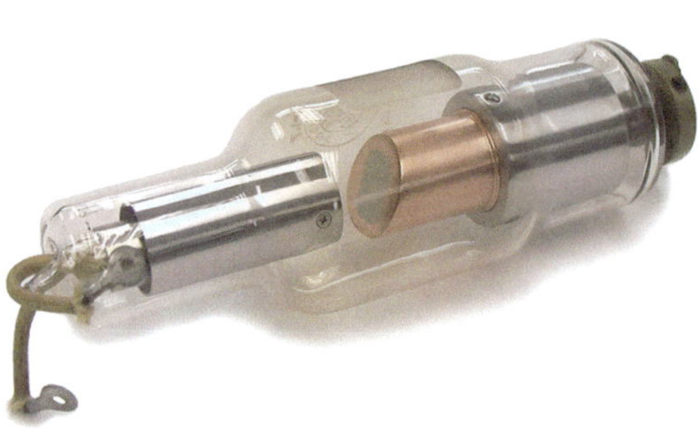

Fig. 2.6 A small general electric diagnostic X-ray tube (D1.7), with "D" denotes "Diagnostic" and "1.7" indicating a fine 1.7 mm focal spot diameter. (Courtesy: The Oak Ridge Associated Universities (ORAU) Museum of Radiation and Radioactivity. Printed with permission)

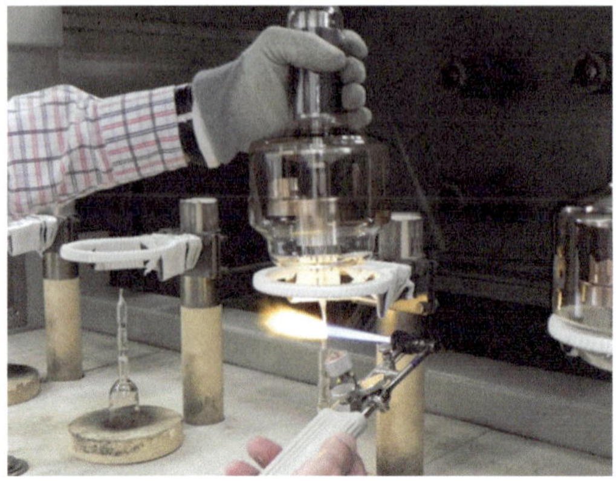

Fig. 2.7 After the exhaust process, a mechanical vacuum pump seals off a glass tube used in general radiography. The vacuum inside is then upheld mainly through ion implantation into electrodes and, to a lesser extent, by a chemical getter. (Image Copyright: Springer Nature [13]. Reprinted with permission)

2.3.3 1918: Goetze's Line Focus

The next big advancement came from surgeon Prof. Dr. Otto Goetze with his patent in 1918, later utilized by C. H. F. Müller in their RÖNTGEN-MÜLLER tubes starting from 1922 [28]. He addressed a key limitation in earlier X-ray tube geometry. Early X-ray tubes often employed a broad filament cathode design. Electrons emitted from the entire broad filament area bombarded the target anode, creating a large focal spot. This large focal spot resulted in limitations for certain X-ray imaging applications:

- Reduced image resolution: The larger focal spot size blurred the details in the resulting X-ray image.
- Increased patient radiation dose: A broader area of the anode was exposed to electrons, potentially leading to a higher radiation dose for the patient.

Goetze's ingenious concept involved modifying the filament design to create a "narrow, line-shaped cathode." This line-shaped filament produced a "much smaller focal spot" on the target anode. This smaller focal spot size offered sharper and more detailed X-ray images enabling improved image resolution with more accurate

Table 2.4 Major milestones in X-ray tube developments

Year	Description
1895	Wilhelm Conrad Röntgen discovered X-rays through meticulous experimentation on 8 November, revolutionizing medical diagnostics and earning the Nobel Prize in Physics in 1901
1896	The first deliberate X-ray image was captured in the United States by O. L. Barringer, E. Hardie, and E. P. Porter at Davidson College, North Carolina, on 12 January
1896	Diagnostic X-rays quickly integrated into medical practice on 03 February, with the first clinical X-ray taken at Dartmouth College in New Hampshire
1896	Commercial production of X-ray tubes begins in response to growing demand, with C.H.F. Müller in Hamburg, Germany, leading the way
1906	British physicist Charles Barkla demonstrated that X-rays are polarized, providing evidence that they are transverse electromagnetic waves [16]
1912	Max von Laue discovered that X-rays are diffracted by crystals, enabling the study of atomic structure [16]
1913	The introduction of thermionic cathodes by W. D. Coolidge marks a significant advancement in X-ray tube technology [17]
1914	Development of two-pulse generator technology
1918	Surgeon Prof. Dr. Otto Goetze patents the line focus, reducing the angle of the anode surface to improve image resolution
1918	Development of shockproof Dental X-ray Machine [15]
1925	Philips introduced the Metalix tube, which solved the problems of X-ray emission in all directions and the hazard of high-voltage cables [18]
1926	J.E. Lilienfeld developed early field-emission X-ray tubes [19]
1928	Introduction to the first portable X-ray apparatus by the Philips [18]
1929	Albert Bouwers from Philips commercializes the rotating anode tube, leading to significant potential for increased instantaneous input power
1959	High-speed tubes "The Super Rotalix (SRO) tube" introduced by the Philips [18]
1962	Rhenium-alloyed tungsten composite anode tube by General Electric [20]
1969	Mammography unit with molybdenum anode [21]
1976	General Electric introduced a three-layer anode composed of a tungsten, rhenium, and molybdenum alloy [22]
1979	Introduction of all metal-ceramics and spiral groove bearing tubes, improving tube reliability and performance
1982	Development of electron beam computed tomography (EBCT) scanners for high-speed cardiac imaging
1989	Direct anode cooling with noiseless rotor [23]
1989	Development of helical CT [24]
1998	Development of grid control rotating anode for angiography by Toshiba [25]
2002	High-speed rotational bearing rotating anode tube for angiography [26]
2003	Siemens introduced a rotating frame tube, enabling fast focal track speeds and improved CT imaging [27]
2005	GE introduces the largest commercial anode with carbon backing, prioritizing efficiency in CT imaging with a diameter of 200 mm [28]
2006	Introduction of STRATON X-ray tube by Siemens
2007	Philips introduces the iMRC® tube with segmented metal anode and spiral-groove bearings, enhancing power density in CT scans [28]
2018	GE unveils the Quantix 160® X-ray tube with groundbreaking cathode technology for spectral CT imaging, allowing rapid tube current adjustment [29]
2019	Researchers from New Zealand developed the MARS spectral CT scanner for 3D color X-ray imaging [16]
2020	Multisource X-ray tube to reduce imaging duration in digital breast tomosynthesis
2023	Line-focus X-ray tube for microbeam radiotherapy with very high dose rates

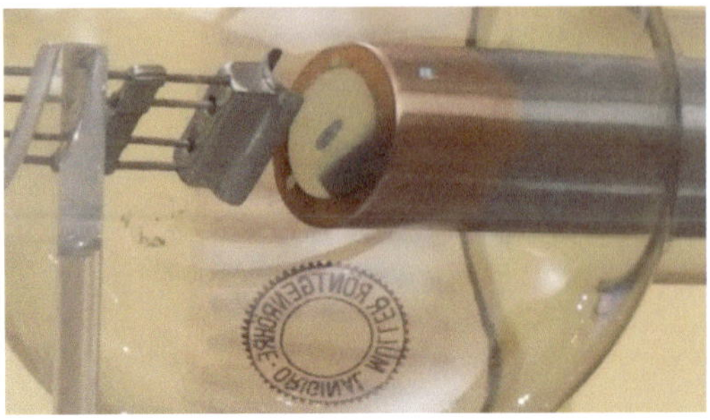

Fig. 2.8 Focusing components of a fixed anode tube with a linear focal spot, designed following O. Goetze's concept, manufactured by C.H.F. Mueller in Hamburg, Germany. The molten structure on the somewhat overheated anode delineates the linear focal spot. (Image originally published in [29]. Republished with permission)

diagnosis of medical conditions. This approach "reduced patient radiation dose" as a more concentrated area on the anode was bombarded by electrons, potentially reducing the overall radiation dose to the patient.

Furthermore, advancements in electron emitters, shaped as lengthy coils of tungsten wire, allowed for higher tube current densities without exceeding space charge limits. Siemens patented a dual focal spot tube 1924, optimizing spatial and contrast resolution. Despite these advancements, the performance of stationary anode tubes eventually plateaued due to thermal limitations, even with improvements in cooling methods such as tungsten-in-copper brazed structures and water coolers (Fig. 2.8).

2.3.4 1925: The Philips Metalix Tube

Early X-ray devices faced challenges such as emitting undesired radiation in all directions and posing hazards with exposed high-voltage cables. Professor Albert Bouwers from the Philips Research Laboratory addressed these issues by developing a cylindrical X-ray tube with a grounded metal canister, a glass window, and a lead layer, simplifying X-ray procedures and removing operator risks. This design ensured controlled emission of X-rays through the special glass window, safeguarding patients and physicians from hazardous radiation while reducing the tube size compared to conventional spherical tubes [18].

It is available in five sizes and features a chrome-iron alloy construction, ensuring a perfect vacuum seal even at high temperatures. An incandescent cathode filament and insulated anticathode electrode created a focused X-ray spot inside. The emitted X-rays passed through a window, with any remaining rays absorbed by internal lead and brass walls. This design offers complete protection without external shielding and boasts increased X-ray output. The "Metalix" tube was recognized for its reliability, with a lifespan of up to 3 years [30] (Figs. 2.9 and 2.10).

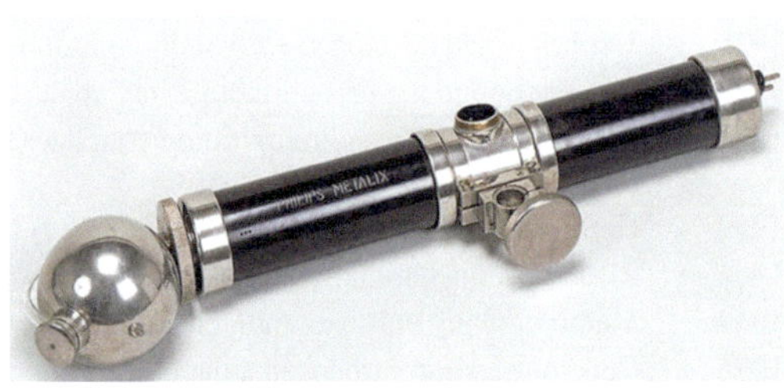

Fig. 2.9 Philips Metalix X-ray tube. (Image Courtesy: "Royal Philips/Philips Company Archives" [31], printed with permission)

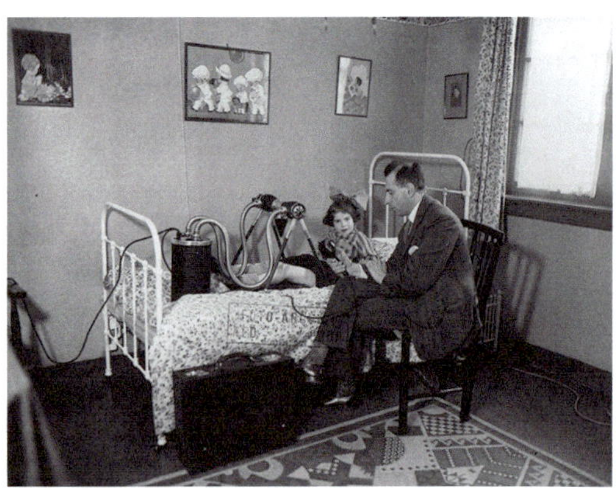

Fig. 2.10 Mobile Metalix X-ray tube (1930). (Image Courtesy: "Royal Philips/Philips Company Archives" [31], printed with permission)

2.3.5 1926: J.E. Lilienfeld's Pioneering Work in Solid-State Field-Effect Amplification

J.E. Lilienfeld further refined early electronic device concepts by proposing one of the first solid-state field-effect amplifier designs in 1926 [19]. Lilienfeld's work laid the foundation for modern electronic devices, leveraging the solid-state principles to control electron flow through a semiconductor, a fundamental aspect of electronic circuitry. His invention was described in his patent application rather than in a published paper. The patent application titled "Method and Apparatus for Controlling Electric Currents" was filed on October 8, 1926, and granted as U.S. Patent No. 1,745,175 on January 28, 1930 [19]. This patent laid the groundwork for solid-state transistor concepts and its applications in electronic amplification.

The contributions of Coolidge and Lilienfeld marked a significant advancement in X-ray and early solid-state electronic technology, enabling the development of more reliable and versatile X-ray equipment for medical diagnostics, industrial testing, and scientific research (Fig. 2.11).

2.3.6 1929: The Introduction of Rotating Anode Tubes

In April 1927, Prof. Albert Bouwers, working at the newly established Philips "Natuurkundig Laboratorium (Physics Laboratory)" in Eindhoven, the Netherlands, aimed to innovate X-ray tube technology while avoiding infringing on Coolidge patents [32]. Bouwers devised the Philips Metalix, the first successful metal center section tube, to shield against harmful X-rays [28]. This design featured a grounded metal center section around the focal spot, pushing glass insulation to the ends, similar to later ceramic insulator designs.

Bouwers also adopted the concept of the rotating anode X-ray tube, initially proposed by an

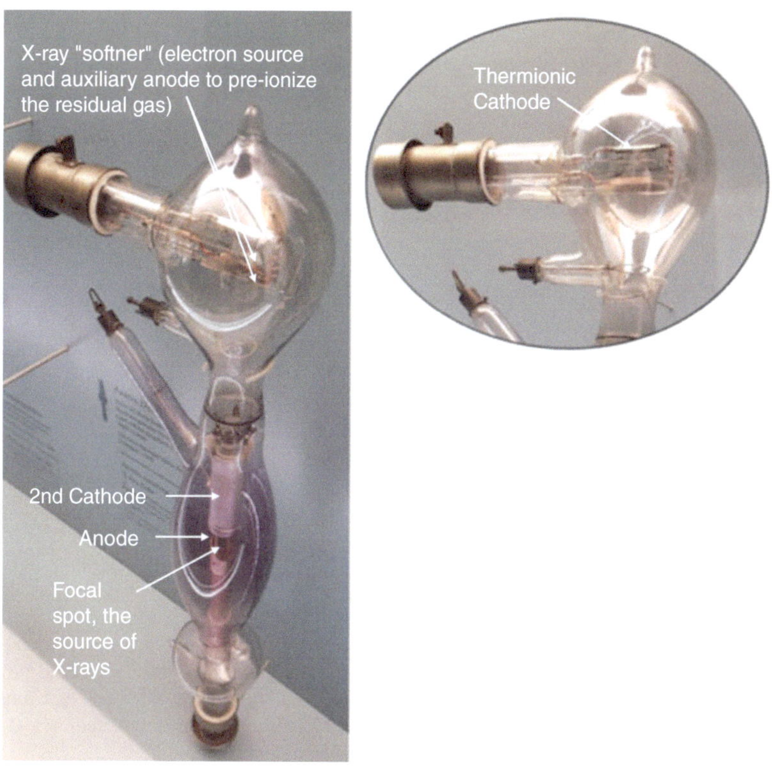

Fig. 2.11 Lilienfeld tube displayed at the German Röntgen Museum, Remscheid-Lennep, Germany. (Image Copyright: Springer Nature [13]. Republished with permission)

earlier concept in 1921 by other researchers. Bouwers oversaw its commercialization by Philips in 1929, based on the METALIX tube design. This innovation introduced a rotating copper anode with a tungsten target surface, offering significant potential for increased instantaneous input power. However, Bouwers encountered reliability issues initially, attributed to the complexity of integrating multiple new technologies into one product platform.

Despite these challenges, Bouwers foresaw promising applications, such as rapid heart imaging, with potential exposure times as short as 0.02 s. However, technical challenges persisted, such as heat transfer issues and the durability of components in high vacuum environments. Bouwers' subsequent patents addressed these concerns, but issues like short bearing lifetimes and lubrication limitations continued to pose obstacles (Fig. 2.12).

Over time, advancements in rotating anode technology addressed some of these challenges. Siemens introduced the all-tungsten anode 1932, enabling higher temperatures and more efficient cooling. Innovations like grid control of electron emission and compound anode materials further improved performance and durability.

Post-World War II, rotating anode tubes became widespread, facilitating shorter exposure times and enabling a series of exposures. Siemens and Philips introduced further refinements, such as the Trinodex all-metal tube and graphite-backed anodes, marking significant advancements in X-ray tube technology.

2.3.7 1959: High-Speed Tubes—The Super Rotalix (SRO) Tubes by Philips

The growth of specialized medical applications involved prolonged imaging sessions requiring heavier tube loads. This could only be accomplished by increasing the rotation speed and diameter of the rotating anode. Due to the inertia of a large tungsten anode, achieving this was challenging. As a result, the bulky tungsten anode disk was substituted with one featuring a com-

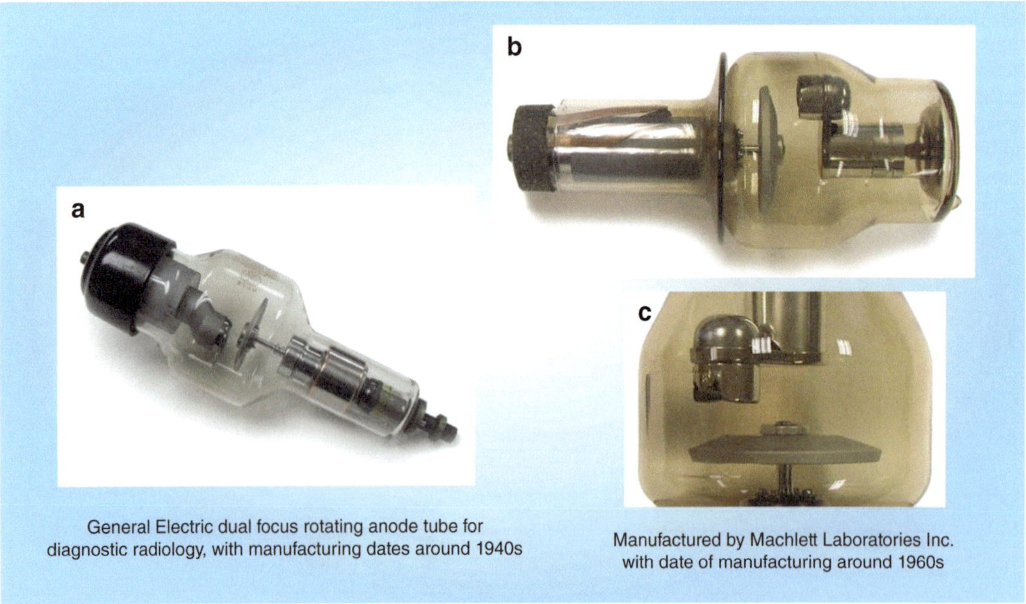

Fig. 2.12 The rotating anode tubes for diagnostic radiology. (**a**) The General Electric dual-focus rotating anode tube has a probable manufacturing date of around 1940. (**b**) The Machlett Laboratories Inc. manufactured rotating anode tubes around the 1960s. (**c**) Close-up image of two cathode filaments and rotating anode. (Image courtesy: Museum of Radiation and Radioactivity. Published with permission)

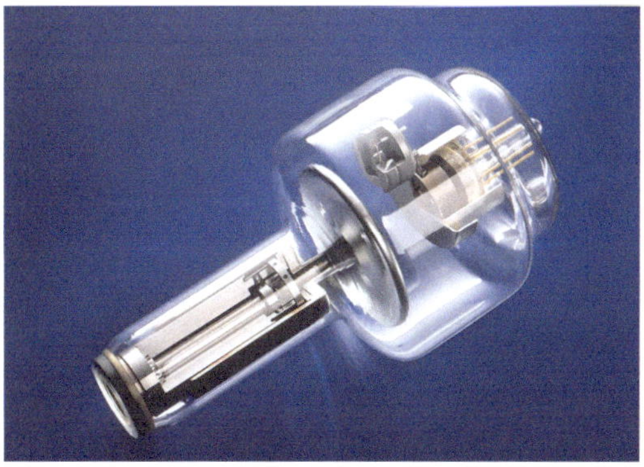

Fig. 2.13 The Super Rotalix (SRO) tube, featuring a fully glass envelope. The "Super" designation signifies the ISO-Hz alternating voltage supply for the induction motor, an upgrade from the 50-Hz supply in earlier models. (Image courtesy: Philips Tech Review [33]. Republished with permission)

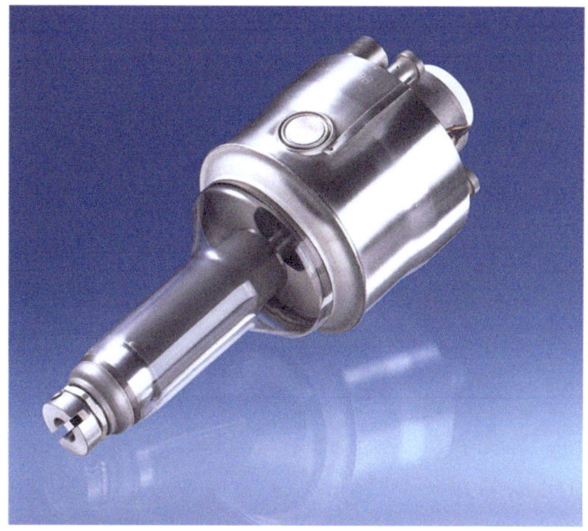

Fig. 2.14 The Super Rotalix Metal tube (SRM), where part of the glass envelope is substituted with metal at ground potential. (Image courtesy: Philips Tech Review [33]. Republished with permission)

posite molybdenum substrate, known for its high melting point but low relative density, topped with a layer of tungsten. In doing so, engineers could enlarge the anode disk to 90 mm and triple the rotational speed upto 9000 revolutions per minute (RPM), resulting in a roughly 70% increase in output with the same focal spot size. Philips introduced this new tube, the Super Rotalix (SRO), to the market in 1959. It remains a staple in universal fluoroscopy and bucky systems to this day [18] (Fig. 2.13).

2.3.8 1973: The Super Rotalix Metal (SRM) X-Ray Tube by Philips

As X-ray technology advanced, there was a need for even stronger output from the X-ray tube. While improvements in the anode design were made, the glass envelope became a problem. Continuous exposure to electrons and ions and metal particle buildup from both electrodes altered the envelope's insulation and affected the tube's high-voltage stability. The solution was to use a different material for the tube envelope. Philips followed the path laid out by Albert Bouwers in 1925 with the Metalix tube by using a metal housing around the anode and cathode. X-rays could exit through a beryllium window in this metal housing. In 1973, Philips introduced the Super Rotalix Metal (SRM), a tube with metal and ceramic envelops, offering higher load capacity than existing SRO tubes [18] (Fig. 2.14).

2.3.9 1979: The Super Rotalix Ceramic (SRC) X-Ray Tube

The need for higher X-ray output persisted, posing challenges due to limited heat capacity, especially in lengthy cardiac examinations. Despite introducing metal tube envelopes, existing technology offered little room for improving maximum output, heat capacity, and tube lifespan. In 1979, Philips introduced a game-changing X-ray tube: the Super Rotalix Ceramic (SRC). Unlike its predecessor, the SRC tube featured a fully metal-ceramic envelope, allowing for a more compact design. With a large anode diameter of 120 mm with bearings on both sides, the SRC tube offered significantly higher load capacity, reducing wait times between acquisitions, which is particularly beneficial for continuous and large series of examinations [18].

The SRC tube constructed entirely of metal and ceramic, introduces significant enhancements compared to earlier Philips Rotalix tubes. The metal casing efficiently conducts secondary electrons away, allowing the tube to handle higher loads and improving image contrast. Despite an increased diameter of the rotating anode, the external dimensions of the tube remain unchanged. Analytical and computer calculations demonstrate optimal temperature distribution within the anode, with tungsten-rhenium alloy and molybdenum combination proving superior in practice. A new motor design with a toroidal winding stator accelerates the anode effectively, overcoming its larger moment of inertia compared to previous tube types by adjusting the supply voltage frequency during start-up for maximum torque [33] (Fig. 2.15).

2.3.10 1987: Enhanced Heat Transfer Rotating Anode X-Ray Tubes with Interleaved Fins by Varian Medical Systems Inc

In 1986, Varian Medical Systems Inc. developed an innovative solution to address the thermal energy generated in the anode of rotating anode X-ray tubes. Patented in 1987 [34], this solution involved integrating heat-dissipating fins on the anode structure. These fins were strategically interleaved with heat-receiving fins attached to the vacuum envelope. This design facilitated superior heat transfer from the anode to the surrounding environment through effective cooling mechanisms.

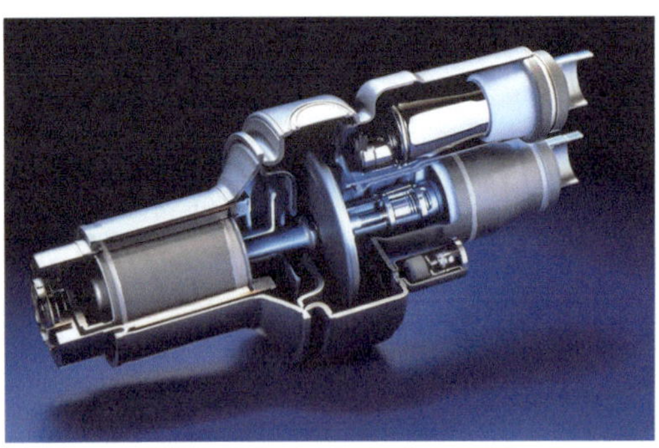

Fig. 2.15 The Super Rotalix Ceramic (SRC) incorporates ceramic instead of glass for high-voltage insulation. With an increased external diameter of the anode to 120 mm (compared to 90 mm in the SRO tube and 100 mm in the SRM tube), the power that can be momentarily applied to the tube has been boosted by 40% compared to the SRO tube. (Image courtesy: Philips Tech Review [33]. Republished with permission)

2.3.11 1989: Maximus Rotalix Ceramic (MRC)

In 1989, Philips made a big leap in X-ray tube technology by swapping out the traditional ball bearings for a spiral groove bearing, which used a special liquid-metal alloy as a lubricant. This upgrade significantly reduced the noise, increased the lifespan, and improved the tube's heat dissipation and current flow.

This innovative bearing, when combined with the advanced SRC tube technology, created the compact MRC tube. It boasted a quietly rotating anode, perfect for long-term use with the ability to be turned on in the morning and off in the evening, ensuring an extended lifespan. The superior heat dissipation the liquid metal lubricant provided gave the MRC tube significantly improved cooling capacity compared to its predecessor, the SRM tube, especially during cine examinations. The introduction of this groundbreaking tube marked a huge advancement in performance and user convenience, particularly benefiting cardiology and vascular systems (Fig. 2.16).

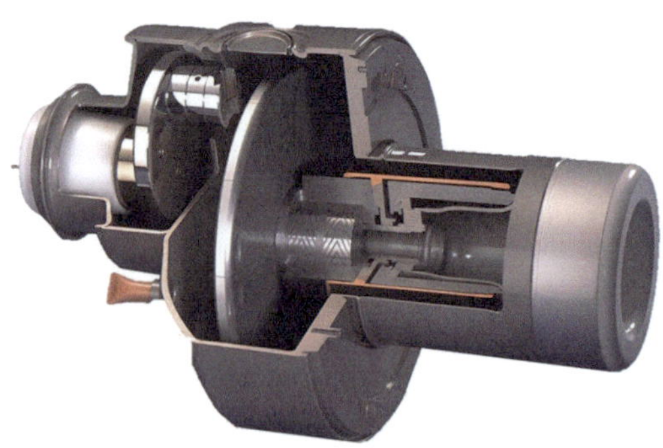

Fig. 2.16 Philips MRC™ 200 series for cardiology and angiography. First rotating anode tube with liquid bearing and 200 mm anode disk. (Image copyright: Rolf Behling, republished with permission [8])

2.3.12 1996: Rotating Anode Cooled by High Thermal Conductivity Fluid by Varian Medical Systems Inc

A rotating X-ray tube's anode was cooled by a liquid metal or metal film circulating in a gap between the anode and a fixed structure. The liquid metal flowed through a labyrinth, magnetic structure, or wick to be trapped in the gap. The recirculated liquid metal was cooled inside or outside the tube in a heat exchanger. A heat exchanger within the tube was in contact with the recirculating liquid metal and contained multiple passages for a cooling fluid, such as water. A high thermal conductivity path was established between the electron projection region and the central region of the tube where heat was extracted. This was achieved using a pyrolytic graphite structure with high thermal conductivity along its radial axis and low thermal conductivity perpendicular to it [35].

2.3.13 2003: Rotating Frame X-Ray Tubes by Siemens

Motivated by the increasing significance of CT, companies made substantial investments. In the mid-1990s, a team at Siemens embarked on reviving the concept of a rotating frame tube by drawing inspiration from a patent dating back to 1915 [36] by William D. Coolidge. The team devised a design that fulfilled higher scan power demand, shorter rotation times, quicker cooldown periods, and smaller focal spots. They presented a new tube technology that meets all these requirements by employing an innovative cooling method and beam control system. Unlike traditional tubes relying on radiative cooling, the Straton® X-ray tube exclusively employed convective cooling, rendering large heat storage capacities of the anode disk unnecessary. With an unprecedented cooling rate of 4.8 MHU/min, waiting times due to anode cooling in clinical workflow were eliminated. Furthermore, an electronic beam deflection system enabled precise control over focal spot position and size, facilitating advanced applications. Additionally, the tube demonstrated exceptional resilience to g-forces exceeding 20 g generated by fast-rotating gantries (Fig. 2.17).

2.3.14 2005: The GE Breakthrough: Largest Commercial Anode

In the 1990s, development projects for single-slice CT primarily aimed to enhance energy

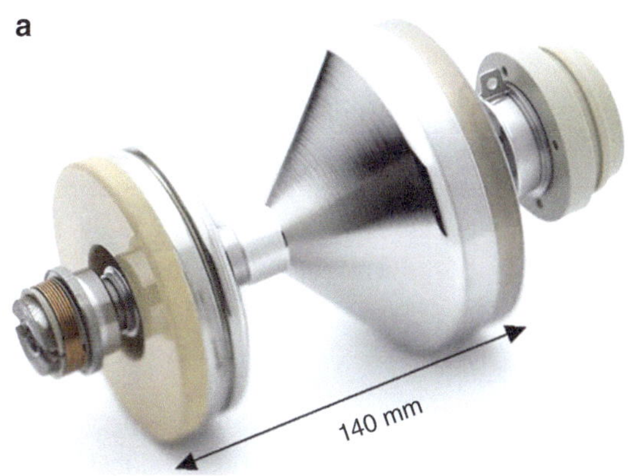

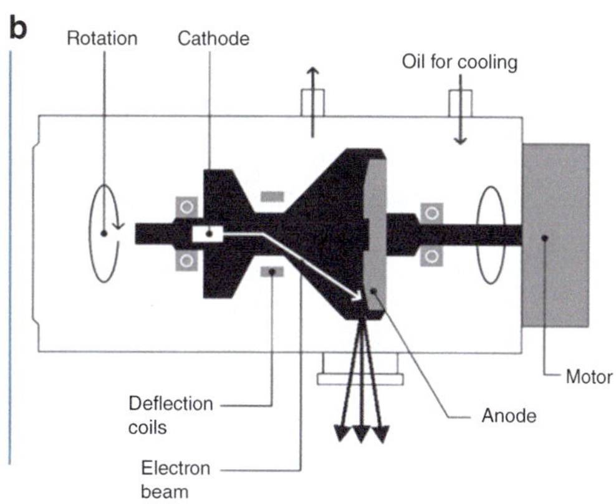

Fig. 2.17 (**a**) The Rotating Envelope tube (RET), that is, the Siemens Straton tube, consists of a cathode and ceramic insulator on the left side, with an anode positioned on the right. The tube had a maximum diameter of 120 mm, with additional installations, including ball bearings and an inductive filament transformer. (**b**) Operation principles and primary components of a RET housing assembly. (Image courtesy: John Wiley and Sons [27]. Reprinted with permission)

throughput per patient, addressing the lengthy scan times typical of that era. One notable outcome of these endeavors was the creation of a high-performance CT tube by GE in 2005, featuring the largest commercial carbon-backed anode at the time, with a diameter of 200 mm. This tube design prioritized efficiency. Unlike conventional setups, where only the cathode has high-voltage potential, in this design, the cathode, housed in a large pancake insulator, was the only component energized. The rest of the tube remained grounded.

An electron trap was integrated to manage backscattered electrons, similar to the Varian tube. However, in the GE tube, some backscattered electrons were reflected to the anode by the cathode. Placing the anode rotor's center of gravity between the ball-bearing raceways ensured balanced load distribution. Additionally, a squirrel-cage motor, positioned in an extension of the tube frame, maximized motor efficiency while connected to ground potential.

2.3.15 2007: Philips' Innovation: The iMRC® Tube for Enhanced Power Density CT Tube

In pursuit of increasing the speed of the focal track, Philips made a significant decision. They abandoned the carbon backing of their premium-tier anode, which would otherwise limit the rotation speed of the anode. This led to the creation of the iMRC® tube (Fig. 2.18).

The iMRC® tube introduced a segmented and gradually recrystallized all-metal titanium-zirconium-molybdenum anode with a tungsten-rhenium top layer. A new generation of spiral groove bearings was introduced, now suspended rigidly on both ends to withstand high centrifugal forces. Designing these bearings posed a challenge. Without countermeasures, the liquid metal "lubricant" had two ends to escape from the bearing members it separated.

The rotor was placed at ground potential along with the anode disk to maximize motor efficiency. The very high focal track speeds achieved resulted in the focal spot's highest available power density capability. A stationary electron trap managed the heat from backscattered electrons. A flat tungsten electron emitter, combined with magnetic focusing and deflection, allowed for relatively high tube currents even at low tube voltage. This innovation is crucial for dose saving in certain CT exams.

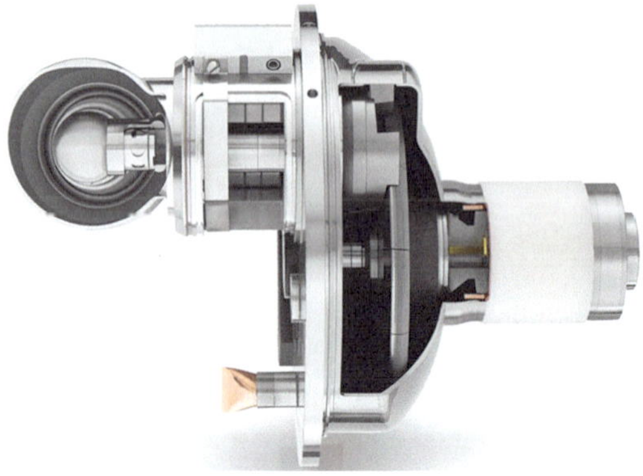

Fig. 2.18 The Philips iMRC tube features monopolar design, ceramic insulation (top left), magnetic focusing and deflection of electron beams, a scattered electron trap (top center), dual suspended hydrodynamic bearings (center right), and a segmented all-metal anode. (Copyright: Springer Nature [37]. Reprinted with permission)

Unlike Siemens, who opted for a rotating frame tube, Philips chose a straight electron drift path and utilized dual magnetic quadrupoles in series, complemented by magnetic dipoles for deflection. These improvements led to a very high electron compression factor. As the detector coverage of the CT system increased, the physical focal spot had to be short to enlarge the anode angle. The high power rating allowed the addition of a relatively thick radiation prefilter of titanium upstream of the patient, reducing the patient's dose despite the higher power.

In late 2014, Siemens launched a very similar tube type with its Vectron® tube, and GE introduced the Quantix 160® tube in 2018, featuring a flat emitter cathode designed for the spectral CT system GE Revolution® CT (Fig. 2.19).

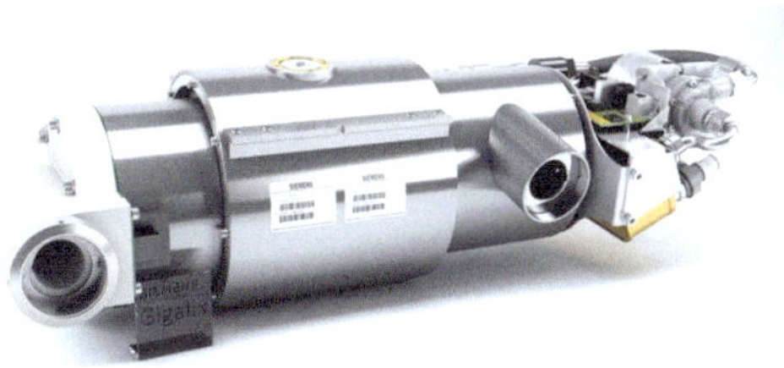

Fig. 2.19 Siemens angiography tube of the Gigalix™series, launched in 2013, with grid switchable flat electron emitter and liquid bearing. (Image copyright: Rolf Behling, republished with permission [8])

2.3.16 2018: GE'S Breakthrough in Cathode Innovation for Spectral CT

In 2018, GE unveiled a groundbreaking advancement in cathode technology by introducing the Quantix 160® X-ray tube for spectral CT. GE's innovation involved using a flat emitters cathode and a pull electrode to generate a variable electric field at the emitter. This mechanism controlled the release of electrons. At low pull field strengths, electronic space charge prevented electron emission to the anode. GE can rapidly adjust the tube current in microseconds by biasing the pull electrode.

The Quantix 160® tube is integrated into the Revolution CT spectral CT system. This system can swiftly modify the tube voltage and measure X-ray attenuation across different "colors" of the X-ray beam to generate spectral data. The tube current is nearly doubled during periods of low tube voltage and X-ray conversion efficiency (Fig. 2.20).

In contrast, Philips utilizes a dual-layer detector for spectral differentiation, while Siemens employs a dual-source system with two spinning X-ray tubes and detector pairs operated at different voltages. This breakthrough in cathode technology marks a significant advancement in spectral CT imaging capabilities (Fig. 2.21).

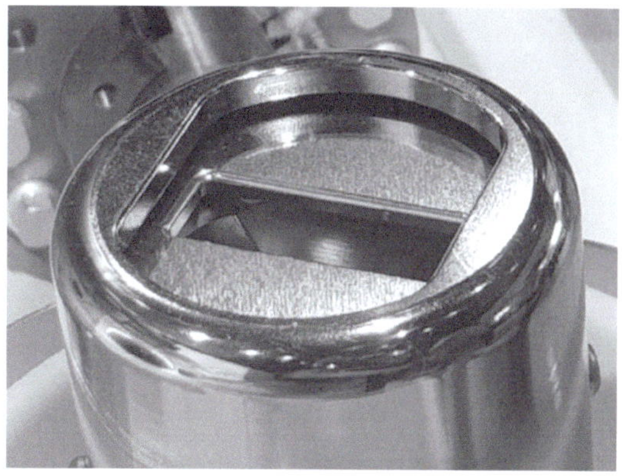

Fig. 2.20 Launched in 2018, the GE Quantix 160® tube features a Pierce-type cathode designed for the spectral CT system GE Revolution Apex. (Image Copyright: Taylor and Francis Group [9]. Reproduced with permission)

2.3.17 2020: Multisource X-Ray Tube to Reduce Imaging Duration in Digital Breast Tomosynthesis

Becker et al. presented the development and assessment of a prototype multi-X-ray-source array (MXA) designed for digital breast tomosynthesis [38]. The MXA consists of an array of tungsten filament cathodes with focus cup grid-controlled modulation and a common rotating anode housed in a single vacuum envelope. Prototypes comprising arrays of three-source elements and eleven-source elements were created and tested. The prototype sources exhibited focal spot sizes of 0.3 mm at 45 kV with 50 mA. The measured X-ray spectra matched the employed tungsten anode with molybdenum filtration, and the tube output (air kerma) ranged from 0.6 mGy/100 mAs at 20 kV to 17 mGy/100 mAs at 45 kV at a distance of 100 cm. Half-value layer (HVL) measurements varied from 0.5 mm Al at 30 kV to 0.8 mm Al at 45 kV, and X-ray pulse widths were adjusted from 20 ms to 110 ms, pri-

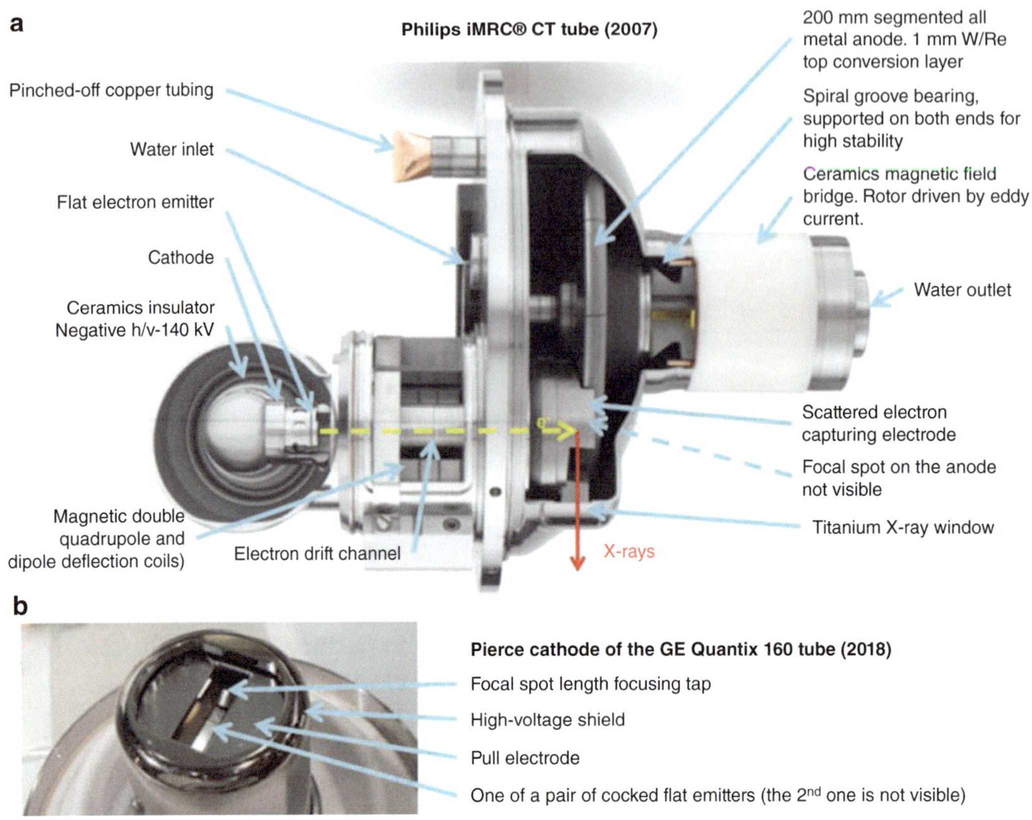

Fig. 2.21 (**a**) Cross-sectional view of the Philips iMRC® X-ray tube. (**b**) The pierce-type cathode of the GE Quantix® tube. (Image Courtesy: Springer Nature [13]. Reprinted with permission)

marily limited by source turn-on/off times of approximately 1 ms. Initial results of reconstructed tomographic data are also provided.

2.3.18 2023: Line-Focus X-Ray Tube for Microbeam Radiotherapy with Very High Dose Rates

Microbeam radiotherapy (MRT) is a cutting-edge approach in radiation oncology, showing promising results in sparing normal tissue while effectively controlling tumors. Using spatially modulated treatment fields, MRT delivers micrometer-wide high-dose peaks and low-dose valleys, enhancing normal tissue resistance to high doses. The line-focus X-ray tube (LFxT) has emerged as a compact clinical source, utilizing an eccentric electron beam to produce X-rays. Monte Carlo simulations suggest accelerating electrons to energies between 300 and 600 keV to achieve the necessary photon energies. The LFxT specifications include a dose rate of 180 Gy/s, an acceleration voltage of 600 kV, and a focal spot width of 50 μm. Challenges include managing emittance for small focal spots and addressing space charge forces. Simulations reveal the feasibility of an electron source and beamline for the LFxT prototype, utilizing a thermal cathode to deliver the required beam current. The LFxT prototype holds promise for providing valuable insights into developing a clinical device with a beam energy of 600 keV [39].

2.4 Basic Principles of X-Ray Tube Operation

Modern X-ray tubes, though based on the fundamental principles of the early Coolidge tubes, have evolved significantly, incorporating advanced technologies to improve performance, reliability, and versatility. The basic principles of X-ray tube operation involve several key components and processes:

The cathode assembly serves as the source of electrons in an X-ray tube and consists of a filament and a focusing cup. The process by which electrons are liberated from the filament is called thermionic emission. Typically made of tungsten due to its high melting point (3422 °C) and robust electron emission properties, the filament is heated to high temperatures (around 1900 °C to 2500 °C). The thermal energy excites electrons, causing them to be emitted from the cathode surface. These electrons are then accelerated toward the anode by a high voltage (ranging from 20 kV to 150 kV), creating the necessary conditions for X-ray production.

The anode serves as the positive electrode in an X-ray tube, converting the kinetic energy of electrons into X-rays through Bremsstrahlung and characteristic radiation processes. The design and material composition of the anode are critical for the efficiency, durability, and performance of the X-ray tube. Many modern X-ray tubes utilize rotating anodes to manage the immense heat generated during X-ray production. These anodes spin rapidly (up to 12,000 rpm), spreading the thermal load over a larger surface area and preventing localized overheating. Typically made from tungsten or a tungsten-rhenium alloy to withstand high temperatures and mechanical stress, these anodes enhance the tube's capacity for higher currents and shorter exposure times (Fig. 2.22).

The high-voltage supply in X-ray tubes is arranged to generate the necessary electric field for accelerating electrons from the cathode to the anode, thereby producing X-rays. High-voltage generators convert mains electricity into the high voltage required for X-ray tube operation, typically ranging from 20 kV to 150 kV for medical applications. Rectifiers convert the alternating current (AC) from the high-voltage transformer into direct current (DC), essential for the proper functioning of X-ray tubes. Silicon-based rectifiers are commonly used due to their efficiency and reliability.

The glass envelope of an X-ray tube maintains a high vacuum environment and provides structural support for the internal elements. Typically made from borosilicate glass due to its excellent thermal and electrical insulation properties, the envelope encases the cathode and anode assemblies. This vacuum environment is essential to

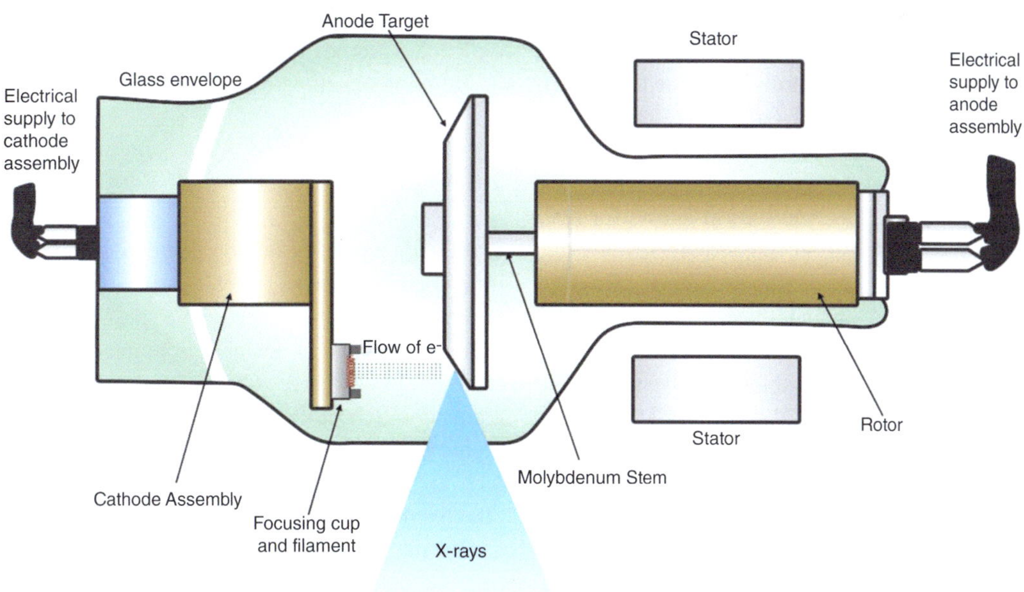

Fig. 2.22 Cross-sectional diagram of an X-ray tube

prevent collisions between the electrons and air molecules, which would otherwise impede the electrons' acceleration from the cathode to the anode, reducing the efficiency of X-ray production. The glass envelope also ensures the integrity of the vacuum over the operational life of the tube, which is vital for consistent performance.

X-ray tube housing plays multiple roles in ensuring the effective, safe, and reliable operation of X-ray tubes. Primarily, it provides radiation shielding by using heavy metals such as lead to confine the emitted X-rays to the intended beam path, minimizing stray radiation. This shielding is essential for protecting both operators and the surrounding environment from unnecessary exposure. The housing also offers mechanical support and protection to the delicate internal components, such as the glass envelope and its internal components such as anode and cathode assemblies, safeguarding them from physical damage during handling and transport. Modern X-ray tube housings are designed to manage heat dissipation effectively, as X-ray tubes generate significant heat during operation, especially at the anode. Cooling systems, including fans, oil, or water circulation, are integrated into the housing to maintain optimal operating temperatures and prevent overheating, thereby extending the tube's lifespan.

Digital integration is a hallmark of modern X-ray tubes, which are fully integrated with digital imaging systems. Digital detectors capture X-ray images and convert them into electronic signals that can be processed, displayed, and stored digitally. This integration allows for real-time image acquisition, immediate review, and advanced image processing techniques, improving diagnostic capabilities and workflow efficiency.

Spectral imaging capability in advanced X-ray tubes, used in modern CT systems, allows for the differentiation of tissues and materials based on their X-ray absorption at different energy levels. By utilizing dual-energy techniques or specialized detectors, these systems provide detailed information about the composition and functionality of scanned tissues, enhancing diagnostic accuracy and enabling new clinical applications.

2.5 Type of X-Ray Tubes

Over the years, X-ray tubes have evolved into highly specialized tools encompassing various X-ray modalities. Worldwide, over 10,000 patents have been filed for innovations in X-ray tube technology [40]. The key attributes of X-ray tubes vary significantly, including X-ray spectra, mechanical interfaces, and energy output. Each is tailored for specific applications and imaging requirements. To meet the diverse needs of users and optimize performance, an extensive range of over hundreds of distinct X-ray tube types are available in the market, each tailored to specific applications and operational requirements [9]. The primary classification of X-ray tubes is based on the type of anode they employ, that is, *stationary and rotating*. The advancement of rotating anode tubes leads to the development of "*rotating envelope X-ray tubes*" and in this, not only the anode but the entire envelope rotates. This design significantly enhances the tube's heat dissipation capacity and allows for higher power outputs, making it suitable for high-demand applications such as advanced medical imaging and high-speed industrial inspections.

Primary Types of X-Ray Tubes

1. Stationary anode X-ray tubes
2. Rotating anode X-ray tubes
3. Rotating envelope X-ray tubes

2.5.1 Stationary Anode X-Ray Tubes

Stationary anode X-ray tubes are used in medical imaging applications, particularly where high power output is not a necessity. These tubes are prominently used in dental radiography, portable radiography, surgery C-arm, and some low-intensity diagnostic procedures. In dental radiography, stationary anode X-ray tubes are favored due to their simplicity, durability, and cost-effectiveness. The fixed anode design ensures a consistent focal spot, which is crucial for obtaining reliable image quality necessary for diagnosing dental issues such as cavities, bone loss, and structural abnormalities. Given the short exposure times and relatively low power requirements in dental applications, the limited heat dissipation capacity of stationary anode tubes is not a significant drawback (Fig. 2.23).

Portable and bedside radiography units also utilize stationary anode X-ray tubes. These units are essential in settings that require mobility and immediate imaging capabilities, such as emergency rooms and intensive care units. The robustness and straightforward design of stationary anode tubes make them ideal for these applications, as they require minimal maintenance and can withstand frequent transport and use. Although stationary anode tubes have a lower power output compared to rotating anode tubes, they provide sufficient imaging capabilities for localized examinations, which are often required in emergency and critical care situations.

The simplicity and cost-effectiveness of stationary anode X-ray tubes make them particularly useful in outpatient settings and smaller medical facilities. For example, in some orthopedic clinics, stationary anode tubes are used for imaging smaller bone structures where high power is not required. The consistent focal spot and reliable performance of these tubes ensure that diagnostic images are of adequate quality for medical evaluation and treatment planning.

2.5.1.1 The Components

The insert, made from evacuated borosilicate glass, encompasses components such as the tungsten wire filament, molybdenum or steel focusing cup, and the copper anode housing the tungsten target. The tungsten, due to its high atomic number and melting point, makes it ideal for the target area whereas copper base helps in effectively conducting heat away from the target area, allowing the anode to cool more efficiently. Enclosed within a steel casing and filled with oil, the tube assembly facilitates the introduction of high-tension cables and provides a reference plane for tube positioning during radiography. Additionally, it serves as an attachment point for accessories like cones and light beam diaphragms. Lead lining within the tube casing attenuates radiation, except for that passing through a radiolucent window. While summarizing, the components can be written as follows:

- Enclosed in a borosilicate glass envelope with an oil-filled casing
- Tungsten wire filament (cathode)
- Molybdenum or steel focusing cup
- Copper anode housing a tungsten target
- Lead lining attenuates radiation (except for the radiolucent window)

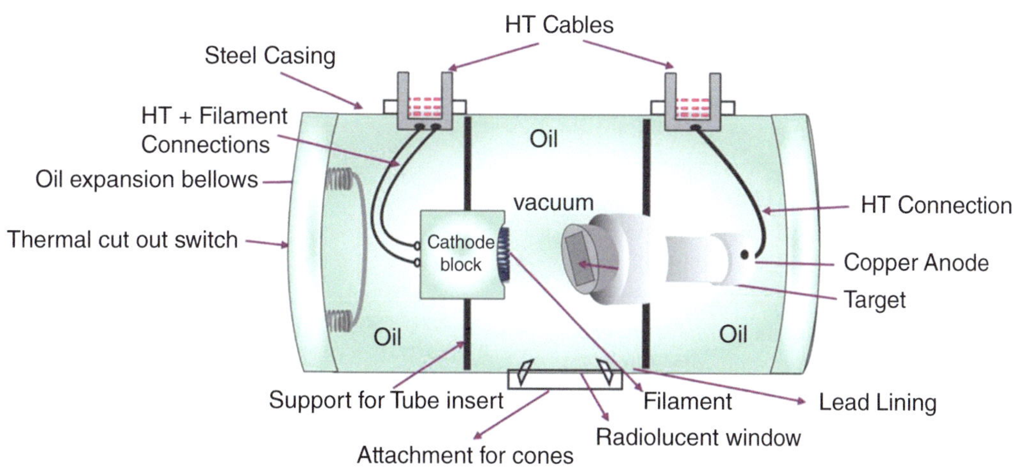

Fig. 2.23 Cross-sectional diagram of stationary anode X-ray tube

2.5.1.2 Operations of Stationary Tubes

During operation, the stationary X-ray tube uses oil for cooling, but as the tube heats up, the oil expands. To prevent this from causing any damage, the design incorporates a bellows mechanism. The bellows mechanism is essentially a stretchy accordion which expands when oil gets hot and needs more space to accommodate it. This prevents pressure buildup and keeps the glass envelope safe from cracking under stress. It is a simple but clever solution for keeping the X-ray tube functioning properly. However, it's crucial to prevent air bubbles from entering the oil, as this may lead to an electrical spark-over and potential damage to the glass envelope.

The oil's primary functions are to provide electrical insulation and transfer heat from the anode to the casing. The fully contracted bellow indicates maximum space creation, signaling the need for cooling to prevent damage or oil leakage. An incorporated cutout switch prevents further exposures until the oil has cooled sufficiently. An external fan can be installed on the tube casing to aid in dissipating heat from the casing to the surrounding air. Additionally, the tube casing is grounded to ensure electrical safety, making it resistant to electric shocks.

In some mobile and all portable units, the X-ray tube assembly integrates not only the insert but also the high-tension transformer and secondary circuit within the oil-filled casing. This configuration simplifies equipment, making it easily maneuverable for bedside radiography.

This type of X-ray tube serves as both a rectifier and an X-ray producer, with a rating based on the maximum safe temperature of the anode for thermionic emission (approximately 2500 °C). To avoid filament destruction and ensure safe operation, the electrical energy responsible for heating must be limited. This is typically achieved by restricting kVp and mA, which affects the rate of heat production at the target. Additionally, exposure time plays a crucial role in controlling target temperature.

2.5.1.3 Advantages and Disadvantages of Stationary Anode Tubes

Advantages

- Simplicity: Fewer components compared to rotating anode systems.
- Compactness: Smaller size due to simpler design.
- Maneuverability: Easier to move and position due to lighter weight and smaller footprint.
- Cost-effectiveness: Generally cheaper to purchase and maintain compared to rotating anode systems (Fig. 2.24).

Disadvantages

- *Limited power output*
  - Temperature limitations of the anode restrict the amount of energy used for X-ray production.
  - Lower power output translates to longer exposure times.
- *Increased risk of motion blur*: Longer exposure times can lead to motion blur if the patient moves during the X-ray acquisition.
- *Filament damage risk.*
  - Backscattered electrons from the anode can damage the filament if not properly controlled.

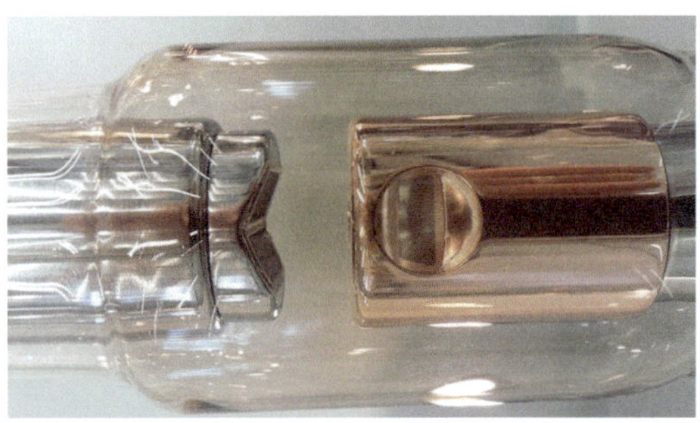

Fig. 2.24 Close-up image of the Philips dual focal spot stationary anode tube FO 17 used in surgical C-arm systems. (Image copyright: Rolf Behling, republished with permission [8])

These limitations underscore the need for careful consideration of operating parameters to achieve optimal imaging outcomes.

2.5.2 Rotating Anode X-Ray Tubes

Rotating anode X-ray tubes have an anode that rotates during operation, spreading the electron impact over a larger surface area. The standard rotating anode X-ray tube features a disk-shaped anode that rotates at high speeds (typically 3000–12,000 RPM). This design allows for better heat dissipation, making them suitable for high-power applications. These tubes offer numerous advantages over stationary anode tubes. They enable higher power and greater heat dissipation, resulting in shorter exposure times and improved image quality in medical imaging applications like CT, fluoroscopy, and general radiography, as well as in industrial and research settings, where prolonged exposures and high imaging demands are typical. The efficiency of energy conversion in X-ray tubes is remarkably low. For example, a CT tube generates light intensity comparable to a consumer LED but requires input power of around 100 kW, with approximately 99% of this energy lost as heat [41]. The rotating motion of the anode spreads heat over a larger surface area, reducing the risk of thermal damage and prolonging the tube's lifespan. Additionally, the ability to adjust the speed of rotation allows for optimized heat distribution and X-ray production, enhancing the versatility and performance of the tube. The anode target is usually made of tungsten, which provides efficient X-ray production due to its high atomic number and melting point (Fig. 2.25).

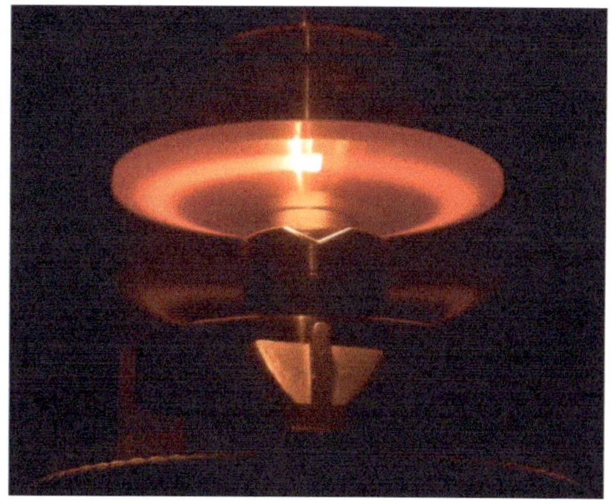

Fig. 2.25 Thermal image of a rotating anode tube during the exhaust process, where the rotating anode shown is facing downward, located about an inch above the cathode at the bottom. (Image copyright: Rolf Behling, republished with permission [8])

2.5.2.1 Subtypes of Rotating Anode X-Ray Tubes

- **High-speed rotating anode X-ray tubes**
  High-speed rotating anode X-ray tubes are a specialized subtype designed for applications requiring rapid imaging sequences, such as advanced CT imaging and dynamic studies. These tubes operate at even higher rotation speeds (up to 12,000–15,000 RPM), enhancing heat dissipation and allowing for shorter exposure times. This capability is crucial for capturing fast-moving anatomical structures, such as the heart, and for reducing motion artifacts in imaging.
- **Liquid metal bearing rotating anode X-ray tubes**
  A more advanced subtype is the liquid metal-bearing rotating anode X-ray tube. Instead of traditional ball bearings, these tubes use liquid metal bearings to support the anode's rotation. Liquid metal bearings offer superior thermal conductivity and reduced mechanical wear, resulting in longer tube life and more stable performance. These tubes are particularly advantageous in high-end CT scanners and other applications **where** prolonged operation and reliability are critical.
- **Mammographic rotating anode X-ray tubes**
  Although primarily used in mammography, these rotating anode tubes have been specifically designed to cater to the unique requirements of breast imaging. They typically feature molybdenum or rhodium targets, which are optimized for producing the lower energy X-rays needed for high-contrast imaging of soft tissues. The rotating anode design

allows for better heat management during the relatively high-intensity exposures required for mammography, ensuring consistent image quality and minimizing thermal damage to the anode.

- **Dual-focus rotating anode X-ray tubes**
  Dual-focus rotating anode X-ray tubes are designed with two different focal spot sizes on the anode target, providing flexibility in imaging. The smaller focal spot size allows for high-resolution images, ideal for detailed examinations, while the larger focal spot can handle higher power loads for general imaging purposes. This dual capability makes them versatile and suitable for a wide range of diagnostic procedures, including detailed studies and routine imaging.

The concept of rotating anode tubes dates back to the late 1920s, with the first functional tube, the "Rotalix," developed by Albert Bouwers and manufactured by Philips in 1929 [42]. Siemens introduced their inaugural rotating anode tube, the "Pantix 60," in 1932, while Machlett followed suit in 1938 [43]. In the late 1930s, General Electric and Eureka also began producing rotating anode tubes in the Americas. These tubes, externally different from their European counterparts, set the standard for X-ray tube industry design. Rotating anode tubes feature glass, glass-metal, or glass-ceramic outer bodies, with high-output tubes often employing a combination of materials, such as the special alloy Kovar. Kovar was developed to address the challenge of creating reliable glass-to-metal seals, essential in electronic devices like light bulbs, vacuum tubes, and cathode ray tubes, as well as in vacuum systems for scientific research. Unlike most metals, Kovar matches the thermal expansion of glass, reducing the risk of joint cracking due to temperature changes [44] (Fig. 2.26).

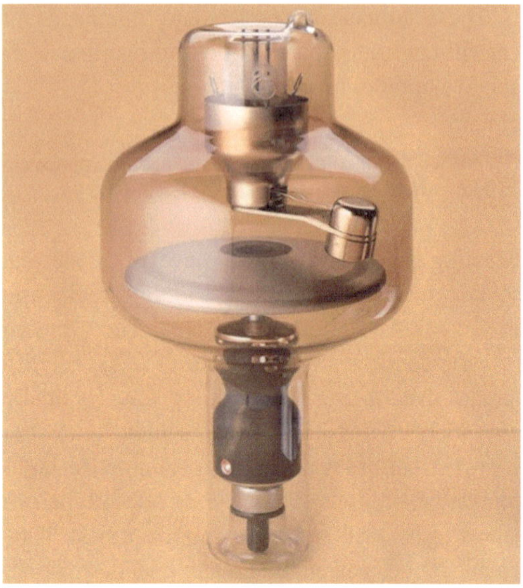

Fig. 2.26 The first rotating anode tube target structure was made principally of graphite coated with tungsten and rhenium. (Image Courtesy: Rolf Behling [8])

The key component of a rotating anode tube is the anode assembly, typically made of tungsten-rhenium alloy, chosen for efficient X-ray production and mechanical robustness. The anode disk, mounted on a spindle, rotates at high speeds, often reaching several thousand RPM. Modern high-power tubes may utilize different anode target materials, predominantly tungsten-based, with variations like rhenium-tungsten, molybdenum-backed, or graphite-backed targets. Most rotating anode X-ray tubes are immersed in insulating oil within a lead-lined tube head to absorb heat and provide cooling, though some modern designs use alternative cooling methods (Fig. 2.27).

During operation, electrons emitted from the cathode are accelerated toward the rotating anode by high voltage. When electrons strike the anode surface, they rapidly decelerate, converting kinetic energy into X-ray photons. The rotating motion helps distribute heat generated by the electron beam impact, preventing localized overheating and damage. Rotating anode X-ray tubes are crucial components of modern X-ray systems, providing high-power beams for medical diagnosis, industrial inspection, and scientific research, driving advancements in various imaging applications.

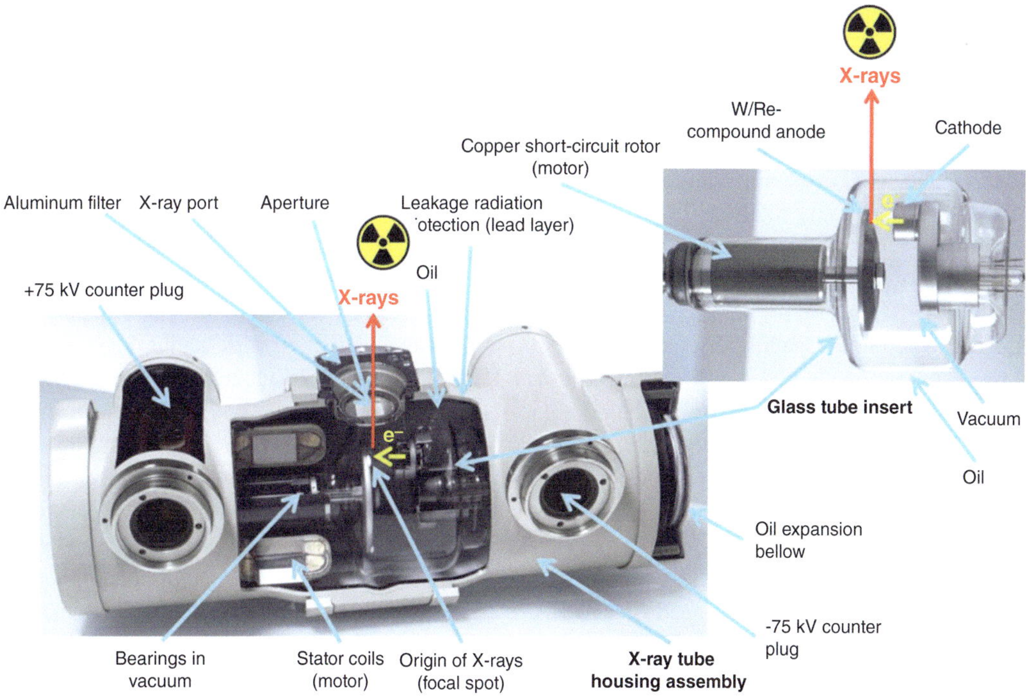

Fig. 2.27 Function and major components of a rotating anode general radiographic X-ray tube assembly. (Image copyright: Rolf Behling, republished with permission [8])

2.5.3 Rotating Envelope X-Ray Tubes

The rotating envelope X-ray tube (RET), also known as the rotation frame tube, revolutionizes heat dissipation, offering specific advantages for various applications. These tubes feature both the anode and cathode within a rotating envelope, enabling higher tube currents and improved heat dissipation, making them valuable in high-power industrial and medical X-ray systems.

Siemens first implemented this concept in 2003, based on a 1915 patent [45], producing rotating frame tubes for CT scans. These tubes have a small rotating anode, approximately 120 mm in diameter, surrounded by oil for cooling. The close connection to the oil prevents excessive temperature rise, although significant temperature differences exist between the focal spot and the backside where it contacts the oil [28] (Fig. 2.28).

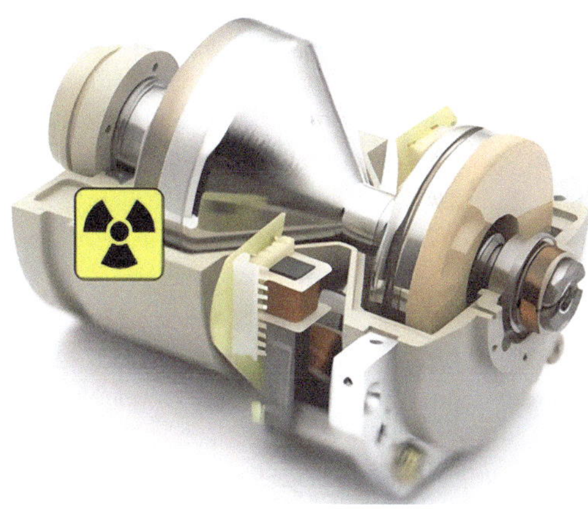

Fig. 2.28 Siemens' Straton® rotating frame tube features the entire tube insert rotating within the tube housing assembly. (Image copyright: Rolf Behling [8]. Republished with permission)

In RETs, electrons emitted from a flat electron emitter at the center of the tube are accelerated along the tube axis. A magnetic dipole field stabilizes the X-ray focal spot, while an electrically controlled magnetic quadrupole field shapes the electron beam. The electron trajectories are deflected outward by the dipole field, impacting the anode about 5 cm off-axis.

Siemens claimed that this tube meets future requirements for CT imaging, featuring increased scan power, shorter rotation times, quicker cooldown periods, and smaller focal spots through innovative cooling and beam control systems [27]. The Straton® X-ray tube utilizes convective cooling exclusively, achieving an unprecedented cooling rate of 4.8 MHU/min, eliminating waiting times due to anode cooling during clinical procedures. Additionally, an electronic beam deflection system allows precise control of focal spot position and size, enabling advanced applications [27].

The RET system rotates the entire tube around its anode axis at a maximum speed of 150 Hz, comprising four main subsystems: the tube envelope, the electron emission cathode, magnetic deflection, and cooling. The tube envelope, made of nonmagnetic stainless steel, connects directly to the anode disk and includes an annular or circular window with a 0.2 mm thickness. The anode disk, primarily composed of tungsten (90%) and rhenium alloyed with tungsten-zirconium-molybdenum (TZM) (10%), boasts a melting point of approximately 3400 °C for tungsten and 2623 °C for TZM [40].

The electron emission cathode system features a tungsten filament within a circular, flat focusing cup. The magnetic deflection system comprises three coils: the R-coil, deflecting the electron beam radially onto the anode's focal spot; the Q-coil, focusing the electron beam; and the Phi-coil, deflecting the flying focal spot tangentially [40].

For cooling, a convective system is used, with the anode disk in direct contact with cooling oil. Turbine flow rotates mineral oil, with flow rates during exposure and pumping set at 25 and 8 liters per minute, respectively [40].

Recent advancements in focusing technology for medical X-ray tubes have significantly reduced space charge limitations, a common issue in legacy X-ray tubes with thermionic emitters. Siemens commercialized flat, directly heated tungsten sheet emitters on a broader scale, initially for mammography tubes and later for the rotating frame CT tube Straton® and angiography tubes. Philips enhanced the emitter size further and added a magnetic double quadrupole focusing system. Unlike Siemens' single quadrupole system in the Straton® tube, the double quadrupole concept of Philips' iMRC® tube allows for a high electron trajectory compression factor [13].

Siemens adopted this technology in the Vectron® tube for CT, launched in 2014. In 2018, GE presented the Quantix 160 tube, featuring a flat emitter cathode for the premium GE Revolution® CT system, which allows for tube voltage switching for spectral X-ray imaging. Extending the basic design of Philips and later Siemens, it comprises a system of pull and focusing electrodes enabling tube current modulation in a matter of microseconds by modulating the space charge in front of a single tungsten flat emitters. This system allows for maintaining constant tube power and focal spot size during modulation of the tube voltage between 80 and 140 kV, with Siemens producing dual-source-dual-detector systems and Philips employing detector-based spectral CT imaging [13] (Fig. 2.29).

The double quadrupole system, even considering mechanical tolerances, produces unprecedented focal spot sizes down to the order of 0.3 mm width on the anode and a length of 3 mm without compromising beam current. As X-rays are taken off in the central beam at a small angle of 7°–12° from the anode, the large physical length of 3 mm translates to an X-ray optical length in the order of the width. The cathodic space charge limitation is practically eliminated, even at low tube voltages. The beam from the flat emitter is first accelerated, then widened by the first magnetic quadrupole, and finally compressed by the second. Z-deflection in focal spot length direction along the tube rotor axis, oriented parallel to the patient axis in a CT system, and x-deflection by energizing extra dipole coils enhance the in-plane spatial resolution in a CT system, reducing image artifacts. The advanced

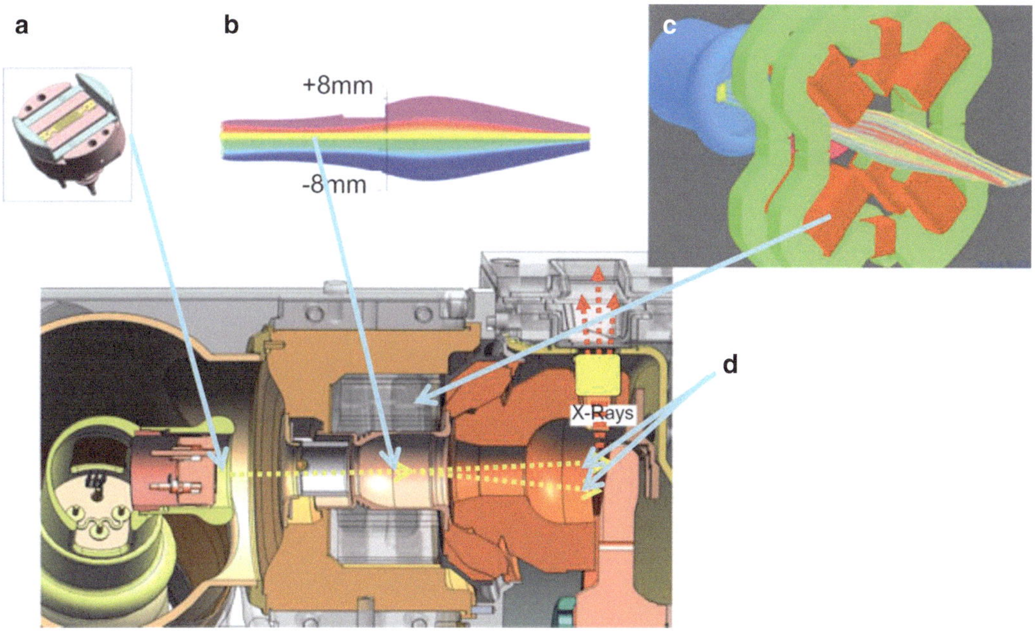

Fig. 2.29 Modern magnetic focusing serves as an advanced alternative to the simpler electrostatic focusing concept. Electrons (**d**) are released by a flat electron (**a**) emitter connected to the negative terminal of the high-voltage source. These electrons accelerate between the cathode and the grounded drift tube funnel, passing through a focusing quadrupole and a deflecting dipole magnet system before striking the anode. Electron trajectories are illustrated in (**b**). The magnet system is shown in (**c**). As depicted in (**d**), the electron beam can be deflected to adjust the X-ray source area. Unlike electrostatic focusing and coil emitters, magnetic focusing significantly reduces space charge limitations. (Image copyright Springer Nature BV [13]. Reprinted with permission)

control of the magnetic quadrupole focusing field, though more complex, offers superior performance [13].

Advantages of Rotating Envelope X-Ray Tubes

- ***Multiple focal spot sizes***: Provides imaging flexibility.
- ***Enhanced heat dissipation***: Ensures stability by managing heat.
- ***High temporal resolution***: Captures dynamic processes.
- ***Suitability for high kV and high mA techniques***: Enables quality imaging in demanding scenarios.
- ***Extended tube lifespan***: Reduces maintenance costs and downtime.

2.6 Components Used in X-Ray Production

The production of X-rays involves several key components within an X-ray tube, which can be broadly divided into the X-ray tube insert assembly and the X-ray tube housing assembly (Fig. 2.30). Each component has its role in ensuring the efficient generation and control of X-rays for medical imaging and industrial applications. A broad outline of these components are as follows:

- **X-ray tube insert assembly**
  - Cathode assembly
    - Filament
    - Focusing cup

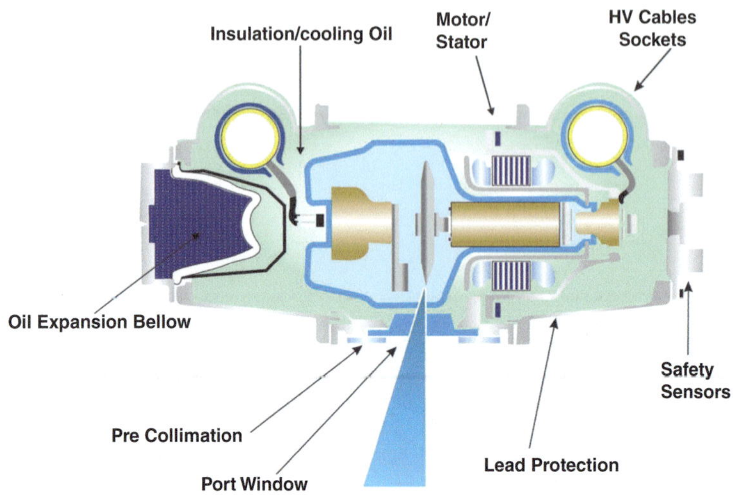

Fig. 2.30 Cross-sectional diagram of X-ray tube insert and housing assembly

- Anode assembly
  - Anode target and focal spot
    - Anode angle and line-focus principle
    - The heel effect
    - Crazing of the anode surface
  - Anode disk and stem
  - Bearing and lubrication
  - Heat dissipation system
- Tube envelope
  - Glass envelope
  - Metal-ceramic envelope
  - Use of metal in X-ray tube envelopes
- **X-ray tube housing assembly**
  - Lead shielding
  - High-tension voltage cable sockets
  - Stator electromagnetic coils
  - Beam pre-collimation
  - X-ray radiation port and window
  - Radiation control timer circuit
  - Bellows
  - Cooling system components

2.6.1 X-Ray Tube Insert Assembly

2.6.1.1 Cathode Assembly

The cathode assembly is responsible for the generation of electrons, which are necessary to produce X-rays. The main elements of the cathode assembly include the filament, focusing cup, and associated electrical connections.

Filament

The filament in X-ray tubes is typically made of tungsten due to its high melting point (around 3422 °C or 6192 °F) and excellent thermionic emission properties. When an electric current of several amperes passes through the tungsten filament, it heats up the filament to temperatures ranging from 1900 °C to 2500 °C, causing it to emit electrons through a process known as thermionic emission. This heating creates an electron cloud around the filament, which is traditionally referred to as the "cathode" [9].

The filament, having diameter ranges from 0.1 to 0.3 mm is encased within an electrostatic focusing "cup," often made of solid metal (Fig. 2.26). When a voltage between 20 kV (for mammography) and 150 kV is applied, a current flow between the cathode and the anode, causing the electrons to achieve velocities that approach relativistic speeds but remain below half the speed of light. To prevent tungsten evaporation, the filament temperature is carefully controlled, staying lower except during exposure (Fig. 2.31).

During the process of thermionic emission, electrons are liberated from a material when it is heated, allowing them to overcome the material's work function—the energy barrier that must be surpassed for electrons to escape. Tungsten has a work function of about 4.5 eV, which varies with crystalline orientation. Nanocrystalline tungsten may reduce the work function by approximately 0.2–0.8 eV, depending on surface properties. The micro-topology of the emitter surface also influences electron emission.

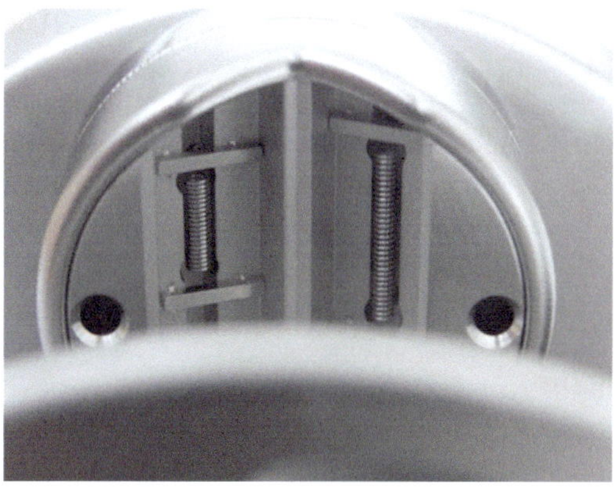

Fig. 2.31 Close-up look at the thermionic cathode showcasing the overlapping focal spots of a Philips SRO™ 33100 tube. (Image copyright: Rolf Behling, republished with permission [8])

The focused beam of electrons is accelerated toward the positively charged anode by the high-voltage potential difference between the cathode and anode. This high-voltage supply can range from tens of kilovolts (kV) to over a hundred kV, depending on the application. Upon striking the anode, the high-energy electrons interact with the anode material (usually tungsten), causing the sudden deceleration of electrons. This interaction results in the production of X-rays through processes such as Bremsstrahlung and characteristic radiation (Fig. 2.32).

Tungsten as Cathode Material

Tungsten wire or flat tungsten sheets are commonly used in X-ray tubes due to their reliability in challenging environments. These environments include high temperatures near the melting point of the target material and gas desorption from the anode. Positioned just a few centimeters from the cathode, the anode contributes to the demanding conditions. Tungsten emitters must endure evaporation and ion bombardment, and their longevity is impacted by residual gas effects. The quality of tungsten emitters is maintained through careful production processes, including attention to grain orientation and stress relief.

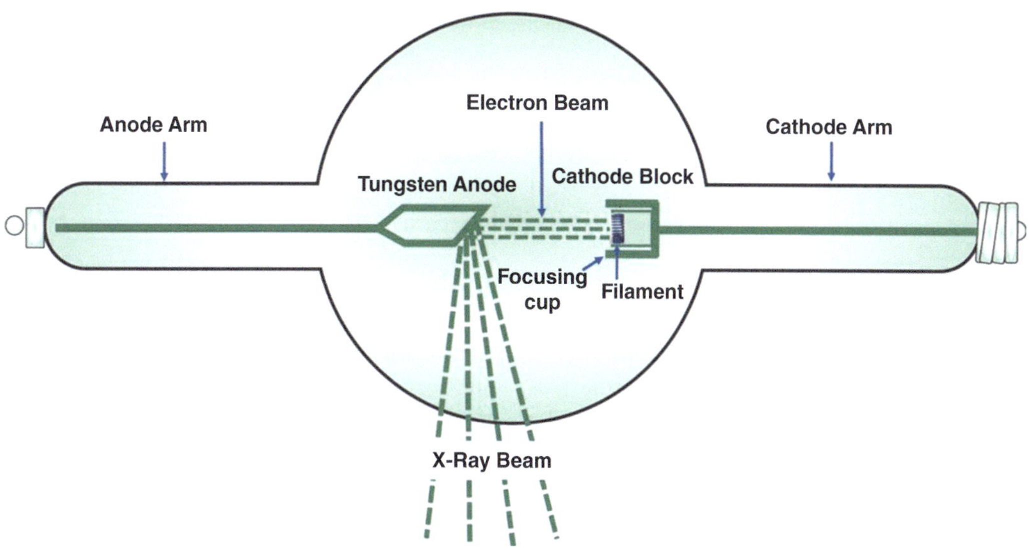

Fig. 2.32 Cross-sectional diagram of Coolidge X-ray tubes

Alternatives to Tungsten Cathodes

To reduce the work function and improve cathode performance, several alternatives to tungsten have been explored. Thorium monolayers on tungsten substrates can significantly lower the work function by nearly 2 eV, though thorium isotopes are radioactive. Dispenser cathodes can reduce the work function to approximately 1.8–2.2 eV, but their reliability in X-ray tubes is still a challenge due to residual gas and ion bombardment. Field emitters like carbon nanotubes (CNTs) offer high mechanical strength and current densities but face issues such as sublimation and thermal resistance. Photoelectric emitters have been explored but struggle with vacuum maintenance and pollution challenges.

Focusing Cup

The focusing cup is typically made of molybdenum or nickel. These materials are chosen for their ability to withstand high temperatures and their effectiveness in shaping the electron beam. It is a negatively charged, concave structure that surrounds the filament. Its role is to direct and focus the electrons emitted from the filament into a narrow, well-defined beam. This focused beam is then accelerated toward the anode. The focusing cup ensures that the electron beam is concentrated on a small area of the anode, which is crucial for producing sharp X-ray images.

Electrical Connections

- **Power supply:** The filament is heated by an electric current supplied through dedicated electrical connections. This current is typically controlled by a low-voltage power supply.
- **Bias voltage:** The focusing cup may also have an applied bias voltage to enhance its ability to focus the electron beam. The bias voltage is usually slightly negative relative to the filament, helping to repel electrons toward the anode.

Variants of Cathode Assemblies

Based on electron emission mechanism, cathodes can be divided into as follows:

(i) Cold cathode (Crookes tube)
(ii) Hot cathode (Coolidge tube)
(iii) Cold field emission (carbon nanotube (CNT))

(i) ***Cold cathodes***

These cathodes were used in Crookes Tube and were called "first-generation cathodes," pioneered by William Crookes in 1875. These cathodes were concave-shaped, made of aluminum, and operated as cold. An anticathode is aligned with the anode, with the cathode positioned between them.

When a high DC voltage (around 100 kV) is applied across the anode and cathode, gas atoms in the tube become ionized, generating positive ions. These ions then strike the cathode, causing it to emit electrons at higher speeds. These electrons subsequently strike a small focal spot on the inclined anode (approximately 1 mm), producing an X-ray from a concentrated source.

X-rays are produced through either bremsstrahlung or X-ray fluorescence processes. A heat sink dissipates the heat generated when electrons strike the anode. This type of tube was in use until the 1920s. However, it had several drawbacks, including relatively low X-ray intensity (about 5 mA), unreliability and instability due to dependency on gas content, inability to control X-ray intensity and energy independently, and susceptibility to overheating following prolonged X-ray exposure.

(ii) ***Hot cathode tube (Coolidge tube)***

William Coolidge introduced significant enhancements to the Crookes tube in 1913, leading to the development of the "second-generation cathodes." This X-ray tube configuration consists of a spherical tempered borosilicate (Pyrex) tube operating under high vacuum conditions (10^{-6} Torr) [40]. It featured two cylindrical arms serving as the cathode and anode. Tungsten, embedded in copper, is employed as the anode material, which can be shaped as circular, square, or rectangular, with thickness and size typically ranging from 2 to 3 mm and 2 to 10 mm, respectively. The anode angle varies between 6° and 20°, with a typical angle of 12°–17°.

Initially, the cathode filament is heated by an electric current, reaching a red-hot state (above 1000 °C) and emitting free electrons through thermionic emission. After applying a high voltage between the cathode and anode, these electrons are accelerated and strike the anode, producing bremsstrahlung and characteristic X-rays. The X-ray output power typically ranges from 1 to 4 kW. This tube design is the precursor to modern X-ray tubes in use today. However, this design has certain technical limitations, including the thermionic cathode's slow temporal response time and high power consumption. Additionally, high temperatures can cause the failure of the cathode metal filament, reducing the X-ray tube's lifespan.

Special anode designs, such as rotating anode systems, manage this focused electron barrage's intense heat and wear. The power output of these tubes ranges from 0.5 to 30 kW [40]. The setup of these tubes involves the filament, focusing cup, anode surface, and tube voltage generators. The tube voltage generates an electric field that drives electrons toward the focal spot on the anode. X-ray tubes with dual focal spots usually employ separate filament/cup assemblies, known as cathode blocks, to control focusing. The focusing level is adjusted by varying the potential difference or bias voltage between the filament and the focusing electrode. Increasing the negative bias voltage reduces the focus size until the electron current ceases, facilitating electronic focus size control or rapid anode current switching, such as in pulsed fluoroscopy. Bias is achieved through a high-resistance grid leak resistor connecting the filament and cup, enabling emitted electrons to charge the cup, which then discharges through the resistor, maintaining a negative potential difference.

(iii) ***Cold field electron emitter***

The conventional thermionic cathode presents inherent limitations such as randomness in electron emission, difficulty controlling emission, and the inability to operate in pulsed mode. To overcome these challenges, cold cathodes based on field-emitting principles offer a promising alternative. Carbon nanotubes (CNTs), known for their remarkable mechanical and electrical properties, exhibit exceptional field-emission characteristics, boasting brilliance levels significantly higher than traditional electron sources.

Given their superior performance, CNT-based field emitter cold cathodes emerge as natural contenders for enhancing X-ray sources. Globally, there is a growing interest in developing CNT-based X-ray sources, with some commercially available CNT cathodes already in existence. However, existing approaches typically involve the random deposition of CNTs through methods like electrophoresis, lacking precise control over their size and dimensions.

The carbon nanotube (CNT) has many tall, thin, sharp tip tubes arranged vertically on a conductive substrate (cathode). As it has a high aspect ratio and physical and chemical inertness, it is used as the electron emitter for the X-ray tube. A gate mesh structure (anode) is coupled to an electrode inside the tube wall, positioned slightly above the sharp tips of the CNTs [9].

When an electric field is given at room temperature between the grid mesh and substrate, it generates more pulsed electron beams at the tips of the CNTs. These electrons are accelerated toward the anode to produce X-rays. This tube has overcome some of the limitations of the conventional hot filament X-ray tube. Its merits are listed as follows: (i) miniaturized X-ray source, (ii) pulsed and shaped X-ray source, (iii) nanoengineered, and (iv) controlled electron beam.

Despite extensive research spanning several decades, carbon nanotubes (CNTs) have yet to find widespread use in commercial tubes for medical imaging. The challenges associated with their integration into such applications include issues such as carbon sublimation in overloaded CNTs, field elongation, rupture at imperfections, and thermal and electrical resistances.

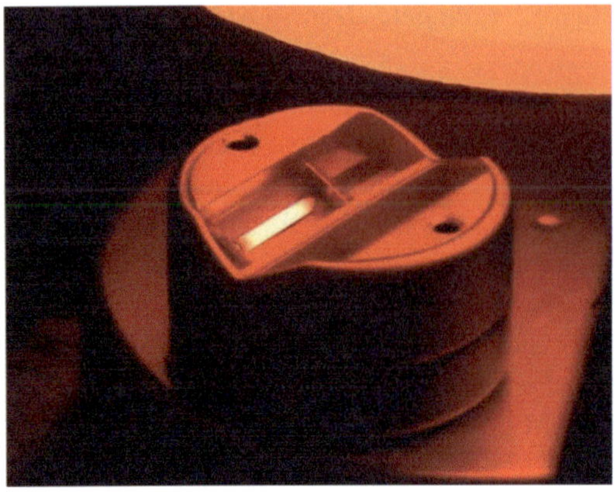

Fig. 2.33 Heated cathode right after turning off the heating current and the high voltage. (Image Courtesy: Title: 9780367546922 | Modern Diagnostic X-Ray Sources 2ed by Rolf Behling [9]. Reproduced by permission of Taylor & Francis Group)

Overheating at certain points further complicates their implementation, ultimately limiting the applicable electric field and the current per nanotube [9].

However, CNTs demonstrate their potential in micro-focus tubes with stationary targets, particularly those designed to operate within a narrow range of tube voltages. In this context, they offer improved stability and the ability to generate higher macroscopic currents from the edges of graphene. This holds the promise of enhanced field enhancement factors, which could significantly benefit the performance of such tubes (Fig. 2.33).

Historical Changes and Current Trends in Cathode Technology

Building upon Crookes' prior concept, Mueller in Hamburg, Germany, enhanced spatial image resolution shortly after Röntgen's discovery by developing the "focus tube." This tube featured a concave cathode plate that emitted electrons perpendicular to its surface upon ion impact. The Victor X-ray Company of Chicago, later acquired by General Electric (GEXCO, now GE Healthcare), used helium or other inert gases inside the tube to reduce sputtering effects. They also implemented a ring-shaped pull electrode connected to the anode to boost electron current [29].

Larger focusing electrodes were introduced to improve focal spot definition amid varying tube current and voltage. However, higher tube currents led to space charge effects and focal spot "blooming" [29].

Modern dual focal spot cathodes of rotating anode tubes have coiled tungsten wires in the cathode head, shaping the electric field and focusing electrons into the desired spot. Siemens introduced a flat tungsten sheet emitter in 1998, refining electron starting conditions. In 2018, GE launched the Quantix 160® X-ray tube for spectral CT, a breakthrough in cathode technology. Unlike previous cathodes operating mainly in saturation, flat emitter cathodes generate an abundance of electrons internally in this system. GE utilizes this tube in the Revolution Apex® spectral CT system, which allows rapid tube voltage alteration and acquisition of spectral data. Conversely, Philips and Siemens employ different approaches in their spectral CT systems, highlighting diverse cathode design and application advancements [29].

2.6.1.2 Anode Assembly

The anode determines the X-ray tube's performance and pricing and is usually the most expensive component of the X-ray tube [9]. There are mainly two types of anodes, viz., stationary anode and rotating anodes apart from modern-day rotating envelope X-ray tubes and micro-focus X-ray tubes. The envelope or housing surrounding the anode also rotates in rotating envelope X-ray tubes. This design allows for a larger surface area to dissipate heat and helps maintain the integrity of the X-ray tube during prolonged use. Micro-focus X-ray tubes are designed to produce a very small focal spot size, which is advantageous for high-resolution imaging applications such as microscopy and industrial inspection. The anode is stationary to achieve this, allowing precise control over the electron beam and minimizing mechanical vibrations that could affect image quality.

Examples of stationary anodes are dental X-rays, mobile/portable X-ray machines, and some low-power X-ray tubes, for example, used in research or low-power medical imaging. The rotating anodes are used in conventional radiography tubes, mammography tubes, grid control X-ray tubes, computed tomography machines, etc. The rotating envelope X-ray tubes are used again in computed tomography X-ray tubes.

In a simple rotating anode tube, the anode is typically a solid disk made of tungsten or a rhenium tungsten alloy with a diameter of 50–120 mm. The anode rotates at approximately 3000–12000 revolutions per minute and is commonly used for general radiography. The whole anode assembly includes several key parts, each with specific functions to ensure efficient X-ray production and heat management. Below is a detailed explanation of the anode assembly's structure and function.

Historical Changes in Anode Technology

The development of anode technology in X-ray tubes has evolved significantly over the years. Initially, early rotating anode designs faced challenges due to the properties of tungsten, which was known for its high density and brittleness. The initial practical use of the rotating anode traces back to the endeavors of Dutch engineer Albert Bouwers. In 1929, Bouwers engineered the pioneering commercial X-ray tube, ROTALIX, for clinical applications at Philips. This tube, founded on the concept of a rotating anode, initially proposed by William D. Coolidge in 1915, followed numerous prior unsuccessful endeavors to harness this principle for achieving elevated tube outputs [46]. It was understood that heat dissipation from a surface escalates exponentially with the fourth power of the absolute temperature.

The initial implementation of high-temperature radiation cooling was introduced by Siemens engineers in 1932. He incorporated this cooling method in the Siemens PANTIX tube, which featured a focal spot of 1.2–2.0 mm at 10–30 kW, coupled with an 80 mm diameter disk made of tungsten [46]. The anode disk was driven by a starter at 3000 rpm, marking the inception of nearly limitless fluoroscopy and radiography operation, considering the requisite cooling intervals [46].

For example, Siemens' Pantix tube from 1932 encountered issues with tungsten anodes breaking in cool conditions [29]. Despite tungsten's ability to withstand high temperatures beyond 2000 °C and its excellent heat radiation properties, preheating was necessary to prevent rupture from thermomechanical stress.

In the 1960s, anode durability was notably improved with the introduction of molybdenum-backed rhenium-tungsten compound anodes. These anodes featured a top layer of rhenium-tungsten (RT) alloy supported by a thick powder-sintered titanium-zirconium-molybdenum (TZM) body, marking a significant advancement in durability [29] (Fig. 2.34).

Thomson-CGR, later GE, introduced graphite-target vascular X-ray tubes in the beginning of 1960s, incorporating lightweight targets. These tubes utilized metal-coated graphite anodes to reduce mass and improve bearing life.

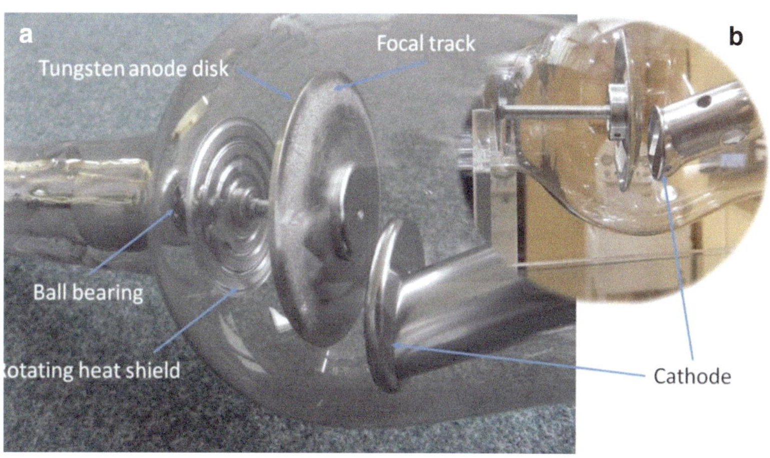

Fig. 2.34 (**a**) The rotating anode mechanism in a Siemens PantixTM tube, featuring an all-tungsten high-temperature disk, was manufactured by Siemens-Reiniger-Werke AG in Rudolstadt, Germany, starting in 1933. (**b**) Earlier version of rotating anode without a heat shield. (Image Courtesy: Rolf Behling [8])

Graphite's excellent thermal emissivity further enhanced performance in these tubes. Meanwhile, Philips developed its Trinodex™ compound produced via high-pressure forging in Eindhoven, characterized by extreme mechanical strength and low porosity, resulting in improved focal track durability [29].

For heavy-duty angiography applications, Siemens and later Varian introduced RT-TZM anodes (tungsten-rhenium coated RT alloy backed by TZM alloy), which enabled improved heat dissipation and reduced thermomechanical erosion of the focal track, in line with standard rotating-anode design improvements. Additionally, rotating anode metal center section tubes utilized stationary structures to trap backscattered electrons, preventing them from heating the anode [29].

Liquid-bearing technology emerged in 1990, further enhancing heat dissipation efficiency by dissipating heat rather than storing it in the anode. These advancements have significantly contributed to X-ray tubes' durability, efficiency, and performance across various applications [29] (Figs. 2.35 and 2.36).

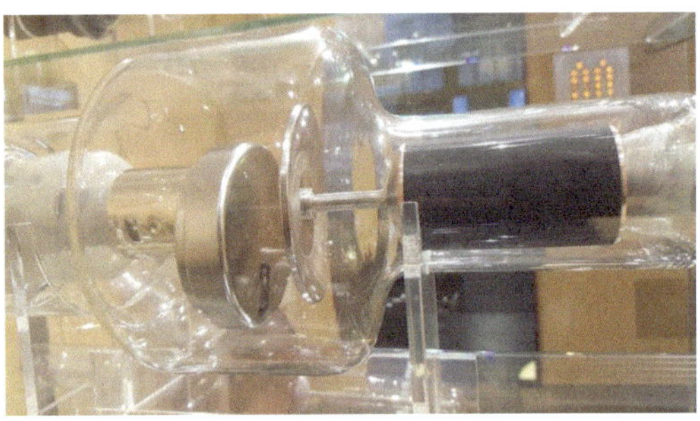

Fig. 2.35 Rotating anode. (Image courtesy: Rolf Behling [8])

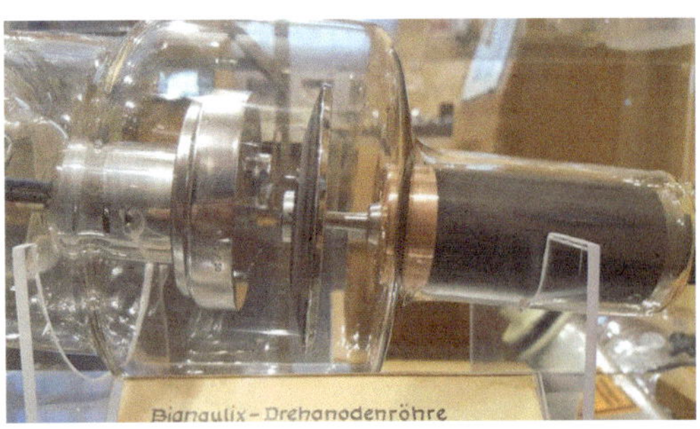

Fig. 2.36 Siemens BiangulixTM tube. Its anode features two distinct focal spot tracks with varying anode angles. (Image Courtesy: Rolf Behling [8])

Components of the Anode Assembly

(i) Anode target and focal spot
(ii) Anode disk and stem
(iii) Rotating mechanism
(iv) Bearing and lubrication system
(v) Heat dissipation system

2.6.1.2.1 Anode Target and Focal Spot

The anode target is the specific area on the anode disk where the electron beam from the cathode is directed and focused. This is the interaction site where the high-energy electrons collide with the anode material, resulting in the production of X-rays. Tungsten is the most commonly used material for the anode target due to its high atomic number (which enhances X-ray production efficiency) and its high melting point (which allows it to withstand the extreme temperatures generated during electron bombardment). Sometimes, a thin layer of rhenium is added to tungsten to improve its mechanical properties and enhance its thermal performance. Tungsten is chosen as the target material for several reasons:

- It has a high atomic number (74), increasing X-ray production efficiency.
- It has a high melting point (3422 °C) and evaporating point (5555 °C), allowing it to withstand the high temperatures generated during an exposure.
- Tungsten's characteristic radiation contributes significantly to the X-ray beam.
- It possesses good thermal conductivity, crucial for transferring heat from the focal areas to the anode's mass.
- It has a reasonable thermal capacity.
- It maintains a low vapor pressure at high temperatures, preserving the vacuum within the insert.

Focal Spot

The focal spot in an X-ray tube refers to the specific area on the anode target where the electron beam from the cathode is focused. This area is crucial because it directly influences the resolution and quality of the X-ray images produced. There are several important characteristics and considerations related to the focal spot:

- **Size**: The size of the focal spot can vary depending on the application. Smaller focal spots provide higher-resolution images, which are particularly important in detailed diagnostic procedures like mammography or fine bone imaging. However, smaller focal spots also concentrate heat in a smaller area, which can lead to overheating and damage if not properly managed.
- **Shape**: The shape of the focal spot can also affect image quality. Ideally, the focal spot should be as close to a point source as possible to reduce image blurring. However, practical designs often result in a slightly rectangular or elliptical shape.
- **Dual focus**: Many X-ray tubes have a dual-focus design, providing two different focal spot sizes that can be selected based on the imaging requirements. This flexibility allows for balance between high-resolution imaging and efficient heat dissipation by offering two distinct focal spot sizes within the same tube.

In 1923, Siemens patented a dual focal spot tube, which allowed optimizing the spatial resolution in the image [8]. Many tubes feature dual focal spots, such as 1.2 mm and 2.0 mm, 0.6 mm and 1.2 mm, 0.3 mm and 2.0 mm, among others [47]. These filaments can be arranged either side by side or in line, as seen in biangular tubes. The sizes of focal spots of different modalities are as follows (Table 2.5).

The key features and benefits are as follows:

- **Enhanced image resolution**: The primary advantage of having a dual focus system is the ability to achieve high-resolution images when necessary. The smaller focal spot in a dual-focus X-ray tube produces finer detail, which is particularly important in applications requiring high precision, such as mammography, angiography, and imaging of small anatomical structures.
- **Thermal management**: Smaller focal spots concentrate the electron beam onto a smaller area of the anode target, leading to higher heat density. This can risk overheating the anode and potentially damaging the X-ray tube. In contrast, the larger focal spot spreads the electron beam over a wider area, reducing heat density and allowing for longer exposure times

Table 2.5 The sizes of focal spots of different modalities

Application	Focal spot sizes (mm)	Technology
Dental and mammography	0.1–0.3 (0.1–0.15 for magnification; ~0.3–0.4 for contact imaging)	X-ray tube with filament and anode
Fluoroscopy, general radiography	Fluoroscopy: ~0.6; General radiography: 0.6–1.2	X-ray tube with filament and anode
Angiography, interventional radiology	0.8–1.0	X-ray tube with filament and anode
CT scan	0.5–2.0 (typical range for fine to large focal spots)	X-ray tube with rotating anode
Constant potential[a]	1.2–1.5	X-ray tube with filament and anode **(not typical for modern applications)**
Radiotherapy[b] for superficial tissues	Not applicable	Linear accelerators generating kV X-rays
Radiotherapy for deep-seated tumors	Not applicable	Linear accelerators generating MV X-rays

[a]**Constant potential X-ray:** Constant potential X-ray machines were used historically; they are not typical in modern medical imaging due to limitations in efficiency and image quality

[b]**Radiotherapy:** Instead of a focal spot size, linear accelerators used in radiotherapy use concept called the penumbra. The penumbra refers to the edge region of the radiation beam where the intensity falls off from the central axis

without overheating. This makes the larger focal spot ideal for general radiographic procedures where heat load management is critical.

- **Operational flexibility**: Dual focus tubes provide operational flexibility, allowing the radiologist or technician to switch between focal spot sizes depending on the diagnostic need. For high-detail imaging, the smaller focal spot can be used. For general imaging or scenarios requiring longer exposures, the larger focal spot can be selected to prevent thermal overload.
- **Improved patient throughput**: The ability to switch between focal spots can improve patient throughput in busy clinical settings. By optimizing the focal spot size for different types of exams, radiologists can achieve high-quality images efficiently, reducing the time needed for each patient and increasing the overall throughput of the imaging facility.
- **Technical design**: Dual-focus X-ray tubes incorporate two filaments of different sizes within the cathode assembly. These filaments are aligned such that each can be independently heated and used to generate the corresponding focal spot size on the anode target. Advanced control mechanisms within the X-ray generator system allow seamless switching between the two filaments, ensuring consistent and reliable performance.
- **Clinical application**: In clinical practice, the dual focus capability is particularly useful in diagnostic procedures where a range of image resolutions is required. For instance, in chest radiography, a larger focal spot can be used to capture broad images of the thorax, while in detailed bone imaging, a smaller focal spot can provide the necessary detail to identify fine fractures or bone anomalies.

2.6.1.2.2 Anode Angle and Line Focus Principle

The anode angle, also known as the target angle, is the angle between the surface of the anode target and the vertical line perpendicular to the electron beam. This angle has a significant impact on the X-ray production process and the characteristics of the resulting X-ray beam. Typically ranging from 6° to about 20° with approximately 12° being most common in diagnostic tubes. These angles are important in determining the effective focal spot size, which directly influences image resolution and heat management. A smaller anode angle results in a smaller effective focal spot, enhancing image sharpness but concentrating heat more intensely on a limited area of the anode. Conversely, a larger anode angle distributes the electron impact over a wider area, improving heat dissipation but potentially reducing image resolution. This balance between image quality and thermal management is essential for the optimal performance of X-ray tubes, particularly in medical imaging where both high-resolution images and reliable operation are critical (Fig. 2.37).

The anode angle is critical in determining the apparent focal spot size and the beam's coverage area at a given focal film distance. For general-purpose tubes, the anode angle is typically around 12–15° [15]. In cases where a smaller field is required, such as in skull units or image intensifiers, a narrower anode angle of about 7°–9° may be used. Biangular tubes are employed when two different field sizes are needed. When the anode currents are high, it is important for the area of the anode hit by electrons to be large, keeping power density in check.

The line focus principle is employed to balance heat dissipation and achieve a small focal spot size. This principle involves angling the anode so that the electrons from the cathode strike it at a specific spot, which, due to the angle, appears as a line when viewed from the perspective of the X-ray beam's direction. By using the line focus principle, X-ray tubes can maintain a small effective focal spot for better image resolution while spreading the heat generated over a larger area of the anode, thereby improving heat management. Anode angles in diagnostic tubes typically vary from 6° to 22°, with 10° to 17° being common for general purposes. Factors like the filament coil diameter and the focusing cup design also play crucial roles in determining the focal spot size.

Historically, Röntgen's initial anode design consisted of an X-ray transparent glass sheet at an "anode angle" of approximately 90° [8]. This primitive setup has evolved significantly, with

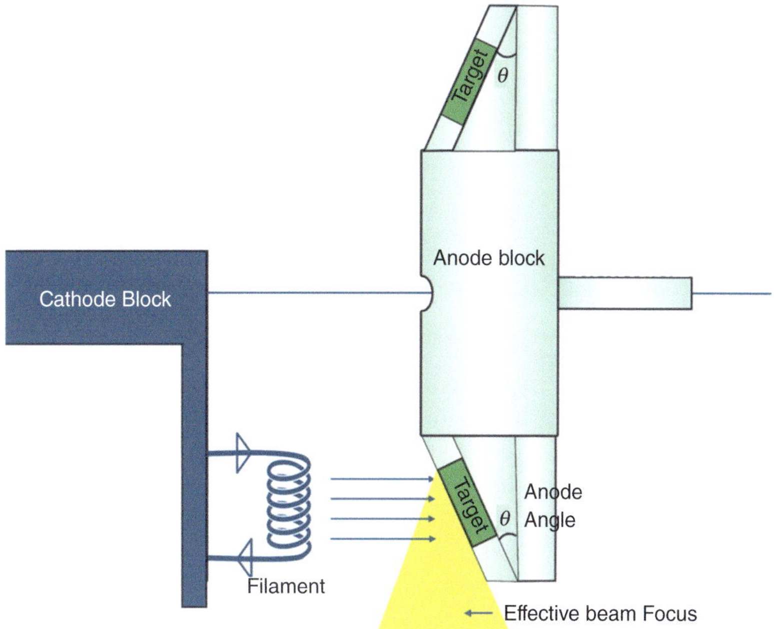

Fig. 2.37 Cathode, rotating anode, and Anode angle

modern designs carefully optimizing the anode angle to enhance both image quality and operational durability.

2.6.1.2.3 The Heel Effect

The heel effect refers to the phenomenon where X-rays produced deeper within the anode material of an X-ray tube experience absorption loss as they pass through the anode. As a result, X-rays emerging near the anode side of the X-ray beam have higher absorption losses than those emerging from the cathode side.

This effect leads to an uneven X-ray intensity distribution across the beam, with higher intensity on the cathode side and lower intensity on the anode side. In projection radiography, the heel effect can sometimes be observed as a slight variation in X-ray intensity across the image. However, it is often barely noticeable in standard radiographs.

In mammography, the heel effect is intentionally utilized to match the decreased organ thickness from the chest wall to the nipple. A more uniform image density can be achieved by positioning the thicker part of the breast closer to the cathode side of the X-ray beam, where the X-ray intensity is higher.

While the line focus principle aims to concentrate the X-ray beam, the anode heel effect introduces variation in its intensity. However, both factors influence the overall performance and quality of X-ray imaging.

2.6.1.2.4 Development of Fine Cracks on the Surface of the Anode (Crazing of the Anode Surface)

During exposure, the target area's surface reaches extremely high temperatures, creating significant temperature differences within the metal. This variance leads to stress accumulation, resulting in surface irregularities known as crazing. These irregularities reduce radiation output from the tube, as the photons must penetrate a thicker metal layer.

To address this issue, a rhenium tungsten alloy (consisting of 10% rhenium and 90% tungsten) is used as the target material. This alloy minimizes crazing, thereby maintaining higher radiation output levels and extending the X-ray tube's lifespan.

Furthermore, high-speed, large-diameter compound anodes are employed to increase loading capacity on the focal area. However, the elevated temperatures experienced by these anodes can

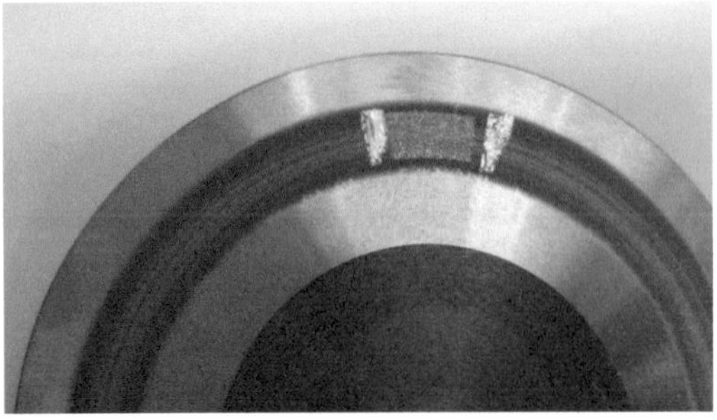

Fig. 2.38 Eroded focal track of a rotating anode. (Image Courtesy: Rolf Behling [8])

induce thermal stresses, potentially distorting the target angle or even causing anode cracking. To mitigate these risks, deliberate cracks or slits are sometimes introduced along the anode's periphery, allowing for stress relief. Alternatively, grooves on either side of the focal track may be incorporated to accommodate expansion and contraction, reducing internal tensions within the anode. Additionally, the edge of the anode is often beveled to optimize the line focus principle (Fig. 2.38).

2.6.1.2.5 Anode Disk and Stem

The anode disk, also referred to as the anode plate, serves as the substrate that supports the anode target. The disk is generally made of the same material as the target area, such as tungsten or a tungsten-rhenium alloy. In some designs, the anode disk might be a composite structure, where a tungsten-rhenium layer is bonded to a base made of molybdenum or graphite to manage thermal expansion and improve durability. The anode disk is designed to rotate in rotating anode X-ray tubes, which helps to distribute the heat generated over a larger surface area, reducing the risk of localized overheating and increasing the lifespan of the tube.

The anode stem acts as the supporting structure for the anode disk and plays a crucial role in heat dissipation. Typically made from materials with excellent thermal conductivity, such as molybdenum, the stem efficiently conducts heat away from the anode disk. Molybdenum is chosen because it not only has excellent thermal conductivity but also maintains structural integrity under high thermal loads. The anode stem is connected to a rotor, which is part of an induction motor system that enables the rotation of the anode disk. This rotation is critical in high-performance X-ray tubes, as it allows the anode to maintain its integrity and functionality even under the high thermal loads generated during prolonged X-ray production.

In rotating anode X-ray tubes, the stem and rotor assembly are enclosed within the tube envelope, which is usually made of glass or metal-ceramic. The rotor is driven by electromagnetic fields generated by the stator coils located outside the envelope. This design not only facilitates the rotation of the anode but also ensures that the anode disk's temperature is managed effectively by distributing the heat over a larger area.

2.6.1.2.6 Rotating Mechanism

The rotating mechanism of anodes in X-ray tubes significantly enhances the performance and longevity of the tube. The primary purpose of rotating anodes is to manage the immense heat generated during X-ray production. In a stationary anode, the electron beam continuously strikes the same spot, which can lead to localized overheating and damage. A rotating anode, however, spreads the electron impact over a larger surface area, thereby distributing the heat more evenly and allowing for higher tube currents and longer exposure times without damaging the anode.

To achieve rotation, the anode is attached to a rotor assembly within the tube. The rotor consists of a copper cylinder, which acts as an armature, connected to the anode stem. Surrounding the rotor outside the vacuum envelope are stator coils, which generate a rotating magnetic field when supplied with alternating current. This magnetic field induces a torque on the rotor, causing it to spin. The design of these electromagnetic stators and their control circuitry is crucial for precise and reliable operation.

The speed of rotation is carefully controlled to optimize heat dissipation. Typical rotation speeds range from 3000 to 12,000 revolutions per minute (RPM). At these speeds, the centrifugal forces ensure that the heat is distributed over a larger area, effectively lowering the temperature at any given point on the anode. Faster rotations allow for greater heat management but require more robust engineering to prevent mechanical failure and to manage the gyroscopic effects that could affect tube alignment.

Additionally, modern X-ray tubes may utilize rotor designs that incorporate spiral groove bearings, often lubricated with gallium-indium-tin (liquid metal), rather than generic hydrodynamic bearings. These bearings create a hydrodynamic film that reduces friction and wear, thereby enhancing the lifespan and reliability of the rotating mechanism. This sophisticated bearing technology allows for smoother rotation and minimizes the noise and vibration associated with high-speed anode rotation.

2.6.1.2.7 Bearing and Lubrication System

The evolution of bearing technology in X-ray tubes has significantly enhanced their performance, reliability, and lifespan. This progression includes the transition from traditional ball bearings to advanced designs such as spiral groove bearings, liquid metal bearings, and hybrid bearings. Additionally, magnetic bearings have been explored, although they present unique challenges.

(a) ***Ball bearings***

Ball bearings were among the first types of bearings used in rotating anode X-ray tubes. E. Pohl publicly demonstrated a rotating anode tube in 1928 in Stockholm, Sweden [8]. Following this, Albert Bouwers of Philips commercialized the technology under the name Rotalix™ in 1929, introducing a rotating copper anode with a tungsten inlay [8]. However, uncoated ball bearings in a vacuum faced the issue of cold welding, which caused the rotors to block or "freeze." Bouwers addressed this by using highly refined grease for lubrication. This early design had limitations in heat dissipation due to the copper anode's temperature cap of around 400 °C [8] (Fig. 2.39).

Since the 1940s, significant improvements have been made to ball-bearing systems. Philips started coating the balls and raceways with lead

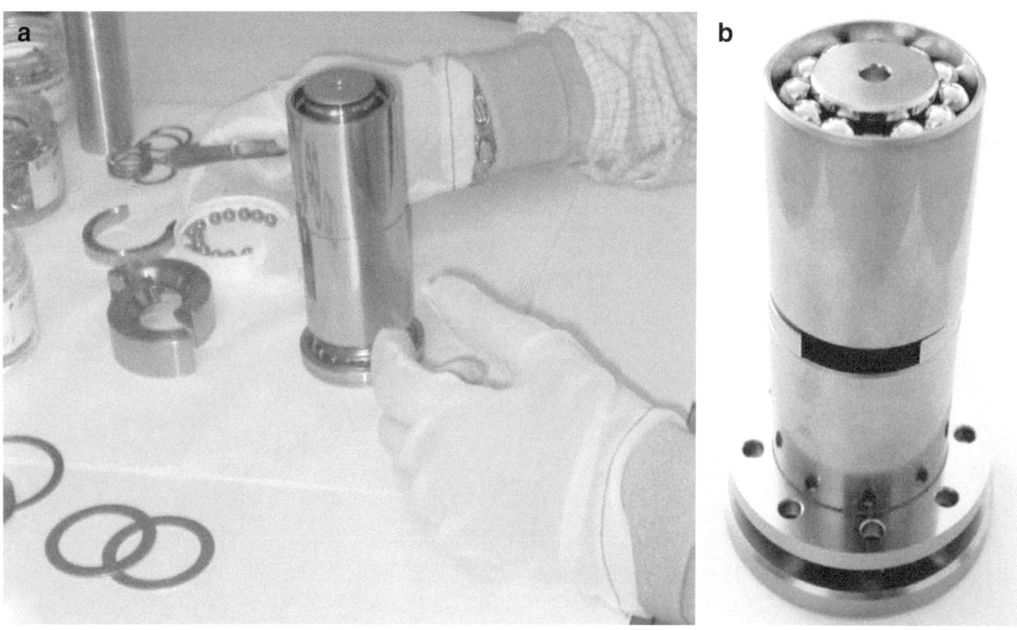

Fig. 2.39 (**a**) Assembly of a high-performance ball-bearing system for CT imaging. (**b**) Shows the entire high-performance unit, designed to support a 200 mm graphite-backed compound anode spinning at over 7200 rpm, experiencing approximately 30 g of centrifugal acceleration. (Image copyright: Springer Nature BV [9]. Reproduced with permission)

(via thin soft-metal film) to reduce wear, and from the 1980s, they used silver or lead films applied by specialized techniques for selected tube types, such as the Super Rotalix Ceramic™ (SRC 120) and earlier Rotalix models [8]. Initially, lead was applied using a suspension of lead particulates in Vaseline™, but by the 1990s, ion coating technology introduced by Varian (now Varex) became the standard [8].

Philips also tackled rotor noise and vibration by implementing a radial spring suspension system for one of the individual bearings, enabling the anode rotor to spin nearly force-free about its intrinsic axial axis of inertia. This design, which was applied to the straddle-type bearing of the SRC tube, helped balance the radial load. This concept was later adapted by Siemens for the Akron™ tube series, GE for the Performix CT tube series, and Varian (now Varex) for the MCS 70xx CT tube series [8].

Despite these advancements, the rotor life of ball-bearing tubes is limited to several hundred hours of rotation time, making it essential to stop the rotation after each exposure to prevent damage.

(b) ***Dry-lubricated ball bearings***

One significant advancement in X-ray tube technology was the introduction of dry-lubricated ball bearings. Unlike traditional ball bearings that require oil or grease lubrication, dry-lubricated bearings eliminate the need for external lubricants, reducing maintenance requirements and improving operational efficiency. These bearings also offered advantages such as reduced friction and enhanced resistance to contamination, resulting in smoother rotation and extended lifespan for X-ray tubes.

Manufacturers utilized various designs and lubrication methods, carefully safeguarding their proprietary details. Variations included spring-loaded and non-spring-loaded bearings, with or without bearing cages, lubricated with materials such as molybdenum disulfide, lead, silver, or a combination thereof [46]. Different methods were employed to apply the lubricants, including sputtering, physical coating, galvanic processes, or run-in processes under powder [46]. These diverse designs and manufacturing processes significantly impacted key properties such as achievable rotation velocity, operational lifespan, and noise levels. Some manufacturers achieved exceptional tube lifetimes despite higher operating noise levels, while others experienced the opposite [46]. By selecting the most suitable lubrication material for specific applications, manufacturers could optimize the performance and reliability of ball-bearing systems in X-ray tubes (Fig. 2.40).

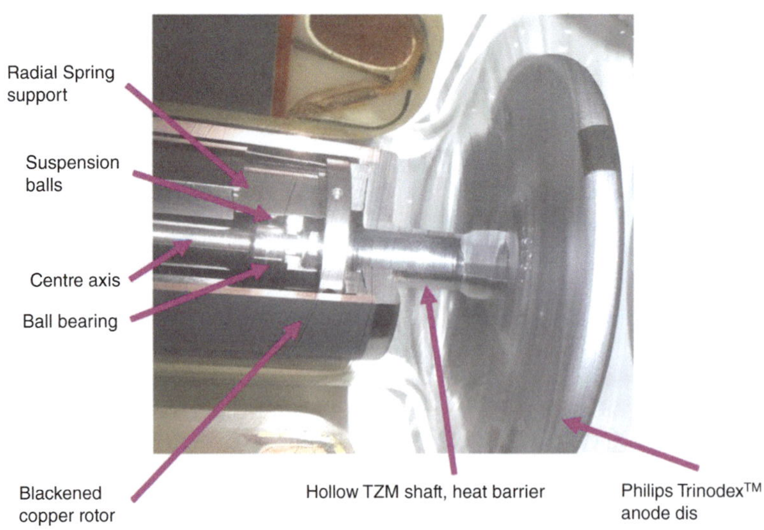

Fig. 2.40 In a Philips glass tube, there is a radial spring-supported ball-bearing system known for its low noise. (Image Courtesy: Rolf Behling [8]. Reprinted with permission)

(c) **Magnetic bearings**

Magnetic bearings were explored as an alternative to traditional ball-bearing designs. These bearings use magnetic fields to levitate the rotor, eliminating physical contact and thus reducing wear and friction. However, controlling the magnetic suspension and current transfer in a high-vacuum environment proved challenging. Magnetic bearings offer potential benefits such as virtually frictionless operation and excellent heat management. However, the complexity of these systems, including difficulties in maintaining stable magnetic suspension and effective current transfer, has limited their widespread adoption in X-ray tubes.

One significant challenge for both ball and magnetic bearing systems is managing the residual enthalpy in the anode. After a patient has been X-rayed and the anode cools down, the residual heat can affect the tube's performance.

(d) **Spiral groove bearings**

Spiral groove bearings were introduced to address the limitations and challenges posed by ball bearings in X-ray tubes. These bearings operate based on the principle of hydrodynamic lubrication. In this system, a thin film of lubricant is maintained within the spiral grooves during the rotation of the anode, creating a pressure differential that significantly reduces friction and wear. This lubrication method ensures a stable and efficient operation of the bearing system, resulting in lower operational noise and longer service life compared to traditional ball bearings.

The introduction of spiral groove bearings in the Philips Maximus Rotalix Ceramic™ (MRC) tube in 1989 marked a significant advancement in X-ray tube technology [8]. These bearings provided enhanced stability and extended operational life, which was particularly beneficial for cardiology and angiography applications where continuous and reliable performance is crucial. The hydrodynamic lubrication achieved by spiral grooves allows for smooth and consistent rotation of the anode, improving the overall efficiency and durability of the X-ray tube.

(e) **Liquid metal bearings**

The introduction of liquid metal bearings represented a groundbreaking advancement in X-ray tube technology, offering unparalleled performance, durability, and reliability. Originating from research pioneered by E.A. Muijderman in the early 1960s, the clinical application of liquid metal bearings began with Philips introducing such tubes in 1989 with the Maximus Rotalix Ceramic™ tube [46].

Liquid metal bearings utilize a gallium-indium-tin alloy as the lubricant, providing nearly frictionless operation and exceptional heat dissipation. This fluidlike metallic alloy enables smooth, continuous rotation of the anode without physical contact, thus minimizing friction and wear. Unlike traditional ball bearings that rely on mechanical contact, liquid metal bearings operate silently, producing minimal vibrations and audible sounds, which enhances the overall user experience (Fig. 2.41).

Anodes equipped with liquid metal spiral groove bearings achieve continuous rotation, eliminating the need for braking and subsequent acceleration required by ball-bearing systems. This operational efficiency minimizes waiting times between imaging cycles. Additionally, they support large anodes with high momentum of inertia, eliminating the need for rotor spin-up times and enabling continuous operation without audible noise. This feature is particularly advantageous in clinical settings where rapid and reliable imaging is essential.

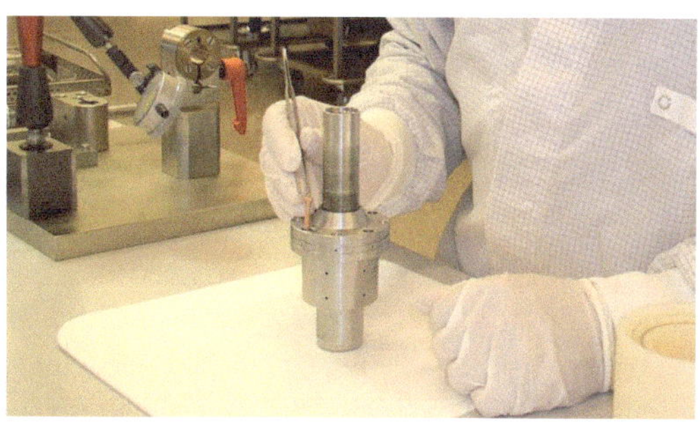

Fig. 2.41 Liquid metal bearing system assembly of a for the Philips MRC™ 200 angiography tube series. (Image Courtesy: Rolf Behling [8]. Reprinted with permission)

Key among their advantages is their exceptional heat dissipation capability. The metallic alloy lubricant efficiently transfers heat from the rotating anode to the cooled tube housing assembly, mitigating the risk of overheating and thermal damage to critical components. This efficient thermal coupling allows heat dissipation capacities ranging from a few hundred watts to two or three kilowatts, contingent on anode temperature and geometrical design. The enhanced heat dissipation extends the lifespan of X-ray tubes and ensures consistent performance over time, even under demanding operating conditions.

Moreover, liquid metal bearings offer superior heat dissipation and shorter cooling periods than conventional ball-bearing tubes. Their efficient thermal coupling of the anode to the cooled tube housing assembly through liquid metal allows for faster and more effective cooling. This advantage significantly reduces the risk of overheating and thermal damage to the X-ray tube, thereby extending its lifespan and ensuring consistent performance even under heavy usage.

Liquid metal bearings also exhibit remarkable durability and reliability. They are resistant to wear, corrosion, and oxidation, making them well-suited for long-term use in X-ray imaging systems. This durability reduces maintenance requirements and minimizes downtime, enhancing operational efficiency and cost-effectiveness. The implementation of liquid metal bearings has accelerated clinical workflows and increased the durability and efficiency of X-ray systems, making them a preferred choice for high-demand medical imaging applications.

(f) **Hybrid bearings**

Hybrid bearings combine the advantages of different bearing types, such as spiral grooves and liquid metal bearings, to optimize the performance of X-ray tubes. These advanced bearing designs aim to achieve the best balance of lubrication, heat management, and durability. By integrating the hydrodynamic lubrication features of spiral grooves with the exceptional heat conduction properties of liquid metal bearings, hybrid bearings provide a comprehensive solution to the challenges faced by X-ray tube manufacturers.

The use of hybrid bearings allows for the benefits of both technologies to be realized in a single system. The hydrodynamic lubrication from the spiral grooves ensures smooth and stable rotation of the anode, reducing friction and wear, while the liquid metal provides excellent heat dissipation, enhancing the thermal management capabilities of the X-ray tube. This combination results in a bearing system that offers extended operational life, reduced maintenance requirements, and improved overall performance. Hybrid bearings have become increasingly popular in modern X-ray tube designs, providing a reliable and efficient solution for the demanding needs of medical imaging.

The advancements in bearing technologies, from spiral groove bearings to liquid metal and hybrid bearings, have significantly improved the performance, reliability, and lifespan of X-ray tubes. These innovations have addressed the limitations of traditional ball bearings, offering superior lubrication, heat management, and durability, which are essential for high-performance medical imaging applications.

(g) **Lubrication system**

Proper lubrication is essential for maintaining the performance and longevity of X-ray tube bearings. Lubricants are selected based on their ability to withstand high temperatures and pressures while providing adequate lubrication to reduce friction and wear. Regular lubrication maintenance is necessary to replenish lost or degraded lubricant and ensure optimal bearing performance.

One approach is the **automatic lubrication mechanism**, which ensures a continuous supply of lubricant to the bearings during operation. This system maintains the optimal level of lubrication, preventing excessive friction and wear on the bearing surfaces. Synthetic oils, which have high thermal stability, low volatility, and excellent lubrication properties, are often used in automatic systems. These oils provide consistent lubrication over a wide temperature range and reduce the frequency of maintenance. Greases, with their high viscosity and good adherence to surfaces, offer long-lasting lubrication, especially suitable for applications where relubrication is difficult. Additionally, graphite-based lubricants, known for their high thermal conductivity and low friction coefficient, are effective in high-temperature environments and provide solid lubrication, reducing the risk of lubricant depletion.

Another approach is **temperature-dependent lubrication**, which adjusts the rate of lubricant delivery based on the operating temperature of the bearings. By optimizing lubrication according to temperature, this system helps dissipate heat effectively, preventing overheating and ensuring smooth operation. High-temperature lubricants, such as polyalphaolefin (PAO) oils, perfluoropolyether (PFPE) oils, and silicone-based lubricants, maintain viscosity and lubrication properties at elevated temperatures, ensuring effective heat dissipation and preventing overheating. Solid lubricants, including molybdenum disulfide (MoS2), tungsten disulfide (WS2), and graphite, provide lubrication in extreme temperatures where liquid lubricants may fail, reducing wear and extending bearing life. Metallic lubricants, like the gallium-indium-tin alloys used in liquid metal bearings, offer nearly frictionless operation and exceptional heat dissipation, crucial for high-performance demands in modern X-ray systems.

Several key considerations must be taken into account for effective lubrication. The lubrication rate must be adjusted based on the operating temperature to ensure optimal lubrication and prevent overheating. Effective lubrication helps dissipate heat generated during operation, maintaining smooth and reliable performance. Regular lubrication maintenance is necessary to replenish lost or degraded lubricant, ensuring the bearings' optimal performance.

The advantages of effective lubrication are manifold. Both spiral grooves and liquid metal bearings minimize friction between moving parts, reducing wear and extending the lifespan of the rotating mechanism. The combination of advanced bearing technology and effective lubrication systems enhances the overall durability and reliability of the anode assembly, even under high-speed operation. By ensuring smooth and reliable rotation, the bearing and lubrication system contributes to the overall performance and efficiency of the X-ray tube, resulting in high-quality diagnostic imaging.

The bearing and lubrication system of anodes in X-ray tubes plays a crucial role in supporting the smooth and reliable rotation of the anode assembly. Advanced bearing technologies, such as spiral grooves and liquid metal bearings, offer superior performance and durability, contributing to the overall efficiency and lifespan of modern X-ray tubes. Regular maintenance and lubrication are essential to ensure the optimal performance and longevity of the bearing system.

2.6.2 Tube Envelope/Tube Frame

The tube envelope is a cover around the cathode and anode assembly which maintains a high vacuum environment, protects internal elements, facilitates heat dissipation, and ensures structural integrity. Its primary function is to house the cathode and anode assemblies within a vacuum-sealed enclosure, crucial for the efficient generation of X-rays. The high vacuum within the tube envelope is essential to minimize electron collisions with air molecules. This ensures that the electrons emitted from the cathode can travel unimpeded to the anode, where X-rays are generated. Any presence of air molecules would cause scattering and energy loss, significantly reducing the efficiency of the X-ray tube. The tube envelope also serves to protect the delicate internal components from external contaminants and mechanical damage. It ensures that the cathode, anode, and associated structures are kept in a controlled environment, free from dust, moisture, and other potentially harmful substances.

During operation, X-ray tubes generate significant amounts of heat, particularly at the anode. The tube envelope must be designed to facilitate effective heat dissipation to prevent overheating and damage. Advanced materials and design considerations are employed to enhance thermal management and prolong the lifespan of the tube. The structural integrity of the tube envelope is critical, especially under the high stress and thermal conditions encountered during X-ray production. The envelope must withstand significant mechanical stresses and thermal cycles without compromising its vacuum seal or structural stability.

Materials Used

X-ray tube envelopes are often constructed from glass or ceramic, and depending on specific application requirements the window for X-ray exit is commonly made from beryllium due to its low absorption properties. Glass has traditionally been preferred as it provides an excellent vacuum seal and is easy to manufacture. However, standard glass frames can cause undesired X-ray filtration of low-energy X-rays (hardening the beam), which is problematic in applications like mammography, where lower photon energy is necessary for optimal contrast-to-noise ratio in imaging soft tissue with fine details such as calcifications and therefore beryllium windows were attached to the glass frame [9]. Beryllium, with its low atomic number and density, provides the lowest absorption coefficient of any material suitable for X-ray windows. This property makes it ideal for minimizing the loss of X-ray intensity, allowing for clearer imaging. The first use of beryllium plates in X-ray tubes occurred in Germany and the United States in the early 1930s, initially as internal hoods around the target to prevent bombardment of the tube walls by secondary electrons [48].

The development of malleable beryllium and the production of thin, vacuum-tight sheets led to the first commercially produced X-ray tubes with beryllium windows in the external envelope in 1942, primarily for X-ray diffraction work [48].

Ceramics offer superior thermal and electrical insulation, making them advantageous in high-voltage applications. They can withstand higher operating temperatures, which is beneficial for thermal management and extending the tube's operational life.

This combination of materials—glass or ceramic envelopes with beryllium exit windows—ensures efficient, high-quality X-ray production suitable for a range of specialized applications. Let us discuss the advantages and disadvantages of glass and ceramic tube envelopes:

Glass

Traditionally borosilicate glass has been the material of choice for X-ray tube envelopes due to its excellent insulating properties, ability to withstand thermal and mechanical stresses, and transparency for visual inspection of internal components. Borosilicate glass is highly resistant to thermal shock and can endure rapid temperature changes, making it suitable for high-energy applications. If the cooling system fails, the pressure within the glass envelope can rise significantly. For instance, in an angiography system, if the cooling fluid flow is blocked, the oil pressure can increase to the system's safety limit. Under such conditions, a glass tube might implode due to the loss of yield strength from overheating, leading to a complete system failure.

Limitations Despite its advantages, glass has several limitations. Under extreme conditions, such as high stress or thermal loads, glass envelopes can be prone to implosion. Additionally, glass is sensitive to the buildup of conductive layers, such as tungsten, which can lead to electron backscattering and material degradation. Advances in materials science have led to the development of more robust alternatives to address these limitations (Fig. 2.42).

Ceramics

Ceramic materials, including alumina (Al_2O_3) and zirconia (ZrO_2), have become increasingly popular in modern X-ray tube designs. Ceramics offer superior thermal and mechanical properties compared to glass, including higher resistance to radiation damage and greater overall durability. This can withstand higher operating temperatures, which is beneficial for thermal management and extending the tube's operational life. They are also more resistant to mechanical shock and radiation damage, making them ideal for high-performance applications. They also have excellent electrical insulating properties, preventing electrical currents from leaking through the envelope. This is crucial for maintaining the integrity of the electron flow from the cathode to

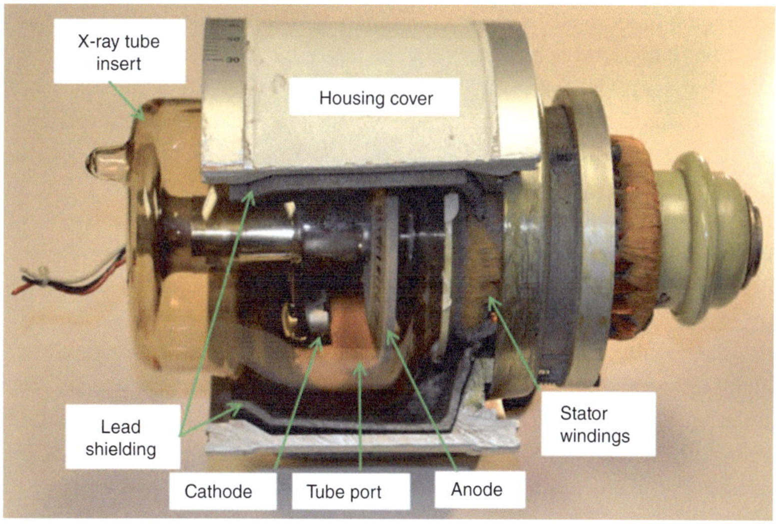

Fig. 2.42 An illustration of an X-ray tube insert, along with a partially cutaway housing, reveals the various components within the X-ray tube. In this particular housing, the lead shielding has a thickness of 2 mm. (Image originally published in reference [49]. Reprinted with permission)

the anode in X-ray tubes. Despite their brittleness, ceramics are incredibly hard and can withstand mechanical stresses that would deform or damage other materials. This makes them highly durable under normal operating conditions. The examples of ceramic tube uses are Siemens SOMATOM Definition Edge and GE Revolution CT which are designed for high-performance imaging, efficient heat management, enhanced image quality and system reliability.

Limitations Ceramics, while strong under compression, are inherently brittle and can fracture under tensile stress or impact. This brittleness makes them susceptible to sudden failure without significant prior deformation, posing reliability issues in applications where mechanical shocks are possible. The manufacturing process for ceramic components is more complex and costly compared to metals and glass. The sintering process, necessary to form dense ceramic parts, requires precise control of temperature and atmosphere, which can increase production costs and time. Although ceramics can withstand high temperatures, their thermal conductivity is generally lower than that of metals. This can limit their efficiency in heat dissipation, which is critical for maintaining the performance and longevity of X-ray tubes under continuous high-power operation. Achieving a vacuum-tight seal with ceramic materials can be challenging. Ceramics require special sealing techniques, such as brazing with metals, which can be complex and costly. Ensuring a durable and leak-free joint is crucial but technically demanding.

Use of Metal in X-Ray Tube Envelopes

The Straton X-ray tubes by Siemens use non-magnetic stainless steel for the tube envelope, known for their innovative design that integrates the anode, rotor, and stator within a single housing. This integration simplifies construction, enhances thermal management, and improves reliability. The stainless steel envelope in Straton tubes allows for efficient cooling, reducing thermal stress on components and enabling higher performance and longer exposure times without compromising the tube's integrity.

Before Siemens launched the Straton® rotating frame tube in 2003, Dunlee (then Aurora, IL, USA) explored a rotating frame tube concept with a larger anode and a stationary focal spot maintained by a magnet. However, this complex design was abandoned in favor of the Philips iMRC® tube after Philips acquired Dunlee and introduced heat-conducting spiral groove bearings [9].

Driven by the importance of CT, Siemens revitalized Wood's 1896 idea of a rotating frame tube, leveraging modern electron optics simulation and electron emission technology [9]. Inspired by Waterton and Metropolitan-Vickers' mid-1940s patent, Siemens set the entire tube frame, including the cathode, insulation, and anode, into motion [9]. The electron beam was steered and focused by a magnetic quadrupole and dipole system, with ball bearings lubricated by oil. The anode disk became part of the tube envelope, with the cathode spinning on a flat ceramic insulator. A circular flat electron emitter connected to the negative high-voltage potential directed the electron beam toward the focal spot track on the rotating anode, guided by a stationary magnetic dipole field. A quadrupole magnetic lens shaped the focal spot, and a pair of dipoles allowed for focal spot deflection. Despite its compact 12 cm anode diameter, the design achieved substantial heat conduction to oil, enabling high-end performance. Challenges such as hydrodynamic friction and cavitation were mitigated with copper casting to prevent cracks from thermal gradients. This compact design facilitated the creation of a dual-source CT system [9].

2.6.3 X-Ray Tube Housing Assembly

2.6.3.1 Lead Shielding

The housing of the X-ray tube is lined with lead to prevent radiation leakage, ensuring that X-rays are directed only toward the target area and protecting operators from unnecessary exposure. Lead shielding within X-ray tubes is essential for protecting patients and staff from about 99% of the emitted bremsstrahlung, which would not be detected by an image receptor. The X-ray tube and its subcomponents reduce unwanted radiation through various means, including the anode disk, which shields about half of the space angle, and a cathode head positioned close to the focal spot. Copper and iron frames of metal center section tubes significantly attenuate X-rays. Additionally, radiation can emerge from landing spots of backscattered electrons at the back of the anode, field-emitted electrons on the inner surfaces of the vacuum envelope and scattering and fluorescence radiation from materials exposed to high-energy radiation.

These aspects are best managed by a dedicated radiation shield, which also serves functions such as electrical insulation, guidance, and encasing of cooling fluid and mechanical interfacing. Protective tube housings are usually compatible with a variety of tubes that may differ slightly by focal spot dimension and anode angle. Although they appear similar, tubes with different anode angles may require different leakage protection around the X-ray window. Certified manufacturers should handle X-ray tube replacement and matching with a collimator to ensure proper shielding and functionality.

Leakage radiation from the diagnostic source assembly should not exceed 0.88 milligray (mGy) air kerma (100 milliroentgens (mR) exposure) in 1 h when the X-ray tube is operated at the leakage technique factors [9]. The US 21 CFR Part 1020 (2005) outlines these factors as the maximum-rated peak tube potential and continuous tube current for the maximum-rated peak tube potential. Most manufacturers distribute the burden of radiation protection equally between the tube housing and the collimator. Typically, the tube housing assembly is designed to emit a maximum of 440 μGy in 1 h, with the collimator potentially emitting an additional 440 μGy in 1 h, mainly from scattered radiation [9].

Lead, with its large atomic number and malleability, is preferred for leakage protection. Despite the restriction of hazardous substances (RoHS) directive excluding lead from most electronic equipment, its use in medical devices and equipment is exempt, provided reuse occurs in auditable closed-loop systems. Efforts are ongoing to find alternatives, such as molded emulsions of tungsten and molybdenum powder in polymers [9]. The outer shell of protective structures should be made from materials with the lowest K-edge to capture fluorescence radiation from upstream materials with the highest atomic numbers [9]. Quality manufacturers inspect all products individually and report results to governmental agencies to ensure compliance and safety.

2.6.3.2 High-Tension Voltage Cable Sockets

High-tension (HT) voltage cable sockets provide essential connections for high-voltage cables, ensuring the safe and effective delivery of power necessary for X-ray production. These components are meticulously designed to handle substantial electrical loads and maintain system safety and stability.

HT cable sockets are typically made from materials that offer superior electrical insulation and thermal resistance, such as high-grade plastics and ceramics. These materials can withstand the high voltages and thermal stresses encountered in X-ray systems. The connectors are often made from durable metals like stainless steel to ensure robust mechanical connections and grounding.

These sockets facilitate the transmission of high voltage from the generator to the X-ray tube, typically in the range of 40–150 kV. They are designed for durability and reliability, capable of withstanding repeated high-voltage cycles with minimal wear. Effective thermal management is also crucial, and HT cable sockets often include features like heat sinks or cooling mechanisms to dissipate excess heat, ensuring stable electrical connections and preventing overheating.

In modern X-ray systems, particularly in mobile and compact units like C-arms and mammography systems, the high-voltage generator and X-ray tube are often integrated into a single housing known as a monoblock. This integration eliminates the need for separate high-voltage cables, simplifying the design and enhancing reliability. In monoblocks used in CT, mammography, and mobile X-ray equipment, components such as the high-voltage transformer, rectifier diodes, smoothing capacitors, and cooling mechanisms are all integrated within a single housing. While this integration simplifies the system, it imposes limitations on peak power rating and continuous heat dissipation due to restricted space and cooling surface area.

Proper installation of HT cable sockets is essential for securing connections and preventing electrical hazards. Technicians must follow precise procedures to avoid gaps or loose connections that could lead to arcing or power loss. Regular maintenance is crucial to ensure the ongoing performance and safety of HT cable sockets, including inspecting insulation and checking connections.

Safety is paramount when dealing with high-voltage components. HT cable sockets must comply with stringent industry standards and regulations, such as those set by the International Electrotechnical Commission (IEC), which specify the required electrical insulation, mechanical strength, and thermal properties.

2.6.3.3 Stator Electromagnetic Coils

In rotating anode tubes, stator coils generate a magnetic field that interacts with the rotor attached to the anode, causing it to spin. This rotation spreads the heat over a larger area of the anode, improving thermal management. The stator is located outside the vacuum envelope of the X-ray tube, while the rotor is situated inside.

Components and Construction

The stator is composed of several electromagnetic coils arranged around the X-ray tube's glass or ceramic envelope. These coils, typically made from copper wire due to their excellent electrical conductivity, are wound around laminated iron cores to form electromagnets. The number of coils can vary but usually includes two or more sets of windings positioned to create a rotating magnetic field. The windings are insulated to prevent short circuits and to ensure efficient operation. The iron cores are laminated to reduce eddy currents and associated losses, enhancing the efficiency of the magnetic field generation.

The coils are encased in a protective housing that is mounted around the X-ray tube. This housing is typically made from materials that provide mechanical protection and electrical insulation.

Functioning

The primary function of the stator electromagnetic coils is to generate a rotating magnetic field. This field interacts with the rotor (anode) located inside the X-ray tube, causing it to rotate. The stator coils are energized by an alternating current (AC) power supply, creating alternating magnetic fields. The arrangement of the coils and the alternating current produce a rotating magnetic field, with the speed of rotation depending on the frequency of the AC supply and the configuration of the stator windings.

The rotating magnetic field induces currents in the rotor, which acts as a conductor. According to the principles of electromagnetic induction, these induced currents generate their magnetic fields, interacting with the stator's rotating field. This interaction produces a torque on the rotor, causing it to spin. The rotation of the rotor spreads the heat generated by the electron bombardment over a larger surface area, reducing the risk of damage and allowing for higher tube currents and shorter exposure times.

Design Considerations

- *Thermal management*
  The stator coils can generate significant heat during operation. Proper thermal management, including cooling systems such as forced air or liquid cooling, is essential to maintain the performance and longevity of the stator.
- *Electrical insulation*
  The insulation of the stator windings must be robust to withstand the high voltages and currents involved in the operation. Insulation materials must also be resistant to thermal degradation.
- *Mechanical stability*
  The stator housing and the positioning of the coils must be mechanically stable to ensure consistent performance and to prevent vibrations that could affect the X-ray tube's function.
- *Control systems*
  Modern X-ray systems incorporate sophisticated control systems to manage the operation of the stator. These systems regulate the AC power supply to the stator coils, allowing precise control over the speed and stability of the anode rotation.

2.6.3.4 Beam Collimation

Beam collimation is designed to shape and narrow the X-ray beam before it exits the tube assembly. This precise shaping serves several essential purposes. Firstly, collimation allows X-rays to be directed more accurately toward the area of interest, which provides high-quality diagnostic images and ensures that radiation exposure is confined to the targeted region.

By limiting the X-ray beam to the desired field of view, collimation reduces scatter radiation, which occurs when X-rays deviate from their original path due to interactions with matter. Scatter radiation can degrade image quality and increase unnecessary radiation exposure to patients and staff. Minimizing scatter radiation enhances image contrast by ensuring that less scatter reaches the image receptor, resulting in clearer and more accurate diagnostic images.

Further, a well-collimated beam leads to better image quality, which is vital for proper medical evaluation and treatment planning. By reducing the volume of tissue exposed to radiation, collimation not only improves the clarity of the images but also enhances patient safety by limiting unnecessary radiation exposure.

Components of Beam Collimation

- **Pre-collimators**: These devices shape the X-ray beam before it exits the tube assembly. They are the first line of beam restriction, ensuring that the beam is narrowed down as it exits the tube.
- **Adjustable collimators**: Located near the X-ray source, these devices further refine the shape and size of the X-ray beam. They often include adjustable shutters or blades that can be manipulated to match the size of the area being imaged.
- **Filter slots**: Often integrated into the X-ray system's housing or the collimator assembly itself, these components provide additional beam shaping and may include filtration elements to remove lower energy X-rays that do not contribute to image formation but increase patient dose.

- **Light field collimators**: These are often used in conjunction with mirrors to project a light field that corresponds to the X-ray field. This visualization helps technicians accurately position the patient and the X-ray beam, ensuring that the area of interest is properly targeted.

Regulatory and Safety Considerations

Beam collimation is not only a technical requirement but also a regulatory one. Standards such as the IEC 60601-1-3 mandate that X-ray systems include adequate filtration and collimation to ensure patient safety and image quality. According to these standards, the total filtration equivalent must be at least 2.5 mm of aluminum to ensure that the X-ray beam is adequately hardened, reducing patient dose and improving image quality.

2.6.3.5 X-Ray Radiation Port and Window

The X-ray radiation port and window are designed to facilitate the efficient and safe emission of X-rays from the tube while maintaining the integrity and performance of the system. The port is the exit point for X-rays from the tube housing. A radiolucent window, typically made of beryllium, covers this port to protect the tube while allowing X-rays to pass through with minimal attenuation.

X-Ray Radiation Port

The radiation port is an aperture in the X-ray tube housing that directs the emitted X-rays toward the target, such as a patient or an imaging detector. This port is precisely aligned with the focal spot on the anode to ensure that the X-ray beam is accurately directed. The size and shape of the radiation port are designed to match the intended beam profile, minimizing unnecessary radiation exposure to adjacent areas and optimizing the quality of the radiographic image.

Proper shielding around the radiation port is crucial to prevent leakage of radiation, which can pose a hazard to both patients and medical personnel. This shielding is typically made of high-density materials like lead or tungsten, which have high atomic numbers and are highly effective at attenuating X-rays. The design of the radiation port also includes collimators or shutters, which can be adjusted to control the size and shape of the X-ray beam, further enhancing the safety and precision of the X-ray emission.

X-Ray Window

The X-ray window is a thin, specialized barrier located at the radiation port that allows X-rays to pass through while maintaining the vacuum seal of the X-ray tube. The material of the window must have a low atomic number to minimize the absorption of X-rays, ensuring that a maximum amount of radiation exits the tube. Common materials used for X-ray windows include beryllium and borosilicate glass.

Beryllium is frequently chosen due to its combination of low atomic number, high strength, and excellent thermal properties. It is capable of withstanding the thermal and mechanical stresses associated with high-energy X-ray production. However, due to its toxicity, handling and manufacturing of beryllium components require strict safety protocols.

The X-ray window must be thick enough to maintain the structural integrity of the vacuum envelope and withstand the internal pressure differences, yet thin enough to allow efficient transmission of X-rays. Typically, window thickness ranges from a few micrometers to a few millimeters, depending on the specific application and energy range of the X-rays being produced.

Integration and Function

In practice, the X-ray window and radiation port work together seamlessly to ensure the controlled release of X-rays. The design must account for thermal expansion and mechanical stresses, as the window will experience significant heating during operation. Advanced materials and manufacturing techniques are employed to create windows that are not only transparent to X-rays but also durable and resistant to long-term wear.

Moreover, the alignment of the X-ray tube, window, and radiation port must be precisely calibrated during manufacturing and installation to ensure optimal performance. Misalignment can lead to reduced image quality and increased radiation exposure.

2.6.3.6 Radiation Control Timer Circuit

The primary function of the radiation control timer circuit is to precisely control the exposure time. Accurate timing is vital because it directly influences the dose of radiation the patient receives, and the clarity of the image produced. Overexposure can lead to unnecessary radiation doses to the patient, while underexposure can result in poor image quality, necessitating repeat exposures and further radiation exposure.

Components and Operation

The radiation control timer circuit typically consists of several key components, including a timer, relays, and safety interlocks, integrated into the X-ray system's control console. Modern X-ray systems often employ digital timers for greater accuracy and reliability. The timer can be preset to the desired exposure time based on the specific imaging requirements, which are determined by factors such as the type of examination, the part of the body being imaged, and the patient's size and condition.

When an X-ray exposure is initiated, the timer circuit activates the high-voltage generator, which in turn energizes the X-ray tube. The circuit then maintains the tube in an active state for the preset duration. Upon reaching the end of the specified exposure time, the timer circuit deactivates the high-voltage generator, terminating the X-ray emission. This process ensures that the exposure time is tightly controlled, contributing to consistent imaging results and enhanced patient safety.

Safety Mechanisms

In addition to timing control, the radiation control timer circuit incorporates multiple safety mechanisms. These include fail-safes that prevent the X-ray tube from being exposed for longer than the set time, thus protecting against accidental overexposure. Furthermore, interlocks are often included to ensure that the system cannot be activated unless all safety conditions are met, such as the proper positioning of the patient and the closure of protective doors in the imaging room.

Integration with Other Systems

The timer circuit is integrated with other components of the X-ray system, such as the automatic exposure control (AEC) system, which adjusts exposure parameters in real-time to achieve optimal image quality based on the patient's anatomy and density. This integration allows for dynamic adjustment of exposure times, contributing to improved diagnostic capabilities while minimizing radiation dose.

Technological Advances

Advancements in microprocessor technology have significantly enhanced the functionality of radiation control timer circuits. Modern systems use sophisticated algorithms and digital interfaces to allow for precise control and easy adjustment of exposure times. These systems often feature programmable settings and preset protocols for different types of examinations, which streamline the imaging process and reduce the potential for human error.

2.6.3.7 Bellows in X-Ray Tubes

The bellows mechanisms accommodate changes in volume due to temperature fluctuations within the tube, preventing mechanical stress and potential damage to the tube assembly. These flexible and expandable components primarily serve as mechanical seals that manage movement and pressure changes while maintaining a vacuum or controlled environment. They are essential for maintaining the integrity of the vacuum system and the proper functioning and longevity of the tube. A bellows enables mechanical coupling to the tube's internal structures while maintaining a completely vacuum-tight enclosure and all joints can be hard soldered or brazed together, allowing the entire system to be baked at high temperatures during pump-down [50].

Function and Importance

The primary function of the bellows in X-ray tubes is to compensate for thermal expansion and contraction of the tube components, particularly the anode assembly of the insulating oil in the tube housing. The oil, which is subjected to intense heat during X-ray production, expands and contracts as it heats up and cools down. Bellows provide the necessary flexibility to accommodate these dimensional changes without compromising the tube. This ensures that the environment inside the X-ray tube is maintained consistently, which is critical for the efficient generation of X-rays and the prevention of contaminants that could impair tube performance. This dynamic response to temperature changes helps prevent mechanical stress on the tube components, reducing the risk of damage and extending the operational lifespan of the tube.

By accommodating the thermal expansion and contraction of the oil assembly, the bellows help to prevent pressure buildup in the tube's components. This prevention mitigates the risk of localized overheating and associated mechanical stress, which can lead to premature failure of the tube. Additionally, the bellows can be part of a larger cooling system that includes heat sinks and cooling fluids to further manage the thermal environment within the tube.

Design and Materials

They are typically made from materials that exhibit high flexibility, durability, and resistance to extreme conditions within the X-ray tube. Common materials include stainless steel and other high-grade alloys that offer excellent thermal and mechanical properties. The design of the bellows involves a series of convolutions or folds that allow them to expand and contract with minimal stress on the material. This design ensures that the bellows can endure repeated cycles of movement and thermal expansion without suffering from fatigue or failure.

Advances in Technology

Recent advancements in materials science and manufacturing techniques have led to the development of bellows with enhanced performance characteristics. Innovations such as improved alloy compositions and precision fabrication methods have resulted in bellows that offer greater durability, flexibility, and resistance to high temperatures and mechanical stress. These advancements contribute to more reliable and efficient X-ray tubes, capable of operating under increasingly demanding conditions.

2.6.3.8 Heat Dissipation System

Managing the significant heat generated during X-ray production has been a critical challenge since the inception of X-rays. A substantial amount of electrical energy must be transferred to the X-ray tube, but only a small fraction, typically less than 1%, is converted into X-rays; the majority is dissipated as heat. This presents a critical limitation as excessive heat can damage the tube, such as causing a melted anode or ruptured tube housing.

In typical CT tubes with 4 cm patient coverage, the surrounding focal track can reach approximately 1000–1200 °C, while the focal spot can peak around 2000–2800 °C. In extreme cases, such as during sequential imaging of trauma patients in CT scans, the temperature may exceed 3000 °C, despite the critical temperature for many tubes being around the melting point of the anode material (around 3400 °C for tungsten, but operational limits are lower to prevent evaporation and cracking) [28, 47]. Innovations like rotating anodes have been implemented to prevent overheating, though they introduced challenges such as bearing lubrication and rapid acceleration requirements [33]. Heat dissipation methods have evolved to include air convection and, in some cases, water circulation.

Traditional and Modern Cooling Methods

Traditionally, ball-bearing technology and air convection cooling dominated the X-ray tube market. Manufacturers increased the heat storage capacity of rotating anodes, measured in mega heat units (MHU), to improve CT workflow. Anode heat content (AHC) measures the total heat stored within the anode during operation and affects its ability to dissipate heat. Excessive heat buildup can lead to overheating and failure of the X-ray tube.

Heat loading on X-ray tubes varies, with quantification achieved through heat units (HU). This is calculated by multiplying kilovolt peak, tube current, exposure time, and a constant multiplier dependent on the voltage waveform. Average anodes typically have a heat capacity of around 250,000 HU, while heavy-duty anodes may exceed 1000,000 HU. The anode dissipates heat primarily through radiation to the tube housing. Excessive heat buildup can damage performance and shorten the tube's lifespan.

Heat is generated when high-voltage electricity accelerates electrons from the cathode to the anode. The heat generated at the anode target can be quantified using the formula:

$$\text{Total heat units} = \text{kVp} \times \text{mA}(\text{average}) \times \text{time}(\text{seconds})$$

To prevent exceeding critical temperature thresholds, kVp and mA must be controlled and heat efficiently transferred away from the anode target.

Fans or oil circulators are employed to enhance cooling efficiency. Heat loading varies significantly depending on application, with chest radiographs generating around 200–500 HU and cine exposures up to 200,000 HU. Rating charts from X-ray manufacturers detail operating limits for tubes, including instantaneous heat capacity, continuous-load heat capacity (for fluoroscopy), and cooling rates for anodes and tube housings. Modern systems include computer monitoring to alert operators to potential damage risks and prompt delays to prevent overheating. With the advent of liquid metal bearing technology, the focus shifted from mega heat units (MHUs) to new standards. The International Electrotechnical Commission (IEC) introduced a new standard, IEC 60613:2009, retiring discussions around anode heat content and related heat units [51].

Heat Dissipation Mechanisms

Heat dissipation in X-ray tubes occurs through several mechanisms:

- **Conduction**: Heat is transferred from the anode target to the anode assembly through conduction. The anode assembly, typically a rotating disk made of high-thermal-conductivity materials like molybdenum or tungsten, spreads heat radially from the focal spot.
- **Radiation**: Heat is removed from the anode through thermal radiation. As the anode heats up, it emits infrared radiation that carries heat energy away to the surrounding environment.
- **Convection**: In rotating anode X-ray tubes, convection currents help dissipate heat from the anode surface to the environment. Despite advancements, air convection remains the primary cooling method. In high-volume facilities, air convection is augmented with fans and external heat exchangers. Remote heat exchangers offer heat dissipation capacities ranging from 500 to 3500 watts, while attached heat exchangers can handle 2500–6000 watts.

Cooling Systems

X-ray tubes employ various cooling systems to enhance heat dissipation:

- **Rotating anode**: Modern X-ray tubes feature a rotating anode disk, which spreads the heat load over a larger area, allowing for more efficient heat dissipation.
- **Coolant circulation**: Internal cooling systems circulate a coolant, such as oil or water, within the anode assembly to absorb and transfer heat away from the target.
- **External cooling**: Systems like fans or water-cooled housings dissipate heat from the X-ray tube assembly to the environment. In fluoroscopy environments, small water coolers enhance cooling capacity compared to air convection alone.

Temperature Monitoring and Regulation

Temperature sensors in X-ray tubes monitor critical components like the anode target. If temperatures exceed safe limits, the X-ray generator may reduce exposure time or shut down to prevent thermal damage. Some manufacturers use numerical simulation and computational models for online monitoring and temperature prediction. Safety measures include thermal or pressure hardware switches that automatically shut off power in emergencies.

Safety Measures to Prevent Implosion and Explosion

Protection against potential hazards such as delamination, bursting, or debris expulsion is crucial. Glass tubes risk implosion, while metal center section tubes may explode if oil leaks. Tube housings and envelopes must protect users and patients. Rigorous type tests under worst-case scenarios ensure tube integrity. An onion-like concentric design, with ductile metal and tube housing materials, is preferred to capture expelled parts and dissipate kinetic energy.

Advances in Heat Exchanger Technology

Recent advancements in heat exchanger technology for X-ray tubes focus on improving heat transfer efficiency, reducing thermal resistance, and enhancing the durability of the components. Innovations include:

- **Microchannel heat exchangers**: Providing greater surface area for heat transfer in compact spaces.
- **Advanced coolants**: New coolants with higher thermal capacities and lower viscosities for improved efficiency.
- **Smart thermal management systems**: Integrating AI and IoT for predictive maintenance and real-time cooling optimization.

These innovations ensure X-ray tubes operate at safe temperatures, maintaining performance and extending equipment life.

2.7 Special X-Ray Tubes

2.7.1 Dental X-Ray Systems

Equipment for dental radiography includes a simple self-rectified unit, the orthopantomography unit (OPG), and the cephalostat or craniostat. The dental unit, primarily used for intraoral radiography of teeth, consists of a self-rectified tube head mounted to provide a high degree of maneuverability. This unit can be either wall-mounted or mobile. The dental units have a basic stationary anode design (Fig. 2.45) and require low power, such as 7–10 mA at 60–70 kVp, and can be sufficient for the radiography of teeth. The focal spot size is typically small, around 0.4–0.7 mm. The timer can be either clockwork or electronic, with a range of times from 0.02 up to 1.0 s, in increments of 0.01–0.1 s (Fig. 2.43).

The proximity between the X-ray source and the image receptor in dental X-ray systems allows for the use of low tube voltages and lower power ratings, particularly in single-shot dental applications. The filament position within the X-ray tube is closer to the anode to improve efficiency. Figure 2.46 provides an internal view of a Philips Oralix™ dental tube housing assembly, which includes vital components such as a high-voltage transformer and rectifying circuitry for stable operation. Dental units typically operate at tube voltages between 60 and 90 kV, with FDA recommendations for optimal operation between 60 and 70 kV. Compliance with these regulations ensures a minimum distance between the X-ray source and the patient's skin, typically 10 and 18 cm, which must be maintained using a compatible beam-limiting device (Fig. 2.44).

The first X-ray images of teeth were taken in 1896 by Otto Walkhoff, a dentist from Braunschweig, and shortly after, physicist Walter König from Frankfurt became the first dentist to take dental radiographs, despite the lack of suitable film material at the time [52]. In 1905, Reiniger, Gebbert, and Schall introduced the "Record" as the first dental X-ray unit, and their product line soon expanded into electromedical

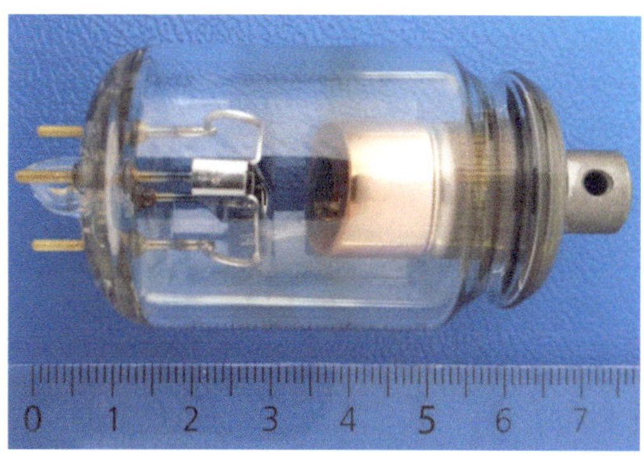

Fig. 2.43 Philips dental tube FO12 for the OralixTM tube head and centimeter ruler. (Image Courtesy: Rolf Behling [8])

equipment and this company eventually evolved into Siemens AG [52]. By 1914, dental radiography had gained enough prominence to be featured in Bennett's "Science and Practice of Dental Surgery," which included a 15-page chapter on the subject by Charles Alexander Clark of the Royal and National Dental Hospitals [52]. More detailed historical changes have been discussed in Chap. 8.

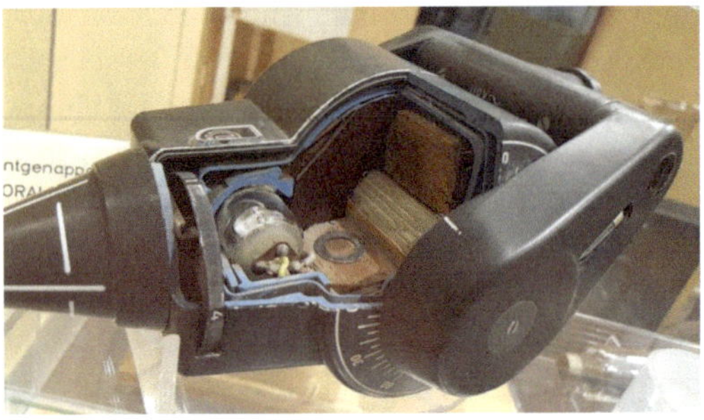

Fig. 2.44 The internal view of a Philips OralixTM dental tube head reveals how tube current and focal spot size were maintained through the utilization of a Wehnelt electrode and self-regulated resistive biasing. (Image Courtesy: Rolf Behling [8])

The tube design for dental X-ray systems incorporates a Wehnelt electrode, typically made of metal, to focus emitted electrons into a narrow beam. Tube current and focal spot size are regulated through self-controlled resistive biasing, ensuring consistent performance of the X-ray tube. This integration enables the production of high-quality dental images while maintaining reliability and efficiency.

Technological advancements have transitioned dental radiography from film-based techniques to digital imaging on computer screens. These advancements have been crucial for clinical diagnoses and treatments of various dental problems. Effective heat management, digital imaging compatibility, and regulatory compliance further enhance the reliability and efficiency of modern dental X-ray systems, ensuring high-quality imaging and patient safety in contemporary dental practices. Table 2.6 summarizes the key differences in X-ray tube design parameters in conventional radiography X-ray tubes versus dental radiography.

Table 2.6 X-ray tube design parameters: conventional radiography versus dental radiography

X-ray tube design parameter	Conventional radiography	Dental radiography
Operating peak voltage (kVp)	40–120 kVp	60–90 kVp
Tube current (mA)	100–800 mA	7–15 mA
Anode material	Tungsten	Tungsten
Tube exit window	Glass or beryllium	Beryllium
Added filtration	Aluminum or copper	Aluminum
Focal spot size	0.6–1.2 mm	0.4–1.0 mm
Beam focusing	Standard	Precision for small focal spot
Beam limiting device	Collimator	Diaphragm or collimator
Applications	General radiography	Dental imaging
Spatial resolution	Moderate to high	High
Heat dissipation	Standard cooling	Limited due to low power
Filament position	Standard	Closer to the anode for some designs to improve efficiency
Tube lifespan	Standard	Long due to low power and usage
Anode heat capacity	250,000–1000,000 HU	20,000–60,000 HU
Cooling method	Air convection, oil cooling	Air convection
Characteristic X-ray production	Bremsstrahlung dominant	Bremsstrahlung dominant
Radiation dose control	Moderate to precise	Very precise
Operation mode	Single-shot, continuous	Single shot
Exposure time	Short	Very short
Heat management	Standard cooling	Efficient heat dissipation systems for high-frequency use
Generator power rating	30–80 kW	0.5–2 kW

2.7.2 Mammography Tubes

High contrast and high spatial resolution are essential for optimal mammography; therefore, standard radiographic equipment is unsuitable for this examination. Mammographic equipment and techniques differ from standard radiography in several ways. The anode material in most of the dedicated film-screen mammography units is molybdenum because it generates lower-energy X-rays. Since the inherent contrast among breast structures is minimal, low-kilovolt photons are important for creating high-contrast images. Some units also utilize rhodium anodes to enhance contrast in denser breasts while maintaining lower radiation doses and short exposure times. Full-field digital mammography units often use more efficient tungsten anodes, have better longevity, and can result in lower radiation doses compared to molybdenum anodes.

Full-field digital mammography (FFDM) units have been commercially available since 2000 and now dominate the mammography market [53]. FFDM utilizes an electronic system for capturing and displaying images, offering higher contrast resolution and better dynamic range compared to film-screen mammography. While FFDM has a slightly lower spatial resolution, it has superior contrast resolution which ensures the production of high-quality images. The radiation dose from FFDM is comparable to that of film-screen mammography for smaller breasts and may be lower for larger breasts [53].

The tubes utilize a rotating anode design, where electrons from the cathode strike the anode target material at a slight angle from normal incidence. In modern equipment, the typical nominal focal spot size for contact mammography is 0.3 mm, while a smaller focal spot of 0.1 mm is primarily used for magnification purposes. The nominal focal spot size is defined relative to the effective spot size at a reference axis, which may vary between manufacturers, usually specified at some midpoint in the image. The X-ray tube is positioned in such a way that the cathode side is adjacent to the patient's chest wall, as it provides the highest intensity of X-rays and compensates for the greater X-ray attenuation near the chest wall. Different target angles and tube angulations may be employed based on the choice of focal spot size and target material, especially in breast imaging.

Most mammography tubes use beryllium exit windows to minimize X-ray attenuation, and no oil is present in the radiation path exiting the tube, as materials like oil, glass, or other metals would excessively attenuate useful X-ray energies. Similar to general radiography, the spectral shape in mammography is adjusted by varying the tube voltage, target material, and the type and thickness of metallic filters placed between the X-ray tube and the breast. Using monoenergetic models, the optimum energy for film imaging is suggested to be between 15 and 25 keV, depending on breast thickness and composition.

The filament in the mammography tube is positioned much closer to the anode than in conventional tubes, allowing a given mA to be achieved at a lower filament temperature. This reduces tungsten evaporation, which is significant for mammography tubes producing low-energy radiation, as any deposited tungsten on the inner surface of the tube would absorb this low-energy radiation more readily than the high-energy beams from conventional tubes. Table 2.7 compares key design parameters for X-ray tubes used in mammography versus fluoroscopic and angiographic X-ray tubes.

2.7.3 Fluoroscopic and Angiographic X-Ray Tubes

The advancements in fluoroscopic and angiographic X-ray tubes were driven by the need for high-resolution, real-time imaging with precise dose control and efficient heat management. Fluoroscopic tubes needed to handle both continuous and pulsed operations for prolonged imaging sessions without overheating, which was addressed by advanced cooling systems and precise dose control mechanisms. Angiographic tubes, on the other hand, required high-power capabilities and rapid image acquisition for capturing detailed vascular structures, achieved

Table 2.7 X-ray tube design parameters: mammography versus fluoroscopic and angiographic X-ray tubes

X-ray tube design parameter	Mammography	Fluoroscopic X-ray tubes	Angiographic X-ray tubes
Operating peak voltage (kVp)	25–35 kVp	50–110 kVp	50–110 kVp
Tube current (mA)	20–100 mA	1–5 mA (pulsed and continuous)	500–1000 mA (pulsed)
Anode material	Molybdenum or rhodium	Tungsten or molybdenum	Tungsten
Tube exit window	Beryllium	Glass or Beryllium	Glass or Beryllium
Added filtration	Molybdenum or rhodium	Aluminum or copper	Copper or specialized filters
Focal spot size	0.1–0.3 mm	0.3–0.6 mm	0.3–1.0 mm
Beam focusing	High precision	Standard	High precision
Applications	Breast imaging	Real-time imaging, guidance during procedures	Real-time vascular imaging, angiography
Spatial resolution	Very high	High	Very high
Heat dissipation	Advanced cooling (oil, air)	Advanced cooling (liquid, air)	Advanced cooling (liquid, air)
Tube lifespan	High due to specialized use	High due to intermittent use	High due to pulsed use
Anode heat capacity	200,000–500,000 HU	300,000–1,500,000 HU	300,000–1,500,000 HU
Cooling method	Forced air, liquid cooling	Forced air, liquid cooling	Forced air, liquid cooling
Characteristic X-ray production	Characteristic peaks significant	Bremsstrahlung dominant	Bremsstrahlung dominant
Radiation dose control	Very precise, real-time adjustment	Very precise, real-time adjustment	Very precise, real-time adjustment
Operation mode	Single-shot, high-frequency	Continuous or pulsed	Pulsed
Exposure time	Very short	Long (minutes)	Very short (milliseconds)
Generator power rating	3–10 kW	50–100 kW	80–120 kW

through pulsed operation, high tube currents, and advanced beam focusing technologies. The use of beryllium windows and specialized filters in both types of tubes enhanced image quality by optimizing the X-ray spectrum and minimizing unwanted radiation.

Fluoroscopic X-ray tubes, operating at peak voltages of 50–110 kVp, are designed for real-time imaging and procedural guidance. These tubes use lower tube currents of 1–5 mA in continuous mode to provide prolonged imaging sessions with minimal patient dose. For pulsed fluoroscopy, higher tube currents may be used to achieve better image quality while still controlling the radiation dose. The anode material remains tungsten or molybdenum, similar to conventional tubes, but the exit window is primarily beryllium to minimize attenuation of low-energy X-rays essential for detailed imaging. Fluoroscopic tubes utilize aluminum or copper filtration to optimize the X-ray beam quality. The focal spot size is smaller, ranging from 0.3 to 0.6 mm, to achieve the higher spatial resolution necessary for real-time imaging. Advanced cooling techniques, such as forced air and liquid cooling, are employed to manage the increased heat load from prolonged use. These tubes also feature very precise radiation dose control and real-time adjustment capabilities to ensure patient safety. The operational mode can be continuous or pulsed, with longer exposure times suitable for extended procedures. The generator power rating for fluoroscopic systems is typically between 40 and 80 kW, supporting the continuous and pulsed imaging demands. Dual-focus tubes are commonly used in radiography and fluoroscopy systems. A small focal spot (0.6 mm) is utilized for fluoroscopy to maximize geometric sharpness, while either the small or large focal spot (1.0–1.2 mm) can be selected for image recording when high tube currents are required. Additionally, a micro-focus (0.3 mm) may be available for applications demanding very high resolution, such as interventional neuroradiology.

Angiographic X-ray tubes are specialized for real-time vascular imaging and angiography, operating at peak voltages of 50–110 kVp and higher tube currents of 500–1000 mA in pulsed mode. In modern angiography X-ray tubes, flat emitters can replace coiled filaments. These flat emitters enable smaller quadratic focal spots, enhancing the visibility of small vessels by reducing blur and improving image sharpness in all directions. The pulsed mode can be achieved using a grid-controlled or grid-switched X-ray tube instead of operating the generator in pulsed mode. In a grid-controlled X-ray tube, a negatively biased grid near the filament halts the flow of electrons from the cathode to the anode between radiation pulses, preventing unwanted X-ray production. This grid control pulsing allows parameters (kV, mA, and ms) to be adjusted within the duration of a single pulse, eliminating unnecessary soft radiation emitted during ramping.

A grid-biased tube features a focusing cup that is electrically isolated from the cathode filament and maintained at a more negative voltage. When the bias voltage is sufficiently large, the resulting electric field stops the tube current. Turning off the grid bias allows the tube current to flow and X-rays to be produced. Grid biasing requires approximately −4000 V applied to the focusing cup concerning the filament to switch the X-ray tube current off [49]. The grid-biased tube is used in applications such as pulsed fluoroscopy and cine-angiography, where rapid X-ray pulsing is necessary. However, biased X-ray tubes are significantly more expensive than conventional, nonbiased tubes.

These tubes commonly use dual-focus tungsten anodes for their high efficiency and durability under intense usage. The exit window is made of beryllium to reduce attenuation and maintain the integrity of the X-ray beam. Copper or specialized filters are used to fine-tune the X-ray spectrum for optimal contrast and image quality in vascular imaging. The focal spot size in angiographic tubes varies from 0.3 to 1.0 mm, with high-precision beam focusing to enhance the visibility of small vessels and reduce image blur. Advanced cooling methods, including forced air and liquid cooling, are necessary to dissipate the substantial heat generated during rapid image acquisition. These tubes feature a high anode heat capacity of 300,000 to 1,500,000 HU to accommodate the intense heat load from high-frequency pulsed imaging. Angiographic X-ray tubes offer very precise radiation dose control with real-time adjustments to minimize patient exposure. The exposure times are very short, typically in milliseconds, to capture high-resolution images of dynamic vascular structures. The generator power rating for angiographic systems ranges from 65–100 kW, reflecting the high power requirements for rapid and precise imaging during interventional procedures.

The combination of grid pulse and flat emitter technology offers a sharp temporal pulse profile, reducing additional doses from high-voltage cable discharge and minimizing both dose and blur. An essential characteristic of X-ray tubes used in angiography and interventional procedures is heat capacity. Due to rapid image recording requirements, heat can accumulate quickly. To address this, high-speed rotational anodes with frequencies up to 200 Hz are utilized, along with circulating water or oil heat exchangers equipped with cooling fans to enhance heat dissipation.

In dedicated angiography or interventional system X-ray tubes, maximum field of view (FOV) size requirements may impose limitations on heat capacity or the minimum usable focal spot size. When a large FOV is necessary, the anode angle must be sufficient to provide adequate coverage without beam intensity cutoff. However, for the same effective focal spot size, a larger anode angle results in a reduced focal spot width, diminishing heat dissipation rates and lowering the tube's heat capacity.

Historical Context and Technological Evolution

In the realm of angiography and cardiology applications, the increasing utilization of fluoroscopy during the 1970s presented challenges for traditional glass tubes [8]. The need to acquire sequences of images during cardiology and angiography procedures, rather than single exposures, surpassed the technical capabilities of glass tubes at that time. Tube longevity was deemed unacceptable, and the limited thermal energy that the tubes could endure per patient proved inadequate, ultimately hindering both image quality and workflow efficiency.

To address these shortcomings, GE introduced a graphite target. This innovation, while not completely resolving the issues, did reduce the rotor starting time and enhanced the durability of the ball bearings during prolonged angiographic procedures. Philips addressed the challenge by launching the Super Rotalix Ceramic™ tube SRC 1200610 [8]. This innovative tube featured a sizable anode suspended on a radially spring-supported straddle bearing system, with a rotating ceramics insulator to optimize motor efficiency. The demand for countermeasures against high patient and staff doses associated with on-site angiographic diagnostics and therapy led to the need for enhanced X-ray filtration to narrow the spectrum. A robust tube like the MRC™ was essential to leverage hard filtration without introducing image noise or prolonged cooling times [8].

Another significant advancement was the implementation of a tube current switch that operated without altering the tube voltage. Philips introduced this feature for angiography and cardiology tubes of the MRC™ series in 1992 [8]. Subsequently, it was integrated into SRM™ metal center section tubes used in radiography/fluoroscopy systems, known as grid-controlled fluoroscopy GCF™[8]. Siemens had already introduced grid control of electron emission back in 1937, resembling current modulation in radio valves [8].

2.7.4 Interventional Fluoroscopy and Computed Tomography Tubes

X-ray tubes for interventional fluoroscopy and CT require high instantaneous X-ray output, high heat loading, and rapid cooling. These demands arise from the need for high-resolution, real-time imaging and the mechanical stresses involved in CT imaging, particularly during rapid tube rotations as fast as 0.3 s per complete rotation. The mechanical forces on the CT tube during these rapid rotations necessitate advanced design features. Planar surface cathode emitters, which differ from the common helical filaments, and enhanced bearing support for the rotating anode are often used to meet these requirements.

Innovative designs, such as the integration of the cathode and anode into a metal vacuum enclosure attached to externally mounted bearings and a drive motor, enhance the tube's durability and performance under significant mechanical forces encountered during rapid rotations. This design ensures stability and efficiency during high-speed operations.

Dynamic steering of the electron beam within the tube is achieved using external electromagnetic deflection coils. These coils direct the electrons to distinct focal spots on the anode, allowing for the production of slightly different projections and improving data sampling during CT acquisition. This technique enhances image quality and resolution by providing more comprehensive data for reconstruction.

In addition to these mechanical innovations, advanced cooling techniques are employed. Direct anode cooling is achieved by circulating oil within the housing, providing extremely high cooling rates and eliminating the need for high anode heat storage capacity. This efficient cooling system significantly reduces the need for imaging interruptions to allow anode cooling, ensuring continuous and efficient clinical examinations with advanced X-ray tubes.

Interventional fluoroscopy and CT tubes operate in both continuous and pulsed modes (for fluoroscopy) and require fast rotation (for CT). Fluoroscopy exposure times can be long to accommodate extended procedures, while CT exposure times are very short, often in milliseconds, to capture high-speed sequences. The cathode emitter designs, including planar surface emitters, are specifically engineered to withstand the high demands of these imaging modalities, ensuring optimal performance and durability (Table 2.8).

2.7.5 Micro- and Nano-Focus X-Ray Tubes

These specialized tubes produce X-ray beams with extremely small focal spots, enabling high-resolution imaging of small objects or features. They are essential for applications such as microelectronics inspection, materials science research, and high-resolution medical imaging. Micro-CT scanners demonstrate versatility in their application across a diverse array of materials, encompassing fossil and non-fossilized teeth and bones,

Table 2.8 X-ray tube design parameters for conventional radiography versus interventional fluoroscopy and computed tomography (CT) tubes

X-ray tube design parameter	Conventional radiography	Interventional fluoroscopy and CT tubes
Operating peak voltage (kVp)	40–150 kVp	80–140 kVp
Tube current (mA)	100–800 mA	100–1200 mA
Anode material	Tungsten or molybdenum	Tungsten
Tube exit window	Glass or beryllium	Beryllium
Added filtration	Aluminum or copper	Copper or specialized filters
Focal spot size	0.5–2.0 mm	0.3–1.0 mm
Beam focusing	Standard	High precision
Applications	General radiography	Real-time imaging, guidance during procedures, CT
Spatial resolution	Moderate to high	Very high
Heat dissipation	Standard cooling (oil immersion)	Advanced cooling (liquid, air, direct anode cooling)
Tube lifespan	Standard	Designed for durability under intense heat loads with rapid cooling, though often shorter overall due to usage stress
Anode heat capacity	100–500 kHU	1,000–8,000 kHU
Cooling method	Air convection, oil cooling	Forced air, liquid cooling, direct anode cooling
Characteristic X-ray production	Bremsstrahlung dominant	Bremsstrahlung dominant
Radiation dose control	Moderate to precise	Very precise, real-time adjustment
Operation mode	Single shot	Continuous or pulsed (fluoroscopy), fast rotation (CT)
Exposure time	Short	Long (fluoroscopy), very short (milliseconds, CT)
Generator power rating	20–80 kW	50–150 kW
Cathode emitter design	Helical filaments	Planar surface emitters
Bearing support	Standard	Enhanced for rotating anode
Anode rotation speed	Up to 10,800 RPM	Up to 12,000 RPM (CT)
Electromagnetic deflection coils	Not used	Used for dynamic electron beam steering (CT)

Table 2.9 X-ray tube design parameters: conventional radiography versus micro- and nano-focus X-ray tubes

X-ray tube design parameter	Conventional radiography	Micro-focus X-ray tubes	Nano-focus X-ray tubes
Operating peak voltage (kVp)	40–120 kVp	10–160 kVp	10–160 kVp
Tube current (mA)	100 800 mA	0.05–1.0 mA	0.001–0.1 mA
Anode material	Tungsten or molybdenum	Tungsten or specialized materials	Tungsten or specialized materials
Tube exit window	Glass or beryllium	Beryllium	Beryllium
Added filtration	Aluminum or copper	Aluminum or custom filters	Aluminum or custom filters
Focal spot size	0.5–2.0 mm	1–50 μm	<1 μm (sub-micron to nm)
Beam focusing	Standard	Highly focused	Extremely highly focused
Applications	General radiography	High-resolution imaging, microimaging	Ultrahigh resolution imaging, nano-imaging
Spatial resolution	Moderate to high	High to ultrahigh	Ultrahigh
Heat dissipation	Standard cooling	Advanced cooling techniques	Advanced cooling techniques
Tube lifespan	Standard	Long due to low power usage	Long due to low power usage
Anode heat capacity	100–500 kHU	Very low (e.g., <50 kHU)	Very low (e.g., <50 kHU)
Cooling method	Air convection, oil cooling	Forced air or liquid cooling	Forced air or liquid cooling
Characteristic X-ray production	Bremsstrahlung dominant	Enhanced characteristic X-ray production	Enhanced characteristic X-ray production
Radiation dose control	Moderate to precise	Extremely precise	Extremely precise

small metal items, jewelry, ceramics, prehistoric pottery, stone, and a spectrum of organic materials, including wood, charcoal, textiles, and archeological remnants of food [54]. An X-ray tube capable of producing a focal spot size with a diameter smaller than 50 μm is referred to as a micro-focus X-ray tube. These tubes are categorized into two types: (i) solid metal anode tubes and (ii) liquid metal jet alloy tubes (Table 2.9).

2.7.6 Solid Metal Anode Micro-Focus X-Ray Tubes

Solid metal anode micro-focus X-ray tubes are specialized devices designed for high-resolution imaging applications such as nondestructive testing, electronics inspection, and material science analysis. These tubes operate based on the Coolidge tube principle, which involves a heated filament (cathode) emitting electrons that are accelerated toward a solid metal anode, where X-rays are produced upon impact. Again, the solid metal anode in these tubes is made of tungsten because of the same high melting point and excellent thermal conductivity properties.

One of the distinguishing features of solid metal anode micro-focus X-ray tubes is their ability to produce a very fine focal spot. The focal spot size typically ranges from 5 to 20 μm, but these tubes are capable of producing even smaller focal spots, sometimes below 1 μm. This fine focal spot size is crucial for achieving high spatial resolution in imaging, allowing for the detailed inspection of small and intricate features in various materials.

These tubes operate at very low power levels, usually ranging from 0.4 to 0.8 W/μm, depending on the material of the anode and the desired focal spot size. The low-power operation is necessary to prevent the anode from melting due to the high power density of the focused electron beam. This means that while these tubes are excellent for high-resolution imaging, their overall X-ray output is limited compared to conventional X-ray tubes, making them suitable for applications where precision is more critical than high power.

A significant advantage of using solid metal anode micro-focus X-ray tubes is the improved image quality resulting from the sharp and precise X-ray beam produced by the fine focal spot. This high-resolution capability is essential for applications such as

1. **Nondestructive testing (NDT)**: Used to detect internal flaws in materials without damaging them, crucial for quality control in manufacturing processes.
2. **Electronics inspection**: Allows for detailed examination of electronic components, circuit boards, and semiconductor devices to identify defects or ensure proper assembly.
3. **Material science analysis**: Facilitates the study of the internal structure and composition of various materials, aiding in research and development.

However, the primary drawback of these tubes is their low operating power. The need to keep the electron beam power density below a maximum threshold to prevent anode melting limits their overall X-ray output. This limitation makes them less suitable for applications requiring high-intensity X-rays but ideal for scenarios where high resolution and precision are paramount.

2.7.7 Liquid Metal Jet Alloy Anode Micro-Focus X-Ray Tube

Liquid metal jet alloy anode micro-focus X-ray tubes represent a significant advancement in X-ray technology, designed for applications requiring extremely high resolution and precision. These tubes utilize an innovative anode composed of a eutectic alloy typically consisting of gallium (68–95%), indium (5–25%), and tin (0–10%). The alloy is responsible for generating X-rays, while the continuous flow of the liquid jet serves as a coolant to manage the heat produced during operation.

The defining feature of these X-ray tubes is their capability to produce a much smaller focal spot compared to conventional X-ray tubes. Typically, the focal spot size is between 5 and 20 μm, which is approximately 50–200 times smaller than that of traditional X-ray tubes. This remarkably small focal spot enables the generation of X-rays with an exceptionally high power density, ranging from 3 to 6 W/μm. This high power density facilitates the acquisition of high-resolution images and allows for faster imaging processes, making these tubes ideal for applications demanding detailed and rapid imaging.

In the context of nano-focus X-ray tubes, the focal spot size is further reduced to the order of 150 nm. These tubes operate at very low power levels to prevent overheating, ensuring the anode does not melt despite the intense electron beam targeting such a small area. The extremely small focal spot size of nano-focus tubes allows for unparalleled image resolution, suitable for the most demanding and precise imaging applications.

The primary uses of liquid metal jet alloy anode micro-focus X-ray tubes include:

1. **Semiconductor inspection**: These tubes enable the detailed examination of semiconductor devices, allowing for the detection of minute defects and ensuring the integrity of electronic components.
2. **Detailed material analysis**: The high resolution provided by these tubes is essential for studying the internal structure and properties of materials, contributing to advancements in material science.
3. **Sophisticated nondestructive testing (NDT)**: These tubes are used to inspect critical components and structures without causing damage, providing valuable insights into potential flaws or failures in materials.

One of the main advantages of using a liquid metal jet alloy anode is its ability to handle the high heat load generated by the concentrated electron beam. The liquid nature of the anode allows for efficient heat dissipation, with the through continuous circulation and regeneration of the jet surface to maintain stable operation. This efficient cooling system ensures continuous operation without the risk of overheating, thereby enhancing the reliability and performance of the X-ray tube (Table 2.10).

Table 2.10 X-ray tube design parameters: solid metal anode micro-focus X-ray tubes versus liquid metal jet alloy anode micro-focus X-ray tubes

X-ray tube design parameter	Solid metal anode micro-focus X-ray tubes	Liquid metal jet alloy anode micro-focus X-ray tubes
Anode material	Solid metal (commonly tungsten)	Liquid metal alloy (typically eutectic of gallium (68–75%), indium (20–25%), tin (5–10%))
Operating peak voltage (kVp)	20–150 kVp	20–150 kVp
Tube current (mA)	0.1–1 mA	0.1–1 mA
Focal spot size	Typically, 5–20 μm, sometimes below 1 μm	Typically, 5–20 μm, nano-focus down to 150 nm
Power density	0.4–0.8 W/μm	3–6 W/μm
Tube exit window	Beryllium	Beryllium
Beam focusing	Standard	High precision
Operating power	Very low to prevent anode melting	Higher power capability due to efficient cooling
Spatial resolution	High	Extremely high
Cooling mechanism	Limited by the solid anode's heat capacity	Efficient heat dissipation with liquid metal cooling
Tube lifespan	Moderate	High due to efficient cooling
Typical applications	High-resolution imaging such as nondestructive testing, electronics inspection, and material science analysis	Advanced imaging applications requiring high resolution and precision such as semiconductor inspection, detailed material analysis, and sophisticated nondestructive testing
Advantages	Fine focal spots for high-resolution imaging	Extremely small focal spots, high power density, and efficient cooling for continuous operation
Drawbacks	Low operating power to avoid overheating, limited heat capacity	Higher complexity and cost due to advanced design and cooling system

2.8 X-Ray Tube Accessories

Each X-ray tube component plays a vital role in generating and controlling X-ray radiation, ensuring accurate imaging while maintaining safety for both patients and operators. Let us now discuss key components in detail:

2.8.1 X-Ray Generator

The X-ray generator is responsible for supplying the electrical power needed for the X-ray tube, allowing the adjustment of X-ray energy, quantity, and exposure duration. The conventional term "generator" does not accurately describe the role of X-ray generator devices. In medical diagnostic applications, the X-ray generator does not inherently generate electrical energy; instead, it transforms AC mains power into high-voltage DC output, often complementing X-ray tubes with additional signals and electrical support. X-ray generators function as sophisticated voltage step-up and current step-down electronics, providing the tube voltage for X-ray production and other power-related functions. They are responsible for producing the electrical energy required to generate X-ray beams for diagnostic and therapeutic purposes. These generators serve as the interface between the operator and the X-ray system, enabling precise control over parameters such as tube voltage, tube current, and exposure time (Fig. 2.45).

Hospitals and diagnostic facilities typically receive a three-phase power supply at 415 volts (360–440 V) and a single-phase power supply at 230 volts (207–253 V). However, diagnostic X-ray tubes operate at much higher voltages,

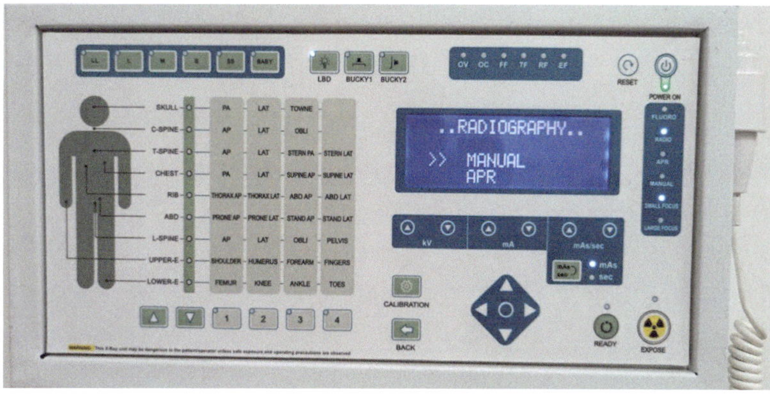

Fig. 2.45 Control panel of the radiographic X-ray generator

ranging from 20 kilovolts to 150 kilovolts. Therefore, local transformers and rectifiers are utilized within the X-ray generators to raise the supplied voltage to the required level. X-ray generators have several main components, including transformers, rectifiers, circuits, diodes, filament and stator circuits, timer switches, and kilovolt and milliampere meters. Transformers are used to step up the voltage from the power supply to the high voltages required by the X-ray tube, while rectifiers convert the AC (alternating current) from the power supply to DC (direct current) necessary for the X-ray tube operation. Diodes are essential for rectification, ensuring current flows in the correct direction. Filament and stator circuits control the X-ray tube filament's heating and the anode's rotation, respectively. Timer switches regulate the duration of the X-ray exposure, and kilovolt and milliampere meters measure and display the tube voltage (kV) and tube current (mA).

Automatic control systems within the generator, such as the phototimer and automatic brightness control, enhance the functionality and safety of X-ray imaging. The phototimer measures radiation exposure at the image receptor, providing immediate feedback to ensure optimal radiographic film densities. Automatic brightness control adjusts fluoroscopic image brightness to maintain consistent image quality. Operators can control the generator settings at the control console, including tube voltage (kV), tube current (mA), exposure time, phototimer film density, spot film acquisition, and fluoroscopic parameters. Tube voltage adjusts the energy of the X-rays produced, tube current controls the quantity of X-rays, and exposure time sets the duration for which X-rays are emitted. Phototimer film density adjusts the density of the radiographic film automatically, while spot film acquisition allows the capture of high-quality static images during fluoroscopy. Fluoroscopic parameters include settings for continuous imaging during diagnostic procedures (Fig. 2.46).

Let us discuss transformers and rectifiers used in X-ray generators.

2.8.1.1 Transformers

Transformers are used to change the potential differences of the incoming electric energy to the appropriate level. They consist of two wire coils wrapped around a closed core. The circuit containing the first coil (connected to the available electric energy source) is called the primary circuit. The circuit containing the second coil (from which the modified electric energy) is called the secondary circuit. In an X-ray circuit, the transformer assembly is a ground metal box filled with oil, and it contains a low-voltage transformer for the filament circuit (step-down transformer), a high-voltage transformer, and a group of rectifiers for the high-voltage circuit (step-up transformer). The autotransformers, which act as both a step-up and step-down transformer, depending on the connection configuration, are used for the voltage selection, where the operator can select

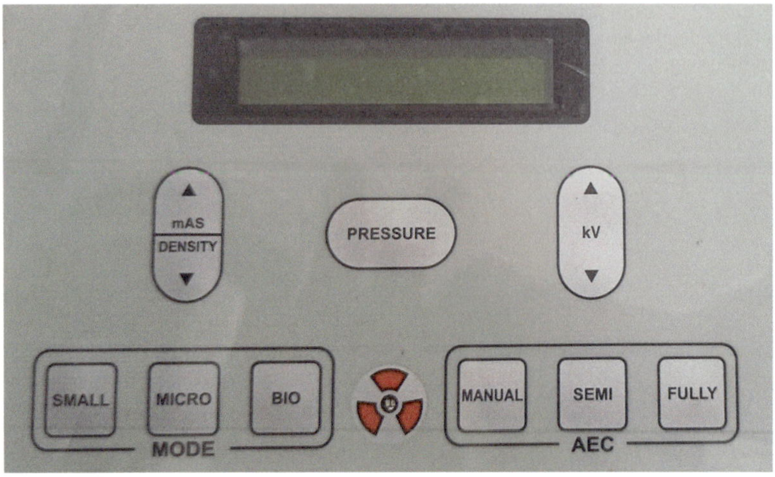

Fig. 2.46 Control panel of mammography X-ray generator

the desired peak kilovoltage (kVp) for adjusting the X-ray exposure. The explanation of these are as follows:

High-Voltage Transformer (Step-Up Transformer) It takes the incoming electrical supply, typically AC voltage (around 230 V or 440 V depending on the region), and significantly increases (steps-up) the voltage to a much higher level, ranging from 20,000 volts (20 kV) to 150,000 kV (150 kV). This high voltage accelerates the electrons within the X-ray tube from the cathode to the anode to produce X-rays.

Filament Circuit Transformer (Step-Down Transformer) It takes a relatively high voltage to step down to a much lower voltage, typically around 10 volts. This lower voltage powers the filament circuit within the X-ray tube. As the filament heats up, it releases electrons through a thermionic emission process. These electrons form a cloud around the filament and become the source electrons for X-ray generation.

Autotransformer An autotransformer is a special type of transformer with a single winding. Depending on the connection configuration, it can act as both a step-up and step-down transformer. In X-ray tube generators, autotransformers are used for voltage selection by adjusting the tapping points on the autotransformer winding. With this, the operator can select the desired peak kilovoltage (kVp) for the X-ray exposure (Fig. 2.47).

2.8.1.2 Rectifiers

The anode must have a positive voltage compared to the cathode to make electrons move toward the anode in an X-ray tube. However, the standard AC voltage power supply switches direction periodically between positive and negative, which will allow the anode to be positive only half the time, and this is undesired in X-ray tubes for continuous X-ray production. Rectifiers solve this problem by allowing current to flow in only one direction. They essentially "rectify" the alternating current, converting it into a unidirectional flow. This ensures that the anode in the X-ray tube remains consistently positive relative to the cathode, accelerating a continuous stream of electrons toward the anode. There are different types of rectifiers used in X-ray tubes, such as:

- **Half-wave rectifiers** allow current to flow only during one-half of the AC cycle. They are simple but less efficient compared to full-wave rectifiers.
- **Full-wave rectifiers**: These rectifiers allow current to flow during both halves of the AC cycle, doubling the output voltage frequency compared to half-wave rectifiers. They are more efficient and provide smoother DC output (Fig. 2.48).

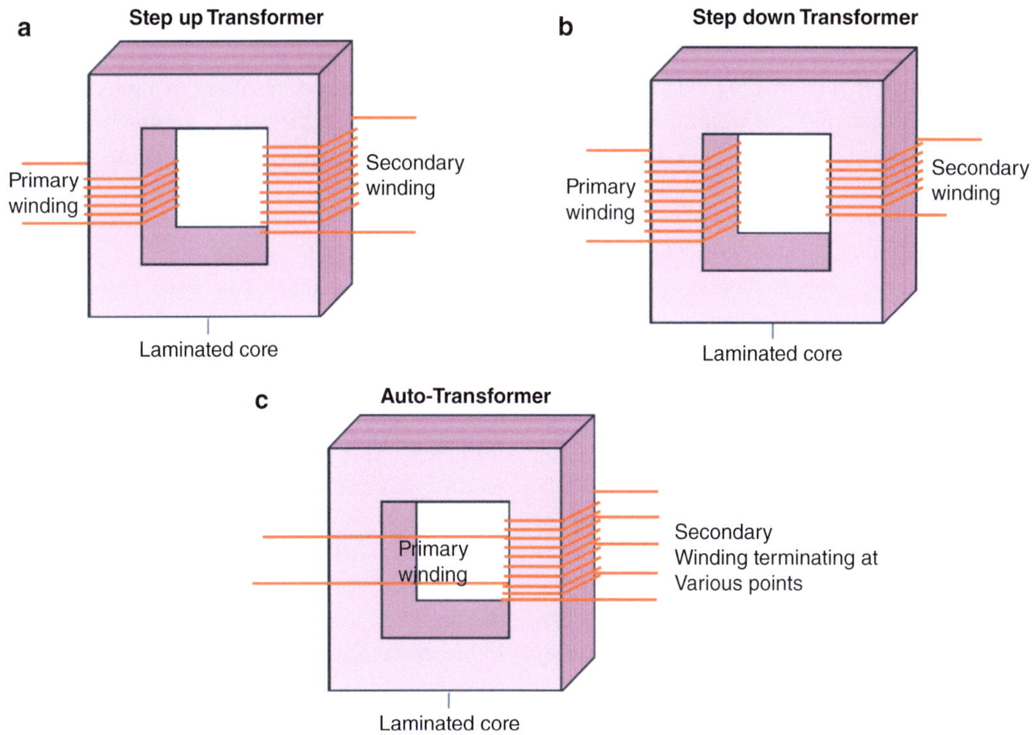

Fig. 2.47 (**a**) Step-up transformer, (**b**) step-down transformer, (**c**) autotransformer, with one wire wound around a core which serves as both the input and output of the transformer to select different voltages

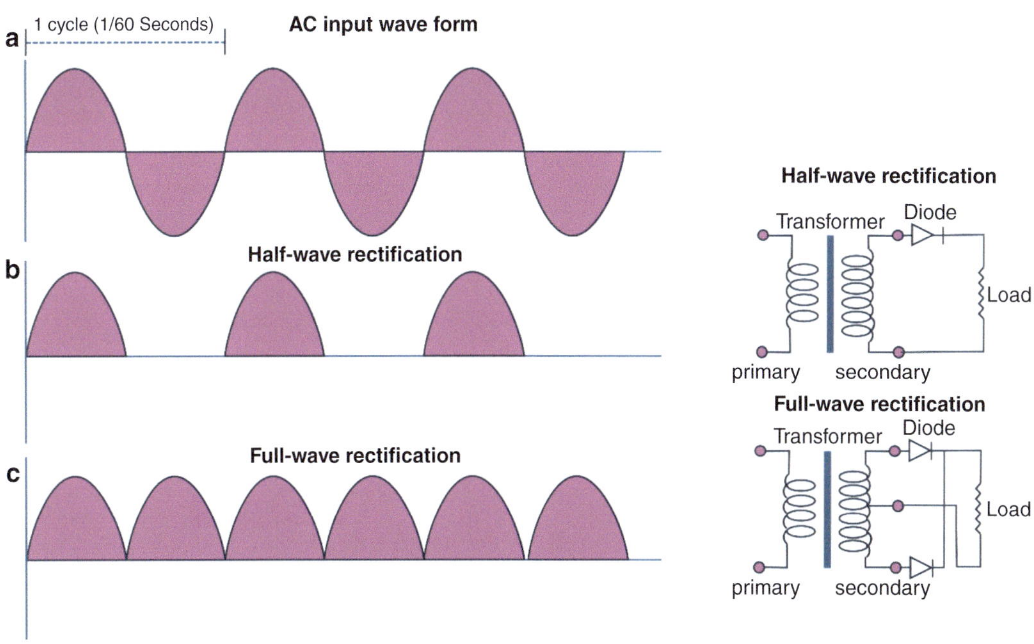

Fig. 2.48 (**a**) Input AC supply, (**b**) half-wave rectification, (**c**) full-wave rectification

Single-Phase and Three-Phase Power Supply and Rectifiers

Again, the supplied alternating current (AC) can be a single-phase and three-phase supply. In a single-phase power supply, electricity flows in a single waveform, oscillating between positive and negative values. Single-phase power supplies are commonly used in smaller medical facilities or clinics, such as portable, dental, and veterinary X-ray machines. These systems are simpler and more economical, but they have some limitations. With a single-phase power supply, there are moments during each cycle when the voltage drops to zero, leading to periods of reduced X-ray output. This can impact image quality and efficiency, especially for high-speed imaging or demanding procedures.

In a three-phase power supply, electricity flows in three separate waveforms, each offset by 120° from the others. This arrangement provides more consistent power delivery and is more efficient and used in most of the commonly used X-ray machines as they provide smoother and more continuous X-ray output, resulting in higher image quality and faster imaging times (Fig. 2.49).

Rectifiers for Single-Phase Power Supply

Half-wave rectifiers utilize only one-half of the AC input waveform, resulting in a pulsating DC output. Therefore, they are less common in modern X-ray machines due to inefficiency and higher ripple in the output voltage. They are also called "one-pulse rectifiers" and have a higher ripple in the output voltage.

On the other hand, full-wave rectifiers use both halves of the AC input waveform to produce a smoother DC output compared to half-wave rectifiers. They offer improved efficiency and stability, improving image quality and system performance. They are referred to as "two-pulse rectifiers" (Fig. 2.50).

Another full-wave rectifier is the bridge rectifier, which is widely used in modern X-ray systems due to its high efficiency and compact design. They provide smooth DC output with low ripple, ensuring reliable X-ray production. Bridge rectifiers utilize a configuration of four diodes arranged so that current can flow through the load during both halves of the AC input waveform. This configuration allows for efficient rectification of the AC input, resulting in smoother DC output compared to half-wave rectifiers.

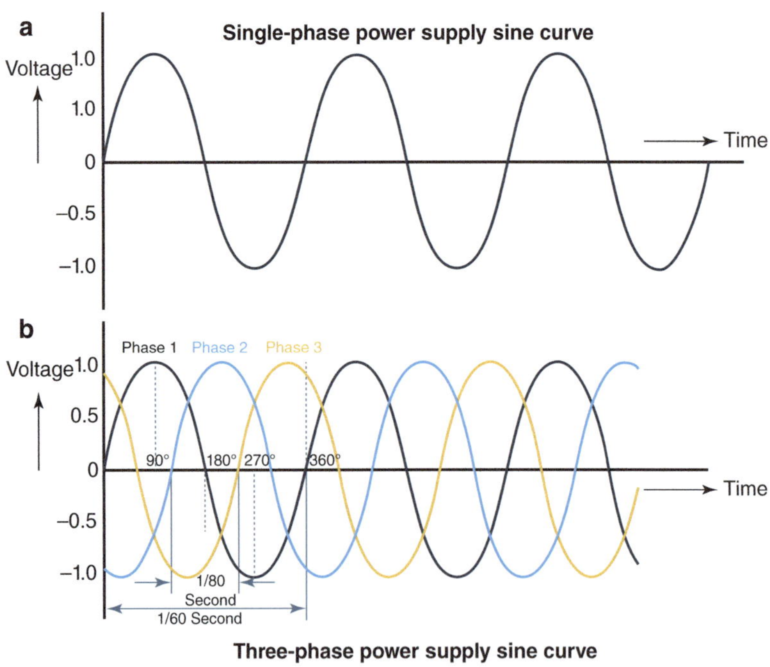

Fig. 2.49 Single-phase and three-phase power supply

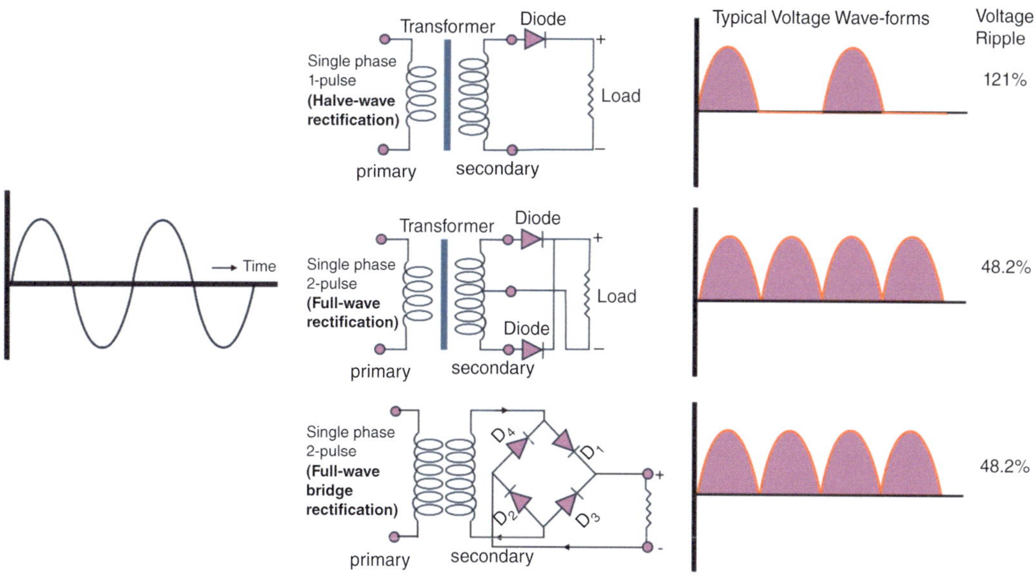

Fig. 2.50 Single-phase half-wave, full-wave, and full-wave bridge rectifiers and their outputs

When we convert AC to DC with the help of rectifiers, the output current is not as smooth as pure DC and produces pulsating DC. The unwanted AC component in the DC makes the output current wavy, known as ripple. Ideally, the ripple should be 0%, but a half-wave rectifier produces 121% ripple, meaning it has more AC than DC, making it less suitable. Full-wave rectifiers with two diodes and full-wave bridge rectifiers (with four diodes) produce 48.2% ripple.

The primary benefits of a full-wave bridge rectifier are twofold: it exhibits reduced AC ripple compared to a half-wave rectifier under the same load conditions and requires a smaller reservoir or smoothing capacitor. Consequently, the fundamental frequency of the ripple voltage doubles compared to the AC supply frequency (100 Hz), whereas in a half-wave rectifier, it remains equal to the supply frequency (50 Hz).

The advantage of using full-wave rectifiers with bridge diodes is that they do not need the center tap on the secondary of the transformer, reducing the cost and allowing for a smaller transformer. However, the disadvantage of bridge rectifiers is that they use two extra diodes, leading to a higher total voltage drop and potentially poorer voltage regulation.

Rectifiers for Three-Phase Power Supplies

In modern X-ray machines, three-phase power supplies are commonly used because they provide more stable and efficient power. Three-phase rectification is essential for converting AC to DC, and the use of six-pulse and twelve-pulse rectifiers, as well as delta and wye configurations, significantly enhances the performance and reliability of these machines.

Six-Pulse Rectifiers

Six-pulse rectifiers are the most basic form of rectification for three-phase power supplies. They consist of six diodes arranged in a bridge configuration, typically forming two sets of three-phase full-wave rectifiers. Each set handles one-half of the three-phase AC input waveform.

Advantages

- **Improved efficiency**: Six-pulse rectifiers utilize all three phases of the AC input, providing a more efficient conversion than single-phase rectifiers.
- **Reduced ripple**: The ripple frequency in a six-pulse rectifier is six times the fundamental frequency of the AC supply, resulting in lower ripple content in the DC output.

- **Cost-effective**: They balance performance and cost well, making them suitable for many X-ray machine applications.

Operation: During each cycle, two diodes conduct simultaneously, ensuring that each phase contributes to the DC output. This results in a smoother DC voltage with a frequency of 300 Hz for a 50 Hz AC supply (Fig. 2.51).

Twelve-Pulse Rectifiers

Twelve-pulse rectifiers enhance performance by using twelve diodes arranged in two six-pulse bridge configurations. These are typically fed by transformers with secondary windings configured in delta and wye connections.

Advantages

- **Lower ripple**: The ripple frequency in a twelve-pulse rectifier is twelve times the fundamental frequency of the AC supply, significantly reducing the ripple content in the DC output.
- **Better performance**: Provides a much smoother DC output, which is crucial for the precision required in X-ray imaging.
- **Improved power factor**: Twelve-pulse rectifiers offer better power factor correction than six ones, improving overall system efficiency.

Operation: The twelve-pulse rectifier operates by combining the outputs of two six-pulse rectifiers. This is achieved through phase shifting, where one set of three-phase inputs is shifted by 30°. The result is a higher frequency ripple that is easier to filter out, producing a cleaner DC output.

Delta and Wye Rectifiers

Delta and wye rectifiers refer to the configurations of the transformer windings that feed the rectifiers. These configurations impact the phase relationships and the performance of the rectification process.

Delta Configuration

- **Phase shift**: A delta configuration introduces a 30-degree phase shift between the primary and secondary windings.
- **Higher efficiency**: Typically used with wye configurations to create twelve-pulse rectifiers, enhancing overall efficiency.
- **Application**: Delta configurations are often used to balance loads and reduce harmonics in the system.

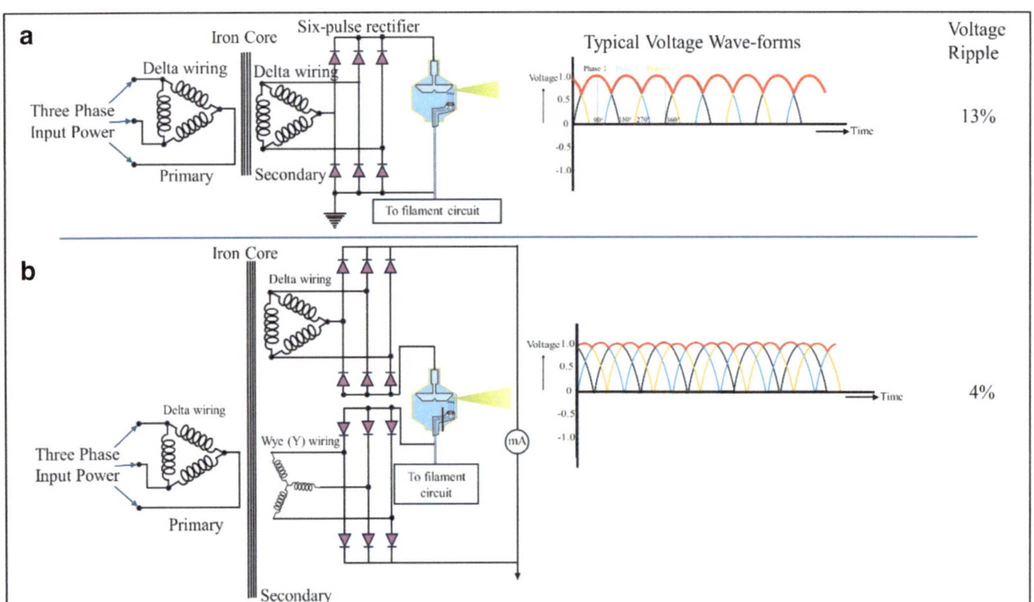

Fig. 2.51 (**a**) Six-pulse rectifier and (**b**) twelve-pulse rectifiers

Wye Configuration

- **Neutral point**: Wye configurations provide a neutral point, which can benefit grounding and safety.
- **Balanced loads**: Helps in balancing the load across phases, which is critical for the stable operation of X-ray machines.
- **Application**: Commonly used in conjunction with delta configurations to form twelve-pulse rectifiers.

Combination of Delta and Wye

- **Twelve-pulse rectification**: A twelve-pulse rectification process is achieved using both delta and wye configurations. This involves using a transformer with a delta primary winding and a wye secondary winding (or vice versa), ensuring phase shifting and combining outputs to reduce ripples and improve efficiency.

To summarize, six-pulse rectifiers offer a good balance of performance and cost, while twelve-pulse rectifiers provide superior performance with lower ripple content and improved power factor. Delta and wye configurations are crucial in enhancing the rectification process, ensuring stable and reliable DC output for high-quality X-ray imaging.

2.8.2 Basic Functionality and Type of X-Ray Generators

Various types of generators, such as single-phase, three-phase, high-frequency, and constant potential generators, produce different voltage waveforms and X-ray beam spectra. The selection of generator power and options depends on the specific clinical application. The applied voltage, known as kilovolt peak (kVp), determines the energy of the X-ray photons produced, with higher kVp settings resulting in higher energy X-rays capable of penetrating denser tissues. Advanced generators can rapidly vary the tube voltage (known as "kVp-switching") to optimize image quality and reduce patient dose during procedures like digital subtraction angiography. Additionally, generators incorporate a filament transformer, acting as a step-down transformer to provide the appropriate low voltage for the X-ray tube filament. The filament current, measured in milliamperes (mA), heats the filament, causing it to emit electrons through thermionic emission, with the tube current controlling the number of electrons and, consequently, the intensity of the X-ray beam.

Accurate exposure time control, crucial for achieving the correct image density and minimizing patient dose, is managed by the generator's timing circuits. Modern generators use electronic timers for precise control. They also include mechanisms to protect against and recover from tube arcing, a phenomenon where an electrical discharge forms inside the X-ray tube, potentially damaging it. The generator can dampen these discharges and rapidly restore normal operation.

Furthermore, X-ray generators supply a heating current to the tube's filament, ensuring consistent electron emission and stable X-ray production. In grid-controlled X-ray tubes, they provide a grid voltage to modulate the electron beam, allowing precise control over X-ray emission and rapid switching in pulsed X-ray systems. For rotating anode X-ray tubes, the generator supplies power to the stator coils, which spread the heat generated by electron impact, allowing for higher tube currents and prolonged tube life.

Continuous monitoring of tube voltage and current is another essential function of X-ray generators. Kilovolt and milliampere meters provide real-time feedback to ensure the tube operates within safe parameters. Generators are also equipped with safety interlocks to prevent operation under unsafe conditions, such as excessive voltage or current, which could damage the X-ray tube or pose a risk to the patient.

By converting low-voltage AC power into high-voltage DC power, regulating voltage and current, controlling exposure timing, protecting against arcing, and providing necessary feedback and safety interlocks, the generators enable precise control over X-ray production, contributing to high-quality medical imaging and patient safety.

2.8.2.1 Design Variants

Various X-ray generator designs, each with different levels of complexity and associated costs, are currently utilized in medical imaging. X-ray generator power ratings vary significantly. The highest ratings, ranging from 80 to 120 kW, are found in interventional radiology and cardiovascular fluoroscopic imaging suites, while modern multirow detector CT scanners typically have generators rated between 85 and 100 kW. General radiographic or radiographic/fluoroscopic systems usually use generators providing 30–80 kW. Lower-powered generators, ranging from 5 to 30 kW, are commonly found in mobile radiography and fluoroscopy systems, dental X-ray systems, and other systems with fixed anode X-ray tubes. It is essential to consider the clinical application and ensure the power ratings of the X-ray tube's large focal spot match those of the generator.

The design variants include the single-phase generator, three-phase generator, constant potential generator, high-frequency generator and capacitive discharge generators. Despite their differences, these generator types share high-voltage transformers, filament transformers, autotransformers, rectifier circuits, kilovolt meters, and milliampere meters. Different designs of X-ray tube generators tailored to specific imaging applications are as follows:

2.8.2.1.1 Single-Phase Generators

Single-phase generators are commonly used in general radiography, dental imaging, and portable X-ray systems. They operate with a simplified full-wave-rectified circuit. The circuit diagram of a single-phase full-wave-rectified generator with key components of the generator is shown in references [49, 55]. This type of generator is designed to use a single-phase AC power source. Its primary circuit comprises various components and includes:

- The autotransformer
- Line voltage compensator
- Kilovolt selector
- Kilovolt meter
- Filament transformer
- Focal spot selector
- Exposure switch

Due to the mechanical contact switch in their primary circuits, exposure times with single-phase generators are typically limited to multiples of 1/20 s.

On the secondary side of the generator, the high-voltage and filament transformers provide isolation from the primary circuit. The filament transformer regulates relatively low voltage and high current, while the high-voltage transformer produces a precisely known tube potential. In conventional generators, the output of the high-voltage transformer is "center-tapped" to the ground, ensuring safety by evenly dividing the potential difference. The milliampere meter measures tube current in the secondary circuit, providing additional safety measures despite being in a high-voltage circuit (Fig. 2.52).

Single-phase generators utilize a bridge rectifier circuit composed of four diodes to ensure that electrons flow consistently from the cathode to the anode. These generators may have "two-pulse" or "one-pulse" output configurations, with the former typically employing a longer exposure time for equivalent radiation output compared to the latter. While single-phase generators have higher voltage ripple, resulting in slightly higher patient dose and potentially poorer image quality, they are still widely used in various medical imaging applications.

2.8.2.1.2 Three-Phase Generators

Three-phase generators are configured typically as either a six-pulse or twelve-pulse generator, and a significant benefit of utilizing them compared to a single-phase generator is the considerable reduction in tube voltage ripple, and this reduction allows for significantly higher X-ray tube loading and a greater portion of its capacity to be utilized [56]. These generators are found in high-throughput imaging environments such as hospitals and medical centers. They utilize three-phase AC waveforms, offering smoother and more consistent X-ray output. Three-phase generators rely on three separate input lines, each sharing identical frequency and

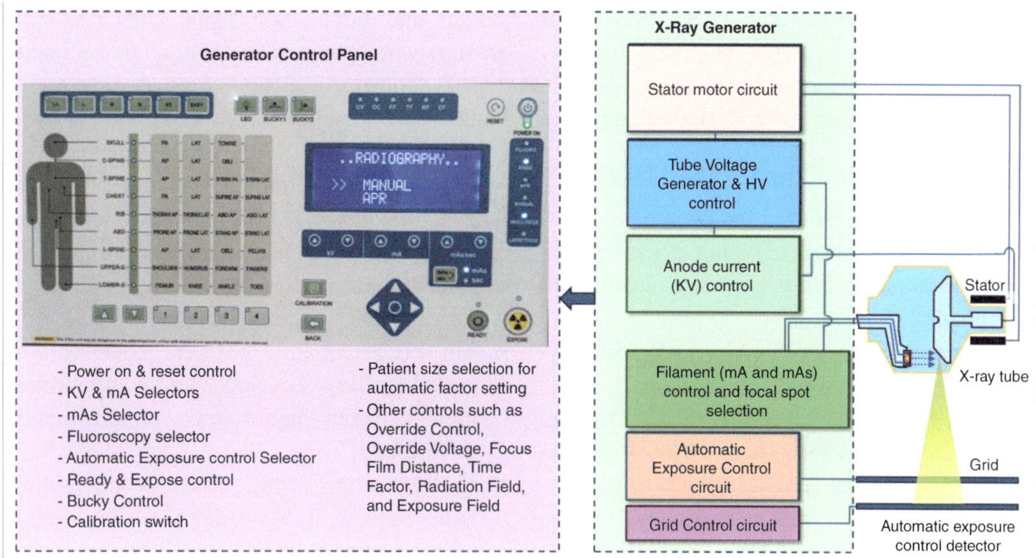

Fig. 2.52 Schematic representation of basic X-ray generator components

voltage amplitude but differing in phase. The phase represents the delay between sinusoidal waveforms relative to a starting point, typically measured in degrees. For instance, a single AC waveform completes a cycle starting from 0°, reaching its maximum peak at 90°, passing through 0 V at 180°, reversing the polarity, hitting a negative peak at 270°, and returning to the origin at 360°.

- Combining these three-phase power supplies yields an overall reduction in voltage variation in the rectified output. This is achieved through separate transformation of individual line voltages, rectification of high-voltage output, and combination of the output rectified waveform, resulting in minimal voltage ripple.
- The efficiency of three-phase generators in X-ray production is increased, and higher tube output is achieved as the average applied voltage during exposure closely matches the peak voltage.
- A three-phase, six-pulse generator consists of two delta configurations of transformers, each with three interconnected transformers operating independently with line voltages of different phases. A bridge rectifier circuit ensures correct polarity and electron flow through the X-ray tube, resulting in a voltage variation of 13–25% compared to single-phase generators.

A more sophisticated three-phase 12-pulse generator includes an input delta configuration and two secondary groups of transformers configured in a delta and a wye. This arrangement doubles the number of output pulses per cycle, resulting in 12 pulses per cycle with an applied voltage variation of 5–10% of the peak voltage.

Three-phase generator designs require high-powered mode circuits on the secondary side to control X-ray exposures. These switches enable precise on-off control of the X-ray beam within extremely short times for accurate exposure control.

However, despite desirable voltage ripple and fast exposure control, three-phase generators are more expensive, require more hardware and electronics, have longer installation times, and occupy more floor space than single-phase systems.

2.8.2.1.3 Constant Potential Generator

Constant potential generators derive their name from their ability to produce a high-voltage waveform with minimal voltage ripple, akin to

DC or "constant potential." This waveform is preferred as it ensures electrons are uniformly accelerated throughout the exposure, resulting in a higher effective energy beam and greater tube output.

- The waveform from constant potential generators is essentially DC, ensuring an even potential difference during exposure, leading to optimal performance.
- These generators are more intricate and bulkier compared to three-phase systems.
- Constant potential generators incorporate two high-voltage electron tubes (triodes or tetrodes) within the secondary circuit, controlling exposure and high voltage. They enable precise tube voltage switching on and off with about 20–50 μs accuracy and adjustment capability.
- Voltage dividers measure actual kilovoltage, which is compared with reference kilovoltage in a comparator circuit to control the grid electrode of the tubes, ensuring rapid adjustment in kilovoltage and a nearly ripple-free waveform.
- Fast electronic adjustment facilitates repetition rates of 500 frames per second or more.

While constant potential generators produce superior voltage waveforms and have the highest output power compared to other types, their high hardware cost, operational expenses (e.g., calibrations), and large space requirements have reduced their popularity for new or replacement radiographic systems.

2.8.2.1.4 High-Frequency Generators

The high-frequency generators employ advanced electronic circuitry to generate high-frequency AC power, resulting in enhanced image quality, reduced patient dose, and improved exposure reproducibility. They represent the forefront of technology in diagnostic radiographic systems and have undergone significant advancements. Its operation involves converting a low-frequency, low-voltage input into a high-frequency, low-voltage waveform, ultimately resulting in a high-frequency, high-voltage output waveform. Both single- and three-phase input lines can offer greater overall power. The AC input power undergoes rectification and smoothing to form a low-voltage DC waveform, followed by an inverter circuit that converts it into a high-frequency AC square wave. Upon transformation by the high-voltage transformer, this high-frequency AC waveform produces a high-voltage output with minimal voltage ripple.

- The high-frequency inverter generator converts low-frequency, low-voltage input into a high-frequency, high-voltage output with minimal ripple.
- It can operate using single- or three-phase input lines, with the latter providing higher overall power.
- The inverter circuit transforms the AC input power into a low-voltage DC waveform, which is then transformed into a high-frequency AC square wave.
- The resulting high-frequency AC waveform is further transformed to produce a high-voltage output with minimal voltage ripple (Fig. 2.53).

In addition to the described components, high-voltage capacitors in the secondary circuit play a crucial role in producing a voltage across the X-ray tube. The generator operates using a closed-loop regulation circuit, which ensures rapid adjustments in kilovoltage and tube current during exposures. Variations in kilovoltage and milliamperes are monitored and corrected instantaneously through feedback circuits. The design of the high-frequency inverter generator offers several advantages, including its versatility with both single- and three-phase input lines, precise regulation of kilovoltage and tube current, and efficient operation of transformers at high frequencies.

- High-voltage capacitors in the secondary circuit produce a voltage across the X-ray tube.
- The generator employs a closed-loop regulation circuit to ensure accurate kilovoltage and tube current adjustments during exposures.
- Its design offers versatility, precise regulation, and efficient operation of transformers at high frequencies.

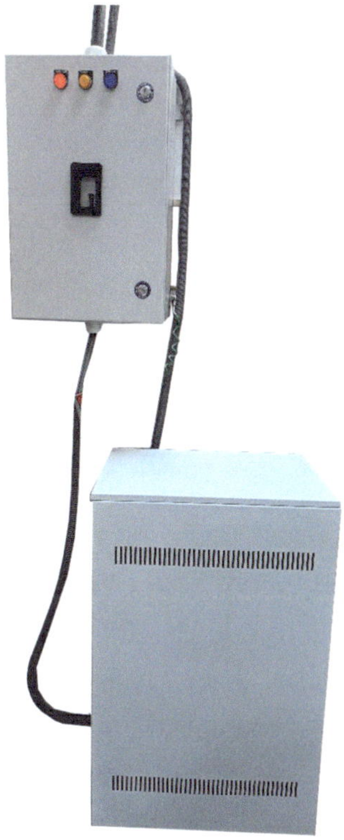

Fig. 2.53 X-ray generator and three-phase power supply

While high-frequency inverter generators are the preferred choice for most applications due to their efficiency and accuracy, constant potential generators may still be considered for specific needs, such as extremely high power requirements or fast kilovoltage switching. However, high-frequency inverter generators generally offer an excellent service record, ease of repair, and reliability, making them the preferred option for modern radiographic systems.

2.8.2.1.5 Capacitive Discharge Generators

In areas with insufficient power supply or remote settings, capacitor-discharge generators prove to be invaluable. Before each exposure, a capacitor is charged to a high voltage, ensuring a rapid energy release when needed. The capacitor is then swiftly connected to the X-ray tube, with the start and duration of the exposure precisely controlled by a grid mechanism. This setup enables the generation of high tube currents and short exposure times, which is ideal for capturing clear images efficiently. However, the discharge of a capacitor leads to a gradual decrease in tube voltage throughout the exposure. It's common for the voltage to drop approximately 1 kV per milliampere-second (mAs) during this process. This voltage drop can pose challenges, particularly when imaging thick body parts, as the decrease in voltage affects the delivered kerma, potentially impacting image quality and diagnostic accuracy.

2.8.2.2 Safety Features and Service Functions by the X-Ray Generators

X-ray tube generators incorporate several safety mechanisms to protect patients, operators, and equipment:

- **Thermal monitoring**: Continuously monitors the temperature of the X-ray tube to prevent overheating, which can lead to tube damage or failure.
- **Arcing detection**: Automatically detects and shuts off the generator in case of electrical arcing within the X-ray tube, preventing potential hazards.
- **Main fuse protection**: Safeguards against power surges or electrical faults by interrupting the circuit in the event of excessive current flow.
- **Internal safety interlocks**: Interlocks ensure that the X-ray tube can only be energized when all safety conditions are met, minimizing the risk of accidental exposure.

They offer service-related functionalities to facilitate maintenance and troubleshooting:

- **Error logging and display**: Records and displays error codes or diagnostic messages to assist service technicians in identifying and resolving issues.
- **Remote access**: Enables remote monitoring and diagnostics, allowing service personnel to troubleshoot equipment problems without being physically present.

- **Application logging**: Logs system performance data and usage statistics, aiding in preventive maintenance and optimization.

The X-ray tube generators provide precise control over imaging parameters, ensuring patient safety and facilitating maintenance and service tasks to maintain optimal system performance.

2.8.3 Filament Circuit

In the intricate system of an X-ray generator, the filament circuit plays a crucial role in ensuring stable and efficient operation. An isolated transformer supplies the necessary heating current to the filament, a crucial element within the X-ray tube. This current is meticulously adjusted by the generator programmed to match the specific requirements dictated by the characteristics of the tube in use. The isolated transformer supplies filament heating current, whereas programmed adjustment adjusts the heating current based on tube characteristics.

Heating currents can vary significantly, reaching up to 10 amperes, typically with voltages under 15 volts AC. To mitigate thermal stress and enhance durability, the filament is preheated to a temperature with negligible thermionic emission, ensuring stable operation even under varying conditions. However, the thermal inertia of the filament imposes limitations on the speed at which tube current can change, especially during scenarios such as falling load conditions. Thermal time constants typically fall within the range of 50–200 ms, influencing the response time of the filament to changes in heating current.

In systems operating at 100 or 120 Hz frequencies, some degree of tube current ripple may occur due to temperature fluctuations induced by the heating cycles. Nonetheless, high-frequency generators benefit from the thermal inertia of the filament, which helps suppress fluctuations in thermionic emission, contributing to overall stability and consistency in X-ray output.

2.8.4 Exposure Control in X-Ray Tubes by the X-Ray Generator

Most single-phase generators and low-power X-ray systems use mechanical switches coupled with mechanical or electronic timers to manage the circuit on the primary side of the high-voltage transformer. The minimum exposure time for these systems is typically 1/120 s (8 ms) because once the switch closes, it remains closed as long as power is applied. During each half-cycle, the voltage and power in the circuit drop to zero, allowing for easy release of the mechanical switch. Therefore, exposure times are generally in increments of 1/120 s.

In contrast, three-phase and constant potential generators use high-voltage triode, tetrode, or pentode switches to control the exposure on the secondary side of the circuit, managed by an electronic timer or phototimer feedback connected to the grid electrode. A small negative voltage bias on the grid (e.g., −1000 V) creates an electric field that overpowers the large potential difference (e.g., 100,000 V), as the grid is close to the cathode of the thyratron (gas-filled triode) or thyristor (solid-state triode) switch. This setup allows the switch to open and close independently of the power in the circuit, enabling exposure times as short as 1 ms or less.

High-frequency inverter generators typically use electronic switching on the primary side of the high-voltage transformer. Their high-frequency waveform characteristics allow for rapid switching, with exposure times as short as 2 ms.

2.8.5 Phototimers

Phototimers replace manual exposure settings by measuring the exposure incident on the X-ray receptor (e.g., screen-film detector) and turning off the X-rays when the proper optical density is achieved. A well-calibrated phototimer ensures consistent film optical density and compensates for patient thickness and attenuation variations.

A phototimer system includes a radiation detector, amplifier, density selector, comparator circuit, termination switch, and backup timer. X-rays passing through the patient generate a small signal in an ionization chamber or other radiation-sensitive device, amplified and integrated. When the accumulated signal reaches a preset reference value, a pulse terminates the exposure. Adjustments to the reference voltage via a density selector switch on the generator control panel can modify the optical density by ±10–20%.

In mammographic systems, the ionization chamber of the phototimer is placed behind the screen-film cassette to avoid artifacts. For general diagnostic imaging, phototimer sensors are placed before the detector because the high kilovolt spectrum makes the chamber transparent to X-rays. A backup timer ensures the X-ray exposure is terminated after a set time if the phototimer fails, preventing overexposure.

2.8.6 Automatic Exposure Controls

Automatic exposure control (AEC), another term for phototimers, is integral to most modern X-ray generators. AEC circuitry consists of detectors measuring the exposure incident on the X-ray receptor, providing feedback to the timing switch of the generator. Preset sensitivity settings are matched to the speed of the X-ray receptor, ensuring optimal radiographs by terminating the power to the X-ray tube after the necessary exposure.

Three sensors are typically used in chest or table cassette stands with AEC capability to account for varying X-ray penetration through different anatomical structures. Depending on the application, the technologist can select signals from one, two, or all three sensors. For example, in chest radiography, the outside sensors might be activated to prevent lung burnout by measuring the transmitted X-ray flux through the lungs, avoiding the high attenuation of the mediastinum.

2.8.7 Fluoroscopic Systems

Fluoroscopic systems use automatic brightness control (ABC), similar to AEC, to maintain optimal kilovolt and milliampere settings for dynamic imaging. ABC ensures consistent image brightness on the display monitor by adjusting the fluoroscopic parameters to compensate for patient thickness and composition changes during the procedure.

2.8.8 Falling Load Generators

Using phototimers or AEC systems, falling load generators minimize exposure time by delivering the maximum possible tube current for the selected tube potential. The generator's circuitry determines the maximum power load limit of the X-ray anode and reduces power continuously during exposure to avoid exceeding the anode's heat load limit. This method allows optimal film density to be achieved in the shortest exposure time, reducing image blurring from patient motion.

2.9 Manufacturing of X-Ray Tubes

The components of an X-ray tube assembly are divided into two main sections: the inner structure, known as the X-ray tube insert assembly, and the outer structure, referred to as the X-ray tube housing assembly. Within the X-ray tube insert assembly, essential parts include the anode structure, cathode structure, and envelope, which can be constructed from either glass or metal-ceramic materials. Meanwhile, the X-ray tube housing assembly comprises components such as lead shielding, high-tension voltage cable sockets, cathode filament circuit, stator electromagnetic coils, insert cooler, beam pre-collimation, X-ray radiation port and window, radiation control timer circuit, bellow, and various heat exchanger parts. For a comprehensive understanding of this classification, refer to the detailed explanation provided by M. Anburajan and J. K. Sharma in reference [40]. Additionally, the primary raw materials necessary for manufacturing X-ray tubes include nickel, copper, tungsten, aluminum, lead, glass, stainless steel (SS), mild steel (MS), and graphite.

The manufacturing process of X-ray tube assembly consists of several steps:

- Processing and cleaning of X-ray tube insert parts.
- Assembly processing of X-ray tube insert parts (anode and cathode).
- Processing of glass or metal-ceramic envelope.
- Degassing of the X-ray tube insert.
- Seasoning of the X-ray tube insert.
- X-ray tube assembly processing.
- Final testing of the X-ray tube assembly.
- Quality control of the X-ray tube assembly.

2.9.1 Processing and Cleaning of X-Ray Tube Insert Parts

To maintain the required high vacuum inside the X-ray tube, meticulous cleaning of the X-ray tube insert parts is essential. This involves thorough washing under pressure to remove any dust, rust, oil, particles, residual product, or carbonaceous surface contamination. After cleaning, the parts must be adequately dried to ensure they are free from water. Typically, an automatic, heavy-duty washing system is utilized for this purpose, employing cleaning agents such as detergent and various cleaning techniques like ultrasound vibration, isopropyl alcohol (IPA) washing, acid etching, vacuum degassing, and nitrogen drying.

2.9.2 Processing of X-Ray Tube Insert Parts Assembly

Within a controlled, clean room environment, the meticulously cleaned anode copper disk, featuring a tungsten target, is meticulously attached to the rotor stem. This rotor employs specially designed bearing balls with surface treatments, applied with nonvolatile lubricants. Concurrently, the cleaned arm of the cathode assembly is joined with an electrostatic focusing cup, connected to a nickel tube. This assembly incorporates both small- and large-sized cathode tungsten filaments, precisely spot-welded into position with micro-precision. Following assembly, both the anode and cathode structures undergo sealing procedures.

2.9.3 Processing of Glass or Metal-Ceramic Envelope

The anode and cathode structures are aligned at the appropriate distance and then carefully positioned within the cleaned envelope, whether made of glass or metal-ceramic material. Any strain in the envelope is corrected as needed.

2.9.4 Degassing of X-Ray Tube Insert

The completed X-ray tube insert undergoes thorough evacuation of all gases using a high vacuum turbo-molecular pump. Subsequently, the insert is subjected to elevated temperatures to eliminate residual gases and is then sealed to maintain the vacuum. Getter materials inside the insert are activated to ensure optimal performance.

2.9.5 Seasoning of X-Ray Tube Insert

The assembled X-ray tube insert is rigorously tested at higher voltages to ensure precise performance and reproducibility. Gradually increasing the tube current and voltage helps eliminate any remaining gases and ensures uniform potential distribution. Following recommended seasoning protocols helps extend the tube's lifespan and prevent potential damage.

2.9.6 X-Ray Tube Assembly

The X-ray tube insert is integrated into the X-ray tube housing assembly, with various subassemblies and accessories meticulously assembled to ensure quality and safety standards are met.

2.9.7 Final Testing of X-Ray Tube Assembly

The completed X-ray tube assembly undergoes visual inspection and rigorous testing under normal and heavy load conditions to ensure all performance metrics are within specified limits. Testing includes focal spot examination, noise assessment, and vacuum level verification.

2.9.8 Quality Assurance/Quality Control of X-Ray Tube Assembly

Quality assurance (QA) is important for ensuring the safety, reliability, and effectiveness of radiographic imaging systems. This process involves a series of comprehensive tests and assessments designed to verify that the technical variables of X-ray machines meet the stringent tolerance values set by regulatory authorities. The regulatory authorities recommend specific tolerance levels for various parameters measured by diagnostic X-ray machines. These include the accuracy of applied X-ray tube potential and linearity of X-ray tube current loading stations for different types of X-ray machines such as general radiography, fluoroscopy, computed tomography, mammography, and dental X-ray machines. The recommended tolerance values for accuracy and linearity vary for each type of machine, with strict criteria to ensure reliable and precise imaging. These standards are established to maintain optimal performance and safety for both patients and medical personnel.

Key Components of Quality Assurance in Diagnostic X-Rays

(i) **Voltage and current characteristics**: Bench tests are conducted to measure the accuracy of the applied X-ray tube potential (kVp) and the linearity of the X-ray tube current (mA). Accurate calibration of these parameters is essential for consistent image quality and patient dose management. Discrepancies in voltage or current can lead to suboptimal imaging or increased radiation exposure.

(ii) **Leakage radiation tests**: Leakage radiation refers to any unintended radiation escaping from the X-ray tube housing. These tests ensure that the level of leakage radiation is within acceptable limits to protect both patients and healthcare workers from unnecessary exposure. This is critical for compliance with safety regulations and maintaining a safe environment in radiological facilities.

(iii) **Noise level tests**: The noise generated by X-ray equipment can interfere with the clarity of diagnostic images. Noise level tests are conducted to ensure that the acoustic noise produced by the X-ray tube and associated equipment remains within acceptable limits. Reducing noise is important for enhancing image quality and ensuring the comfort of patients during imaging procedures.

(iv) **Vibration tests**: Vibration can affect the stability of the X-ray tube housing and the alignment of the imaging components. Vibration tests verify that the housing remains stable during operation, preventing any potential image distortions or mechanical failures. This ensures the longevity of the equipment and consistent image quality.

(v) **Focal spot size and centering assessments**: The focal spot size and its precise positioning on the anode are critical for image resolution and sharpness. These assessments ensure that the X-ray tube's focal spot is correctly sized and centered, providing high-resolution images necessary for accurate diagnosis. Misalignment or improper focal spot size can result in blurred images and diagnostic errors.

2.9.9 Regulatory Tolerance Levels

Regulatory authorities, such as the U.S. Food and Drug Administration (FDA) and similar bodies worldwide, provide specific tolerance levels for various parameters measured by diagnostic X-ray machines. These tolerance levels ensure that the equipment operates within safe and effective limits.

- **Accuracy of applied X-ray tube potential**: The accuracy of the applied voltage (kVp) must fall within a specified range of the set value. For example, general radiography machines might have a tolerance of ±5%, while more stringent requirements apply to specialized equipment like mammography machines.
- **Linearity of X-ray tube current**: The linearity of the X-ray tube current (mA) ensures consistent radiation output across different exposure settings. This linearity is crucial for dose management and achieving uniform image quality across various examinations. The tolerance for linearity typically ranges within ±10% of the expected value.

Implementing rigorous quality assurance protocols for diagnostic X-ray equipment ensures that all technical variables meet or exceed the established tolerance levels. This systematic approach not only enhances the quality and reliability of diagnostic images but also safeguards patient and operator safety. By adhering to regulatory standards and conducting regular comprehensive assessments, healthcare facilities can maintain the optimal performance of their X-ray systems, ultimately contributing to better clinical outcomes and patient care.

2.10 X-Ray Tube Maintenance and Safety

2.10.1 Recommendations to Maximize X-Ray Tube Life

To extend the operational life of X-ray tubes, consider the following recommendations:

- **Minimize filament boost "prep" time**: Limit the filament boost "prep" time to reduce tungsten evaporation and prevent tube failure due to unstable operation and arcing.
- **Optimize tube current and exposure time**: Use lower tube currents with longer exposure times to reduce thermal load on the anode and filament.
- **Avoid high technique factors for extended periods**: Refrain from using high kV and mAs settings for prolonged periods to avoid overheating and damage to the anode and bearings.
- **Follow the manufacturer's warm-up procedures**: Adhere to proper warm-up procedures to ensure even thermal expansion and prevent anode damage.
- **Limit rotor start and stop operations**: Reduce rotor operations and incorporate delays between exposures to avoid overheating and mechanical wear.
- **Regularly monitor tube performance**: Perform routine checks on tube performance to detect and address issues early.
- **Maintain optimal cooling**: Ensure the cooling system operates efficiently to prevent overheating and preserve tube integrity.
- **Handle with care during installation and maintenance**: Follow proper installation and handling procedures to prevent physical damage.

2.10.2 Filtration in X-Ray Imaging

Filtration in X-ray imaging involves both inherent and added filtration to enhance image quality and patient safety:

- **Inherent filtration**: Attenuation of X-rays by the X-ray tube materials, including glass or aluminum, which filters out lower-energy X-rays not useful for imaging.
- **Added filtration**: Additional metal sheets like aluminum or copper are used to remove low-energy X-rays, improving image quality and reducing patient dose.
- **Compensation filters**: Used to equalize X-ray exposure across different areas of the patient, improving image quality and dose distribution. Examples include wedge filters and "bow-tie" filters in CT.
- **Safety and optimization**: Filtration enhances patient safety by reducing unnecessary radiation exposure and focusing on energies useful for imaging.

2.10.3 X-Ray Generator Safety Measures

To ensure safety in the radiology department, follow these guidelines:

- **Training and certification**: Ensure all personnel have proper training and certification.
- **Radiation protection equipment**: Use lead aprons, thyroid shields, and gloves during scans.
- **Exposure time and dose optimization**: Apply the ALARA principle and use automatic exposure control (AEC) to minimize radiation exposure.
- **Control access and radiation signs**: Restrict access to the X-ray room and be aware of radiation signs to prevent accidental exposure.

2.10.4 X-Ray Tube Rating Chart

X-ray tube rating charts are vital for safe operation:

- **What is an X-ray tube rating chart?**: A graphical representation of the safe operating limits for an X-ray tube, including maximum tube current and voltage.
- **Components of an X-ray tube rating chart**: Includes kVp range (*X*-axis), mA range (*Y*-axis), and exposure times.
- **Importance of X-ray tube rating charts**: Ensures safety by preventing overheating and damage, optimizes image quality, and minimizes patient dose.
- **Interpreting the X-ray tube rating chart**: Radiographers must understand the specific chart for their X-ray tube model and follow manufacturer guidelines.

2.10.5 Safety Measures for Installing an X-Ray Unit

Consider these factors during X-ray unit installation:

- **Electric power supply**: Ensure a stable power supply.
- **Power backup source**: Provide a reliable backup for outages.
- **Room layout**: Design with proper lead protection and shielding.
- **Floor capacity**: Verify the floor can support the equipment's weight.
- **Ventilation and cooling**: Install adequate ventilation and cooling systems.
- **Lighting setup**: Provide appropriate lighting for operation.
- **Emergency off switches**: Equip the room with accessible emergency switches.
- **Proper earthing**: Ensure proper electrical grounding.

2.10.6 X-Ray Tube Overload Protection Circuits

Overload protection circuits are essential for safeguarding X-ray tubes:

- **Role of overload protection circuits**: Monitor and control tube current, voltage, and exposure time to prevent damage.
- **Key components**
  - **Current monitoring**: Detects and limits excess current.
  - **Voltage monitoring**: Prevents excessive voltage and heat production.
  - **Time control**: Limits exposure duration.
  - **Temperature sensors**: Monitor temperature and activate protective measures.
  - **Interlock systems**: Trigger shutdowns to ensure safety.

2.11 Common X-Ray Tube Failures

X-ray tubes have been a proven and cost-effective method for generating X-radiation, useful in medical, inspection, and scientific applications. Over the past century, advancements in materials, processing equipment, and design have significantly improved X-ray tubes. Today, two main types dominate the market: rotating anode tubes, primarily used in medical applications ranging from 25 kilovolts (kV) to 150 kV, and stationary anode tubes, used in inspection industries from 25 kV to over 400 kV, with some reaching the million-volt range.

- **Rotating anode tubes:** These are used primarily in a pulsed mode, handling currents above 1000 milliamperes with exposure times ranging from 1 ms to 10 s.
- **Stationary anode tubes:** These typically operate at 1–20 milliamperes and are designed for nearly continuous use, often running for many hours at a time.

Producing a high-quality X-ray tube involves controlling various scientific disciplines, including thermodynamics, heat transfer, materials science, vacuum technology, high voltage, electronics, atomic/radiation disciplines, and manufacturing processes. Effective integration and control of the X-ray tube and generator are essential for achieving desired technical results and prolonging tube life.

Factors Affecting X-Ray Tube Performance

(i) **Normal aging**
- Normal filament burnout
- Accelerated filament burnout
- Slow leaks
- Inactivity
- Glass crazing
- Arcing
- Target microcracking
- Accidental damage
- Bearings

(ii) **Deficiencies in manufacturing**
- **Immediate failures**
  - Weed out by test
  - Hold period
  - Improper materials
  - Process failures
- **Latent failures**
  - Process optimization
  - Marginal/poorly understood processes
  - Failure analysis/untraceable causes

(iii) **Application mismatch**
- Low kV/high mA emission
- Temperature/life

(iv) **Improper drive by the power supply**
- Supply impedance
- DC/AC filament
- High frequency
- Rotational speed/brake
- Filament boost
- Logic circuits
- Filament limit/filament preheat settings

(v) **Tube enclosure considerations**
- Dielectric (oil) leak
- Overheating
- Ambient temperatures
- Housing attitude
- Cable/ground connections
- Dielectric expansion requirements
- Rating discipline

Proper management of these factors is crucial for maintaining the functionality and longevity of X-ray tubes, ensuring they continue to be effective tools in various scientific and medical fields.

2.11.1 Normal Aging of X-Ray Tubes

X-ray tubes age and have a limited lifespan due to the gradual degradation and consumption of their materials, which leads to a decline in performance over time. This section details the various factors that contribute to the normal aging process of X-ray tubes.

2.11.1.1 Normal Filament Burnout

The electron beam in an X-ray tube is generated by a tungsten filament, a material chosen for its durability and ability to emit electrons effectively. Despite experiments with other materials like dispenser cathodes, lanthanum hexaboride, and thorium-doped tungsten, pure tungsten remains the best option. The tungsten filament is shaped into a helix to strengthen it and increase its surface area for better electron emission.

Over time, the tungsten filament slowly evaporates, especially at higher temperatures, leading to the formation of hot spots that accelerate the burnout process. Typically, a 10% reduction in the filament's wire mass, equating to about a 5.13% decrease in diameter, is considered the end of its useful life.

2.11.1.2 Accelerated Filament Burnout

Several factors can accelerate filament burnout, including:

- **High tube current:** Increasing the tube current raises the filament temperature, speeding up tungsten evaporation.
- **Low tube voltage:** Lower voltages at high currents also increase filament temperature and evaporation rates. For example:
- Operating at 160 kV and 5 mA reduces filament life by 21 times compared to 160 kV and 1 mA.
- Operating at 40 kV and 5 mA reduces filament life by 43 times compared to 160 kV and 1 mA.

Filament failures due to high operating temperatures are common, with tungsten evaporating non-uniformly, forming hot spots that grow and accelerate burnout.

2.11.1.3 Slow Leaks

X-ray tubes require a high vacuum to function properly. Over time, glass-to-metal seals and metallic brazed joints can fatigue and allow minute amounts of gas to enter, increasing gas pressure and reducing tube performance through materials evaporation and high-voltage arc-over.

2.11.1.4 Inactivity

Lack of use can cause gases to accumulate within the tube. When the tube is re-energized, this can lead to arc-over, especially at higher voltages. Manufacturers often recommend a warm-up procedure after periods of inactivity, although sometimes more extensive "seasoning" is required to restore proper function.

2.11.1.5 Glass Crazing

The glass vacuum wall of X-ray tubes serves as an insulator for the tube electrodes. Over time, metal from the anode and filament can evaporate onto the glass, causing arc-over and tube failure. This condition, known as "crazing" or "etching," can be mitigated by techniques like sandblasting the glass, using hooded anodes, and incorporating metal or ceramic components to reduce metal deposition.

2.11.1.6 Arcing

Arcing is common in high-voltage systems and can be caused by high gas levels, metal evaporation on insulator surfaces, and the crazing of insulators. It can also result from small particles within the tube that generate conductive films on insulators, causing focused electron beams that trigger arcs.

2.11.1.7 Target Microcracking

When power is supplied to the tube, the temperature at the target surface rises rapidly, causing stress and minute cracks. In stationary anode tubes, target temperatures are lower, but in rotating anode tubes, which handle much higher power, microcracking is more severe. This reduces radiation output and increases tungsten evaporation onto the glass, leading to higher failure rates.

2.11.1.8 Accidental Damage

Accidental damage can occur from improper handling during installation and operation. Adhering to recommended protocols and double-checking procedures can prevent such incidents.

2.11.1.9 Bearings

In rotating anode tubes, bearing failure is a significant issue. High temperatures and speeds reduce bearing life. Over time, lubricants wear off, leading to steel-to-steel contact and eventual failure. Choosing the appropriate tube type based on operational requirements can help mitigate this risk.

Understanding and managing these factors can extend the life and improve the performance of X-ray tubes, ensuring their continued effectiveness in medical, inspection, and scientific applications.

2.11.2 Manufacturing Deficiencies in X-Ray Tubes

2.11.2.1 Immediate Failures

Even with meticulous manufacturing processes, not all X-ray tubes are identical, and small differences can impact their operation.

(a) **Weed out by testing:** After production, each tube undergoes extensive testing to ensure it meets performance standards. This includes high-voltage stability tests where the tube is subjected to voltages 15% higher than its maximum operating voltage. This process removes gases and particles and conditions surfaces for high-voltage operation. Performance tests check for high-voltage stability, cathode emission, filament characteristics, focal spot size, and thermal loading. Rotating anode tubes also undergo tests for noise, vibration, and rotor and bearing performance. Tubes that fail these tests are scrapped, and the causes of failure are analyzed to improve manufacturing processes.

(b) **Hold period:** Tubes that initially pass tests may degrade over 2–4 weeks due to undetectable vacuum leaks that allow gas to enter, impairing high-voltage performance. This can be revealed through extended idle times or normal inventory rotations.

(c) **Improper materials:** Modern materials like oxygen-free copper, cobalt alloys, and high-temperature ceramics have improved tube performance, but maintaining material quality is crucial. Sometimes, substandard materials, such as extruded copper bars with stringers causing vacuum leaks, slip through quality checks. These issues are usually caught in-house before reaching customers.

(d) **Process failures:** Advanced processes like vacuum-remelted metals, turbo-molecular pumps, and high-temperature vacuum processing enhance tube performance. However, if these processes fail or lose control, it can lead to marginal or rejected tubes.

2.11.2.2 Latent Failures

Latent or unpredictable failures may occur over time and are often unforeseen.

(a) **Process optimization:** Manufacturing processes have evolved over years of experience, and manufacturers are hesitant to change them without clear evidence due to potential unknown consequences. For example, outgassing processes for anode assemblies must balance adequate removal of gases without causing hidden damage. Finding the right balance between conservatism and aggressiveness is challenging, and once a process is successful, it is often left unchanged.

(b) **Marginal or poorly understood processes:** Some failures result from poorly understood processes. For instance, the lubrication on rotating anode bearings, usually applied by chemical or physical evaporation, may require a "run-in" to distribute the lubricant uniformly. The optimal thickness is crucial; too thin compromises bearing life, while too thick causes rough operation and jamming. Historical data and trial and error guide these processes, but the underlying reasons are not always well understood.

(c) **Failure analysis/untraceable causes:** Failure analysis is crucial for identifying the causes of failures. While some issues are obvious, others require extensive analysis. However, many failures remain untraceable due to the destruction of evidence during failure or disassembly. A common issue in long-lived tubes is arcing, often caused by high residual gas pressure, insulator degradation, and field emission from microscopic particles. These particles can create minute electrical currents that induce arcing, puncture insulators, or accelerate and cause impact damage.

To mitigate particulate contamination, manufacturers stress cleanliness, assembling tubes in clean rooms and using ultrasonic cleaning or electropolishing. New tubes undergo "seasoning" at high voltage to burn off or move particulates to inactive areas. However, this process is not always perfect, and achieving a tube that never arcs is extremely difficult.

Understanding and addressing these manufacturing deficiencies are vital to improving the reliability and performance of X-ray tubes in various applications.

2.11.3 Application Mismatch in X-Ray Tubes

Early mammography illustrates how using an ill-suited X-ray tube can lead to poor results. Initially, standard diagnostic tubes were used for mammograms, resulting in subpar images and radiation burns. Over time, it was discovered that molybdenum radiation at approximately 30 kV with very small focal spots was effective for early breast cancer diagnosis. New tubes designed to meet these specifications are now the gold standard for early detection.

(a) **Low kV/high mA emission**

A common mismatch occurs when a tube designed for high-voltage use is operated at lower voltages (typically half or less of the maximum). The filament must run at a higher current to maintain sufficient emission. For example, a rotating anode tube operating at 125 kV and 300 mA needs 16% more power to function properly at 50 kV and 300 mA. This small 3.8% increase in filament temperature results in the tungsten evaporating at about three times the rate, reducing filament life by a factor of three. Higher tube currents exacerbate this issue, leading to even shorter filament life. Often, manufacturers are reluctant to create special designs for limited sales, resulting in this type of mismatch.

(b) **Temperature and tube life**

A fundamental rule for X-ray tubes is that higher temperatures shorten tube life. More power leads to higher temperatures, causing increased filament evaporation and unwanted metallic deposits that can lead to insulator arc over. Operating the target at higher temperatures also causes target evaporation and changes in radiation quality due to microcracking.

Thermomechanical stresses are another concern. Glass-to-metal seals experience increased stress with higher temperatures, potentially causing fine cracks and mechanical fatigue from thermal cycling. The more cycling, the quicker fatigue develops. Higher power accelerates fatigue. Therefore, operating X-ray tubes at the lowest usable power extends their life.

Understanding and addressing these mismatches is crucial to ensure optimal performance and longevity of X-ray tubes in various applications.

2.11.4 Improper Power Supply Operation in X-Ray Sources

In an X-ray source, the power supply is crucial for operating the tube, including the filament and often the rotor for a rotating anode tube. It also contains the logic and interlocks necessary for system operation, making it an integral part of the X-ray source. Both the tube and power supply must work in harmony.

(a) **Supply impedance**

One critical characteristic of the power supply is its impedance. For stationary anode tubes operating at a few hundred watts, a high impedance (high resistance) minimizes damage to the tube and sensitive electronics during an arc. Arcing is extinguished when the supporting voltage is reduced. In high impedance supplies, the resistance increases the voltage across it, thereby reducing the voltage on the tube and other parts of the high-voltage circuitry, protecting the system.

However, high impedance may not provide enough energy to clear up the cause of arcing, such as particles or field emissions, allowing the arcing to continue.

For rotating anode tubes, which operate at much higher power (up to over 100 kW), the supply cannot have a high impedance as it would hinder the required power. The stored energy must be limited to typically less than 10 joules to avoid tube damage during an arc. High-voltage cables and voltage multiplier capacitors store energy, and at higher voltages, the stored energy increases due to its proportionality to the voltage squared.

(b) **DC vs AC filament operation**

Filaments typically operate under alternating current (AC) conditions due to three main reasons:

1. Historical ease of control and supply.
2. Avoiding grain growth that occurs with direct current (DC), which makes filaments brittle and shortens their life.
3. Preventing focal spot distortion caused by a small fixed potential at one end of the filament under DC conditions.

With AC, any bias alternates between both ends of the filament, eliminating distortion. Under DC, especially for thin filaments, tungsten ions can form and deposit unevenly, creating "notches" that cause hotspots, increased evaporation, and eventual burnout. Filament life can be reduced by two to ten times with DC operation. Modern power supplies using DC filaments incorporate high-frequency converters, adding a low amplitude high-frequency ripple to minimize notching effects.

(c) **High-frequency effects**

Glass-to-metal seals in tubes are made from magnetic alloys such as Kovar (iron, nickel, and cobalt). Under high frequency, these materials suffer from magnetic hysteresis, eddy currents, and the skin effect, which sap energy from the current flow. This necessitates more power from the supply to overcome these losses, especially at higher frequencies, which can heat the feedthroughs and cause mechanical stress. Currently, frequencies up to 40 kHz are used. For cathode and anode supplies, high-frequency, high-voltage systems are rectified to DC.

(d) **Rotation speed and braking**

For rotating tubes, bearing life and filament evaporation are critical for tube longevity. When an exposure is needed, stator power is applied to achieve a specific rotation speed. Speeds are standardized based on commercial power frequencies: 3600 rpm (60 Hz) or 10,800 rpm (triple speed) and 3000 rpm (50 Hz) or 9000 rpm (triple speed). Due to friction and incomplete magnetic coupling, actual speeds are slightly lower, with manufacturers specifying minimum speeds like 3000, 9500, 2800, and 8500 rpm to account for slip.

Upon exposure, stator power is applied for a set time to reach minimum speed, depending on the anode's moment of inertia, stator voltage, and frequency. Rotor "boost" time typically ranges from 1.5 to 6 s. After boosting, the stator enters "run" mode, maintaining speed with reduced voltage. Following exposure, braking is applied to quickly reduce rotor speed, avoiding the damaging effects of passing through resonance frequencies (about 4000 to 5000 rpm). This sequence includes exposure initiation, stator boost, filament boost, exposure, filament idle, and anode braking. Modern power supplies allow adjustments for these sequences.

(e) **Filament boost**

When not producing X-rays, the filament is in idle mode, with current below the emission point. For exposures, the filament current is "boosted" to allow tube current flow when high voltage is applied. After exposure, the filament returns to idle. Boost times range from 0.5 to 1 s, which is crucial for rotating anode tubes with high tube currents to minimize filament evaporation. For continuous pulsed systems, the filament may run in boost mode throughout to handle high repetition rates.

(f) **Logic circuits**

The logic sequencing and performance are critical, involving interlocks, imaging sequences, radiographic requirements, and system reliability. Tube arcing can cause transients, producing circuit failures in logic. Modern power supplies use isolated logic circuits to protect sensitive electronics from transients during normal operation and arcing.

(g) **Filament limit and preheat settings**

The filament limit setting protects the filament by capping the maximum output current from the power supply, ensuring it does not exceed the manufacturer's specification. This setting should be 10–15% higher than the current needed for maximum emission at the lowest kV setting, providing headroom and better response.

The filament preheat (or standby) current, supplied during standby conditions, is typically around 1–2 amps but should not exceed 50% of the filament limit specification. It can be set to zero if fast emission current ramping is not needed.

By adhering to these guidelines, the performance and lifespan of X-ray tubes can be optimized.

2.11.5 Considerations for X-Ray Tube Enclosures

The X-ray tube must be enclosed in a suitable container to prevent X-rays from emitting in all directions, provide high-voltage insulation, and allow cooling of the tube and system. For standalone X-ray tubes, this container is referred to as the housing, tube assembly, or radiation source. When the power supply is combined with the tube, it is usually called a Monoblock® (a registered trademark of Spellman).

(a) **Dielectric (oil) leak**

The dielectric, typically oxidation-inhibited transformer oil, provides high-voltage insulation to prevent arcing from high-voltage surfaces. If oil leaks occur, air can also enter the housing, leading to arc-overs. Continuous arcing can cause carbon from the disintegrated oil to coat surfaces, which cannot be restored. Oil seals are often made with "O" rings, with Buna N rubber being suitable for inhibited oil, while materials like neoprene are not, as they swell in this oil. Manufacturers recommend compressing O rings about 5–10%, but in practice, 25% compression is used to account for high temperatures causing the O rings to lose resilience and start seeping.

The oil contains absorbed gases that must be removed by vacuum treatment to prevent their release in the housing, increasing dielectric strength, measured in volts per distance (typically over 30 kilovolts per inch). Plastic insulators inside the housing can leach chemicals, degrading dielectric strength, especially at higher temperatures. Careful testing of materials used inside the housing is essential, even for new manufacturing lots.

(b) **Overheating**

Overheating can cause arcing in both the tube and the housing. Many systems use heat exchangers with fans, and sometimes pumps, to circulate the oil. These exchangers must be kept clean, as dust can inhibit both natural and forced air convection, leading to overheating. Establishing a maintenance schedule is crucial.

(c) **Ambient temperatures**

Ambient temperatures should adhere to the manufacturer's specifications, typically around 25–30 °C. Under high load conditions, the housing can rise to 75–80 °C. If the ambient temperature is higher than specified, this increase will add to the housing temperature, causing overheating. Enclosures used to stop radiation leakage can raise ambient temperatures above recommendations. Additionally, plastic or cloth covers intended to protect equipment can obstruct airflow and lead to overheating.

(d) **Housing orientation**

The tube housing, with or without a heat exchanger, can become hot at the top due to the convection currents of the dielectric cooling oil, which rise like smoke and carry heat to the top. It is essential to ensure the best housing orientation for operation. Thermocouples can help identify hot areas, but they require good thermal contact for accurate measurements.

(e) **Cable and ground connections**

Good electrical connections are essential, especially for grounding and connections such as stators, over-temperature switches, and high-voltage cables. Tight screw connections without frayed contacts and wires are a must. High-voltage cable connections are critical; air in these connections can ionize and arc through the insulation. High-voltage grease is typically used to seal out air and ensure intimate contact between surfaces. Once arc trails start, they are irreparable. Follow the manufacturer's recommendations for cable insulator installation closely.

(f) **Dielectric expansion**

As the oil heats, it expands, requiring sufficient volume in the system to accommodate this expansion. Conversely, during shipping or cold conditions, volume for contraction must be allowed. This expansion and contraction are usually managed with a flexible diaphragm, allowing volume changes. A safety factor of at least 25% is advisable. Setting the neutral point in the expansion excursions is also crucial, ensuring the diaphragm can accommodate the expected expansion and contraction. These are key design and manufacturing requirements.

(g) **Rating discipline**

Operating within the published ratings is vital for tube longevity. Familiarity with and planning around high voltage and filament power are crucial to avoid long-term overheating and short-term anode overpower, which can cause focal spot melt. Ensure the heat exchanger operates unencumbered, especially for rotating anode tubes where proper rotation must be maintained. Adhere to individual exposure ratings to ensure the correct focal spot is energized, the appropriate speed chart is used, and proper pulse times are chosen. Coordinate charts with filament emission and volt-ampere characteristics to prevent overloads. Always double-check the charts to avoid misreading them.

By following these guidelines, the performance and lifespan of X-ray tubes can be optimized, ensuring safe and effective operation.

2.12 Advancements in X-Ray Tube Technology

Recent advancements in X-ray tube technology have led to significant improvements in overcoming existing limitations and enhancing the capabilities of X-ray imaging systems. These developments encompass innovations in design, materials, and control mechanisms, contributing to the efficiency, reliability, and performance of X-ray tubes. Here are the key advancements:

2.12.1 Advancements in Rotating Anode X-Ray Tube Technology

- **Modified shape of the glass envelope**: The shape of the glass envelope has been optimized to better accommodate various types of electrodes and the rotating assembly. This redesign allows for improved spatial arrangement, enhancing the stability and durability of the X-ray tube. These modifications lead to better heat dissipation, reduced risk of electrical arcing, and increased overall tube lifespan.
- **Use of dry lubricants**: The introduction of dry lubricants such as silver and lead in the anode rotation mechanism has significantly reduced wear and tear on the bearings. Dry lubricants minimize friction and enhance the smooth operation of the rotating anode, leading to lower maintenance requirements and longer operational life.
- **Electromagnetic induction for anode rotation**: Anode rotation is achieved through the process of electromagnetic induction within the rotor and stator assembly, eliminating the need for mechanical connections. This method reduces wear and mechanical failure points, allowing for precise control over the anode's rotational speed, and improving the consistency and quality of X-ray production. It also enables faster acceleration and deceleration of the anode, optimizing operational efficiency.
- **Offset cathode cup and filament design**: The cathode cup and filament are strategically offset to position the target track near the periphery of the beveled anode track, which is angled at 6–20°. This offset design allows for a smaller focal spot size without compromising the thermal load capacity, resulting in higher-resolution imaging. The angled anode track also improves heat distribution, reducing the risk of localized overheating.
- **Anode stem material**: The anode disk is connected to the anode stem, which is typically made of molybdenum (Mb). Molybdenum is chosen for its excellent thermal conductivity and low thermal expansion properties. Using molybdenum helps in efficiently conducting heat away from the anode, preventing overheating and enhancing the overall durability of the X-ray tube. It also supports higher anode rotation speeds without deformation.
- **Enhanced cooling systems**: Modern rotating anode X-ray tubes incorporate advanced cooling systems, including liquid cooling and improved air-cooling designs, to manage the significant heat generated during operation. Enhanced cooling mechanisms allow for higher power loads and longer operational times, reducing the risk of thermal damage and extending the life of the X-ray tube.
- **Improved material composition**: Innovations in the composition of the anode target materials, such as alloying tungsten with rhenium, have improved its thermal and mechanical properties. These advancements provide greater resistance to thermal cracking and wear, leading to more reliable performance and higher image quality.
- **Vibration and noise reduction**: Implementation of vibration-dampening techniques and noise reduction materials within the X-ray tube housing. These improvements lead to quieter operation and reduced mechanical stress on the rotating components, enhancing the user experience and prolonging equipment life.
- **Advancements in target (anode) design**: Modern anode designs incorporate different angles between 6° and 20° along with designs of biangular focus to optimize X-ray beam geometry and improve image resolution. These designs enhance imaging flexibility and allow for more precise diagnostic capabilities. Incorporation of materials like graphite-backed tungsten and molybdenum-rhenium alloys provides improved thermal performance and durability.

- **Spiral groove bearings**: The use of spiral groove bearings in the anode rotation mechanism reduces friction and wear, enhancing operational smoothness and extending the lifespan of the rotating anode system.
- **Blackening of anode disk**: Blackening the anode disk improves thermal emissivity, allowing for better heat dissipation. This reduces the risk of overheating and enhances the efficiency and lifespan of the anode.
- **Increased speed of anode rotation**: Advancements in rotor design allow for increased anode rotation speeds up to 15,000 rpm, reducing the thermal load on any single point and improving overall heat management and X-ray production efficiency [57].
- **Metal-ceramic tubes technology**: Metal-ceramic tubes combine the thermal and electrical advantages of metal with the insulating properties of ceramics. This technology enhances tube performance, durability, and reliability under high-stress conditions.

2.12.2 Grid-Controlled X-Ray Tubes

Grid-controlled X-ray tubes provide enhanced control over the X-ray beam, allowing for rapid switching and precise modulation of exposure times. This improves image quality and reduces patient dose.

2.12.3 High-Power X-Ray Tubes

Technical advances have been made to achieve high power levels and address issues of target temperature, heat storage, and heat dissipation:

- **Redesigned tube envelope, cathode, and anode assemblies**: Including anode rotation and target design improvements.
- **Increased anode heat capacities**: Anode heat capacities have increased by up to five times, preventing cooling delays during most clinical procedures, with tubes now capable of 5–8 million heat units.
- **Improved heat dissipation rate**: Enhancements in the heat dissipation rate have significantly increased the heat storage capacity of modern X-ray tubes.
- **Thick graphite backing of target disks**: Use of thick graphite backing, large anode diameters (200 mm or more), improved high-temperature rotor bearings, and metal housings with ceramic insulators.
- **Extended tube lifespan**: Modern tubes offer a working life ranging from 10,000 to 40,000 h, compared to the 1000 h typical of conventional CT tubes.

2.12.4 Dose Management

- **Automatic exposure control (AEC) systems**: GE, Siemens, Toshiba along with other companies have expanded their AEC systems to vary the X-ray tube current in response to patient attenuation, improving dose management and image quality.

The continuous advancements in X-ray tube technology have significantly improved their performance, reliability, and lifespan. Innovations in the shape of the glass envelope, the use of dry lubricants, electromagnetic induction for rotation, offset cathode cup and filament design, and the use of molybdenum for the anode stem have collectively enhanced the efficiency of these critical medical imaging components. Additionally, improvements in cooling systems, material composition, and vibration and noise reduction further contribute to the technological evolution of rotating anode X-ray tubes, ensuring they meet the demanding requirements of modern medical imaging. With the increasing use of artificial intelligence, these advancements will further progress at a more rapid pace, ushering in a new era of enhanced diagnostic capabilities and patient care.

Exercise

Multiple-Choice Questions

1. What is the primary material used for the filament in X-ray tubes due to its high melting point and thermionic emission properties?
   A. Platinum
   B. Tungsten
   C. Molybdenum
   D. Graphite
2. Which X-ray tube modality typically operates at tube voltages between 20 and 45 kV?
   A. General radiography
   B. Computed tomography
   C. Mammography
   D. Fluoroscopy
3. In which application is X-ray technology used to detect contaminants and pesticide residues?
   A. Automotive
   B. Food and agro
   C. Nanotechnology
   D. Aerospace
4. What key characteristic of X-rays makes them useful for medical diagnostics?
   A. High energy density
   B. Ability to penetrate solid objects
   C. Ability to emit visible light
   D. Low cost of production
5. Which scientist is credited with the discovery of X-rays in 1895?
   A. Wilhelm Conrad Röntgen
   B. William Crookes
   C. Michael Faraday
   D. John Hittorf
6. What was a major issue faced by Crookes tubes in early X-ray production?
   A. Difficulty in liberating electrons from the electrode
   B. Inconsistent gas pressure
   C. Inefficient electron emission
   D. High risk of tube explosion
7. What advancement did William D. Coolidge introduce in 1913 that revolutionized X-ray technology?
   A. The rotating anode
   B. The hot cathode X-ray tube
   C. The line focus tube
   D. The Metalix tube
8. What was a key feature of Goetze's line focus tube introduced in 1918?
   A. Broad filament cathode design
   B. Line-shaped filament
   C. High-pressure gas environment
   D. Tungsten anode
9. What was the primary material used in the anode of the Philips Metalix tube introduced in 1925?
   A. Tungsten
   B. Chromium-iron alloy
   C. Molybdenum
   D. Carbon
10. What was a major innovation of the Super Rotalix (SRO) tube introduced by Philips in 1959?
    A. Use of a composite molybdenum substrate
    B. Introduction of rotating anodes
    C. Improved vacuum insulation
    D. Use of liquid metal for cooling
11. What is the primary function of the filament in an X-ray tube?
    A. To focus the electron beam
    B. To convert X-rays into electrical signals
    C. To generate electrons through thermionic emission
    D. To cool the anode
12. Which material is commonly used for the filament in X-ray tubes due to its high melting point and efficient electron emission?
    A. Copper
    B. Molybdenum
    C. Tungsten
    D. Lead
13. What is the main advantage of a rotating anode X-ray tube compared to a stationary anode tube?
    A. Simplicity in design
    B. Better heat dissipation and higher power output
    C. Lower cost
    D. Reduced risk of filament damage

14. Which type of X-ray tube is specifically designed for high-speed imaging sequences and rapid rotation?
    A. High-speed rotating anode X-ray tube
    B. Mammographic rotating anode X-ray tube
    C. Liquid metal bearing rotating anode X-ray tube
    D. Dual-focus rotating anode X-ray tube
15. What is the purpose of the glass envelope in an X-ray tube?
    A. To provide electrical insulation and maintain a vacuum
    B. To enhance the X-ray image resolution
    C. To cool the cathode and anode
    D. To focus the electron beam on the anode
16. What is the primary function of the filament in the X-ray tube's cathode assembly?
    A. To focus the electron beam on the anode
    B. To generate high voltage across the cathode and anode
    C. To emit electrons through thermionic emission
    D. To support the anode during rotation
17. Why is tungsten commonly used as the material for the filament in X-ray tubes?
    A. It has a low work function
    B. It has a high melting point and excellent thermionic emission properties
    C. It is inexpensive and easy to manufacture
    D. It provides a high atomic number for increased X-ray production
18. What is the main advantage of a rotating anode in X-ray tubes?
    A. It increases the focal spot size for better image resolution
    B. It enhances the heat dissipation by spreading the heat over a larger surface area
    C. It reduces the cost of manufacturing X-ray tubes
    D. It allows the use of lower voltage in the X-ray tube
19. Which bearing technology uses a thin film of lubricant maintained within spiral grooves?
    A. Ball bearings
    B. Liquid metal bearings
    C. Spiral groove bearings
    D. Magnetic bearings
20. What effect does the anode angle have on the X-ray beam?
    A. It increases the X-ray tube's operational voltage
    B. It affects the effective focal spot size and heat management
    C. It enhances the cathode's thermionic emission properties
    D. It controls the rotation speed of the anode disk
21. What is the primary function of the tube envelope in an X-ray tube?
    A. To enhance the X-ray beam intensity
    B. To house the cathode and anode assemblies within a vacuum-sealed enclosure
    C. To filter the X-ray beam
    D. To dissipate heat from the X-ray tube
22. Why is beryllium commonly used for the X-ray window in X-ray tubes?
    A. It has a high atomic number
    B. It has excellent thermal conductivity
    C. It provides low absorption of X-rays
    D. It is cost-effective
23. Which material is preferred for the construction of high-tension (HT) cable sockets in X-ray systems due to its electrical insulation properties?
    A. Glass
    B. Aluminum
    C. Stainless steel
    D. Ceramic
24. What is the main purpose of beam collimation in X-ray systems?
    A. To increase the intensity of the X-ray beam
    B. To direct the X-ray beam toward the area of interest and reduce scatter radiation
    C. To shield the X-ray tube from external damage
    D. To manage the thermal load of the X-ray tube
25. What is the role of the stator electromagnetic coils in rotating anode X-ray tubes?
    A. To provide electrical insulation
    B. To generate a rotating magnetic field that causes the anode to spin

C. To support the X-ray tube mechanically
D. To regulate the X-ray exposure time
26. Which anode material is commonly used in film-screen mammography units to generate lower-energy X-rays?
A. Tungsten
B. Rhodium
C. Molybdenum
D. Beryllium
27. In dental X-ray systems, what is the typical focal spot size?
A. 1.0 mm
B. 0.8 mm
C. 0.5 mm
D. 0.3 mm
28. Which of the following features is NOT typically associated with fluoroscopic X-ray tubes?
A. High-precision beam focusing
B. High tube currents of 500–1000 mA
C. Use of tungsten or molybdenum anodes
D. Long exposure times in continuous mode
29. What is the primary reason for using beryllium exit windows in mammography X-ray tubes?
A. To enhance image contrast
B. To minimize X-ray attenuation
C. To increase X-ray beam intensity
D. To improve anode cooling
30. In which X-ray tubes is the focal spot size typically around 5 μm?
A. Conventional radiography tubes
B. Micro-focus X-ray tubes
C. Nano-focus X-ray tubes
D. Angiographic X-ray tubes
31. What is the primary function of the X-ray generator?
A. To directly produce X-rays from electrical energy
B. To convert AC mains power into high-voltage DC output for the X-ray tube
C. To control the filament heating in the X-ray tube
D. To capture X-ray images
32. What type of rectifier is used to ensure that the anode in an X-ray tube remains positive relative to the cathode?
A. Half-wave rectifier
B. Full-wave rectifier
C. Bridge rectifier
D. Three-phase rectifier
33. Which component of an X-ray generator is responsible for stepping up the voltage to the high levels required for X-ray production?
A. Filament transformer
B. High-voltage transformer
C. Autotransformer
D. Rectifier
34. What is the key advantage of using a twelve-pulse rectifier in X-ray machines?
A. Lower ripple frequency in the DC output
B. Simpler circuit design
C. Lower operational costs
D. Higher energy consumption
35. Which type of X-ray generator is typically used for high-throughput imaging environments due to its smooth and consistent X-ray output?
A. Single-phase generator
B. Capacitive discharge generator
C. Three-phase generator
D. High-frequency generator
36. What is the primary purpose of the degassing process in X-ray tube manufacturing?
A. To clean the X-ray tube insert
B. To remove all gases and activate getter materials
C. To season the X-ray tube insert
D. To assemble the anode and cathode structures
37. Which component is not part of the X-ray tube housing assembly?
A. Lead shielding
B. Cathode filament circuit
C. Beam pre-collimation
D. X-ray tube envelope
38. What is the purpose of quality assurance (QA) in the context of diagnostic X-ray machines?
A. To enhance image quality only
B. To verify that the equipment meets regulatory standards and safety requirements
C. To test the mechanical stability of the X-ray tube
D. To calibrate the X-ray tube voltage and current

39. In X-ray tube maintenance, which of the following is a recommended practice to maximize tube life?
    A. Use high kV and mAs settings for extended periods
    B. Minimize filament boost “prep” time
    C. Avoid regular performance monitoring
    D. Skip warm-up procedures
40. What is the primary role of added filtration in X-ray imaging?
    A. To improve image resolution
    B. To reduce patient dose by removing low-energy X-rays
    C. To enhance the X-ray tube’s cooling efficiency
    D. To stabilize the X-ray tube housing
41. What is a primary factor in accelerating filament burnout in X-ray tubes?
    A. High filament temperature
    B. High ambient temperature
    C. Low filament voltage
    D. Excessive dielectric oil
42. Which material is most commonly used for the filament in X-ray tubes due to its durability and electron emission properties?
    A. Lanthanum hexaboride
    B. Thorium-doped tungsten
    C. Dispenser cathodes
    D. Pure tungsten
43. What is the main consequence of high tube currents in X-ray tubes?
    A. Reduced filament temperature
    B. Increased filament life
    C. Accelerated tungsten evaporation
    D. Decreased target microcracking
44. In rotating anode X-ray tubes, what is one of the advancements used to improve heat dissipation?
    A. Increased ambient temperatures
    B. Enhanced cooling systems
    C. Reduced anode rotation speeds
    D. Decreased filament temperature
45. What is a key factor in preventing arcing in high-voltage X-ray tubes?
    A. High filament current
    B. Low impedance power supply
    C. High-frequency operation
    D. High ambient temperature
46. Which component is typically included in a dental X-ray unit to enhance its functionality?
    A. High-voltage transformer
    B. Rotating anode
    C. Beryllium exit window
    D. Liquid metal jet anode
47. For mammography, which anode material is most commonly used due to its ability to generate lower-energy X-rays?
    A. Tungsten
    B. Rhodium
    C. Molybdenum
    D. Beryllium
48. What is the primary reason for using beryllium as the exit window material in mammography tubes?
    A. To enhance X-ray beam quality
    B. To minimize X-ray attenuation
    C. To increase tube lifespan
    D. To improve anode heat capacity
49. In angiographic X-ray tubes, what is the purpose of the grid-controlled X-ray tube?
    A. To enhance image resolution
    B. To enable real-time image adjustments
    C. To stop electron flow between radiation pulses
    D. To minimize heat generation
50. Which cooling method is commonly used in interventional fluoroscopy and CT tubes to manage the high heat load?
    A. Air convection
    B. Liquid cooling
    C. Forced air
    D. Oil cooling

Short Questions

1. Explain the significance of Wilhelm Conrad Röntgen’s discovery of X-rays and how it impacted medical diagnostics.
2. Describe the main operational differences between X-ray tubes used for mammography and those used for computed tomography (CT).
3. Describe the key improvements introduced by the Coolidge tube compared to the Crookes tube.

4. How did the introduction of the rotating anode tube in 1929 impact X-ray technology?
5. Describe the role of the focusing cup in the X-ray tube's cathode assembly.
6. What are the benefits of using a tungsten-rhenium alloy for the anode target in X-ray tubes?
7. Explain why ceramics are becoming increasingly popular in modern X-ray tube designs compared to glass.
8. Describe the function of the radiation control timer circuit in an X-ray system.
9. Describe the significance of the filament position in dental X-ray tubes and its effect on efficiency.
10. Explain the advantage of using a rotating anode in mammography X-ray tubes.
11. Describe the role of autotransformers in X-ray generators and how they adjust the peak kilovoltage (kVp) for X-ray exposure.
12. Explain the significance of using phototimers in X-ray systems and how they contribute to consistent film optical density.
13. Describe the steps involved in the assembly processing of X-ray tube insert parts.
14. Explain how X-ray tube rating charts help ensure safe operation of X-ray equipment.
15. Describe how "glass crazing" affects the performance of X-ray tubes and how it can be mitigated.
16. Explain the role of "dry lubricants" in modern rotating anode X-ray tubes.
17. Describe the primary difference in focal spot size requirements between mammography and conventional radiography X-ray tubes.

Long Question

1. Discuss the historical development of X-ray technology, highlighting key experiments and advancements from the seventeenth to the early twentieth century. Include the contributions of early scientists, the evolution of X-ray tubes, and the rapid integration of X-ray technology into medical practice following Wilhelm Conrad Röntgen's discovery.
2. Discuss the evolution of X-ray tube technology from the early Crookes tubes to the modern Super Rotalix Ceramic (SRC) tube. Highlight key technological advancements and their impact on X-ray imaging performance and clinical applications.
3. Discuss the significance of the heel effect in X-ray imaging and explain how it can be managed to optimize image quality, particularly in mammography.
4. Discuss the various heat dissipation mechanisms employed in X-ray tubes and explain how advancements in technology have improved the efficiency of these mechanisms. Include the role of rotating anodes, coolant circulation, and modern cooling systems in managing heat during X-ray production.
5. Discuss the advancements in X-ray tube design that address the needs of high-resolution imaging in computed tomography (CT) and interventional fluoroscopy. Include in your discussion the role of cooling systems, tube current specifications, and focal spot sizes. How do these advancements contribute to the performance and reliability of modern X-ray imaging systems?
6. Discuss the differences between single-phase and three-phase X-ray generators in terms of their efficiency, voltage ripple, and typical applications. Include how each type of generator affects the quality of X-ray imaging and its suitability for different clinical settings.
7. Discuss the comprehensive quality assurance procedures for diagnostic X-ray machines and their importance in maintaining optimal performance and safety. Include an explanation of key components such as voltage and current characteristics, leakage radiation tests, and noise level tests.
8. Discuss the impact of "slow leaks" in X-ray tubes on their performance and lifespan. Include the mechanisms by which slow leaks affect tube performance and outline the preventive measures that can be taken to address this issue.

MCQ Answers

1. B. Tungsten
2. C. Mammography
3. B. Food and Agro
4. B. Ability to penetrate solid objects
5. A. Wilhelm Conrad Röntgen
6. A. Difficulty in liberating electrons from the electrode
7. B. The hot cathode X-ray tube
8. B. Line-shaped filament
9. B. Chromium-iron alloy
10. A. Use of a composite molybdenum substrate
11. C. To generate electrons through thermionic emission
12. C. Tungsten
13. B. Better heat dissipation and higher power output
14. A. High-speed rotating anode X-ray tube
15. A. To provide electrical insulation and maintain a vacuum
16. C. To emit electrons through thermionic emission
17. B. It has a high melting point and excellent thermionic emission properties
18. B. It enhances the heat dissipation by spreading the heat over a larger surface area
19. C. Spiral groove bearings
20. B. It affects the effective focal spot size and heat management
21. B. To house the cathode and anode assemblies within a vacuum-sealed enclosure
22. C. It provides low absorption of X-rays
23. D. Ceramic
24. B. To direct the X-ray beam toward the area of interest and reduce scatter radiation
25. B. To generate a rotating magnetic field that causes the anode to spin
26. C. Molybdenum
27. B. 0.8 mm
28. D. Long exposure times in continuous mode
29. B. To minimize X-ray attenuation
30. B. Micro-focus X-ray tubes
31. B. To convert AC mains power into high-voltage DC output for the X-ray tube
32. B. Full-wave rectifier
33. B. High-voltage transformer
34. A. Lower ripple frequency in the DC output
35. C. Three-phase generator
36. B. To remove all gases and activate getter materials
37. D. X-ray tube envelope
38. B. To verify that the equipment meets regulatory standards and safety requirements
39. B. Minimize filament boost "prep" time
40. B. To reduce patient dose by removing low-energy X-rays
41. A. High filament temperature
42. B. Thorium-doped tungsten
43. C. Accelerated tungsten evaporation
44. B. Enhanced cooling systems
45. B. Low impedance power supply
46. A. High-voltage transformer
47. C. Molybdenum
48. B. To minimize X-ray attenuation
49. C. To stop electron flow between radiation pulses
50. B. Liquid cooling

References

1. INTELL IQ. 2024–2031 Global and Regional Rotating Anode X-ray Tubes Industry Status and Prospects Professional Market Research Report Standard Version. 2024. https://www.linkedin.com/pulse/rotating-anode-x-ray-tubes-market-research--report-provides-thorough/.
2. Heilbron JL. Electricity in the 17th and 18th centuries: a study of early modern physics. University of California Press; 1979.
3. Hollenback KL, Bell CL, Brian SM. Draw the lightning down: Benjamin Franklin and Electrical Technology in the age of enlightenment. University of California Press; 2003.
4. Mould RF, The early history of x-ray diagnosis with emphasis on the contributions of physics 1895–1915; 1995.
5. Jousten K. The history of vacuum science and vacuum technology. In: Handbook of vacuum technology. Wiley; 2016. p. 1–18. https://doi.org/10.1002/9783527688265.ch1.
6. Macnalty A, Ashworth Underwood E. Section of the history of medicine and the early development of radiology. Proc R Soc Med. 1945;
7. Philips CES. Bibliography of X-ray literature and research (1896–1897). Nature. 1897;
8. Behling R. X-RAY Tubes development - IOMP History of Medical Physics. 2018. [Online]. Available: https://commons.wikimedia.org/w/index.php?curid=3068002.

9. Behling R. Modern diagnostic X-ray sources; technology, manufacturing, reliability, 2nd edn; 2021.
10. Nascimento MLF. Brief history of X-ray tube patents. World Patent Inf. 2014;37:48–53. https://doi.org/10.1016/j.wpi.2014.02.008.
11. Meggitt G. Taming the rays: a history of radiation and protection. 2nd ed. Pitchpole Books; 2018. ISBN-978-0957554986
12. Dyson NA. X-rays in atomic and nuclear physics; 1990.
13. Gaertner G, Knapp W, Forbes RG. Modern developments in vacuum electron sources; 2021. [Online]. Available: http://www.springer.com/series/560
14. Frankel R. Articles Centennial of Rontgen's Discovery of X-rays; 1995.
15. Paul S. Biomedical engineering and its applications in healthcare. Springer Singapore. 2019; https://doi.org/10.1007/978-981-13-3705-5.
16. Prabhu S, Naveen DK, Bangera S, Subrahmanya Bhat B. Production of X-RAYS using X-RAY tube. J Phys Conf Ser (IOP Publishing Ltd). 2020; https://doi.org/10.1088/1742-6596/1712/1/012036.
17. Robinson RC, Moore CN. Manufacture Coolidge-X-ray-tube; 1920.
18. Hofman JAM. The art of medical imaging: Philips and the evolution of medical X-ray technology; 2010.
19. Lilienfeld JE. Method and apparatus for controlling electric currents, Patent No. 1,745,175; 1926.
20. Gibeaut WA, Ogden HR, Ratliff JL. Tungsten research and development review: 1960–1962. Columbus: Defence Metals Information Centre; 1963.
21. Haus Arthur G. Historical-technical-developments-in-mammography. Technol Cancer Res Treat. 2002;1(2):119–26. ISSN 1533-0346
22. William REH, Love D. X-ray tube anode with alloyed surface and method of making the same- Patent US4109058; 1976.
23. Behling R. The MRC 200: A new high-output X-ray tube. 1990. [Online]. Available: https://www.researchgate.net/publication/293424361
24. Kalender WA. Principles and applications of spiral CT. Nucl Med Biol. 1994;21(5):693–9. https://doi.org/10.1016/0969-8051(94)90039-6.
25. Ltd. Canon Electron Tubes & Devices Co., Company History – Canon.
26. Robert IK, Kim H. Thin rotating plate target for X-Ray tube US6560315, US – Patents. 2002.
27. Schardt P, et al. New x-ray tube performance in computed tomography by introducing the rotating envelope tube technology. Med Phys. 2004;31(9):2699–706. https://doi.org/10.1118/1.1783552.
28. Paolo R. Handbook of X-ray imaging. New York: CRC Press/Taylor & Francis Group; 2018.
29. Behling R. X-ray sources: 125 years of developments of this intriguing technology. Phys Med. 2020;79:162–87. https://doi.org/10.1016/j.ejmp.2020.07.021.
30. The Phillips. Phillips metalix x-ray tubes, London; 1925. https://doi.org/10.1016/S0140-6736(01)42484-6.
31. Philips Museum. Metalix and Rotalix: pioneering innovations in X-ray technology. https://www.philips.nl/en/a-w/philips-museum/stories/metalix-rotalix.html.
32. Boersma K. Tensions within an industrial research laboratory: the Philips Laboratory's X-ray Department between the wars. Enterp Soc. 2003;4(1):65–98. https://doi.org/10.1017/s1467222700012453.
33. Hart W, Peter D, Reiber K. A metal/ceramic diagnostié X-ray tube; 1983.
34. Parker TS. Varian rotating anode fin patent 1986. 1987.
35. W. A.-A. J. T. G. A. J. J. Anderson. X-ray tube with rotating anode cooled by high thermal conductivity uid; 1996.
36. Coolidge William ID. X-Ray Apparatus – US1215116. 2017. [Online]. Available: https://patents.google.com/patent/US1215116A/en. Accessed 12 Apr 2024.
37. Shefer E, et al. State of the art of CT detectors and sources: a literature review. Curr Radiol Rep. 2013;1(1):76–91. https://doi.org/10.1007/s40134-012-0006-4.
38. Becker AE, Hernandez AM, Boone JM, Schwoebel PR. A prototype multi-X-ray-source array (MXA) for digital breast tomosynthesis. Phys Med Biol. 2020;65(23):235033. https://doi.org/10.1088/1361-6560/abc305.
39. Matejcek C, Winter J, Aulenbacher K, Dimroth A, Natour G, Bartzsch S. A novel electron source for a compact x-ray tube for microbeam radiotherapy with very high dose rates. Phys Med. 2023;106:102532. https://doi.org/10.1016/j.ejmp.2023.102532.
40. Anburajan M, Sharma JK. Overview of X-ray tube technology. In: Biomedical engineering and its applications in healthcare. Singapore: Springer Singapore; 2019. p. 519–47. https://doi.org/10.1007/978-981-13-3705-5_21.
41. Behling R. Chapter 2: X-ray tube physics and technology. In: Russo P, editor. Handbook of X-ray imaging, physics and technology. 1st ed. Taylor & Francis Group, LLC; 2018.
42. Kemerink GJ, et al. Forgotten electrical accidents and the birth of shockproof X-ray systems. Insights Imaging. 2013;4(4):513–23. https://doi.org/10.1007/s13244-013-0238-8.
43. Grigg ERN. The trail of the invisible light: from X-Strahlen to radio(bio)logy; 1965.
44. Wikipedia. Kovar. https://en.wikipedia.org/wiki/Kovar#:~:text=Kovar%20(trademark%20of%20CRS%20Holdings,allow%20a%20tight%20mechanical%20joint.
45. William ID. Coolidge, "X-Ray apparaus," 1,215,116; 1917.
46. Ammann E, Kutschera W. X-ray tubes-continuous innovative technology. Br J Radiol. 1997;
47. Forster E. Equipment for diagnostic radiography. Springer Netherlands; 1985. https://doi.org/10.1007/978-94-009-4930-0.

48. Rogers TH. High-intensity radiation from beryllium-window X-ray tubes. Radiology. 1947;48(6):594–603. https://doi.org/10.1148/48.6.594.
49. Bushberg JT, Seibert JA, Leidholdt EM, Boone JM. The essential physics of medical imaging. 4th ed. Lippincott Williams & Wilkins (LWW); 2020.
50. Anderson WA. High intensity X ray source using bellows – European Patent Office; 1989. Accessed 7 June 2024. [Online]. Available: https://patentimages.storage.googleapis.com/a0/f3/72/55a0332a1645a1/EP0330336A2.pdf
51. IEC 60613 INTERNATIONAL STANDARD NORME INTERNATIONALE Electrical and loading characteristics of X-ray tube assemblies for medical diagnosis Caractéristiques électriques et de charge des gaines équipées pour diagnostic médical. 2010. [Online]. Available: www.iec.ch/searchpub/cur_fut-f.htm
52. Burke FJT, et al. 125 years of developments in dentistry, 1880–2005 part 3: dental equipment and materials. Br Dent J. 2005;199(6):365–9. https://doi.org/10.1038/sj.bdj.4812696.
53. Brant WE, Helms CA. Fundamentals of diagnostic radiology. 4th ed. Wolters Kluwer/Lippincott Williams & Wilkins; 2012.
54. Morigi MP, Casali F. Radiography and computed tomography for works of art. In: Russo P, editor. Handbook of X-ray imaging: physics and technology, vol. 1. CRC Press; 2018.
55. Anthony S. X-ray generators AAPM 1997; 1997.
56. Heinz M. US3939351 three phase generators, Feb. 1976.
57. M. D. R. O. (Plantsville, C. Joseph W. Motz Gaithersburg), X-ray tube having transmission anode, Patent number: 7978824; 2011.

3 Digital Radiography Systems: Principles of Operation, Clinical Applications, and Quality Control

Learning Objectives

Section A	**Section B**
Introduction, History, and Classification: Computed Radiography What factors should be taken into consideration when deciding to plan a CR installation? History of CR technology CR working principle Overview of computed radiography Benefits of computed radiography CR instrumentation CR cassette CR imaging plate CR digitizer CR dynamic range CR clinical applications Advantages of a CR system CR Artifacts CR: Quality control Quality control of CR imaging plates Visual inspection Screen cleaning maintenance Uniformity test QC precautions CR: Top manufacturers	History, Introduction, and Classification: DR Major components of a digital radiography imaging system DR instrumentation DR flat-panel detectors—direct and indirect detector technology Advantages of FPDs in digital radiography include: DR—charge-coupled devices and detectors (CCD) Classification of flat-panel detectors Woking principles: indirect vs direct flat-panel detectors CCD detectors Flat-panel TFT detectors DR clinical applications DR artifacts Types of flat-panel detector artifacts Addressing flat-panel detector artifacts Subclassification of DR artifacts DR: Quality control Tools and equipment needed Implementing the QC tests Recent technological advancements in digital radiography

D. Prakash, R. P. Kotian, *Fundamentals of X-ray Imaging*,
https://doi.org/10.1007/978-981-96-7328-5_3

3.1 Section A: Computed Radiography Systems

3.1.1 Introduction, History, and Classification: Computed Radiography

Computerized radiography (CR) systems with photostimulable phosphors (PSP) image detectors were commercially available in 1983. As a result of their ability to offer cost-effective transitions from film-based imaging to digital imaging, radiology departments accepted these systems, which allowed them to keep and use existing radiography equipment in place of digital radiography (DR). The shift to digital imaging was complete with the addition of CR readers and the switch from film to image plate cassettes.

CR is a digital imaging technique used in medical imaging to produce detailed, high-quality images. An X-ray beam is focused on an image plate coated with a photostimulable storage phosphor in CR. A CR reader reads the plate, stimulating the phosphor with a laser to create a digital image that can be viewed and modified on a computer.

CR is more efficient and has a higher image quality and the capability of storing and transferring images electronically when compared to classic film-based radiography. It is commonly used in hospitals, clinics, and imaging centers for several diagnostic purposes, including the detection of fractures, cancers, and other abnormalities [1].

3.1.1.1 What Factors Should Be Taken into Consideration When Deciding to Plan a CR Installation?

Computed radiography can be viewed as a digital alternative on traditional X-ray film. Imaging plates are utilized with the same radiographic examination procedures and techniques as film, and they come in a variety of system classes (the image quality) with varying exposure lengths. However, in computed radiography, it is not only the imaging plate type that influences image quality; the scan settings utilized by the scanner are also important. The scanner's resolution capabilities (basic spatial resolution, or SRb) are particularly significant in determining image quality.

The first scanner created was equipped to attain 30 μm spatial resolution with a laser focus of only 12.5 μm (when using high-resolution image plates). The imaging governing authorities at that time certified this performance through certification. The scanners variable laser focus size allows it to be easily changed for inspection tasks that require less demanding fundamental spatial resolution. This system had a fixed laser focus of 50 μm, which was extremely useful for low-resolution applications.

Overall, computed radiography is a valuable technology that has revolutionized the field of medical imaging, providing healthcare providers with the tools they need to make accurate diagnoses and provide the best possible care for their patients and is still currently used despite the invent of digital radiography techniques [2].

3.1.1.2 History of CR Technology

Computed radiography (CR) has a rich history spanning several decades, including technological developments and substantial advances in medical imaging. Here is a summary of the main milestones in the development of CR:

1. **Invention of the photostimulable phosphor (PSP) plate (1976)**
   Dr. Yoshihiro Nishikawa and his colleagues at Fuji Photo Film Co., Ltd. in Japan invented the photostimulable phosphor (PSP) plate, which served as the cornerstone for computed radiography. PSP plates are coated with photostimulable phosphors, which can absorb and store X-ray radiation.
2. **Introduction of the first CR systems (1981)**
   The first commercial CR system was released by Fuji in 1981, which signaled the start of the mainstream use of digital radiography technology. These early systems collected X-ray images using PSP plates, which were subsequently processed by specialized CR readers.
3. **Continued technological advancements (1980s–1990s)**

The image quality, speed, and practicality of CR technology significantly improved over the 1980s and 1990s. Compact and efficient CR systems were developed by manufacturers like Fuji, Agfa, and Kodak, enabling healthcare facilities of various sizes to have greater access to digital imaging.

4. **Integration with picture archiving and communication systems (PACS) (1990s)**
   The radiology department workflow was further improved in the 1990s with the integration of CR systems with Picture Archiving and Communication Systems (PACS). PACS replaced conventional film-based archives by enabling the electronic storage, dissemination, and retrieval of digital images.
5. **Transition to digital radiography (2000s)**
   CR was a major factor in the extensive switch from film-based radiography to digital radiography that occurred in the 2000s. Compared to traditional film, digital radiography had many advantages, such as higher image quality, faster image acquisition, and more advanced image processing tools.
6. **Continued evolution and innovation (2010s–present)**
   With improvements in sensor technology, image processing algorithms, and connection features, CR technology has developed further in the years that have followed. Manufacturers have released CR systems that are lighter, more portable, and have better workflow efficiency and image resolution.
7. **Hybrid imaging systems (PET/CT, SPECT/CT) incorporating CR (2000s–present)**
   In order to enable the simultaneous acquisition of anatomical and functional images, computed radiography has also been included into hybrid imaging systems like PET/CT and SPECT/CT. More thorough diagnostic assessments are made possible by these hybrid systems, which integrate CR's diagnostic powers with those of other imaging modalities.

In the history of computed radiography, there has always been an element of invention and technological advancement, which finally led to the widespread use of digital imaging in radiology imaging all over the world. CR is still a crucial part of contemporary medical imaging procedures, providing physicians with better patient care and increased diagnostic capacity [3].

3.1.2 Computed Radiography Working Principle

In radiology, computed radiography is a digital imaging technique used to obtain X-rays. It transformed traditional film-based radiography by replacing the laborious and time-consuming film development procedure with a more efficient digital workflow. A phosphor plate replaces typical X-ray film in CR, retaining energy when exposed to X-rays. Digital images are created when this stored energy is released during scanning. CR uses photostimulable phosphor as an image receptor. A typical film screen shell houses the image receptor. Using the photostimulable luminescence method, computed radiography captures electrons at high energy levels using radiation absorption. By utilizing conventional radiography equipment for digital radiography, CR facilitates the transition from conventional radiography to digital radiography [4].

Electron Storage Capability

Photostimulable phosphor is a thin layer of phosphor grains on computed radiography plates. A plate is exposed to X-ray radiation, which excites the phosphor and traps electrons in the lattice until the second cycle of illumination excites them again.

Analog to Digital Conversion

A tiny, high-intensity laser (usually generating 680 nm red light) is used to cause previously trapped electrons to return to their respective valence bands and generate violet light (400–450 nm). Using an analog-to-digital converter (ADC), this violet light will be translated into an electric signal by a photomultiplier tube (PMT). The computed radiography plate can be "reset" with a white light, allowing it to be reused multiple times (typically 40,000–50,000 exposures) if handled properly.

Workflow Process: CR Readout Process

An imaging plate, constructed of barium fluor halide and based on photostimulable phosphor (PSP), is used to acquire images. Each exposure is recorded on a single imaging plate. The image plate is housed in a cassette, like a screen film cassette. Radiographic equipment is then used to expose the plate to X-rays. Figure 3.1 illustrates how electrons trapped in the phosphor plate are stimulated to higher energy levels during exposure, which produces a latent picture. In a CR reader or digitizer, the imaging plate is processed and retrieved to reveal this latent picture.

Processing of Image

The image is processed using the following procedures. First, the cassette is opened in the CR reader, then the imaging plate is released. As the rollers move, the image plate is scanned with a laser beam. By stimulating trapped electrons to release themselves and return to a lower energy state, laser light emits light photons. The wavelengths of the two light sources (laser and emitted light photons) are used for clinical image retrieval. With the CR digitizer (or reader), the digital image signal differs from laser light in that it has a shorter wavelength and higher energy than the laser light. This allows the photomultiplier tube (PMT) to identify higher-energy and shorter-wavelength light photons.

A fiber-optic light guide collects the light released by the imaging plate and sends it to a PMT, which generates an electronic signal. In the fifth step, the electronic signal is digitized, displayed on a monitor, and transmitted to a PACS. Finally, a high-intensity halogen lamp is used to remove any remaining energy from the previous exposure. An image plate is returned to its cassette when it is ready to be reused. In the CR image workflow, artifacts can appear at any stage [5]. In general, CR artifacts fall into two categories: acquisition artifacts and processing artifacts.

3.1.2.1 Overview of Computed Radiography

1. **Exposure:** CR, like standard radiography, begins with the patient being exposed to X-rays. The X-rays penetrate the body of the patient and are attenuated by different tissues, resulting in varying intensity patterns.
2. **Phosphor plate:** Instead of film, X-rays are aimed at a phosphor plate. This plate is made up of layers of X-ray-sensitive phosphor crystals. As a result of exposure to X-rays, the phosphor atoms in the plate become excited and store energy.
3. **Image formation:** A latent image is left on the phosphor plate after exposure. After the plates are removed from the X-ray machine, they are placed in the CR reader. The plate is scanned using a laser beam inside the reader. Figure 3.2 illustrates how the phosphor crystals convert stored energy into visible light.
4. **Signal conversion:** Phosphor plates generate light that is detected by photomultiplier tubes

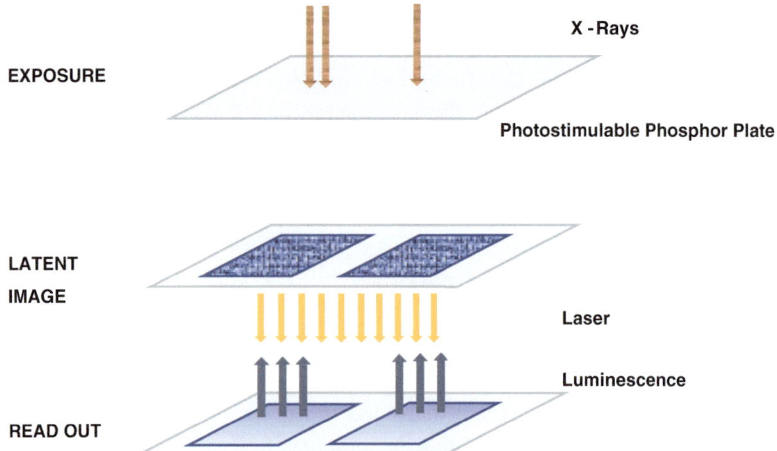

Fig. 3.1 CR readout illustration

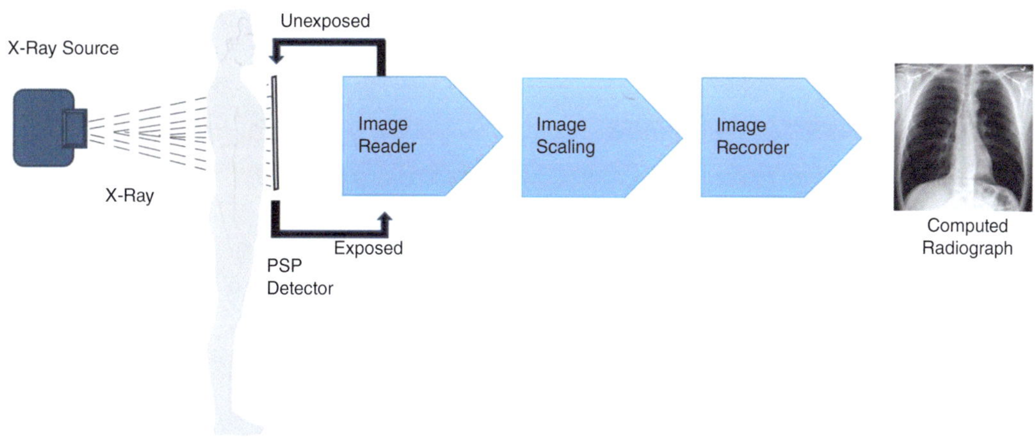

Fig. 3.2 PSP image acquisition and processing

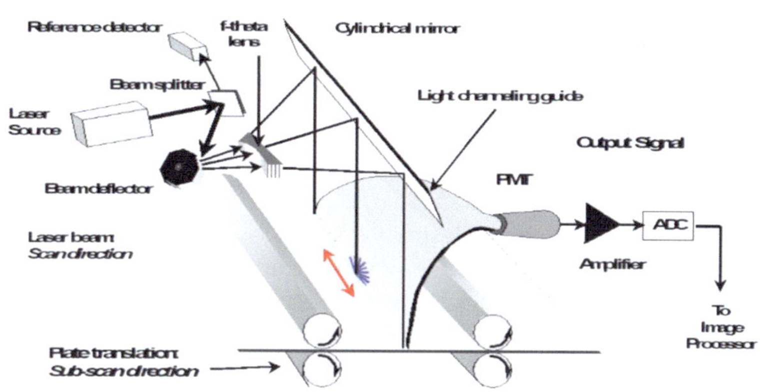

Fig. 3.3 Internal operation of CR reader

or charge-coupled devices (CCDs) within CR readers. The circuits in the reader transform the analog signal to a digital signal as depicted in Fig. 3.3.

5. **Digital image:** A high-speed computer processes the digital signal and produces a high-resolution grayscale image that is presented on a high-resolution medical imaging monitor. Radiologists and technologists can then alter images to highlight specific areas of interest, change contrast and brightness, and annotate findings.

3.1.2.2 Benefits of Computed Radiography

- Digital workflow: CR removes chemical processing and film storage, speeding the radiography process and lowering environmental impact.
- Image quality: CR produces digital images with higher resolution and dynamic range than traditional film-based radiography. This can result in better diagnostic accuracy.
- Image viewing: Radiologists can use software tools to improve digital images and extract diagnostic information.
- Efficient storage and retrieval of digital images improves accessibility and collaboration among healthcare practitioners.

Overall, computed radiography has altered the field of radiology by providing a faster, more efficient, more adaptable way to capture and interpret X-ray images [6–8].

3.1.3 Computed Radiography Instrumentation

The CR unit comprises of the following components

A. **CR cassette**
B. **CR imaging plate**
C. **CR digitizer**

A. **CR cassette**

A computed radiography (CR) cassette is an essential component of the CR imaging process, which captures X-ray images in medical imaging. Unlike standard X-ray films, which require chemical processing, CR systems digitize X-ray images, allowing them to be stored and manipulated electronically. A photostimulable phosphor plate (PSP) replaces the standard film in the CR cassette. Latent images are produced when the phosphor substance is exposed to X-rays. Lasers scan the plate after the cassette is exposed in a CR reader, releasing the trapped energy. A photomultiplier tube or a solid-state detector captures the produced light, converts it into a digital signal, and then processes it using specialized software to create a digital image.

CR cassettes come in a variety of sizes to meet different imaging requirements, ranging from small cassettes for extremities to bigger ones for chest or belly imaging. They are built to last and reusable with carbon fibre components, with protective layers to keep the fragile phosphor plate from being damaged. The CR image plates are stored in cassettes. They are entirely compatible with normal radiography cassettes and come in such sizes. A CR cassette serves two functions: it holds and protects the IP (image plate) while also receiving and storing image identification data. Cassettes include the image plates. The CR cassette also houses the memory chip as depicted in Fig. 3.4. The memory chip will hold all patient-related data, including patient demographics and image quality. Ther writing of data to the memory chip is done via radio transmission to the antenna card integrated into the cassette [6, 9–11].

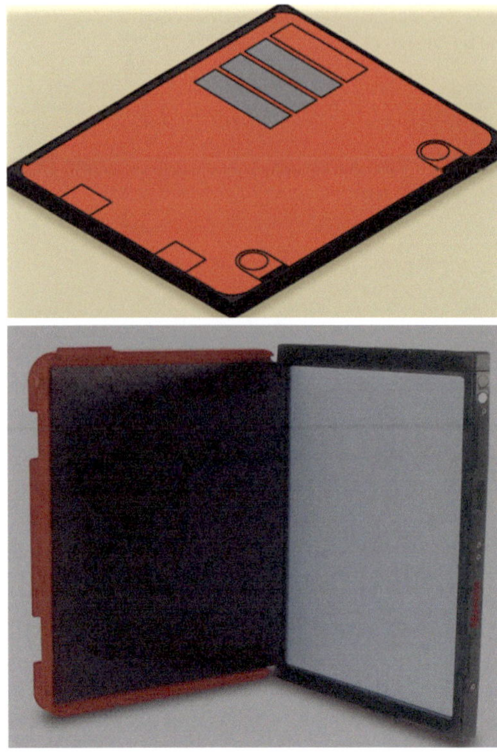

Fig. 3.4 Typical CR cassette

Primary functions of the CR cassettes

- Holding the IP plates
- Protecting the IP plates against mechanical damage, electrostatic charging, dust, and dirt.
- IP plates have a rigid structure with ribbed structure and rubber-protected corners with its inner lining made of felt, protecting the image plate against mechanical damage, dust, antistatic charging, and lead backed to avoid backscatter.
- Holding the image identification data with memory chip, which contains all image-relevant data, patient demographics, image quality-related data, and speed credentials.
- The writing information is embedded into the memory chip contactlessly via radio transmission to the antenna card built into the cassette plates.

CR cassette available sizes

35 × 43 cm (14 × 17″)
35 × 35 cm (14 × 14″)
24 × 30 cm

18 × 24 cm
8 × x 10″
10 × 12″
15 × 30 cm dental
18 × 24 cm and 24 × 30 cm for mammography

B. **CR imaging plate**

Computed radiography (CR) imaging plates are an essential component of the CR imaging system, a digital imaging technology used in medical imaging. The image plate in CR systems is essentially a flexible, lightweight screen with a phosphor coating. When exposed to X-rays or other ionizing radiation, the phosphor layer stores energy proportional to the amount of radiation it receives. Once the image plate has been exposed, it is read by a CR reader. CR readers use laser beams to scan image plates, releasing light from the phosphor layer. The light is captured and converted into an electrical signal by a photosensitive detector. A computer digitizes and processes the electronic signal to create a digital image that may be viewed on an LCD screen, altered, and saved digitally.

The benefits of CR imaging plates are their flexibility, reusability (after erasure), and low cost as compared to other digital imaging technologies such as direct digital radiography (DR). However, CR systems often have slower image acquisition and processing durations than DR systems. Despite this, CR remains a popular technique, particularly in contexts where upgrading to DR is not immediately possible or cost-effective.

CR Plate: Technical Considerations

The Image Plate is composed of a phosphor supported by a base material and covered in a protective layer as depicted in Fig. 3.5. The image plate contains phosphor, which is sensitive to X-rays. A transition from one stable state to another occurs when phosphorus is exposed to X-rays. The phosphor returns to its usual state after a delay of about 48 h if not triggered. An X-ray's impact on the phosphor granules determines the amount of excitation. Imaging plates display a wide dynamic range. Upon stimulation, the plate discharges the excess energy received via X-ray excitation. This stimulation is provided by a laser in the digitizer. CR image plates contain latent images until they are scanned in a digitizer. It is very important to protect IP plates from mechanical damage, electrostatic charging, dust, and filth. IP plates feature a strong structure with rubber-protected corners. The felt inner lining protects the image plate from mechanical damage, dust, antistatic charging, and backscatte as it is lead-backed [9, 12–14].

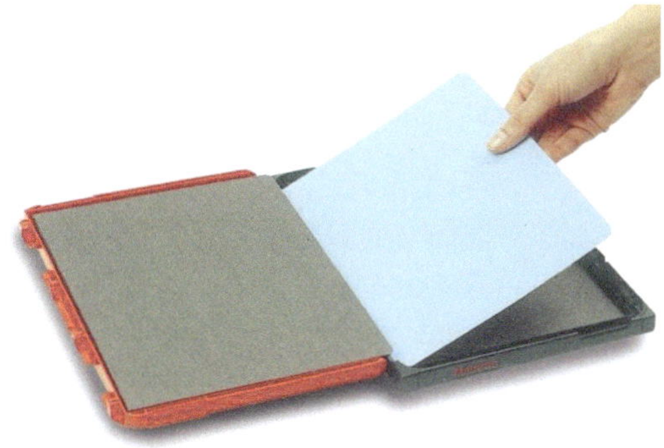

Fig. 3.5 CR imaging plate

Unique characteristics of the storage phosphors used in CR imaging plate

- Storage phosphors have great absorption efficiency, capturing a high percentage of entering X-rays and reducing the needed dose.
- They also provide high sharpness across all spatial frequencies with excellent homogeneity.
- Very wide dynamic range.
- Enables visualization of all the required diagnostic information in one exposure even if wide variety of different materials in the object being examined.
- Less sensitive to variations in the exposure conditions.
- **Consequences**
  - Less retakes required.
  - Option to reduce the dose.
- These phosphors also have exceptional absorption efficiency means that a large percentage of incoming X-rays are effectively

captured, reducing the required dose. Additionally, great homogeneity ensures exceptional sharpness across all spatial frequencies.

- They also display short response time with previous pixel reaction that must fade before the next pixel stimulation.
- Unique features of phosphors, results in higher absorption efficiency and homogeneity with a higher signal-to-noise ratio-Sr and T (BaSrFBrI: Eu) contribute to a larger stimulation range that shifts toward longer wavelengths, peaking at the stimulating laser's wavelength.
- Iodine causes a modest shift in the luminescence spectra longer wavelengths. Its sharpness decreases slightly but remains below the visible threshold with improved signal-to-noise ratio compensates for the loss.

EBC topcoat (electron beam cured)

- This coating ensures long lifetime of the plate and provides efficient protection against mechanical wear as depicted in Figs. 3.6 and 3.7 (during daily operation).
- It also provides protection against chemical cleaning solutions.
- The EBC smooth surface also ensures an optimal signal-to-noise ratio.

Reading the image signal in the digitizer

Following exposure, the ADC cassette is inserted into the digitizer. The plate currently contains a latent picture. A laser beam shall sweep across the plate, scanning it along lines. The image is scanned line by line, and each line has a specific number of pixels. The number of pixels read varies depending on the standard utilized. Meanwhile, the plate shall proceed ahead.

Light is then emitted from the phosphor inside the plate in every direction. As a result, a set of mirrors and a light guide are designed to capture as much emitted light as feasible as depicted in Fig. 3.8. The light is directed into the photomultiplier and then into a fiber-optic cable (or any material that can conduct light). The photomulti-

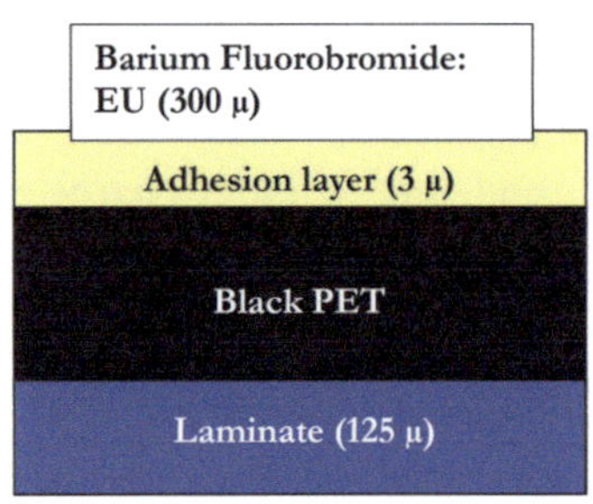

Fig. 3.6 CR imaging plate internal structure

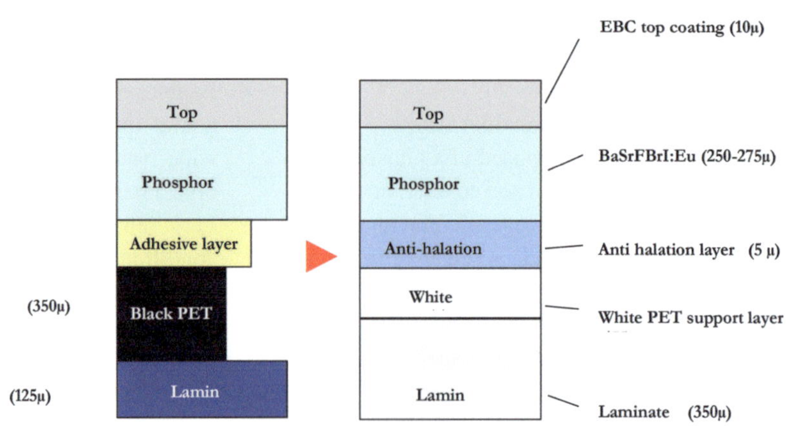

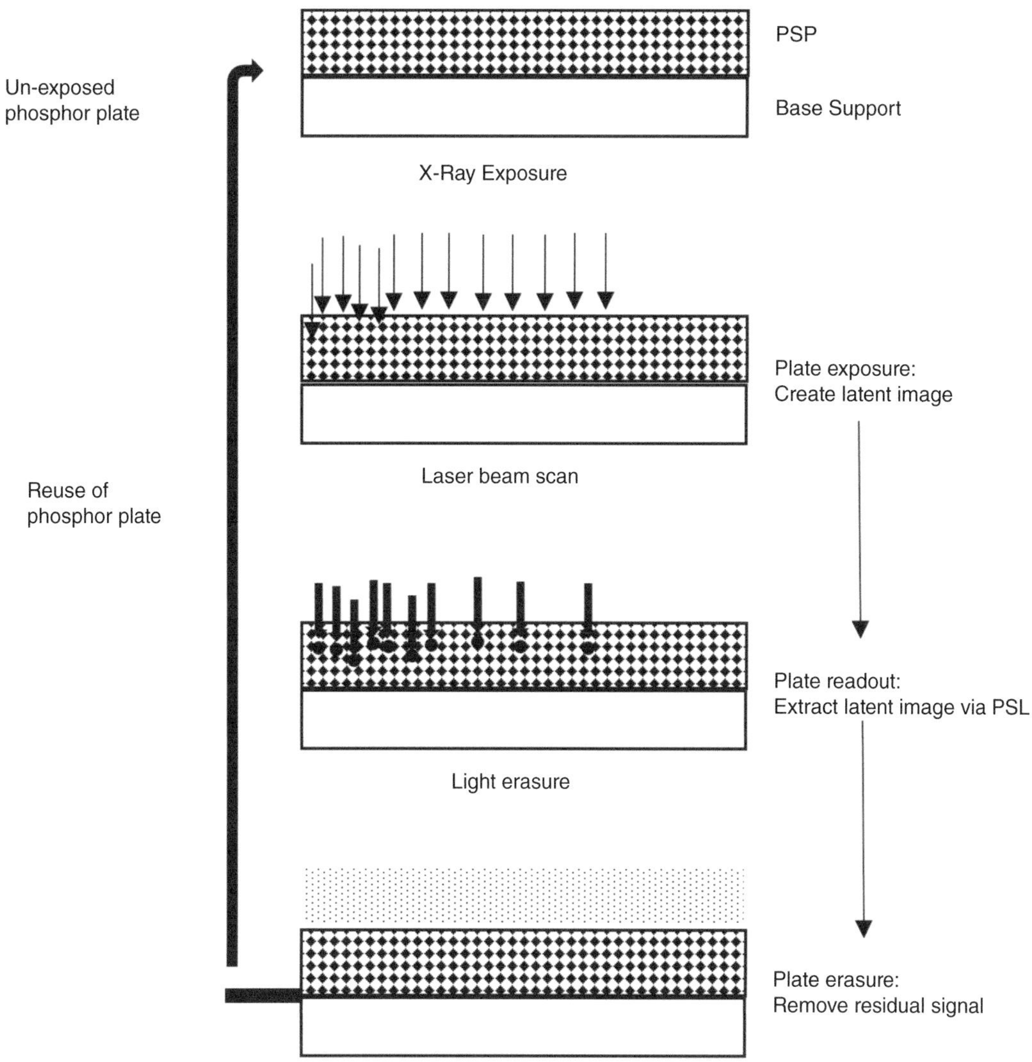

Fig. 3.7 The phosphor plate cycle

plier turns the gathered light into an analog electrical signal, which is then digitized into 12 bits.

C. **CR digitizer**

Workflow in the digitizer

Computed radiography (CR) digitizers are specialized devices used in medical imaging that transform analog X-ray analog images to digital format. Here is a brief explanation of how they work:

1. **Exposure:** The process begins with the patient being exposed to X-rays. As X-rays travel through the body, different tissues absorb the rays differently, leaving a latent image on the imaging plate.
2. **Imaging plate:** CR systems utilize a photostimulable phosphor imaging plate rather than a typical X-ray film. This plate is composed of a substance that stores energy when exposed to X-rays.
3. **Plate scanning:** After exposure, the imaging plate is taken from the patient and placed in the CR digitizer. The CR digitizer comprises both of laser scanning device and a photodetector.

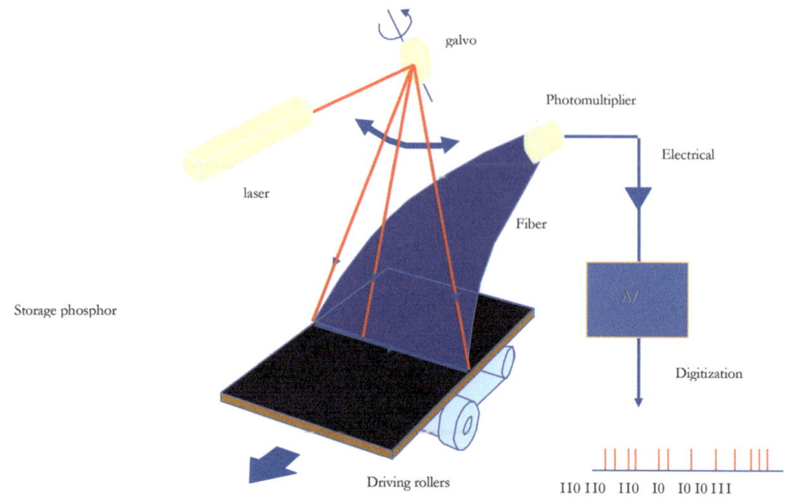

Fig. 3.8 Signal reading process

4. **Laser scanning:** The CR digitizer uses a laser to scan the image plate. The laser triggers the stored energy within the phosphor substance, causing it to generate light.
5. **Light detection:** When the phosphor emits light, a photodetector turns it into an electrical signal. The intensity of light is proportional to X-ray exposure received by the imaging plate.
6. **Digital conversion:** Analog-to-digital converters convert the photodetector's electrical signals into digital data. This digital data depicts the X-ray image acquired on the imaging plate.
7. **Image processing:** Digital data undergoes numerous procedures to improve image quality, correct artifacts, and alter contrast and brightness.
8. **Image display:** Radiologists and medical imaging experts can study the produced digital image on a computer monitor or viewing device.

The greatest advantage of CR digitizers is their ability to manipulate and store digital images, allowing for easy sharing, remote viewing, and integration with hospital information systems (HISs) and picture archiving and communication systems (PACSs). Additionally, CR systems offer a wider dynamic range and higher image quality than traditional X-ray films [15–19].

Digitizer Optimum Throughput

A CR digitizer can process between 86 and 100 plates per hour (depending on their size). Light collection in the scan engine has been improved with better fibre and mirror shape, resulting in higher image quality. The digitizer should have a 50 mW laser diode, which is smaller, faster to start up, and wears less than classic digitizers' with helium-based laser tubes. The erasing unit uses a variety of white light halogen bulbs.

The image seen in the Fig. 3.9 is processed using the techniques outlined below. In the CR reader, the cassette is opened first, then the imaging plate is released. The rollers move the image plate so that the laser beam can scan it. Laser light stimulates trapped electrons to release themselves and return to a lower energy state, resulting in light photons being emitted. The wavelength differences between laser light and emitted light photons are the basis for retrieving pictures.

A photomultiplier tube (PMT) can distinguish light photons with higher energy and shorter wavelengths from laser light, which has a longer wavelength and lower energy than the signal from a CR digitizer (or reader). The fourth step is to collect the light released by the imaging plate and send it to an electronic signal generator in the PMT. The fifth step involves digitizing the signal, storing it in a monitor, and transmitting it. An intense halogen lamp removes residual energy from the image plate in the final step. The image plate is then returned to the cassette as shown in Fig. 3.10. The other internal parts of the digitizer are depicted in Figs. 3.11, 3.12, 3.13, 3.14, 3.15, 3.16, and 3.17.

The CR image workflow can produce artifacts at any stage. A CR artifact can be divided into two types: image acquisition artifacts and image processing artifacts.

1—Cassette input area
2—Casette handling area (Opening, reading, identification, and releasing the plate)
3—Imaging plate transportation area
4—Imaging plate scanning area
5—Imaging plate erasure area
6—Casette plate handling area (insertion and closing)
7—Casette output area

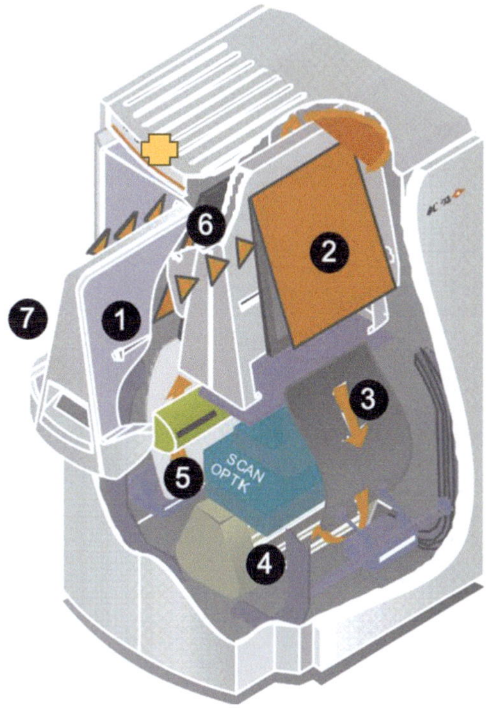

Fig. 3.9 Workflow in a CR digitizer

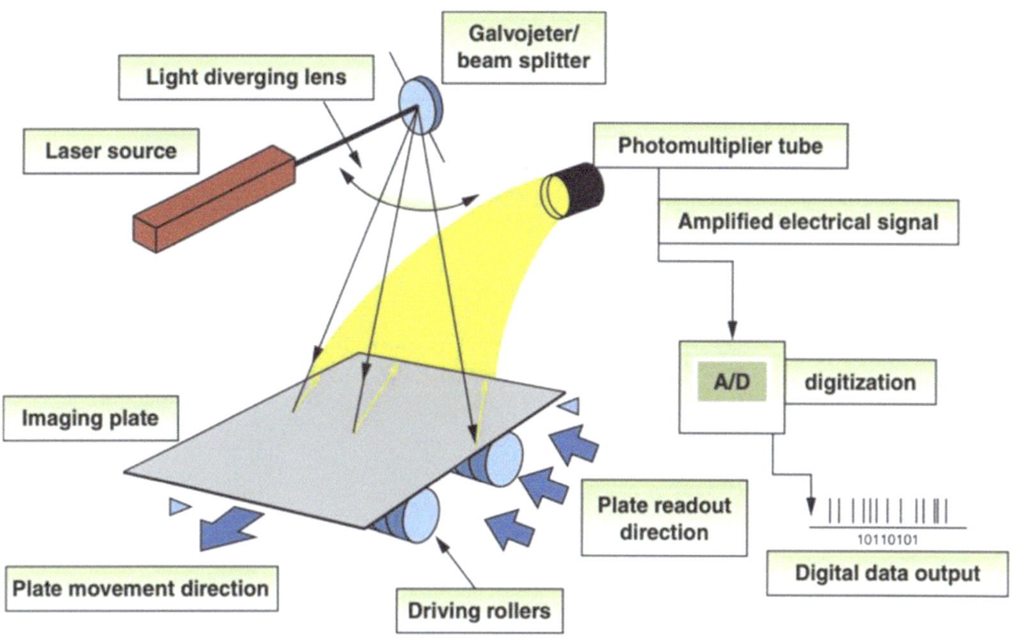

Fig. 3.10 CR digitizer readout

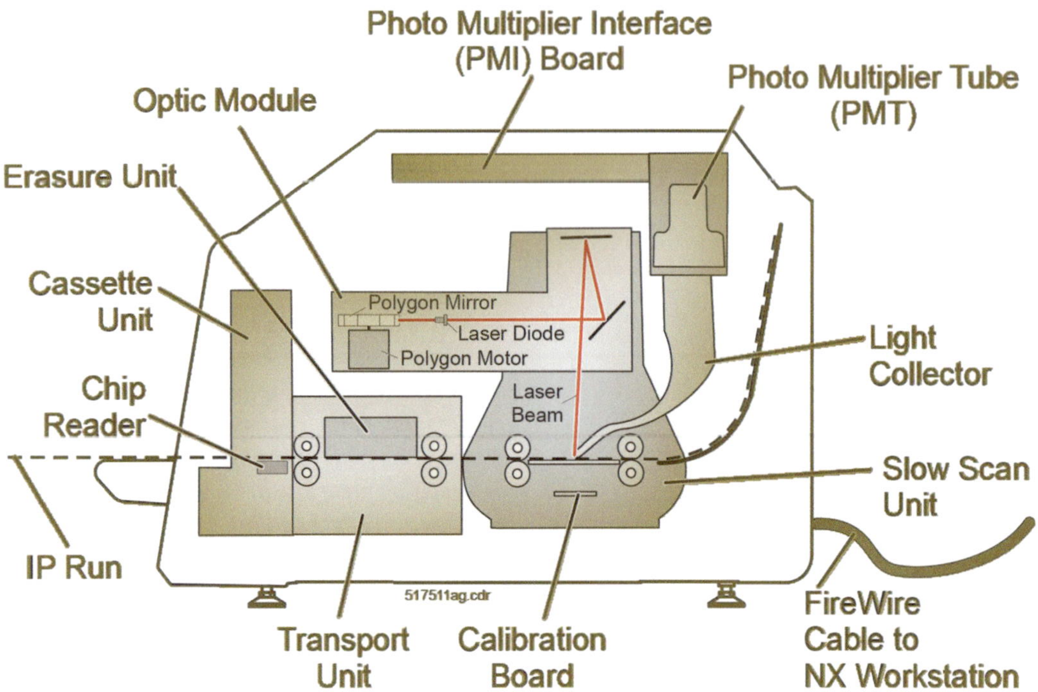

Fig. 3.11 Internal structure and working of a CR digitizer

Fig. 3.12 Internal structure cassette unit

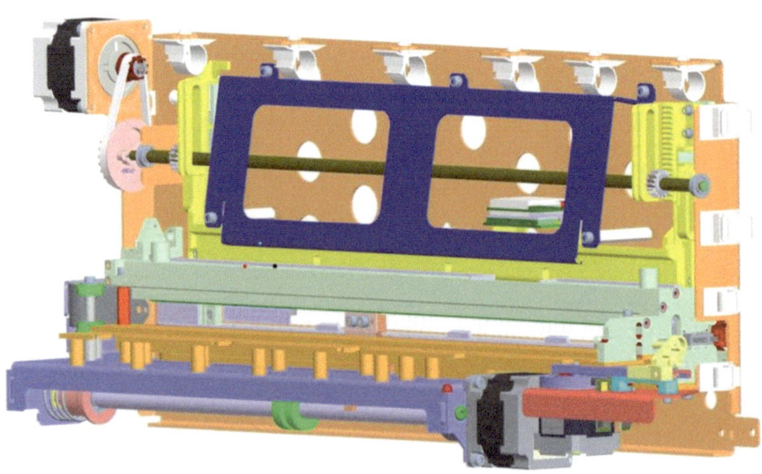

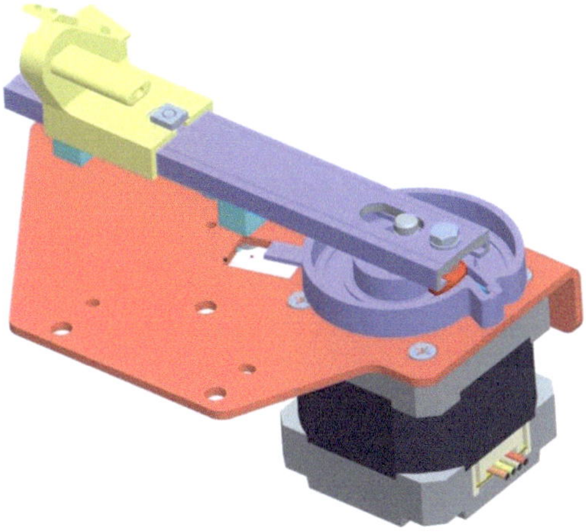

Fig. 3.13 Internal structure cassette locking unit

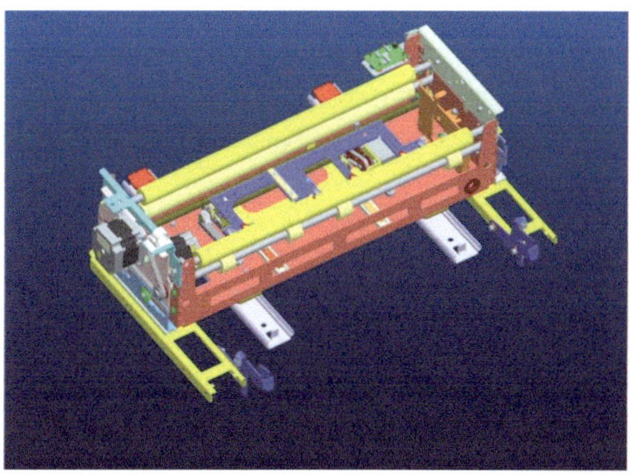

Fig. 3.14 Internal structure transport unit with rollers

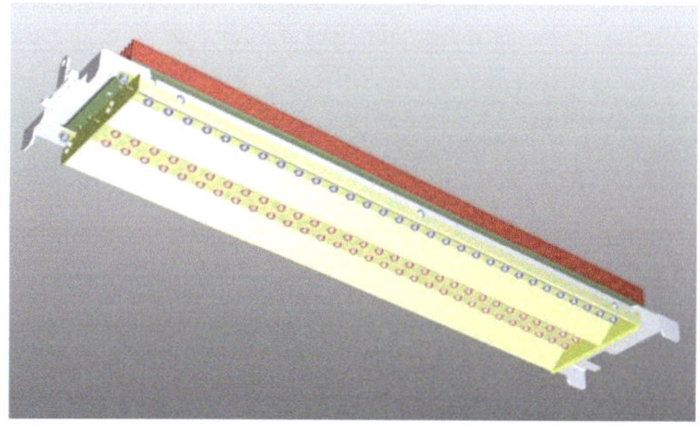

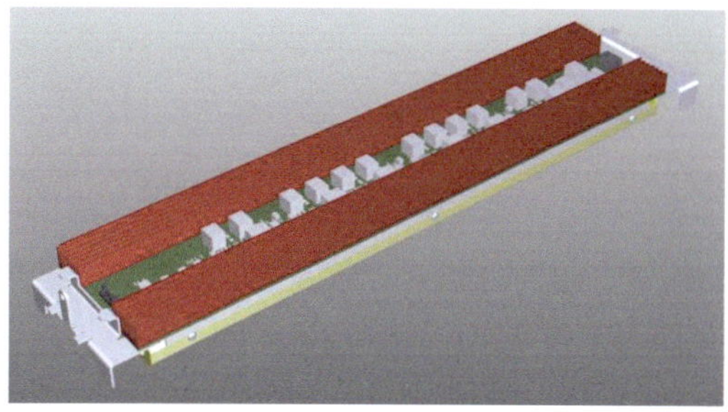

Fig. 3.15 Internal structure erasure unit

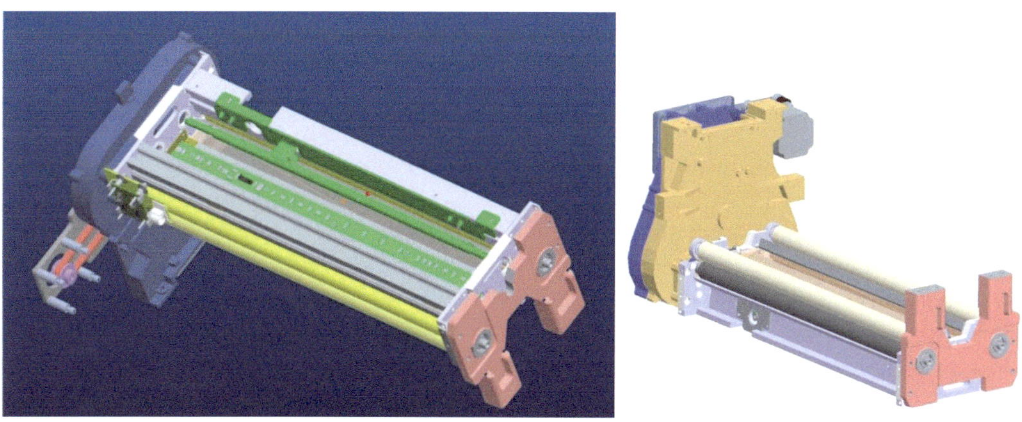

Fig. 3.16 Internal structure scan module

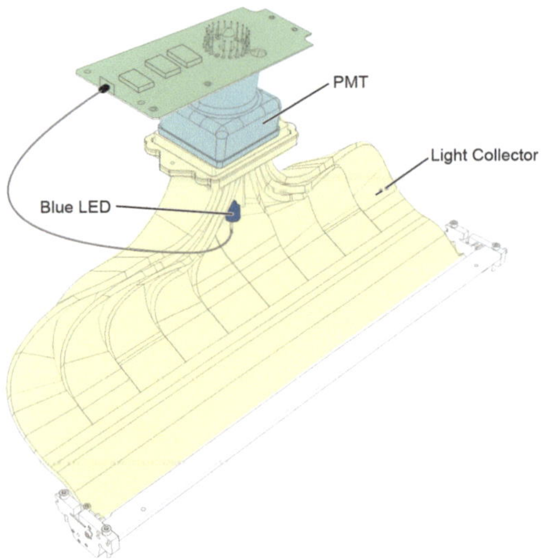

Fig. 3.17 Internal structure PMT

3.1.3.1 CR Dynamic Range

3.1.3.2 CR Dynamic Range

(CR) is a radiology-specific digital imaging technology that produces diagnostic images. A CR system's dynamic range refers to the range of radiation intensities it can detect and record accurately.

In CR systems, the X-ray image is captured using a storage phosphor plate. As X-rays are passed through the plate, the energy is stored, which is then released when a laser or another light source is used to scan the plate. X-ray exposure intensity determines the intensity of emitted light, which is then transformed into digital data.

A CR system's dynamic range is determined by a number of elements, including phosphor plate sensitivity, scanning system resolution, and digital picture bit depth. CR systems typically have a dynamic range of 10,000 to 16,000 shades of gray, which is sufficient to detect the tiny variations in tissue density required for diagnostic imaging.

A broader dynamic range enables better distinction between tissues of different densities, resulting in increased image quality and diagnostic accuracy. However, dynamic range must be balanced with other criteria such as image resolution and noise levels in order to get ideal image quality for diagnostic applications.

3.1.3.3 CR Clinical Applications

Computed radiography (CR) has numerous clinical uses in radiology, providing advantages such as digital image storage, modification, and transmission. Here are some of the most important clincial applications of CR in radiology:

1. General radiography: Common applications for CR include chest, bone, abdomen, and extremities imaging. It provides the benefits of digital imaging, such as immediate image acquisition, post-processing capabilities, and ease of image storage and retrieval.
2. Emergency radiology: CR enables quick image acquisition and interpretation, helping diagnose and manage acute diseases such fractures, dislocations, and trauma-related injuries.
3. Orthopedic imaging: CR is often used to diagnose bone fractures, joint problems, and musculoskeletal traumas. It generates detailed images of bone structures, enabling precise diagnosis and treatment planning.
4. Integrating CR with fluoroscopy equipment allows for real-time imaging during operations like gastrointestinal investigations, arthrography, and vascular treatments. Compared to traditional film-based fluoroscopy, digital fluoroscopy with CR provides higher image quality, lower radiation exposure, and increased post-processing possibilities.
5. Mammography: CR systems tailored for breast imaging can identify and diagnose breast cancer and other problems. Digital mammography with CR provides high-resolution images, increased contrast, and the ability to enhance and edit images to better visualize breast tissue.
6. Dental radiography uses CR to capture intraoral and extraoral images, such as periapical, bitewing, panoramic, and cephalometric X-rays. Digital dental imaging with CR yields high-quality images for identifying dental caries, periodontal disease, and other oral health issues.

7. Portable imaging: CR systems provide bedside imaging for critically ill or immobile patients in intensive care units, emergency departments, and other clinical settings. Portable CR systems offer greater flexibility and simplicity when acquiring diagnostic images at the point of care.

Overall, computed radiography is an important part of modern radiology practice, with several clinical applications that aid in effective diagnosis, treatment planning, and patient care [20–22].

3.1.3.4 Advantages of a CR System

The benefits of CR systems include faster imaging, lower radiation doses, and enhanced image editing. However, they are gradually being replaced by digital radiography (DR) systems, which use digital detectors (such as amorphous selenium or amorphous silicon) and do not require cassettes or readers. Below mentioned bullets are few advantages of CR:

- Computer radiography (CR) is more forgiving than analog film systems. There is no need to be concerned about overexposure or underexposure.
- CR is more practical. It allows you to maximize the value of your existing radiology rooms.
- CR provides greater image quality compared to conventional film.
- The CR system has a compact footprint and can service numerous radiography rooms.
- CR eliminates image degradation by storing images digitally and allowing for easy recovery at any time. There are no chemical abatement difficulties [23, 24].

Practical tips for CR units

How many times can a storage phosphor plate be used?

- Proper handling can extend the life of phosphor plates.
- Physical damage to the plate can shorten its useful life.
- The chemistry of phosphors does not deteriorate with repeated exposure.
- A properly cared-for plate can produce thousands of images.
- A single plate is tested at the factory over a minimum of 10,000 times and remains in good shape.

How to clean the phosphor plates?

- Using anhydrous ethyl alcohol and lint-free wipes to clean phosphor plates.
- Screen cleaners should not be used since they are stronger than ethyl alcohol and may leave residue on the plates.
- To clean a plate, avoid using paper towels or gauze since they can leave lint, dust, and fibers.
- Instead, use ethyl alcohol straight to the plate and wipe it across.
- Before using the plates, allow them to dry for a few minutes. Daily practice is recommended.

How often should the phosphor plates be cleaned?

- When not in use, plates should be cleaned daily and stored in a cassette.
- A good way to ensure that the plates dry well is to clean them at the end of the day.

3.1.4 CR Image Artifacts

Artifacts in images hide or mimic clinical characteristics. Artifacts in radiography images are distracting and can impair proper diagnosis. Computed radiography (CR) images are created using standard imaging equipment such as bucky and grids, as well as x-ray tables and tubes; nevertheless, certain components of CR technology cause artifacts that seem different than those observed in conventional radiography. These artifacts can be traced back to several components of the CR imaging system. These components comprise an imaging plate, a CR reader, an electro-optical system for image development, computer algorithms for raw image processing, and a hard copy output device.

All of these components may serve as origins for artifacts. Understanding how each of these elements contributes to artifacts in the imaging process may help you develop a solution for overcoming such artifacts. Improper posture and motion can both contribute to these distortions. There are several types of artifacts, including transitory phosphor plate faults caused by dust, grime, or failure to erase images. Through screen cleaning and plate erasure, these artifacts can easily be removed. There are certain persistent image plate artifacts, such as scratches or plate aging. Plate replacement is required in these cases. Failure in reading can result in scan line artifacts. Laser strength decreases over time. Though lasers have an estimated life duration, beyond a certain point, it is required to replace the laser subsystem or, in some cases, the optical system. Artifacts can be caused by dust particles on the mirror or in the light guide.

Computed radiography (CR) is a type of medical radiography that uses phosphor plates to produce X-ray images. These plates are then scanned with a CR reader to generate digital images. CR, like any other imaging technique, is susceptible to artifacts, which are irregularities or distortions in the image that can impair diagnostic accuracy. Here are some common artifacts seen in computed radiography.

1. Phantom images: Previous images on the imaging plate can cause artifacts in subsequent images.
2. Foreign particles like dirt, dust, or scratches on the image plate can create artifacts.
3. Scatter radiation: Surrounding objects can reduce visual quality, causing artifacts like low contrast and sharpness.
4. Grid lines: Poor alignment or damage to the grid used to decrease scatter radiation can result in grid lines on images.
5. Moire effect: If the grid used in imaging does not match the digital sampling rate, it might result in a repeating interference pattern.
6. Ghost images: These are weak images of high-contrast objects that were previously captured but not properly deleted from the imaging plate.
7. Light or laser artifacts: Image artifacts may occur due to light leaks or laser malfunction in the CR reader.
8. Quantization noise: The limited number of gray levels in digital images causes a grainy appearance.
9. Image stitching artifacts: When numerous images are stitched together to create a bigger image, misalignment, or distortion may occur.
10. Motion artifacts: Patient movement during image acquisition can result in blurring or distortion.
11. Exposure artifacts: Over or underexposure of the image plate can cause loss of detail or excessive noise.
12. Beam hardening: Different materials absorb X-rays differently, resulting in visual artifacts like streaks or shading.
13. Processing artifacts: Errors in digital image processing, such as faulty calibration or modification, can create artifacts.
14. Aliasing artifacts: When an object's spatial frequency exceeds the Nyquist frequency, it causes distortions like jagged edges and false structures.

These are only a few of the frequent artifacts found in computed radiography. Radiologic technologists and radiologists must understand and recognize these abnormalities to provide a precise interpretation and optimal patient care [25–30].

Artifacts can be developed at any stage of the CR image workflow as discussed earlier in the subsection CR workflow. CR artifacts are extensively divided into two types: A. Image acquisition artifacts and B. Image processing artifacts and summarized and discussed in Tables 3.1, 3.2, 3.3 and Figs. 3.18, 3.19, 3.20, 3.21, 3.22, 3.23, 3.24, 3.25, 3.26, 3.27, 3.28, 3.29, 3.30, 3.31, 3.32, 3.33, 3.34, 3.35, 3.36, and 3.37.

3.1.5 CR: Quality Control

Quality control (QC) in computed radiography (CR) is essential for ensuring the dependability and accuracy of digital radiographic images. Here are some important features of CR quality control:

Table 3.1 Image acquisition artifacts

Artifact	Causes	Appearance	Remedy
Twin duplication artifact	Double exposure to the same imaging plate	Duplication of images	Applications and hands on training of the equipment
Collimation error	Inadequate collimation	Image unsharpness	Accurate collimation matching the anatomy and cassette size
Missed/delayed scanning	Prolonged or missed delay between the image acquisition and read out processing	Image fading	Immediate image plate reading after image acquisition as a standard process
Cassette Back exposure	Improper placement of imaging plate or cassette back damage	Mixed band image shading	Regular quality checks and inspection of cassettes and imaging plates
Inappropriate technical factor error			
Overexposure	Improper kVp and mA/mAs setting	Dark images	User manual recommendations of CR dynamic range to be followed based on patient body weight
Underexposure	Improper kVp and mA/mAs setting	Grainy images	User manual recommendations of CR dynamic range to be followed based on patient body weight
Grid imaging error	Mismatched grid ratio usage	Moire banded effect	Follow user manual specifications matching the CR hardware
Scatter radiation effect	Improper cassette storage	Image quality deterioration when used for clinical imaging	Proper cassette storage and cassette erasure within the CR digitizer before usage if necessary
Image plate misuse	Cassette and plate damage during maintenance	Kink marks	Following standard operating process and QA for CR care and maintenance
Light bulb effect	X-rays that are uncollimated or overweight individuals have more backscattered radiation entering the imaging plate	A darker portion of an image compared to the rest	Using more precise collimation or lowering the peak voltage will minimize back scatter

Table 3.2 Image processing (hardware-related) artifacts

Artifact	Causes	Appearance	Remedy
Artifacts due to image plate cracks, and dust	Damage during transportation and maintenance process	Focal radiopacities as minute spots on the image	Plate replacement and regular maintenance QA checks
Rollers (within the CR digitizer related artifacts)	Roller malfunction, mechanical damage, dust retention, and transport roller defect	Image contrast alteration is seen with half-read images of varying radiopacities	Periodic QA maintenance and cleaning or part replacement
Plate reader artifact	Dust accumulation over the light guide and beam deflector	Radiopaque image appearance	Periodic QA maintenance and cleaning
Cassette related artifact	Cracked lead coating at the back	Radiolucent image appearance	Cassette replacement

Table 3.3 Image processing (software-related) artifacts

Artifact	Causes	Appearance	Remedy
Image transmission artifact—communication error artifact	Failure of power during image transmission	Absent pixel lines on the image	Repeat the radiography
Data cable malfunction	Data cable failure	Mixed bands of radiopaque and radiolucent lines on the image	Cable replacement
Improper erasure artifact	Halogen erasure bulb malfunction	Previous images details seen on the existing image	Replacement of halogen vapor bulbs or proper selection of body parts is required

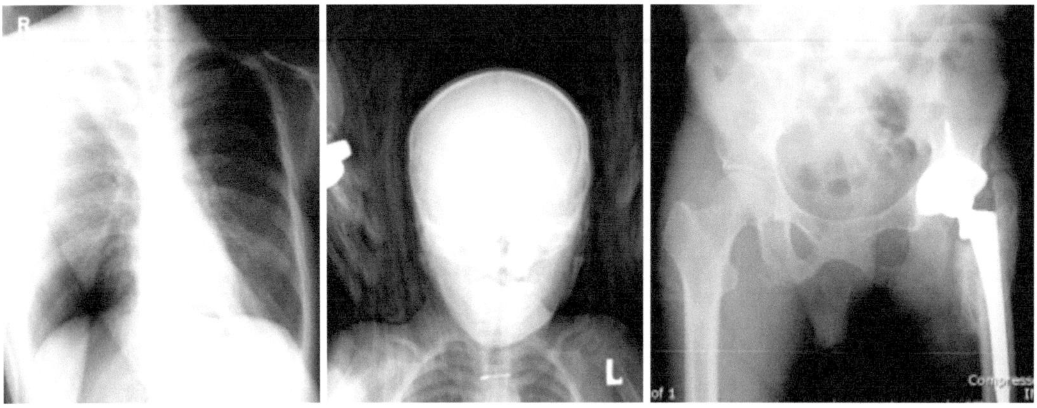

Fig. 3.18 Twin duplication artifact

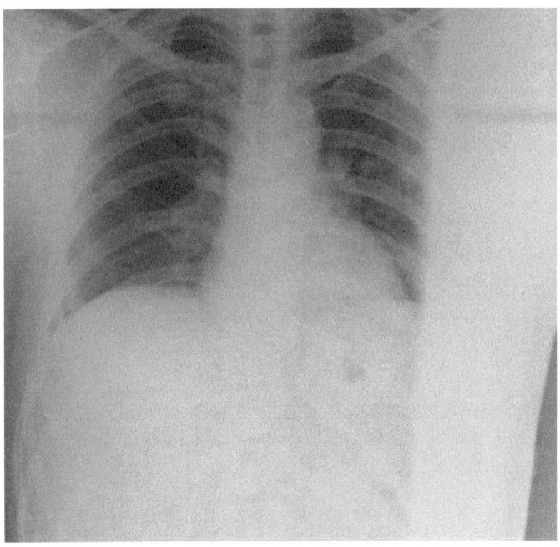

Fig. 3.19 Collimation error

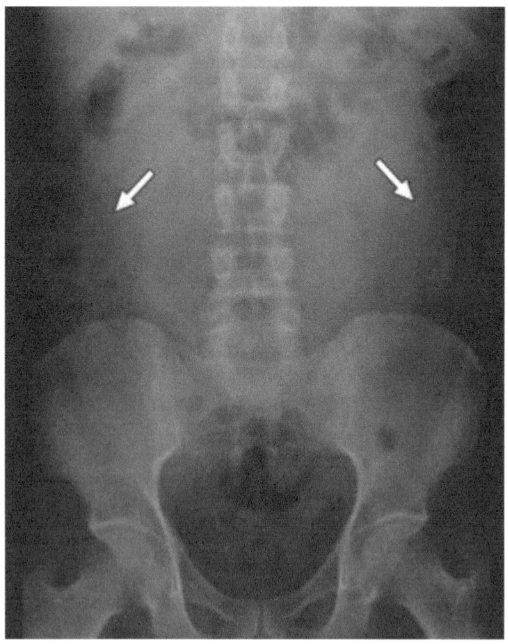

Fig. 3.20 Missed/delayed scanning (greater than 48 h after exposure)

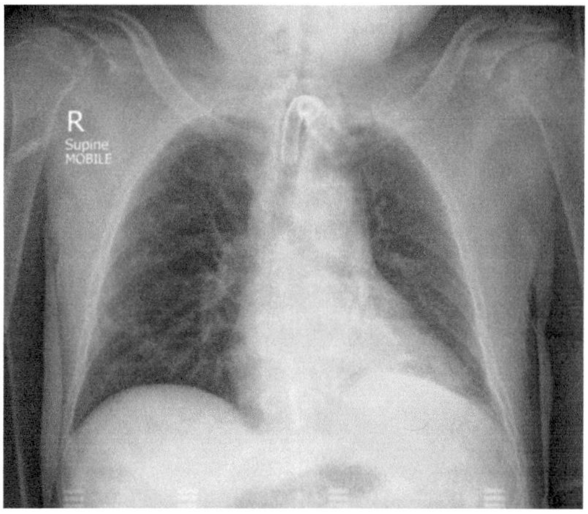

Fig. 3.21 Cassette back exposure

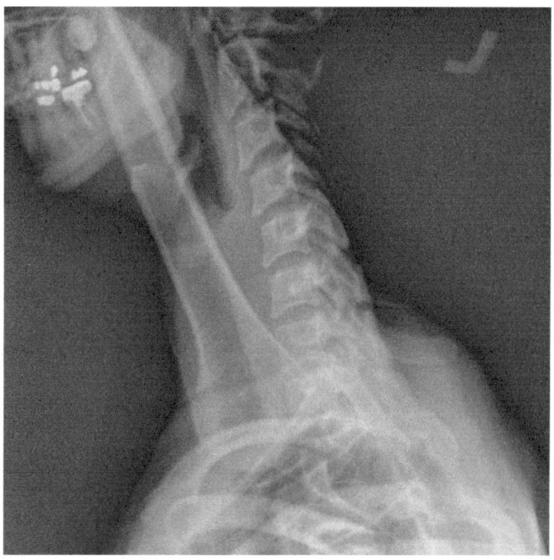

Fig. 3.22 Inappropriate technical factor error—overexposure

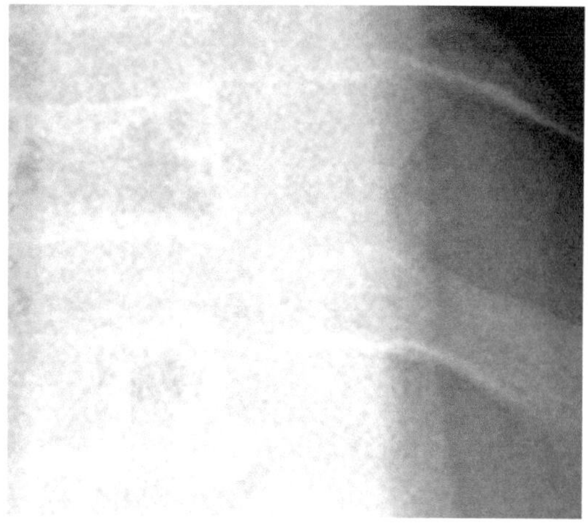

Fig. 3.23 Inappropriate technical factor error—underexposure

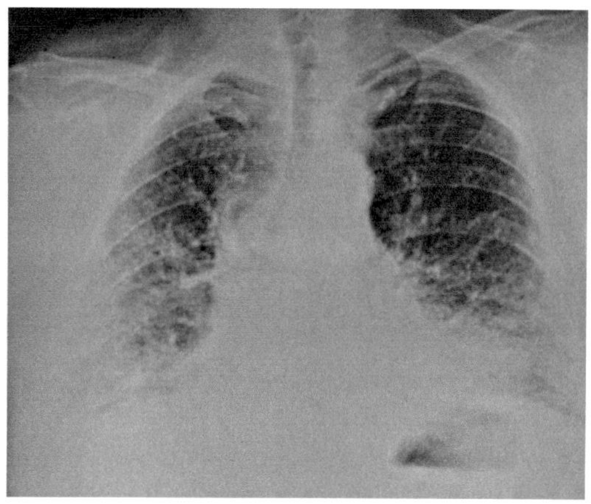

Fig. 3.24 Inappropriate technical factor error—underexposure

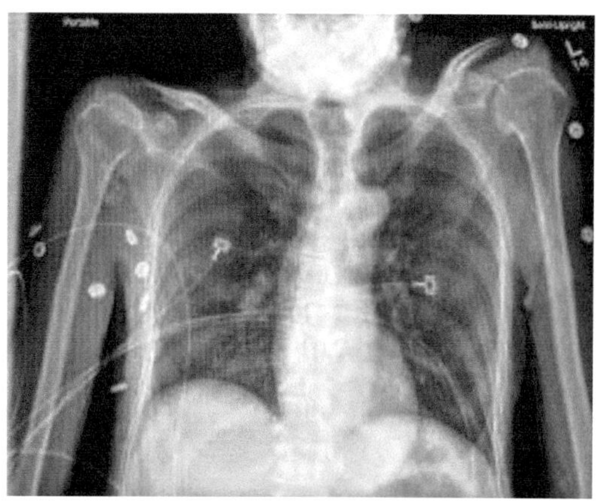

Fig. 3.25 Grid imaging error

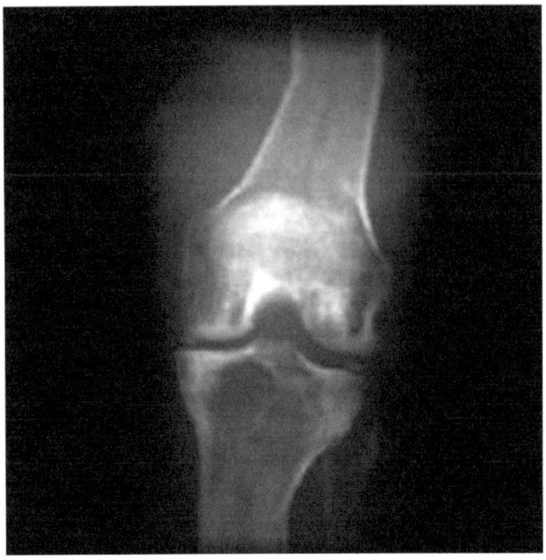

Fig. 3.26 Scatter radiation effect

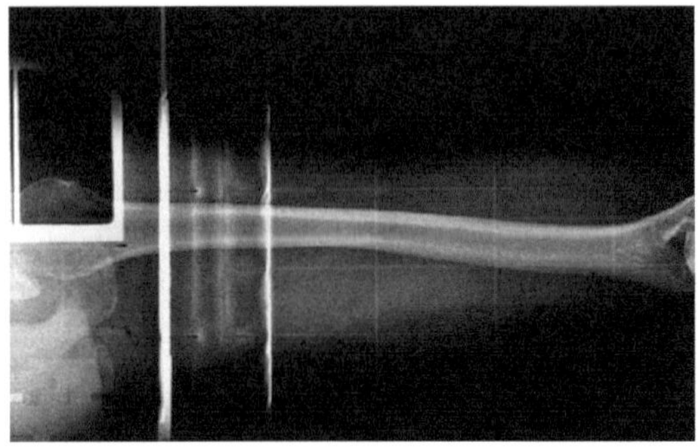

Fig. 3.27 Image plate misuse

Fig. 3.28 Light bulb effect

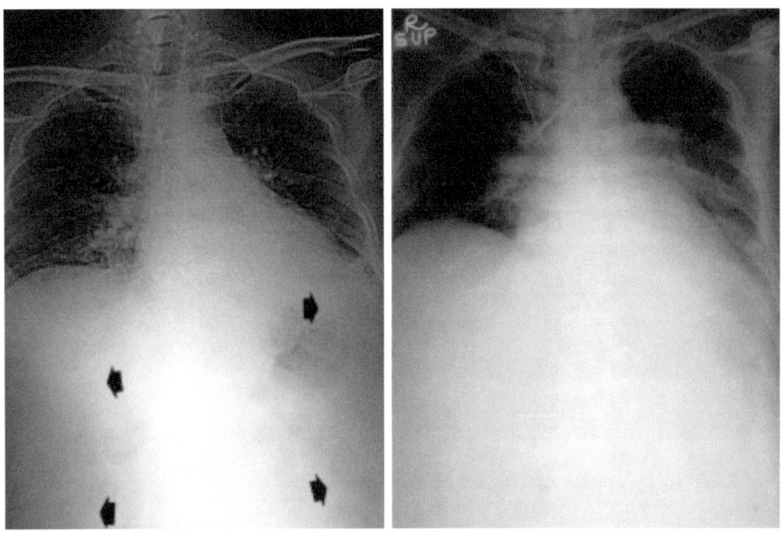

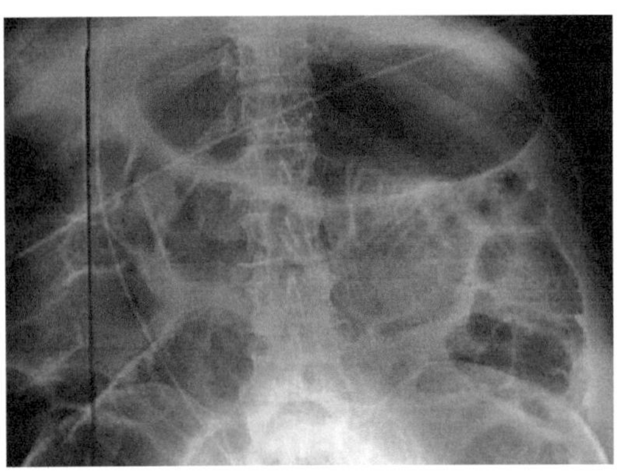

Fig. 3.29 Artifacts due to image plate cracks and dust

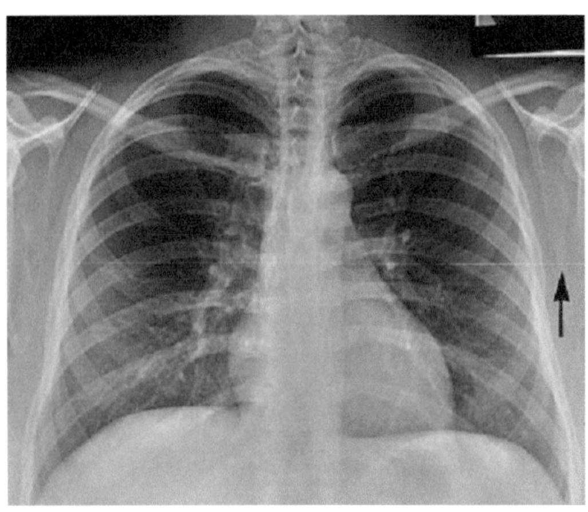

Fig. 3.30 Artifacts due to image plate cracks and dust

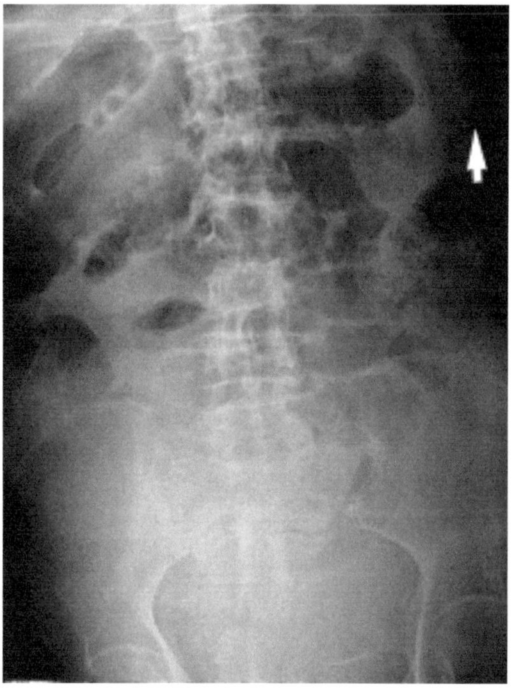

Fig. 3.31 Artifacts due to image plate cracks and dust

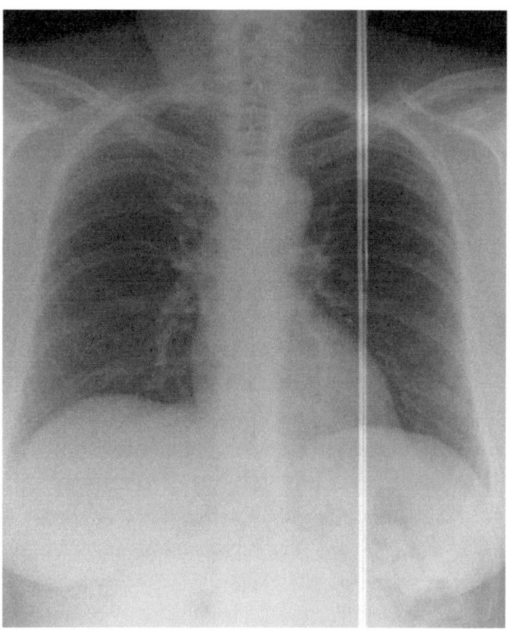

Fig. 3.32 Rollers (within the CR digitizer-related artifacts)

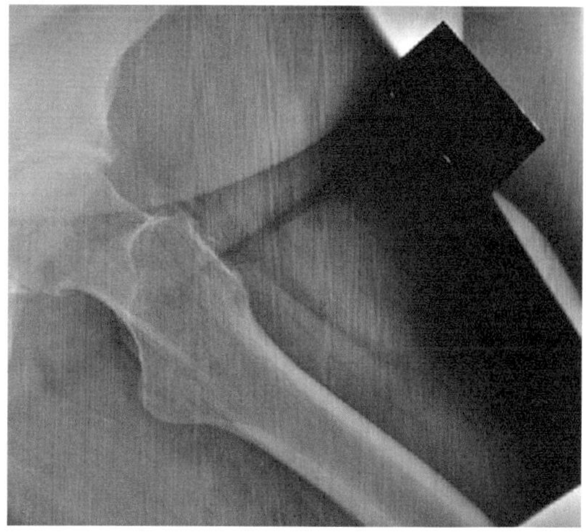

Fig. 3.33 Plate reader artifact

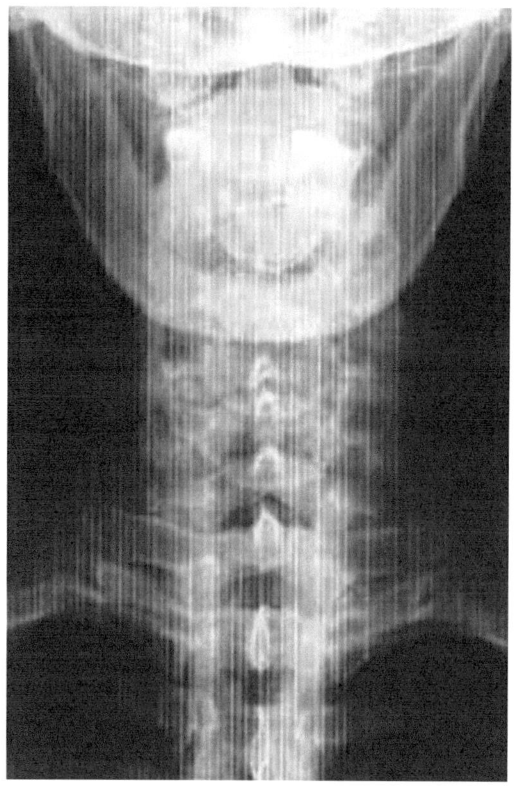

Fig. 3.34 Cassette-related artifact

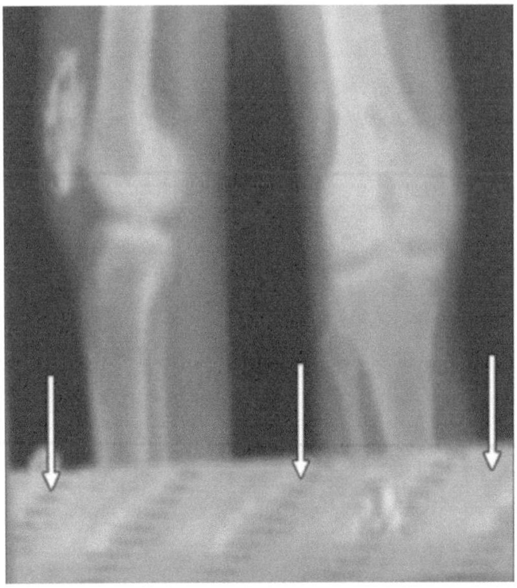

Fig. 3.35 Image transmission artifact—communication error artifact

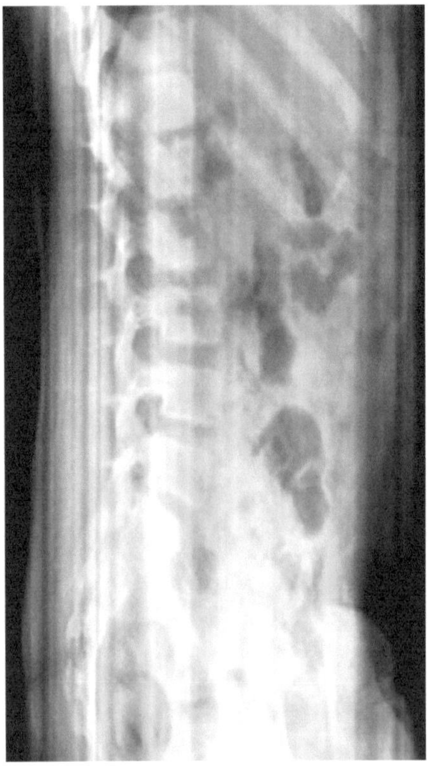

Fig. 3.36 Data cable malfunction

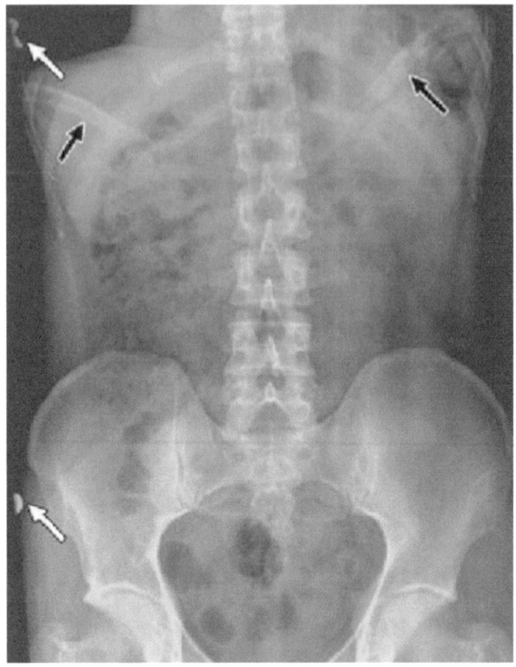

Fig. 3.37 Improper erasure artifact

1. Daily QC checks should be conducted to ensure the CR system is running properly. This includes confirming the CR reader's operation, assuring appropriate calibration of the image plate (IP) reader, and checking for mechanical faults.
2. Regularly clean IP plates to remove dust, dirt, and artifacts that might degrade image quality. To prevent plate damage, follow the manufacturer's cleaning method recommended.
3. Conduct regular sensitivity checks to verify the CR system produces consistent image quality. This entails taking images of a phantom with known densities and evaluating the system's ability to reliably detect them.
4. Regularly inspect CR images for abnormalities, including scratches, stains, and IP plate wear. Investigate the source of any artifacts and take corrective action as needed to avoid recurrence.
5. Calibrate image display monitors routinely for appropriate presentation of CR images.

Monitor brightness, contrast, and spatial resolution to ensure that image quality is constant across all workstations.
6. Monitor exposure indices to monitor radiation dose levels and maintain consistency in exposure parameters. Compare these readings to reference values to find any differences that could indicate incorrect exposure settings.
7. Image rejection analysis: Examine rejected images to determine frequent causes of rejection, such as placement mistakes, motion artifacts, or exposure concerns. Develop solutions to solve these concerns and reduce the risk of image rejection.
8. Implement dose monitoring devices to track radiation levels during each CR examination. Review dosage reports regularly to discover the potential for dose optimization and confirm that dose guidelines are followed.
9. Provide continual training and education to CR technologists to improve their proficiency in CR imaging techniques, artifact recognition, and quality control processes. Stay informed about the latest innovations and best practices in CR technology and imaging standards.
10. Ensure regulatory compliance and accreditation standards for CR imaging facilities. This may entail following criteria published by organizations such as the American College of Radiology (ACR), the Joint Commission, and the Food and Drug Administration (FDA), as well as participating in accreditation programs such as the ACR quality-control manual.

By developing a comprehensive quality control program that addresses these critical areas, CR imaging facilities can maintain high levels of image quality, precision, and patient safety. Regular quality-control tests and constant monitoring are required to identify and address any faults as soon as possible, maintaining the CR system's optimal functioning and delivery of high-quality diagnostic images [31–36].

Quality control of CR imaging plates

In order to control the quality of CR imaging plates, an x-ray source, a display device (soft-copy or hardcopy), and a CR reader must be used. Whenever the images generated from an imaging plate contain too many little white speck artifacts, this technique should be performed every 2 months. It should be noted that cleaning the phosphor screens too frequently or using unapproved cleaning chemicals can cause the phosphor to discolor.

Equipment needed

1. An X-ray source that has been calibrated (with a compliance report).
2. A calibrated hard-copy or soft-copy display (accompanied by a compliance report).
3. CR reader and ID station (with compliance report).
4. Densitometer (if a hard-copy display is used).
5. Aluminum and copper filters (1 mm Al, 1″ Al, and 2.5 mm Cu).
6. Ion chambers.
7. An ion chamber stand.
8. Soft linens and screen cleaning solution.
9. Ethanol anhydride and water should be used as the screen-cleaning solution.
10. Timer.
11. Reduce backscatter by using a lead sheet or apron.
12. Screen-handling gloves that are lint-free.
13. Permanent markers.

Visual Inspection

Visually evaluate all imaging plates for physical flaws. For CR cassettes, ensure that the screen plate is straight and the screen base is not bent. Also, make sure the cassette label matches the type of plate (standard or high resolution) inside.

Screen Cleaning Maintenance

Before proceeding with the testing processes, all image plates should be cleaned and erased. Handle the screens using gloves. Take the screen from the cassette. Pull the screen out gently and parallel to the cassette, as pulling out at an angle can harm the screen's surface.

Remove dust and tiny particles from the screen's surface by gently wiping it with the screen cleaning cloth.

If dirt is resistant to cleaning, use the appropriate cleaning liquid plate cleaning solution and a mixture of ethanol anhydride and water in a circular or straight motion to remove it. Avoid applying excessive pressure. Before inserting the screen back into the cassette, dry the screen surface with a dry cloth. Ensure that the screen is completely dry and residue-free before inserting it back into the cassette.

Stepwise Procedure for Imaging Plate Screen Maintenance

- Collect and stack cassettes for cleaning by the CR ID station.
- "Read" the cassettes. Make that the cassette ID (the number in the top left corner of the screen in the "READ" option) matches the cassette label. If the label is not present or has been erased, write the cassette ID on the tape's label area.
- Check that the number on the back of the cassette matches the one on the screen. If the screen number is not visible or has been erased, write the cassette ID on the back of the screen.
- Repeat steps 1–3 for all cassettes.
- Erase all cassettes.
- Choose a clean, well-lit room with plenty space for a large table. An X-ray room with a tabletop is perfect.
- Clean the tabletop with alcohol and a cloth.
- Put gloves on.
- Remove the screens from the cassettes in an organized method. Place cassettes and screens adjacent to each other to prevent mixing. Avoid touching the screen's white sensitive surface (especially if you have long fingernails).
- Visually check cassettes and screens for any physical faults. Look for chipping, discoloration, bending, and cracks on the displays. Any faults other than dust and minor chippings at the edges should be documented in the log table (you may want to include the location of such problems as well).
- Gently wipe the screen with a cleaning cloth to remove dust and tiny debris.
- To remove stubborn filth, use a moist cloth with cleaning solutions and wipe in a circular or straight motion. Avoid applying excessive pressure. Also, avoid using too much cleaning solution.
- Let the screen dry.
- Clean the cassette's innards with screen-cleaning solution and a cloth, focusing on the tube side.
- Let the cassette dry.
- Place the screen back into the cassette. Before inserting the screen back into the cassette, it should be properly dry and residue-free.
- Proceed with the next step.

Uniformity Test

The plates should be exposed to 10 mR entry exposure with an 80 kVp, 1 mm Al/0.5 mm Cu filter, and a source-to-image distance of 180 cm (SID) as depicted in Fig. 3.38 and Table 3.4. The beam can also be used without filtration, as long as it is done consistently with the same X-ray tube. Do not utilize the bucky for exposures; instead, position the cassette on the bucky or on an elevated platform above the floor (to avoid backscatter). The cassette's long axis must be perpendicular to the tube's axis. Ensure that a consistent and minimal delay is maintained between exposing and reading the plates (1–15 min).

Unless otherwise specified, choose the pattern body component and "raw data" and "no edge enhancement" options, with the level set to Exposure Index and the window to 1024. For all CR systems, utilize a semi-EDR to assess the sensitivity of body parts. The image should be uniform with no artifacts. If the plate is not adequately cleaned, some white specks will appear. The location of such artifacts varies on each plate screen, and they should be removed by cleaning the screen.

Any other artifact is deemed abnormal. Determine the image's average pixel value and its standard deviation (SD). Two times the standard deviation should be within 10% of the average pixel value. A hard-copy display should have an

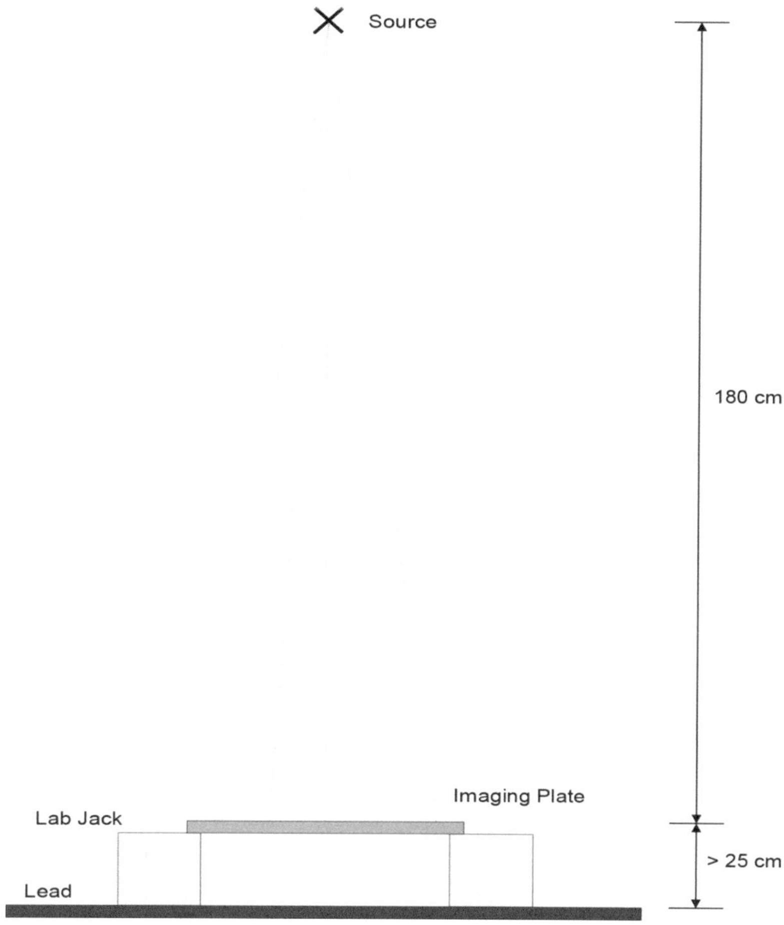

Fig. 3.38 CR QC test exposure setup

optical density within 10% of the average value at the center of each quadrant. There should be no more than 10% variation from plate to plate [37–42].

QC precautions

- Frequent cleaning of phosphor plates might cause discoloration.
- Before usage, delete imaging plates that have not been used in more than 24 h (if applicable, apply secondary erase).
- Remove overexposed plates from clinical usage for 24 h and erase before reuse (primary erase for plates if applicable).

Additional QC Tests—Perfomed as per Company Recommendations and Guidelines

- Dark noise
- IP uniformity
- Linearity and calibration
- Pixel size (spatial accuracy)
- Ghost imaging
- Laser beam function
- High-contrast resolution and resolution uniformity

3.1.5.1 CR: Top Manufacturers

As of 2023, numerous businesses are well-known for producing computed radiography (CR) equipment. Here are some of the leading manufacturers worldwide:

1. Fujifilm medical systems: A top manufacturer of medical imaging equipment, including CR systems. Their CR systems are renowned for their dependability, image quality, and innovative functionality.
2. Carestream Health provides several medical imaging technologies, including CR systems for digital radiography. Their CR systems are

Table 3.4 CR plate QC logsheet

Cassette size	Cassette no.	Date	Visual defects	Cleaning (√)	Nonuni-formities	Exposure level	Comments
14 × 17							
``							
``							
``							
``							
``							
``							
``							
``							
``							
``							
``							
``							
``							
``							
10 × 12							
``							
``							
``							
``							
``							
``							
``							
``							
``							
``							
``							
``							
``							
``							
8 × 10							
``							
``							
``							
``							
``							
``							
``							
``							
``							
``							
``							
``							
``							
``							

widely utilized in a variety of healthcare settings and are renowned for their ease of use and adaptability.
3. Agfa HealthCare is a major leader in the medical imaging business, providing CR systems and other digital radiography products. Their CR systems are designed to give high-quality images.

1. Koninklijke Philips N.V. (Philips Healthcare) offers a wide range of medical imaging equipment, including CR systems. Their CR systems are intended to suit the requirements of healthcare practitioners for digital radiography imaging.
2. Canon Medical Systems Corporation (previously Toshiba Medical Systems Corporation) manufactures medical imaging devices, such as CR systems. Their CR systems are intended to produce high-resolution images and improve process efficiency.
3. Hitachi Healthcare Americas (previously Hitachi Medical Systems) provides various medical imaging technologies, including CR systems. Their CR systems are renowned for their dependability, performance, and sophisticated imaging capabilities.
4. Konica Minolta Healthcare Americas offers digital radiography solutions, including CR systems, for healthcare facilities. Their CR systems produce images of excellent quality and provide effective workflow solutions.

These are some of the world's leading producers of computed radiography systems, while other firms also make CR systems or provide digital radiography solutions. When selecting a CR system, healthcare facilities must consider their individual needs and requirements, including image quality, workflow efficiency, reliability, and support services.

CR has evolved to be a universal imaging technique for imaging the chest, abdomen, musculoskeletal system, and pediatric anatomy. As a result of its complex function, CR is both lauded and derided by ordinary technologists because it requires extensive ongoing training. As a result of the separation of detector, display, and archive in digital radiography, plain radiographic images can be moved, stored, printed, and viewed with greater flexibility than when using screen-film technology. The electronic and digital revolution in medicine has made CR technology a viable option for people. Technologists and radiologists prefer CR imaging because of its ability to improve pathology and reveal concealed anatomy, despite its lower spatial resolution. An experienced CR technician can provide high-quality diagnostic images when using this new modality.

3.2 Section B: Digital Radiography Systems

3.2.1 History, Introduction, and Classification: Digital Radiography

Over the last two decades, many radiology departments have gradually replaced screen and film radiography with digital radiography. This technology is also becoming widely accepted in human and veterinary care simultaneously. Technical advancements in digital radiography have been rapid, and in nearly every case, the cost of these equipment has decreased. Another factor influencing the pricing of digital radiography equipment is the rising number of vendors, summit industries, and (Agfa, Fuji, Kodak in health) who are interested in this market [43–45].

This subsection provides an overview of digital radiography (DR). First, digital radiography is defined, followed by a summary of the critical components of digital radiography imaging systems. The last topic explains flat-panel digital radiography (FPDR) in detail. In this chapter, we will provide a detailed overview of the components of digital radiography imaging systems.

Digital radiography (DR) has transformed medical imaging by replacing traditional film-based radiography and computed radiography with digital technologies. Here is a quick summary of its history:

- During the late twentieth century, digital radiography emerged as a concept. Researchers and engineers began digitizing images from X-rays for better storage, retrieval, and manipulation.

- Computed radiography (CR) era (1980s–1990s): CR was a pioneering digital radiography technology that gained widespread adoption. CR systems acquire X-ray images through imaging plates covered with photostimulable phosphors. These plates are then scanned, yielding digital images. Compared to traditional film-based radiography, CR systems offer faster image acquisition, electronic storage, and digital enhancement and manipulation capabilities.
- Introduction of direct digital radiography (DDR) (late 1990s–early 2000s): DDR systems provided improved image quality and workflow efficiency. DDR systems recorded X-ray images directly using digital detectors such amorphous silicon or selenium, eliminating the need for intermediate imaging plates.
- Sensor technology advancements from 2000 to present:
  In the 2000s, developments in digital sensor technology resulted in advanced DR systems with higher resolution, sensitivity, and faster picture acquisition. Manufacturers introduced digital detectors, such as flat-panel detectors (FPDs), which are now widely used in DR systems due to their high image quality and efficiency.
- Integration with PACS: Integrating digital radiography equipment with PACS enables seamless picture storage, retrieval, and sharing within healthcare facilities. PACS integration leads to speedier diagnosis, enhanced communication among healthcare providers, and better patient care.
- Mobile and portable DR systems are becoming increasingly popular, allowing for imaging in clinical situations such as bedside examinations, emergency departments, and operating rooms.
  Portable DR systems provide flexibility, convenience, good image quality, and diagnostic accuracy.
- Digital radiography continues to innovate through ongoing research and development, including advancements in detector technology, dose optimisation, AI integration for image analysis, and improved workflow automation.

Digital radiography has impacted medical imaging techniques, providing various advantages such as improved image quality, greater diagnostic capabilities, increased workflow efficiency, and lower radiation exposure for patients and healthcare personnel [46–49].

This chapter describes the technological features of flat-panel digital radiography (FPDR). Several aspects of wireless digital detectors require a description, including FPDR, its components, types of FPDR systems, design characteristics, operating principles, image processing and imaging performance characteristics, artifacts, and basic aspects of wireless digital detectors. This type of system uses amorphous silicon (a-Si) and amorphous selenium (a-Se) to create digital images using a set of electrical components specifically designed to produce digital images different from computed radiography (CR). There are two types of FPDR systems: indirect and direct digital detectors. X-ray scintillators (X-ray conversion layer) are used in the former, followed by amorphous silicon (a-Si) photodiode flat-panel layer with a thin-film transistor (TFT) array to read out the electrical charges. In the latter, X-ray photons from a patient are detected and converted directly into electric charges by a photoconductor like amorphous selenium (a-Se).

The TFT array and associated circuits collect and store changes for later reading. EI is also a feature of FPDR systems. It provides a visual indication of the amount of exposure used for each examination and whether the exposure meets the manufacturer's requirements. Furthermore, raw data are presented during preprocessing and postprocessing as "for processing" and "for presentation," respectively [50–54].

3.2.2 DR Instrumentation: Major Components of a Digital Radiography Imaging System

According to the American Association of Physicists in Medicine (AAPM), digital radiography refers to the use of images produced by photostimulable storage phosphors (computed radiography, or CR), amorphous silicon, amorphous selenium, charge-coupled devices, or metal oxide semiconductor field effect transistors. Compared with film-screen radiography, these technologies can generate acceptable images across a wider range of exposure conditions [55, 56].

A digital radiography (DR) imaging system typically consists of several major components, including:

1. **X-ray Source:** This component generates X-rays used to create radiographic images. X-ray tubes and high-voltage generators are usually included to provide the necessary imaging energy.
2. **Detector:** In digital radiography, the detector captures the X-rays after they pass through the patient. There are two main types of detectors:
   - Flat-panel detectors (FPD): These are the most common type in modern DR systems. They consist of a large, flat panel that directly converts X-rays into electrical signals. Charge-coupled devices: In digital radiography, CCD (charge-coupled device) technology is often used as an image receptor. CCDs are semiconductor devices that convert light into electrical charges. In digital radiography, X-rays interact with a scintillator material, which emits light in response. This light is then captured by the CCD.
3. **Image Processing Software:** This software is used to enhance and manipulate the digital images captured by the detector. It may include features such as image stitching, noise reduction, contrast enhancement, and image annotation tools.
4. **Control Console:** The control console is the user interface where radiologic technologists can adjust exposure settings, review images, and perform other system operations. It typically includes a monitor for image display and controls for adjusting parameters such as X-ray tube voltage, current, and exposure time.
5. **Image Display and Storage**: Digital radiography systems often include high-resolution monitors for viewing images in real time. A Picture Archiving and Communication System (PACS) or a Radiology Information System (RIS) is also used to store the images digitally for easy access, retrieval, and long-term storage.
6. **Networking Infrastructure:** DR systems are often integrated into hospital or clinic networks to facilitate image sharing, remote viewing, and access to patient records. This infrastructure includes servers, routers, and other networking components.
7. **Power Supply and Cooling Systems:** X-ray sources and detectors require stable power sources and cooling systems to operate reliably and maintain image quality. These components may include transformers, power regulators, and cooling fans or liquid cooling systems.

These components work together to capture, process, display, and store digital radiographic images, providing healthcare imaging professionals with valuable diagnostic information for patient care as depicted in Fig. 3.39 [57, 58].

3.2.3 DR Flat-Panel Detectors: Direct and Indirect Detector Technology

Flat-panel detectors (FPDs) are an essential component of digital radiography systems, providing numerous advantages over traditional film-based or computed radiography (CR) systems. Here's how they operate and why they're preferred:

1. **Structure:** FPDs are made up of two primary components: a scintillator layer and a collection of photodiodes or thin-film transistors (TFTs). The scintillator layer transforms X-rays to visible light, which is then converted into electrical impulses by photodiodes or TFTs.
2. **X-ray absorption and conversion:** The FPD's scintillator layer produces light photons when X-rays travel through the patient's body.

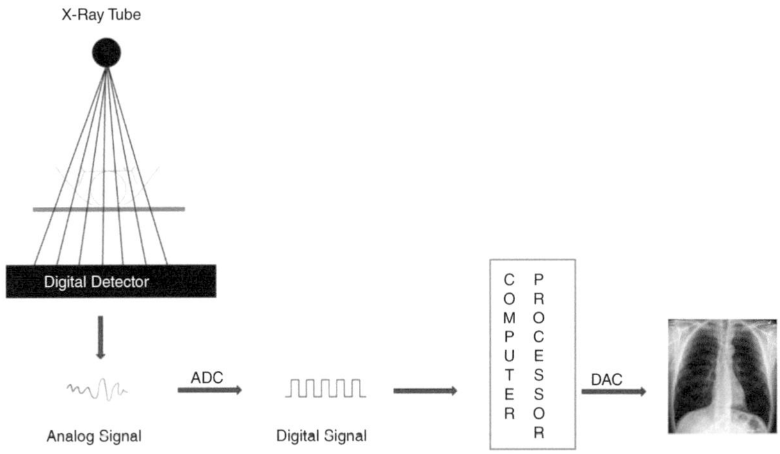

Fig. 3.39 Technical components of digital radiography

3. **Light detection:** The FPD's photodiodes, or TFTs, detect light photons and transform them into electrical charges.
4. **Charge collection and readout:** The photodiode or TFT array collects electrical charges, which are then read pixel by pixel. Each pixel represents a specific place on the detector and contains data about the X-ray intensity that struck it.
5. **Analog-to-digital conversion:** The electrical signals from each pixel are then transformed from analog to digital format, resulting in a digital representation of the X-ray attenuation across the patient's body.
6. **Image processing and display:** The digital image data is processed in several processes to improve image quality before being shown on a monitor for interpretation by a radiologist.

3.2.3.1 Advantages of FPDs in Digital Radiography Include

- High image quality: FPDs offer excellent spatial resolution and contrast sensitivity, allowing for detailed and accurate images.
- Real-time imaging: FPDs enable real-time imaging for procedures such as fluoroscopy, providing immediate feedback to clinicians.
- Wide dynamic range: FPDs can capture a wide range of X-ray intensities, allowing for imaging of both dense and less dense tissues without overexposure or underexposure.
- Dose efficiency: FPDs require lower radiation doses compared to film-based systems, making them safer for patients while still producing high-quality images.
- Convenience: FPDs produce digital images that can be easily stored, transmitted, and manipulated, improving workflow efficiency in healthcare settings.

Overall, flat-panel detectors play a crucial role in modern digital radiography, offering improved image quality, efficiency, and versatility compared to traditional imaging technologies [59–62].

Digital radiography (FPDR) was developed as a solution to the shortcomings of conventional radiography (CR). There is a fundamental difference between the digital detector (IP) and the CR detector (flat panel). There are currently two types of flat-panel digital radiography imaging systems, based on the type of detector used:

1. **Indirect conversion digital radiography systems**
2. **Direct conversion digital radiography systems**

Figures 3.40, 3.41, and 3.42 show the essential components of these detectors and the procedures involved in producing an image for indirect and direct conversion systems. Figures 3.40, 3.41, and 3.42 shows how X-rays are converted into light using cesium iodide as a phosphor. When the phosphor produces light, it strikes a matrix array

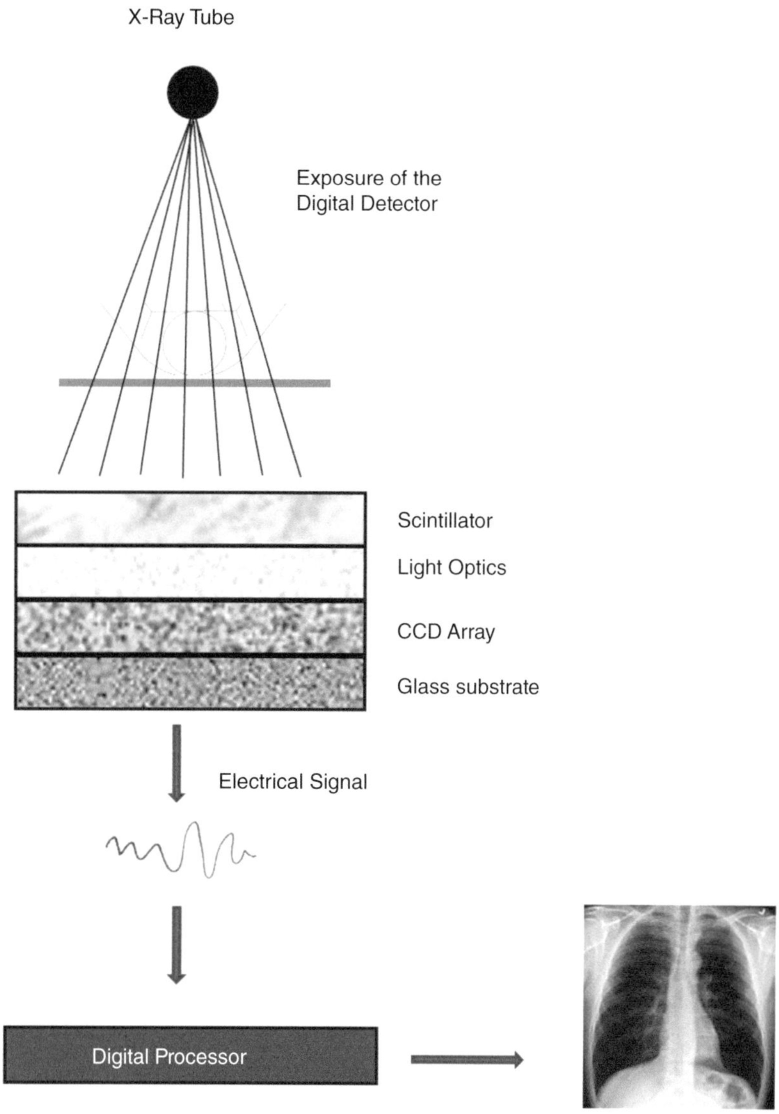

Fig. 3.40 Indirect flat-panel detector using CCD array

of electronic devices, generating and storing electrical charges directly proportional to the exposure to X-rays. In order to create an image, the charges generate electrical impulses that are then digitized and processed by a digital computer [61–63].

A direct conversion digital radiography system converts X-rays directly into electronic signals. In Fig. 3.42, X-rays strike a photoconductor (such as selenium) that generates electrical signals when connected to a matrix array of electronic devices. A digital computer digitizes and processes these impulses to produce an image. Figure 3.40 illustrates the second type of indirect conversion detector. An array of charge-coupled devices (CCDs) is used instead of an array of electrical elements as in the counter part type. As indicated, the CCDs are connected to a scintillator phosphor cesium iodide. An image is created when X-rays strike the phosphor, producing light that is directed to a CCD array, which converts light into electrical signals that are digitized and processed by a digital computer.

A flat-panel digital detector can be erased and reused after all electrical charges have been read out. In addition, flat-panel detectors have numerous advantages, including excellent DQE and

Fig. 3.41 Indirect flat-panel system

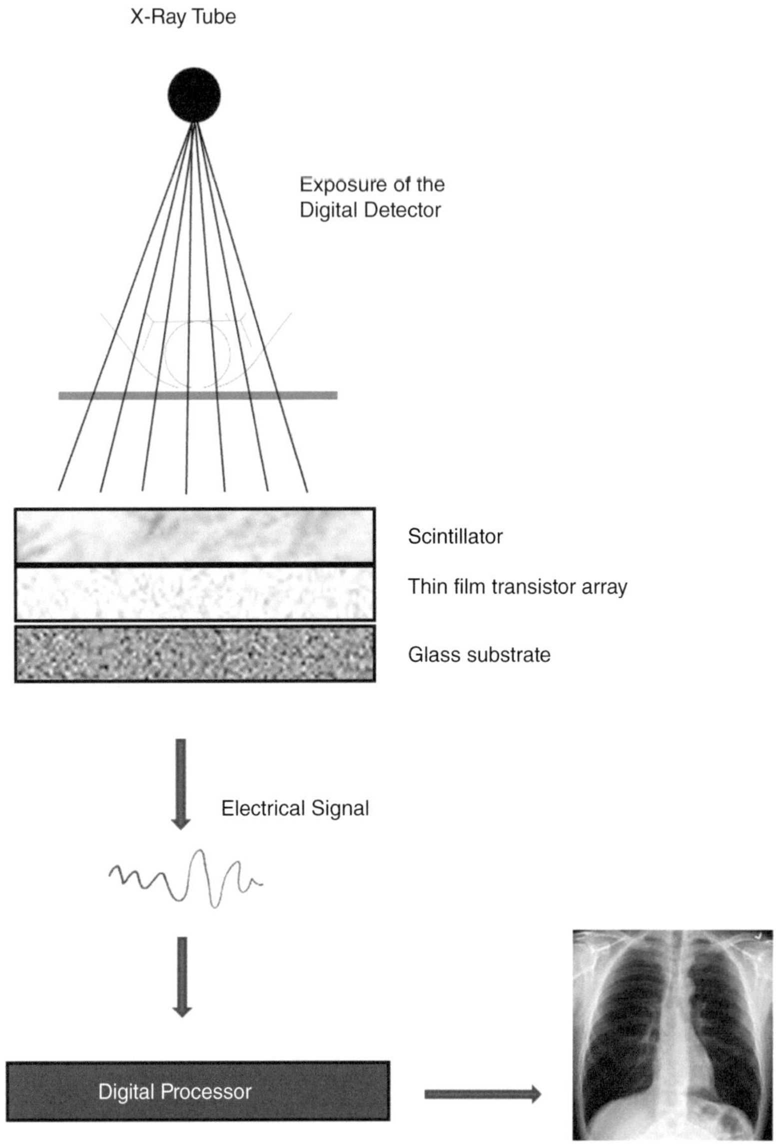

spatial resolution comparable to that of CR detectors [64–68].

3.2.3.2 DR: Charge-Coupled Devices and Detectors (CCD)

Here's a simple description of how CCD works in digital radiography:

1. X-ray exposure: X-rays penetrate through the body and interact with a scintillator material, converting energy into visible light.
2. Light conversion: The scintillator produces light, which is directed toward the CCD.
3. Charge generation: The CCD generates electric charges based on the intensity of the light.
4. Charge transfer: Electric charges are transported pixel by pixel through the CCD chip to a readout register.
5. Analog-to-digital conversion: Charges from the readout register are converted into digital signals.
6. Image reconstruction: Digital signals are processed and reconstructed to create a displayable image.

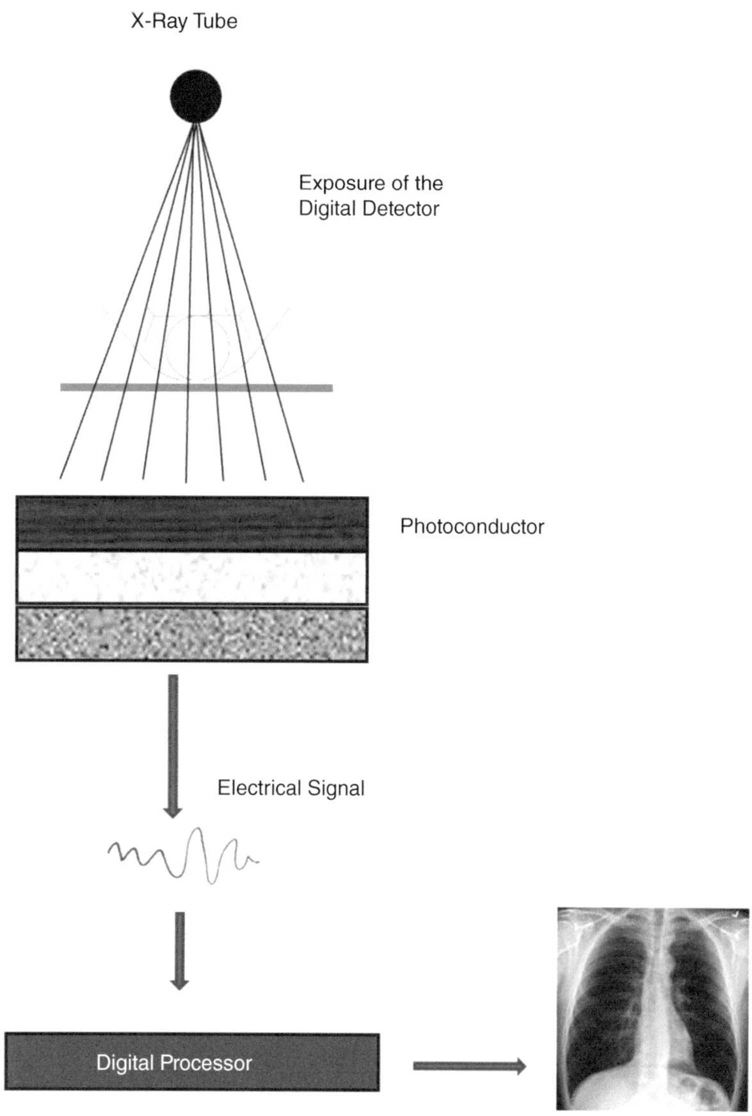

Fig. 3.42 Direct flat-panel system

CCD technology provides various benefits in digital radiography, including great sensitivity to light, low noise levels, and reasonably high resolution. However, CCDs have limitations, such as restricted dynamic range and blooming (charge overflow into adjacent pixels).

In addition, the characteristic curve of digital detectors used in CR and flat-panel digital radiography differs significantly from that of film. Digital detector output signals are proportional to radiation dose input. As a result of this linear response, the film characteristic curve has a wider range of exposure latitudes (determined by its slope). Herein lies a major advantage of digital detectors. Regardless of the input exposure, the wide exposure latitude of the digital detector produces acceptable photos. Film-screen radiography produces light images when exposed low, whereas dark images when exposed high. It would be necessary to repeat these images in order to get an acceptable film density, increasing the radiation exposure to the patient [69].

3.2.3.3 Classification of Flat-Panel Detectors

Flat-panel detectors have been broadly classified into (A) **indirect detector** and (B) **direct detector** types, as illustrated in Fig. 3.43.

Indirect digital detector: technical considerations

Figure. There are two types of indirect digital detectors: the charge-coupled device (CCD) digital detector (Fig. 3.40) and the thin-film transistor (TFT) digital detector (Fig. 3.41). Both types of detectors are distinguished by the technical component that converts light into electrical impulses.

A. **Indirect CCD digital detectors**

CCD digital detectors convert light to electrical charge indirectly via a CCD chip. As a commercially available technology, the CCD digital detector is not considered a flat-panel digital detector (as the title suggests technically); however, it will be discussed in this chapter.

Figure 3.40 depicts the key technical components of a CCD-based digital radiography detector, which include an X-ray absorber, light optics, and a CCD sensor (chip) for capturing light. Additionally, CCDs are electrical charge readout devices that combine many CCDs to expand the detection area. The scintillation screen (which detects and converts X-rays into light), the light collection optics, and the array of CCDs, or CCD cameras, are also important components. CCD detectors can be fiber-optic-coupled, lens-coupled, or fiber-optic-coupled scanning arrays.

Indirect TFT Flat-Panel Detectors

An indirect flat-panel digital detector operates on an indirect conversion mechanism, using many physical components to convert X-rays into light, which is then turned into electrical charges. These components consist of an X-ray scintillator (X-ray conversion layer), an amorphous silicon (a-Si) photodiode flat-panel layer, and a thin-film transistor (TFT) array for reading out the photodiode array's electrical charges. The organization of these components is shown in Fig. 3.41.

In flat-panel digital detectors, cesium iodide (CsI) or gadolinium oxysulfide (Gd2O2S) is commonly used as the X-ray scintillator layer. It is not the first time these phosphors have been used in X-ray imaging; they were previously applied to image intensifiers (CsI) and rare-earth intensifying screens (Gd2O2S). An interesting design feature is the method by which these phosphors are placed into the a-Si photodiode array. In contrast, Gd2O2S crystals are deposited as powdered particles rather than needle-like patterns in CsI crystals (structured phosphor) [66, 67, 70–72].

Structured scintillators are often referred to as structured scintillators, while unstructured scintillators are known as unstructured scintillators. Furthermore, powdered phosphors cause light to spread laterally, destroying the image's spatial resolution. Structured phosphors, such as CsI needles, reduce lateral light dispersion, increasing picture spatial resolution. The effect is clearly shown in Fig. 3.41.

An a-Si photodiode flat-panel array follows the X-ray scintillator (X-ray detection medium). A silicon layer is deposited on a thin glass substrate (typically 0.7 mm) by plasma-enhanced chemical vapor deposition. "Needle-like" design reduces lateral spread of light, improving spatial resolution. Electrical charges are generated by converting light from the X-ray detector scintillator to the a-Si photodiode layer. In addition to a-Si photodiode, thin-film transistors (TFTs), storage capacitors, and accompanying electronics are located nearby. The capacitor captures and stores the electrical charge generated by the array of a-Si photodiodes. TFT digital detectors are often referred to as indirect conversion flat-panels in this context.

B. **Direct digital detector: technical considerations**

Figure 3.42 depicts the cross section of a direct flat-panel TFT digital detector. A high voltage source, a top electrode, a dielectric layer, photoconductors, collection electrodes, TFTs, storage capacitors, and a glass substrate make up this detector.

In addition to amorphous selenium (a-Se), other photoconductors can also be used, such as lead oxide, lead iodide, thallium bromide, and gadolinium compounds. The use of a-Se is common today because of its outstanding X-ray photon detection characteristics and high spatial resolution. X-ray photons are detected by the photoconductor and converted directly into electrical charges. For later reading, the TFT and accompanying circuitry (such as capacitors) collect and store the changes.

A focus is placed on the design (or framework) of the flat-panel TFT digital detector (especially with regard to indirect and direct flat-panel TFTs). Photoconductors detect and convert X-ray photons directly into electrical charges. Charges are gathered and stored by the TFT and related electronics (e.g., capacitors) [57–59, 71–79].

Flat-panel TFT digital detectors are constructed as matrices of detector elements called pixels, with each element equivalent to one pixel. An integrated circuit with a large area is called a large-area integrated circuit. Matrix arrays, also known as active matrix arrays, are composed of rows and columns that address and read signals from pixels.

According to the Figs. 3.43 and 3.44, each pixel has a TFT (switch), a storage capacitor, and a sensing area. Direct flat-panel TFT detectors detect X-ray photons passing through the patient, while indirect flat-panel TFT detectors detect light emitted by a CsI scintillator. In indirect flat-panel TFT detectors, photodiodes (photosensitive storage elements) are used, whereas direct flat-panel TFT detectors use a-Se photoconductors.

A flat-panel detector also includes other electronic components besides the pixel matrix. Each row of pixels is activated by switching circuits, while each column is read by electronic amplifiers (multiplexers). The electronic signal (analog signal) is then converted to digital form using an

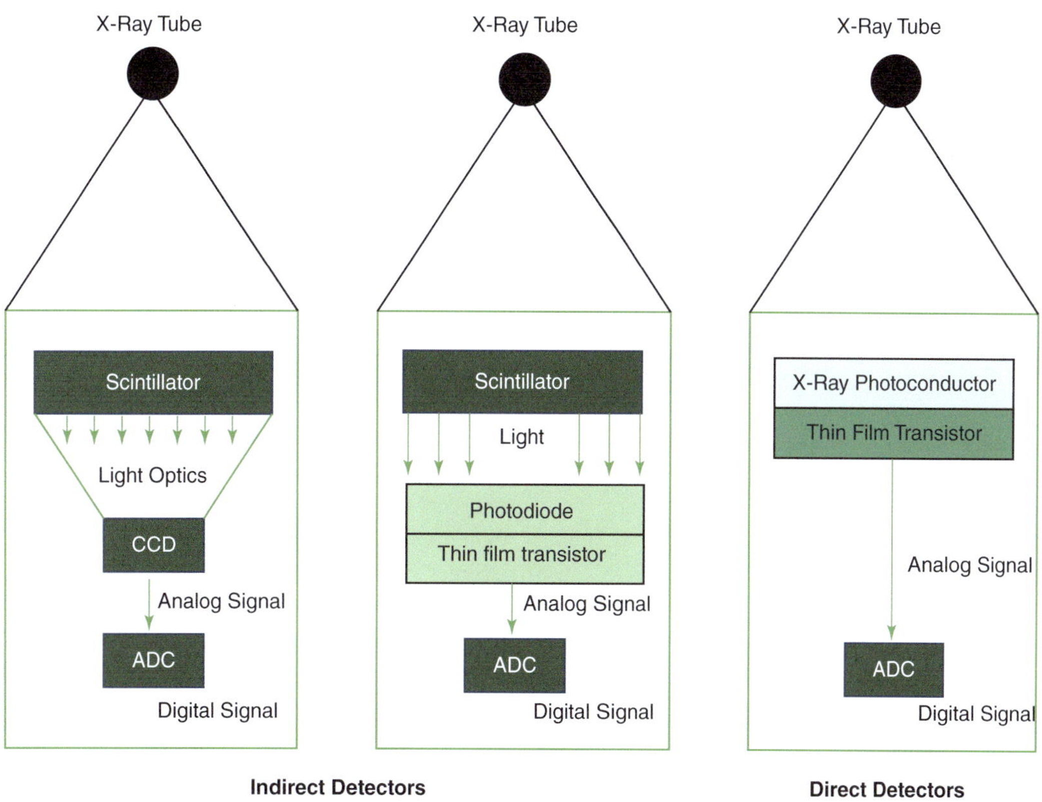

Fig. 3.43 Flat-panel digital radiography detectors (indirect vs direct): design configuration considerations

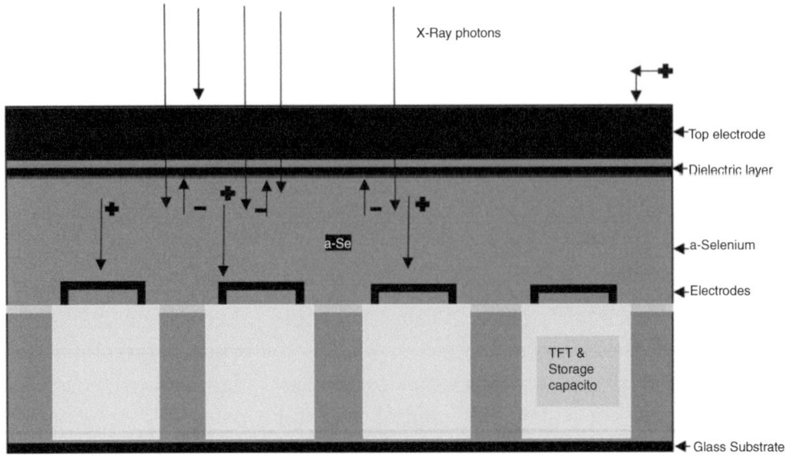

Fig. 3.44 Components of an amorphous-Se (a-SE) TFT direct flat-panel digital detector

analog-to-digital converter (ADC). ADCs are also integrated into flat-panel detectors. For image processing, the digital data stream is routed to a digital computer.

3.2.3.4 Woking Principles: Indirect vs Direct Flat-Panel Detectors

General principles

It is necessary to understand the physics of scintillation phosphors, photoconductors, semiconductors, and electronics in order to understand the principles of digital detectors using CCD and flat-panel technologies. In addition, some of the technical aspects of these detectors are proprietary, so only a general description of how they work will be provided.

CCD detectors and flat-panel detectors will be discussed in this section (from the exposure of the detector to the detection of latent images generated by electrical charges). Also covered will be the exposure latitude, the indication of exposure, and the processing of images generated by flat-panel digital detectors.

3.2.3.5 CCD Detectors

CCD digital detectors have a variety of design topologies. Figure depicts indirect conversion detectors that use a CCD to gather light from a scintillator. CCD silicon chips consist of millions of individual pixels arranged into a matrix array. The scintillator produces electron-hole pairs (charges) based on the amount of light falling on each pixel. A bucket brigade of the system electronics transfers the charge from each pixel in a row to the next row, then down all of the columns to the last row of the readout. For digitalization, the charge pattern from the readout row of pixels is transferred to the ADC. Digital images are created by processing digital data streams in a digital computer.

A limitation of the CCD digital detector is the use of light optics (lenses, mirrors, and fiber optics) to connect the X-ray scintillator to the CCD silicon chip. CCD arrays shrink the output image from scintillator phosphors to the size of the optical system. Consequently, the signal-to-noise ratio is reduced when images are minified or demagnified. Attempts are being made to create additional CCD detectors to deal with image quality degradation caused by small-area CCD detectors. These detectors require more research to determine their objective imaging performance.

3.2.3.6 Flat-Panel TFT Detectors

As previously stated in the chapter, there are two types of flat-panel TFT digital detectors for radiographic imaging. It is possible to use either indirect or direct flat-panel TFT detectors as depicted in Figs. 3.44 and 3.45. In direct detectors, an amorphous-Se (a-Se) photoconductor converts X-rays directly into electrical charges, while indirect detectors use a light-sensitive photodiode (to catch light from the scintillator phosphor, such as CsI).

These detectors are notable for their widespread use in radiography, fluoroscopy, and angi-

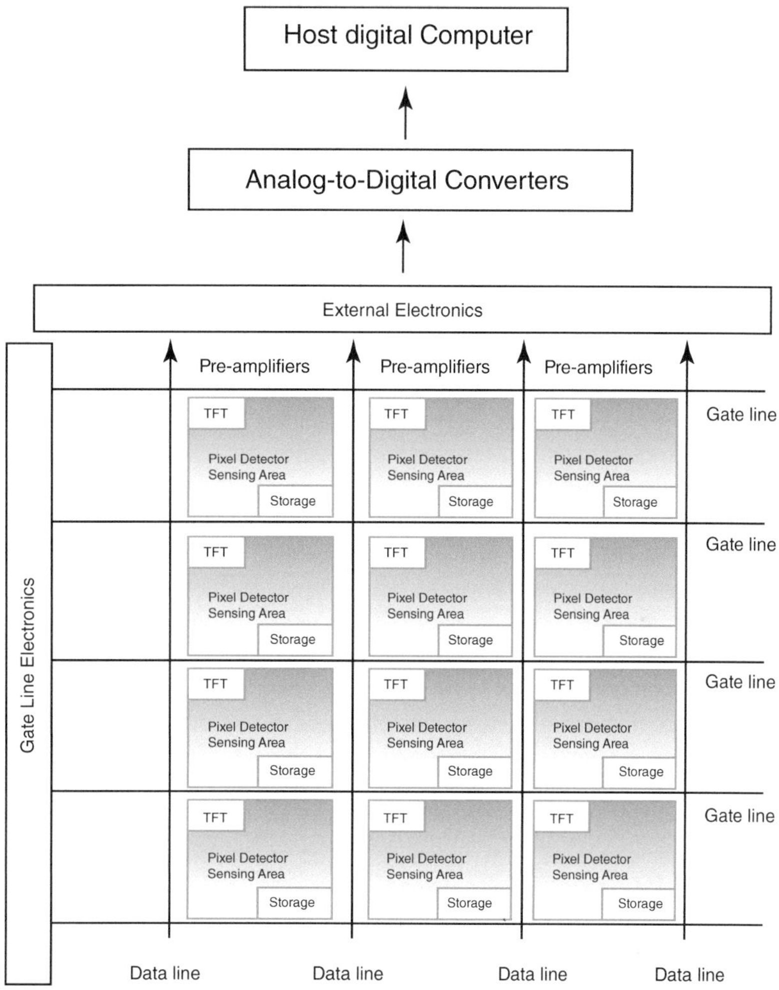

Fig. 3.45 Basic construction of a flat-panel digital detector

ography procedures that employ the Brems or continuous X-ray spectrum. With this spectrum, a wide range of voltages can be used (such as 50 kVp to 140 kVp) to scan various types of body parts. In addition, flat-panel detectors are used in digital mammography, where a dedicated X-ray tube generates an optimized spectrum for imaging the breast (distinct or discrete spectrum). It is important to note that mammographic kV might vary from 26 kV to 32 kV.

The Z for CsI is approximately 54 (Z for Cs = 55; Z for I = 53), and the CsI scintillator layer thickness is around 600 μm. Due to these characteristics, it is suitable for angiography, fluoroscopy, and radiography. In order to achieve the best results when imaging mammograms, it is essential to use a thinner layer of CsI (approximately 150 mm) and a specific X-ray spectrum. For mammography, a thickness of approximately 250 mm is required and 1000 mm for radiographic and angiographic imaging are required for a-Se digital detectors. Apart from the K-edge characteristic, which plays an important role in X-ray absorption, another important factor is the K-edge characteristic. Detecting X-rays and converting them into electrical charges and then reading them are the operational principles of flat-panel digital detectors. These two methods will now be described in more detail [80].

An indirect flat-panel TFT digital detector converts X-ray photons into light photons by using a scintillator layer, such as CsI. A-Si photodiodes convert light photons into electrical charges when they strike the a-Si layer. Digital detectors with a-Se photoconductors stacked on top of a-Si TFTs receive X-ray photons in contrast to direct flat-panel detectors. TFT components and the top electrode of this detector are connected by an electric field. An electric field moves electrical charges generated by X-rays toward the TFT components when they encounter a-Se. These two techniques represent latent images as matrix arrays of pixels with charge distributions. There must be a reading of all accusations at this point. This is accomplished using readout electronics.

TFT digital detectors use complex electronic circuitry to read electrical charges from matrix arrays. Active matrix readout involves row-by-row reading of pixels in a highly methodical manner. It is necessary to prepare the flat-panel detector before using it for an X-ray examination. This preparation is known as startup. Compared to radiography, fluoroscopy uses flat-panel TFT digital detectors that differ in their readout processes and circuitry. A radiograph produces a static image, whereas a fluoroscopy images are dynamic and depict motion throughout [81].

3.2.4 DR Clinical Applications

Due to its wide clinical uses in a variety of healthcare professions, digital radiography (DR) has emerged as a cornerstone in medical imaging. Here are some major clinical applications of digital radiography:

- **General radiography:** Digital radiography is commonly utilized for X-rays of the chest, skeletal system, abdomen, and extremities. It generates comprehensive images of bones, soft tissues, and organs, which aid in the detection of fractures, infections, tumors, and other disorders.
- **Digital fluoroscopy:** Real-time X-ray imaging is commonly utilized for GI tests, barium enemas, and cardiac catheterizations. When compared to traditional fluoroscopy equipment, digital fluoroscopy provides higher image quality, lower radiation doses, and a more efficient workflow.
- **Mammography:** Digital mammography is an essential tool for breast cancer screening and diagnosis. It provides high-resolution images of breast tissue, enabling the detection of microcalcifications, masses, and architectural abnormalities. Digital mammography also allows computer-aided detection (CAD) technologies to help breast radiologists spot probable problems.
- Digital radiography is ideal for pediatric imaging as it produces high-quality images with low radiation exposure. It is utilized in a variety of pediatric examinations, such as chest X-rays, skeletal surveys, and abdomen imaging, to help diagnose congenital anomalies, traumas, and developmental issues.
- Digital radiography is essential in orthopedic imaging for evaluating bone fractures, joint injuries, and musculoskeletal problems. It enables exact visualization of bone architecture and alignment, which informs treatment decisions and surgical planning.
- Trauma imaging: Digital radiography is critical for assessing fractures, dislocations, and soft tissue injuries. It offers quick imaging in emergency departments, trauma centers, and critical care units, allowing for more timely diagnosis and management of trauma patients.
- Dental imaging: Digital radiography is commonly utilized in both intraoral and extraoral dental imaging. It produces precise images of the teeth, gums, and surrounding structures, which aid in the diagnosis of dental caries, periodontal disease, and oral pathology. When compared to traditional film-based procedures, digital dental radiography has several advantages, including lower radiation exposure and improved image quality.
- Pulmonary imaging: Digital radiography evaluates lung pathology, including pneumonia, edema, and nodules. Chest X-rays and digital chest radiography are typical methods for evaluating respiratory problems and tracking disease development in individuals with lung illnesses.

Overall, digital radiography offers a wide range of clinical applications in medical imaging, providing healthcare providers with valuable diagnostic information for patient care across various specialties and clinical settings.

3.2.5 DR Artifacts

Digital radiography can be hampered by image artifacts, which are anomalies or distortions in the final image that can impair diagnostic accuracy. Understanding these artifacts is critical for imaging technologists and radiologists in detecting and correcting them. Here are some typical and most common digital radiography image artifacts:

1. Scatter radiation artifacts: X-rays encounter patient tissues and scatter in multiple directions before reaching the detector. This can cause dispersed photons to contribute to visual development, resulting in diminished contrast and increased image noise.
2. Grid cutoff: Artifacts occur when the X-ray grid is not aligned with the beam or detector. This can cause grid lines to emerge on the image, resulting in image deterioration and lower diagnostic quality.
3. Moiré patterns: Grid lines can interfere with the detector's pixel pattern, creating a noticeable pattern on the image. This artifact can conceal the underlying anatomy and alter image interpretation.
4. Backscatter artifacts: When dispersed radiation interacts with the detector, it creates ghost images or streaks on the final image. This can happen when the X-ray beam is not properly collimated or positioned.
5. Beam hardening artifacts: When an X-ray beam travels through thick tissues, like bone, it becomes more penetrating. This can produce streaking or cupping artifacts in the image, especially in locations with high tissue density.
6. Aliasing artifacts: When high-frequency information in an image exceeds the detector's Nyquist frequency, it causes pixelation and distortion. This can produce jagged edges or moiré patterns in the final image.
7. Quantization noise arises when the detector's analogue signal is digitized into discrete levels, resulting in pixel-level changes in image intensity. This might cause a grainy look or loss of clarity in low-contrast sections of an image.
8. Motion artifacts: When patients or X-ray equipment move during image acquisition, it causes blurring or distortion. This may compromise image sharpness and diagnostic accuracy.
9. Detector artifacts: Defective or malfunctioning detectors might result in visual artifacts like dead pixels, bright or dark patches. These artifacts might mimic pathology or hide important anatomy.
10. Software processing artifacts: Improperly performed image processing algorithms such as noise reduction, contrast enhancement, and reconstruction can result in artifacts. This may result in fake features or distortions in the final image.

Radiographers and radiologists should be familiar with these digital radiography image artifacts in order to detect and reduce their impact on diagnostic image quality. Proper placement, collimation, exposure technique, and image processing settings are critical for minimizing artifacts and delivering high-quality diagnostic images [27, 30, 82].

Flat-panel detectors (FPDs) are critical components of digital radiography systems, noted for producing high-quality images with minimal radiation exposure. However, as with any technology, they are susceptible to a variety of artifacts, which can compromise image quality and potentially lead to diagnostic mistakes. Radiologists and technologists must understand the causes of these artifacts, as well as mitigation techniques [83–87].

3.2.5.1 Types of Flat-Panel Detector Artifacts

1. **Gain variations**

   Description: Inconsistencies in the gain (sensitivity) of detector elements as depicted in Fig. 3.46.

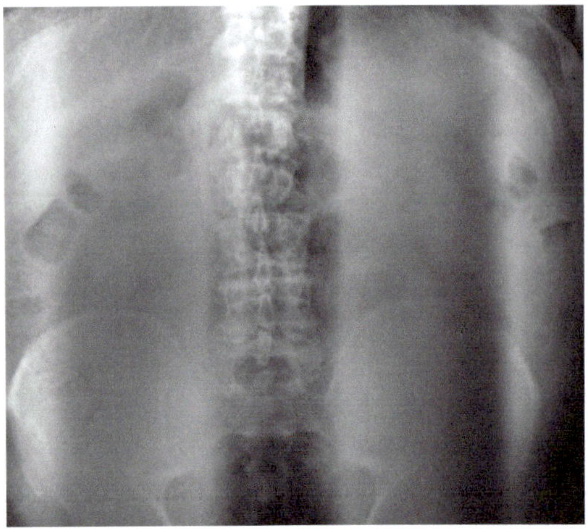

Fig. 3.46 Gain variation artifact

Cause: Variations in manufacturing or aging of detector elements.

Appearance: The image may show non-uniform brightness or banding.

Corrective action: Regular calibration and uniformity corrections can mitigate this artifact.

2. **Dead pixels/clusters**

   Description: Pixels or clusters of pixels that do not react to X-ray irradiation as depicted in Fig. 3.47.

   Possible causes include physical damage or flaws in the detector array.

   Appearance: Black spots or lines on the image.

   Corrective action: Dead pixel repair techniques can interpolate data from adjacent pixels to disguise faults.

3. **Offset drift**

   Description: Temporal variations in the electronic baseline signal as depicted in Fig. 3.48. Possible causes include temperature changes and electronic noise.

   Appearance: This may cause gradual changes in image brightness or contrast.

   Corrective action: Regularly calibrate the detector to adjust the baseline offset.

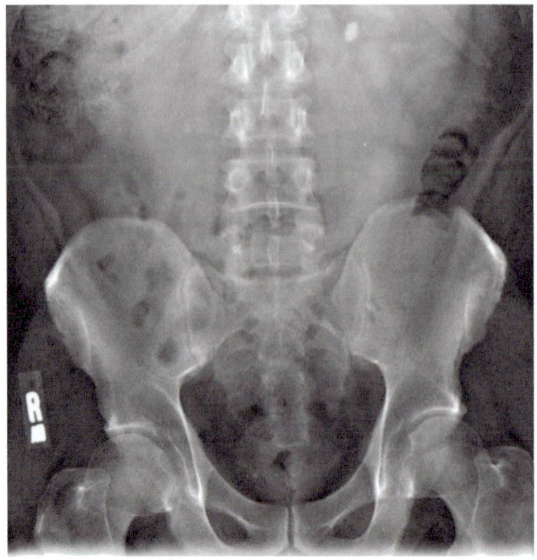

Fig. 3.47 Dead pixels artifact

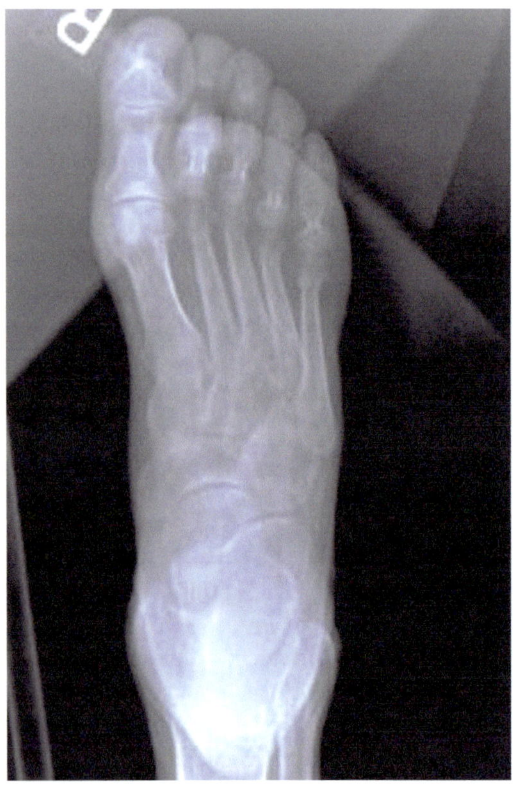

Fig. 3.48 Offset drift artifact

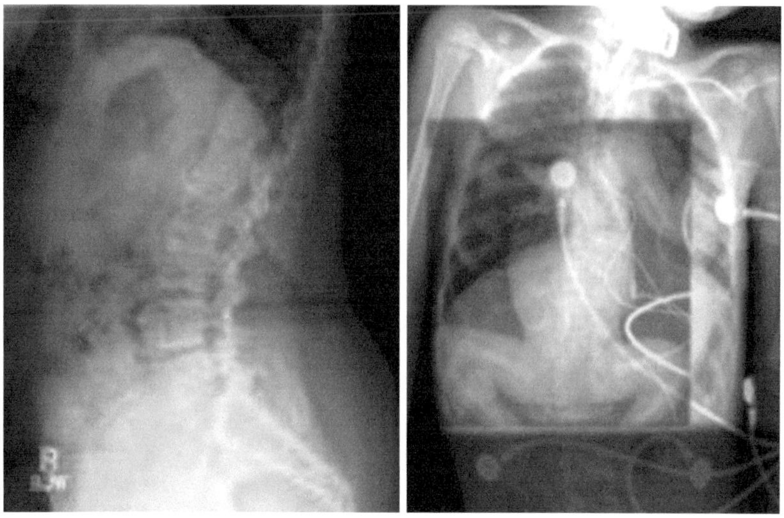

Fig. 3.49 Image lag artifact

4. **Image lag**
   Description: The retention of a previous image in the current frame as depicted in Fig. 3.49 with a lead marker shadow from the previous image.
   The cause is an incomplete resetting of detector elements between exposures.
   Appearance: Ghosting or leftover images overlap the present image.
   Corrective action involves allowing enough time between exposures for a complete reset and utilizing appropriate correction algorithms.
5. **Mechanical artifacts**
   Description: Artifacts caused by physical damage or movement during image acquisition as depicted in Fig. 3.50 on a test device image.
   Causes include detector damage, patient movement, or mechanical vibrations.
   Appearance: Variable, with blurring or repeated patterns.
   Mitigation measures include proper detector handling and maintenance, as well as patient and equipment stabilization during imaging.
6. **Environmental interference**
   Description: Artifacts created by external electromagnetic waves.
   Cause: Proximity to EMI-emitting gadgets.
   Image appearance may include random noise or patterned artifacts as depicted in Fig. 3.51.
   Mitigation involves shielding the detector and keeping it away from probable sources of electromagnetic interference (EMI).

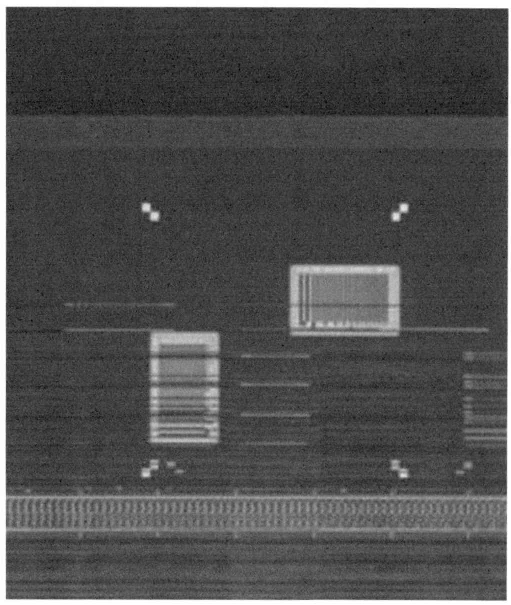

Fig. 3.50 Mechanical artifact

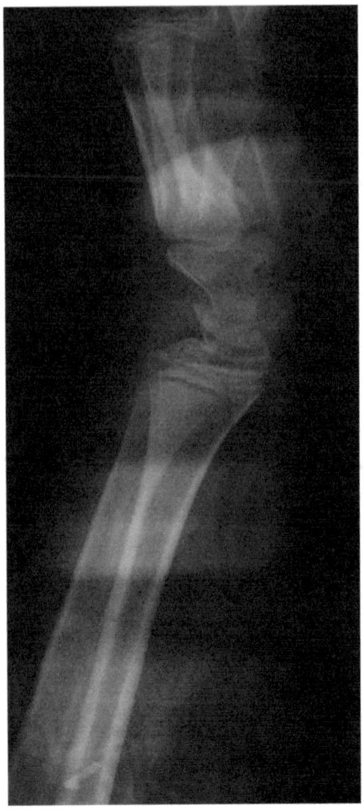

Fig. 3.51 Environmental interference artifact

3.2.5.2 Addressing Flat-Panel Detector Artifacts

Effective management of FPD artifacts involves a combination of routine maintenance, regular calibration, and the use of advanced software algorithms designed to correct or mitigate artifacts. Radiology departments should implement quality-control programs that include:

- Routine calibration: Regular calibration procedures help maintain the uniformity and sensitivity of the detector.
- Quality assurance testing: Periodic testing to identify and correct potential issues before they affect clinical imaging.
- Software updates: Keeping imaging software up to date to leverage the latest correction algorithms and enhancements.
- Training and education: Ensuring that radiology personnel are well-trained to recognize artifacts and understand the steps required to address them.

Table 3.5 DR Flat-panel artifact with classification

Category	Artifact
Pre-exposure	A. Memory B. Dead pixels C. Calibration mask
Exposure	A. Grid cutoff B. Double exposure C. Quantum mottle D. Saturation E. Paradoxic exposure effect F. Planking G. Radiofrequency interference
Reading	A. Moire
Workstation	A. Faulty transfer B. Border detection C. Diagnostic specifier D. Clipping E. Density threshold

By proactively managing these artifacts, radiology departments can ensure high-quality imaging, accurate diagnostics, and optimal patient care.

3.2.5.3 Subclassification of DR Artifacts

A digital artifact can be classified based on the step at which it was created. The primary categories include preexposure, exposure, postexposure, reading, and workstation artifacts (Table 3.5). Identifying the step at which an artifact was formed is critical for rectifying the error and reducing its occurrence in future investigations. The approaches for diagnosing digital artifacts differ from those used for CR.

DR—quality control

With the introduction of digital imaging, conventional quality assurance processes have expanded beyond the typical domains of medical imaging with screen-film radiographic image sensors. Quality assurance (QA) and quality-control (QC) methods are excellent tactics for ensuring the continual quality improvement of a medical imaging device. Radiology's QA/QC rules, methods, and related activities are all aimed at

1. Use the ALARA (as low as reasonably attainable) principle to ensure that patients receive the least amount of radiation possible.

2. Establish the optimum image quality for diagnosis.
3. Reduce the cost of radiological procedures.

For digital radiography systems, QA and QC are constantly evolving, and dedicated tools are now available to test the operation of digital imaging equipment as well as PACS components [88–98]. For example, QC testing for DR systems, such as dark noise and exposure index calibration, is becoming more widespread, with engineers executing these tests regularly (AAPM, 2006).

Quality-control (QC) testing for flat-panel detectors (FPDs) in digital radiography are critical for ensuring that the imaging system produces high-quality images and functions properly. The following are some of the most common quality-control tests:

1. **Visual inspection**
   - **Frequency:** Daily
   - **Purpose:** Check for physical damage, cleanliness, and proper connections.
   - **Procedure:** Inspect the FPD for any visible damage, ensure it is clean, and check all cables and connectors.
2. **Detector calibration**
   - **Frequency:** As recommended by the manufacturer or if image quality issues occur.
   - **Purpose:** Ensure the detector is functioning correctly and producing accurate images.
   - **Procedure:** Calibrate according to the manufacturer's specifications. This often entails taking images of a consistent phantom and altering settings based on the findings.
3. **Dark noise/offset test**
   - **Frequency:** Weekly or monthly
   - **Purpose:** Evaluate the detector's electronic noise level without x-ray exposure.
   - **Procedure:** Take an image without X-rays and evaluate its homogeneity and noise level.
4. **Flat-field test**
   - **Frequency:** Weekly or monthly.
   - **Purpose:** Evaluate the detector's reaction to a uniform X-ray field.
   - **Procedure:** Acquire an image of a uniform phantom (e.g., a flat field phantom) and check for uniformity. Look for artifacts, nonuniform areas, or defective pixels.
5. **Contrast-to-noise ratio (CNR) and signal-to-noise ratio (SNR)**
   - **Frequency:** Monthly or quarterly.
   - **Purpose:** Evaluate the detector's capacity to distinguish between minor variations in X-ray attenuation.
   - **Procedure:** Use a phantom with known contrast objects, acquire images, and calculate CNR and SNR, as depicted in Fig. 3.52.
6. **Spatial resolution test**
   - **Frequency:** Monthly or quarterly.
   - **Purpose:** Assess the detector's ability to resolve fine details.
   - **Procedure:** Use a high-resolution phantom (e.g., line pair or bar pattern phantom) and analyze the spatial resolution, as depicted in figure above.
7. **Detective quantum efficiency (DQE)**
   - **Frequency:** Annually.
   - **Purpose:** Measure the efficiency of the detector in converting X-ray energy into an image.
   - **Procedure:** Requires phantoms and software. Evaluate the output signal and noise

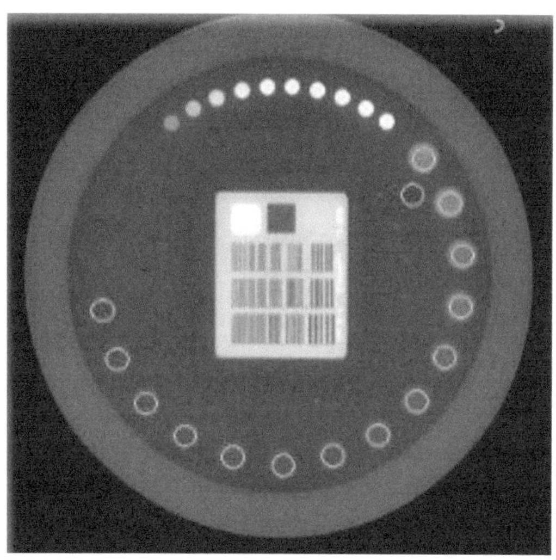

Fig. 3.52 Test tool phantom for SNR and CNR

characteristics with the input X-ray signal and noise.

8. **Image artifacts**
   - **Frequency:** Daily or weekly.
   - **Purpose:** Identify undesirable artifacts that may affect image quality.
   - **Procedure:** Regularly check clinical images for artifacts. If artifacts are identified, run more testing.
9. **Exposure index verification**
   - **Frequency:** Quarterly.
   - **Purpose:** Ensure the exposure index values are accurate and within acceptable limits.
   - **Procedure:** Use a calibrated dosimeter to measure exposure and compare it with the detector's exposure index readout.
10. **Overall system performance**
    - **Frequency:** Annually.
    - **Purpose:** Comprehensive evaluation of the entire digital radiography system.
    - **Procedure:** Includes many of the above tests, plus additional checks as recommended by the system manufacturer.

General recommendations

- **Documentation:** Keep detailed records of all QC tests, results, and any corrective actions taken.
- **Training:** Ensure that personnel performing QC tests are properly trained.
- **Manufacturer guidelines:** Always follow the manufacturer's recommendations for QC procedures and frequencies.

Quality-control (QC) tests for flat-panel detectors (FPDs) in digital radiography require a variety of specialized tools and equipment. Here is a list of commonly used tools and equipment for performing these tests:

3.2.5.4 Tools and Equipment Needed

- **Phantoms:** Various types, including uniformity, resolution, and contrast-detail phantoms.
- **Software:** Analysis software for measuring DQE, CNR, SNR, and other parameters.
- **Dosimeter:** For verifying exposure indices.
- **Visual inspection tools:** Cleaning materials, magnifying glass, etc.

Implementing a regular and thorough QC program helps maintain the performance of FPDs in digital radiography, ensuring reliable and high-quality diagnostic imaging.

1. **Phantoms**
   - **Uniformity phantoms:** Used to test the uniformity of the detector response. Typically made of a material that mimics the attenuation properties of human tissue as depicted in Fig. 3.53.
   - **Resolution phantoms:** Such as line pair or bar pattern phantoms, used to assess spatial resolution.
   - **Contrast-detail phantoms:** Used to evaluate the contrast-to-noise ratio (CNR) and signal-to-noise ratio (SNR). These phantoms contain objects of varying sizes and contrast levels.

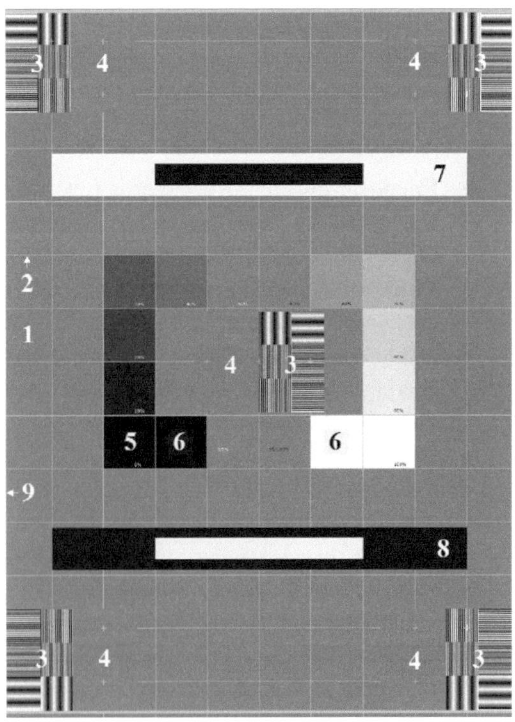

Fig. 3.53 Classical tool for DR quality control

- **Multipurpose phantoms:** Comprehensive phantoms that include a variety of test patterns for multiple QC tests, such as the Leeds test objects or AAPM (American Association of Physicists in Medicine) test phantoms.

2. **Software and Analysis Tools**
   - **QC software:** Often provided by the detector or imaging system manufacturer. Used for analyzing images and calculating metrics such as DQE, MTF (modulation transfer function), and NPS (noise power spectrum).
   - **Image analysis software:** General-purpose software that can analyze image quality parameters, such as ImageJ, MATLAB, or specific radiology QC software like RadiaSoft.
3. **Dosimeters**
   - **Ionization chambers:** Used to measure the dose delivered to the detector.
   - **Solid-state detectors:** Provide fast and accurate dose measurements and are often used for routine QC checks.
   - **Photodiode dosimeters:** Another type of dosimeter used for measuring the exposure delivered to the detector.
4. **Test tools and devices**
   - **Edge devices:** For measuring the modulation transfer function (MTF).
   - **Step wedges:** For assessing contrast resolution and dynamic range.
   - **Pinholes or slit cameras:** For precise measurements of focal spot size, which can impact spatial resolution.
5. **Visual inspection tools**
   - **Magnifying glass or loupe:** For detailed visual inspections of the detector surface.
   - **Cleaning materials:** Nonabrasive cloths, cleaning solutions recommended by the manufacturer, and compressed-air canisters to remove dust and debris.
6. **Radiographic markers**
   - **Lead markers:** Used to mark specific points or areas on the phantom or detector for reference in QC images.
7. **Calibration tools**
   - **Light meter:** For verifying the calibration of the monitor used for image review.
   - **Colorimeter or spectrophotometer:** For calibrating the display monitor to ensure accurate grayscale and color representation.
8. **Environmental monitors**
   - **Temperature and humidity monitors:** To ensure the detector is operating within the manufacturer's specified environmental conditions.
   - **Vibration monitors:** To detect any vibrations that could affect the performance of the detector.
9. **Documentation tools**
   - **QC logs and checklists:** For recording test results and ensuring that all required tests are performed at the appropriate intervals.
   - **Digital recordkeeping systems:** Software solutions for maintaining comprehensive QC records, which can be crucial for regulatory compliance and quality assurance.
10. **Communication tools**
    - **Calibration and service reports:** Tools or software for generating detailed reports on the status and performance of the detector after QC tests and servicing.

3.2.5.5 Implementing the QC Tests

Ensure that the personnel conducting the QC tests are properly trained in the use of these tools as depicted in Fig. 3.53 and understand the procedures for each test. Following manufacturer guidelines and industry standards (such as those from the AAPM or IEC) is crucial for accurate and effective quality control [90–98].

Regular QC testing using the appropriate tools helps maintain the performance and reliability of FPDs in digital radiography, ensuring high-quality diagnostic images and patient safety.

3.2.6 Recent Technological Advancements in Digital Radiography

Recent advances in digital radiography have greatly improved imaging capabilities, efficiency, and patient safety. Here are some important developments:

1. Direct capture detectors, including amorphous selenium (a-Se) detectors, are increasingly used. These detectors convert X-rays directly to electrical impulses, eliminating the need for a separate scintillator layer, resulting in higher image quality and dose efficiency.
2. Wireless digital radiography detectors are increasingly popular due to their flexibility and simplicity. They provide easy positioning and movement throughout the imaging area, decreasing patient pain and increasing workflow productivity.
3. Dual-energy imaging: Digital radiography systems capture images at two energy levels, improving tissue characterization and detecting anomalies such as bone fractures and lung nodules.
4. AI integration in digital radiography systems helps radiologists with image interpretation, workflow optimization, and quality assurance. AI can assist detect and highlight problems, shorten interpretation times, and increase diagnostic accuracy.
5. Iterative reconstruction algorithms minimize image noise and artifacts while maintaining detail in digital radiography. These algorithms enhance image quality, especially at lower radiation doses, making imaging safer for patients.
6. Portable and handheld digital radiography devices are designed for use in emergency rooms, intensive care units, and other point-of-care environments. These little gadgets enable bedside imaging and speed up patient care by eliminating the requirement for patient transportation to radiology departments.
7. Advanced quantitative imaging techniques, including digital tomosynthesis and spectral imaging, offer three-dimensional and spectrum data on tissue composition. These approaches improve the visualization of anatomical features and diseases, resulting in higher diagnostic accuracy.
8. Dose monitoring and optimization: Digital radiography systems now include real-time dose monitoring tools to track radiation exposure for patients and imaging professionals. This enables dosage optimization and adherence to ALARA (As Low As Reasonably Achievable) guidelines, which reduce radiation dangers.

These improvements all contribute to the continued growth of digital radiography, allowing healthcare practitioners to provide high-quality imaging services while improving efficiency, safety, and diagnostic accuracy.

Exercise

Multiple-Choice Questions (MCQs)

1. What is the key technology that replaced traditional X-ray film in computed radiography (CR)?
   A. Computed tomography (CT)
   B. Photostimulable phosphor (PSP) plates
   C. Digital signal processor (DSP)
   D. Magnetic resonance imaging (MRI)
2. Who invented the photostimulable phosphor (PSP) plate, the cornerstone of computed radiography?
   A. Dr. Robert Ledley
   B. Dr. Paul Lauterbur
   C. Dr. Yoshihiro Nishikawa
   D. Dr. Raymond Damadian
3. In the CR system, what is used to scan the imaging plate to release the stored energy?
   A. X-rays
   B. High-intensity halogen lamp
   C. Laser beam
   D. Ultraviolet light
4. What year was the first commercial CR system released by Fuji, marking the start of digital radiography?
   A. 1976
   B. 1981
   C. 1983
   D. 1990
5. What component is used to convert the violet light into an electric signal in CR?
   A. Photostimulable phosphor
   B. Photomultiplier tube (PMT)
   C. Digital-to-analog converter (DAC)
   D. Fiber-optic light guide

6. What happens to the phosphor atoms in the CR plate when exposed to X-rays?
   A. They become ionized
   B. They become excited and store energy
   C. They emit light immediately
   D. They undergo fission
7. What is the main function of the CR reader in the imaging process?
   A. To capture X-ray images
   B. To convert digital signals to analog
   C. To scan the plate and convert stored energy to visible light
   D. To store patient data
8. Which component in the CR reader detects the light generated by the phosphor plates?
   A. Photomultiplier tubes
   B. Laser beam
   C. X-ray tube
   D. Memory chip
9. What type of data does the memory chip in a CR cassette store?
   A. X-ray images
   B. Patient demographics and image quality data
   C. Radiation dose information
   D. CR reader settings
10. What is the primary benefit of the EBC (electron beam cured) topcoat on CR imaging plates?
    A. Enhances image sharpness
    B. Protects the plate from mechanical wear and cleaning solutions
    C. Increases the plate's sensitivity to X-rays
    D. Improves the efficiency of light emission
11. What type of imaging plate is used in CR systems instead of typical X-ray film?
    A. Selenium plate
    B. Silicon plate
    C. Photostimulable phosphor plate
    D. Silver halide plate
12. What triggers the stored energy in the phosphor substance during the CR digitization process?
    A. Heat
    B. Laser
    C. UV light
    D. Magnetic field
13. Which of the following is NOT an advantage of CR systems over traditional X-ray films?
    A. Digital image manipulation
    B. Higher radiation exposure
    C. Easier image storage and sharing
    D. Wider dynamic range
14. What is the typical dynamic range of CR systems?
    A. 1,000 to 2,000 shades of gray
    B. 5,000 to 8,000 shades of gray
    C. 10,000 to 16,000 shades of gray
    D. 20,000 to 30,000 shades of gray
15. What type of artifact is caused by improper kVp and mA/mAs settings leading to dark images?
    A. Underexposure
    B. Overexposure
    C. Collimation error
    D. Scatter radiation effect
16. What should be included in the daily QC checks for a CR system?
    A. Image rejection analysis
    B. Dark noise test
    C. CR reader operation confirmation
    D. High-contrast resolution
17. Which material is recommended for cleaning CR imaging plates?
    A. Ethanol anhydride and water
    B. Soap and water
    C. Alcohol and water
    D. Sodium hydroxide solution
18. What is the primary purpose of conducting regular sensitivity checks on CR systems?
    A. To verify CR system produces consistent image quality
    B. To enhance the color resolution of images
    C. To improve the sharpness of the image display monitors
    D. To check for mechanical faults in the CR reader
19. What is used to reduce backscatter during imaging plate maintenance?
    A. Copper filters
    B. Lead sheet or apron
    C. Ion chambers
    D. Soft linens

20. Which company is not mentioned as a top manufacturer of CR equipment?
    A. Fujifilm Medical Systems
    B. Canon Medical Systems Corporation
    C. Siemens Healthineers
    D. Hitachi Healthcare Americas
21. What does the American Association of Physicists in Medicine (AAPM) define digital radiography as?
    A. Use of film-screen radiography
    B. Use of images produced by photostimulable storage phosphors, amorphous silicon, amorphous selenium, CCDs, or MOSFETs
    C. Use of traditional X-ray films
    D. Use of ultrasound imaging
22. What is the primary function of the X-ray source in a digital radiography system?
    A. Displaying images
    B. Generating X-rays for creating radiographic images
    C. Storing digital images
    D. Processing digital images
23. Which component of a digital radiography system captures X-rays after they pass through the patient?
    A. X-ray source
    B. Control console
    C. Detector
    D. Power supply
24. Which of the following is NOT an advantage of flat-panel detectors (FPDs) in digital radiography?
    A. High image quality
    B. Real-time imaging
    C. High radiation dose requirement
    D. Wide dynamic range
25. In direct conversion digital radiography systems, what material is typically used as the photoconductor?
    A. Cesium iodide
    B. Amorphous silicon
    C. Selenium
    D. Scintillator phosphor
26. What are the two broad classifications of flat-panel detectors?
    A. Indirect and CCD detectors
    B. CCD and direct detectors
    C. Indirect and direct detectors
    D. TFT and direct detectors
27. Which material is commonly used as a photoconductor in direct digital detectors?
    A. Amorphous silicon (a-Si)
    B. Cesium iodide (CsI)
    C. Amorphous selenium (a-Se)
    D. Gadolinium oxysulfide (Gd2O2S)
28. What is the main advantage of using structured phosphors like CsI needles in indirect TFT flat-panel detectors?
    A. Increased radiation dose
    B. Increased image noise
    C. Reduced lateral light dispersion and increased spatial resolution
    D. Increased light dispersion
29. What is the role of the analog-to-digital converter (ADC) in flat-panel detectors?
    A. To store electrical charges
    B. To convert electrical charges into light photons
    C. To convert analog signals into digital data
    D. To generate X-ray photons
30. Which artifact is caused by patient or equipment movement during image acquisition?
    A. Moiré patterns
    B. Motion artifacts
    C. Scatter radiation artifacts
    D. Grid cutoff
31. What is the primary cause of gain variations in flat-panel detectors?
    A. Variations in manufacturing or aging of detector elements
    B. Dead pixels
    C. Temperature changes
    D. Patient movement
32. What corrective action is suggested for offset drift in flat-panel detectors?
    A. Dead pixel repair
    B. Regular calibration
    C. Detector replacement
    D. Increasing exposure time
33. What is the appearance of mechanical artifacts in digital radiography images?
    A. Black spots or lines
    B. Variable, with blurring or repeated patterns

C. Ghosting or leftover images
D. Uniform brightness

34. Which artifact is caused by external electromagnetic waves?
A. Gain variation
B. Dead pixels
C. Environmental interference
D. Image lag

35. Which tool is used to assess the contrast-to-noise ratio (CNR) in digital radiography?
A. Ionization chamber
B. Multipurpose phantom
C. Step wedges
D. Pinhole camera

36. What causes gain variations in flat-panel detectors?
A. Physical damage
B. Manufacturing variations or aging
C. Temperature changes
D. Electromagnetic interference

37. How do dead pixels or clusters appear in an image?
A. Nonuniform brightness
B. Gradual changes in brightness or contrast
C. Black spots or lines
D. Ghosting or leftover images

38. What is a common cause of offset drift in flat-panel detectors?
A. Electromagnetic interference
B. Physical damage
C. Temperature changes and electronic noise
D. Patient movement

39. Which of the following can help mitigate mechanical artifacts in flat-panel detectors?
A. Regular calibration
B. Dead pixel repair techniques
C. Allowing enough time between exposures
D. Proper detector handling and maintenance

40. What is a benefit of AI integration in digital radiography systems?
A. Improved mechanical stability
B. Assistance in image interpretation and workflow optimization
C. Increased exposure time
D. Reduced need for calibration

Short Questions

1. Explain the role of the CR reader in the computed radiography process.
2. What advancements in CR technology occurred between the 1980s and 1990s?
3. Explain the function of the phosphor layer in a CR imaging plate.
4. What are the benefits of using CR imaging plates compared to traditional X-ray films?
5. Describe the main components involved in the CR digitization process from exposure to image display.
6. List at least three common clinical applications of CR in radiology.
7. Describe the process for visual inspection of CR cassettes and imaging plates.
8. Explain the importance of monitoring exposure indices in CR systems.
9. Describe the primary difference between direct and indirect flat-panel TFT digital detectors.
10. What are the common clinical applications of digital radiography?
11. Explain the role of image processing software in a digital radiography system.
12. Describe the main difference between direct and indirect conversion digital radiography systems.
13. Explain the importance of routine calibration in managing flat-panel detector artifacts.
14. Describe the corrective actions that can be taken to mitigate image lag artifacts in digital radiography.
15. Explain the appearance and corrective action for image lag in flat-panel detectors.
16. Describe the importance of routine calibration in addressing flat-panel detector artifacts.

Long Question

1. Describe the workflow process of CR readout, from the exposure of the imaging plate to the final digital image display. Include details on the image processing steps, and explain the significance of each component involved in this process.

2. Describe the process of image acquisition and processing in computed radiography, including the roles of the CR cassette, imaging plate, and reader. Discuss how the system converts X-rays into a digital image and the significance of each component in the workflow.
3. Discuss the various artifacts associated with CR imaging systems, including their causes, appearances, and potential remedies. Explain how these artifacts can impact diagnostic accuracy and patient care.
4. Discuss the various quality-control procedures and maintenance practices that should be implemented in a CR imaging facility to ensure optimal performance and safety.
5. Discuss the structure, operation, and advantages of flat-panel detectors (FPDs) in digital radiography systems. Include details on the process from X-ray absorption to image display.
6. Discuss the various types of image artifacts that can occur in digital radiography and how they impact diagnostic accuracy. Include specific examples and suggest potential mitigation strategies.
7. Discuss the various quality-control (QC) tests necessary for flat-panel detectors (FPDs) in digital radiography, including their purposes and the tools required for each test.
8. Discuss the various quality-control (QC) tests for flat-panel detectors (FPDs) in digital radiography and explain the purpose and procedures for at least three of these tests.

Answers for MCQs

1. B. Photostimulable phosphor (PSP) plates
2. C. Dr. Yoshihiro Nishikawa
3. C. Laser beam
4. B. 1981
5. B. Photomultiplier tube (PMT)
6. B. They become excited and store energy
7. C. To scan the plate and convert stored energy to visible light
8. A. Photomultiplier tubes
9. B. Patient demographics and image quality data
10. B. Protects the plate from mechanical wear and cleaning solutions
11. C. Photostimulable phosphor plate
12. B. Laser
13. B. Higher radiation exposure
14. C. 10,000 to 16,000 shades of gray
15. B. Overexposure
16. C. CR reader operation confirmation
17. A. Ethanol anhydride and water
18. A. To verify CR system produces consistent image quality
19. B. Lead sheet or apron
20. C. Siemens Healthineers
21. B. Use of images produced by photostimulable storage phosphors, amorphous silicon, amorphous selenium, CCDs, or MOSFETs
22. B. Generating X-rays for creating radiographic images
23. C. Detector
24. C. High radiation dose requirement
25. C. Selenium
26. C. Indirect and Direct Detectors
27. C. Amorphous selenium (a-Se)
28. C. Reduced lateral light dispersion and increased spatial resolution
29. C. To convert analog signals into digital data
30. B. Motion Artifacts
31. A. Variations in manufacturing or aging of detector elements
32. B. Regular calibration
33. B. Variable, with blurring or repeated patterns
34. C. Environmental interference
35. B. Multi-Purpose Phantom
36. B. Manufacturing variations or aging
37. C. Black spots or lines
38. C. Temperature changes and electronic noise
39. D. Proper detector handling and maintenance
40. B. Assistance in image interpretation and workflow optimization

References

1. Sonoda M, Takano M, Miyahara J, Kato H. Computed radiography utilizing scanning laser stimulated luminescence. Radiology. 1983;148(3):833.
2. Pongnapang N. Practical guidelines for radiographers to improve computed radiography image quality. Biomed Imaging Interv J. 2005;1(2):e12.
3. da Silveira Gatto LB, Braz D, Pacifico L, Travassos P, Magalhaes LA. Comparison of x-ray spectra and mean glandular dose estimations in computed radiog-

raphy systems for mammography: simulations versus measurements. Radiat Phys Chem. 2024;216:216.
4. Marolf A, Blaik M, Ackerman N, Watson E, Gibson N, Thompson M. Comparison of computed radiography and conventional radiography in detection of small volume pneumoperitoneum. Vet Radiol Ultrasound. 2008;49(3):227.
5. Zelviani S. Kualitas citra pada direct digital radiography dan computed radiography. Jurnal Teknosains. 2017;11(1):59–62.
6. James JJ, Davies AG, Cowen AR, O'Connor PJ. Developments in digital radiography: an equipment update. Eur Radiol. 2001;11(12):2616.
7. Johnston RF, Pickett SC, Barker DL. Autoradiography using storage phosphor technology. Electrophoresis. 1990;11:5.
8. Kuramoto T, Takarabe S, Okamura K, Shiotsuki K, Shibayama Y, Tsuru H, et al. Effect of differences in pixel size on image characteristics of digital intraoral radiographic systems: a physical and visual evaluation. Dentomaxillofac Radiol. 2020;49(6):20190378.
9. van Langen H, Castelijn T. Durability of imaging plates in clinical use. Phys Med. 2009;25(4):207.
10. Ho BKT. Automatic acquisition interfaces for computed radiography, CT, MR, US, and laser scanner. Comput Med Imaging Graph. 1991;15(3):135.
11. Sones RA, Barnes GT. A method to measure the MTF of digital x ray systems. Med Phys. 1984;11(2):166.
12. Andriole KP. Anatomy of picture archiving and communications systems: nuts and bolts – image acquisition: getting digital images from imaging modalities. J Digit Imaging. 1999;12(2 SUPPL. 1):216.
13. Kumar S, Nayak KP, Hareesha KS. Improving visibility of stereo-radiographic spine reconstruction with geometric inferences. J Digit Imaging. 2016;29(2):226.
14. Amemiya Y, Matsushita T, Nakagawa A, Satow Y, Miyahara J, Chikawa J, ichi. Design and performance of an imaging plate system for X-ray diffraction study. Nucl Instrum Methods Phys Res A. 1988;266(1–3):645–53.
15. MacMahon H, Xu XW, Hoffmann KR, Giger ML, Yoshimura H, Doi K, et al. Clinical experience with an advanced laser digitizer for cost-effective digital radiography. Radiographics. 1993;13(3):635.
16. Yoshimura H, Xu XW, Doi K, MacMahon H, Hoffmann KR, Giqer ML, et al. Development of a high quality film duplication system using a laser digitizer: comparison with computed radiography. Med Phys. 1993;20(1):51.
17. Huda W, Honeyman JC, Palmer CK, Frost MM, Staab EV. Computed radiography and film digitizer inputs to an intensive care unit teleradiology system: an image quality comparison. Acad Radiol. 1996;3(2):110.
18. Salazar AJ, Romero JA, Bernal OA, Moreno AP, Velasco SC, Díaz XA. Noninferiority and equivalence evaluation of clinical performance among computed radiography, film, and digitized film for telemammography services. Int J Telemed Appl. 2016;2016:1.
19. Buchanan A, Ghosh S, Kalathingal S, Dalsania H, Raina R. Effect of 3 different disinfection methods on the image quality of photostimulable phosphor plates. Oral Surg Oral Med Oral Pathol Oral Radiol. 2024;137(2):172.
20. Fellner C, Pötter R, Knocke TH, Wambersie A. Comparison of radiography- and computed tomography-based treatment planning in cervix cancer in brachytherapy with specific attention to some quality assurance aspects. Radiother Oncol. 2001;58(1):53.
21. Nanavaty P, Alvarez MS, Michael AW. Lung cancer screening: advantages, controversies, and applications. Cancer Control. 2014;21(1):9.
22. Ge H, Wang Z, Zhang J. X-ray, digital tomographic fusion, CT, and MRI in early ischemic necrosis of the femoral head. Medicine. 2024;103(2):e36281.
23. Erdelyi RA, Duma VF, Sinescu C, Dobre GM, Bradu A, Podoleanu A. Dental diagnosis and treatment assessments: between X-rays radiography and optical coherence tomography. Materials. 2020;13(21):4825.
24. Fujita S, Tanaka M, Hirota S, Fuji T. Clinical application of computed radiography in orthopedic surgery. J Digit Imaging. 1995;8(1 Supplement):51.
25. Urban T, Noichl W, Engel KJ, Koehler T, Pfeiffer F. Correction for X-ray scatter and detector crosstalk in dark-field radiography. IEEE Trans Med Imaging. 2024;43:2646.
26. Jeon D, Kim W, Cho H, Park M. Removing grid artifacts from a two-dimensional crisscrossed grid in cone-beam computed tomography to enhance image quality. J Instrum. 2024;19(3):C03037.
27. Honey ID, MacKenzie A. Artifacts found during quality assurance testing of computed radiography and digital radiography detectors. J Digit Imaging. 2009;22(4):383.
28. Bhondwe S, Tivaskar S, Luharia A, Dhande R, Pathade A. Artifacts IN computed radiography-a review article. J Pharm Negat Results. 2022;13(8):133–9.
29. Hammerstrom K, Aldrich J, Alves L, Ho A. Recognition and prevention of computed radiography image artifacts. J Digit Imaging. 2006;19(3):226.
30. Shetty CM, Barthur A, Kambadakone A, Narayanan N, Kv R. Computed radiography image artifacts revisited. Am J Roentgenol. 2011;196:W37.
31. Samei E, Seibert JA, Willis CE, Flynn MJ, Mah E, Junck KL. Performance evaluation of computed radiography systems. Med Phys. 2001;28(3):361.
32. Shepard SJ, Wang J, Flynn M, Gingold E, Goldman L, Krugh K, et al. An exposure indicator for digital radiography: AAPM task group 116 (executive summary). Med Phys. 2009;36(7):2898.
33. Uffmann M, Schaefer-Prokop C. Digital radiography: the balance between image quality and required radiation dose. Eur J Radiol. 2009;72(2):202.
34. Humphrey LL, Teutsch S, Johnson M. Lung cancer screening with sputum cytologic examination, chest radiography, and computed tomography: an update for the U.S. Preventive Services Task Force. Ann Intern Med. 2004;140:740–53.

35. Seeber M, Lederer KA, Rowan C, Strohmayer C, Ludewig E. Image processing setting adaptions according to image dose and radiologist preference can improve image quality in computed radiography of the equine distal limb: a cadaveric study. Vet Radiol Ultrasound. 2024;65(1):19.
36. Horn-Lodewyk J, van der Merwe B, Kali GM, Munro L. Evaluating the knowledge and training of forensipathologists and registrars performing forensic radiography at a forensic pathology mortuary in the Free State province, South Africa. Health SA Gesondheid. 2022;27:2014.
37. Mora P, Pfeiffer D, Zhang G, Bosmans H, Delis H, Razi Z, et al. The IAEA remote and automated quality control methodology for radiography and mammography. J Appl Clin Med Phys. 2021;22(11):126.
38. Patel I, Natarajan T, Hassan SS, Kirby MC. The use of computed radiography for routine linear accelerator and simulator quality control. Br J Radiol. 2009;82(982):827.
39. Ningtias DR, Wahyudi B, Harsoyo IT. Comparative test of the effect of X-ray tube current analysis and exposure time on CR (computed radiography) image quality. J Inf Telecommun Eng. 2022;6(1):267–75.
40. Ropolo R, Rampado O, Isoardi P, Izzo A, Savio L, Cammarota T, et al. Automated quality control in computed radiography. Radiol Med. 2006;111(8):1156.
41. Ningtias DR, Suryono S, Susilo S. Pengukuran Kualitas Citra digital computed radiography Menggunakan Program Pengolah Citra. J Pendidik Fis Indon. 2016;12(2):161.
42. Rampado O, Isoardi P, Ropolo R. Quantitative assessment of computed radiography quality control parameters. Phys Med Biol. 2006;51(6):1577.
43. Leblans P, Vandenbroucke D, Willems P. Storage phosphors for medical imaging. Materials. 2011;4:6.
44. Spoor F, Jeffery N, Zonneveld F. Using diagnostic radiology in human evolutionary studies. J Anat. 2000;197:61.
45. Huda W, Nickoloff EL, Boone JM. Overview of patient dosimetry in diagnostic radiology in the USA for the past 50 years. Med Phys. 2008;35:5713.
46. Mulherin BL. History, physiology, modality options, and safety for diagnostic imaging of the oral cavity. In: Veterinary oral diagnostic imaging. John Wiley & Sons, Inc; 2024.
47. Tay YX, McNulty JP. Radiography education in 2022 and beyond – writing the history of the present: a narrative review. Radiography. 2023;29:391.
48. Yoshida M, Yoshihara H, Honda E. History of digital detectors in intraoral radiography. Dent Health Curr Res. 2018;04(02):1–5.
49. Serindere G, Gündüz K. Digital imaging and dental record. J Clin Exp Med. 2021;38:113.
50. Krug B, Stützer H, Schuhmacher P, Winnekendonk G, Zähringer M, Goßmann A, et al. Vergleich der digitalen direkten flachdetektor- und der analogen film-folien-technik in der darstellung normaler anatomischer strukturen der weiblichen brust. Geburtshilfe Frauenheilkd. 2006;66(2):171.
51. Nguyen VH, Tran NL, Vu PT, Le TL, Pham NH. Development of digital image processing software for Vikomed X-ray equipment. In: BME-HUST 2016 – third international conference on biomedical engineering; 2016.
52. Bloomquist AK, Yaffe MJ, Mawdsley GE, Hunter DM, Beideck DJ. Lag and ghosting in a clinical flat-panel selenium digital mammography system. Med Phys. 2006;33(8):2998.
53. Fahrig R, Jaffray DA, Sechopoulos I, Webster SJ. Flat-panel conebeam CT in the clinic: history and current state. J Med Imaging. 2021;8(05):052115.
54. Woodland M, Pack L, Rist P, Crane B. Comparison of digital radiography, ultrasonography, and positive contrast vaginourethrography for determining reproductive status of female cats. Vet Radiol Ultrasound. 2014;55(4):368.
55. Yaffe MJ, Rowlands JA. X-ray detectors for digital radiography. Phys Med Biol. 1997;42:1.
56. Suetens P. Fundamentals of medical imaging. Cambridge University Press; 2017.
57. Floyd J, Warp RJ, Dobbins JT, Chotas HG, Baydush AH, Vargas-Voracek R, et al. Imaging characteristics of an amorphous silicon flat-panel detector for digital chest radiography. Radiology. 2001;218(3):683.
58. Fernandez A, Raposo V, Miquelez S, Caudepon F, Fuentemilla N, Bragado L, et al. Characterization of the spectral response of CsI flat panel detectors in digital radiography. Phys Med. 2021;92:S104.
59. Zhao W, Blevis I, Germann S, Rowlands JA, Waechter D, Huang Z. Digital radiology using active matrix readout of amorphous selenium: construction and evaluation of a prototype real-time detector. Med Phys. 1997;24(12):1834.
60. Kasap SO, Rowlands JA. X-ray photoconductors and stabilized a-Se for direct conversion digital flat-panel X-ray image-detectors. J Mater Sci Mater Electron. 2000;11(3):179–98.
61. Zhao W, Ristic G, Rowlands JA. X-ray imaging performance of structured cesium iodide scintillators. Med Phys. 2004;31(9):2594.
62. Kasap SO, Rowlands JA. Direct-conversion flat-panel X-ray image sensors for digital radiography. Proc IEEE. 2002;90(4):591–604.
63. Spahn M, Strotzer M, Völk M, Böhm S, Geiger B, Hahm G, et al. Digital radiography with a large-area, amorphous-silicon, flat-panel x- ray detector system. Investig Radiol. 2000;35(4):260.
64. Ono K, Yoshitake T, Akahane K, Yamada Y, Maeda T, Kai M, et al. Comparison of a digital flat-panel versus screen-film, photofluorography and storage-phosphor systems by detection of simulated lung adenocarcinoma lesions using hard copy images. Br J Radiol. 2005;78(934):922.
65. Moreira EV, Fritz MC. Flat-panel detectors are accepted for digital radiography in place of conventional radiography in pipeline weld inspection. Methods. 2007;2004(1):1–13.
66. Khalil T, Monteiro F, Dandache A, Salame C. Review of flat panel detectors technique for medical imaging

quality improvement. In: AIP conference proceedings. AIP Publishing; 2020.
67. Borasi G, Samei E, Bertolini M, Nitrosi A, Tassoni D. Erratum: contrast-detail analysis of three flat panel detectors for digital radiography. Med Phys. 2006;33:1707.
68. Cowen AR, Kengyelics SM, Davies AG. Solid-state, flat-panel, digital radiography detectors and their physical imaging characteristics. Clin Radiol. 2008;63:487.
69. Krug KB, Stützer H, Frommolt P, Boecker J, Bovenschulte H, Sendler V, et al. Image quality of digital direct flat-panel mammography versus an indirect small-field CCD technique using a high-contrast phantom. Int J Breast Cancer. 2011;2011:1.
70. Sun C, Ge J, Sun K. Optimization on calibration of flat panel detector in digital radiography. Nucl Tech. 2018;41(9):27–34.
71. Williams MB, Krupinski EA, Strauss KJ, Breeden WK, Rzeszotarski MS, Applegate K, et al. Digital radiography image quality: image acquisition. J Am Coll Radiol. 2007;4:371.
72. Mothiram U, Brennan PC, Lewis SJ, Moran B, Robinson J. Digital radiography exposure indices: a review. J Med Radiat Sci. 2014;61:112.
73. Lewin JM, Isaacs PK, Vance V, Larke FJ. Dual-energy contrast-enhanced digital subtraction mammography: feasibility. Radiology. 2003;229(1):261.
74. Leonard RL, Berkowitz DT, Thomas A, Howansky A, Lubinsky AR, Johnson JA. Scintillating glass-ceramic substrates for indirect flat panel detectors in digital radiography. J Am Ceram Soc. 2020;103(12):6893.
75. Borasi G, Nitrosi A, Ferrari P, Tassoni D. On site evaluation of three flat panel detectors for digital radiography. Med Phys. 2003;30(7):1719.
76. Borasi G, Samei E, Bertolini M, Nitrosi A, Tassoni D. Contrast-detail analysis of three flat panel detectors for digital radiography. Med Phys. 2006;33(6):1707.
77. Zhou Z, Teng S, Jiang W, An Z. X-ray flat-panel-detector-based digital radiography and its image calibration. Beijing Hangkong Hangtian Daxue Xuebao/J Beijing Univ Aeronaut Astronaut. 2004;30(8):698–701.
78. Takashima Y, Suganuma N, Sakurazawa H, Itoh H, Hirano H, Shida H, et al. A flat-panel detector digital radiography and a storage phosphor computed radiography: screening for pneumoconioses. J Occup Health. 2007;49(1):39.
79. Kotter E, Langer M. Digital radiography with large-area flat-panel detectors. Eur Radiol. 2002;12(10):2562.
80. Kim HK, Cunningham IA, Yin Z, Cho G. On the development of digital radiography detectors: a review. Int J Precis Eng Manuf. 2008;9:86–100.
81. Haruta Y, Kawakami M, Nakano Y, Kundu S, Wada S, Ikenoue T, et al. Scalable fabrication of metal halide perovskites for direct X-ray flat-panel detectors: a perspective †. Chem Mater. 2022;34:5323.
82. Walz-Flannigan A, Magnuson D, Erickson D, Schueler B. Artifacts in digital radiography. Am J Roentgenol. 2012;198(1):156.
83. Walz-Flannigan AI, Brossoit KJ, Magnuson DJ, Schueler BA. Pictorial review of digital radiography artifacts. Radiographics. 2018;38:833.
84. Jiménez DA, Armbrust LJ, O'Brien RT, Biller DS. Artifacts in digital radiography. Vet Radiol Ultrasound. 2008;49(4):321.
85. Dixon J, Biggi M, Weller R. Common artefacts and pitfalls in equine computed and digital radiography and how to avoid them. Equine Vet Educ. 2018;30:326.
86. Chris C, Vicky G. Identification and valuation of archaeological artefacts: developments using digital X-radiography. J Inst Conserv. 2018;41(2):128.
87. Willis CE, Thompson SK, Shepard SJ. Artifacts and misadventures in digital radiography. Appl Radiol. 2004;33(1):11.
88. Valentin J. Managing patient dose in digital radiology. Ann ICRP. 2004;34:1–73.
89. Mengel R, Kruse B, Flores-de-Jacoby L. Digital volume tomography in the diagnosis of Peri-implant defects: an in vitro study on native pig mandibles. J Periodontol. 2006;77(7):1234.
90. Meertens H, Van Herk M, Weeda J. A liquid ionisation detector for digital radiography of therapeutic megavoltage photon beams. Phys Med Biol. 1985;30(4):313.
91. The use of dental radiographs: update and recommendations. J Am Dent Assoc. 2006;137(9):1344.
92. Freedman M, Steller D, Jafroudi H, Mun SK. Quality control of storage phosphor digital radiography systems. J Digit Imaging. 1995;8(2):67.
93. Durán EJ, Salas LF, Benavides SO, Bolanos G. Quality control implementation on digital radiography equipment at Fundación Valle Del Lili. J Phys Conf Ser. 2019;1247:012007.
94. Nyathi T, Chirwa TF, Van Der Merwe DG. A survey of digital radiography practice in four South African teaching hospitals: an illuminative study. Biomed Imaging Interv J. 2010;6(1):e5.
95. Chotas HG, Floyd CE, Johnson GA, Ravin CE. Quality control phantom for digital chest radiography. Radiology. 1997;202(1):111.
96. Nitrosi A, Bertolini M, Borasi G, Botti A, Barani A, Rivetti S, et al. Application of QC-DR software for acceptance testing and routine quality control of direct digital radiography systems: initial experiences using the Italian association of physicist in medicine quality control protocol. J Digit Imaging. 2009;22(6):656.
97. Jones AK, Heintz P, Geiser W, Goldman L, Jerjian K, Martin M, et al. AAPM no 151: ongoing quality control in digital radiography. Med Phys. 2015;42(11):6658.
98. Jones AK, Heintz P, Geiser W, Goldman L, Jerjian K, Martin M, et al. Ongoing quality control in digital radiography: report of AAPM imaging physics committee task group 151. Med Phys. 2015;42(11):6658.

Mammography: Physics, Principle of Operation, Quality Control, and Safety

4

Learning Objectives

Introduction Historical evolution of Mammography Understanding breast anatomy for mammography Mammography Equipment & its Components X-ray Tube *Cathode* *Anode* *Anode heel effect* Tube Housing Filters Protective Shroud X-ray tube generator Face Shield Collimator Compression Device Breast Support and Grid Assemblies Image Receptor & Automatic Exposure Control *Film-Based Mammography* *Digital Mammography* *Automatic Exposure Control (AEC)* Foot Pedals and Digital Display for Compression Magnification Stand Radiation Output Digital Breast Tomosynthesis Principles of Digital Breast Tomosynthesis Advantages of DBT Limitations and Disadvantages of Digital Breast Tomosynthesis (DBT) Quality Control in Mammography History of QC in mammography Quality Control Tests for Digital Mammography (2D and DBT) Role of professionals, test procedures and frequency	Quality control tests Mammography Equipment Evaluation (MEE) ACR DM Phantom Image Quality DBT Z Resolution Spatial Resolution DBT Volume Coverage Automatic Exposure Control System Performance Average Glandular Dose Unit Checklist Acquisition Workstation Monitor QC Radiologist Workstation Monitor QC Film Printer QC (if applicable) Evaluation of Site's Technologist QC Program Evaluation of Display Device Technologist QC Program ACR DM Phantom Image Quality Computed Radiography Cassette Erasure (if applicable) Compression Thickness Indicator Visual Checklist Acquisition Workstation Monitor QC Radiologist Workstation Monitor QC Film Printer QC (if applicable) Viewbox Cleanliness (if applicable) Facility QC Review Compression Force Manufacturer Calibrations (if applicable) Repeat Analysis (Optional) System QC for Radiologist (Optional) Radiologist Image Quality Feedback (Optional)

D. Prakash, R. P. Kotian, *Fundamentals of X-ray Imaging*,
https://doi.org/10.1007/978-981-96-7328-5_4

4.1 Introduction

Breast cancer is a significant global health concern, currently accounting for approximately 1 in 8 cancer diagnoses and totalling around 2.3 million new cases annually across both sexes combined [1]. It represents about a quarter of all cancer cases in females and was the most commonly diagnosed cancer among women in 2020 [2]. In 2020, an estimated 685,000 women succumbed to breast cancer, making up 16% or 1 in every 6 cancer deaths among women [3]. The future outlook indicates a troubling trend, with the number of newly diagnosed breast cancer cases projected to increase by over 40%, reaching approximately 3 million cases per year by 2040 [4]. Correspondingly, deaths from breast cancer are expected to rise by more than 50%, from 685,000 in 2020 to 1 million in 2040 [4].

Given these alarming statistics, early detection and diagnosis can greatly enhance treatment outcome and survival rates. Mammography, a specialized medical imaging technique, plays a crucial role in identifying breast cancer at an early, more treatable stage. Early detection can significantly improve survival rates and reduce the need for extensive treatment, thereby improving the quality of life for patients. The rising prevalence and projected increase in breast cancer cases and mortality underscore the urgent need for widespread access to mammography and other preventive measures.

Mammography is a specialized medical imaging technique that uses low-dose X-rays to create detailed images of breast tissue. It is primarily utilized as a screening tool to detect breast cancer at an early stage, often before symptoms appear. The main purpose of mammography is to identify abnormalities such as tumors, microcalcifications, and other changes in the breast tissue that may indicate the presence of cancer [5].

The sensitivity and specificity of mammography refer to its accuracy in correctly identifying breast cancer. Sensitivity measures the test's ability to correctly detect individuals who have the disease, while specificity measures its ability to correctly identify those who do not have the disease. Mammography along with adjunctive ultrasonography has a sensitivity rate of about 70% to 97%, which means it successfully identifies a significant proportion of breast cancer cases, though it may miss some, particularly in women with dense breast tissue [6–8]. Its specificity typically ranges from 85% to 90%, indicating a high likelihood of accurately identifying individuals without breast cancer, although false positives can occur, leading to additional tests and procedures [5, 9, 10]. Despite its drawbacks, such as painful breast compression, exposure to radiation, and the need for extensive infrastructure and specialized personnel, mammography remains the gold standard for breast cancer screening [11].

Mammography is widely used not only for screening but also for diagnostic purposes. In the context of screening, it is recommended for women at average risk of breast cancer, typically starting at the age of 40 to 50, depending on guidelines and personal risk factors [12, 13]. For diagnostic purposes, mammography is utilized to investigate specific breast problems, such as lumps, pain, or nipple discharge, and to further evaluate abnormalities found during a screening mammogram. Its use in both screening and diagnostic settings is vital for early detection, which is crucial for successful treatment and improved survival outcomes [14].

4.2 Historical Evolution of Mammography

The evolution of mammography dates back to 1913, with the first known use of radiography in breast imaging, when Albert Salomon performed X-ray examinations of mastectomy specimens. His work demonstrated that both normal breast anatomy and various types of tumors, including circumscribed and infiltrative tumors, could be visualized using radiographs, laying the groundwork for mammographic imaging [15] (Fig. 4.1). In 1927, German surgeon Otto Kleinschmidt and his mentor Erwin Payr documented the first use of mammography, emphasizing its critical importance in the early detection of breast cancer [16] (Fig. 4.1). In 1930, Stafford Warren, an

American radiologist, extended this research by performing X-rays on women's breasts in vivo before mastectomy. Out of 119 women who underwent surgery, 54 were correctly diagnosed preoperatively, achieving an accuracy rate of 93% [17]. During the 1930s through the 1950s, further advancements were made by American radiologist Jacob Gershon-Cohen (Fig. 4.2) and pathologist Helen Ingleby [18]. They conducted radiologic-pathologic correlations of breast lesions, reported on the interval growth of tumors on mammography, and highlighted the potential for mammographic screening [19]. Meanwhile, Raul Leborgne, a radiologist from Uruguay, made significant contributions by associating radiographic calcifications with breast cancer. He also improved mammographic techniques by employing breast compression, beam collimation, and spot compression views to better assess suspicious areas [19]. His insights have now become an integral part of the standard clinical practice in mammography [20].

The 1960s marked a pivotal era for mammography. Initially, radiologists used general-purpose X-ray tubes without breast compression, capturing images on direct-exposure films. These images were often low in contrast, and areas near the chest wall were underexposed, making results inconsistent across different locations [21, 22]. The widespread acceptance of mammography is largely credited to Robert Egan, an American radiologist who refined the technique by using industrial film with fine grain emulsion, along with high milliampere-seconds (mAs) and low kilovolt peak (kVp) settings [22]. In 1965, Egan produced a video detailing his standardized mammographic technique, which played a crucial role in disseminating his method [23]. The following year, Charles Gros (Fig. 4.2) of Compagnie Générale de Radiologie (CGR) in France developed the first dedicated mammography unit, known as the "Senographe" (Fig. 4.3). This unit featured a molybdenum target instead of tungsten, a small focal spot, and built-in breast compression, significantly optimizing the mammographic technique [24]. General Electric later acquired CGR and continues to sell modernized versions of the "Senographe" [18].

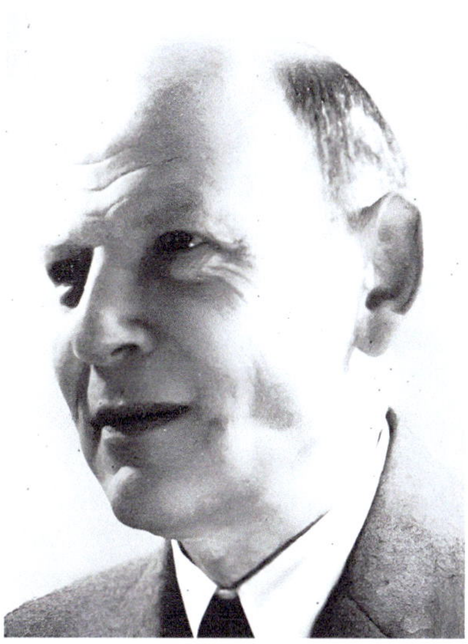

Albert Salomon
(8 December 1891 - 18 December 1966)

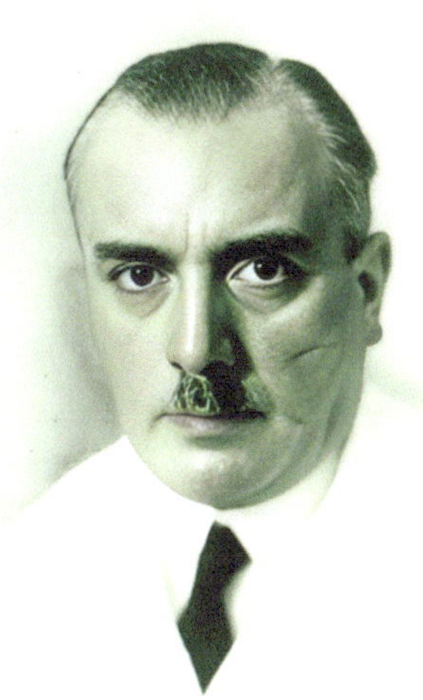

Otto Kleinschmidt
(31 Jul 1880 - 5 Jun 1948)

Fig. 4.1 Albert Solomon who did first known use of radiography in breast imaging ("Figure used with permission of Saunders, an imprint of Elsevier Inc., from Breast Imaging. Lawrence W. Bassett, Mary Catherine Mahoney, Sophia Kim Apple, Carl J. D'Orsi. 1st ed. 2011. ISBN 978-1-4160-5199-2; permission conveyed through Copyright Clearance Center, Inc.") and German surgeon Otto Kleinschmidt who documented first use of mammography. (Courtesy: Wikimedia, published under creative commons license)

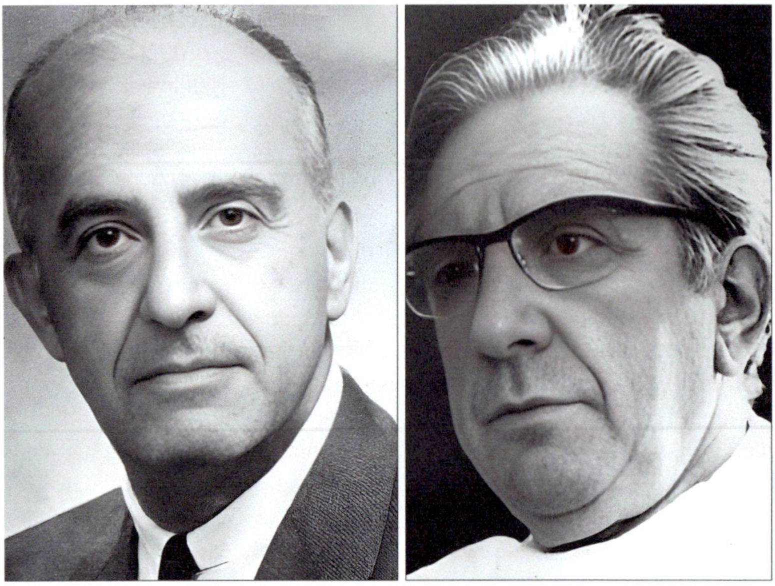

Fig. 4.2 Jacob Gershon-Cohen who correlated radiologic-pathologic of breast lesions. (Courtesy: American Journal of Roentgenology [25]). Charles Gros who developed the first dedicated mammography unit ("Figure used with permission of Saunders, an imprint of Elsevier Inc., from Breast Imaging. Lawrence W. Bassett, Mary Catherine Mahoney, Sophia Kim Apple, Carl J. D'Orsi. 1st ed. 2011. ISBN 978-1-4160-5199-2; permission conveyed through Copyright Clearance Center, Inc.")

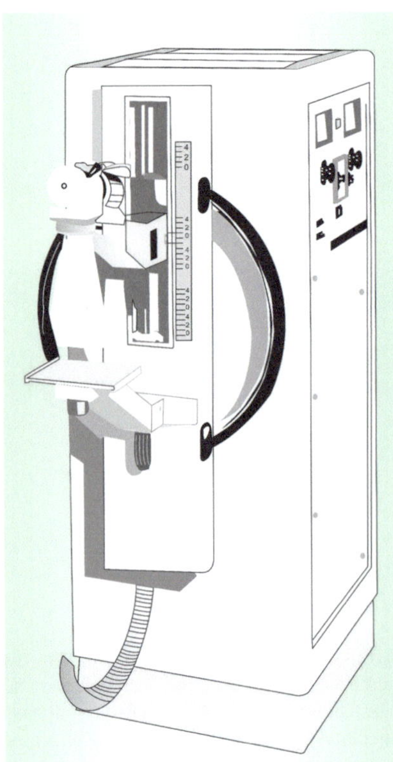

Fig. 4.3 First dedicated mammography machine "Senographe"

Several other key developments from the 1960s through the 1990s contributed to the widespread adoption of mammography. Mobile vans equipped with mammography units brought the technology to a broader public. In 1963, Strax and his team conducted a large-scale breast cancer screening of 62,000 New York women using a mobile X-ray van and an efficient process with multiple changing cubicles, resulting in a nearly 30% reduction in breast cancer deaths among participants compared to the control group, and highlighting the critical role of radiologists in early detection and treatment [26]. The 1970s also saw the introduction of screen-film mammography cassettes, which combined high-resolution intensifying screens with single-emulsion X-ray film in a vacuum-sealed cassette. This innovation allowed for faster imaging processing, better image contrast, and reduced radiation exposure [27]. Additionally, the development of the wire localization technique enabled more precise surgical excision of non-palpable mammographic abnormalities [28].

In 1972, Siemens introduced the "Mammomat" system, which simplified the configuration of

X-ray equipment, featured an optimized X-ray tube for breast diagnostics capable of visualizing structures as small as 0.1 millimeters, and was deemed suitable for cancer screening due to its ease of operation, high image quality, and low radiation dose [29]. In 1978, the introduction of the moving grid for mammography reduced scattered radiation and enhanced intrinsic image contrast, enabling companies to develop more advanced equipment capable of producing more detailed images [30]. During the 1980s and 1990s, additional randomized controlled trials corroborated the findings of the HIP trial, further validating the effectiveness of mammography for early breast cancer detection and encouraging its broader use [31]. These advancements, along with continuous improvements in imaging technology and techniques, have made mammography a cornerstone of breast cancer screening programs worldwide, significantly contributing to the early detection and treatment of breast cancer, ultimately improving patient outcomes and reducing mortality rates.

Using dedicated complex physical models, such as the Monte Carlo model, was introduced in the 1980s to reduce the radiation burden while producing high resolution images [32]. This led to anti-scatter grid technology that improved spatial resolution and reduced dose, while recent virtual grid software has further minimized exposure and enhanced image contrast [33].

From 1985 onwards, mammography underwent significant advancements, both in technology and regulation. Between 1986 and 1992, the U.S. federal and state governments implemented laws mandating the use of dedicated mammography machines in hospitals, establishing stringent quality standards, and requiring periodic inspections of equipment. These regulations aimed to ensure the reliability and safety of mammographic imaging [34]. One notable technological development during this period was the introduction of the mediolateral oblique (MLO) view as a standard projection in mammography. This view, along with the adoption of automated breast compression systems, improved the visualization of the mammary gland and its structures, enhancing diagnostic accuracy [34]. These innovations paved the way for the development of digital mammography, which was approved by the U.S. Food and Drug Administration (FDA) in 2000 [35] (Table 4.1).

Table 4.1 Summary of important events in the evolution of mammography

Year	Event	Description
1913	First Use of Radiography in Breast Imaging	Albert Salomon used X-ray examinations on mastectomy specimens, demonstrating visualization of breast anatomy, tumors spread, and microcalcifications associated with malignancy.
1927	First Use of Mammography for Early Detection	Otto Kleinschmidt and Erwin Payr emphasized the importance of mammography of a living patient, highlighting the role of mammography in early breast cancer detection.
1930	In Vivo X-rays for Breast Cancer Diagnosis	Stafford Warren conducted X-rays on women's breasts before mastectomy, achieving 84% diagnostic accuracy.
1930s–1950s	Radiologic-Pathologic Correlations	Jacob Gerson Cohen and Helen Ingleby reported on tumor growth and the potential for mammographic screening.
1949	Association of Radiographic Calcifications with Breast Cancer	Raul Leborgne linked calcifications with breast cancer and improved mammographic techniques.
1960s	Refinement of Mammographic Techniques	Robert Egan improved imaging contrast and reduced underexposure, establishing a standardized mammographic technique.
1965	Development of Dedicated Mammography Unit	Charles Gros developed the "senographe," featuring optimized X-ray technology and built-in breast compression.
1963	Large-Scale Breast Cancer Screening	Strax conducted screenings using mobile X-ray vans, resulting in a significant reduction in breast cancer deaths.

(continued)

Table 4.1 (continued)

Year	Event	Description
1970s	Introduction of Screen-Film Mammography Cassettes	Enhanced image processing, contrast, and reduced radiation exposure.
1972	Introduction of the MAMMOMAT System	Siemens introduced a system capable of visualizing small structures, suitable for cancer screening.
1978	Introduction of the Moving Grid for Mammography	Improved image contrast by reducing scattered radiation.
1980s–1990s	Validation of Mammography for Early Breast Cancer Detection	Additional trials corroborated the effectiveness of mammography, encouraging broader use.
1980s	Introduction of Monte Carlo Model and Anti-Scatter Grid Technology	Reduced radiation dose and improved image resolution.
1985–1992	Implementation of Mammography Regulations	U.S. laws required dedicated mammography machines, quality standards, and periodic inspections.
2000	FDA Approval of Digital Mammography	Digital mammography provided high-quality images with lower radiation doses.
1997	Proposal of Digital Breast Tomosynthesis (DBT)	Dr. Loren T. Niklason et al. introduced DBT to create 3D images and improve detection in dense breasts.
2003	First Clinical Use of Contrast-Enhanced Mammography (CEM)	Jong et al. demonstrated the effectiveness of CEM in identifying breast lesions.
2011	FDA Approval of CEM	CEM showed superior performance in detecting breast lesions compared to traditional mammography.
Recent	Integration of AI and Radiomics in Mammography	AI and radiomics enhance diagnostic accuracy, predict lesion characteristics, and improve patient comfort and care.

Digital mammography represented a major shift from traditional film-based methods. In this technology, the transmitted radiation is captured by an electronic image detector rather than film. This change decouples image acquisition from image storage, allowing for better data management and analysis. The primary advantage of digital mammography is its ability to obtain high-quality images with lower radiation doses, making the process safer for patients. Digital detectors produce signals based on absorbed energy, which are then converted into images. Full-field digital mammography (FFDM) was found to have significantly higher accuracy in identifying breast lesions compared to traditional screen-film mammography [36].

Digital Breast Tomosynthesis (DBT) emerged to address the limitations of conventional mammography, especially in dense breasts where tissue overlap can obscure lesions. The application of DBT was proposed in 1996 (patent filed) and clinically implemented in 1999 by Dr. Loren T. Niklason et al. at Massachusetts General Hospital. They pioneered DBT, which creates three-dimensional (3D) sectional images of the breast, offering a clearer view by reducing anatomical noise and tissue overlap [37]. It works by acquiring multiple low-dose X-ray projections from different angles around the breast, which are then reconstructed into thin slices. This method improves the visualization of nodules, architectural distortions, and other abnormalities, enhancing the detection of malignancies [38]. Clinical studies showed DBT increases cancer detection rates from 6.1 to 8.0 per 1000 examinations and a reduction in the false-positive rate from 10.3% to 8.5% [39] along with other confirmatory studies [40–42]. Despite these promising results, DBT faces challenges such as additional radiation exposure compared to full-field digital mammography (FFDM) and ongoing debate over its efficacy in detecting microcalcifications and lesions in very dense breasts [43].

Contrast-Enhanced Mammography (CEM) represents a significant advancement in breast imaging, combining contrast-enhanced techniques with traditional mammography to improve the visualization of breast lesions. The first clinical use of CEM was reported by Jong et al. in 2003, demonstrating its effectiveness in identifying breast lesions [44]. General Electric subsequently developed a dual-energy subtraction mammography prototype, with Dromain et al. publishing the first study using this device in 2011 [45]. FDA approval of CEM in the United States occurred later (2011 for prototypes; broader clinical acceptance followed gradually in the 2010s), showing superior performance in lesion detection compared to traditional mammography [46].

CEM uses dual-energy exposure (26–33 kVp and 44–50 kVp) following contrast injection, providing detailed breast structure visualization with minimal radiation exposure, in line with European screening guidelines [47]. Recent studies have highlighted CEM's diagnostic strengths, particularly in dense breasts where traditional methods may falter. CEM offers several benefits over MRI, including faster execution, lower cost, reduced psychological impact, fewer false positives, and suitability for patients who cannot undergo MRI [48, 49]. CEM has proven effective in defining lesion extent preoperatively, supporting conservative surgery, and reducing unnecessary biopsies for benign conditions [50, 51]. It excels in distinguishing malignant from benign lesions, offering a good balance of false positives and negatives [52].

Recent advancements in mammography emphasize the integration of artificial intelligence (AI) and radiomics, reflecting a broader trend toward precision and personalized medicine. AI, with its capacity to emulate human decision-making processes, and radiomics, often referred to as the "genetics of the image," are transforming how breast lesions are detected and interpreted. These technologies enhance diagnostic accuracy by reducing false-positive and false-negative interpretations, and by improving overall reliability of clinical assessments [53, 54].

Radiomics allows the extraction of specific intrinsic image characteristics, which can be correlated with clinical outcomes through complex mathematical algorithms. This capability is particularly valuable for predicting the benignity or malignancy of breast lesions, potentially optimizing biopsy requests. Additionally, radiomics can predict crucial prognostic information, such as receptor status of breast neoplasms, before biopsy, and even anticipate biopsy underestimation [55–58].

Moreover, recent technological advances in mammography have focused on improving patient comfort during diagnostic procedures. This includes designing equipment that minimizes discomfort and considers the patient's overall experience, not just the clinical aspects. As mammography continues to advance, the emphasis will likely shift towards more patient-centric diagnostic methods, ensuring a holistic approach to patient care [59]. These advancements in technology, combined with evolving quality standards and regulations, have contributed to the widespread adoption of mammography as a crucial tool for early breast cancer detection, improving diagnostic precision and patient outcomes.

4.3 Understanding Breast Anatomy for Mammography

Understanding breast anatomy aids in identifying normal structures and potential abnormalities. The breast comprises various tissues, each serving a distinct function, and can be broadly categorized into external and internal structures.

Externally, the breast includes the nipple and the areola. The nipple is the central point from which milk is secreted during lactation, surrounded by the areola, a pigmented area containing small glands (Montgomery's glands) that secrete lubricating and protective substances. The skin over the breast connects to underlying breast tissue via an anterior fascial layer and superficial fibrous extensions known as Cooper's ligaments, named after Sir Astley Cooper, who made significant contributions to the understanding of breast anatomy in his 1840 treatise "On the Anatomy of the Breast" [60].

Internally, the breast consists of lobes, lobules, ducts, fibrous tissue, adipose tissue, blood vessels, and the lymphatic system. The human breast is a modified apocrine exocrine gland derived from specialized skin structures, composed of overlying skin and subcutaneous tissue, breast parenchyma (including ducts and lobules), and supporting stroma. The breast is divided into 15–20 sections called lobes, each containing smaller structures known as lobules, which are responsible for milk production and are connected to ducts that transport milk to the nipple [61]. The ducts converge at the nipple, facilitating milk release during breastfeeding. Typically, between 15 and 20 main milk ducts exit at the nipple, although anatomical studies show considerable variation in duct number, course, and branching, without a perfectly radial arrangement [62]. The mammary gland is most effectively examined by dividing it into four quadrants using imaginary vertical and horizontal lines that intersect at the nipple. These regions are identified as the upper outer quadrant, upper inner quadrant, lower inner quadrant, and lower outer quadrant [63].

Fibrous tissue, including Cooper's ligaments, provides structural support to the breast, maintaining its shape and attaching it to the skin and chest wall. The deep parenchymal tissues are enveloped by both an anterior and posterior fascial layer. The breast overlies the pectoralis major muscle superiorly, serratus anterior muscle laterally, and upper abdominal oblique muscles inferiorly. The female breast is generally larger than the male breast and contains a greater volume of fibroglandular tissue, whereas the male breast predominantly consists of adipose tissue with rudimentary ducts (Fig. 4.4).

The proportion of adipose tissue, which surrounds the lobes and ducts and provides cushioning, can vary significantly among individuals and undergo dynamic changes with age, body mass index, and hormonal influences (e.g., puberty, pregnancy, lactation, and menopause). The breast's lymphatic system consists of a network of lymphatic vessels that drain into lymph nodes, primarily located in the axilla (underarm area) and secondarily in the supraclavicular and internal mammary (parasternal) regions. The lymphatic system plays a crucial role in the immune response and is also the principal pathway for metastatic spread of breast cancer.

On a mammogram, different tissues appear with varying densities. Fibroglandular tissue, including ducts, lobules, and supporting fibrous tissue, appears white due to its density and is most abundant in younger women. This density decreases with age, as the proportion of adipose tissue, which appears radiolucent (gray to dark on mammograms) on mammograms, increases.

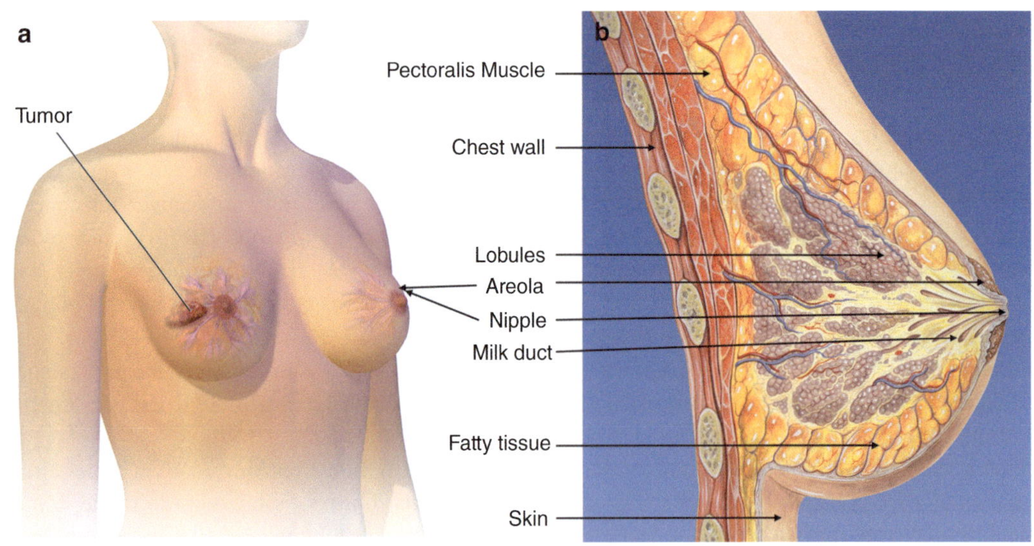

Fig. 4.4 The anatomy of the female breast includes the nipple and areola on the external surface. Internally, it comprises pectoralis muscle, lobules, milk duct, fatty tissue, lymph nodes, and other components. (Image copyright: (**a**) Bruce Blaus and (**b**) Patrick J. Lynch. Printed under creative commons license)

The skin is usually visible as a white edge, and striated chest wall muscle and reniform axillary lymph nodes are commonly seen on the mammographic craniocaudal and mediolateral oblique (MLO) views [62].

Breast density is a key consideration in mammography, as the proportion of glandular to fatty tissue can affect the sensitivity of the imaging. Dense breasts, characterized by a higher proportion of fibroglandular tissue, reduce sensitivity for detecting lesions, particularly small masses or microcalcifications, due to tissue masking [6–8]. Factors like age, hormonal status, pregnancy, lactation, and prior surgeries influence breast density and structure [62]. For instance, pregnancy and lactation typically markedly increase glandular tissue volume and vascularity in the breast, which regresses after lactation ceases, sometimes resulting in asymmetry if one breast was preferentially used during feeding [62].

Digital mammography, the most commonly used imaging tool for the breast, benefits from an improved dynamic range over the historically used screen-film mammography. This advancement enhances the visualization of different breast tissues and structures, providing a more detailed and accurate assessment. A sound knowledge of breast anatomy is therefore essential for accurately interpreting mammograms, distinguishing between normal structures and potential abnormalities, and determining the most appropriate imaging techniques and follow-up procedures for each patient.

4.4 Mammography Equipment

Mammography is one of the most technically demanding radiographic examinations, requiring precise control of various factors to achieve optimal image quality. These factors include patient positioning and compression, equipment selection, technique, exposure factors, and image processing [64]. Ensuring the technical quality of the mammographic image depends heavily on equipment design and performance, image processing capabilities, the training of technologists, and the guidance provided by medical physicists.

4.4.1 Components of a Mammography Unit

4.4.1.1 X-ray Tube

In mammography units, stationary anode X-ray tubes are typically used due to their ability to handle the specific demands of breast imaging. Instead of rotation, mammography anodes (often molybdenum or rhodium) use careful design of the anode angle and material to balance heat dissipation and beam quality. The relatively low kV (25–35 kV) and limited mA settings mean that stationary anodes are sufficient for clinical use. This is particularly important in mammography where precise imaging of small structures, such as microcalcifications, is needed. Because of the lower heat load in mammography compared to general radiography, stationary anodes remain durable and clinically efficient.

4.4.1.1.1 Cathode

The cathode emits electrons, via a filament typically made of tungsten, chosen for their durability and high melting points. These characteristics are essential for withstanding the high temperatures generated during thermionic emission, a process where the filament is heated by an electrical current, causing it to release electrons into the tube. These electrons are then accelerated towards the anode, where they generate X-ray photons. A distinctive feature of mammography X-ray tubes is the dual-focus design of the cathode, which includes two filament sizes. This design allows for different focal spot sizes, providing flexibility in imaging. The smaller focal spot, around 0.1 mm, is ideal for high-resolution imaging, crucial for detecting small structures like microcalcifications. In contrast, the larger focal spot, approximately 0.3 mm, is used for faster image acquisition, which is particularly beneficial during routine screenings. Heat management is less critical at the cathode than at the anode, but robust filament design ensures tube stability and longevity (Fig. 4.5).

4.4.1.1.2 Anode

The anode is target for the accelerated electrons produced by the cathode. Modern mammography

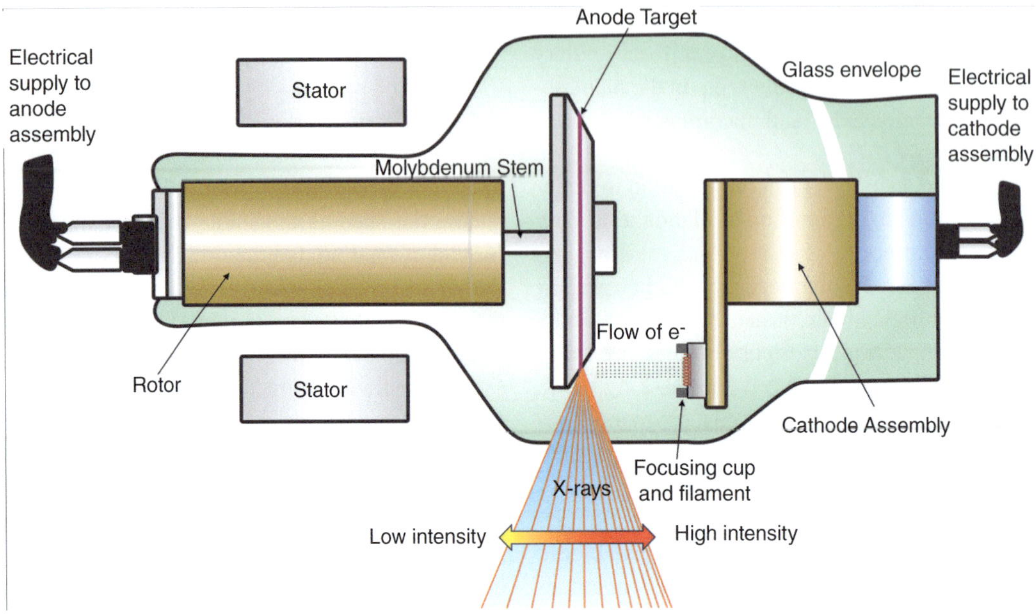

Fig. 4.5 Mammography X-ray tube and anode heel effect

units predominantly utilize a stationary anode design, since the relatively low tube loading in breast imaging does not require rotation for heat dissipation. The stationary design is sufficient to maintain high image quality at the low kV and mA settings used in mammography. Typically, the anode is made from **molybdenum**, a material known for generating K characteristic X-rays in the optimal energy range of 17.4–19.9 keV. This energy range provides excellent contrast and detail necessary for accurately identifying breast tissue abnormalities, such as tumors and microcalcifications. Molybdenum's emission spectrum aligns well with the absorption properties of breast tissue, ensuring effective imaging with relatively low radiation doses.

In addition to molybdenum, some mammography systems use **rhodium** anodes, which produce X-rays with slightly higher energies (20–23 keV). Rhodium anodes offer improved penetration and image quality, which is particularly beneficial for imaging dense or thick breast tissues. The anode's effective target angle in mammography is typically much smaller (around 6–16 degrees), which provides a thin, uniform X-ray beam and minimizes focal spot blur. Tube orientation and beam geometry are carefully designed to ensure coverage of the breast, including the chest wall and peripheral tissue. This design ensures thorough assessment and detailed imaging across the entire breast tissue.

4.4.1.1.3 Anode Heel Effect

The anode heel effect is a fundamental phenomenon in X-ray imaging that arises due to the geometry and physics of the X-ray tube. It plays a particularly significant role in mammography, where precise imaging of the breast tissue is crucial. This effect refers to the variation in X-ray intensity emitted from the anode, depending on the direction of the beam relative to the anode's surface. Specifically, X-rays emitted closer to the anode's surface (the "heel" of the anode) have to travel through more of the anode material itself, causing greater attenuation and resulting in lower X-ray intensity compared to those emitted perpendicular to the anode surface.

In mammography, the anode heel effect is not merely a technical nuance but an aspect that can be leveraged to optimize image quality. The setup typically involves positioning the X-ray tube above the patient, with the X-ray beam directed downwards towards the breast and image receptor. The X-ray tube is oriented so that the cathode side is closest to the patient's chest wall, while the anode side is nearer to the nipple. This arrangement is strategic: the anode heel effect naturally results in a higher X-ray intensity on the cathode side compared to the anode side. Since the breast is generally thicker near the chest wall, the increased intensity from the cathode side helps to penetrate this denser tissue, providing a clearer and more uniform image across the entire breast (Fig. 4.6).

The practical implications of the anode heel effect in mammography are multifaceted. Firstly, it aids in achieving consistent image quality by compensating for the variations in breast thickness. The gradient in X-ray intensity—from higher near the chest wall to lower near the nipple—ensures that even the denser, posterior regions of the breast receive adequate exposure. This careful balancing act helps to prevent underexposure of the thicker parts and overexposure of the thinner regions, which could otherwise obscure critical diagnostic details. Moreover, the anode heel effect's influence extends to the choice of effective target angle (typically 6–16° in mammography) and tube angulations. By manipulating these parameters, manufacturers can fine-tune the distribution of X-ray intensity to match the specific needs of different breast sizes and compositions.

4.4.1.2 Tube Housing

The tube housing serves multiple essential functions such as providing structural support, effective heat dissipation, and radiation shielding for the X-ray tube. Inside the housing, insulating oil absorbs heat generated during X-ray production and provides electrical insulation. This cooling is vital, as the anode still dissipates heat even in stationary anode designs used in mammography, though not to the same extreme as rotating-anode tubes in general radiography. The housing is lined with lead or other radiation-absorbing materials to contain stray radiation, ensuring that only the intended X-ray beam is directed towards

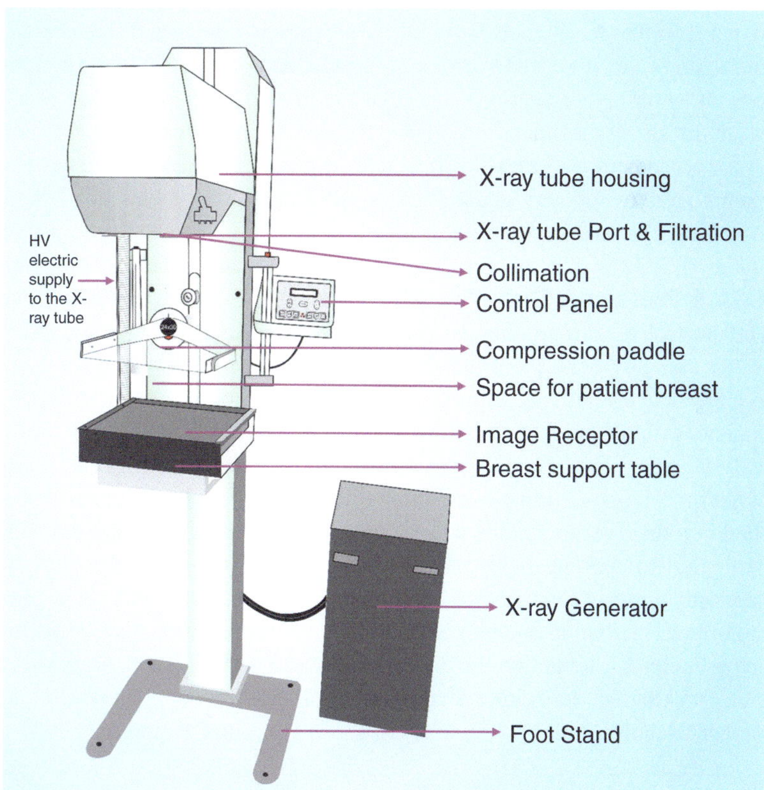

Fig. 4.6 Mammography machine and its components

the patient's breast. This shielding is crucial for protecting both the patient and healthcare personnel from unnecessary radiation exposure, while also safeguarding the surrounding environment.

4.4.1.3 Filters

Filters are designed to shape the X-ray spectrum and optimize the quality of the images. In mammography, the energy of the X-rays must be finely tuned to achieve the best contrast between different tissues, particularly between glandular and adipose tissues. Filters made from materials like molybdenum (Mo), rhodium (Rh), and in some digital systems, silver (Ag) or aluminum (Al) as additional options are used to selectively absorb lower-energy photons that contribute to patient dose without improving image quality. By filtering out these lower-energy photons, the remaining X-ray beam is hardened, enhancing image contrast and reducing noise.

The selection of the filter material is patient-specific, often depending on factors like breast density and thickness. For example, molybdenum filters are generally used for thinner breasts or when softer X-rays are required, while rhodium filters are preferred for denser breasts as they allow for higher-energy X-rays that can penetrate thicker tissues more effectively. Silver filters are sometimes used in full-field digital mammography for very dense breasts, offering even higher beam energies (up to ~30 keV range).

4.4.1.4 Protective Shroud

The protective shroud that encases the X-ray source assembly serves multiple functions. It acts as a physical barrier, protecting the delicate components within from dust, moisture, and mechanical damage. The shroud also contributes to radiation safety, providing an additional layer of shielding that prevents radiation leakage. This is particularly important in ensuring that only the necessary dose is delivered to the patient, thus minimizing radiation exposure. Moreover, the shroud helps to streamline the appearance of the unit, making it less intimidating and more patient-friendly.

4.4.1.5 X-ray Tube Generator

Mammography requires specialized X-ray generators that operate at low kilovoltage to achieve adequate tissue contrast, typically within the range of 25–50 kVp depending on the image receptor type. These generators must produce accurate and consistent low kilovoltage to ensure high-quality imaging. Additionally, to facilitate relatively short exposure times, the tube currents available should be relatively high. A critical feature of mammography X-ray generators is the sharp rise and fall times on the voltage waveform, which are necessary for precise timing and efficient X-ray production [65].

High-frequency generators, which can operate at multiple thousands of cycles per second compared to the 60 cycles per second characteristic of full-wave and three-phase systems, are particularly beneficial in mammography. These high-frequency generators produce a low-ripple waveform, approximating a constant potential waveform, which is ideal for this application. Low-ripple systems offer numerous advantages, including lower patient dose, shorter exposure times, and greater heat-loading capacity. The consistent high voltage of these systems enhances X-ray production efficiency by generating fewer low-energy photons and allowing more photons to reach the image plane, thus reducing patient absorption and shortening exposure times.

The ability to use relatively high milliamperage values further reduces exposure times, minimizing patient motion and associated image-degrading effects. Low-ripple systems also have greater heat-loading capacity in their focal spots, enabling the use of submillimeter focal spots that are crucial for magnification techniques requiring the visualization of small details. This capacity also allows for the use of grids to suppress scattered radiation without increasing exposure times, as grids typically double the heat load for each exposure. Additionally, larger source-to-image distances (SIDs) can be implemented without adversely affecting exposure times, further improving image quality.

Modern mammography units use high-frequency generators (not three-phase), since they provide superior low-ripple performance compared to older three-phase supplies. A robust quality assurance program is essential for these generators, periodically checking the accuracy and reproducibility of kilovoltage, as well as the performance of the phototimer or milliampere-second timer. Systems with phototimers should yield consistent film density regardless of breast thickness and kilovoltage setting [65].

4.4.1.6 Face Shield

Both screen-film mammography (SFM) and full-field digital mammography (FFDM) units feature a protective barrier or face guard designed to prevent patients from leaning into the X-ray beam during exposure. This shield helps avoid image artifacts and unnecessary radiation exposure. The U-arm is controlled via multiple sets of buttons located on the gantry, allowing technologists to adjust the U-arm's position, rotate it for oblique imaging, and operate the compression devices. These controls are strategically placed to ensure ease of use and efficiency during the imaging process.

Mammography units are designed with a source-to-image distance (SID) of approximately 60 to 66 cm (commonly standardized at 65 cm), which provides a balance between good patient accessibility and image quality. Longer SIDs can increase tube loading, while shorter SIDs may restrict patient access and affect image quality, particularly during magnification procedures. Proper alignment of the X-ray beam with the chest wall edge of the compression paddle is crucial for maximizing the imaging of chest wall breast tissue.

4.4.1.7 Collimator

The collimator in mammography determines the X-ray field of view (FOV), ensuring that the X-rays are precisely directed at the area of interest. This precision is essential for both image quality and patient safety, as it helps achieve high-quality images while minimizing radiation exposure. Collimators can be either motor-driven or manually adjusted, with the choice between high-end and less expensive units depending on the facility's specific needs and budget. Both approaches aim to provide accurate and efficient imaging.

In high-end mammography units, the collimator blades are motor-driven, allowing for automatic adjustment to the size of the image receptor. This feature enables operators to reduce the FOV to two or more smaller sizes with the press of a button, offering enhanced convenience and accuracy without the need for manual intervention. Conversely, less expensive units use an automatic switching mechanism between two standard FOV sizes, typically 18 × 24 cm and 24 × 30 cm. These units may require manual switching of diaphragms for small focal spots, magnification, and coned-down views. Some units require manual diaphragm switching between small and large FOVs, providing a practical and cost-effective solution for varying imaging needs.

The collimator edge cuts off the anode side of the beam, resulting in a straight edge along the original beam center that aligns with the patient's chest wall. The cathode side of the tube is typically located on the chest wall side of the patient. In some systems, the tube is angled to further emphasize the anode region of the X-ray field. Fixed-aperture collimators, usually used in mammography, consist of four blades forming a rectangle and can be chosen for specific sizes and the desired SID. Some systems have a fifth blade that allows for collimating the beam closer to the actual breast outline, although it may be advantageous not to use this fifth blade and allow the full X-ray field to fall on the film receptor. This technique blackens the non-breast areas of the image, reducing light glare from the view box and adding only negligible scatter to the image.

Despite these differences, the operational distinction between high-end and less expensive units is minimal, especially in those where the collimator automatically switches between different FOV sizes. Both types of units maintain convenience, as grid and magnification stands are adjusted, making the process straightforward regardless of the collimation method used (Fig. 4.7).

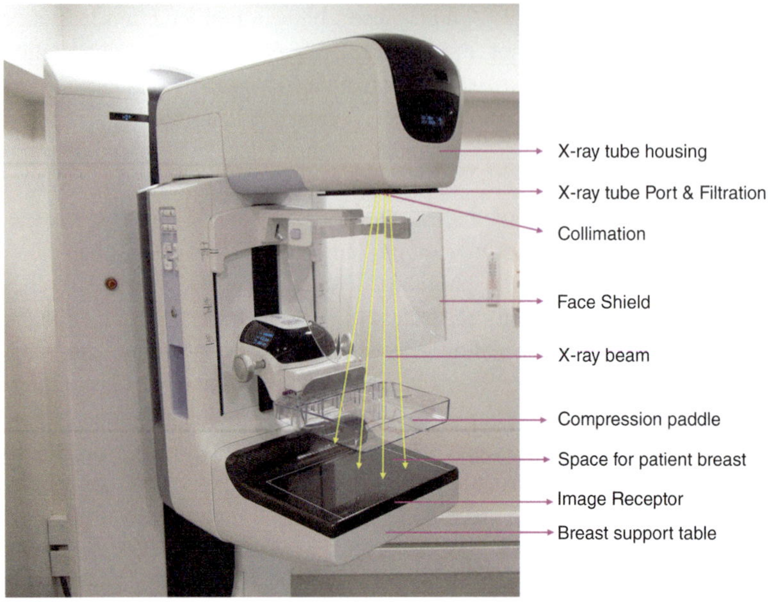

Fig. 4.7 The mammography unit and its different parts. (Image by Elías Alarcón from Pixabay)

4.4.1.8 Compression Device

The compression device in a mammography machine is critical for enhancing image quality and ensuring patient safety. Each unit includes mechanical drive components within the vertical section of the U-arm and various paddles. According to the Mammography Quality Standards Act (MQSA) regulations, the compression must be power-driven and operable by a foot switch or hand controls accessible from the technologist's side, with manual fine-adjustment controls also accessible from from at least one side of the unit.

Compression devices come with various-sized paddles that correspond to all full-field image receptors. The chest wall edge of the paddles must be straight and parallel to the edge of the image receptor. Typically, a mammography unit is equipped with multiple paddles for different techniques, including small, large, spot grid, and magnification paddles. Screening units generally require only small and large grid paddles.

Design and function are governed by strict regulations. The central ray, orthogonal to the image receptor, should project parallel to the chest wall, with the paddle lip aligned accordingly. The paddle lip must not extend beyond the chest wall of the film by more than 6 mm, ideally not exceeding 3 mm to ensure proper imaging of tissue near the chest wall. The chest wall edge of the compression paddle should be straight and parallel to the image receptor; additional 3 cm lip height is not specified in MQSA. MQSA regulations also stipulate that the paddle must remain flat and parallel to the breast support cover, with no more than a 1.0 cm (10 mm) deflection under compression. The initial power-driven compression force must be between 11 and 20 kg (approximately 25 and 45 pounds). Paddles not designed to be flat must meet specific manufacturer specifications, and a deflection of about 2 cm is generally acceptable for patient comfort.

Newer "flex" paddles improve tissue visualization and patient comfort by reducing motion and providing even compression with a rounded edge at the chest wall side (commonly 2–5 mm radius depending on manufacturer). The compression plate should be stiff, transparent plastic, forming a sharp 90° angle with the chest wall.

Compression in mammography reduces geometric and motion unsharpness by pushing breast structures closer to the receptor plane, reducing tissue volume, and thereby decreasing scattered radiation and enhancing subject contrast. Thinner breasts require less exposure time, further reducing motion unsharpness. Compression decreases patient dose since less exposure is needed for a thinner breast. Additionally, it helps delineate tissue borders better.

4.4.1.9 Breast Support and Grid Assemblies

These components are integral to supporting the breast during imaging. The grid assemblies help reduce scatter radiation, thereby improving image clarity. According to the Mammography Quality Standards Act (MQSA), grid use is not mandated by MQSA; magnification mammography is performed without a grid, and some digital breast tomosynthesis (DBT) systems achieve dose efficiency without one. These assemblies, typically mounted on the U-arm's mounting plate, consist of a breast support plate, a grid, a grid drive motor, associated electronics, an image receptor, and a bottom plate. The grids, usually with a ratio of 4:1 or 5:1, control scatter radiation by preferentially absorbing scattered X-rays, thus enhancing the image contrast. The use of high-transmission cellular (HTC) grids has further improved image contrast by controlling scatter in two directions, resulting in better performance compared to traditional linear grids (Fig. 4.8).

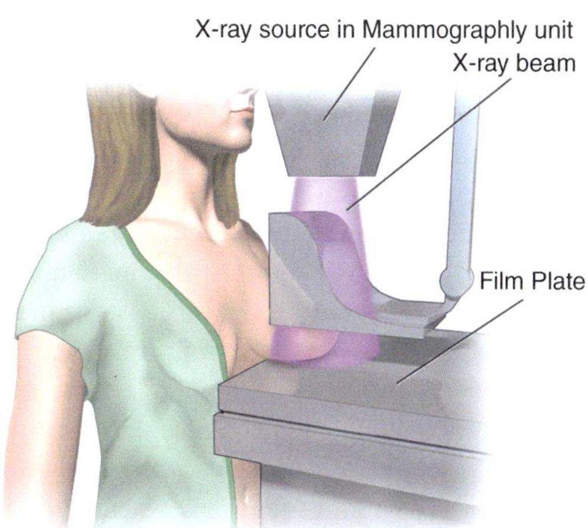

Fig. 4.8 Performing mammography. (Image copyright: BruceBlaus. Published under creative commons license)

4.4.1.10 Image Receptor and Automatic Exposure Control

In mammography, image receptors capture X-ray images of breast tissue, with two primary types: *film-based* and *digital detectors*. Each type has unique characteristics, affecting image quality, diagnostic accuracy, patient comfort, and clinical workflow. Additionally, Automatic Exposure Control (AEC) systems are integrated into these receptors to ensure optimal image quality and patient safety by adjusting exposure parameters based on breast thickness and tissue density.

4.4.1.10.1 Film-Based Mammography

Film-based mammography, or screen-film mammography (SFM), has been a standard for many years. It utilizes intensifying screen cassettes and single emulsion film designed specifically for mammography. The film consists of silver bromide grains in a gelatin matrix coated onto a polyester base, with a typical emulsion layer thickness of 10 μm and a polyester base of 180 μm. The intensifying screen, often made from rare-earth phosphors such as gadolinium oxysulfide ($Gd_2O_2S{:}Tb$) or similar materials, enhances the film's sensitivity by emitting light when struck by X-rays, which then exposes the film.

SFM systems typically offer high spatial resolution, crucial for detecting fine details such as microcalcifications. However, they have a limited dynamic range, making it challenging to differentiate subtle differences in breast tissue density. The chemical process of film development involves multiple steps, including immersion in developing and fixing solutions, which significantly impacts the image's speed and contrast. While high-speed screens are commonly used, medium-speed screens are sometimes employed for specific techniques, like magnification and imaging dense breasts, despite a slight increase in image noise and decrease in spatial resolution.

4.4.1.10.2 Digital Mammography

Digital mammography employs various digital detectors, including flat-panel detectors (FPDs) and computed radiography (CR) systems. These detectors capture X-rays and convert them into electronic signals, which are then digitized. Several types of digital detectors are used, such as slot-scanning systems with a scintillator and charge-coupled device (CCD) array, flat-panel systems using amorphous silicon (a-Si) with cesium iodide (CsI) or amorphous selenium (a-Se), and computed radiography systems using photostimulable phosphor plates. For example, flat-panel phosphor systems use CsI crystals deposited on a matrix of light-sensitive diodes and thin-film transistors, which convert absorbed X-ray photons into visible light, subsequently detected and converted into a digital signal. The CsI crystals' columnar structure helps contain the light, improving quantum efficiency. The a-Se systems directly convert X-ray energy into an electric charge, which is then read out and digitized, offering high X-ray absorption and spatial resolution.

Digital mammography offers several advantages over film-based systems. It provides a wider dynamic range, allowing for enhanced visualization of subtle abnormalities, particularly in dense breast tissue. However, while digital mammography has greater dynamic range and contrast resolution, its limiting spatial resolution (≈5–7 lp/mm for flat panels) is generally lower than that of SFM (≈15 lp/mm). The ability to adjust image contrast and brightness helps in detecting and analyzing potential issues more accurately. Additionally, digital systems integrate seamlessly with computer-aided detection (CAD) software, assisting radiologists in identifying suspicious areas and improving diagnostic accuracy.

One of the key benefits of digital mammography is the potential to optimize radiation dose: average glandular dose is comparable to or slightly lower than SFM when properly calibrated, but not universally reduced. This is particularly advantageous for younger women and those who need frequent mammograms, as it minimizes their exposure to radiation. The digital format also eliminates the need for film processing, which streamlines the workflow and reduces the time spent on manual handling and image retrieval. Digital images can be stored electronically and easily transmitted for remote consultations, facilitating faster access to specialist opinions. Moreover, the elimination of physical film storage saves space and reduces administrative tasks, contributing to overall efficiency in clinical settings.

4.4.1.10.3 Automatic Exposure Control (AEC)

In SFM, the AEC system includes a sensor located in the U-arm mounting plate behind the image receptor. This sensor detects X-rays that penetrate the breast and the screen-film cassette, generating a current proportional to the detected X-ray energy. The current charges a capacitor, and when the voltage across the capacitor matches a reference value, the exposure is terminated. Modern SFM AECs apply corrections for factors such as beam hardening and film reciprocity law failure, ensuring consistent film density as breast thickness and X-ray tube potentials vary. The Mammography Quality Standards Act (MQSA) regulations mandate that the AEC maintain film density within ±0.15 optical density (OD) of the average OD as breast phantom thickness varies from 2.0 to 6.0 cm. In fact, MQSA requires that the optical density be within ±0.15 OD of the mean for phantom thicknesses between 2–6 cm at 28 kVp with Mo/Mo target-filter, using a standard phantom (21 CFR 900.12(e)(5)(iii))

In full-field digital mammography (FFDM), the AEC sensor is typically integrated into the digital detector. The system often performs a short "pre-exposure" to evaluate factors such as breast thickness and density, subsequently determining the optimal exposure parameters for the final image. This ensures accurate and consistent signal intensity across varying conditions. An effective AEC system must cover an adequate region of the breast to account for its variability. For SFM, a sensor with a sensitive area of approximately 1–5 cm^2 (depending on design, typically around 2–3 cm^2 for commercial units) or an array of smaller sensors can achieve this, providing consistent film OD. The system should also support separate density calibrations for grid and magnification techniques and offer multiple exposure steps for precise control over film OD.

The choice between film-based and digital mammography depends on various factors, including the clinical setting, patient demographics, and available resources. While film-based systems have been reliable and provide high spatial resolution, digital systems offer greater flexibility, efficiency, and image quality. Continuous advancements in digital technologies are improving mammographic imaging, leading to better breast cancer detection and diagnosis. The integration of AEC systems in both film-based and digital systems ensures optimal image quality and patient safety, making them indispensable in modern mammography practices.

4.4.1.11 Foot Pedals and Digital Display for Compression

Both SFM and FFDM units are equipped with two methods for providing compression to the compression paddle. Foot pedals, located on either side of the U-arm, are used for initial compression, allowing a maximum force of approximately 45 decanewtons (daN), equivalent to about 100 pounds, as recommended by the Mammography Quality Standards Act (MQSA) and aiding the technician during patient positioning. Additionally, a manual knob at the compression paddle allows for fine-tuning the amount of compression. A digital display near the base or top of the U-arm shows the compression force, thickness, and angle of the U-arm, helping technologists optimize patient positioning for better image quality.

4.4.1.12 Magnification Stand

Diagnostic mammography units are required by MQSA regulations to have radiographic magnification capabilities for noninterventional problem-solving procedures. To perform magnification imaging, the grid between the X-ray source and the image receptor is removed and replaced with a magnification stand on the U-arm's mounting plate. The regulations stipulate that the system must provide at least one magnification value within the range of 1.4–2.0, and the unit must also have a small focal spot to meet resolution requirements.

Magnification is used to enhance the visualization of specific areas within the breast. The process improves image quality by enhancing system spatial resolution and increasing the number of X-ray photons used to image the structure of interest, resulting in a significant decrease in effective noise. Systems typically offer magnification values between ×1.5 and ×2.0, with a focal spot size of 0.1 mm (or smaller, such as 0.05 mm) being recommended for optimal resolution. Higher magnification (e.g., ×1.7) requires a smaller focal spot to maintain image sharpness and accurately delineate microcalcifications.

Magnification also benefits from lower kVp and shorter exposure times, which enhance subject contrast and reduce the likelihood of patient motion. The smaller the field of view (FOV), the lower the relative intensity of scatter, improving image clarity. However, excessively small FOVs can complicate positioning and reduce the ability to orient the image. A 12 × 18-cm FOV at the image plane is a practical compromise, balancing improved image contrast with manageable positioning and orientation.

4.4.1.13 Radiation Output

MQSA regulations require mammography units to produce a minimum radiation output rate of at least 7.0 mGy air kerma per 100 mAs at 28 kVp, measured at 4.2 cm above the breast support in the standard Mo/Mo target-filter mode. This requirement ensures that the system delivers sufficient output to achieve diagnostic image quality under standard test conditions. Modern units typically exceed this minimum output, with some capable of producing significantly higher output levels, enabling shorter exposure times and improved imaging performance, allowing shorter exposure times and better image quality, particularly for dense breasts.

4.5 Digital Breast Tomosynthesis

Digital Breast Tomosynthesis (DBT) is a three-dimensional (3D) imaging technique that reconstructs tomographic images of the breast from multiple low-dose projection images. These images are acquired by moving the X-ray tube over a limited angular range, which helps overcome the limitations of traditional two-dimensional (2D) mammography, where overlapping fibroglandular tissue can obscure lesions and complicate the differentiation between benign and malignant features. DBT is particularly useful in dense breast tissues, offering better tissue structure differentiation and improved diagnostic accuracy.

Numerous studies, especially from the United States, have demonstrated that combining full-field digital mammography (FFDM) with DBT enhances sensitivity, specificity, and reader performance compared to 2D mammography alone [40–42, 66]. Large-scale prospective trials, such as the Oslo Tomosynthesis Screening Trial and the STORM screening study, have shown significant improvements in cancer detection rates and reductions in false-positive recall rates with DBT [67, 68]. These findings are supported by other research, including the Malmö Breast Tomosynthesis Screening Trial and the TOMMY Trial, which highlight the potential of DBT to improve breast cancer screening outcomes across various populations [69].

4.5.1 Principles of Digital Breast Tomosynthesis

4.5.1.1 Image Acquisition and Reconstruction

In a DBT exam, the patient's breast is compressed between two plates, similar to conventional mammography. An X-ray tube moves in an arc over the breast, capturing multiple low-dose X-ray projections at various angles, typically ranging from 15° to 50° depending on the manufacturer and system design [70]. Wider arcs provide more tomographic information, enhancing the separation of breast tissue into distinct layers. The X-ray detector collects the transmitted X-rays, which are reconstructed into a series of thin, high-resolution slices, usually about 1 mm thick. These slices can be viewed on specialized workstations or imaging software, allowing radiologists to scroll through the images and gain a clearer view of the breast structures. This detailed layer-by-layer imaging reduces the impact of overlapping tissue, making it easier to identify abnormalities and improve diagnostic accuracy.

4.5.1.2 Angular Range and Resolution

- **Narrow Angular Range (15°):** Requires fewer projections but results in less distinct separation of breast planes, potentially causing more overlap in the images.
- **Wide Angular Range (60°):** Requires more projections, providing better vertical (z-axis) resolution and improved detection of closely spaced structures.

One concern with DBT is the increased radiation dose compared to traditional 2D mammography. To mitigate this, synthetic mammography (SM) has been developed, which reconstructs 2D images from the DBT dataset, potentially replacing the need for FFDM. This reduces overall acquisition time and radiation exposure while maintaining cancer detection rates and positive predictive values. However, SM may result in reduced conspicuity of microcalcifications compared to FFDM and can introduce various imaging artifacts, such as metallic artifacts, bright-band artifacts, blurring of the axilla, and truncation artifacts [71] (Fig. 4.9).

4.5.1.3 Integration into Clinical Practice

DBT is used in both screening and diagnostic settings. In screening, DBT can reduce recall rates by providing clearer images, thus better distinguishing between benign and suspicious findings. In diagnostic contexts, it aids in further evaluating and characterizing lesions detected during screening or clinical examinations. Despite challenges like increased radiation dose and potential artifacts, DBT represents a significant advancement in breast imaging, offering a promising balance between diagnostic accuracy and patient safety.

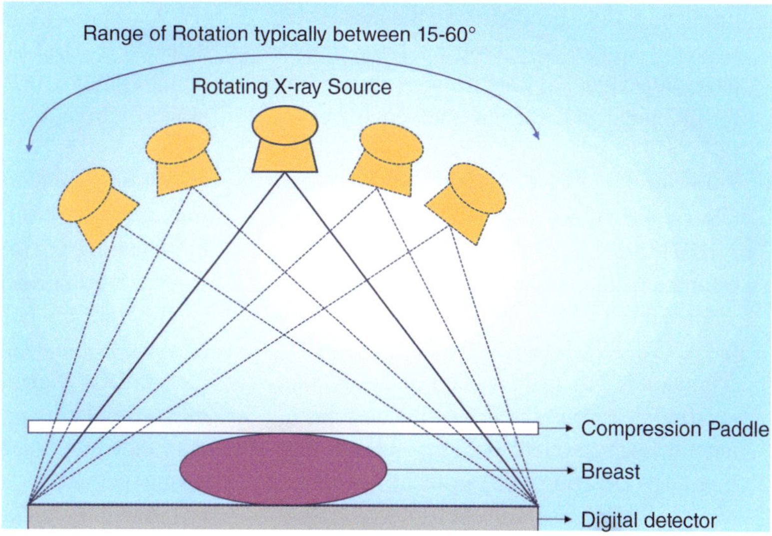

Fig. 4.9 Image sampling in digital breast tomosynthesis

4.5.2 Advantages of DBT

1. **Improved Cancer Detection Rate (CDR)**

   DBT has been shown to significantly enhance the CDR when used alongside 2D mammography. For instance, the Oslo Tomosynthesis Screening Trial (OTST) reported an increase in CDR from 6.1 to 8.0 [67], and the STORM trial showed an increase from 5.3 to 8.1 [72]. Another observational study by Friedewald et al. found a 27% increase in CDR, especially in dense breasts, by improving lesion conspicuity [73]. This improvement is particularly notable in detecting invasive cancers with relatively good prognosis, such as tubular, papillary, and mucinous subtypes.

2. **Reduction in Recall Rates (RR)**

   DBT has been associated with a reduction in RR for further evaluation, as it offers better mass characterization. This decrease in RR can reduce the need for additional imaging tests, such as ultrasound (USG) or MRI, thereby reducing patient anxiety and healthcare costs. Studies have reported up to a 15–30% relative reduction in recall rates, along with an increase in the positive predictive value (PPV) of recalls by approximately 15–20% [74].

3. **Decreased Need for Supplemental Views**

   The 3D nature of DBT allows for better visualization of breast structures, often eliminating the need for supplemental views like spot compressions and tangential views. Philpotts et al. concluded that incorporating tomosynthesis led to fewer images per diagnostic case, which in turn resulted in a quicker diagnostic workup for patients and improved patient throughput and resource utilization [75].

4. **Enhanced Lesion Localization and Depth Determination**

   DBT is particularly useful for localizing lesions that are visible in only one view. The ability to scroll through contiguous sections helps in determining the exact location and depth of a lesion, aiding in targeted ultrasound and guided biopsy. It also helps avoid unnecessary workup for skin-localized lesions by accurately identifying their location within the breast tissue [76].

5. **Better Evaluation of Architectural Distortion and Asymmetries**

   DBT can better reveal architectural distortions, often a sign of malignancy, which are sometimes missed in 2D mammography. This "decamouflaging" effect enhances the visibility of these distortions and asymmetries, improving the specificity of diagnoses and reducing unnecessary biopsies [70]. Studies have shown that DBT has a higher probability-for-malignancy detection rate compared to FFDM [77].

6. **Superior Mass Detection and Characterization**

   DBT has been found more accurate size estimation than FFDM and in some studies comparable to MRI for certain mass assessments [78, 79]. It provides better margin discrimination due to thin slice reconstruction, making it easier to discern suspicious characteristics such as spiculations and microlobulation [70]. DBT also aids in identifying areas of fat within masses, such as fat necrosis, lipomas, and hamartomas, although these findings alone do not rule out malignancy [70].

4.5.3 Limitations and Disadvantages of Digital Breast Tomosynthesis (DBT)

1. **Radiation Dose**

   The mean glandular dose (MGD) in DBT is generally higher compared to full-field digital mammography (FFDM) [80]. The addition of two tomosynthesis views to a standard 2D mammogram approximately doubles the total radiation dose compared with FFDM alone, although it remains below the 3 mGy/view limit set by the Mammography Quality Standards Act (MQSA)/FDA. While synthesized mammograms can reduce this dose by approximately 40–45%, concerns about radiation exposure persist, particularly in patients with dense breast tissue [81]. Additionally, the use of antiscatter grids and post-processing scatter-reduction software helps maintain image quality, which can complicate the imaging process [82].

2. **Detection of Complex Sclerosing Lesions**

   DBT increases the detection of both benign and malignant complex sclerosing lesions, often unmasking pathology not seen on FFDM. However, the positive predictive value (PPV) of biopsies for architectural distortions detected by DBT is lower (10–15%, in a particular study 10.2%) compared to FFDM alone (around 40%, in a particular study 43.4%) [70]. Despite this, persisting distortions without a history of surgery or trauma should still be sampled due to their high malignancy risk [83].

3. **Artifacts from Surgical Staples**

   High-density objects such as surgical clips or markers can create blurring and ripple artifacts in DBT images. These artifacts make the margins of clips appear ill-defined and thicker than they are, potentially obscuring or mimicking pathology. This issue arises from a phenomenon similar to volume averaging in CT imaging, especially when the number of acquired projections is lower relative to the number of reconstructed slices [84].

4. **Limitations in Detecting Calcifications**

   DBT alone is not as reliable for detecting or characterizing microcalcifications. Individual DBT sections may only show a limited number of calcifications, making it less effective than FFDM with spot magnification views for detailed assessment. Consequently, FFDM (particularly magnification views) remains the preferred method for evaluating calcifications [85, 86].

5. **Storage and Data Management**

   DBT generates significantly larger files than 2D FFDM, with sizes ranging from 200 to 450 MB compared to 8 to 24 MB for FFDM. The increased data size poses challenges for storage and requires more advanced workstations with rapid scrolling and cine capabilities, adding to costs and logistical considerations for healthcare facilities [87].

6. **Increased Reading Time**

   The necessity for radiologists to interpret a separate set of DBT data can significantly increase the reading time for each study. This additional time requirement may impact productivity, particularly in large-scale screening programs, with studies reporting up to a 1.5–2 fold increase in interpretation time per case [40].

The American College of Radiology considers digital breast tomosynthesis (DBT) an appropriate modality for breast cancer screening for all women, with studies indicating cost benefits when added to screening programs. In countries, where formal screening programs are lacking and healthcare resources are unevenly distributed, DBT could be particularly beneficial given the high incidence of breast cancer in premenopausal women with dense breasts. While ultrasonography serves as a useful adjunct in dense breast imaging, the limited availability of trained radiologists poses a challenge. DBT could be selectively used, potentially guided remotely by radiologists, to enhance screening effectiveness.

4.6 Quality Control in Mammography

4.6.1 History of QC in Mammography

As mammography became more widely adopted in the latter part of the twentieth century, concerns grew over the variability in the quality of mammograms. These concerns included inconsistencies in technical image quality, radiation dose, and interpretation accuracy. In 1985, the U.S. Food and Drug Administration (FDA) conducted the Nationwide Evaluation of X-ray Trends (NEXT) survey, revealing more than one-third (36%) of mammograms were of unacceptable quality [88]. This finding underscored the need for improved standards and oversight in breast imaging practice.

To address these issues, the American College of Radiology (ACR) launched a voluntary mammography accreditation program in 1987. This program aimed to standardize quality and safety in mammography. Despite its voluntary nature, the program's initial results were concerning, with 30% of applicants failing their first accreditation attempt [18]. In response, Dr. Gerald Dodd and a committee of experts developed a practical, step-by-step manual for mammography quality control under the ACR's auspices, culminating in the publication of the first ACR Mammography Quality Control Manual in 1990 [89]. This manual provided essential guidelines for radiologic technologists, medical physicists, and radiologists.

Recognizing the need for mandatory regulations, the U.S. Congress passed the Mammography Quality Standards Act (MQSA) in 1992 as amended in 1998 and 2004 [90]. The MQSA established comprehensive guidelines for mammography facilities, including requirements for equipment performance, radiation dose limitations, personnel qualifications, and standardized reporting. It mandated that all mammography facilities in the USA be accredited by an approved accreditation body and undergo annual inspections. In its first year, the MQSA revealed that 26% of facilities had significant violations [18]. However, the act has been highly effective in improving standards; today, fewer than 1% of facilities have level 1 violations, the most serious category [18]. Furthermore, image quality scores have improved, and radiation doses have decreased significantly.

In 1992 and 1994, the ACR published updated editions of the Mammography Quality Control Manual, incorporating new guidelines such as the Positioning and Compression Guide. These manuals were pivotal in setting the standards for mammography practices in the USA. The ACR's manual was referenced in the FDA's Interim Rules for Mammography Facilities and later aligned with the MQSA Final Rules in the 1999 edition, which included additional sections such as "Clinical Image Quality" [89] (Table 4.2).

Similar quality monitoring programs have been established worldwide. Australia implemented the BreastScreen Australia National Accreditation Standards in 2015, while Europe has been guided by the European Guidelines for Quality Assurance in Breast Cancer Screening and Diagnosis, now in its fourth edition. These guidelines have been instrumental in ensuring high-quality breast cancer screening services.

The advent of digital mammography and digital breast tomosynthesis has brought further advancements and challenges in quality maintenance. The Digital Mammographic Imaging Screening Trial demonstrated overall equivalence

Table 4.2 Key historical milestones and reports in mammography quality assessment

Timeline	Key activities and findings
1974	*Initial Survey*: Bicehouse HJ conducted a survey on mammographic exposure levels and techniques in Eastern Pennsylvania.
1976	*Nationwide Report*: Butler PF and Jensen JE reported on nationwide trends in breast exposure and mammographic quality assurance programs.
1980	*Internal Report*: The Bureau of Radiological Health provided a report on nationwide trends in breast exposure.
1985, 1988, 1992	*National Surveys*: Conway BJ and colleagues conducted national surveys of mammographic facilities, published in Radiology (1994) [91].
1987	*ACR Quality Control Initiative*: Dr. Gerald Dodd and a committee of experts initiated the creation of a manual for mammography quality control under the auspices of the ACR [18].
1990	*ACR Mammography Quality Control Manual*: The first edition of the ACR manual was published, providing guidelines for technologists, physicists, and radiologists, funded by the ACR and American Cancer Society.
1992	*Second Edition of ACR Manual:* The ACR released an updated version of the manual, including the Positioning and Compression Guide.
1992	*Mammography Quality Standards Act (MQSA):* Legislation enacted to standardize mammography practices in the U.S., mandating quality control measures aligned with the ACR manual.
1994	*Third Edition of ACR Manual*: Further updates were made, enhancing the guidance for quality control tests and incorporating more stringent criteria.
1995 to Present	*MQSA Implementation*: Ongoing inspections and regulations under MQSA, including radiation dose measurements and quality control standards.
1999	*Revised ACR Manual*: The manual was updated to align with MQSA Final Rules, including a new "Clinical Image Quality" section [89].
2016	*Digital Mammography QC Manual*: FDA approved the ACR's new Digital Mammography Quality Control Manual and Phantom for routine QC of digital mammography equipment.
2018	*Digital Breast Tomosynthesis QC Procedures*: The FDA approved QC procedures for digital breast tomosynthesis (DBT) in the updated Digital Mammography Quality Control Manual, integrating DBT with full-field digital mammography systems.

in accuracy between digital and film-screen mammography. Digital breast tomosynthesis, in particular, has shown promise in improving cancer detection rates with better specificity compared to digital mammography alone. These technological advancements have introduced new challenges, such as ensuring detector quality control, optimizing image display and printing, and managing data storage. In 2016, the FDA approved the ACR's new Digital Mammography Quality Control Manual and Phantom for routine QC of digital mammography equipment. By 2018, the FDA also approved QC procedures for digital breast tomosynthesis, allowing the updated manual to be used for both full-field digital mammography and DBT systems [92].

4.6.2 Quality Control Tests for Digital Mammography (2D and DBT)

Before a facility QC technologist may start using the procedures in the ACR Digital Mammography QC Manual for the first time on a unit, the medical physicist must first conduct an annual survey of the digital mammography unit and display devices using the manual and the ACR Digital Mammography Phantom. This is important to provide testing techniques and procedures for the QC technologist to use during routine QC. After this is done, the QC technologist may start performing routine QC using the ACR Digital Mammography QC Manual.

The tests designated for DBT must be conducted in addition to the applicable tests for the 2D full-field digital mammography system. Applicable 2D tests must be performed whether or not the system is used for 2D imaging since they test system components which may impact DBT performance. If the DBT system employs an "add-on" device, applicable 2D tests must be repeated with the "add-on" device in place.

4.6.3 Role of Professionals, Test Procedures, and Frequency

Quality Assurance (QA) and Quality Control (QC) ensures the safety, accuracy, and reliability of mammographic imaging. These processes are essential to comply with regulatory standards, such as the Mammography Quality Standards Act (MQSA) and country-specific codes to maintain high-quality diagnostic services.

4.6.3.1 Role of the Medical Physicist

The medical physicist plays an important role in the QA/QC process, particularly in the initial setup and ongoing maintenance of digital mammography systems. Before use of mammography unit and display devices, a set of tests are to be carried out as acceptance tests and established as base line. Thereafter an annual survey is required to be conducted to measure any deviations from the baseline reading. All the deviations are to be corrected before any clinical use of the equipment. The annual survey ensures that the equipment is functioning correctly.

The medical physicist's responsibilities include:

- **Acceptance test or Mammography Equipment Evaluation (MEE)**: Conducted before clinical use to ensure compliance with MQSA requirements.
- **Annual Quality Control Tests**: These include ACR DM Phantom Image Quality, DBT Resolution, Spatial Resolution, DBT Volume Coverage, and others. These tests ensure that the equipment continues to meet necessary standards.
- **Evaluation of Automatic Exposure Control System Performance**: This involves checking the system's ability to adjust radiation dose based on breast density.
- **Assessment of Average Glandular Dose**: Ensuring the radiation dose remains within safe limits.
- **Review of Technologist and Display Device QC Programs**: Annual evaluation to ensure compliance and effectiveness.

4.6.3.2 Role of the QC Technologist

The QC technologist is responsible for the day-to-day quality control of the mammography equipment. After the medical physicist's initial evaluation, the technologist performs routine QC tests as specified in the ACR Digital Mammography QC Manual. These tests are designed to identify any deviations from the established baseline performance and to ensure that the equipment operates within safe and optimal parameters.

The QC technologist's responsibilities include:

- **Weekly Tests**: ACR DM Phantom Image Quality and Computed Radiography Cassette Erasure.
- **Monthly Tests**: Compression Thickness Indicator, Visual Checklist, Acquisition Workstation Monitor QC, Radiologist Workstation Monitor QC, Film Printer QC, and Viewbox Cleanliness.
- **Semiannual Tests**: Compression Force.
- **Optional Tests**: Repeat Analysis, System QC for Radiologist, and Radiologist Image Quality Feedback.

4.6.3.3 Documentation and Compliance

Facilities must maintain records of all procedures, test results, and corrective actions. These records can be stored in hardcopy or electronic formats and must be readily available for review by MQSA inspectors and accreditation bodies. Documentation should include:

- **Assigned Responsibilities**: Clearly defined roles for all staff involved in QA/QC.
- **Procedures and Test Results**: Detailed records of all QA/QC activities, including tests performed and their outcomes.
- **Corrective Actions**: Documentation of any issues found during testing and the steps taken to resolve them.
- **Equipment Service and Maintenance**: Logs of routine and non-routine maintenance activities (Table 4.3).

Table 4.3 Quality control tests for digital mammography (2D and DBT)

Test	Frequency	Corrective action timeframe	Responsible person
Mammography Equipment Evaluation (MEE)	Before clinical use	Before clinical use	Medical Physicist
ACR DM Phantom Image Quality	Acceptance and then Annual	Before clinical use	Medical Physicist
DBT Z Resolution	Acceptance and then Annual	Within 30 days	Medical Physicist
Spatial Resolution	Acceptance and then Annual	Within 30 days	Medical Physicist
DBT Volume Coverage	Acceptance and then Annual	Before clinical use	Medical Physicist
Automatic Exposure Control System Performance	Acceptance and then Annual	Within 30 days	Medical Physicist
Average Glandular Dose	Acceptance and then Annual	Before clinical use	Medical Physicist
Unit Checklist	Acceptance and then Annual	Critical: before clinical use; less critical: within 30 days	Medical Physicist
Acquisition Workstation Monitor QC	Acceptance and then Annual	Within 30 days; before clinical use for severe defects	Medical Physicist
Radiologist Workstation Monitor QC	Acceptance and then Annual	Within 30 days; before clinical use for severe defects	Medical Physicist
Film Printer QC (if applicable)	Acceptance and then Annual	Before clinical use	Medical Physicist
Evaluation of Site's Technologist QC Program	Annual	Within 30 days	Medical Physicist
Evaluation of Display Device Technologist QC Program	Annual	Within 30 days	Medical Physicist
ACR DM Phantom Image Quality	Weekly	Before clinical use	QC Technologist
Computed Radiography Cassette Erasure (if applicable)	Weekly	Before clinical use	QC Technologist
Compression Thickness Indicator	Monthly	Within 30 days	QC Technologist
Visual Checklist	Monthly	Critical: before clinical use; less critical: within 30 days	QC Technologist
Acquisition Workstation Monitor QC	Monthly	Within 30 days; before clinical use for severe defects	QC Technologist
Radiologist Workstation Monitor QC	Monthly	Within 30 days; before clinical use for severe defects	QC Technologist
Film Printer QC (if applicable)	Monthly	Before clinical use	QC Technologist
Viewbox Cleanliness (if applicable)	Monthly	Before clinical use	QC Technologist

(continued)

Table 4.3 (continued)

Test	Frequency	Corrective action timeframe	Responsible person
Facility QC Review	Quarterly	Not applicable	QC Technologist
Compression Force	Semiannual	Before clinical use	QC Technologist
Manufacturer Calibrations (if applicable)	Manufacturer Recommendation	Before clinical use	QC Technologist
Optional—Repeat Analysis	As Needed	Within 30 days after analysis	QC Technologist
Optional—System QC for Radiologist	As Needed	Within 30 days; before clinical use for severe artifacts	QC Technologist
Optional—Radiologist Image Quality Feedback	As Needed	Not applicable	QC Technologist

This structured approach to QA/QC in mammography ensures that all aspects of imaging—from equipment functionality to image quality—are consistently monitored and maintained. This comprehensive framework not only meets regulatory requirements but also enhances the overall quality of patient care.

4.7 Quality Control Tests

A detailed explanation of each quality control test has been provided in the ACR QC Manual 2018 for mammography and it is an open source document available freely on internet at link https://www.acr.org/-/media/ACR/Files/Clinical-Resources/QC-Manuals/Mammo_QCManual.pdf. A brief outline is mentioned below:

4.7.1 Mammography Equipment Evaluation (MEE) and Annual Surveys

The MEE is performed before a mammography system is used clinically and during annual surveys to ensure the continued compliance of the equipment with safety and performance standards. Conducted by a qualified medical physicist, the MEE includes a thorough inspection of the system's hardware, software, and safety mechanisms. Key aspects of this evaluation include:

1. **System Motion and Stability**: The tube-image receptor assembly must be capable of being fixed in any operational position without unintended motion, even during power interruptions.
2. **Image Receptor Sizes and Magnification Capability**: The system must accommodate different receptor sizes, including the removal of grids for magnification procedures. It should also provide radiographic magnification capabilities, typically within a range of 1.4–2.0 times, necessary for detailed imaging during problem-solving procedures.
3. **Light Field and Illumination**: Any system with a light beam passing through the X-ray beam-limiting device must maintain an average illumination of not less than 160 lux at a distance of 100 cm or the maximum SID.
4. **Focal Spot and Target Selection**: The system must clearly indicate the selected focal spot and target material prior to exposure. In cases where these are determined by an algorithm based on the exposure, the system should display the selected settings after the exposure.
5. **Compression**: The evaluation ensures that the compression device operates effectively, providing power-driven compression and fine adjustments from both sides of the patient. The compression paddles must match the size of the image receptors and be flat and parallel, with specific allowances for slight deflections and patient comfort adjustments at the chest wall edge.

6. **Technique Factor Selection and Display**: The system should allow for manual selection of exposure parameters (kVp, mA, and time) and display the selected factors before exposure. In AEC mode, the system must display the actual kVp and mAs used.
7. **Safety Features**: Including the presence of special lights for film illumination, known as hot lights, and film masking devices to limit the illuminated area to the exposed portion of the film, facilitating accurate interpretation by radiologists.

The MEE utilizes the ACR Digital Mammography Phantom to simulate patient tissue, verifying the system's capability to reproduce small details and contrasts accurately. This comprehensive evaluation is crucial to minimize radiation exposure, ensure high diagnostic image quality, and confirm the system's readiness for clinical use. Any identified issues must be addressed before the system is approved for patient imaging, ensuring compliance with all relevant standards and maintaining patient safety and diagnostic efficacy.

4.7.2 ACR Digital Mammography Phantom Image Quality

The ACR DM Phantom Image Quality test uses a specialized phantom that mimics the properties of breast tissue, providing a standardized way to evaluate the system's imaging capabilities. During the test, images of the phantom are taken and analyzed for the visibility of critical features like fibers, specks, and masses. These features are representative of potential abnormalities that could appear in actual clinical images.

The evaluation process includes checking various image quality parameters such as contrast, resolution, and noise levels. By assessing these factors, the test ensures that the system can consistently produce high-quality images necessary for accurate diagnosis. The phantom used in the test represents a standard breast with 50% glandular and 50% adipose tissue, compressed to 4.2 cm, which helps in maintaining consistency across different equipment.

Each feature in the image, such as fibers, specks, and masses, is scored based on its visibility, with specific criteria for full or partial points. The number of visible features determines the system's performance, with a required minimum score to pass. If the system fails to meet the tolerance levels, it indicates that the image quality may not be sufficient for reliable diagnostics, and corrective actions must be taken to address the issues.

This test is conducted regularly, including during the initial Mammography Equipment Evaluation and annual surveys.

4.7.3 DBT Z Resolution

The DBT Z Resolution test assesses the ability of a digital breast tomosynthesis (DBT) system to resolve structures along the Z-axis, which refers to depth. This test ensures that the system can distinguish between closely spaced structures, improving the detection and characterization of lesions in the breast. The evaluation is performed using a phantom or test object with known dimensions, and the resulting images are analyzed to measure the system's Z-axis resolution.

The process involves acquiring a DBT image from the ACR Digital Mammography (DM) Phantom Image Quality test and using the image to evaluate the Z resolution. The test includes scrolling through the image slices to find the one where a specific speck group appears most in focus, measuring signal data across different slices, and calculating the full width at half maximum (FWHM) value, which represents the system's Z resolution. This value is typically measured in line pairs per millimeter (lp/mm), indicating the system's ability to separate structures at different depths.

For accurate assessment, the test requires determining the baseline FWHM from the initial measurement or the oldest annual survey if the MEE is unavailable. The results help ensure that any blurring in the Z-direction is not excessive, as excessive blurring can obscure details and reduce diagnostic accuracy. If the measured Z resolution does not meet the manufacturer's specifications or baseline values, adjustments or repairs are necessary to restore optimal performance.

This test is conducted annually, during the MEE of new units, and after relevant servicing to maintain the high-quality imaging standards required for effective breast cancer screening and diagnosis.

4.7.4 Spatial Resolution

The Spatial Resolution test evaluates a mammography system's ability to display fine details, essential for detecting small calcifications and subtle tissue changes. This test uses a resolution pattern or phantom to assess the system's capacity to distinguish closely spaced objects. It measures the highest number of line pairs per millimeter (lp/mm) that the system can resolve, reflecting the system's resolving power.

The test involves creating a test patient and turning off all image processing to acquire a "for processing" (raw) image. A compression paddle is installed, and the ACR Digital Mammography (DM) Phantom is placed on the breast support with the wax insert facing up and away from the chest-wall edge, rotated 180° from its normal orientation. A line pair pattern is then placed on the phantom at a 45° angle and lightly compressed to keep it secure during exposure.

The system makes one exposure using a manual technique close to the ACR DM Phantom technique. This process is repeated for any other clinically used targets, including the magnification stand and paddle in the system's most frequently used clinical magnification mode. The procedure is also repeated in the DBT imaging mode and, if applicable, in 2D mode with an add-on device for DBT.

At the acquisition station, each image is viewed using full resolution and the greatest zoom available. The highest frequency at which at least half the length of the lines can be continuously resolved is recorded, ensuring that the polarity of the lines does not reverse. If reversal occurs, the limiting resolution has been surpassed.

The expected standards for spatial resolution are a minimum of 4.0 lp/mm for 2D images, 6.0 lp/mm for 2D magnification mode images, and 2.0 lp/mm for DBT images. If the system does not meet these criteria, maintenance or calibration is required, with corrections needing to be completed within 30 days to maintain reliable diagnostic performance.

4.7.5 DBT Volume Coverage

The DBT Volume Coverage test ensures that the digital breast tomosynthesis (DBT) system adequately images the entire breast volume during a scan. The incomplete coverage can lead to missed lesions and incomplete diagnostic information. The procedure involves measuring the field of view provided by the DBT system to confirm that it encompasses the entire breast tissue area. This is verified using a known object or phantom, ensuring that all breast areas, including the edges, are visualized without gaps.

To conduct the test, an exam is initiated at the acquisition workstation, and a system for naming and identifying QC images is used to match the mammography unit to the printed image. The largest available image receptor size and corresponding paddle are used for acquiring the ACR DM Phantom image. The phantom is positioned on the breast support surface, with specific positioning criteria: the pink wax insert facing up and away from the chest-wall edge, the phantom centered left-to-right, and the edge of the phantom aligned with the chest wall edge of the digital image receptor.

Two 0.1-mm thick sheets of aluminum are placed on top of and below the DM phantom, and the paddle is manually compressed to 5 decanewtons or 12 pounds of compression force, ensuring consistent compression force for each test. An exposure is made in the DBT mode using a manual technique similar to the ACR DM Phantom DBT technique. The image set is then reviewed at the acquisition workstation, scrolling through the thinnest slices available to determine if both the top and bottom aluminum sheets are well-defined and in focus.

If the system fails the test, the positioning of the aluminum sheets is verified, and the test is repeated. Each aluminum sheet must be well-defined within one slice to confirm that the entire breast volume is being imaged. Any deficiencies must be corrected before the system can be used clinically, ensuring accurate diagnosis and effective patient management.

4.7.6 Automatic Exposure Control System Performance

The Automatic Exposure Control (AEC) System Performance test evaluates the AEC system's capability to maintain consistent image quality across varying breast thicknesses. The AEC system automatically adjusts exposure parameters to optimize image quality while minimizing radiation dose, ensuring images are neither overexposed nor underexposed. This test involves imaging phantoms of different thicknesses to assess the consistency of image quality and radiation dose.

To perform the test, a test patient is created on the acquisition workstation, and compression paddles along with tissue-equivalent attenuators (e.g., acrylic, BR-12, BR-50) are used. The attenuators, which vary in thickness (2, 4, 6, and 8 cm), are placed on the image receptor and positioned to cover the AEC area. The small size paddle is installed if available; otherwise, the large size paddle is used. The compression paddle is lowered to a specific thickness, and the AEC mode, density control, and other relevant settings are selected. An image is acquired using the AEC mode employed clinically, and the technique information (AEC Mode, Density Setting or Exposure Compensation, target, filter, kVp, mAs, and indicated average glandular dose) is recorded.

The process is repeated for each phantom thickness and in different imaging modes, including magnification and DBT modes. If an add-on device is used for DBT, the steps are repeated in 2D mode with the DBT fixture in place.

The system's performance is evaluated by calculating the signal-to-noise ratio (SNR) for each mode and attenuator. The SNR is calculated using the mean signal value and standard deviation of the background signal, taking into account any DC offset provided by the manufacturer. The results are compared against the SNR from the last MEE or the oldest annual survey if the MEE data is unavailable. The acceptable SNR variation is typically within ±15% of the last MEE's SNR.

If the AEC system's performance does not meet the established criteria, adjustments or corrective actions are required. The facility must contact an authorized service representative to address any issues, and corrective actions must be documented. Failures must be corrected within 30 days, and for MEEs, the corrections must be made before clinical use. This ensures the system's reliability and safety, providing consistent and optimal image quality for all patients.

4.7.7 Average Glandular Dose

The Average Glandular Dose (AGD) test measures the radiation dose absorbed by the glandular tissue in the breast during mammography. This test helps minimize radiation exposure while ensuring adequate image quality for accurate diagnosis. AGD is calculated based on the exposure parameters, breast thickness, and tissue composition, often using a standard breast phantom representing a 4.2 cm thick compressed breast composed of 50% glandular and 50% adipose tissue.

To conduct the test, a dosimeter is positioned at a height of 4.2 cm above the breast support, just under the compression paddle, and centered approximately 4 cm from the chest wall edge of the image receptor. The setup aims to simulate the typical clinical conditions for a standard breast. The X-ray system settings, such as target material, filtration, and kVp, are adjusted according to the ACR Digital Mammography (DM) Phantom Image Quality test technique. A manual exposure is then made, and the exposure value is recorded. This process is repeated multiple times to ensure consistency.

The AGD is computed using the entrance exposure (K) and a series of correction factors (g, c, and s) that account for breast composition and X-ray spectra differences. The AGD should not exceed 3.0 mGy per view for a standard breast. If the calculated AGD is above this threshold, immediate corrective actions are required to reduce the dose. Furthermore, if the mammography unit provides an indicated AGD, it must be within ±25% of the calculated value.

The results from this test help verify that the mammography system operates within safe dose limits, thereby protecting patients from unnecessary radiation exposure. If any discrepancies or excessive doses are detected, the issues must be resolved before the equipment is used clinically. This test is performed as part of the MEE for new units, annually, and after relevant service, ensuring consistent and safe operation of the system.

4.7.7.1 Collimation Assessment

Collimation Assessment ensures that the X-ray field is correctly aligned with the imaging detector, which is important for minimizing patient radiation exposure and enhancing image quality by reducing scattered radiation. This test involves verifying that the X-ray field matches the size and position of the imaging detector, ensuring that the entire area of interest is covered while avoiding unnecessary exposure outside this area. Proper alignment is required, with allowable misalignment typically within 2% of the source-to-image distance (SID). Discrepancies in collimation can result in incomplete imaging or unnecessary radiation exposure, necessitating corrections to maintain optimal imaging and patient safety.

The assessment procedure includes several steps. First, a test object or phantom is used to set up the equipment. The compression paddle is removed, and the largest field of view (FOV) is selected. For digital breast tomosynthesis (DBT) systems, the test is performed in 2D mode. The collimation test tool, or a combination of radiopaque objects like coins, is placed on the breast support and aligned with the X-ray field's edges. The paddle is then replaced and positioned 4–6 cm from the breast support, followed by making an exposure. This process is repeated for different anode tracks and field sizes as needed.

Evaluation involves measuring the distance between the light field and the radiation field and checking the alignment of the collimator with the image receptor's edges. Discrepancies should be corrected to ensure the radiation field does not exceed the edges of the light field by more than 2% of the SID. Additionally, the chest-wall edge of the compression paddle should align closely with the chest-wall edge of the image receptor, not extending beyond by more than 1% of the SID. If significant misalignment is found, a qualified service engineer should be contacted to address the issue promptly. Failures must be corrected within 30 days, and for MEEs, corrections should be made before clinical use.

4.7.7.2 Evaluation of Site's Technologist QC Program

The Evaluation of Site's Technologist QC Program reviews the effectiveness and compliance of the facility's quality control program as implemented by technologists. This evaluation ensures that technologists adhere to QC protocols, maintaining consistent image quality and patient safety. Conducted by a medical physicist, the review assesses the frequency, accuracy, and documentation of the QC tests performed by technologists. Compliance with the ACR QC Manual and MQSA standards is verified, ensuring all necessary tests are regularly conducted and issues are promptly addressed. Proper documentation of test results and corrective actions is vital for maintaining accreditation and providing high-quality care. The evaluation ensures the facility meets all required standards and corrects any deficiencies to maintain compliance and quality.

4.7.8 Unit Checklist

The Unit Checklist ensures that all locks, detents, angulation indicators, and mechanical support devices for the X-ray tube and breast support assembly are functioning correctly. This checklist is part of the mammography equipment evaluation (MEE) for new units, conducted annually, and after relevant service. The critical aspects include verifying the mechanical stability of the unit, ensuring smooth movement of all parts, checking the proper functioning of locks and detents, and confirming that the detector or image receptor holder assembly is free from wobble or vibration during normal operation. It also involves checking the security and orientation of cassette-based systems, the integrity of compression paddles, and ensuring that there are no sharp edges or other hazards, including electrical risks.

Furthermore, the checklist requires verification of the cleanliness of the mammography area, the adequacy of radiation shielding for the operator, the proper functioning of indicators, the operation of automatic decompression systems (if available), and the manual release of compression in case of power failure. The audible exposure indicator's volume level and the movement range of the DBT assembly are also checked. Additionally, current and accurate technique charts should be posted, and any unit-specific checks should be included as necessary.

Critical items identified as hazardous, inoperative, or malfunctioning must be repaired or replaced by appropriate service personnel before clinical use. Less critical issues must be addressed within 30 days or, for MEEs, before clinical use.

4.7.9 Acquisition Workstation Monitor QC

The Acquisition Workstation Monitor QC involves checking the monitor used for acquiring and processing mammographic images. This test ensures the monitor displays images with correct brightness, contrast, and resolution. Accurate monitor performance is critical, as discrepancies can lead to misinterpretation of images and missed diagnoses. Typically performed monthly by the QC technologist, the test uses a test pattern to assess grayscale display, geometric distortion, and luminance uniformity. Tolerance levels are specified for various parameters, with any deviations requiring calibration or replacement of the monitor to maintain image quality.

4.7.10 Radiologist Workstation Monitor QC

Radiologist Workstation Monitor QC is similar to the Acquisition Workstation Monitor QC but focuses on monitors used by radiologists for diagnostic interpretation. Given the critical role these monitors play in patient diagnosis, this test ensures display quality meets high standards required for clinical decision-making. The test includes evaluating grayscale accuracy, luminance response, and uniformity. It aims to ensure subtle details essential for diagnosing breast cancer are visible without distortion. The test is conducted monthly, with any issues requiring immediate attention to maintain diagnostic accuracy.

4.7.11 Film Printer QC (If Applicable)

Film Printer QC is conducted to ensure film prints accurately reflect the quality and details of the original digital data. This is important in facilities where film is still used for image storage or review. The QC technologist checks the printer for correct film density, contrast, and resolution. The process involves printing a test image and comparing it to the original digital file to ensure fidelity. This test is typically performed monthly, and any deviations from quality standards require corrective actions to maintain consistency in image quality.

4.7.12 Evaluation of Display Device Technologist QC Program

The Evaluation of Display Device Technologist QC Program assesses the QC procedures for all display devices used in the facility, including those by technologists and radiologists. This evaluation ensures display devices meet necessary standards for image quality, critical for accurate diagnosis and patient care. Conducted annually by a medical physicist, the evaluation includes reviewing QC tests for luminance, resolution, and geometric accuracy. This ensures all display devices function optimally, with any deviations corrected promptly to maintain diagnostic precision.

4.7.13 Computed Radiography Cassette Erasure (If Applicable)

Computed Radiography Cassette Erasure QC is crucial for facilities using computed radiography systems. The test ensures imaging plates are properly erased between exposures, preventing ghost images from previous scans. The process involves exposing the cassette to a test pattern, erasing it, and reading the plate again to ensure no residual image is present. This test, typically performed weekly, requires corrective actions if any residual images are detected. Proper erasure maintains image quality and patient safety.

4.7.14 Compression Thickness Indicator

The Compression Thickness Indicator test ensures the compression paddle accurately reflects the actual thickness of the compressed breast. Accurate measurements are crucial for optimizing image quality and ensuring consistent radiation doses. The test uses a known thickness gauge or object to check the paddle's measurement accuracy. The QC technologist compares the indicated thickness with the actual thickness, with discrepancies required to be within a specified tolerance, typically ±5 mm. This test, conducted monthly, ensures any inaccuracies are immediately corrected for diagnostic accuracy and patient comfort.

4.7.15 Visual Checklist

The Visual Checklist is a routine inspection of the mammography room and equipment for cleanliness, proper function, and safety. The QC technologist checks the condition of the compression paddles, the cleanliness of the X-ray tube housing, and the overall condition of the imaging area. The checklist also includes verifying the presence and condition of safety equipment, such as protective lead aprons. This inspection helps identify and rectify issues that could affect image quality or patient safety. Critical items must be addressed before clinical use, while less critical items should be resolved within 30 days.

4.7.16 Viewbox Cleanliness (If Applicable)

The Viewbox Cleanliness test is necessary for facilities using film for reviewing mammographic images. This test ensures lightboxes used to display films are clean and provide uniform illumination. Dust or smudges on the viewbox can obscure details in mammographic images, potentially leading to missed diagnoses. The QC technologist checks the viewbox for cleanliness and ensures all bulbs are functioning correctly. This test, typically performed monthly, requires resolution of issues before clinical interpretation.

4.7.17 Facility QC Review

The Facility QC Review is a comprehensive assessment of the entire mammography quality control program at the facility. This review includes evaluating all QC tests, documentation, and compliance with ACR and MQSA standards. Typically conducted quarterly by a medical physicist, the review ensures the facility adheres to all necessary protocols and procedures. It also includes assessing record-keeping practices, ensuring all QC tests and corrective actions are documented properly. This review is essential for maintaining accreditation and ensuring high-quality patient care.

4.7.18 Compression Force

The Compression Force test measures the force applied by the mammography machine's compression paddle during imaging. Proper compression is crucial for achieving optimal image quality and minimizing radiation dose. The test uses a calibrated force gauge to measure the maximum force applied by the paddle. The force must be within a specified range, typically between 11 and 20 decanewtons (daN), ensuring sufficient compression without causing patient discomfort. This test is performed semiannually, with deviations from the acceptable range requiring correction to ensure patient safety and diagnostic accuracy.

4.7.19 Manufacturer Calibrations (If Applicable)

Manufacturer Calibrations involve periodic checks and adjustments recommended by the equipment manufacturer. These calibrations ensure the mammography system operates according to the manufacturer's specifications, maintaining optimal performance. The process may include recalibration of the X-ray generator, adjustment of image processing algorithms, and verification of system settings. The frequency and scope of these calibrations depend on the manufacturer's guidelines. Proper calibration is essential for maintaining image quality, ensuring accurate radiation dose delivery, and complying with regulatory requirements. Any identified issues must be promptly addressed.

4.7.20 Repeat Analysis (Optional)

The Repeat Analysis test is an optional quality control measure that involves analyzing the frequency and causes of repeated mammographic images. This analysis helps identify patterns or issues contributing to image repeats, such as equipment malfunctions, technologist errors, or patient movement. The goal is to minimize repeat exposures, reducing radiation dose to patients and improving workflow efficiency. Conducted as needed by the QC technologist or medical physicist, the analysis typically reviews a sample of cases over a specific period. Corrective actions may include additional technologist training, equipment adjustments, or protocol modifications.

4.7.21 System QC for Radiologist (Optional)

The System QC for Radiologist test is another optional measure, focusing on the quality control of systems used specifically by radiologists for image interpretation. This test ensures all components of the radiologist's workstation, including monitors and image processing software, function correctly and provide optimal image quality. Conducted as needed by the QC technologist or medical physicist, the evaluation checks for issues such as monitor calibration, software updates, and system integration. Proper system QC is crucial for accurate and efficient image interpretation.

4.7.22 Radiologist Image Quality Feedback (Optional)

The Radiologist Image Quality Feedback process is optional and involves gathering feedback from radiologists regarding the quality of mammographic images. This feedback helps identify issues with image quality not apparent through routine QC tests. Radiologists can provide insights into issues such as image sharpness, contrast, and artifacts, affecting their diagnostic ability. Feedback is typically collected periodically and reviewed by the QC technologist and medical physicist. The information gathered can lead to adjustments in imaging protocols, equipment settings, or technologist training to improve image quality.

Exercise

Multiple Choice Questions (MCQs)

1. What percentage of all cancer cases in females does breast cancer represent?
   A. 10%
   B. 25%
   C. 50%
   D. 75%

2. By how much is the number of newly diagnosed breast cancer cases expected to increase by 2040?
   A. 10%
   B. 25%
   C. 40%
   D. 50%
3. What is the primary use of mammography?
   A. Treatment of breast cancer
   B. Screening and diagnostic purposes
   C. Prevention of breast cancer
   D. None of the above
4. What was the significant contribution of Robert Egan to the field of mammography?
   A. Development of the first dedicated mammography unit
   B. Introduction of the wire localization technique
   C. Refinement of mammographic techniques for better imaging contrast
   D. First clinical use of Contrast-Enhanced Mammography (CEM)
5. What is Digital Breast Tomosynthesis (DBT) primarily used for?
   A. Creating 3D images of the breast
   B. Reducing radiation dose during imaging
   C. Screening for cardiovascular diseases
   D. Treating breast cancer
6. Which of the following advancements in mammography helps in distinguishing malignant from benign lesions?
   A. Traditional mammography
   B. Radiomics
   C. Full-field digital mammography (FFDM)
   D. Contrast-Enhanced Mammography (CEM)
7. What was the historical significance of Albert Salomon's work in 1913?
   A. Introduced Digital Breast Tomosynthesis
   B. Conducted the first use of radiography in breast imaging
   C. Developed the first dedicated mammography unit
   D. Created the "senographe" mammography machine
8. What structure is responsible for milk production in the breast?
   A. Ducts
   B. Lobes
   C. Lobules
   D. Areola
9. What does the mammary gland predominantly consist of in females compared to males?
   A. Adipose tissue
   B. Fat
   C. Muscle
   D. Fibroglandular tissue
10. What does the appearance of fibroglandular tissue on a mammogram indicate?
    A. Dark areas due to low density
    B. White areas due to high density
    C. Dark edges of the skin
    D. Absence of lymph nodes
11. What is the primary purpose of using rotating anode X-ray tubes in mammography?
    A. To increase patient comfort
    B. To enhance heat dissipation and allow higher tube currents
    C. To provide a constant potential waveform
    D. To reduce radiation exposure to healthcare personnel
12. Which material is commonly used for the anode in mammography units to produce K characteristic X-rays in the optimal energy range?
    A. Tungsten
    B. Rhodium
    C. Molybdenum
    D. Aluminum
13. What effect is leveraged in mammography to optimize image quality by compensating for variations in breast thickness?
    A. Inverse square law
    B. Anode heel effect
    C. Photoelectric effect
    D. Bremsstrahlung

14. What is the typical kilovoltage range used in mammography to achieve adequate tissue contrast?
    A. 10–20 kVp
    B. 25–50 kVp
    C. 50–100 kVp
    D. 100–150 kVp
15. Which type of mammography detector is associated with a wider dynamic range and the ability to adjust image contrast and brightness?
    A. Screen-film
    B. Digital
    C. Intensifying screen cassette
    D. Phosphor plate
16. What is the primary function of filters in mammography equipment?
    A. To enhance image contrast and reduce noise
    B. To increase radiation dose to the patient
    C. To provide a barrier against mechanical damage
    D. To absorb high-energy photons
17. Which component in a mammography unit helps in reducing geometric and motion unsharpness?
    A. Anode
    B. Cathode
    C. Compression device
    D. X-ray generator
18. What minimum radiation output rate is required by MQSA regulations for mammography units at 28 kVp in the standard Mo/Mo target-filter mode?
    A. 500 mR/s
    B. 600 mR/s
    C. 800 mR/s
    D. 1000 mR/s
19. What is the primary advantage of Digital Breast Tomosynthesis (DBT) over traditional 2D mammography?
    A. Lower radiation dose
    B. Enhanced visualization of overlapping tissue
    C. Shorter examination time
    D. Elimination of the need for compression
20. Which of the following trials reported a significant increase in cancer detection rates with DBT?
    A. STORM trial
    B. Oslo Tomosynthesis Screening Trial
    C. Malmö Breast Tomosynthesis Screening Trial
    D. All of the above
21. What is a concern associated with DBT in comparison to 2D mammography?
    A. Reduced sensitivity
    B. Increased radiation dose
    C. Limited usefulness in dense breasts
    D. Lack of availability
22. Which of the following is a limitation of DBT in detecting breast abnormalities?
    A. Difficulty in detecting calcifications
    B. Poor image resolution
    C. High rate of false positives for masses
    D. Inability to detect complex sclerosing lesions
23. What is the purpose of synthetic mammography (SM) in DBT?
    A. To increase the radiation dose
    B. To replace the need for full-field digital mammography
    C. To provide better visualization of microcalcifications
    D. To eliminate the need for radiologists
24. What percentage of mammograms were deemed unacceptable in the 1985 NEXT survey?
    A. 10%
    B. 25%
    C. 36%
    D. 50%
25. When did the U.S. Congress pass the Mammography Quality Standards Act (MQSA)?
    A. 1985
    B. 1990
    C. 1992
    D. 1999

26. Which professional is responsible for conducting the Mammography Equipment Evaluation (MEE)?
    A. Radiologist
    B. Medical physicist
    C. QC technologist
    D. Radiologic technologist
27. Which test ensures that a digital breast tomosynthesis (DBT) system adequately images the entire breast volume during a scan?
    A. Spatial Resolution
    B. DBT Volume Coverage
    C. ACR DM Phantom Image Quality
    D. Average Glandular Dose
28. How often is the ACR DM Phantom Image Quality test performed by the QC technologist?
    A. Monthly
    B. Semiannually
    C. Weekly
    D. Annually
29. What is the maximum allowable average glandular dose (AGD) per view for a standard breast in mammography?
    A. 1.0 mGy
    B. 2.0 mGy
    C. 3.0 mGy
    D. 4.0 mGy
30. Which country implemented the BreastScreen Australia National Accreditation Standards in 2015?
    A. United States
    B. United Kingdom
    C. Canada
    D. Australia

Short Questions

1. Explain the significance of early detection in breast cancer and the role of mammography in achieving it.
2. Describe the role of radiomics in breast cancer detection and diagnosis.
3. What are the benefits of Digital Breast Tomosynthesis (DBT) over traditional mammography?
4. Explain the role of Cooper's ligaments in the breast anatomy.
5. What is the purpose of the cathode's dual-focus design in mammography X-ray tubes?
6. How do rhodium anodes differ from molybdenum anodes in terms of X-ray production?
7. Explain the role of Automatic Exposure Control (AEC) in mammography.
8. Describe the image acquisition process in Digital Breast Tomosynthesis.
9. What are some of the benefits of using DBT in breast cancer screening?
10. Describe the role of the medical physicist in the QA/QC process for mammography.
11. What was the primary aim of the American College of Radiology's (ACR) voluntary mammography accreditation program launched in 1987?
12. Explain the importance of the Average Glandular Dose (AGD) test in mammography.

Long Questions

1. Discuss the historical evolution of mammography from its inception to modern-day practices, highlighting key milestones and technological advancements.
2. Explain the integration of artificial intelligence (AI) and radiomics in modern mammography and their impact on diagnostic accuracy and patient care.
3. Describe the components and functions of a mammography unit, highlighting the significance of each component in ensuring optimal image quality and patient safety.
4. Discuss the differences between screen-film mammography (SFM) and full-field digital mammography (FFDM), including their respective advantages and disadvantages
5. Discuss the limitations and disadvantages of Digital Breast Tomosynthesis (DBT) and how they impact its clinical use. Include considerations of radiation dose, detection capabilities, artifacts, and practical challenges.

6. Discuss the evolution and impact of quality control regulations in mammography, from the ACR's voluntary accreditation program to the implementation of the MQSA.
7. Outline the key quality control tests for digital mammography (2D and DBT), including their purposes, frequency, and responsible personnel.

Answers to MCQs

1. B. 25%
2. C. 40%
3. B. Screening and diagnostic purposes
4. C. Refinement of mammographic techniques for better imaging contrast
5. A. Creating 3D images of the breast
6. D. Contrast-Enhanced Mammography (CEM)
7. B. Conducted the first use of radiography in breast imaging
8. C. Lobules
9. D. Fibroglandular tissue
10. B. White areas due to high density
11. B. To enhance heat dissipation and allow higher tube currents
12. C. Molybdenum
13. B. Anode heel effect
14. B. 25–50 kVp
15. B. Digital
16. A. To enhance image contrast and reduce noise
17. C. Compression device
18. C. 800 mR/s
19. B. Enhanced visualization of overlapping tissue
20. D. All of the above
21. B. Increased radiation dose
22. A. Difficulty in detecting calcifications
23. B. To replace the need for full-field digital mammography
24. C. 36%
25. C. 1992
26. B. Medical physicist
27. B. DBT Volume Coverage
28. C. Weekly
29. C. 3.0 mGy
30. D. Australia

References

1. Sung H, et al. Global cancer statistics 2020: GLOBOCAN estimates of incidence and mortality worldwide for 36 cancers in 185 countries. CA Cancer J Clin. 2021;71(3):209–49. https://doi.org/10.3322/caac.21660.
2. Heer E, Harper A, Escandor N, Sung H, McCormack V, Fidler-Benaoudia MM. Global burden and trends in premenopausal and postmenopausal breast cancer: a population-based study. Lancet Glob Health. 2020;8(8):e1027–37. https://doi.org/10.1016/S2214-109X(20)30215-1.
3. Anderson BO, et al. The Global Breast Cancer Initiative: a strategic collaboration to strengthen health care for non-communicable diseases. Lancet Oncol. 2021;22(5):578–81. https://doi.org/10.1016/S1470-2045(21)00071-1.
4. Arnold M, et al. Current and future burden of breast cancer: global statistics for 2020 and 2040. Breast. 2022;66:15–23. https://doi.org/10.1016/j.breast.2022.08.010.
5. D'Orsi CJ, Sickles EA, Mendelson EB, Morris EA. ACR BI-RADS atlas: breast imaging re-porting and data system. American College of Radiology, 2013.
6. Ohuchi N, et al. Sensitivity and specificity of mammography and adjunctive ultrasonography to screen for breast cancer in the Japan Strategic Anti-cancer Randomized Trial (J-START): a randomised controlled trial. Lancet. 2016;387(10016):341–8. https://doi.org/10.1016/S0140-6736(15)00774-6.
7. Zeeshan M, Salam B, Khalid QSB, Alam S, Sayani R. Diagnostic accuracy of digital mammography in the detection of breast cancer. Cureus. 2018; https://doi.org/10.7759/cureus.2448.
8. https://www.cancer.gov/types/breast/hp/breast-screening-pdq, Breast Cancer Screening (PDQ®)–Health Professional Version.
9. Nishikawa RM. Current status and future directions of computer-aided diagnosis in mammography. Comput Med Imaging Graph. 2007;31(4–5):224–35. https://doi.org/10.1016/j.compmedimag.2007.02.009.
10. Pisano ED, et al. Diagnostic accuracy of digital versus film mammography: exploratory analysis of selected population subgroups in DMIST. Radiology. 2008;246(2):376–83. https://doi.org/10.1148/radiol.2461070200.
11. Fitzjohn J, Zhou C, Chase JG. Critical assessment of mammography accuracy. IFAC-PapersOnLine. 2023;56(2):5620–5. https://doi.org/10.1016/j.ifacol.2023.10.472.
12. Practice bulletin number 179: breast cancer risk assessment and screening in average-risk women. Obstet Gynecol. 2017;130(1):e1–e16. https://doi.org/10.1097/AOG.0000000000002158.
13. Schünemann HJ, et al. Breast cancer screening and diagnosis: a synopsis of the European breast guidelines. Ann Intern Med. 2020;172(1):46. https://doi.org/10.7326/M19-2125.

14. Tabar L, Yen MF, Vitak B, Tony Chen HH, Smith RA, Duffy SW. Mammography service screening and mortality in breast cancer patients: 20-year follow-up before and after introduction of screening. Lancet. 2003;361(9367):1405–10. https://doi.org/10.1016/S0140-6736(03)13143-1.
15. Salomon A. Über die Lokalisierung und Verbreitungsweise der Mammakarzinome (on the localization and dissemination of breast carcinomas). Archiv für Klinische Chirurgie. 1913;101:573–91.
16. Brustdruse O, Kleinschmidt I. In: Zweife P, Payr E, Hirzel S, editors. Die Klinik der Bosartigen Geschwulste. Leipzig: Von Hirzel; 1927. p. 5–90.
17. Warren SL. A Roentgenologic study of the breast. Am J Roentgenol Radium Ther. 1930;24:1131–41.
18. Feigin K. Quality assurance in mammography: an overview. Eur J Radiol. 2023;165 https://doi.org/10.1016/j.ejrad.2023.110935.
19. Cohen JG, Ingleby H. Breast lesions; a study of their clinical, pathologic and radiologic correlations. JAMA J Am Med Assoc. 1950;142(11):857–64.
20. Nicosia L, et al. History of mammography: analysis of breast imaging diagnostic achievements over the last century. MDPI; 2023. https://doi.org/10.3390/healthcare11111596.
21. Wolfe J. Breast patterns as an index of risk for developing breast cancer. Am J Roentgenol. 1976;126(6):1130–7. https://doi.org/10.2214/ajr.126.6.1130.
22. Egan RL. Experience with mammography in a tumor institution. Radiology. 1960;75(6):894–900. https://doi.org/10.1148/75.6.894.
23. Egan RL. Mammography technique, 1965.
24. Wolfe JN. Breast patterns as an index of risk for developing breast cancer. Online; 1976. Available: www.ajronline.org
25. Hermel MB. Jacob Gershon-Cohen, MD, DSc. (Med.), 1899–1971. Am J Roentgenol Radium Ther Nucl Med.1971;112(2):417–9. https://doi.org/10.2214/ajr.112.2.417
26. Strax P. Results of mass screening for breast cancer in 50,000 examinations. Cancer. 1976;37(1):30–5. https://doi.org/10.1002/1097-0142(197601)37:1<30::AID-CNCR2820370105>3.0.CO;2-V.
27. Cooperman SACREHCBEJAM. Preoperative localization of occult lesions of the breast. Surg Gynecol Obstet. 1976;142(6):917–9.
28. Hall FM, Kopans DB, Sadowsky NL, Homer MJ. Development of wire localization for occult breast lesions: Boston remembrances. Radiology. 2013;268(3):622–7. https://doi.org/10.1148/radiol.13121943.
29. Ingo Zenger of Siemens Healthineers AG ©2024, "The history of mammography, https://www.medmuseum.siemens-healthineers.com/en/stories-from-the-museum/history-mammography.
30. Barnes GT, Brezovlch IA. The intensity of scattered radiation in mammography. Radiology. 1978;126(1):243–7. https://doi.org/10.1148/126.1.243.
31. Ballard-Barbash RKCPEBMCEAFJBFRGSS. Breast cancer screening in 21 countries delivery of services, notification of results and outcomes ascertainment. Eur J Cancer Prev. 1999;8(5):417–26.
32. Chan HP, Frank PH, Doi K, Iida N, Higashida Y. Ultra-high-strip-density radiographic grids: a new antiscatter technique for mammography. Radiology. 1985;154(3):807–15. https://doi.org/10.1148/radiology.154.3.3969487.
33. Chen H, Danielsson M, Xu C, Cederström B. On image quality metrics and the usefulness of grids in digital mammography. J Med Imaging. 2015;2(1):013501. https://doi.org/10.1117/1.JMI.2.1.013501.
34. Feig SA. Mammography equipment: principles, features, selection. PMID: 3306772. Radiol Clin North Am. 1987;25(5):897–911.
35. White J. FDA approves system for digital mammography. J Natl Cancer Inst. 2000;92(6):442. https://doi.org/10.1093/jnci/92.6.442.
36. Pisano ED, et al. Diagnostic performance of digital versus film mammography for breast-cancer screening. Online; 2005. Available: www.nejm
37. Niklason LT, et al. Digital Tomosynthesis in breast imaging. Radiology. 1997;205(2):399–406. https://doi.org/10.1148/radiology.205.2.9356620.
38. Lynge E, Vejborg I, Andersen Z, von Euler-Chelpin M, Napolitano G. Mammographic density and screening sensitivity, breast cancer incidence and associated risk factors in Danish breast cancer screening. J Clin Med. 2019;8(11):2021. https://doi.org/10.3390/jcm8112021.
39. Tirada N, et al. Digital breast Tomosynthesis: physics, artifacts, and quality control considerations. Radiographics. 2019;39(2):413–26. https://doi.org/10.1148/rg.2019180046.
40. Skaane P, et al. Comparison of digital mammography alone and digital mammography plus Tomosynthesis in a population-based screening program. Radiology. 2013;267(1):47–56. https://doi.org/10.1148/radiol.12121373.
41. Skaane P, et al. Prospective trial comparing full-field digital mammography (FFDM) versus combined FFDM and Tomosynthesis in a population-based screening programme using independent double reading with arbitration. Eur Radiol. 2013;23(8):2061–71. https://doi.org/10.1007/s00330-013-2820-3.
42. Ciatto S, et al. Integration of 3D digital mammography with Tomosynthesis for population breast-cancer screening (STORM): a prospective comparison study. Lancet Oncol. 2013;14(7):583–9. https://doi.org/10.1016/S1470-2045(13)70134-7.
43. McDonald ES, Oustimov A, Weinstein SP, Synnestvedt MB, Schnall M, Conant EF. Effectiveness of digital breast Tomosynthesis compared with digital mammography. JAMA Oncol. 2016;2(6):737. https://doi.org/10.1001/jamaoncol.2015.5536.

44. Jong RA, et al. Contrast-enhanced digital mammography: initial clinical experience. Radiology. 2003;228(3):842–50. https://doi.org/10.1148/radiol.2283020961.
45. Dromain C, et al. Dual-energy contrast-enhanced digital mammography: initial clinical results. Eur Radiol. 2011;21(3):565–74. https://doi.org/10.1007/s00330-010-1944-y.
46. Sogani J, Mango VL, Keating D, Sung JS, Jochelson MS. Contrast-enhanced mammography: past, present, and future. Elsevier Inc; 2021. https://doi.org/10.1016/j.clinimag.2020.09.003.
47. Zanardo M, et al. Technique, protocols and adverse reactions for contrast-enhanced spectral mammography (CESM): a systematic review. Springer Verlag; 2019. https://doi.org/10.1186/s13244-019-0756-0.
48. Cozzi A, Magni V, Zanardo M, Schiaffino S, Sardanelli F. Contrast-enhanced mammography: a systematic review and meta-analysis of diagnostic performance. Radiological Society of North America Inc; 2022. https://doi.org/10.1148/radiol.211412.
49. Łuczyńska E, et al. Comparison between breast MRI and contrast-enhanced spectral mammography. Med Sci Monit. 2015;21:1358–67. https://doi.org/10.12659/MSM.893018.
50. Nicosia L, et al. Contrast-Enhanced Spectral Mammography and tumor size assessment: a valuable tool for appropriate surgical management of breast lesions. Radiol Med. 2022;127(11):1228–34. https://doi.org/10.1007/s11547-022-01561-x.
51. Nicosia L, et al. Contrast-enhanced spectral mammography in the evaluation of breast microcalcifications: controversies and diagnostic management. Healthcare (Switzerland). 2023;11:4. https://doi.org/10.3390/healthcare11040511.
52. Nicosia L, et al. A score to predict the malignancy of a breast lesion based on different contrast enhancement patterns in contrast-enhanced spectral mammography. Cancers (Basel). 2022;14(17) https://doi.org/10.3390/cancers14174337.
53. Becker AS, Marcon M, Ghafoor S, Wurnig MC, Frauenfelder T, Boss A. Deep learning in mammography diagnostic accuracy of a multipurpose image analysis software in the detection of breast cancer. Investig Radiol. 2017;52(7):434–40. https://doi.org/10.1097/RLI.0000000000000358.
54. Morgan MB, Mates JL. Applications of artificial intelligence in breast imaging. Radiol Clin North Am. 2021;59(1):139–48. https://doi.org/10.1016/j.rcl.2020.08.007.
55. Nicosia L, et al. Radiomic features applied to contrast enhancement spectral mammography: possibility to predict breast cancer molecular subtypes in a non-invasive manner. Int J Mol Sci. 2022;23(23):15322. https://doi.org/10.3390/ijms232315322.
56. Wang G, Shi D, Guo Q, Zhang H, Wang S, Ren K. Radiomics based on digital mammography helps to identify mammographic masses suspicious for cancer. Front Oncol. 2022;12 https://doi.org/10.3389/fonc.2022.843436.
57. Kuhl CK. What the future holds for the screening, diagnosis, and treatment of breast cancer. Radiology. 2023;306(3) https://doi.org/10.1148/radiol.223338.
58. Chitalia R, et al. Radiomic tumor phenotypes augment molecular profiling in predicting recurrence free survival after breast neoadjuvant chemotherapy. Commun Med. 2023;3(1):46. https://doi.org/10.1038/s43856-023-00273-1.
59. Mendat CC, Mislan D, Hession-Kunz L. Patient comfort from the technologist perspective: factors to consider in mammographic imaging. Int J Women's Health. 2017;9:359–64. https://doi.org/10.2147/IJWH.S129817.
60. Cooper AP. On the anatomy of the breast. In: Anatomy of the breast. London, UK: Longman, Orme, Green, Browne, and Longmans; 1840.
61. Khan YS, Fakoya AO, Sajjad H. Anatomy, thorax, mammary gland. Online; 2023. Available: https://www.ncbi.nlm.nih.gov/books/NBK547666/
62. Jesinger RA. Breast anatomy for the Interventionalist. Tech Vasc Interv Radiol. 2014;17(1):3–9. https://doi.org/10.1053/j.tvir.2013.12.002.
63. McGhee DE, Steele JR. Breast biomechanics: what do we really know? American Physiological Society; 2020. https://doi.org/10.1152/physiol.00024.2019.
64. Lawrence W Bassett, Mary C. Mahoney, Sophia Apple, Carl D'Orsi. Breast imaging: expert radiology series. ISBN-978-1416051992, vol. 1. Saunders; 2010.
65. Balter S. Tutorial generators, X-ray tubes, and exposure geometry in mammography1, 1990.
66. Caumo F, et al. Incremental effect from integrating 3D-mammography (tomosynthesis) with 2D-mammography: increased breast cancer detection evident for screening centres in a population-based trial. Breast. 2014;23(1):76–80. https://doi.org/10.1016/j.breast.2013.11.006.
67. Skaane P, et al. Digital mammography versus digital mammography plus Tomosynthesis in breast cancer screening: the Oslo Tomosynthesis screening trial. Radiology. 2019;291(1):23–30. https://doi.org/10.1148/radiol.2019182394.
68. Bernardi D, et al. Breast cancer screening with Tomosynthesis (3D mammography) with acquired or synthetic 2D mammography compared with 2D mammography alone (STORM-2): a population-based prospective study. Lancet Oncol. 2016;17(8):1105–13. https://doi.org/10.1016/S1470-2045(16)30101-2.
69. Gilbert FJ, Tucker L, Gillan MGC, Willsher P, Cooke J, Duncan KA, Michell MJ, Dobson HM, Lim YY, Strudley C, Astley SM, Morrish O, Young KC, Duffy SW, Purushothaman H. The TOMMY trial: A comparison of TOMosynthesis with digital MammographY in the UK NHS Breast Screening Programme – a multicentre retrospective reading study comparing the diagnostic performance of digital breast tomosynthesis and digital mammography with digital mammography alone NIHR Journals Library. 2015;19(4):1–136. https://doi.org/10.3310/hta19040

70. Dhamija E, Gulati M, Deo SVS, Gogia A, Hari S. Digital breast Tomosynthesis: an overview. Indian J Surg Oncol. 2021;12(2):315–29. https://doi.org/10.1007/s13193-021-01310-y.
71. Chikarmane SA, Offit LR, Giess CS. Synthetic mammography: benefits, drawbacks, and pitfalls. Radiographics. 2023;43(10) https://doi.org/10.1148/rg.230018.
72. Houssami N, et al. Interval breast cancers in the 'screening with Tomosynthesis or standard mammography' (STORM) population-based trial. Breast. 2018;38:150–3. https://doi.org/10.1016/j.breast.2018.01.002.
73. Shapiro S. Evidence on screening for breast cancer from a randomized trial. Cancer. 1977;39(6):2772–82. https://doi.org/10.1002/1097-0142(197706)39:6<2772::AID-CNCR2820390665>3.0.CO;2-K.
74. Rose SL, Tidwell AL, Bujnoch LJ, Kushwaha AC, Nordmann AS, Sexton R. Implementation of breast Tomosynthesis in a routine screening practice: an observational study. Am J Roentgenol. 2013;200(6):1401–8. https://doi.org/10.2214/AJR.12.9672.
75. Philpotts LE, Crenshaw J, Kalra VB, Butler RS. How tomosynthesis optimizes patient work-up, throughput, and resource utilization [Abstract SSK01-09]. In Scientific assembly and annual meeting of the radiological society of North America, 2013.
76. Roth RG, Maidment ADA, Weinstein SP, Roth SO, Conant EF. Digital breast Tomosynthesis: lessons learned from early clinical implementation. Radiographics. 2014;34(4):E89–E102. https://doi.org/10.1148/rg.344130087.
77. Zuley ML, et al. Digital breast Tomosynthesis versus supplemental diagnostic mammographic views for evaluation of noncalcified breast lesions. Radiology. 2013;266(1):89–95. https://doi.org/10.1148/radiol.12120552.
78. Luparia A, et al. Accuracy of tumour size assessment in the preoperative staging of breast cancer: comparison of digital mammography, Tomosynthesis, ultrasound and MRI. Radiol Med. 2013;118(7):1119–36. https://doi.org/10.1007/s11547-013-0941-z.
79. Mann RM, Veltman J, Barentsz JO, Wobbes T, Blickman JG, Boetes C. The value of MRI compared to mammography in the assessment of tumour extent in invasive lobular carcinoma of the breast. Eur J Surg Oncol. 2008;34(2):135–42. https://doi.org/10.1016/j.ejso.2007.04.020.
80. Feng SSJ, Sechopoulos I. Clinical digital breast Tomosynthesis system: Dosimetric characterization. Radiology. 2012;263(1):35–42. https://doi.org/10.1148/radiol.11111789.
81. Sechopoulos I, Suryanarayanan S, Vedantham S, D'Orsi C, Karellas A. Computation of the glandular radiation dose in digital Tomosynthesis of the breast. Med Phys. 2007;34(1):221–32. https://doi.org/10.1118/1.2400836.
82. Sechopoulos I, Suryanarayanan S, Vedantham S, D'Orsi CJ, Karellas A. Scatter radiation in digital Tomosynthesis of the breast. Med Phys. 2007;34(2):564–76. https://doi.org/10.1118/1.2428404.
83. Pujara AC, Hui J, Wang L. Architectural distortion in the era of digital breast tomosynthesis: Outcomes and implications for management. Clin.l Imaging. 2019;54:24–9. https://doi.org/10.1016/j.clinimag.2019.01.004.
84. Hu Y, Zhao B, Zhao W. Image artifacts in digital breast Tomosynthesis: investigation of the effects of system geometry and reconstruction parameters using a linear system approach. Med Phys. 2008;35(12):5242–52. https://doi.org/10.1118/1.2996110.
85. Spangler ML, et al. Detection and classification of calcifications on digital breast Tomosynthesis and 2D digital mammography: a comparison. Am J Roentgenol. 2011;196(2):320–4. https://doi.org/10.2214/AJR.10.4656.
86. Tagliafico A, et al. Characterisation of microcalcification clusters on 2D digital mammography (FFDM) and digital breast tomosynthesis (DBT): does DBT underestimate microcalcification clusters? Results of a multicentre study. Eur Radiol. 2015;25(1):9–14. https://doi.org/10.1007/s00330-014-3402-8.
87. Hooley RJ, Durand MA, Philpotts LE. Advances in digital breast Tomosynthesis. Am J Roentgenol. 2017;208(2):256–66. https://doi.org/10.2214/AJR.16.17127.
88. Bicehouse HJ. Survey of mammographic exposure levels and techniques used in eastern Pennsylvania. 7th Annual National Conference on Radiation Control, DHEW Publication (FDA) 76–8026; 1975.
89. Hendrick RE, et al. Quality control manual radiologist's section clinical image section radiologic technologist's section. Medical Physicist's Section American College of Radiology Committee on Quality Assurance in Mammography Mammography; 2004.
90. Mammography Quality Standards Act (MQSA).
91. Conway BJ, Suleiman OH, Rueter FG, Antonsen RG, Slayton RJ. National survey of mammographic facilities in 1985, 1988, and 1992. Radiology. 1994;191(2):323–30. https://doi.org/10.1148/radiology.191.2.8153301.
92. Berns EA, et al. Quality control manual and digital breast Tomosynthesis radiologist's section radiologic technologist's section medical physicist's section. American College of Radiology Subcommittee on Quality Assurance in Mammography of the Committee on Mammography Accreditation Digital Mammography; 2018.

5 Fluoroscopy: Physics, Principle of Operation, and Quality Control

Learning Objectives

The Early Era of Fluoroscopic Imaging Techniques Unknown Facts about Fluoroscopic Imaging Special demands for Fluoroscopic imaging Mechanism of action in fluoroscopy Fluoroscopy Instrumentation: Image intensifier an image intensifier a fluoroscopic X-ray tube a spot film device and bucky slot a viewing camera radiation protection devices Fluoroscopy - Radiation Protection Devices Modes of operation and Automatic brightness control Clinical applications of fluoroscopy	Digital Fluoroscopy Classification of flat panel detectors in digital fluoroscopy Choosing the right scintillator for flat panel detectors Working Principle of Indirect TFT Flat Panel Detector Working Principle of Indirect CCD Flat Panel Detector Working Principle of Direct Flat Panel Detector Radiation dose considerations and radiation protection in Fluoroscopy Room design for Fluoroscopy Equipment, practice, and Image Quality Image quality control in Fluoroscopy Technological Advancements in Fluoroscopy Fluoroscopy image related artefacts Quality control in Fluoroscopy Learning outcomes

5.1 The Early Era of Fluoroscopic Imaging Techniques

The term fluoroscopy dates to the 1920s, when shoe salespeople used it to visualize the bones of the feet, which was mostly used for children's shoe shopping as depicted in Fig. 5.1. This method was later dubbed the shoe-fitting fluoroscope manufactured by Adrian Shoe Fitter in Washington D.C. However, due to the harmful effects of radiation reported in young children, the use of this technique was completely discontinued in the 1950s. For a 20-second exposure, the typical direct radiation doses to the feet were several rads, and the scatter radiation doses to the abdomen were 100–200 millirem [1–3]. A typical shoe-fitting fluoroscopy device is depicted in Fig. 5.2.

The fluoroscopic era began on November 8, 1895, when Sir Wilhelm Conrad Roentgen accidentally discovered a barium platinocyanide screen that emitted light when exposed to X-rays. The first fluoroscopes were created and widely available worldwide not long after the revolution-

D. Prakash, R. P. Kotian, *Fundamentals of X-ray Imaging*,
https://doi.org/10.1007/978-981-96-7328-5_5

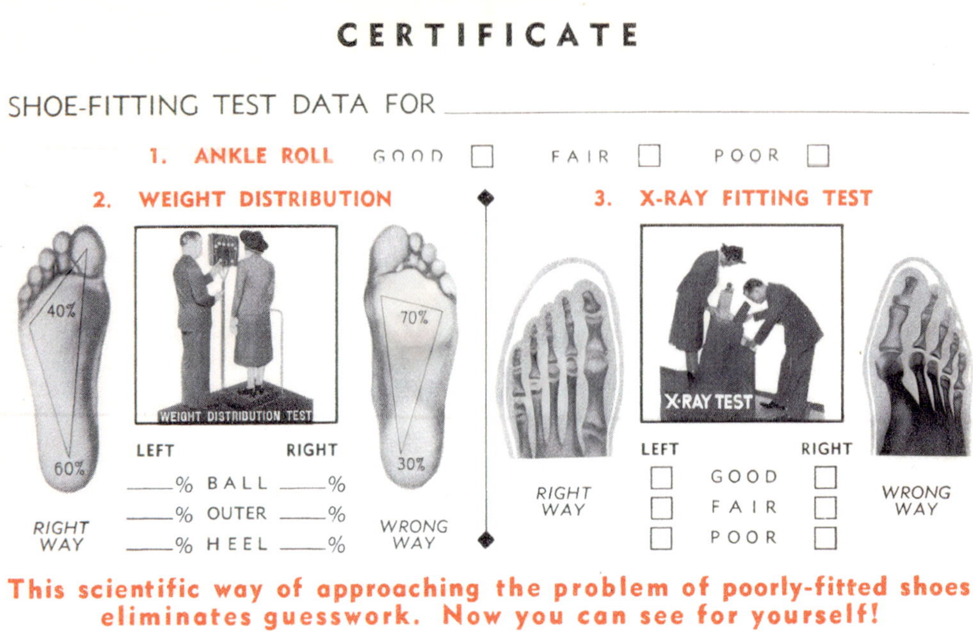

Fig. 5.1 Typical shoe-fitting datasheet

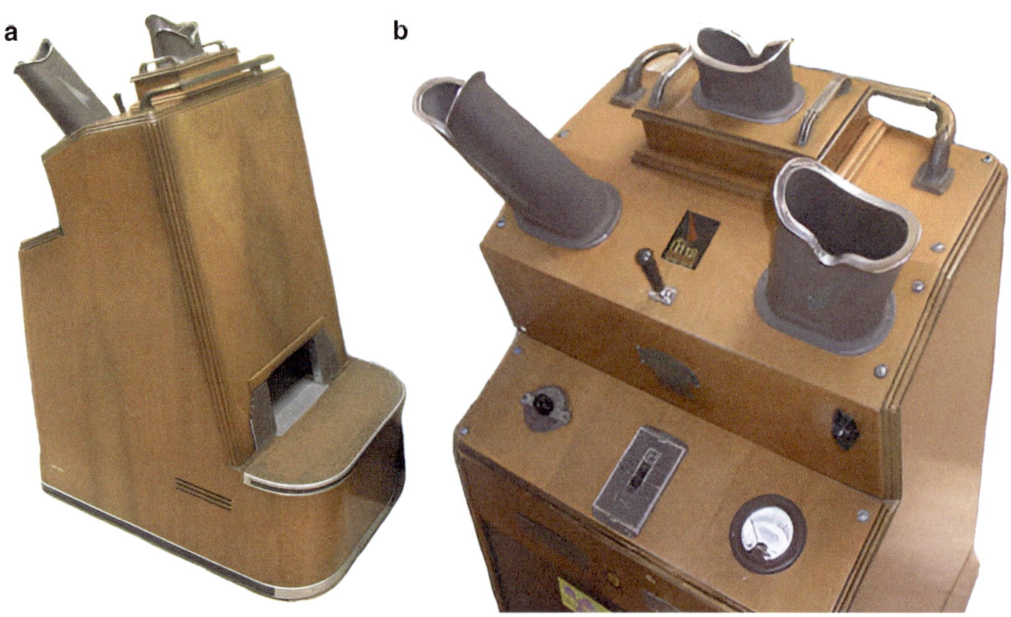

Fig. 5.2 Ancient shoe-fitting fluoroscope

ary discovery of X-rays. The first fluoroscope was invented in 1896 by Sir Enrico Salvioni. The first fluoroscopes were cardboard tunnels covered in a layer of fluorescent metal salts with a viewing eyepiece used by the radiologist to visualize the fluoroscopic live images. However, this technique produced extremely faint radiographic images. Hence, the radiologist would spend a brief period in a dark room before the imaging procedure for adapting his eyes to perceive these weak faint images. This problem of dark room adaption was solved by the invention of red goggles by Sir Wilhelm Trendelenburg.

On the other hand, Sir Thomas Edison's discovery of calcium tungstate screens in the late 1890s produced brighter images than the first-generation fluoroscopes. The early prediction that live fluoroscopic images would eventually replace still X-rays was proven incorrect, as the latter produced images with superior diagnostic resolution [4, 5]. Fluoroscopy successfully produced live images of the body's internal structure for many decades and was not recorded until the late 1960s. However, as technology progressed, live imaging and recording became the norm.

Early scientists wrongly projected that still X-ray images would be replaced by moving images from fluoroscopy, but the latter's better diagnostic value prevented this. Early radiologists had to sit in a dark room behind the fluorescent screen because of the screens' limited light and a lack of knowledge about the dangers of X-rays. There were high radiation doses as a result. Additionally, scientists and medical imaging professionals frequently place their hands directly in the X-ray beam, resulting in radiation burns and even more significant health problems. In reality, the risky levels of exposure caused the cancer death of Edinson's lab assistant at the age of 39.

The 1950s saw the invention of the television camera and the X-ray picture intensifier, which completely changed fluoroscopy. The fluorescent screen's light output may be boosted by the picture intensifier, making it possible to see it even in a well-lit space, also the inclusion of a camera that allowed for image viewing on a monitor. Now, the radiologist could see the radiographs from a different room without having to worry about getting exposed to radiation.

Since then, advancements in image intensifiers, flat panel detectors, and screen phosphors have made it possible to improve image quality while exposing patients and personnel to less radiation.

5.2 Unknown Facts About Fluoroscopic Imaging

Some lesser-known facts about fluoroscopic imaging are listed below:

1. **History:** Thomas Edison invented fluoroscopic imaging in the late 1800s, using a luminous screen to visualize X-rays.
2. **Radiation exposure:** Ionizing radiation, which can be hazardous to the human body, is used in fluoroscopic imaging. As a result, fluoroscopic imaging is carefully regulated and controlled to reduce radiation exposure.
3. **Contrast agents:** In fluoroscopic imaging, contrast agents are frequently employed to make interior structures more visible. Depending on the location of the body being scanned, these drugs can be supplied orally, intravenously, or via other means.
4. **Applications:** Fluoroscopic imaging is employed in a variety of medical treatments, such as surgeries, cardiac interventions, and orthopedic procedures. It can also be used to diagnose illnesses like gastrointestinal issues and lung disorders.
5. **Imaging technologies**: New fluoroscopic imaging techniques, such as digital fluoroscopy and cone-beam computed tomography (CBCT), have been developed as a result of advances in imaging technology. These technologies provide better image quality while reducing radiation exposure.
6. **Interventional radiology:** Fluoroscopic imaging is an important technique in interventional radiology, which uses minimally invasive treatments to diagnose and treat a variety of medical disorders. Fluoroscopic imaging is used by interventional radiologists to guide catheters, wires, and other devices through the body to specific regions for diagnosis or therapy.
7. **Limitations:** While fluoroscopic imaging is an important diagnostic technique, it has limits. It generates 2D visuals that can be difficult to read, and it can't tell you how internal structures work. As a result, additional imaging modalities such as MRI and CT scans may be required to provide accurate images of a patient's condition.

5.3 Special Demands for Fluoroscopic Imaging

Fluoroscopy is a medical imaging procedure that uses X-rays to create real-time images of the inside structures of the body. Because of the nature of this technique, certain special requirements must be met to obtain optimum-quality images while also ensuring the safety of both the patient and the imaging staff. Two of the most important special requirements of fluoroscopy are:

A. **Illumination:**

Increased image brightness was the traditional advantage of image intensifier fluoroscopic imaging over conventional fluoroscopic imaging. The illumination of the imaging room, on the other hand, is critical in interpreting and reading fluoroscopic images. Lumens per square meter, or lux, are commonly used to measure illumination.

The amount of light that falls on a surface or per unit area is measured in lux, which is the amount of light that falls on a surface or per unit area. Lumens per square meter (1 m/m^2) are the units of measurement. As a result, lux and lumens per square meter are nearly interchangeable. In fluoroscopy imaging, this is used to calculate the intensity of light passing through a surface and being perceived by the human eye. Fluoroscopic images are viewed with illumination levels ranging from 100 to 1000 lux. These levels of illumination that are visible to the human eye must be explored.

B. **Human sight:**

"The components in the eye that are culpable for vision are known as rods and cones. Light has to travel through the cornea, a clear protective layer, and then the lens, where it appears on the retina. The iris is placed between the cornea and the lens and controls the quantity of light that enters the eye in the same way that the diaphragm of a photographic camera does. When exposed to bright light, the iris contracts, limiting the amount of light that enters. The iris dilates when exposed to low light conditions, such as a dimly lit digital radiography reading room. When light enters the retina, the rods and cones recognize it. Rods and cones are tiny structures that number over 1 lakh per square centimeter of the retina. The cones are concentrated in the fovea centralis, which is located in the retina's core. Rods, on the other hand, are found in greater abundance on the retina's periphery. There are no rods in the fovea centralis. The rods activate when they are exposed to low light as they are sensitive to it. The rod vision threshold is about two lux. On the other hand, Cones are less light sensitive; their vision threshold is only around a hundred lux, but cones may respond to high light levels that rods cannot. As a result, cones are used for daytime and rods for night-time vision respectively. This component of visual physiology explains why dim objects appear brighter when not directly viewed. As radiologists and imaging professionals know, a dim object is best examined peripherally, where rod vision predominates. Cones can see much smaller objects than rods. The ability to discern fine detail is referred to as visual acuity. Cones are also considerably better at differentiating between different levels of brightness. Contrast perception is the name given to this eyesight characteristic. Cones can detect a wide range of light wavelengths. Colour is perceived by cones, whereas rods are colourblind. The eye's sensitivity is greatest under scotopic conditions in the green area of the bandwidth."

5.4 Mechanism of Action in Fluoroscopy

To understand how fluoroscopy works, it is critical to first compare it to visible light. The naked eye can perceive visible light directly because it does not penetrate through an object; however, X-rays can penetrate through a wide range of objects that are not visible to the human eye. To overcome this process of image visualization of the internal structure of the human body using X-rays, the X-ray intensity must be converted into a form that is visible using traditional film-based radiography and, more recently, digital detectors. Classic fluoroscopy, on the other hand, accomplishes this by utilizing the fluorescence property of certain crystals, which converts

X-rays into visible light. The use of fluorescent crystals gave rise to the term "fluoroscopy."

X-rays are reflected or attenuated as they traverse the patient's body, rendering a shadow on the fluorescent screen of radio-opaque tissue such as thick bone. On fluoroscopy imaging, the bone appears black. Fluoroscopy's primary application is in the visualization of the cavity, hollow, and moving structures within the body; it is not useful in bone imaging. Images produced on the fluorescent screen by photoelectric interaction of X-ray with matter produced by mildly unattenuated X-rays from radiolucent tissues produce good images. We are now in the digital era of medical imaging, and all forms of digital imaging use electronic detectors such as flat panel detectors to convert X-ray energy directly into electrical signals [6, 7].

5.5 Fluoroscopy Instrumentation: Image Intensifier

The process of acquiring fluoroscopic images consists of a series of controlled processes and coordinated event sequences. The major hardware requirements for fluoroscopy would include the following as depicted in Fig. 5.3:

1. An image intensifier
2. A fluoroscopic X-ray tube
3. A spot film device and bucky slot
4. A viewing camera
5. Radiation protection devices

5.5.1 Image Intensifier

In fluoroscopy, an image intensifier converts X-ray photons into visible light photons, which can then be used to create an image on a TV screen monitor. The image intensifier is made up of a vacuum tube with several components such as an input phosphor, an X-ray converter, a photocathode, a series of electron optics, and an output phosphor [8].

X-rays interact with the X-ray converter, which is commonly constructed of cesium iodide or gadolinium oxysulfide when they pass through the input phosphor. This substance absorbs X-rays and turns them into photons of visible light.

Cesium and antimony compounds are used to make the photocathode. The photocathode, which is placed near the X-ray converter, absorbs pho-

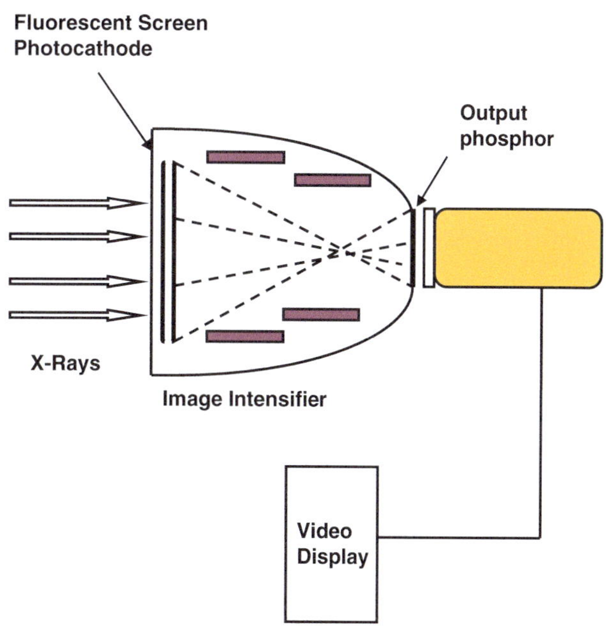

Fig. 5.3 Fluoroscopy components

tons of visible light and produces electrons in reaction. These electrons are then accelerated and focused by a series of electron optics, which direct them toward the output phosphor.

The output phosphor is coated with a silver-coated zinc cadmium sulphate material that emits visible light in response to electron bombardment. This results in a clear, visible image that can be viewed on a screen or recorded for later analysis [9, 10].

Overall, the image intensifier allows for a more detailed and accurate view of the body's internal structures during fluoroscopy, making it a valuable diagnostic tool.

5.5.2 Fluoroscopy X-ray Tube

Fluoroscopy X-ray tubes include special design elements that enable them to continuously emit X-rays with relatively high intensity. A fluoroscopy X-ray tube's main design components include some of the following:

1. **Anode:** The X-ray tube's anode, which receives electron bombardment to produce X-rays, is a component. Typically, tungsten or similar high-density metal that can survive the intense heat produced during continuous operation is used as the anode in fluoroscopy. For heat dissipation and tube protection, the anode is typically formed like a disk or a cone.
2. **Cathode:** The X-ray tube's cathode, when heated by a filament, emits electrons. The cathode in fluoroscopy is often comprised of a thin tungsten wire that has been wound around a filament. The filament heats up and emits electrons that are propelled toward the anode when a current is supplied to it.
3. **Focusing cup:** The cathode is surrounded by a small metal cup called the focusing cup, which aids in concentrating the electrons on the anode. The X-ray beam's intensity and directionality can be impacted by the size and form of the focusing cup.
4. **Cooling system:** Since the X-ray tube used in fluoroscopy produces a lot of heat, it needs a cooling system to keep it from overheating and suffering damage. This could include a system for cooling liquid or air, as well as additional devices like heat sinks or fans.
5. **Collimators:** The X-ray beam can be shaped and directed with the aid of collimators. Collimators can be used in fluoroscopy to change the angle and direction of the beam or to reduce the shape and size of the X-ray field.

A fluoroscopy X-ray tube's design is tailored for high-intensity, continuous operation while minimizing the danger of tube damage or overheating.

5.5.3 Spot Film and Bucky Device

A spot film and bucky device are used in fluoroscopy to capture static images of the area being examined.

A spot film is a type of X-ray film that can be exposed quickly during a fluoroscopy procedure to capture an image of the anatomy. It is used to capture a high-quality still image of a particular area of interest within the body. The spot film is usually placed behind the patient and exposed when the radiologist or the imaging technologist activates the exposure with a foot pedal or another control device.

A bucky device is a mechanism that keeps the spot film in place during exposure. It consists of a film tray or cassette and a movable grid that helps to reduce scatter radiation and improve image quality. Before the exposure, the bucky device is placed between the X-ray tube and the patient, and the spot film is placed in the tray or cassette.

The spot film and bucky device, when used together, allow the radiologist or imaging technologist to capture a static image during a fluoroscopy procedure, allowing the radiologist to better evaluate the anatomy and any potential abnormalities.

5.5.4 Fluoroscopy Viewing Camera

A fluoroscopy viewing camera is a specialized camera used in medical imaging to view the fluoroscopic image produced by the X-ray machine. The camera is placed behind the patient and records the image that is projected onto a fluorescent screen. The image is then sent to a video monitor, where the radiologist and imaging technologist can view the internal structures of the body in real-time.

Fluoroscopy cameras are typically equipped with zoom, focus, and brightness adjustments, allowing for a clearer and more detailed image. Some cameras can also capture still images or video footage of the fluoroscopic exam for later review or analysis.

A fluoroscopy viewing camera is essential for guiding interventional procedures like cardiac catheterization, gastrointestinal studies, and orthopedic surgeries. It enables the healthcare provider to monitor the administration of contrast agents or other therapeutic substances as well as the position and movement of instruments. Overall, the fluoroscopy viewing camera is critical to the safety and accuracy of numerous medical procedures.

A scintillation crystal, a lens system, and a charge-coupled device (CCD) or complementary metal-oxide-semiconductor (CMOS) sensor are typical components of the latest generation viewing camera. The X-ray beam is transformed into visible light by the scintillation crystal, which is focused on the CCD or CMOS sensor by the lens system. The visible light is then converted by the sensor into a digital signal, which is then transmitted to the computer or monitor for display as depicted in Figs. 5.4 and 5.5.

The viewing camera's quality is critical for obtaining high-quality fluoroscopic images. To capture the full range of X-ray intensities, a high-quality camera should have a high spatial resolution, low noise, and a wide dynamic range. Furthermore, the camera should have a high frame rate to capture quick movements and changes in the patient's anatomy.

Internal Structure and Working Principles of Fluoroscopy Camera System

The television monitoring system for a fluoroscopic image is developed in such a way that the image-intensifier tube's output phosphor is directly connected to a television camera tube. A vidicon is a type of television camera tube that is frequently used in fluorescence imaging. It has a sensitive input surface that is the same size as the image-intensifier tube's output phosphor. The television camera tube turns the light images from the image intensifier's output phosphor into an electrical signal that is sent to the television monitor and rebuilt as an image on the television. One significant benefit of television monitoring is the ability to electronically control brightness and contrast. Using television monitoring, several radiologists can simultaneously view the fluoroscopic image. It is even common for moni-

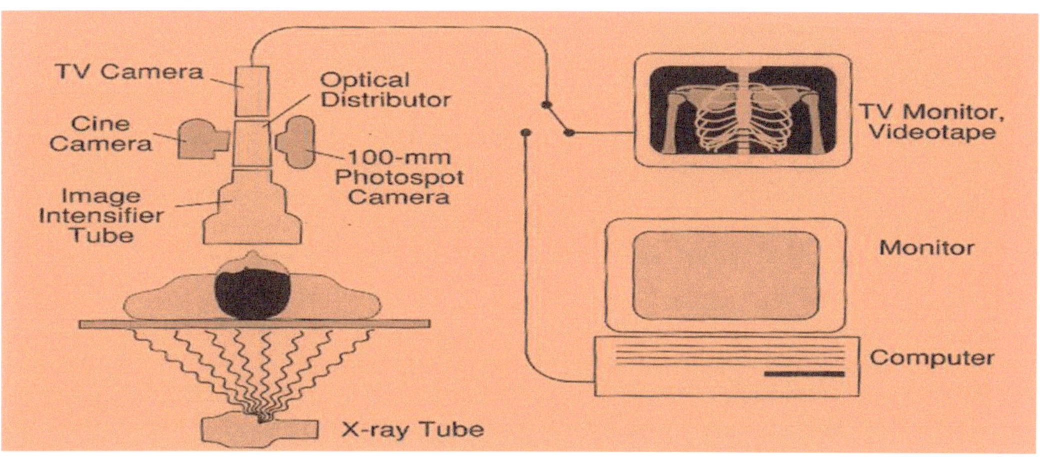

Fig. 5.4 Typical fluoroscopic system using an X-ray image intensifier and video camera

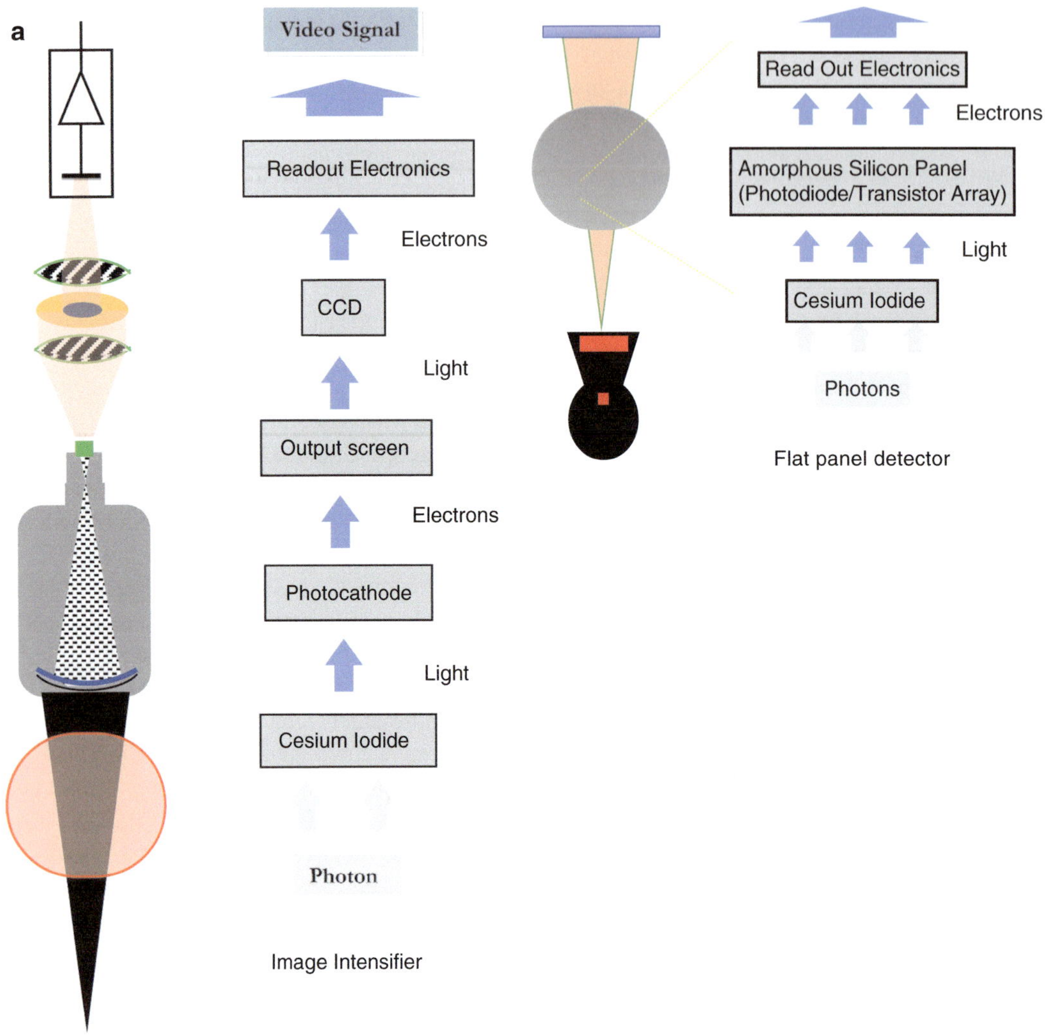

Fig. 5.5 (**a**) Image intensifier vs (**b**) Digital flat panel detector

tors to be installed remotely in the examination room for the benefit of others. Television monitoring also allows for the electronic storage of images for later viewing and manipulation.

Television Camera

The visual image on the image intensifier's output phosphor is converted into an electrical signal using two approaches. The thermionic television camera tube and the solid-state charge-coupled device (CCD) are two examples.

The television camera is comprised of a cylindrical housing that measures around 15 mm in diameter and 25 cm in length and houses the television camera tube's heart. It also has electromagnetic coils that aid in the direction of the electron beam within the tube. For television fluoroscopy, there are several different television camera tubes, but the vidicon and its modified variant, the Plumbicon, are the most widely used. The glass envelope serves the same function as the X-ray tube in that it maintains a vacuum while also provide the interior components with mechanical support. The cathode, its electron cannon, several electro-static grids, and a target assembly that functions as an anode are among the internal components. A heated filament emits a continuous stream of electrons via thermionic emission in an electron cannon. The control grid accelerates electrons to the anode by producing an electron beam. Additional electrostatic grids speed up and focus the electron beam. Deflection coils, focusing coils, and alignment coils are external electromagnetic coils that regulate the size and location of the electron beam. A wire mesh-like structure connects the electron beam to the target assembly at the tube's anode end.

The target assembly is made up of three layers that are layered on top of each other. The window is the small piece of glass that is attached to the glass envelope's outside. The signal plate is a thin metal or graphite coating applied to the interior of the glass. The signal plate is sufficiently thin to convey energy effectively while remaining thick enough to transmit light. The term derives from the fact that it transmits the visual signal from the tube to the external video circuit. An antimony trisulfide photoconductive layer coats the inside of the signal plate. This layer, known as the target, is swept by the electron beam. While exposed to light, antimony trisulfide conducts electrons; while exposed to darkness, it serves as an insulator. The target's mechanism is complex, however, it can be easily summarized as follows. When light strikes the window from the image-intensifier tube's output phosphor, it is directed to the target through the signal plate. When the electron beam strikes the same point on the target repeatedly, some of its electrons flow through the target to the signal plate and then out of the tube as the video signal. No visual signal is produced if that area of the target is dark. The magnitude of the video signal is related to the light intensity [11].

Coupling to the Image Intensifier

Image intensifiers and television camera tubes are designed so that the image intensifier tube's output phosphor is the same width as the television camera tube's window, which is commonly 2.5 or 5 cm, as demonstrated in Fig. 5.5. For connecting the image-intensifier tube to the television camera tube, there are two popular approaches. The simplest approach is to employ a fiberoptic bundle. The Fiberoptics bundle is only a few millimeters thick, but per square centimeter, it is packed with thousands of glass fibers. The image-intensifier tower can be easily relocated due to the compact assembly of this type of coupler. This connector is robust and can endure severe handling. The main disadvantage is that it cannot fit the additional lenses needed by devices like cine or photo spot cameras. Lens coupling is necessary to accept a cine or photo spot camera. This type of connection results in a much larger assembly that must be handled with care. Because misalignment results in a hazy image, the lenses and mirror must remain completely calibrated.

The light from the output phosphor is absorbed by the objective lens and converted into a parallel beam. When an image is recorded on film, a beam-splitting mirror interrupts the beam, allowing only a portion of it to be broadcast to the television camera and the remainder to be reflected by a film camera. The fluoroscopist can view the image as it is being recorded in this mode. When not in use, the beam-splitting mirror is generally detached from the beam. Lenses on both the television and film cameras concentrate the parallel light beam onto the film and the targets of the respective cameras. These camera lenses are critical components in the optical chain in terms of alignment. While portrayed as simple convex lenses, the lenses are complex lens systems made up of numerous separate lens elements [12].

Television Monitor

"The video signal is amplified and sent via cable to the television monitor, where it is transformed into a viewable image. The television monitor is one end of a closed-circuit television system. The television camera tube, also known as a CCD, is at the other end. Closed-circuit television fluoroscopy differs from home television in two ways: there is no audio and no channel selection. Typically, the radiological technologist works with only two controls: contrast and brightness. The cathode ray tube, often known as the television image tube, is at the heart of the television display. It is similar to the television camera tube in several ways: A glass envelope, electron cannon, and external coils are used to focus and steer the electron beam. Its anode assembly is larger than a television camera tube and consists of a fluorescent screen and a graphite liner. The magnitude of the video signal obtained by the television camera tube is proportional to the intensity of the light received by the television camera tube. The electron beam of the television image tube, unlike the television camera tube, varies in strength depending on how the video signal is encoded. A control grid connected to the electron gun modulates the electron stream's intensity. The external coils focus this electron beam onto the fluorescent output screen. A flash of light results from an interaction between electrons and an output phosphor. To reduce lateral dispersion, the phosphor is composed of linear crystals that are oriented perpendicular to the glass envelope. It frequently rests on a thin layer of aluminium that transmits electron beams but deflects light.

Television Image

Despite being complicated, the image on the television monitor is simple to describe. It requires converting the output phosphor's visible light image from the image-intensifier tube into an electrical video signal created by the steady electron beam from the television camera tube. The video signal then modulates the electron beam of the television picture tube, converting it into a viewable image on the fluorescent screen of the picture tube. Both the continuous electron beam in the television camera tube and the modified electron beam in the television picture tube are extremely focused pencil beams that are simultaneously and accurately directed by the external electromagnetic coils of each tube. Because they are constantly moving in the same direction and being in the same position at the same time, these beams are synchronous. Although this explanation is for a television image tube, keep in mind that the same electron beam pattern occurs in a television camera tube. The electron beam moves from the upper left to the upper right corner of the screen, generating a line of varying light intensity along the way. This is referred to as an active trace. The image then shifts back to the left side of the screen as the electron beam is blanked or turned off. This is an example of a horizontal retracement. Up until the electron beam hits the bottom of the screen, a succession of active traces are then followed by horizontal retraces.

This is very similar to how writing a line of information in word processing behaves. (The active trace): The process continues to the bottom of the page once the cursor returns (the horizontal retrace). An electron beam creates a television field as one person finishes a page. However, the similarities end there because you would keep word processing. Before retracing vertically to the top of the screen, the electron beam is blanked once more. With the exception of the fact that each active trace of the first field is located in between two adjacent active traces of the second field, the electron beam now defines a second television field that is comparable to the first one. Two interlaced television fields combine to produce a single field, and the movement of the electron beam is referred to as interlacing. Earlier the United States used to run on a 60 Hz power supply, which produced 60 television fields and 30 television frames each second. This is advantageous since home films or old films, which are filmed at 16 frames per second, lack any flickering on the television. The human eye cannot distinguish flickering at rates more than 20 frames per second. With a frame rate of 30 frames per second, each frame lasts for 33 milliseconds.

The signal is erased as the electron beam scans the optical signal in the television camera tube. The electron beam instantly fades as it produces the television optical signal in the television picture tube, hence the term fluorescent screen. As a result, every new television frame contains 33 milliseconds of fresh data. Since each frame contains 525 active trace lines, standard broadcast and closed-circuit televisions are referred to as 525-line systems. Due to the time required for retracing, only about 480 lines are used per frame. Better spatial resolution is achieved by other specialized systems, which contain 875 or 1024 lines per frame. These high-resolution technologies are extremely beneficial in digital fluoroscopy.

The creation of a television frame with equal horizontal and vertical resolution is the aim of television designers. Commercial television systems have a bandpass of about 3.5 MHz. The bandpass of fluoroscopy systems is roughly 4.5 MHz, while the bandpass of 1000-line high-resolution systems is about 20 MHz. The television screen continues to be the image-intensified fluoroscopy system's weakest link. Although the picture intensifier is effective up to about 5 lp/mm, a 525-line system has a spatial resolution of roughly 1 lp/mm. To capture the image's increased resolution produced by the image intensifier, it must be captured on film using an optically linked photographic camera [13]."

5.6 Fluoroscopy—Radiation Protection Devices

Fluoroscopy is a medical imaging technique that uses X-rays to produce real-time images of the body's internal structures. Because X-rays can be harmful in high doses, radiation protection devices should be used to reduce radiation exposure to both the patient and the medical imaging staff. The following are some of the most commonly used radiation protection devices in fluoroscopy:

1. **Lead aprons and thyroid shields:** These are lead-based protective garments worn by medical personnel during the procedure to shield their bodies from radiation. The torso is covered by the lead apron, while the thyroid shield is worn around the neck to protect the thyroid gland. Lead aprons should be at least 0.5 mm thick lead equivalent, and thyroid shields should be at least 0.25 mm thick lead equivalent.
2. **Gonadal shields:** These are lead shields placed over the patient's reproductive organs during the procedure to protect them from radiation exposure. Gonadal shields should be at least 0.25 mm thick in lead equivalent.
3. **Collimators:** Collimators are devices that aid in the shaping and direction of the X-ray beam. Collimators can reduce the amount of radiation exposure to the patient and the medical imaging staff by narrowing the field of view and limiting the size and shape of the X-ray beam.
4. **Dose monitoring devices:** These are devices that can measure how much radiation the patient and medical imaging staff are exposed to during the procedure. This data can be used to fine-tune the procedure parameters and reduce the radiation dose.
5. **Image intensifiers**: Image intensifiers are devices that amplify and convert the X-ray signal into a visible image. Image intensifiers can reduce the amount of radiation exposure required to obtain an optimal-quality image by increasing the sensitivity of the imaging system.
6. **Automatic exposure control:** This is a feature of modern fluoroscopy systems that allows the X-ray dose to be automatically adjusted based on the size and density of the body part being imaged. Automatic exposure control can reduce the amount of radiation exposure required to obtain a diagnostic image by optimizing the dose for each patient.

Overall, radiation protection devices are an important part of fluoroscopy procedures and can help to reduce the risks of X-ray exposure [14–28].

Modes of Operation and Automatic Brightness Control (ABC) ABC devices use a feedback system based on the amount of light at the image intensifier's output, which signals back to the generator, to calculate the amount of radiation to be incident on the patient. The incident radiation and radiation dose could increase or decrease due to the feedback system.

5.7 Clinical Applications of Fluoroscopy

Fluoroscopy is widely used in clinical applications such as diagnostic tests, surgical procedures, and interventional radiology. The following are some clinical applications of fluoroscopy:

1. **Diagnostic imaging:** Fluoroscopy is commonly used in diagnostic imaging procedures such as upper GI series, barium enema, and voiding cystourethrography. A contrast agent (barium sulphate) is ingested or injected into the body during these procedures, and fluoroscopy is used to produce real-time images of the contrast agent as it moves through the body. This enables the radiologist to see the structure and function of organs and tissues, as well as diagnose conditions like blockages, tumours, and reflux.
2. **Interventional radiology:** In interventional radiology procedures such as angiography, embolization, and biopsy, fluoroscopy is widely used. Fluoroscopy is used to guide a catheter or needle to the site of interest, and then the treatment is administered or tissue samples are collected. Interventional specialists use fluoroscopy to precisely envision the site of interest while avoiding damage to surrounding tissues.
3. **Surgery:** In surgical procedures such as spinal surgery, joint replacement, and orthopedic surgery, fluoroscopy is used. Fluoroscopy is used in these procedures to guide surgical instruments and ensure procedure accuracy. Fluoroscopy is particularly useful in minimally invasive procedures, where the surgeon has limited visibility and must rely on imaging to guide the procedure.
4. **Pain management:** In pain management procedures such as nerve blocks, spinal injections, and radiofrequency ablation, fluoroscopy is commonly used. Fluoroscopy is used in these procedures to precisely guide the injection or ablation to the site of pain, ensuring that the treatment is delivered to the correct location.

Fluoroscopy is a versatile and widely used medical imaging technique with a wide range of clinical applications. Its real-time imaging capabilities make it particularly useful in procedures requiring precision and accuracy, and its low radiation dose and improved imaging technology have made it safer and more effective than ever [29–31].

5.8 Digital Fluoroscopy

Digital fluoroscopy is a medical imaging technique that captures and processes X-ray images in real-time using digital technology. This technique is similar to traditional fluoroscopy in that it uses X-rays to create real-time moving images of internal body structures, but the images are captured and stored digitally rather than on film or the image intensifier.

Compared to traditional fluoroscopy, digital fluoroscopy (DF) has several advantages. One advantage is improved image quality. Higher-resolution images, enabled by digital technology, can provide more detail and clarity, as well as better contrast between different tissues. Because digital systems can use lower radiation doses while still producing high-quality images, digital fluoroscopy can reduce the amount of radiation exposure to the patient. Another advantage of digital fluoroscopy is the ability to electronically store and manipulate images. Images can now be stored on a computer system and accessed from multiple locations, making them more accessible. Digital images can also be enhanced, contrast and brightness adjusted, and measurements or calculations performed using specialized software.

There are two different kinds of DF: one that uses digital flat-panel detectors (FPDs) and the other that employs an image intensifier connected to a digital imaging chain. The former is being phased out in favour of the latter, which can generate dynamic visuals that may be shown and watched in real-time. These detectors are sometimes referred to as dynamic FPDs as a result. The cesium iodide amorphous-silicon (CsI a-Si) TFT indirect digital detector and the a-selenium TFT direct digital detector are the two types of dynamic FPDs now available for digital fluoroscopy. These detectors have high frame rates and quick data transfer rates, which is a significant feature. Frame rates of 15–30 frames per second (fps) or more are feasible with readout speeds of 30–50 ms. Additionally, dynamic FPDs are capable of operating in two different reading modes: continuous X-ray mode and pulsed X-ray mode. The latter's main objective is to lower the dose given to the patient throughout the process.

FPD DF systems provide image magnification in two ways: (a) electronic magnification (zoom) and (b) binning. With the first technique, there is no increase in spatial resolution, and the signal-to-noise ratio (SNR) is the same for the original and magnified images. Binning has the disadvantage of reduced spatial resolution since the effective area of each image pixel is four times bigger than ungrouped pixels, but it has the advantage of lower data rates and less image mottle. FPD DF offers benefits such as distortion-free images, enhanced contrast resolution, high detective quantum efficiency (DQE), and uniform image quality over the entire displayed rectangular image [32, 33].

5.8.1 Classification of Flat Panel Detectors in Digital Fluoroscopy

Digital radiography (DR) detectors are classed as indirect flat panels or direct flat panels based on the fundamental physics of each type of panel. X-rays are transformed into light photons using indirect flat panels, which are then detected by a CCD, Si photodiode, and TFT array. The X-rays are converted into electrons using direct flat panels, which are detected by a TFT. Direct flat screens obtain higher spatial resolution by eliminating the visible light stage, which can blur images as light spreads.

There are both indirect and direct varieties of flat panel detectors. The thin film transistors (TFT) type and the CCD type of indirect flat panels are further separated. In the image and comparison table, the key differences between the CCD and TFT kinds are that the CCD type uses fiber optics and the TFT type uses an array of photodiodes are highlighted. Flat panel detectors are classified into two types: indirect detectors and direct detectors. The indirect flat panels are further classified as thin film transistors (TFTs) and CCDs [34, 35]. The primary distinctions are highlighted in Fig. 5.6 and comparison Table 5.1, which are that the CCD type requires fiber optics and the TFT type uses an array of photodiodes.

The next portion of this chapter will outline the steps each type of detector must take in order to produce an image. While we will use brief image graphics to depict the phases from X-ray interaction to digital signal, it should be noted that all of these interactions take place in flat panels with multiple other detector pieces around them. (i.e., often more than 1024 by 1024 detector elements).

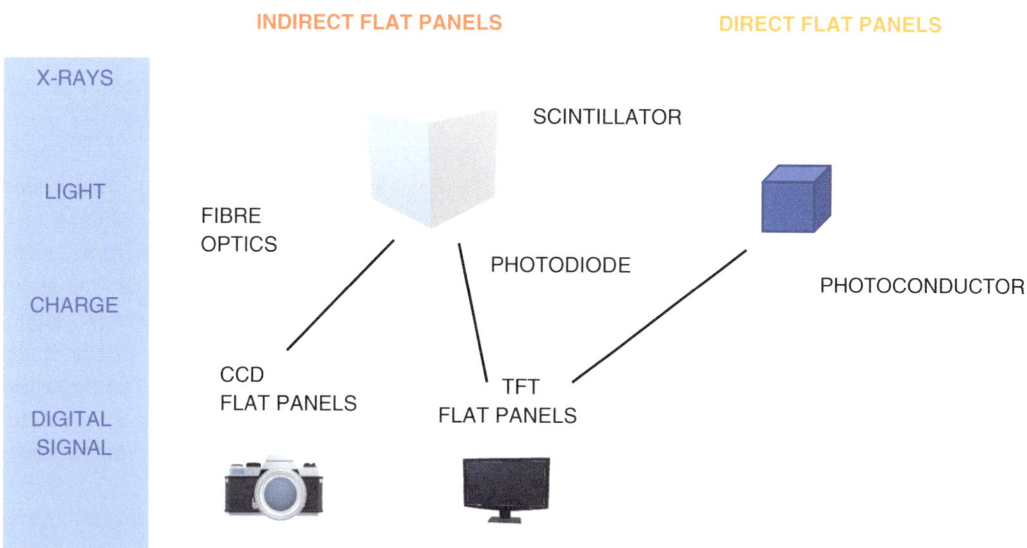

Fig. 5.6 Indirect vs direct flat panels

Table 5.1 Vital comparisons between indirect vs direct flat panel detectors

	Flat panel—indirect (TFT)	Flat panel—indirect (CCD)	Flat panel—direct
Capture capability	Scintillator (CsI) [to light]	Scintillator (CsI) [to light]	Se photoconductor [to electrons]
Light channel guide	Not applicable	Fiber-optics	Not applicable
Light to charge conversion	Si photodiode	CCD	Not applicable
Reading process	TFT	CCD	TFT

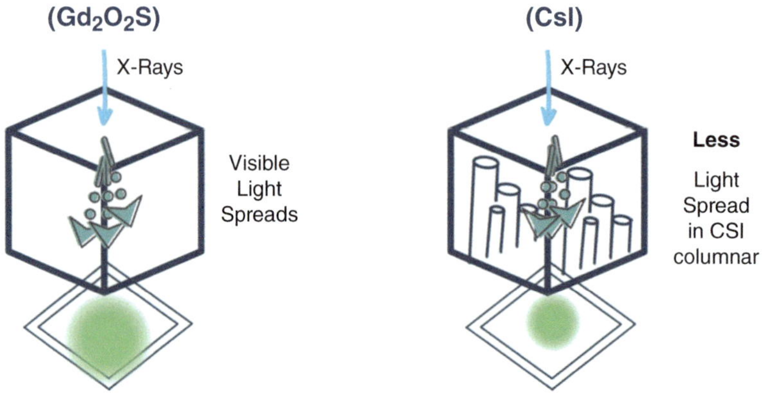

Fig. 5.7 Gd2O2S vs CsI crystals

5.8.2 Choosing the Right Scintillator for Flat Panel Detectors

There are crystals that emit visible light while absorbing X-rays. These are the first component in the production of indirect panels, and they are referred to as scintillators. Gadolinium OxiSulfate, (GOS) and Cesium Iodine(CsI) are the two most commonly utilized compounds for the scintillation layer. While GOS is less expensive and delivers a stronger light output than CsI, the light spreads out and blurs the light signal, which will be tested in later phases. While CsI has a columnar structure, which causes light to follow the columns as it goes through the crystal, it has a smaller light spread. Because of the reduced blurring, CsI-based systems have improved spatial resolution compared with GOS systems.

Furthermore, one sort of flat panel (Indirect CCD type) requires light to be focused down to a smaller size, such as by a fiber optic, in order to be measured on the CCD. GOS's light is likewise more dispersed in the direction, making it difficult to focus. As a result, as shown in Fig. 5.7, CsI is increasingly often used in CCD-type flat panel systems.

Based on the cost against spatial resolution trade-off, both GOS and CsI are appropriate scintillation layer alternatives for general-purpose digital fluoroscopy and radiography systems.

5.8.3 Working Principle of Indirect TFT Flat Panel Detector

"The most typical kind of Digital Fluoroscopy equipment is the indirect flat panel, which is read out with an array of Thin Film transistors (TFTs). TFT flat panels, which share the same fundamental technology as LCDs (Liquid Crystal Displays), are used in many popular flat panel monitors and televisions. Each pixel in an LCD can be turned on and off independently, and each detector element in an X-ray detector may be read out separately, thanks to the TFT array.

Figure 5.8 depicts the early transformation of the incoming X-rays into visible light. Each X-ray is converted into a vast number of light

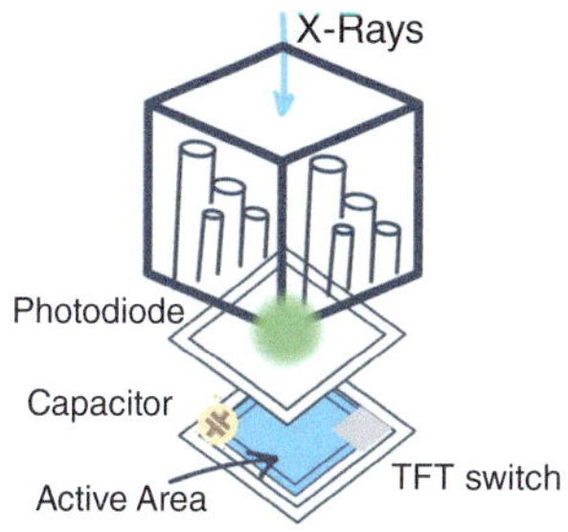

Fig. 5.8 Indirect TFT flat panel detector

photons that scatter as they pass through the screen. As mentioned before, the most prevalent scintillators are based on gadolinium or cesium iodide (CsI). The visible light photons are subsequently counted on a photodiode, which converts the light signal to an electrical signal. Photodiodes frequently employ amorphous Selenium (Si). Electron and hole pairs are produced when light photons impact a photodiode.

The photodiode material (Si) was elected because the light photons emitted by the scintillator combine to form a photocurrent or a current produced by the light energy transferred from the scintillator. The rationale for this is due to material qualities (particularly, the Si bandgap). After the photodiode turns the light into an electrical signal, a TFT (thin film transistor) array is utilized to read out the measured charge. The TFT array is constructed on a glass substrate with silicon acting as a conductor to connect circuit components. Furthermore, silicon dioxide is employed as an insulator in the circuit design to ensure that every electronic component is flat and incorporated into the TFT. Each TFT detector element includes a capacitor to store the charge and a TFT switch or gate to control when the charge is read out. Figure 5.5 depicts the active zone of each detector element (DEL). This is the zone where active change can be deposited. Additional electronics are required, such as a capacitor (to maintain the charge) and a TFT switch (to open when it is time to read the value from that DEL). The ancillary electronics, such as the switch and capacitor, consume space and cannot be as compact as the detection element. As the number of detector elements decreases, the proportion of the DEL that is the active zone, or the fill fraction, decreases. Because the signal is read from the active area, a higher fill percentage is preferable, resulting in a more effective detector because more of the X-rays that travel through the patient contribute to detector readings [32]. This efficiency directly contributes to the dose efficiency of the system. Because we also want to maximize dose efficiency, this factor limits how small each DEL can work efficiently.

Increased fill fraction increases acquisition efficiency. Increasing the fill fraction, on the other hand, has no effect on spatial resolution. Because the effective size of the pixels has a significant impact on spatial resolution, the DEL size must be reduced to increase spatial resolution due to the detector. Any X-ray system's focus spot blurring has an important influence on resolution [36]."

5.8.4 Working Principle of Indirect CCD Flat Panel Detector

"CCDs (Charge Coupled Devices) or CMOS (Complementary Metal-Oxide-Semiconductors), which are commonly used in digital cameras, are another alternative for an indirect flat panel detector. CCDs are well-suited for sensing visible light because they frequently serve as sensors in digital cameras. One additional benefit of CCDs is their capacity to be read out fast. Unfortunately, the size of the CCDs is inconsistent with that of the flat panel detector.

A fiber optic connection can be used as a light funnel to transfer light from the greater size of the scintillator region down to the smaller size of the CCD to connect the visible light from the scintillator to the CCD or CMOS detector, as shown in Fig. 5.9. When compared to the TFT flat screen, there is a slight decline in efficiency since not all of the visible light is directed down to the CCD. Lenses or electron-optic coupling can be used instead of fiber optics to demagnify the signal [37, 38].

CCD and CMOS technology's key advantage is its reading speed, as the electronics in the CCD allow the detector to be read faster than standard TFT arrays. This is notably beneficial for inter-

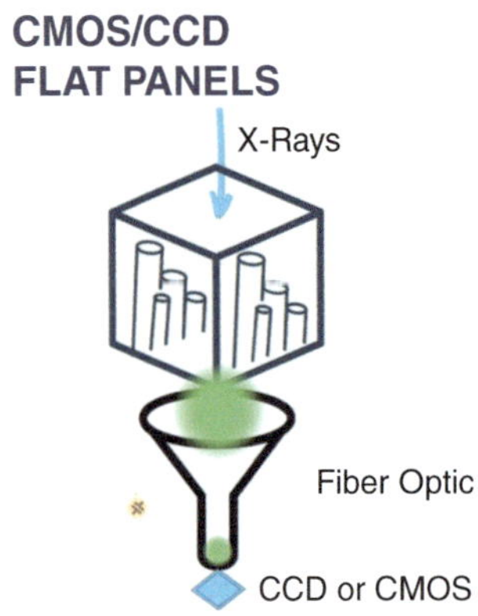

Fig. 5.9 Indirect CCD flat panel detector

ventional and fluoroscopy imaging, which have far higher frame rates (the number of images acquired per second) than normal radiography."

5.8.5 Working Principle of Direct Flat Panel Detector

"To convert X-rays into a measurable signal, direct flat panel detectors employ an entirely separate physical interaction method. The visible light stage required in indirect detectors is bypassed with direct flat panel detectors, and the X-rays are transformed directly into electron and hole pairs. As shown in Fig. 5.10, direct flat panel detectors are designed around flat panels of amorphous selenium (aSe), the substance with which X-rays interact and create electron and hole pairs. CMOS sensors are then added since they may become more common if CCD production declines. Because they are widely utilized, CCD sensors have dominated this industry to date. CCD and CMOS, on the other hand, are related technologies that will be used in an indirect flat panel system that will use fiber optics to funnel down visible light, according to a radiological specialist.

When a voltage is supplied across the detector, electrons move faster towards one side and holes move slower towards the opposite side. The electrons that are directly attracted to the positive side can then be counted. This movement of electrons is also known as an electric current. The captured electrons are then gathered in the active

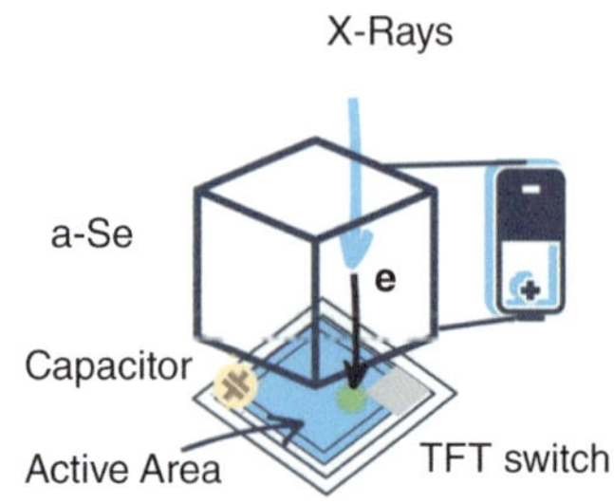

Fig. 5.10 Direct flat panel detector

zone of a TFT array, where the charge is stored in a capacitor for each detector element. The TFT incorporates circuits that amplify and convert an analogue electrical signal to a digital signal. TFTs contain distinct switches or gates at each detector element that allow them to be read individually [37].

The main advantage of direct flat panel detectors is that electrons are not as widely distributed as visible photons. Even when the detector elements are the same size, direct flat panel methods have a higher resolution. The aSe used in direct detectors is less effective at blocking higher-intensity X-rays, such as those used to examine larger patients' abdomens. Direct flat panel detectors are particularly well suited for mammography due to the necessity for exceptionally high spatial resolution and the comparatively weak X-ray beam" [39–44].

5.9 Radiation Dose Considerations and Radiation Protection in Fluoroscopy

While fluoroscopy can provide valuable diagnostic information, it also exposes patients and imaging professionals to ionizing radiation, which can be harmful if not used properly.

Here are some key considerations for radiation dose and radiation protection in fluoroscopy:

1. **Reduce Radiation Dose:** It is critical to use the least amount of radiation necessary to obtain a diagnostic image. This can be accomplished by optimizing the imaging system's technical parameters, such as tube current, voltage, and

exposure time. Furthermore, shielding devices such as lead aprons and thyroid collars can reduce radiation exposure to patients and imaging healthcare personnel [45].
2. **Image Gently and Image Wisely:** These are two initiatives that promote medical imaging safety and appropriateness in children and adults, respectively. They provide recommendations for optimizing radiation dose and employing imaging techniques that reduce radiation exposure while maintaining diagnostic accuracy.
3. **Dose Monitoring:** Regular dose monitoring is required to ensure that the dose remains within acceptable limits. This is possible through the use of dose-tracking software, which can provide feedback on the radiation dose received by the patient and imaging personnel.
4. **Training and Education:** Imaging personnel who perform fluoroscopy should receive appropriate radiation protection training and education, including the safe use of imaging equipment and shielding devices [21, 46].
5. **ALARA principle:** The ALARA principle is a guiding principle in radiation protection that stands for "as low as reasonably achievable." It means that radiation doses should be kept as low as reasonably achievable while taking into account the procedure's benefits and the potential risks associated with radiation exposure [47, 48].

Overall, radiation dose considerations and radiation protection are critical aspects of fluoroscopy that necessitate careful attention and adherence to best practices to ensure the safety of patients and healthcare personnel [16, 49, 50].

5.10 Room Design for Fluoroscopy

Fluoroscopy enables continuous real-time imaging and is commonly used in complex investigations and treatments that necessitate some imaging staff being in close contact with the patient for all or part of the procedure. Others, who do not need to be near the patient, take a seat behind a console. The procedures can be lengthy and involve high doses near the patient. As a result, additional safeguards are generally provided at the table.

The design of a fluoroscopy room is pivotal for the patient and medical imaging technologist personnel's safety as depicted in the fig. A well-designed fluoroscopy room should produce optimum-quality images while exposing patients and staff to as little radiation as possible.

General Guidelines

Overcoach or under-couch X-ray tubes may be used in fluoroscopy systems. Since overcoach tubes are typically operated by remote control from behind a protective screen and have higher quantities of dispersed radiation, this area is under strain. Fluoroscopy remote control equipment may require a smaller examining room and a larger control space. In general, under couch tube systems have higher staff occupancy rates and lower levels of effective dosage from the scatter to imaging personnel. At the tableside, there is usually an exposure control foot switch that should be protected. To prevent unintentional exposure of imaging workers or patients, there should be obvious audible and visual warnings when the X-ray beam is turned on.

In the controlled area, a ceiling-mounted TV display is usually installed so that the operator can view live fluoroscopy images while working close to the patient. As part of the construction or outfitting project, a variety of movable shielding (such as mobile lead screens mounted on the ceiling and lead skirts mounted on tables) should be implemented. Personal protective equipment (such as thyroid collars and lead aprons, for example) should be properly stored in a confined area and have easy access.

Following examinations, patients should have direct access to a toilet, especially in rooms used for barium procedures. It is suggested that changing facilities be clustered together. Radiation shielding estimates for fluoroscopy systems only need to take scattered radiation into account because the principal beam is typically totally intercepted by the image receptor in modern equipment. A second over-couch general tube, however, is frequently placed in fluoroscopy rooms and can be used, for instance, to acquire lateral radiography views during barium examinations. In these circumstances, the room must also be taken into account as a general room, and main radiation shielding must be taken into consideration. Here are some important factors to consider when designing a fluoroscopy room:

1. **Imaging Room size:** The fluoroscopy room should be large enough to accommodate the equipment and medical staff while still allowing for patient movement. To ensure optimum image quality and reduced radiation exposure, the room should be designed to minimize the distance between the X-ray tube and the image receptor.
2. **Shielding:** To protect imaging staff and patients from unnecessary exposure to ionizing radiation, the room should be designed with radiation shielding. To limit the spread of radiation outside the room, shielding materials such as lead should be used in walls, doors, and ceilings.
3. **Equipment placement:** The equipment should be placed in such a way that radiation exposure to the imaging staff and patients are minimized. Positioning the X-ray tube and image receptor should optimize image quality while minimizing exposure to non-target tissues.
4. **Patient positioning:** The fluoroscopy table should be designed to allow the patient to be comfortably positioned during the procedure. The table should be adjustable to accommodate patients of various sizes and designed to limit patient movement during the procedure.
5. **Lighting:** The room should be well-lit to allow for clear visualization of the equipment and communication between medical personnel during the procedure.
6. **Communication system:** To allow staff to communicate with the patient during the procedure, a communication system should be in place. This could be an intercom system or a two-way audio communication system.
7. **Storage area:** The room should have enough space for equipment, supplies, and patient records.

A well-designed fluoroscopy room as depicted in Fig. 5.11 is essential for ensuring patient and

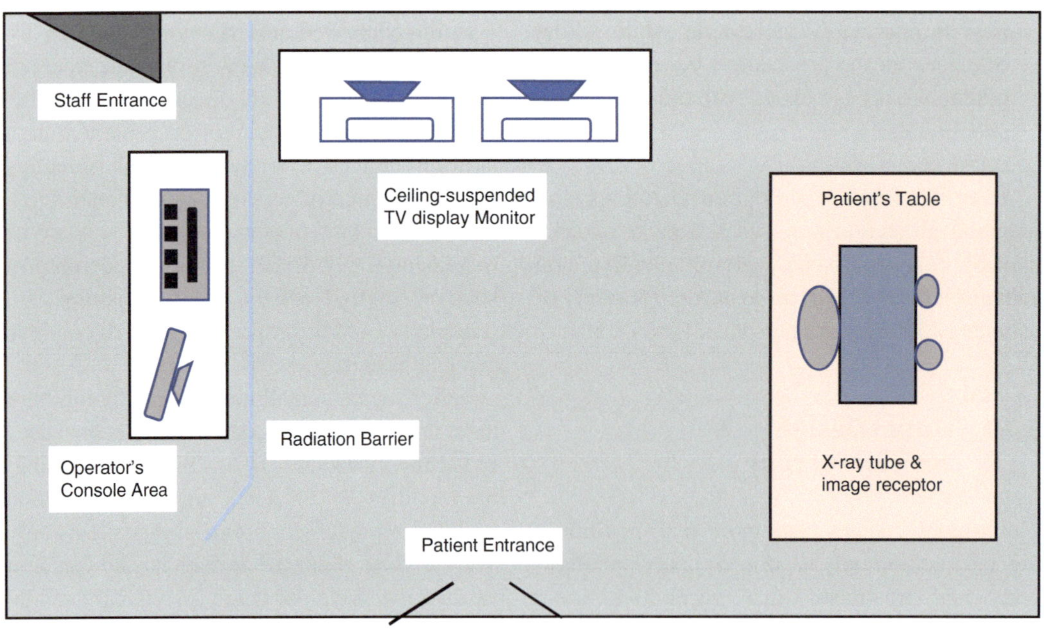

Fig. 5.11 Fluoroscopy general purpose room design

staff safety while maximizing image quality. Radiation shielding, equipment placement, patient positioning, lighting, communication systems, and storage space should all be considered when designing it [36, 51].

5.11 Equipment, Practice, and Image Quality

The image quality obtained during fluoroscopy is critical for accurate diagnosis and treatment planning. Several factors influence fluoroscopy image quality, including:

1. **X-ray beam energy and dose:** The clarity and contrast of the images obtained can be affected by the quality and intensity of the X-ray beam. Higher X-ray energy and dose can provide clearer images but may increase the patient's risk of radiation exposure.
2. **Image intensifier:** An image intensifier is a piece of equipment that converts X-rays into visible light, which is then captured by a camera to create an image. Image resolution and contrast can be affected by the image intensifier's quality and performance.
3. **Camera technology:** The camera used to capture the image from the image intensifier can have an impact on the final image quality. Better images can be produced by high-resolution cameras with low noise levels.
4. **Patient positioning and motion:** Image blurring during fluoroscopy can be caused by patient motion. This effect can be mitigated by proper patient positioning and immobilization.
5. **Image processing:** Digital image processing techniques can be used to improve the quality of fluoroscopy images. These techniques can boost image contrast, reduce noise, and sharpen structure edges.

In summary, several factors influence image quality in fluoroscopy, including X-ray beam energy and dose, image intensifier, camera technology, patient positioning and motion, and image processing techniques. Radiologists, imaging professionals, and treating physicians can obtain optimum-quality images that aid in diagnosis and treatment planning by optimizing these factors.

5.11.1 Image Quality Control in Fluoroscopy

Fluoroscopy is heavily reliant on image quality control. Image quality control ensures that the fluoroscopy system generates images of the highest quality, allowing for accurate diagnosis and treatment planning. Some important factors to consider when controlling image quality in fluoroscopy are as follows:

1. **Image Quality Parameters:** Several parameters influence the quality of fluoroscopic images, including spatial resolution, contrast resolution, temporal resolution, and noise. Regular monitoring of these parameters is required to ensure that the imaging system is operating at peak efficiency.
2. **Technical Performance Testing:** Technical performance testing entails putting the imaging system through its paces to ensure that it meets the manufacturer's image quality specifications. This can be accomplished by testing the X-ray generator, collimators, detectors, and other imaging system components regularly.
3. **Phantom Testing:** Phantom testing entails evaluating image quality using a test object, such as an anthropomorphic phantom or a test pattern. Phantom testing can provide information on image quality parameters such as spatial and contrast resolution, and other parameters.
4. **QA Program:** A QA program is a methodical approach to ensuring that the imaging system is operating at peak performance. Regular monitoring of image quality parameters, technical performance testing, phantom testing, and results documentation should all be part of the program.

5. **User Training:** Image quality control in fluoroscopy relies heavily on user training. Healthcare workers who perform fluoroscopy should receive adequate training in image quality control principles, including the use of test objects and quality assurance programs.

Overall, image quality control is a critical aspect of fluoroscopy that necessitates careful attention and adherence to best practices to ensure accurate diagnosis and treatment planning. Regular monitoring of image quality parameters, technical performance testing, phantom testing, and a quality assurance program can all aid in ensuring that the imaging system is operating at peak efficiency [52–57].

Techniques for Improving Image Quality in Fluoroscopy

1. **Significance of appropriate patient positioning and immobilization:**
   - If a child feels at ease and relaxed (optimum-quality images and shorter screening), they are considerably more inclined to engage.
   - The use of absorbents, sandbags, sheets, or other basic restraint measures with the assistance of attendants is beneficial.
2. **Advantages of proper collimation:**
   - The Light Beam Diaphragm (LBD) can be used to place the patient in an over-couch system.
   - Does away with the necessity for fluoroscopy for positioning.
   - Collimation should be focused on the target region.
   - Don't utilize extremely precise collimation if the equipment has an uncontrolled automatic brightness control (ABC), as this will cause glare, over-contrasted images, and excessively high doses.
3. **Importance of Focus-to-Skin Distance**
   - Position the patient as close to the image intensifier as feasible and the X-ray tube as far away from the patient's table as possible to avoid an excessive skin dose.
   - For optimum image quality and a reduced dose, place the image detector as close to the patient as possible (5 cm) for example the under coach systems.
4. **Anti-scatter Grid**
   - Pediatric equipment, particularly fluoroscopic systems, should have replaceable anti-scatter grids.
   - It is recommended that young children avoid using a grid, which can reduce the dose by up to 50%.
5. **Do's and Don'ts of Magnification**
   - Try to use magnification when absolutely necessary.
   - A field of vision with a diameter of less than 12 cm may result in 4 times the dose of a field with a diameter of 25 cm.
   - Digital radiography allows for post-processing magnification with no increase in dosage.
   - When switching from a wide field of view to a greater magnification, the image intensifier tube's exposure time and the absorbed dose to tissues within the beam increase. Examples:
   - "Field of view, diameter 25 cm; Dose rate = 0.3 mGy/s"
   - "Field of view, diameter 17 cm; Dose rate = 0.6 mGy/s"
   - "Field or view, diameter 12 cm; Dose rate = 1.23 mGy/s"
6. **Exposure factors**
   - Fluoroscopy with a low tube potential (50–60 kV) demonstrates low to moderate contrast studies better, such as those utilising iodinated contrast media or dilute barium.
   - When used with extensive tube filtration of 0.25 mm copper, it can increase quality while decreasing the dose.
   - The dose is proportional to the tube current and beam on time.
   - During the process, it is critical to pay attention to fluoroscopy timing alerts.
7. **Benefits of Filtration**
   - The usage of extra tube filtration may enable overall radiation dose reductions.
   - 0.1 mm Cu should be integrated into all current technologies used in pediatric imaging to lower dosage by 20% without compromising image quality.

- Double-contrast enhanced colon imaging: Adding 0.3 mm Cu may lower the effective dose by 40–45% at 100 Kv tube voltage without affecting image quality significantly.

8. **Automatic Brightness Control (ABC)**
   - In fluoroscopic systems for children, specific kV/mA dose rate curves for automatic brightness control (ABC) should be used.
   - A pre-set regulated tube potential (kV) and variable tube current (mA) with "dose hold" capability should be recommended.
9. **Significance of Pulsed Fluoroscopy**
   - Pulsed fluoroscopy should be standard on all newer technology devices.
   - Variable pulse rates should be a default feature.
   - Using a Grid-controlled pulsed fluoroscopy X-ray tube allows for extremely short exposures, lowering the overall radiation dose to the patient.
   - The lowest pulse rate delivers the lowest dose, depending on whether a compensatory increase in tube current (mA) is used to preserve quality.
   - In some systems, at low pulse rates, the pulse width is increased, resulting in a less significant dosage reduction.
   - Pulse length is lowered from 5 to 20 milliseconds for adults to 2–10 milliseconds for children; pulsed fluoroscopy enables significant patient dose reduction at rates as low as 3 frames/sec.

Advantages of Digital Modern Systems

- Utilizes a low frame rate, lowering the frame rate from 15 frames per second to 3 frames per second, reducing the dose by a factor of 5.
- Using the final image hold and digital spot imaging reduces the dose by 50%.
- Patient dosage reductions are also feasible with cine (digital) and video replay.
- The system stores the most recent cine loop in memory.
- The adult curve is the default characteristic curve on fluoroscopic systems, and it is usually set to 15 f/s.
- Make sure that the application specialist configures the system correctly for pediatric imaging and that the staff of radiology and imaging technologists does not get used to a higher frame rate, which could lead to needless radiation exposure and blurring of quickly moving objects.
- Frame grab technique: During the screening process, the image is taken directly from the image intensifier/digital detector with no additional dose. It is recommended to use this technique appropriately when diagnostic detail is not required [56].

10. **Patient Dose Management Strategy**
    - Document all patient dosing records (adult and pediatric).
    - Following each procedure, the dose data should be noted and checked.
    - The latest patient dose management techniques should be used.
    - As a standard protocol, a calibrated dose area product meter linked with real-time point dosimeters should be developed.
    - While mobile fluoroscopy is useful when a patient is unable to visit the radiology department, it might result in lower image quality and unnecessary staff and patient exposures.
    - Whenever possible, X-ray exams should be performed with fixed units in the Radiology department.
    - Mobile C-Arms should be able to remove the anti-scatter grid and use a calibrated KAP/rate meter.
    - Each imaging technologist should pay special attention to the KAP measurements, fluoroscopic time, and collimation that are displayed.
    - In high-pressure areas such as operating rooms, trained imaging experts should operate C-arms.

5.12 Technological Advancements in Fluoroscopy

Technological improvements in fluoroscopy technology have resulted in improved image quality, radiation safety, and procedural efficiency. Here are some recent fluoroscopy technological advancements:

1. **Flat-panel detectors:** Flat-panel detectors (FPDs) are a relatively new addition to digital fluoroscopy. These detectors provide high-resolution images while emitting low radiation doses, improving patient safety. FPDs are also smaller and more portable than traditional image intensifiers, making them more suitable for use in a variety of medical settings.
2. **Image-guided robotics:** Image-guided robotics (IGR) is the latest invention that guides surgical robots during complex procedures using real-time fluoroscopic imaging. This technology has been used in several surgical procedures such as spine surgery, brain surgery, and joint replacement.
3. **3D printing:** Patient-specific surgical tools and implants have been created using 3D printing for use in fluoroscopy-guided procedures. Surgeons can use 3D printing to create precise tools and implants that fit the patient's anatomy, improving procedural outcomes and decreasing recovery time.
4. **AI-powered image processing:** To improve image processing and analysis in fluoroscopy, artificial intelligence (AI) algorithms have been developed. These algorithms can assist in detecting anomalies in real-time images, improving image quality, and lowering radiation dose.

Overall, technological advances in fluoroscopy have improved patient safety, procedural efficiency, and diagnosis and treatment accuracy.

5.13 Fluoroscopy Image-Related Artefacts

Although fluoroscopy is a valuable diagnostic imaging tool, certain factors can cause artefacts to appear on the viewing screen. Fluoroscopic imaging artefacts are typically caused by image distortions caused by image chain components. The use of an image intensifier creates expected typical artefacts in image-intensified fluoroscopy and photo spot imaging due to geometrical obstacles and internal light scatter [58]. Several common image distortions cause some of the most common fluoroscopy image-related artefacts, including:

1. **Veiling Glare:**
   A common artefact that can occur in fluoroscopy is veiling glare. It is a type of image degradation caused by scattered radiation within the imaging system, and it can result in a loss of contrast and image quality. The following are some important facts about the veiling glare artefact in fluoroscopy:
   - **Cause:** Veiling glare occurs when X-rays scatter within the imaging system, resulting in an increased background signal that reduces image contrast and clarity. This scattering can happen within the patient's body, the imaging equipment, or other components in the imaging environment.
   - **Manifestation effects:** Image quality can suffer as a result of glare, with reduced contrast and sharpness. It can also cause a "haze" or "fog" to appear over the image, which can obscure important details.
   - **Prevention:** There are several strategies for preventing or reducing veiling glare in fluoroscopy. These include the use of collimators and other devices to narrow the field of view and reduce the amount of scattered radiation, the use of high-quality

image intensifiers and other equipment designed to reduce scattering, and the optimization of imaging parameters to reduce radiation exposure.

- **Correction:** Image processing techniques such as digital subtraction angiography can be used to correct veiling glare in some cases. This entails taking two images, one with and one without contrast material, and subtracting the two to produce an image with less background signal and more contrast.

Overall, veiling glare is a common artefact in fluoroscopy, but there are strategies for preventing, reducing, or correcting its effects. It is possible to obtain high-quality images that provide valuable diagnostic information while minimizing the risks associated with X-ray exposure by minimizing the amount of scattered radiation and optimizing the imaging parameters (Fig. 5.12).

2. **Vignetting:**
Another artefact that can occur in fluoroscopy is vignetting, which is more common in systems that use an image intensifier to amplify the X-ray signal. It is a type of image degradation that causes a darkening of the image around the edges, making important details less visible. Here are some important facts about the fluoroscopy vignetting artefact:

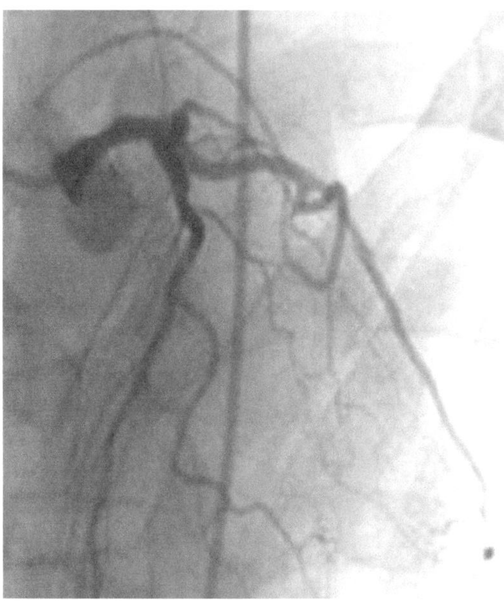

Fig. 5.12 Veiling glare artefact

- **Cause:** Vignetting occurs when the X-ray signal is not amplified uniformly across the image intensifier, resulting in a signal loss at the image's edges. This can be caused by several factors, such as the image intensifier's shape, the position of the X-ray source and detector, and the presence of other components in the imaging environment.
- **Manifestation effects:** Vignetting can degrade image quality by making important details around the image's edges less visible. It can also make measuring the size and location of structures within the body more difficult.
- **Prevention:** There are several strategies for preventing or reducing vignetting in fluoroscopy. These include using larger diameter image intensifiers with more uniform amplification, optimizing the position of the X-ray source and detector, and minimizing the presence of other materials that can scatter or absorb X-rays.
- **Correction:** Vignetting can be corrected in some cases using image processing techniques. This entails using a correction algorithm to adjust the image's brightness and contrast to compensate for signal loss at the edges.

Vignetting is a common artefact in fluoroscopy, particularly in systems that use an image intensifier. However, by employing high-quality imaging equipment, optimizing imaging parameters, and employing correction algorithms, it is possible to obtain high-quality images that provide valuable diagnostic information while minimizing the effects of this artefact (Fig. 5.13).

3. **Blooming:**

Fluoroscopy can produce blooming, which is a type of image artefact. It's caused by an overly bright X-ray signal, which can oversaturate the image intensifier and cause light to bleed into adjacent areas of the image. Here

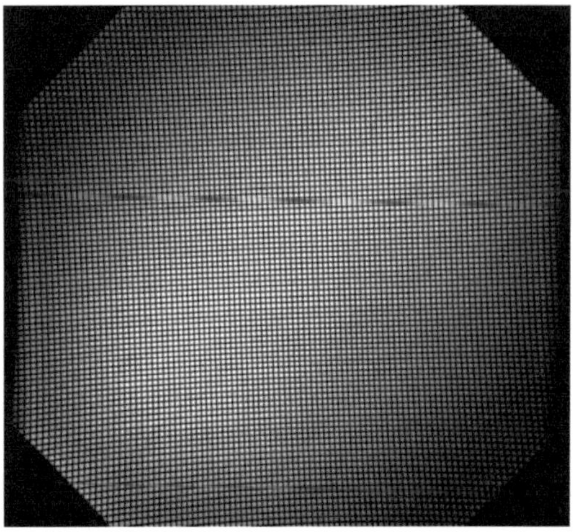

Fig. 5.13 Vignetting artefact

are some important facts about fluorescence blooming artefacts:

- **Cause:** Blooming occurs when the X-ray signal is too intense and exceeds the image intensifier's dynamic range, causing it to saturate. When the X-ray beam is too powerful or the imaging parameters are not optimized, this can occur.
- **Manifestation effects:** Blooming can degrade image quality by reducing the visibility of important details and increasing background noise. It can also cause bright areas to appear around structures that should be darker, making accurate anatomy assessment more difficult.
- **Prevention:** There are several strategies for preventing or reducing blooming in fluoroscopy. Optimizing the X-ray exposure parameters, using collimators to narrow the beam and minimize scatter, and using image intensifiers with higher dynamic ranges are examples of these.
- **Correction:** Blooming can be corrected in some cases using image processing techniques. This entails using a correction algorithm to remove the excess signal from the image's blooming areas, improving the visibility of the underlying anatomy.

Blooming is a common artefact in fluoroscopy that occurs when the X-ray signal is too strong. However, by optimizing imaging parameters, using high-quality equipment, and employing correction algorithms, high-quality images that provide valuable diagnostic information while minimizing the effects of this artefact can be obtained.

4. **Pincushion Distortion:**
Pincushion distortion is a geometric distortion that causes straight lines to appear curved and shaped like a pincushion. The following are some important facts about pincushion distortion artefacts in fluoroscopy:
   - **Cause:** The spherical input phosphor structure and the photocathode electron picture transferred onto the planar output phosphor structure are the two key components that contribute to pincushion distortion. When compared to the centre, the curvature of the input phosphor/photocathode causes more severe distortion and a larger spacing between equidistant points near the image's periphery. Because the curvature of the input phosphor surface is greatest near the image's edges, this distortion is more noticeable when utilising a large FOV. In the image's middle, geometric distortion is reduced.

   The other factor causing pincushion distortion is, when the magnetic fields used to deflect the electron beams in the image intensifier are not uniform, the electrons are deflected more strongly towards the image's edges, resulting in pincushion distortion. This causes the image's shape to be distorted, with straight lines curved.
   - **Manifestation effects:** Pincushion distortion can degrade image quality by obscuring important details and increasing measurement errors. It can also make accurate anatomy assessment more difficult and lead to incorrect diagnoses.
   - **Prevention:** Pincushion distortion can be avoided by using image intensifiers with uniform magnetic fields, optimally positioning the X-ray source and image intensifier, and using high-quality equipment.
   - **Correction:** Image processing techniques can be used to correct pincushion distortion after the fact in some cases. This

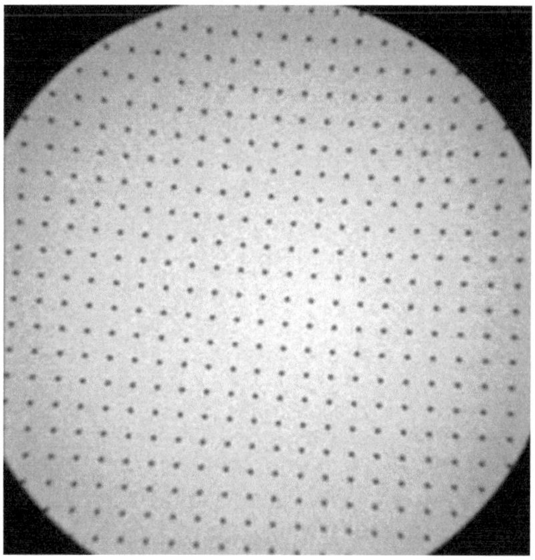

Fig. 5.14 Pincushion artefact

entails using a correction algorithm to map the distortion across the image and correct the line shape. The planar geometry of the scintillator in flat-panel detectors designed for fluoroscopy eliminates pincushion distortion artefacts.

Pincushion distortion is a common artefact in fluoroscopy, especially in systems that use an image intensifier. However, by employing high-quality imaging equipment, optimizing imaging parameters, and employing correction algorithms, it is possible to obtain high-quality images that provide valuable diagnostic information while minimizing the effects of this artefact (Fig. 5.14).

5. **S Distortion:** Image distortions are largely absent in flat panel image receptors. Image artefacts such as S-distortion can occur in fluoroscopy. It is a geometric distortion that causes straight lines to appear S-shaped, with a sinusoidal curve. The following are some important facts about S-distortion artefacts in fluoroscopy:
   - **Cause:** S distortion is a corollary to pincushion distortion caused by the influence of external magnetic fields on electron trajectories from the input phosphor to the output phosphor. As the system rotates, this can cause a time-varying non-linear warping of the image; the distortion can be reduced by shielding it with metal magnetic field attenuators.
   S-distortion occurs when the magnetic fields used in the image intensifier to deflect the electron beams are not uniform, causing the electrons to be deflected more strongly towards one side of the image. This causes the image's shape to be distorted, with straight lines appearing S-shaped.
   - **Manifestation effects:** S-distortion can degrade image quality by reducing the visibility of important details and increasing measurement errors. It can also make accurate anatomy assessment more difficult and lead to incorrect diagnoses.
   - **Prevention:** S-distortion can be avoided by using image intensifiers with uniform magnetic fields, optimally positioning the X-ray source and image intensifier, and using high-quality equipment.
   - **Correction:** S-distortion can be corrected in some cases using image processing techniques. This entails using a correction algorithm to map the distortion across the image and correct the line shape.
   Overall, S-distortion is a common artefact in fluoroscopy, especially in systems with an image intensifier [57, 59–61]. However, by using high-quality equipment, optimizing imaging parameters, and employing correction algorithms, high-quality images that provide valuable diagnostic information while minimizing the effects of this artefact can be obtained (Fig. 5.15).
6. **Motion blur:** The resulting images may appear blurry if the patient or the imaging device moves during the procedure.
7. **Scatter radiation:** When X-rays bounce off an object in the patient's body, they are detected by the imaging device as scatter radiation. This can give the resultant image a grainy appearance.

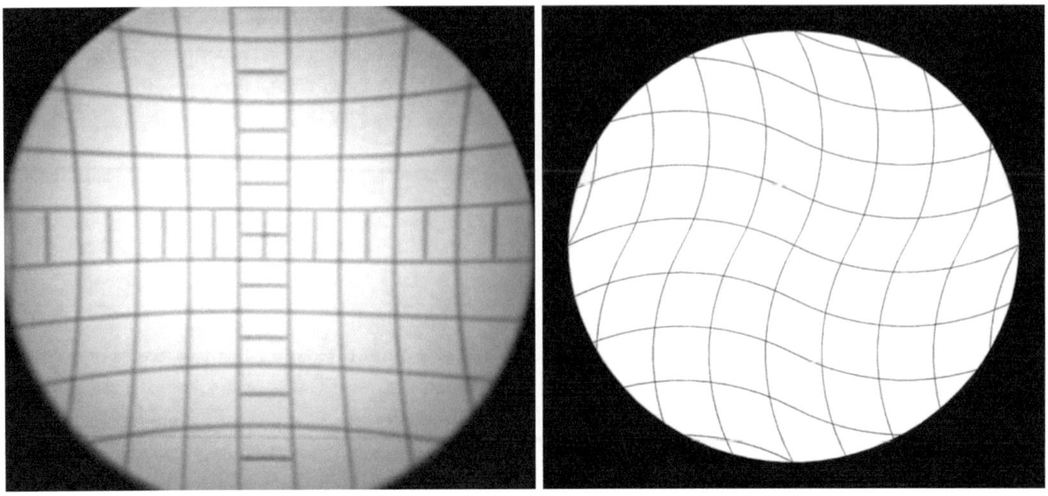

Fig. 5.15 S Distortion artefact

8. **Overexposure:** When too much radiation is used during the procedure, the images produced may be too bright, making it difficult to see details.
9. **Underexposure:** In contrast, if insufficient radiation is used, the resulting images may be too dark, making it difficult to see details.
10. **Dead pixels**: Individual pixels on the imaging device may fail from time to time, resulting in small black or white spots on the screen.
11. **Image lag:** The resulting images may appear distorted or delayed if the imaging device is not fast enough to keep up with the patient's movement.
12. **Grid line artefacts:** Grid lines are used to reduce scatter radiation, but they can sometimes appear on the screen and obscure the image.
13. **Image noise:** Image noise can be caused by several factors, including low radiation levels, electronic interference, or improper imaging device calibration.

To ensure accurate diagnosis and treatment, medical imaging professionals must be aware of these artefacts and take steps to minimize them whenever possible.

5.14 Quality Assurance (QA) and Quality Control (QC) in Fluoroscopy

QA measures to ensure that the machine emits only the amount of X-ray needed to achieve optimum-quality imaging while minimizing the need for repetitive procedures. To ensure the well-being of both patients and imaging technologists, QA testing is undertaken. It also enables scheduled upkeep, which can help to increase the machine's longevity.

QC and QA are important aspects of fluoroscopy imaging to ensure that the images produced are of optimum quality and that the procedure is safe for the patient and the medical imaging staff.

Here are some details about fluoroscopy imaging quality control and quality assurance:

1. **Equipment maintenance:** Regular maintenance of the fluoroscopy equipment is crucial to ensure that it is functioning properly and producing accurate images. The equipment should be calibrated and serviced regularly to ensure that it is working optimally.
2. **Personnel training:** Personnel involved in fluoroscopy procedures should be trained to operate the equipment safely and effectively.

They should be familiar with the safety protocols and techniques for minimizing radiation exposure to patients and staff.
3. **Radiation dose monitoring:** Radiation dose monitoring is essential to quality control in fluoroscopy imaging. The dose of radiation should be monitored for every patient to ensure that it is within safe limits and that the risk of radiation exposure is minimized.
4. **Image QC:** The quality of the images produced by fluoroscopy imaging should be regularly assessed to ensure that they are of high quality and accurate. This can be achieved through regular image evaluations and quality assurance programs.
5. **Patient safety:** Patient safety is crucial to fluoroscopy imaging quality assurance. Patients should be properly prepared for the procedure, and their safety should be monitored throughout the procedure to minimize the risk of adverse events.

Performing quality assurance testing in fluoroscopy varies based on the type of practice and the professional role of the staff namely imaging technologist, medical physicist, or service engineer. Further, it also depends upon the specific policies of the hospital, organization, equipment manufacturer, and geography. The following quality control tests should be performed in fluoroscopy imaging to check for proper functioning:

1. Dose rate
2. kvP and mAs
3. Half Value Layer (HVL)
4. Constancy testing
5. mAs/dose linearity

Typical Scanning Parameters Checked Using the Latest QC Types of Equipment

- "kVp, including waveform plot (R/F sensor)"
- "mAs and mA (mAs sensor option)"
- "Dose (R/F sensor)"
- "Dose rate including waveform plot (R/F sensor)"
- "The max dose rate in automatic mode"
- "HVL (R/F sensor")
- "Time (R/F sensor"
- "Pulse characteristics including pulse frequency and dose per pulse (R/F sensor)"
- "Total Filtration (TF) (R/F sensor)"
- "Grayscale calibration of medical monitors (Light sensor)"
- "Light field intensity and contrast measurements of medical monitors (Light sensor)"
- "X-ray field vs light field position (DXR+)"
- "Tube leakage (Survey sensor)"

Working Principle of a Type RF Sensor Equipment Used for Fluoroscopic Quality Control Test

Connect the detector sensor and turn on the standard base unit.

1. Place the attached sensor in the field, crosshair pointed at the source of the X-ray beam. The measurement result is unaffected by the sensor's angle in the horizontal plane.
2. Expose.
3. Retrieve the result from the base unit. All of the above-mentioned sensor parameters should be gathered during the same exposure.
4. Use the unit software for in-depth analysis.

Local, national, or internationally recognized guidelines, standards, and manufacturer recommendations should all be followed when performing fluoroscopic quality assurance testing. Standards include AAPM (the United States) as an example.

To obtain high-quality photographs during a real diagnostic procedure, a phantom can be utilized to represent a patient's body during exposure. This enables precise measurements of the greyscale, resolution, and other characteristics as depicted in Fig. 5.16.

In summary, quality control and quality assurance are essential aspects of fluoroscopy imaging to ensure that the equipment is functioning properly, the personnel are trained to operate it safely and effectively, and the patient's safety and wellbeing are prioritized [62–67] (Table 5.2).

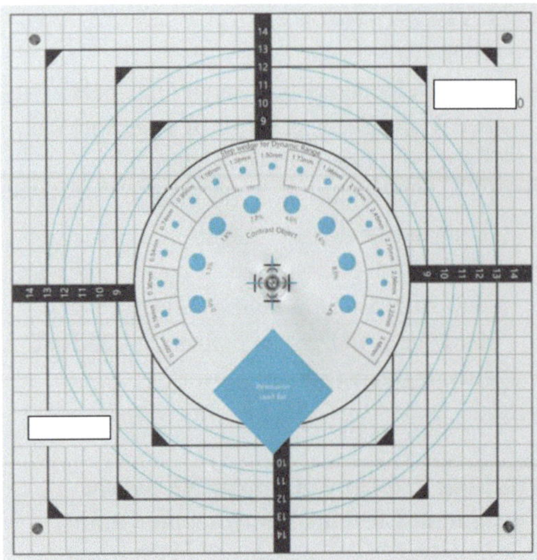

Fig. 5.16 Typical fluoroscopy quality assurance testing device/phantom

5.15 Learning Outcomes

The learning effects of fluoroscopy can vary depending on the level of training and the exact technique being performed. However, some common learning outcomes are as follows:

1. Knowledge of the principles and physics of X-ray imaging and fluoroscopy, as well as radiation safety and dose management.
2. Understanding of the anatomy and physiology of the body part under examination, including variations and anomalies.
3. Understanding of the proper positioning and manipulation of fluoroscopy equipment, including the X-ray source, image intensifier, and viewing system, to obtain optimal images.
4. Ability to interpret fluoroscopic images and identify normal and abnormal findings,

Table 5.2 Fluoroscopic quality control (QC) test summary

Sr. No	QC test	Frequency	Expected results/standard values
1	Equipment Warm-up Procedure	Daily	Warm up the tubes and check that everything is in working order. A fluoroscopy phantom image is comparable to the facility standard.
2	Laser Printer – QC test	Weekly	**1. SMPTE Test Pattern** OD = optical density 0% {patch} - 2.45 ± 0.15 OD 10% {patch} - 2.10 ± 0.15 OD 40% {patch} - 1.15 ± 0.15 OD 90% {patch} - 0.30 ± 0.08 OD **2. Inverted grayscale** 0% {patch} - 2.50 ± 0.15 OD 10% {patch} - 2.25 ± 0.15 OD 40% {patch} - 1.35 ± 0.15 OD 90% {patch} - 0.30 ± 0.08 OD *Note: The 5% patch ought to remain visible just within the 0% patch. The 95% patch ought to be visible only within the 100% patch.
3	Phantom Reading—(Fluoroscopy Video Monitor test)	Monthly	kVp 5%, mA <10% high and low contrast, depending on the phantom utilized
4	Equipment Visual – Quality Assurance test	Initially and quarterly	All test above standard values
5	Lead protective gear test	Initially and annually	No breaks or cracks
6	QC Survey and Quality Assurance Program Review	Initially and annually	As per set hospital standards and guidelines.
7	For spot film and radiography		As per set hospital standards and guidelines.

including identifying potential complications.

5. Understanding of the indications and contraindications for fluoroscopic procedures, as well as the ability to choose the best procedure for a given clinical scenario.
6. Knowledge of medications and contrast agents used in fluoroscopic procedures, including indications, administration, and potential side effects.
7. Effective communication skills with patients, including the ability to explain the procedure, obtain informed consent, and provide appropriate instructions before, during, and after the procedure.
8. Knowledge of the role of fluoroscopy in interventional procedures such as biopsy, drainage, and therapeutic interventions, as well as the ability to carry out these procedures safely and effectively.
9. Understanding of the relevant regulations and guidelines governing the use of fluoroscopy, as well as the ability to keep accurate documentation and procedure records.

Overall, fluoroscopy learning outcomes include a blend of technical skills, clinical knowledge, and patient communication, all to provide safe and effective diagnostic and interventional procedures.

Exercise

Multiple Choice Questions (MCQs)

1. What led to the discontinuation of the shoe-fitting fluoroscope in the 1950s?
   A. It was too expensive to maintain
   B. It provided inaccurate shoe sizes
   C. Harmful effects of radiation exposure in children
   D. Lack of interest from the public
2. Who invented the first fluoroscope?
   A. Sir Wilhelm Conrad Roentgen
   B. Sir Enrico Salvioni
   C. Sir Thomas Edison
   D. Sir Wilhelm Trendelenburg
3. What was the primary purpose of the red goggles invented by Sir Wilhelm Trendelenburg?
   A. To protect eyes from radiation
   B. To enhance the brightness of X-ray images
   C. To adapt radiologists' eyes to perceive faint images
   D. To prevent accidental exposure to X-rays
4. What advancement in the 1950s revolutionized fluoroscopy?
   A. Discovery of calcium tungstate screens
   B. Introduction of digital fluoroscopy
   C. Invention of the television camera and X-ray picture intensifier
   D. Development of red goggles for eye adaptation
5. Which component of the eye is responsible for night-time vision?
   A. Cones
   B. Rods
   C. Iris
   D. Cornea
6. What is the primary function of the image intensifier in fluoroscopy?
   A. To convert X-rays into electrical signals
   B. To convert X-ray photons into visible light photons
   C. To cool the X-ray tube
   D. To reduce scatter radiation
7. What material is commonly used for the anode in a fluoroscopy X-ray tube?
   A. Cesium iodide
   B. Gadolinium oxysulfide
   C. Tungsten
   D. Antimony trisulfide
8. Which component in the television camera tube converts light images into electrical signals?
   A. Input phosphor
   B. Photocathode
   C. Target assembly
   D. Output phosphor
9. What is the purpose of collimators in fluoroscopy?
   A. To capture static images
   B. To amplify the X-ray signal

C. To shape and direct the X-ray beam
D. To convert visible light into electrons

10. Which of the following is NOT a commonly used radiation protection device in fluoroscopy?
A. Lead apron
B. Thyroid shield
C. Fiberoptic bundle
D. Gonadal shield

11. What is one of the key advantages of digital fluoroscopy compared to traditional fluoroscopy?
A. Higher radiation doses
B. Lower image quality
C. Better image storage and manipulation
D. Increased physical storage requirements

12. Which of the following is a feature of dynamic flat-panel detectors (FPDs) in digital fluoroscopy?
A. Slow data transfer rates
B. Frame rates of 15–30 frames per second
C. Use of fiber optics in direct detectors
D. Inability to operate in pulsed X-ray mode

13. What is the primary function of a scintillator in indirect flat panel detectors?
A. Convert X-rays directly into electrical signals
B. Emit visible light when absorbing X-rays
C. Convert visible light into X-rays
D. Store electrical charge for later readout

14. Which of the following is a characteristic of direct flat panel detectors?
A. Use of CCDs to capture images
B. Conversion of X-rays into visible light
C. High resolution due to limited electron spread
D. Requirement for fiber optics

15. What is the purpose of a thin film transistor (TFT) in an indirect TFT flat panel detector?
A. Amplify visible light photons
B. Read out the measured electrical charge
C. Convert electrical signals into digital signals
D. Emit visible light photons

16. What is a key consideration for reducing radiation dose during fluoroscopy?
A. Increasing the tube current
B. Reducing the exposure time
C. Using no shielding devices
D. Increasing voltage

17. The ALARA principle stands for:
A. As Low As Reasonably Achievable
B. As Low As Really Achievable
C. As Light As Reasonably Achievable
D. As Long As Reasonably Achievable

18. Which of the following is NOT mentioned as a factor influencing fluoroscopy image quality?
A. X-ray beam energy and dose
B. Image intensifier
C. Patient diet
D. Camera technology

19. What is recommended for pediatric imaging in terms of anti-scatter grids?
A. Always use anti-scatter grids
B. Avoid using grids to reduce the dose by up to 50%
C. Use fixed anti-scatter grids
D. Use grids to increase dose

20. What does pulsed fluoroscopy help achieve?
A. Increased patient exposure
B. Longer exposure times
C. Reduced radiation dose
D. Continuous imaging

21. What is the primary benefit of flat-panel detectors (FPDs) in fluoroscopy?
A. Higher radiation doses
B. Lower image quality
C. Improved patient safety
D. Increased size and weight

22. What is a common cause of veiling glare in fluoroscopy?
A. Overexposure
B. Patient movement
C. Scattered radiation within the imaging system
D. Uniform amplification across the image intensifier

23. Which artefact in fluoroscopy causes straight lines to appear curved like a pincushion?
A. S Distortion
B. Vignetting
C. Pincushion Distortion
D. Motion Blur

24. What is a recommended method to prevent motion blur in fluoroscopy?
    A. Use of higher radiation doses
    B. Reducing patient and device movement
    C. Increasing the size of the image intensifier
    D. Employing lower resolution detectors
25. What is the purpose of quality assurance (QA) in fluoroscopy?
    A. To increase radiation doses for better imaging
    B. To ensure equipment functions correctly and safely
    C. To minimize patient safety during procedures
    D. To reduce the frequency of equipment maintenance

Short Questions

1. Describe the role of contrast agents in fluoroscopic imaging.
2. Explain the mechanism of action in fluoroscopy and how it differs from visible light.
3. Describe the role of the output phosphor in the image intensifier.
4. Explain the function of automatic exposure control in fluoroscopy.
5. Explain the difference between indirect and direct flat panel detectors in digital fluoroscopy.
6. What are the two types of scintillators used in indirect flat panel detectors, and what are their main characteristics?
7. What are the "Image Gently" and "Image Wisely" initiatives in medical imaging?
8. List three key factors to consider when designing a fluoroscopy room.
9. Describe the role of 3D printing in fluoroscopy-guided procedures.
10. Explain the significance of radiation dose monitoring in fluoroscopy quality control.

Long Question

1. Discuss the historical development of fluoroscopic imaging techniques, highlighting key milestones and technological advancements from the early era to the present day.
2. Discuss the components and working principles of the television monitoring system in fluoroscopy, including the image intensifier and television camera tube.
3. Describe the working principle of indirect TFT flat panel detectors in digital fluoroscopy. Include details about the role of the scintillator, photodiode, and TFT array in the process.
4. Discuss the importance of image quality control in fluoroscopy, including the methods used to ensure high-quality imaging and safe practice. Mention at least five specific techniques or practices that are employed to maintain or improve image quality.
5. Discuss the various types of fluoroscopy image-related artefacts, their causes, and the methods to prevent or correct them. Include examples such as veiling glare, vignetting, blooming, pincushion distortion, and S distortion.

Answers to MCQs

1. C. Harmful effects of radiation exposure in children
2. B. Sir Enrico Salvioni
3. C. To adapt radiologists' eyes to perceive faint images
4. C. Invention of the television camera and X-ray picture intensifier
5. B. Rods
6. B. To convert X-ray photons into visible light photons
7. C. Tungsten
8. C. Target assembly

9. C. To shape and direct the X-ray beam
10. C. Fiberoptic bundle
11. C. Better image storage and manipulation
12. B. Frame rates of 15–30 frames per second
13. B. Emit visible light when absorbing X-rays
14. C. High resolution due to limited electron spread
15. B. Read out the measured electrical charge
16. B. Reducing the exposure time
17. A. As Low As Reasonably Achievable
18. C. Patient diet
19. B. Avoid using grids to reduce the dose by up to 50%
20. C. Reduced radiation dose
21. C. Improved patient safety
22. C. Scattered radiation within the imaging system
23. C. Pincushion Distortion
24. B. Reducing patient and device movement
25. B. To ensure equipment functions correctly and safely

References

1. Williams CR. Radiation exposures from the use of shoe-fitting fluoroscopes. N Engl J Med. 1949;241(9):333–5.
2. Lewis L, Caplan PE. The shoe-fitting fluoroscope as a radiation hazard. Calif Med. 1950;72(1):26.
3. Duffin J, Hayter CR. Baring the sole: the rise and fall of the shoe-fitting fluoroscope. Isis. 2000;91(2):260–82.
4. Rothenberg L. WE-G-213-00: WE-G-213-00: history symposium: radiological physics pioneers: Roentgen and the AAPM Award Eponyms - William Coolidge, Edith Quimby, and Marvin Williams - who were they and what did they do? Med Phys. 2015;42(6Part40):3686–7.
5. DiSantis DJ. Early American radiology: the pioneer years. Am J Roentgenol. 1986;147(4):850–3.
6. Schueler BA. The AAPM/RSNA physics tutorial for residents general overview of fluoroscopic imaging. Radiographics. 2000;20(4):1115–26.
7. Wang J, Blackburn TJ. The AAPM/RSNA physics tutorial for residents: X-ray image intensifiers for fluoroscopy. Radiographics. 2000;20(5):1471–7.
8. Kruger RA, Mistretta CA, Houk TL, Kubal W, Riederer SJ, Ergun DL, Shaw CG, Lancaster JC, Rowe GG. Computerized fluoroscopy techniques for intravenous study of cardiac chamber dynamics. Investig Radiol. 1979;14(4):279–87.
9. Onihashi H, Aida H, No K, Noji T, Murakoshi Y, Ito K, Saito K, Koma J. Flat x-ray image intensifer system for real-time fluoroscopy. In: Medical imaging 2001: physics of medical imaging 2001;4320:509-15.
10. Månsson LG, Kheddache S, Börjesson J, Mattsson S, Schlossman D. Digital chest radiography with a large image intensifier. An ROC study with an anthropomorphic phantom. Eur J Radiol. 1989;9(4):208–13.
11. Kittleson AC, Griewski LR, Whitehouse WM. Two-camera video technique for recording and teaching procedures involving fluoroscopy. J SMPTE. 1966;75(7):652–4.
12. Okkalides D. Assessment of target recovery after TV camera saturation in X-ray fluoroscopy using a personal computer with frame-grabber. Br J Radiol. 1996;69(821):415–21.
13. Luhta R, Rowlands JA. Feasibility of a large area x-ray sensitive vidicon for medical fluoroscopy: Signal and noise factors. Med Phys. 1997;24(5):609–20.
14. Kuon E, Birkel J, Schmitt M, Dahm JB. Radiation exposure benefit of a lead cap in invasive cardiology. Heart. 2003;89(10):1205–10.
15. Durán A, Hian SK, Miller DL, Le Heron J, Padovani R, Vano E. Recommendations for occupational radiation protection in interventional cardiology. Catheter Cardiovasc Interv. 2013;82(1):29–42.
16. Ho P, Cheng SW, Wu PM, Ting AC, Poon JT, Cheng CK, Mok JH, Tsang MS. Ionizing radiation absorption of vascular surgeons during endovascular procedures. J Vasc Surg. 2007;46(3):455–9.
17. Morishima Y, Chida K, Ito O. New radioprotective device that can be used for fluoroscopic exam: possibility to contribute to staff exposure protection during VFSS. Dysphagia. 2022;37(6):1519–24.
18. Cheon BK, Kim CL, Kim KR, Kang MH, Lim JA, Woo NS, Rhee KY, Kim HK, Kim JH. Radiation safety: a focus on lead aprons and thyroid shields in interventional pain management. Korean J Pain. 2018;31(4):244–52.
19. Meisinger QC, Stahl CM, Andre MP, Kinney TB, Newton IG. Radiation protection for the fluoroscopy operator and staff. Am J Roentgenol. 2016;207(4):745–54.
20. König AM, Etzel R, Thomas RP, Mahnken AH. Personal radiation protection and corresponding dosimetry in interventional radiology: an overview and future developments. In: RöFo-Fortschritte auf dem Gebiet der Röntgenstrahlen und der bildgebenden Verfahren. 2019;191(6):512–21. © Georg Thieme Verlag KG.
21. Harstall R, Heini PF, Mini RL, Orler R. Radiation exposure to the surgeon during fluoroscopically assisted percutaneous vertebroplasty: a prospective study. Spine. 2005;30(16):1893–8.
22. Kim KP, Miller DL, De Gonzalez AB, Balter S, Kleinerman RA, Ostroumova E, Simon SL, Linet MS. Occupational radiation doses to operators performing fluoroscopically-guided procedures. Health Phys. 2012;103(1):80–99.
23. Brasselet C, Blanpain T, Tassan-Mangina S, Deschildre A, Duval S, Vitry F, Gaillot-Petit N,

Clement JP, Metz D. Comparison of operator radiation exposure with optimized radiation protection devices during coronary angiograms and ad hoc percutaneous coronary interventions by radial and femoral routes. Eur Heart J. 2008;29(1):63–70.
24. Lange HW, von Boetticher H. Randomized comparison of operator radiation exposure during coronary angiography and intervention by radial or femoral approach. Catheter Cardiovasc Interv. 2006;67(1):12–6.
25. Kim KP, Miller DL, Balter S, Kleinerman RA, Linet MS, Kwon D, Simon SL. Occupational radiation doses to operators performing cardiac catheterization procedures. Health Phys. 2008;94(3):211–27.
26. Yamada R, Saimyo Y, Tanaka K, Hattori A, Umeda Y, Kuroda N, Tsuboi J, Hamada Y, Takei Y. Usefulness of an additional lead shielding device in reducing occupational radiation exposure during interventional endoscopic procedures: an observational study. Medicine (Baltimore). 2020;99(34):e21831.
27. Antić VM. Semi-automatic positioning of the protective screen based on integration with C-arm X-ray device. Nucl Technol Radiat Prot. 2021;36(1):85–90.
28. Koenig AM, Etzel R, Greger W, Viniol S, Fiebich M, Thomas RP, Mahnken AH. Protective efficacy of different ocular radiation protection devices: a phantom study. Cardiovasc Intervent Radiol. 2020;43(1):127–34.
29. Mach JC, Omar A, Barone HE, Harb A, Abujudeh H. Fluoroscopy and MRI induced skin injuries: a review of diagnostic, management, and preventative principles. Curr Radiol Rep. 2021;9(1):1.
30. Johnson RC, Leopold JA, Loscalzo J. Vascular calcification: pathobiological mechanisms and clinical implications. Circ Res. 2006;99(10):1044–59.
31. Zhang R, Niu HM, Guo T, Xie PF, Wu JM, Xie JB, Wang L. Clinical application of special fluoroscopy method in the treatment of distal radius fractures with volar locking plate. Zhongguo Gu Shang= China J Orthop Trauma. 2023;36(2):128–32.
32. Siewerdsen JH, Antonuk LE, El-Mohri Y, Yorkston J, Huang W, Cunningham IA. Signal, noise power spectrum, and detective quantum efficiency of indirect-detection flat-panel imagers for diagnostic radiology. Medical physics. 1998;25(5):614–28.
33. Zhao W, Rowlands JA. X-ray imaging using amorphous selenium: Feasibility of a flat panel self-scanned detector for digital radiology. Med Phys. 1995;22(10):1595–604.
34. Pooley RA, McKinney JM, Miller DA. The AAPM/RSNA physics tutorial for residents: digital fluoroscopy. Radiographics. 2001;21(2):521–34.
35. Sixel KE, Ruschin M, Tirona R, Cheung PC. Digital fluoroscopy to quantify lung tumor motion: potential for patient-specific planning target volumes. Int J Radiat Oncol Biol Phys. 2003;57(3):717–23.
36. Kalender WA, Kyriakou Y. Flat-detector computed tomography (FD-CT). Eur Radiol. 2007;17(11):2767–79.
37. Jain A, Bednarek DR, Rudin S. Micro-angiographic fluoroscope: comparison for different input phosphors. IEEE Trans Nucl Sci. 2014;61(3):1106–11.
38. Krug KB, Stützer H, Frommolt P, Boecker J, Bovenschulte H, Sendler V, Lackner K. Image quality of digital direct flat-panel mammography versus an indirect small-field CCD technique using a high-contrast phantom. Int J Breast Cancer. 2011;2011(1):701054.
39. Kasap S, Frey JB, Belev G, Tousignant O, Mani H, Greenspan J, Laperriere L, Bubon O, Reznik A, DeCrescenzo G, Karim KS. Amorphous and polycrystalline photoconductors for direct conversion flat panel X-ray image sensors. Sensors. 2011;11:5112–57.
40. O'Connell J, Kundu S, Saidaminov M, Bazalova-Carter M. Next generation high resolution perovskite direct conversion detector: Monte Carlo design optimisation and virtual clinical trial. Phys Med Biol. 2023;68(2):025016.
41. Haruta Y, Kawakami M, Nakano Y, Kundu S, Wada S, Ikenoue T, Miyake M, Hirato T, Saidaminov MI. Scalable fabrication of metal halide perovskites for direct X-ray flat-panel detectors: a perspective. Chem Mater. 2022;34(12):5323–33.
42. Miyahara Y, Kitagaki H, Nishimura T, Itakura K, Takahashi S, Yokokawa M, Uchida N, Inomata T. Usefulness of direct-conversion flat-panel detector system as a quality assurance tool for high-dose-rate 192Ir source. J Appl Clin Med Phys. 2015;16(1):121–9.
43. Mizuta M, Sanada S, Akazawa H, Kasai T, Abe S, Ikeno Y, Mitou S. Comparison of anti-scatter grids for digital imaging with use of a direct-conversion flat-panel detector. Radiol Phys Technol. 2012;5(1):46–52.
44. Sharma R, Sharma SD, Sarkar PS, Datta D. Imaging and dosimetric study on direct flat-panel detector-based digital mammography system. J Med Phys. 2018;43(4):255–63.
45. Sturchio GM, Newcomb RD, Molella R, Varkey P, Hagen PT, Schueler BA. Protective eyewear selection for interventional fluoroscopy. Health Phys. 2013;104(2S):S11–6.
46. Sanchez R, Khong PL, Ringertz H. Radiologic protection in pediatric radiology: ICRP recommendations. Pediatr Radiol. 2013;43(8):920–1.
47. Paul J, Jacobi V, Farhang M, Bazrafshan B, Vogl TJ, Mbalisike EC. Radiation dose and image quality of X-ray volume imaging systems: cone-beam computed tomography, digital subtraction angiography and digital fluoroscopy. Eur Radiol. 2013;23(6):1582–93.
48. Boone JM, Seibert JA, Sabol JM, Tecotzky M. A Monte Carlo study of x-ray fluorescence in x-ray detectors. Med Phys. 1999;26(6):905–16.
49. Balonov MI, Shrimpton PC. Effective dose and risks from medical x-ray procedures. Ann ICRP. 2012;41(3–4):129–41.
50. Klingler JH, Hubbe U, Scholz C, Volz F, Roelz R, Beck J, Watzlawick R, Broenner J, Hoedlmoser H, Krueger MT, Hohenhaus M. The impact of imple-

menting a radiation-sparing protocol for percutaneous Kyphoplasty—a prospective Dosemetric study. Glob Spine J. 2023;13(6):1541–9.
51. Elameen EJ, Mohamed MA, Saeed MK, Alameen S, Alamin HJ. Fabricating pediatrics bone tissue equivalent materials for CT quality control evaluation. IJMPCERO. 2025;14(3):75–88.
52. Wu Z, Yang Y, Hu D, Lyu T, Li Y, Tang H, Shu H, Xi Y, Zhang Y, Chen Y. Cone-beam computed tomography limited-angle image reconstruction using planning CT-guided deep diffusion model. IEEE Trans Instrum Meas. 2025.
53. Peng J, Wang T, Xie H, Qiu RL, Chang CW, Roper J, Yu DS, Tang X, Yang X. Optimization-based image reconstruction regularized with inter-spectral structural similarity for limited-angle dual-energy cone-beam CT. Phys Med Biol. 2024.
54. Takiguchi K, Urikura A, Yoshida T, Nakaya Y, Endo M, Aramaki T. Radiation dose and image quality of CT fluoroscopy with partial exposure mode. Diagnostic Interv Radiol. 2020;26(4):333.
55. Tapiovaara MJ, Sandborg M. Evaluation of image quality in fluoroscopy by measurements and Monte Carlo calculations. Phys Med Biol. 1995;40(4):589.
56. Kenny P, Costello D, McCarthy D, Kenny E. A novel quantitative measure of image quality in fluoroscopy. Phys Med. 2020;71:150–60.
57. Monnin P, Viry A, Damet J, Nowak M, Vitzthum V, Racine D. A novel method to assess the spatiotemporal image quality in fluoroscopy. Phys Med Biol. 2021;66(24):245001.
58. Hendee WR. The essential physics of medical imaging. Radiology. 1994;191(3):786.
59. Luo Y, Ma Y, O'Brien H, Jiang K, Kohli V, Maidelin S, Saeed M, Deng E, Pushparajah K, Rhode KS. Edge-enhancement densenet for X-ray fluoroscopy image denoising in cardiac electrophysiology procedures. Med Phys. 2022;49(2):1262–75.
60. Stagni R, Fantozzi S, Cappello A, Leardini A. Quantification of soft tissue artefact in motion analysis by combining 3D fluoroscopy and stereophotogrammetry: a study on two subjects. Clin Biomech. 2005;20(3):320–9.
61. Podsiadło P, Liszka G, Popiela T, Sanak T, Kosiński S, Darocha T. Artifacts in fluoroscopy and changes in radiation dose caused by heating blankets and insulating covers during simulated endovascular treatment. Emerg Radiol. 2021;28(1):9–14.
62. Chida K, Kaga Y, Haga Y, Takeda K, Zuguchi M. Quality control phantom for flat panel detector X-ray systems. Health Phys. 2013;104(1):97–101.
63. Vano E, Gonzalez L. Approaches to establishing reference levels in interventional radiology. Radiat Prot Dosimetry. 2001;94(1–2):109–12.
64. Groenewald A, Groenewald WA. Development of a universal medical X-ray imaging phantom prototype. J Appl Clin Med Phys. 2016;17(6):356–65.
65. Konst B, Nøtthellen J, Nalum Naess S, Båth M. Novel method to determine recursive filtration and noise reduction in fluoroscopic imaging–a comparison of four different vendors. J Appl Clin Med Phys. 2021;22(1):281–92.
66. Spelic DC, Kaczmarek RV, Hilohi MC, Moyal AE. Nationwide surveys of chest, abdomen, lumbosacral spine radiography, and upper gastrointestinal fluoroscopy: a summary of findings. Health Phys. 2010;98(3):498–514.
67. Parelli RJ. Principles of fluoroscopic image intensification and television systems: workbook and laboratory manual. CRC Press; 2020.

Computed Tomography: Physics, Principle of Operation, Quality Control, and Safety

6

Learning Objectives

6.1 An introduction and Overview Computed Tomography
6.2 Historical Perspective of CT
- Pioneering Contributions
- Allan Cormack's Innovations
- Godfrey Hounsfield's Development

6.3 Overview of CT Generations
- First Generation
- Second Generation
- Third Generation
- Fourth Generation
- Fifth Generation
- Slip-Ring Technology
- Spiral/Helical CT
- Multislice CT (MSCT)
- Wide Cone Beam CT

6.4 Advancements in CT Technology
- Dual-Source CT (DSCT)
- Photon Counting CT (PCCT)

6.5 Advantages of CT over Conventional Radiography
6.6 Principles and Working of CT Scanners
- Hounsfield Units and basis for Image Reconstruction
- Beer-Lambert Law and X-ray Attenuation
- Polychromatic X-ray Source Consideration

6.7 Windowing in CT Imaging
- Window Level
- Window width

6.8 CT Instrumentation & Detector Technology
- (i) The Scanning Part: Gantry and the Patient Table
  - X-ray Tubes
  - High-Voltage Generators
  - Collimators
  - Filters
  - Detectors
  - Data Acquisition System (DAS)
  - Gantry Motor and Rotational Mechanism

6.9 Artefacts in CT imaging
- 2D Artifacts
  - Beam Hardening Artifacts
  - Partial Volume Artifacts
  - Motion Artifacts
  - Ring Artifacts
  - Noise
  - Aliasing Artifacts
- 3D Artifacts
  - Metal Artifacts
  - Spiral CT Artifacts
  - Cone Beam Artifacts
  - Zebra Artifacts
  - Staircase Artifacts
  - Out-of-Field Artifacts

6.10 Quality control in CT
- Acceptance Testing for Defect Detection & Establishing Baseline Equipment Performance
- Routine QC for Performance Monitoring & Follow-Up Measurements for Verification
- QC Tests and Their Frequencies
- Quality control procedures
  - Table Travel Accuracy
  - Radiation Beam Width
  - Low-Contrast Performance
  - Spatial Resolution
  - CT Number Accuracy
  - Artifact Evaluation
  - CT Number Uniformity
  - Dosimetry
  - CT Scanner Display Calibration
  - Other Tests as Required by State or Local Regulations
  - Daily Tests
  - Water CT Number and Standard Deviation*
  - Artifact Evaluation
  - Weekly Tests

(continued)

D. Prakash, R. P. Kotian, *Fundamentals of X-ray Imaging*,
https://doi.org/10.1007/978-981-96-7328-5_6

6.1 An Introduction and Overview of Computed Tomography

Computed Tomography (CT) is a revolutionary medical imaging technique that has significantly transformed radiology and healthcare. Initially known as Computed Axial Tomography (CAT) scanners, the term "axial" was later dropped as the technology evolved beyond just axial imaging. CT provides detailed cross-sectional images of the body's internal structures, enabling healthcare professionals to diagnose and evaluate a wide range of medical conditions. Operating on the principle of X-ray absorption, CT employs a rotating X-ray tube and a detector array to capture images from multiple angles around the patient. These images are processed by a computer to reconstruct cross-sectional slices, or "tomograms," of the patient's body. Variations in tissue density result in differences in X-ray absorption, creating contrast in the images: denser tissues, like bones, appear white, while less dense tissues, like organs, appear in various shades of gray.

CT's defining feature is its ability to produce cross-sectional images, providing a three-dimensional view of anatomical structures. These images, often referred to as "slices," allow for precise visualization of organs, blood vessels, bones, and any pathological conditions. Contrast agents, typically iodine-based, can be administered intravenously or orally to improve tissue differentiation and highlight specific structures or abnormalities, enhancing the visibility of blood vessels, tumors, and areas of inflammation.

The term "Computed Tomography" (CT) has evolved through a rich history of development in medical imaging. The concept of tomography, involving imaging specific layers or sections of the body, originated in the early 20th century. Early techniques were described using terms like "body section radiography" and "stratigraphy" (from stratum, meaning "layer"). In 1935, Grossman refined these techniques and introduced the term "tomography" (from the Greek "tomos," meaning "section") [1]. By 1937, Watson had developed transverse axial tomography, producing cross-sectional images, but these early images lacked sufficient detail for clinical use [1].

A significant breakthrough occurred with Godfrey Hounsfield's development of computerized transverse axial scanning (tomography). His work, first demonstrated in 1971 and published in 1973 in the British Journal of Radiology, revolutionized diagnostic radiology [2]. This new technique was initially referred to as "computerized transverse axial tomography," but various other terms emerged, including "computer-assisted tomography" and "computerized axial tomography" (CAT scans). As the technology spread and refinements were made, it became widely known as "Computed Tomography" (CT). Initially, CT scans were also referred to as "EMI scans," reflecting the involvement of EMI, the company where Hounsfield worked. Early CT scanners primarily provided cross-sectional images along a single plane, but advancements in detector technology and computational power soon allowed for the production of highly detailed three-dimensional images. This progression significantly enhanced the diagnostic capabilities of CT scans, making them an indispensable tool in modern medicine. The standardization of the term "computed tomography" was established by the Radiological Society of North America (RSNA) and accepted by the American Journal of Roentgenology [1]. This terminology is now universally recognized and used throughout the radiologic community, highlighting the importance and widespread adoption of CT technology in diagnostic imaging.

CT offers precise imaging capabilities for a wide range of clinical purposes, including head and brain imaging, chest and abdominal assessments, cancer detection and staging, vascular imaging, trauma evaluation, and neurological conditions. CT also guides minimally invasive procedures, assists in pediatric and dental imaging, and plays a pivotal role in oncology, gastrointestinal and urological assessments, orthopedics, sinus and ear diagnostics, and screening programs. It is valuable in medical research and radiation therapy planning by providing accurate anatomical information, enhancing patient care and outcomes.

CT employs ionizing radiation, necessitating careful dose management to minimize patient exposure. Modern CT scanners incorporate dose-reduction techniques and protocols to maintain image quality while ensuring patient safety. The key principles of radiation safety, such as justification, optimization, and dose limitation, are employed in each case. The justification ensures scans are performed only when medically necessary, optimizing techniques to minimize radiation dose, keeping it as low as reasonably achievable (ALARA), conducting scans swiftly while preserving image quality, maintaining a safe distance, shielding patients when needed, and taking special precautions for pediatric and pregnant patients. The cardinal principles of radiation safety—time, distance, and shielding—are also applied when necessary, with special care taken to prevent unjustified or accidental exposures. Staff undergo regular monitoring and training, and machines undergo quality control checks. These practices in CT radiology prioritize patient and staff safety while delivering accurate diagnostics.

Advances in CT technology have significantly transformed medical imaging. Multislice CT (MSCT) scanners enable faster and more detailed 3D imaging, while Dual-Energy CT (DECT) enhances tissue differentiation. Cone-Beam CT (CBCT) is valuable tool in dentistry, and cardiac CT aids in coronary artery disease diagnosis. Low-dose CT with dose reduction techniques reduces radiation exposure, and AI integration automates analysis. Quantitative and functional imaging provide crucial data, while portable CT scanners offer point-of-care convenience. Spectral CT improves material differentiation, and the latest innovation, photon counting CT, provides improved image resolution and contrast by directly measuring the energy of incoming photons, enhancing tissue characterization and potentially lowering radiation doses. These innovations continually enhance CT's diagnostic capabilities across various medical fields.

MDCT scanners have advanced CT technology by enabling the simultaneous capture of multiple slices during a single rotation. Unlike traditional CT scanners that acquire a single slice of an image per rotation, MDCT scanners capture multiple slices simultaneously, significantly improving diagnostic accuracy and speed. This has played a significant role in advancing diagnostic medicine, enabling earlier and more accurate diagnoses and guiding treatment decisions. Ongoing innovations encompass AI integration for improved analysis, personalized medicine with tailored protocols, enhanced quantitative and functional imaging capabilities, and the integration of CT with other modalities. Advancements also focus on reducing artifacts, developing portable CT scanners, and improving spatial resolution. Dose optimization remains a priority, along with research into spectral CT and photon counting CT for better tissue differentiation. These ongoing developments continue to enhance CT's diagnostic precision, accessibility, and patient outcomes.

6.2 Historical Perspective of Computed Tomography

The development of CT imaging is attributed to Sir Godfrey Hounsfield and Allan MacLeod Cormack, who were awarded the Nobel Prize in Physiology or Medicine in 1979 for their pioneering work. With traditional X-ray photographs, structures in three-dimensional space often overlap, making it difficult to distinguish individual components. Additionally, X-ray film cannot provide absolute values for variations in tissue density. The CT imaging overcomes these limitations.

Allan Cormack (23 Feb 1924–07 May 1998), a physicist who worked on cancer therapy at Groote Schuur Hospital in Cape Town, was asked for radiation dose calculations and the method of using conventional X-ray for dosimetry was extremely imprecise (Fig. 6.1). He found the solution and was able to reconstruct a precise cross-section of an object with an irregular shape in a model experiment and this mentioned in his two articles published in 1963 and 1964 [3]. His pioneering work, which involved stating the principles for reconstructing a cross-section of tissues in an organ based on X-ray projections,

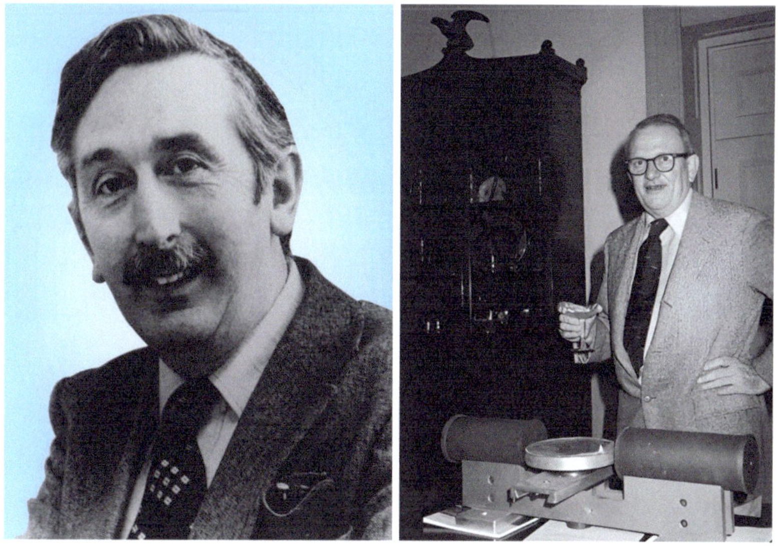

Fig. 6.1 The inventors of CT technology. Left: Sir Godfrey Hounsfield, right: Allan Cormack. (Image courtesy: (**a**) National Institutes of Health and Tufts University, Massachusetts. Reprinted under creative common license)

preceded the actual development by several years and made significant contributions to the development of computer-assisted tomography theory [3]. Although his method had potential benefits, but it was not adopted immediately due to computer limitations at the time.

Godfrey N. Hounsfield (28 August 1919–12 August 2004) on the other hand, living in Britain, was unaware of all these happenings. He initially worked on Radar systems during war time in Royal Air Force as volunteer reservist and rose to the rank of Corporal. Later, he did a diploma from Faraday House Electrical Engineering College, London [4]. He joined Electric and Musical Industries (EMI) in 1951 and worked on Radar systems, got interest in Computers which was still in infancy those days and later transferred to EMI Central Research Laboratories. During the mid-1960s, Hounsfield was exploring pattern recognition of letters. It was during this time that he began to ponder whether he could create a three-dimensional representation of the contents within a box by taking readings through the box at random angles. Hounsfield discovered that it was easier to reconstruct the three-dimensional object within the box as a series of slices, as opposed to treating the content as a whole volume [5].

During a summer vacation in 1967, he met a physician who narrated about the limitations of conventional radiography to him [6]. This was perhaps his first exposure to the challenge of interpreting human anatomy, which he saw as similar to "reading through a box." He began to consider whether it would be possible to create a system that could recognize text in a closed book by shining light across each page from different angles and measuring the resulting output. He simplified the problem of reading a book in three dimensions by dividing it into a series of two-dimensional parallel slices. He believed that with enough data, it would be possible to calculate the contents of a page. By late 1967, he could develop the solution of Computed Tomography reconstruction using simplest possible arithmetic that was compatible with the available computers. All these works were done unfunded, but the idea of "3D x-ray" was generated. By Jun 1968, he initiated for patent disclosure.

He requested funding from the UK Department of Health and Social Security (DHSS) and submitted a proposal and funding request for £10K in August 1968 [6], but it was rejected and advised to improve the scope the work. In October, he submitted a funding application titled "Proposed Project: An Improved Form of

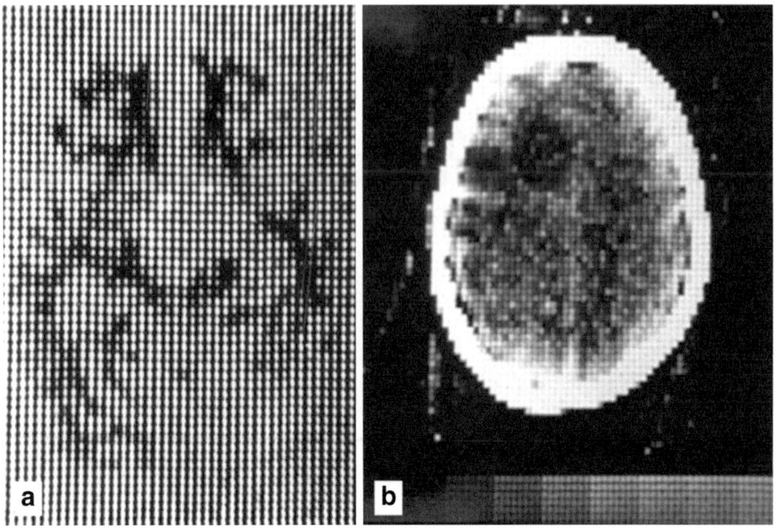

Fig. 6.2 (**a**) Image of brain acrylic model done on prototype CT scanner "lathe bed scanner," (**b**) Brain image of first live patient. (Image © The Nobel Foundation [7] Reprinted with permission)

X-Radiography." The purpose of the project was to explore the use of computers in enhancing information obtained from gamma or X-ray examinations of objects.

On October 28, 1968, the proposal received £2500 DHSS funding and meager funding equivalent to EMI's contribution, which amounted to half of the requested amount. Some additional funding was received later, but despite this, the total funding received was just £69,000 [6]. Incredibly, the first CT image of a live patient was produced in almost exactly 3 years and Hounsfield developed a CT scanner called "the EMI scanner," clinically usable computerized tomography for the head examinations.

Between Nov 1968 and mid-1969, a prototype CT scanner called the "lathe first bed scanner" was created, and the first image reconstruction of a brain acrylic model was generated on 5th Nov 1969 [8]. The first CT scan of a live patient was done on 01st October 1971, under the supervision of Dr. James Ambrose at Atkinson Morley Hospital, London (Fig. 6.2). The continuous development in the technology since then has brought the CT scans which we see today.

Hounsfield was not aware of Cormack's contributions and developed his own method for reconstructing the image. He had a rare combination of vision, intuition, and imagination, and was skilled in selecting the most appropriate physical factors for a challenging system. His findings impressed the medical community with their effectiveness. Later on in 1979, Allan Cormack and Godfrey Hounsfield both were jointly awarded Nobel Prize in Physiology or Medicine.

6.3 An Overview of CT Generations

The development of Computed Tomography (CT) technology can be categorized into several distinct generations, each marked by advancements in imaging speed, resolution, and detector technology (Table 6.1). These successive generations have progressively enhanced diagnostic capabilities, reduced scan times, and improved image quality, cementing CT's role as a critical tool in modern medical diagnostics (Table 6.2).

6.3.1 First Generation CT Scanners

The first CT scanners, developed by Godfrey Hounsfield, are classified as first-generation CT scanners. These pioneering devices played a pivotal role in medical imaging, setting the stage for the evolution of modern CT scanners. First-generation CT scanners utilized a single X-ray

Table 6.1 Timeline in CT technology development

Time period	Event
1963	Particle physicist Allan Cormack established the theoretical framework for CT imaging by publishing research that illustrated the capacity to deduce an object's internal structure from the attenuation line integral passing through it [10].
Summer 1967	Radar operator turned electrical engineer Godfrey Hounsfield met with a physician who conveyed the drawbacks of conventional radiography. He began to think if he could reconstruct a three-dimensional representation of an object from gamma ray transmission measurements taken through the object and used computer simulation to test his theory.
Nov 1967 - Jul 1968	Hounsfield worked on unfunded research to develop his CT scanning theory.
Aug 1968	Hounsfield submitted a project to the UK Department of Health and Social Security (DHSS) requesting £10K for funding.
Oct 1968	Hounsfield submitted a revised and improved project titled "Proposed Project: An Improved Form of X-Radiography." He received fund approval on 28th Oct 1968 for a sum of £2500, with an equivalent amount from EMI [6].
1969	Between Nov 1968 and mid-1969, a prototype CT scanner called the "lathe first bed scanner" was created, and the first image reconstruction of a brain acrylic model was generated on 5th Nov 1969 [8].
1 Oct 1971	The first CT scan of a live patient was conducted at Atkinson Morley Hospital, South-West London, England, under the supervision of Dr. Ambrose, who initially supported Hounsfield by providing a brain acrylic model for testing the prototype "lathe bed scanner" [5]
18 Jun 1973	The first CT scan in the USA was performed at the Mayo Clinic, followed by another scan a month later at Massachusetts General Hospital [6].
Feb 1974	The first whole-body CT scanner was developed and installed by Robert Ledley et al. at Georgetown University, Washington [11].
Dec 1974	Second-generation CT scanners, equipped with 30 detectors covering approximately 10 degrees and a 20-second scan time to reduce motion effects during breath-hold imaging, were installed at Northwick Park Hospital in Middlesex, UK.
Late 1975	Third-generation CT scanners with rotate-rotate only technology, a concept credited to Douglas Boyd of Stanford University, were installed [6].
1975	The first breast imaging scanner was developed by GE and installed at the Mayo Clinic, USA [6].
1977	Fourth-generation CT scanners, developed by separating the CT tube and detectors by John A. Stein and Larry A. Shepp, featured a stationary ring of detectors around the patient with a tube that rotates in the space between the patient and the detector ring.
1979	Allan M. Cormack and Godfrey N. Hounsfield were awarded the Nobel Prize in Physiology or Medicine.
1981	Fifth-generation CT scanners introduced Electron Beam CT (EBCT), an ultrafast scanner with 33–100 milli-second scan duration, paving the way for Coronary Calcium Scoring [6].
1982	A prototype CT-assisted radiotherapy planning system was developed [12].
1986	Electron beam CT machines were enhanced to facilitate more imaging modes such as thorax, abdomen, and pelvis [8]
1987	Introduction of slip-ring technology in CT machines, allowing continuous rotation of the X-ray tube. The first slip-ring scanners were introduced by Siemens and Toshiba.
1989	Helical/Spiral CT scanners were introduced by Siemens and GE [8]
1992	Spiral CT revolutionized CT angiography by enabling volumetric image processing and replacing invasive angiography [13].
1992	Introduction of multi-slice CT scanners, starting with two-slice scanners. The first dual-slice CT scanner (CT-Twin) was introduced by Elscint.
1998	Development of 4-slice CT scanners and Cone Beam CT for dental and maxillofacial imaging [14].
1998	Development of grid control rotating anode for angiography by Toshiba [15]
2002	Introduction of 16-slice CT scanners.

(continued)

Table 6.1 (continued)

Time period	Event
2002	High-speed rotational bearing rotating anode tube for angiography [16]
2003	Siemens introduced a rotating frame tube, enabling fast focal track speeds and improved CT imaging [17].
2005	Development of 64-slice CT scanners
2005	GE introduces the largest commercial anode with carbon backing, prioritizing efficiency in CT imaging with a diameter of 238 mm [18].
2006	Introduction of STATRON x-ray tube by Siemens.
2006	Dual Source CT machines were introduced [8]
2007	Introduction of 128-slice and 256-slice CT scanners.
2007	Philips introduces the iMRC® tube with segmented metal anode and spiral-groove bearings, enhancing power density in CT scans [18].
2008	Development of 320-slice CT scanners.
2013	Introduction of Spectral CT imaging by Philips, which allows differentiation of materials based on their energy-dependent attenuation [19]
2014	Development of iterative reconstruction techniques to significantly reduce radiation dose while maintaining image quality [20]
2018	GE unveils the Quantix 160® X-ray tube with groundbreaking cathode technology for spectral CT imaging, allowing rapid tube current adjustment [21].
2019	AI-powered CT scanners by various manufacturers to enhance image quality, reduce noise, and assist in diagnostic interpretation [22]
Mid-2010s and USFDA approval in 2021	Photon Counting CT machines were developed. Although a prototype system with a 15 cm field of view was introduced by GE in 2007, they gained USFDA approval in 2021 [8]

Table 6.2 Generation wise key differences in CT technology

CT generation/ model advancement	Introduction year	Key features
First	Oct 1971	Translate and rotate with single detector and pencil beam. Scan time: 5.5 minutes, 10-mm slices Completed scan of 10 slices took about 30 minutes to acquire and same time to reconstruct [23] Reconstruct image with 80 × 80 matrix 1° incremental move
Second	Dec 1974	Translate and rotate with multiple detector and small fan beam. Scan time: 20 second 256 × 256 image matrix 6° incremental move
Third	Late 1975	Rotate-rotate only with fan beam. Scan time: 5 second Currently used multi-detector CTs work on modified version of this generation CT machines
Fourth	Concept in March 1976, Shipped first unit in 1977 to Columbia University [6]	Rotate-stationary - Detector stationery in a ring with tube rotates in space between the patient and the detector ring. Scan time: 5 seconds Sub-mm in-plane resolution, 512 × 512 image matrix, and; Slices as thin as 2 mm

(continued)

Table 6.2 (continued)

CT generation/ model advancement	Introduction year	Key features
Fifth generation	1981 [6] Proposal in 1979 [24]	Electron Beam CT machine Scan time: 33–100 ms Designed mainly for cardiac imaging. No moving parts
Spiral or helical CT	1987	Slip ring technology Eliminated of the step-and-shoot scan mode and the resultant inter-scan delay Savings of contrast agent, and Reduction of motion artifact or spatial mis-registration.
Multi-detector CT (MDCT)	Introduction in 1992	Started with twin-slice CT scanner offered by Elscint (Elscint TWIN) in 1992 4-slice scanner in 1998 16-slice scanner in 2002 64-slice scanner in 2005 128-slice scanner in 2007 256-slice scanner in 2007, and 320-slice scanner in 2008
Cone beam CT	Introduced in late 1990s and approved by the FDA for use in the United States in 2001 [25]	Used for dental and maxillofacial imaging. Allows panoramic imaging. Provides high quality, accurate 3D representation of the osseous elements of the maxillofacial region.
Dual-energy CT	2008	Dual-source-dual-detector CT Scan mode at dual peak energies to conduct advanced clinical applications for material differentiation with spectral resolution.
Photon counting CT	Early prototypes in the mid-2010s USFDA Approval 30 Sep 2021	Utilizing a direct conversion X-ray detector [26], Suppressed electronic noise [27] Simultaneous single-tube-potential [28–30]. Multi-energy imaging [28–30] High spatial resolution without loss of dose efficiency [31–33] Radiation dose reduction compared with energy-integrating detector (EID) CT for the same image quality [33, 34] Improved iodine contrast-to-noise ratio [35]

tube and one sodium iodide scintillator detector, arranged in a "translate-and-rotate" mechanism (Fig. 6.3). The X-ray tube and detector would rotate around the patient and simultaneously move linearly along the patient's body to collect data. This method involved taking 180 views over 180 degrees, with the tube and detector translating linearly and then rotating in 1-degree increments (Fig. 6.4). On October 1, 1971, this system acquired two continuous slices per scan, each with an 80x80 matrix of 3 mm × 3 mm × 13 mm voxels, in about 5.5 minutes from a live patient [9]. Image reconstruction in these early scanners relied on the back-projection technique, which was instrumental in pro-

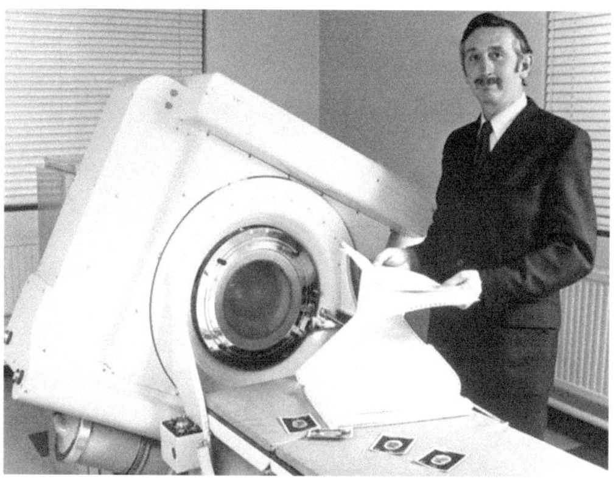

Fig. 6.3 Sir Godfrey N Hounsfield stands beside the EMI-Scanner in 1972. (Image courtesy: European Society of Musculoskeletal Radiology—ESSR. Reprinted with permission)

ducing the initial cross-sectional images of the body.

Despite relatively low image resolution and quality, first-generation CT scanners marked a historic milestone by enabling non-invasive visualization of internal structures and significantly advancing diagnostic capabilities in the medical field. Subsequent generations of CT scanners built upon these foundations, leading to enhanced speed, image quality, and expanded clinical applications.

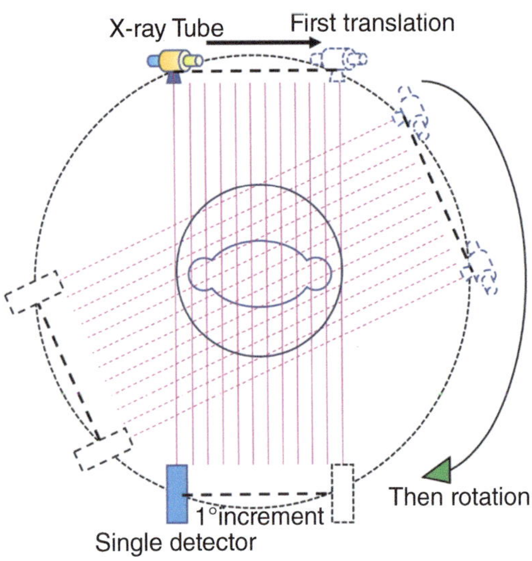

Fig. 6.4 First generation CT Scanners: Narrow beam with translate-rotate motion

6.3.2 Second Generation CT Scanners

Introduced in late 1974, the second-generation CT scanners aimed to reduce data acquisition time, making CT scans quicker and more efficient by increasing the number of detectors while retaining the "translate-and-rotate" motion. By late 1975, the number of detectors increased to 30, reducing acquisition time to 20 seconds. The X-ray tube and detector assembly moved in discrete steps, typically around 6 degrees per step instead of 1 degree (Fig. 6.5). Despite improvements, second-generation CT scanners faced challenges related to the heavy X-ray tube and rapid translational and rotational movements, leading to frequent misalignments and significant image artifacts, which compromised diagnostic quality. This need for improvement paved the way for third-generation CT scanners.

6.3.3 Third Generation CT Scanners

In late 1975, third-generation CT scanners were introduced to eliminate translational motion, relying solely on rotational motion. These scanners featured a fan-beam X-ray covering the entire field of view and used an array of detectors (Fig. 6.6). The acquisition process took less than 5 seconds [9]. During scanning, the X-ray tube

Fig. 6.5 Second generation CT scanners: Multiple-narrow beams with translate-rotate motion

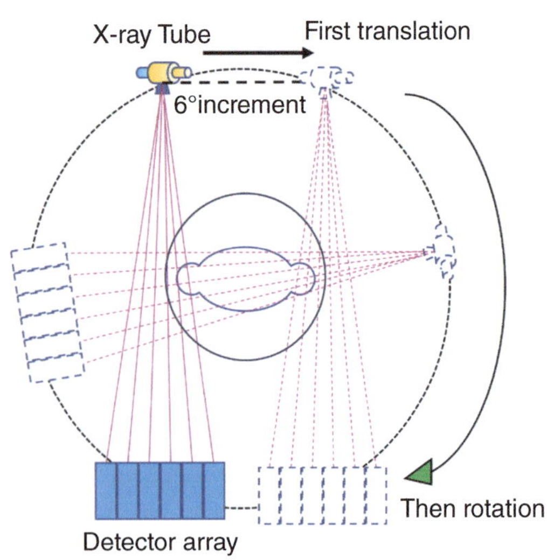

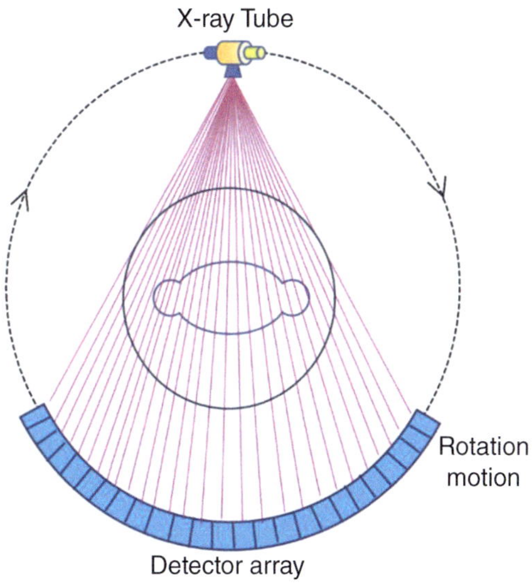

Fig. 6.6 Third generation CT Scanners: Fan-beam, rotate-rotate only

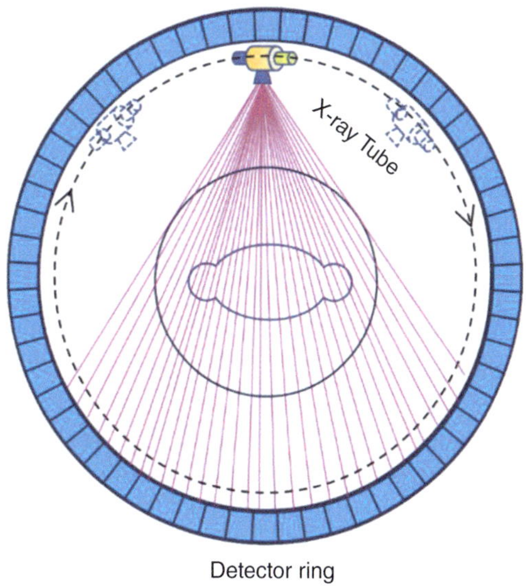

Fig. 6.7 Fourth generation CT Scanners: Fan-beam with stationary circular detector

and detector assembly rotated around the patient without relative movement to each other.

However, these models again had some limitations. They supplied power supply to the X-ray tube with electric cables which restricted the continuous circular motion, forcing the scanner to move clockwise and counterclockwise to acquire adjacent slices. The heavy gantry's continuous acceleration and deceleration limited the scan speed to approximately 2 seconds per rotation, resulting in detector stability issues and image artifacts. These limitations led to the investigation of the 4th generation of CT scanners. Although the third-generation scanners became very popular, today's modern multi-slice CT (MSCT) scanners are still based on the third generation only. However, they feature hardware refinements such as slip-ring technology and multiple-detector rows.

Though the Varian System introduced slip ring in 1976 with third generation CT scanners which supported continuous gantry rotation and transferred high-voltage power, but they had small diameter of slip ring and transferred high power unlike modern CT scanner slip rings that transfer power at low voltage and have a compact high voltage power supply on the gantry [6], but this constant rotation and the ability to perform half-scan reconstructions enabled dynamic scanning with sub-3-second temporal resolution.

6.3.4 Fourth Generation CT Scanners

The fourth generation of CT scanners was first introduced in 1976 and the first unit was shipped to Columbia University in 1977 [4]. These scanners featured an enclosed stationary detector ring with a rotating X-ray tube inside it, achieving scan durations of about 1 second (Fig. 6.7) [5]. However, the tube required a large ring of 170–180 cm to maintain sufficient tube-patient distance. The full-circle detector ring increased the cost of the scanner considerably. Despite spatial resolution improvements to around 4 mm, scatter correction problems remained unsolved in this generation.

6.3.5 Fifth Generation CT Scanners

Proposed in 1979 [24] and introduced in 1981 [6], Electron Beam CT (EBCT) scanners enabled ultrafast scanning with durations between 33 and

100 milliseconds [6], pioneering Coronary Calcium Scoring. The system had no mechanically moving part and was sealed in a vacuum, similar to cathode-ray tubes (Fig. 6.8). The high-speed electron beam is focused and deflected by carefully built coils to sweep around the target ring. The fan-beam X-rays are produced and collimated to the set of detectors positioned in an arc of 216 degrees with 8 cm of coverage along the patient axis is obtained for the heart. Later in 1986, the Electron beam CT machine was added to facilitate more imaging modes such as thorax, abdomen, and pelvis [8]. However, the higher equipment cost and poor image quality for general imaging limit the use of EBCTs.

6.3.6 Slip-Ring Technology

Prior to 1987, CT scanners relied mostly on cables to power the X-ray tubes and transmit detector signals [9]. This setup necessitated a stop in rotation after every 360 degrees, requiring the cables to be looped onto a drum, released during a single rotation, and then spooled back in the opposite direction. This process was time-consuming, taking at least 8–10 seconds for each cycle, with only 1–2 seconds dedicated to data acquisition. As a result, the temporal resolution was poor, which led to longer procedural duration. The modern CT scanner slip rings that transfer power at low voltage and have a compact high voltage power supply on the gantry, was introduced in 1987, which eliminated interscan delays and allowed for continuous nonstop rotation. The slip ring is a circular ring that transfers power and data signals from the stationery to the rotating part of the scanner (Fig. 6.9).

It marked a significant advancement in imaging capabilities and revolutionized the way data and power was transmitted from the rotating X-ray tube to the detectors. This innovation enabled the development of helical or spiral CT scanning, where the X-ray tube and detectors rotate continuously as the patient moves through the scanner, creating detailed 3D images. Slip-ring technology

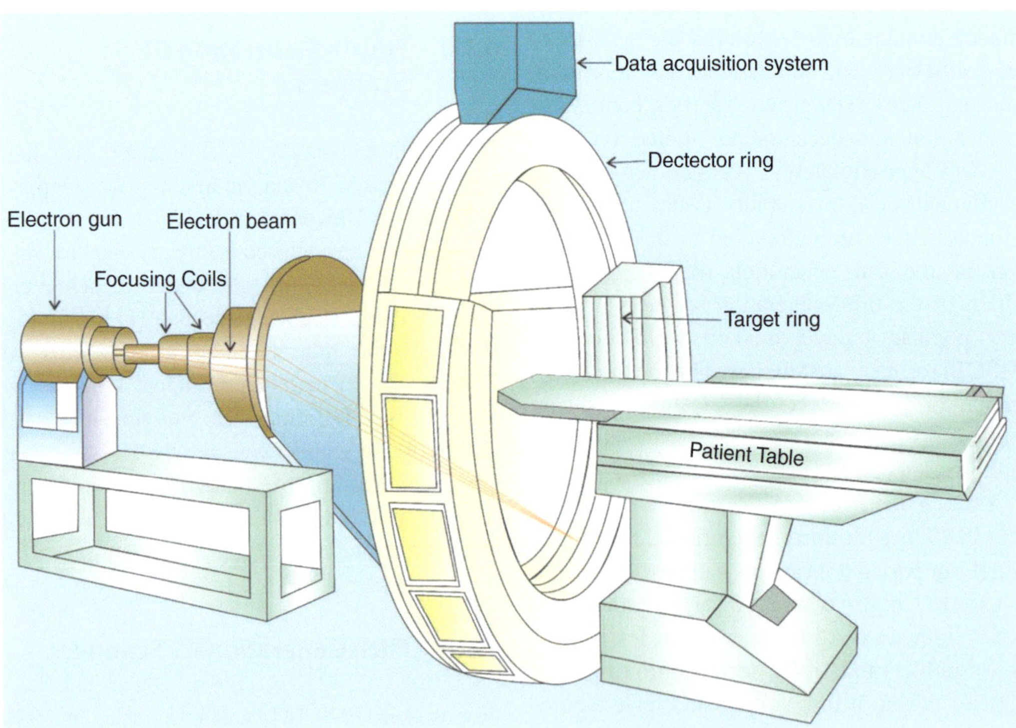

Fig. 6.8 Electron beam CT scanners

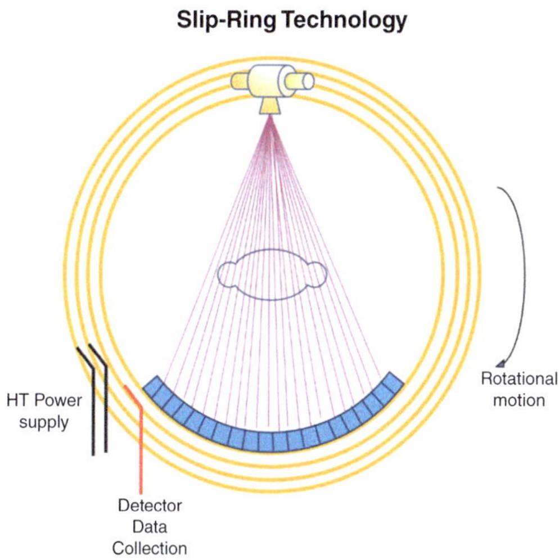

Fig. 6.9 Slip ring technology

greatly improved imaging speed, efficiency, and image quality, making it a foundational element in modern CT scanning technology.

6.3.7 Spiral/Helical CT

The development of slip ring technology led to the creation of spiral or helical CT scanners. There is no practical or technical difference between the two terms; it is simply a matter of how the manufacturer chooses to name the technology. The first of these scanners was introduced in 1990, but it took two more years for it to gain clinical acceptance [26]. In a conventional CT scanner, the X-ray beam is rotated in a circular motion around the patient or object to capture attenuation profiles from multiple angles, which are then used to generate various image planes. The object is then moved slightly within the gantry for the next measurement, and this process is repeated until high-quality images have been created slice by slice. This imaging method is known as axial imaging or the step-and-shoot method, and it takes a long time to complete. During the scan, the patient must remain still to avoid motion artifacts and blurry images. However, shorter scan durations are necessary to prevent motion-related artifacts, which led to the development of spiral (or helical) CT scanners.

In spiral CT scanners, the object is moved continuously through the gantry in the Z-direction, while the X-ray tube and detector assembly move in a circular, rotatory motion in the XY plane to capture images continuously (Fig. 6.10). A single data set represents the volume covered in a specific number of spiral turns. Spiral CT scanners allowed physicians to image entire organs in a single breath-hold.

6.3.8 The Concept of Pitch

In helical CT scans, the concept of "pitch" is used to determine the speed of table movement and the thickness of the slice being scanned. It is calculated by dividing the distance travelled by the table in one 360° gantry rotation by the beam collimation.

Pitch Formula (Single Slice CT)

$$\textbf{Pitch} = \frac{\text{Table Movement per Rotation}}{\text{Slice Thickness}}$$

Pitch Formula (Multi-slice CT)

$$\textbf{Pitch} = \frac{\text{Table Movement per Rotation}}{\text{Number of Slices} \times \text{Slice Thickness}}$$

Where:

- **Table Movement per Rotation** refers to the distance the CT table moves during one complete rotation of the X-ray tube around the patient.
- **Number of Slices** is the number of slices or detectors in the z-axis direction that are simultaneously acquired in one rotation.
- **Slice Thickness** is the thickness of each individual slice being imaged.

The Pitch has no unit.

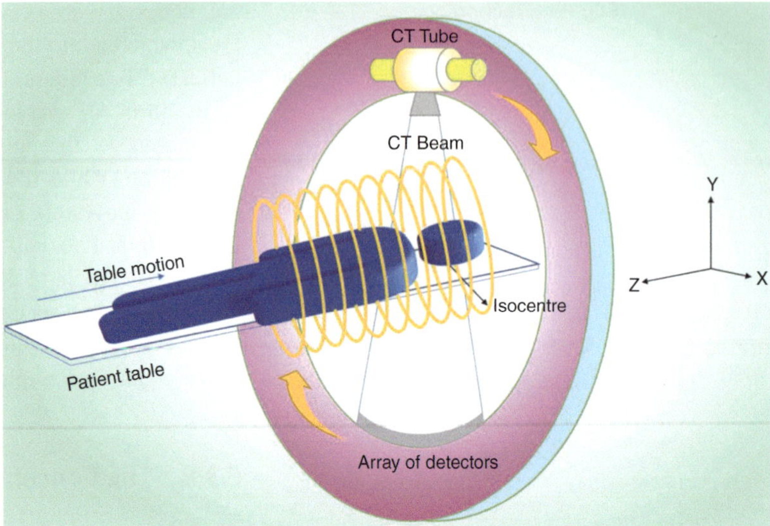

Fig. 6.10 Spiral CT scanners

Practical Examples of Pitch

1. **Pitch = 1:**
   - If the table moves 5 mm per rotation and the slice thickness is 5 mm, then the pitch is 1.
   - This means the table advances exactly one slice thickness per rotation, ensuring the entire X-ray helix is covered without gaps or overlaps.
2. **Pitch > 1:**
   - If the table moves 7.5 mm per rotation and the slice thickness is 5 mm, then the pitch is 1.5.
   - This results in a gap in the X-ray helix, meaning less overlap of X-ray beams. This can speed up the scan and reduce radiation exposure but may compromise image quality due to reduced data density.
3. **Pitch < 1:**
   - If the table moves 4 mm per rotation and the slice thickness is 5 mm, then the pitch is 0.8.
   - This causes an overlap in X-ray exposure, increasing the data density and improving image quality, but also increasing radiation exposure to the patient.

Importance of Pitch

The pitch value affects both the speed of the scan and the quality of the images produced:

- **High Pitch (>1)**: Faster scans, lower radiation dose, but potentially lower image quality due to gaps in data.
- **Low Pitch (<1)**: Slower scans, higher radiation dose, but potentially higher image quality due to more overlap and denser data acquisition.

Balancing pitch is essential for optimizing the trade-off between image quality and radiation exposure. Common pitch values typically range from 0.7 to 1.5, depending on the clinical requirements of the scan.

6.3.9 Multi-slice CTs

The evolution of multi-slice CT (MSCT) technology, also referred to as multiple-detector-row CT (MDCT), marks significant advancements in medical imaging. The concept of MSCT was initially introduced in 1992 with the development of twin CT systems, but it wasn't until late 1998 that the first modern MSCT scanners were introduced [36]. These advanced scanners feature a rotating arc of detectors along with the X-ray tube(s), which allows for volumetric data acquisition using thin slices, thereby improving image resolution and scan efficiency.

In these systems, the detectors are arranged in multiple rows along the z-axis, which is the axis along the length of the patient's body. The earliest MSCT scanners included 16 rows of detector elements, each with a width of either 1.25 mm or 1 mm, providing a total coverage of 20 mm along the z-axis. Manufacturers offered various combinations of detector widths, such as 1.25 mm, 2.5 mm (1.25 mm × 2), 5 mm (1.25 mm × 4), 10 mm (2.5 mm × 4), and 20 mm (5 mm × 4), to form 4-slice data channels, as handling data from 16 slices simultaneously was challenging at the time [36].

The capabilities of MSCT scanners expanded rapidly. Between 2003 and 2004, the market saw the introduction of 6-, 8-, 16-, 32-, and 40-slice models [36]. By 2005, 64-slice models had become available, offering total z-axis coverage of 32–40 mm, depending on slice thicknesses ranging from 0.5 mm to 0.625 mm [36]. These advancements allowed for faster scans and more detailed images. In the years 2007 and 2008, even more advanced models were released, including 128-, 256-, and 320-slice CT scanners, as well as dual-source CT scanners, which could cover up to 16 cm along the z-axis [20].

By 2012, Toshiba Medical (now Canon Medical Systems) introduced a digitally enhanced 640-slice CT scanner. This innovation utilized double-slice technology and the coneXact™ reconstruction algorithm, which improved image quality, although the z-axis coverage remained at 16 cm [37].

Today, the most commonly available CT scanners are those with 16-, 32-, 40-, 64-, and 128-slice configurations. The less commonly available 256- and 320-slice CT scanners are more costly but offer superior imaging capabilities [38]. These advancements allow for the simultaneous acquisition of images of entire organs, such as the heart, brain, blood vessels, and joints, thanks to their larger z-coverage. The best in-plane spatial voxel dimensions reported for state-of-the-art MSCT scanners are between 0.23 mm and 0.4 mm, with z-direction voxel dimensions around 0.3 mm, indicating their high precision and resolution [38]. These technological improvements in MSCT have revolutionized medical imaging by providing faster, more detailed, and higher quality scans, which are crucial for accurate diagnosis and treatment planning.

6.3.10 Wide Cone Beam CT

Wide Cone Beam Computed Tomography (CBCT) is an enhancement of multi-slice CT (MSCT) systems, utilizing a wider X-ray beam and larger detector arrays to capture volumetric data more efficiently. This technology is particularly beneficial for applications requiring comprehensive three-dimensional imaging with high resolution and reduced scan times.

The MSCT enables organ coverage with isotropic spatial resolution, which is crucial for temporally sensitive clinical applications such as coronary computed tomography angiography (CCTA) and traditional 64-row scanners can produce good CCTA images, but their quality is highly dependent on patient heart rate and stability [39]. The typical dimensions of an adult heart include a length of approximately 12 centimeters from base to apex, a width ranging between 8 and 9 centimeters at its broadest transverse diameter, and a depth of about 6 centimeters from anterior to posterior [40]. Covering the entire heart, typically requires multiple rotations and cardiac cycles. Techniques such as step-and-shoot mode and multisector reconstruction have been employed to achieve low-dose cardiac imaging, but they face limitations when dealing with high and variable heart rates [39].

Wide Cone Beam CT addresses these issues by using a large coverage detector that captures the entire heart in a single cardiac cycle and eliminates inconsistencies in cardiac phase and significantly improves image quality [39]. This technology allows for the collection of imaging data within a single heart cycle, ensuring consistent cardiac phase data and suspending X-ray exposure until a regular heart rate is detected, thus achieving excellent image quality despite heart rate instability.

Beyond CCTA, wide cone beam CT provides clinical benefits in volume perfusion and dose reduction. A larger coverage detector enables faster *z*-axis coverage, minimizing patient motion-related issues and relaxing the breath-hold requirement for adults and sedation for pediatric patients. Studies have demonstrated excellent image quality even at high heart rates using wide cone CT systems.

However, wide cone beam CT systems face technical challenges, particularly with scattered radiation and artifacts from large cone angles. The scatter-to-primary ratio increases almost linearly with *z*-axis coverage, necessitating proper compensation through hardware design or algorithmic corrections. For instance, 2D focusing post-patient collimation can effectively reduce scattered radiation along the *z*-axis, significantly suppressing image artifacts.

Additionally, handling artifacts associated with the large cone angle is complex. In step-and-shoot mode, missing frequency-domain information and redundant data from half-scan acquisitions can lead to artifacts. Advanced reconstruction algorithms are essential to compensate for both missing frequency and redundant samples, ensuring accurate image quality. Extensive research into wide-cone reconstruction algorithms has resulted in significant reductions in artifacts, enhancing the overall effectiveness of wide cone beam CT systems.

Despite its challenges, ongoing developments in hardware design and reconstruction algorithms continue to enhance its capabilities, making it a valuable tool in modern medical diagnostics and treatment planning.

6.4 Advancements in CT Technology

6.4.1 Dual-Source CT

Dual-source CT (DSCT) technology, designed for enhanced imaging capabilities, is particularly beneficial for robust coronary CT angiography (CCTA), especially at higher and irregular heart rates. Temporal resolution, crucial for clear imaging, refers to the time required to acquire sufficient data to reconstruct an axial image. In DSCT, this is approximately half the gantry rotation time for image pixels near the isocenter, the typical heart position. Unlike the total scan time, temporal resolution is pivotal for cardiac imaging clarity. Despite advancements in CT systems over the past three decades, achieving gantry rotation times shorter than 0.25 seconds has been challenging due to mechanical constraints from increased centrifugal forces.

DSCT addresses these limitations by utilizing two X-ray tubes and corresponding detectors positioned at a 90-degree angle, enabling simultaneous data acquisition at the same anatomical level (Fig. 6.11). This configuration allows DSCT to achieve a temporal resolution of about a quarter of the gantry rotation time, with third-generation systems reaching 66 milliseconds. This high temporal resolution, independent of the patient's heart rate, contrasts with single-source CT systems, which require multi-sector reconstruction and are dependent on the heart rate-gantry rotation time relationship.

Since its commercial introduction in 2006, DSCT has demonstrated reliability in performing CCTA in patients with high and irregular heart rates, proving accurate in diagnosing significant coronary artery disease. DSCT systems can scan the entire heart within one heartbeat using a high-pitch mode, ensuring gapless volume coverage along the *z*-axis and scan speeds of up to

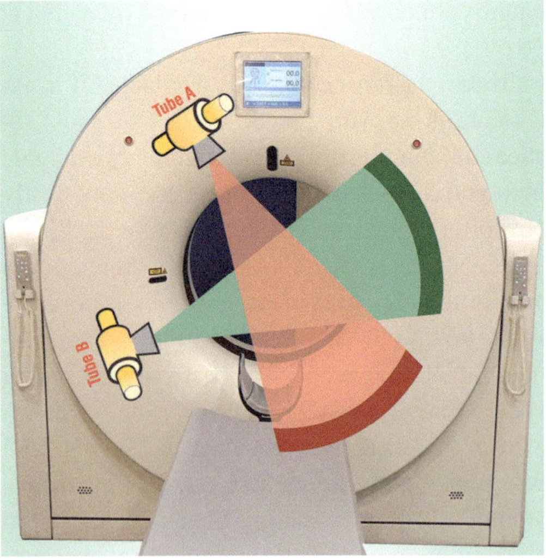

Fig. 6.11 Dual source CT machine

737 mm/s in third-generation systems. This mode, combined with ECG-triggering, allows for rapid, low-dose imaging of the heart in about 160 milliseconds.

High-pitch DSCT scanning is also advantageous for imaging larger anatomical ranges quickly, such as chest CT angiography and aortic scans, and is particularly beneficial in pediatric radiology and emergency settings. DSCT's ability to acquire dual-energy data simultaneously by operating X-ray tubes at different kV settings (e.g., 80 and 140 kVp) enhances material differentiation and reduces radiation dose.

However, DSCT systems face challenges, including data truncation and cross-scattered radiation. Data truncation occurs when one detector's field of view (FOV) is smaller, requiring extrapolation to avoid artifacts. Cross-scattered radiation, resulting from one tube's scattered radiation detected by the opposite detector, degrades image quality and requires correction. Techniques for correction include direct measurement with additional detector elements and model-based methods using Monte Carlo simulations. Despite these challenges, DSCT's high temporal resolution, rapid scan capabilities, and reduced radiation dose make it a valuable tool in modern radiology, particularly for cardiac and emergency imaging.

6.4.2 Photon Counting CT Machine

Photon Counting Computed Tomography (PCCT) represents an innovative technology capable of delivering CT data with exceptionally high spatial resolution, free from electronic noise, and embedded with inherent spectral information [39]. Unlike traditional CT systems that rely on energy-integrating detectors, PCCT utilizes photon-counting detectors (PCDs) to count individual X-ray photons and measure their energy. This detailed and innovative approach provides a host of benefits, making PCCT a promising technology for future clinical applications.

In 2008, GE Healthcare introduced the first preclinical prototype of a PCCT system, utilizing a cadmium-telluride (CdTe) detector with 1×1 mm^2 detector pixels and 2 energy thresholds [41]. Despite its limitations, including the requirement for lower radiation doses than clinically needed, this prototype demonstrated the potential for dual-energy imaging. Subsequently, Siemens Healthcare installed three preclinical prototypes of hybrid dual-source PCCT systems in clinical research environments starting in 2014. These prototypes, based on the SOMATOM Flash clinical dual-source CT, featured CdTe photon-counting detectors with a z-coverage of 16 mm at the isocenter and subpixels with a size of 0.225×0.225 mm^2. They allowed for scanning with typical clinical parameters, such as rotation times of 0.5 seconds and tube currents up to 550 mA, enabling extensive phantom and patient studies [41].

In 2017, Philips Healthcare introduced a single-source PCCT prototype equipped with a cadmium-zinc-telluride (CZT) detector, boasting a pixel size of 0.5×0.5 mm^2 and 5 energy thresholds. This system, later upgraded to a preclinical PCCT with a larger field of view (FOV) and shorter gantry rotation time, facilitated large animal and human studies, including cardiac CT. The year 2020 saw the installation of the second generation of preclinical PCCT systems by Siemens Healthcare, featuring a CdTe detector with subpixels measuring 0.275×0.322 mm^2 (0.151×0.176 mm^2 at the isocenter). These systems offered a 50-cm FOV with a z-coverage of 57.6 mm at the isocenter and various collimation options, contributing to evaluations of PCCT performance and image quality in clinical settings [41].

Finally, in September 2021, Siemens Healthcare commercially introduced the first-generation PCD dual-source CT, marking a significant milestone in the commercialization of PCCT technology. This system, named NAEOTOM Alpha, features two CdTe detectors with subpixel sizes of 0.275×0.322 mm^2 (0.151×0.176 mm^2 at the isocenter) and offers a FOV of 50 cm diameter. With a shortest gantry rotation time of 0.25 seconds and the ability to combine subpixels into macro-pixels, this system provides enhanced temporal resolution for ECG-controlled cardiac examinations. Additionally, it offers data acquisition with various collimation options and multiple energy thresholds for both detectors, further expanding the capabilities of PCCT technology. These advancements underscore the continuous refinement and expansion of PCCT technology parameters, paving the way for its widespread adoption in clinical practice [41].

6.4.2.1 Working Principles of Photon Counting CT

PCCT systems are equipped with PCDs made from semiconductor materials such as cadmium-telluride (CdTe), cadmium-zinc-telluride (CZT), or silicon (Si). These detectors function by applying a high voltage between a large-area cathode electrode and pixelated anode electrodes, creating a strong electric field across the semiconductor layer. When X-ray photons are absorbed by the semiconductor, they generate electron-hole pairs. In CdTe and CZT detectors, the semiconductor layers are relatively thin (1.4–2 mm) due to their high atomic numbers, which facilitate efficient X-ray absorption [41] (Fig. 6.12).

As the electron-hole pairs are separated by the electric field, they migrate towards the anodes, creating short current pulses lasting about a nanosecond. These pulses are then converted into voltage pulses by an electronic pulse shaping circuit, where the pulse height is proportional to the energy of the absorbed X-ray photons. Once the pulses surpass a set threshold energy level (typically 20–25 keV), they are counted by the read-out electronics.

To capture spectrally resolved data, multiple counters operating at different threshold energies are employed. Each counter records a distinct data stream for X-ray quanta exceeding its specific threshold energy, providing detailed spectral information crucial for various diagnostic purposes.

CdTe and CZT-based PCDs are commonly used in both preclinical and clinical PCCT systems due to their effective X-ray absorption and reasonable pulse separation capabilities. However, these detectors can experience inaccuracies in energy registration due to physical effects such as charge sharing at pixel boundaries and fluorescence, potentially leading to errors in spectral data.

Silicon-based PCDs, though offering better spectral separation and reduced charge sharing and fluorescence effects, require higher radiation doses because many X-ray quanta are scattered

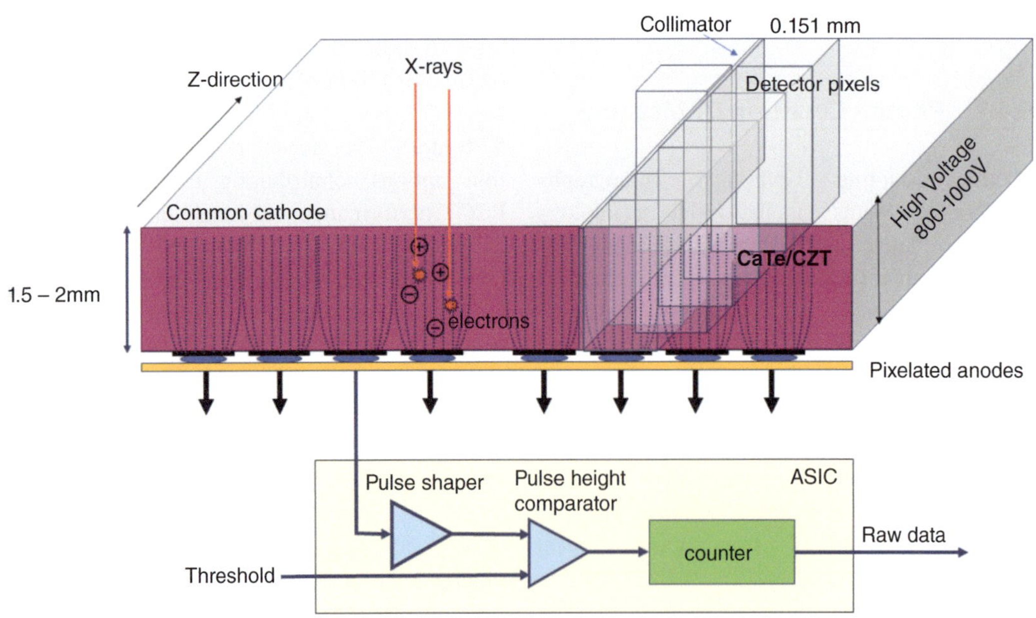

Fig. 6.12 CdTe/CZT PCD and its read-out Application-Specific Integrated Circuit (ASIC)

within the Si crystal and do not contribute to the signal.

A challenge for PCCT systems is pulse pile-up, as medical CTs operate at high X-ray flux rates, reaching up to 10^9 counts per second per mm^2 [39].

6.4.2.2 Advantages over Traditional CT

1. **High Spatial Resolution:** PCCT systems offer superior spatial resolution compared to traditional CT, primarily due to their finely structured photon-counting detectors (PCDs). Unlike Energy-Integrating Detectors (EIDs), which require opaque interlayers between pixels to prevent crosstalk (limiting pixel size and dose efficiency), PCDs are made from semiconductor materials like cadmium-telluride (CdTe), cadmium-zinc-telluride (CZT), or silicon (Si), and do not require such interlayers. This allows for much smaller detector pixels, enhancing spatial resolution.

   PCCT has achieved spatial resolutions as fine as 0.15 mm in the scan plane and 0.41 mm in slice width, with pixel sizes ranging from 0.225×0.225 mm^2 to 0.5×0.5 mm^2 [41]. This increased resolution is particularly beneficial for detailed imaging of small structures, such as those in high-resolution chest CT and temporal bone anatomy. PCCT provides better differentiation of fine structures, improved signal-to-noise ratios, and reduced image noise, even at lower radiation doses.

   Clinical studies have demonstrated PCCT's advantages over EID-CT. In ultra-high-resolution (UHR) temporal bone exams, PCCT showed superior image quality and significant dose savings (mean reduction of 79.3%) [42]. In lung imaging, PCCT improved diagnostic confidence for conditions like interstitial lung disease (ILD) and provided better image quality at lower doses [43]. For coronary CTA, PCCT improved stenosis quantification accuracy and reduced blooming artifacts, enhancing visualization of plaques and vessel lumens [44].
2. **Spectral Information:** PCCT uses detectors that naturally capture spectral information by measuring the energy of each detected photon. This feature allows for multi-energy imaging, which improves the distinction between different tissues and materials, especially in scans using contrast agents. In multi-threshold mode, detectors provide signals based on specific energy thresholds, enabling dual-energy applications like material decomposition into iodine and water. This leads to the creation of virtual monoenergetic images (VMIs), iodine maps, and virtual noncontrast (VNC) images [41].

   VMIs are standardized images that adjust iodine contrast regardless of acquisition conditions. Studies have shown that VMIs from PCCT offer better image quality and contrast-to-noise ratio (CNR) compared to traditional CT images, especially at lower energy levels [45]. For example, in a study with oncologic patients, VMIs at 70 keV from PCCT had lower image noise and higher CNR than traditional CT images, even with similar radiation doses [46]. VMIs also allow for contrast agent dose reduction. Studies have demonstrated sufficient iodine CNR in VMIs at 40 keV with a 50% reduction in contrast agent concentration [47].

   PCCT's ability to reconstruct VMIs at different energies improves diagnostic confidence and reduces radiation exposure. For coronary CTA, VMIs at 50 keV combined with high iterative reconstruction levels provided diagnostic image quality with lower contrast doses [48]. VNC images from PCCT closely match true noncontrast (TNC) images, reducing the need for additional nonenhanced scans.

   In cardiovascular CT, PCCT supports applications like PURE Calcium and PURE Lumen (Siemens Healthineers), which enhance coronary calcium assessment and vessel lumen visualization by removing iodine or calcium from contrast-enhanced images, thus improving image quality and reducing artifacts [49, 50].
3. **Reduced Noise and Improved Contrast-to-Noise Ratio (CNR):** PCCT systems effectively eliminate the electronic noise that affects traditional scintillation detectors,

resulting in clearer images with less noise and fewer artifacts [27]. In Photon Counting Detectors (PCDs), the lowest threshold energy that X-ray quanta must exceed to be counted is typically around 20 keV. This threshold is well above the noise floor of the electronics, so electronic noise does not impact the count rates of PCDs. Consequently, at low X-ray flux, the signal exhibits only the statistical quantum noise of the X-ray photons. In contrast, traditional Energy-Integrating Detectors (EIDs) are dominated by electronic noise at low X-ray flux, leading to increased image noise, noise streaks, and unstable CT values.

The ability of PCCT to reduce electronic noise enhances the contrast-to-noise ratio (CNR), particularly in scans utilizing contrast agents. This improvement in image clarity and stability, even at low radiation doses, underscores PCCT's potential to provide superior diagnostic images while minimizing radiation exposure.

4. **Dose Efficiency:** The geometric dose efficiency of PCCT is higher than that of traditional CT detectors because there are no optical separation layers that absorb X-rays without contributing to the image. This means that PCCT can achieve high-quality images with a lower radiation dose, enhancing patient safety. They provide significantly better, lower-noise images, particularly beneficial for low-dose scans and examinations of obese patients [41]. Studies on preclinical prototypes demonstrated the superior image quality of PCDs at low radiation doses, which is crucial for applications like lung cancer screening [51]. For instance, in a study of 80 patients evaluated for interstitial lung disease (ILD) using both third-generation Dual-Source CT (DSCT) and first-generation Photon Counting DSCT (PCD-DSCT), PCD-CT achieved comparable image quality at a 66% lower radiation dose [52]. Similar dose reduction possibilities with maintained or improved image quality have been reported in pediatric thorax examinations and contrast-enhanced abdominal CT scans of obese patients [53, 54].

5. **Improved Iodine Contrast-to-Noise Ratio in Photon Counting CT**

   PCCT significantly enhances the iodine contrast-to-noise ratio (CNR) compared to traditional Energy-Integrating Detectors (EIDs). In EIDs, lower-energy X-ray quanta produce less light and thus contribute less to the detector signal, which is based on the total X-ray energy registered. Conversely, Photon Counting Detectors (PCDs) count all X-ray quanta above a certain energy threshold equally, making low-energy X-ray quanta, which contain most low-contrast information, more influential.

   Iodine, commonly used in contrast agents, has a K-edge at 33 keV and absorbs X-rays most strongly just above this energy. Consequently, PCCT images exhibit higher iodine contrast than EID-CT images taken with the same X-ray tube voltage (kVp), particularly at higher voltages [35]. This results in a higher iodine CNR at the same radiation dose. A study on a preclinical PCD-CT prototype using anthropomorphic phantoms of various sizes showed mean increases in iodine CNR of 11%, 23%, 31%, and 38% at 80, 100, 120, and 140 kVp, respectively [35].

   Clinically, improved iodine CNR translates into better image quality in contrast-enhanced scans or the potential for reduced radiation or contrast agent doses. An early phantom study achieved a 32% dose reduction due to higher iodine CNR [55]. In an oncological cohort study of 70 patients undergoing routine contrast-enhanced abdominal and pelvic CT, PCCT provided similar or better image quality (higher liver lesion conspicuity) at a 32% lower radiation dose compared to second-generation DSCT [56]. Another study involving 100 oncologic chest patients demonstrated a mean radiation dose reduction of over 40% with maintained image quality using PCCT compared to DSCT [57].

6.4.2.3 Clinical Applications

(PCCT) significantly enhances various imaging applications. In cardiovascular imaging, PCCT improves the visualization of small arteries, stents, and plaques in coronary computed tomography angiography (CCTA), aiding in the assessment of coronary artery disease. PCCT also provides comparable coronary artery calcium scores (CACS) to conventional CT at reduced doses and offers better stent imaging by minimizing blooming artifacts. Its high resolution and spectral capabilities benefit myocardial assessment and extracellular volume quantification. For thoracic imaging, PCCT achieves high-resolution images at lower doses, crucial for frequent scans in lung conditions, and can replace true non-contrast (TNC) scans with virtual non-contrast (VNC) reconstructions. In abdominal imaging, PCCT delivers superior image quality even for obese patients, enhancing the visualization of abdominal pathologies and malignancies through spectral post-processing. Neuroimaging with PCCT offers improved differentiation between gray and white matter and reduces beam-hardening artifacts, enhancing neurovascular assessments. PCCT also excels in temporal bone imaging, providing detailed views of small structures and postoperative changes. In musculoskeletal imaging, PCCT delivers detailed images of trabecular bone and reduces metal artifacts near orthopedic implants, aiding in the evaluation of bone metastases and implant integration [58].

6.4.2.4 Challenges and Future Directions

Despite its advantages, PCCT faces several challenges that limit its full potential. One limitation lies in the current constraints of X-ray tubes, which impose limits on achievable image quality due to factors such as maximum filament current, power, and inadequate focal spot size. Additionally, while PCCT shows promise in reducing radiation doses, achieving non-inferior image quality compared to conventional CT scans is a primary aim of many studies. However, to leverage the spectral properties of PCCT effectively, a relatively wide energy spectrum is required, often necessitating higher tube voltages that may correlate with increased dose and reduced contrast, depending on the clinical task at hand. Moreover, the extensive data generated by PCCT demands significant computational resources for data processing or necessitates meticulous protocol selection and reconstructions to manage the data volume, especially in Ultra-High-Resolution (UHR) mode. Furthermore, while PCCT facilitates the creation of high-quality images and offers opportunities for physician-driven image post-processing, its impact on clinical decision-making remains uncertain. Questions persist regarding whether PCCT will enable earlier diagnosis or potentially make invasive interventions obsolete. These challenges underscore the need for further research to optimize algorithms for accurate calcium scoring, evaluate PCCT's efficacy across various medical applications, and address concerns regarding its impact on clinical decision-making [58].

6.5 Advantages of CT Over Conventional Radiography

Conventional radiography works by passing X-rays through the body and capturing the resulting image on a detector. As the X-rays pass through the body, they are attenuated to varying degrees by different tissues based on their density and composition, resulting in a two-dimensional image where dense tissues like bone appear white and less dense tissues appear in shades of gray or black. However, conventional radiography faces limitations such as superimposition of structures, limited contrast resolution, lack of depth information, and artefacts. Computed Tomography (CT) overcomes these issues by using a rotating X-ray tube and detectors to capture multiple projections from different angles, which are then reconstructed into detailed cross-sectional images. CT offers superior contrast resolution, three-dimensional reconstruction, multiplanar reformatting, quantitative analysis, artefact reduction, functional imaging, and rapid, comprehensive scans. These capabilities allow CT to provide clearer, more detailed images without overlapping structures, facilitating accurate diagnosis and better visualization of internal anatomy. These advantages can be understood through a comparison of their technical aspects and their impact on diagnostic efficacy.

(i) **Detailed Cross-Sectional Imaging**

One of the primary advantages of CT over conventional radiography is its ability to produce detailed cross-sectional images of the body. While conventional radiography provides two-dimensional images that can superimpose different structures, CT scans generate three-dimensional images by taking multiple cross-sectional slices. This is achieved through the rotation of the X-ray tube and detectors around the patient, capturing multiple projections from various angles. The data is then reconstructed into detailed images that allow for better visualization of internal structures without overlapping tissues. This capability is particularly beneficial in diagnosing complex anatomical regions and detecting small lesions that might be obscured in traditional radiographs.

(ii) **Superior Contrast Resolution**

CT imaging offers superior contrast resolution compared to conventional radiography. This means that CT can differentiate between tissues with very similar densities more effectively. The use of Hounsfield Units (HU) in CT imaging (discussed in next section of the chapter) provides a quantitative scale for radiodensity, enhancing the ability to distinguish between different tissue types. For instance, subtle differences between gray and white matter in the brain or between various types of soft tissues can be more easily identified with CT, aiding in more accurate diagnosis and treatment planning.

(iii) **3D Reconstruction and Multiplanar Reformatting**

The advanced reconstruction algorithms used in CT allow for the generation of three-dimensional images and multiplanar reformatting. This means that once the data is acquired, images can be viewed in different planes—axial, sagittal, coronal, or any arbitrary orientation—without the need for additional scans. This multiplanar capability is invaluable for surgical planning, as it provides a comprehensive view of the anatomy, helping surgeons to navigate complex structures with greater precision. In contrast, conventional radiography is limited to predefined planar views, often requiring multiple projections to get a somewhat complete picture, which can still be insufficient for detailed analysis.

(iv) **Quantitative Analysis and Functional Imaging**

CT scanners enable quantitative analysis, allowing for the measurement of tissue densities in Hounsfield Units. This quantification can be critical in assessing the composition of tissues, such as identifying fat content in the liver or measuring the density of calcifications in arteries. Additionally, with the advent of advanced techniques like CT perfusion and CT angiography, functional imaging becomes possible. These techniques can provide information about blood flow, vessel patency, and tissue perfusion, offering insights beyond what is possible with static images. Conventional radiography lacks these advanced capabilities, limiting its use to structural evaluation alone.

(v) **Reduced Artefacts and Enhanced Clarity**

CT imaging reduces the artefacts commonly seen in conventional radiography. Beam hardening, scatter, and overlapping structures often result in artefacts that can obscure important details in radiographic images. CT, on the other hand, uses algorithms to correct for many of these artefacts, providing clearer and more accurate images. The ability to adjust the X-ray beam's energy and the sophisticated detectors used in CT further enhance image clarity by optimizing the signal-to-noise ratio.

(vi) **Rapid and Comprehensive Imaging**

Modern CT scanners are incredibly fast, often completing scans in just a few seconds. This rapid imaging capability is crucial in emergency settings, where quick and accurate diagnosis can be lifesaving. For example, in trauma cases, CT can quickly assess multiple injuries in different parts of the body, providing a comprehensive overview that conventional radiography would take much longer to achieve with multiple separate exposures. The speed and comprehensiveness of CT scans make them indispensable in acute care.

(vii) **Advanced Applications and Versatility**

CT's versatility extends to a wide range of applications, from routine examinations to complex diagnostic challenges. It is used extensively in oncology for detecting and monitoring tumors, in cardiology for assessing coronary artery disease, and in neurology for evaluating stroke and brain injuries. The ability to perform specialized scans, such as virtual colonoscopy and CT-guided interventions, further showcases the adaptability of CT technology. Conventional radiography, while useful for basic imaging, lacks this level of versatility and specialization.

CT's ability to provide detailed cross-sectional images, superior contrast resolution, advanced quantitative and functional imaging, reduced artefacts, rapid scanning, and versatility in applications significantly enhances its diagnostic power compared to conventional radiography. These technical advantages make CT an indispensable tool in modern medical imaging by improving diagnosis and treatment planning.

6.6 Principles and Working of CT Scanners

Computed Tomography (CT) scanners work by using X-rays to create detailed cross-sectional images of the body. The basic principle involves an X-ray tube that emits a fan-shaped beam of X-rays as it rotates around the patient, who is positioned on a motorized table that moves incrementally through the gantry (the circular frame that houses the X-ray tube and detectors). As the X-rays pass through the body, they are attenuated to varying degrees by different tissues. This attenuation is a measure of how much the X-ray beam is reduced in intensity as it passes through a material, depending on the material's density and atomic number.

6.6.1 Hounsfield Units and Basis for Image Reconstruction

The X-rays that pass through the body are detected by an array of sensors positioned opposite the X-ray tube, called CT detectors. These detectors measure the amount of X-ray energy that reaches them and convert this information into electronic signals. CT images are obtained by reconstructing the linear attenuation distribution from its projection acquired with an X-ray detector based on energy integration or photon counting mechanisms. In the energy integration mode, an electric current proportional to the total energy carried by the X-ray fluency impinging upon a detector cell is recorded. In the photon counting mode, the electric pulse generated by an interaction between an X-ray photon and the detector scintillator at each cell is counted, whereby the pulse height is proportional to the energy deposited by the X-ray photon. Consequently, a threshold and range in the pulse height can be set to not only suppress electronic noise but also endow each detector cell with energy resolution. Regardless of whether energy integration or photon counting is used for data acquisition, a CT with a monochromatic X-ray source can be conceived to obtain the 2D distribution of the linear attenuation coefficient, $\mu(x, y; E)$, from its projection, where x, y is the position and E is energy of the X-rays. The data from the detectors is then processed by a computer to reconstruct images of the body's internal structures. This process is known as attenuation mapping. Each pixel in the resulting CT image corresponds to a specific volume element (voxel) within the body and is assigned a value based on the degree of X-ray attenuation.

These values are typically expressed in Hounsfield Units (HU) or CT numbers, a scale named after Sir Godfrey Hounsfield, one of the inventors of CT scanning. The Hounsfield scale is a quantitative measure of radiodensity, with distilled water at standard temperature and pressure (STP) assigned a value of 0 HU and air at STP assigned a value of −1000 HU. Dense materials, such as bone, have positive HU values (e.g., ranging from +1000 HU to +3000

HU, or even higher for metals), while less dense tissues like fat have negative HU values (e.g., typically around −120 to −90 HU [−100 HU]). The use of Hounsfield Units allows for precise differentiation between various types of tissue, enabling detailed and accurate diagnostic images.

The linear attenuation map is generated from the 360° of rotation of the X-ray tube and detectors and used for reconstructing the image in CT technology. The relationship between transmission intensities pre- and post-patient and the linear attenuation coefficient is as follows:

$$I = I_0 e^{-\mu x} \quad (6.1)$$

This equation is called general form of the Beer-Lambert law. Where:

- I is the intensity of the X-ray beam after passing through the material.
- I_0 is the initial intensity of the X-ray beam.
- μ is the linear attenuation coefficient of the material.
- x is the thickness of the material.

The Hounsfield Unit is calculated using the formula:

$$\text{HU}_{\text{material}} = 1000 \times \left(\frac{\mu_{\text{material}} - \mu_{\text{water}}}{\mu_{\text{water}}} \right) \quad (6.2)$$

In most CT systems, CT numbers range from −1000 HU to +3000 HU, and even higher for very dense materials, for different tissues. The lung, mostly filled with air, has HU values between −400 HU and −900 HU. Soft tissues have values around −80 HU to 80 HU, spongy bone (trabecular bones) ranges from 300 HU to 800 HU, and harder cortical bones range from 700 HU to 3000 HU. Metallic implants and iodinated CT contrast agents typically have HU values ranging from +100 HU to +3000 HU, depending on concentration and material. Metallic foreign bodies exhibit higher HU values, including stainless steel (2222 ± 737 HU), titanium (2921 ± 218 HU), gold (2908 ± 325 HU), lead (2758 ± 539 HU), copper (2909 ± 228 HU), and silver (3069 HU), with a mean value of 2633 ± 603 HU. Non-metallic foreign bodies include silicone (278 ± 120 HU), glass (947 ± 523 HU), polyethylene (32 ± 5 HU), polylactide plate (144 ± 16 HU), stone (1320 ± 280 HU), plastic (−47 HU), and wood (−464 HU), with a mean value of 557 ± 526 HU [59]. Table 6.3 provides different substances with their corresponding Hounsfield Units (HU), which are used in CT imaging to measure radiodensity.

6.6.2 Beer-Lambert Law and X-ray Attenuation

The Beer-Lambert law describes how X-rays are attenuated as they pass through a material. The attenuation of the X-ray beam while penetrating the human body is crucial for forming subject contrast in X-ray CT imaging. In the energy range of 20–150 keV used for diagnostic imaging, X-ray attenuation is mainly determined by photoelectric absorption and Compton scatter.

Table 6.3 Substances with their corresponding Hounsfield Units (HU)

Substance	Hounsfield Units (HU)
Air	−1000
Lung (inhaled air)	−700 to −600 (approximately −800 HU for normal lung)
Fat	−100 to −90
Water	0
Cerebrospinal fluid (CSF)	0 to +10
Blood	+13 to +50
Muscle	+10 to +40 (often cited as 35–55)
Kidney	+20 to +40 (Normal parenchyma typically 30–40 HU)
Liver	+45 to +60
Spleen	+40 to +55
Bone (cancellous)	+300 to +800
Bone (cortical)	+700 to +3000
Iodine-based contrast media	+25 to +600
Barium sulfate contrast	+200 to >3000
Calcifications	+100 to +300 (ranges commonly 100–400 HU, but can vary greatly, even up to 1900 HU in some tissues)
Metal (e.g., implants)	> +3000

As discussed earlier, the general form of the Beer-Lambert law is:

$$I = I_0 e^{-\mu x}$$

In CT imaging, the linear attenuation coefficient $\mu(x, y; E)$ depends on both the position and the energy of the X-rays, and is given by:

$$\mu(x,;y,;E) = \alpha(x,y) f_c(E) + \beta(x,y) f_p(E)$$

Where:

- $f_c(E)$ represents the energy dependency of Compton scatter (Klein-Nishina Function).
- $f_p(E) \approx \frac{1}{E^{3.2}}$ represents the energy dependency of photoelectric absorption.
- $\alpha(x, y)$ and $\beta(x, y)$ are characteristic coefficients of the material at location (x, y):
  - $\alpha(x,y) \approx K_1 \frac{Z^{3.8}\rho}{A}$
  - $\beta(x,y) \approx K_2 \frac{Z\rho}{A}$
  - Z denotes the atomic number, A the mass number, and ρ the mass density of the material.
  - K_1 and K_2 are constants.

For a given material, Z/A is nearly constant for a material, $\alpha(x, y)$ is primarily determined by the atomic number, while $\beta(x, y)$ is dominantly determined by mass or electron density [60].

CT images are reconstructed from the linear attenuation distribution using projection data acquired with an X-ray detector based on energy integration or photon counting mechanisms. In the energy integration mode, an electric current proportional to the total energy carried by the X-ray fluence impinging upon a detector cell is recorded. In the photon counting mode, the electric pulse generated by an interaction between an X-ray photon and the detector scintillator at each cell is counted, with the pulse height proportional to the energy deposited by the X-ray photon. This mode allows for energy resolution and the suppression of electronic noise.

The linear attenuation coefficient $\mu(x, y; E)$ can be obtained from its projection using:

$$\int_L \mu(x,;y,;E)\,dl = \int_L \begin{bmatrix} \alpha(x,y) f_c(E) \\ +\beta(x,y) f_p(E) \end{bmatrix} dl$$

Where $\int_L dl$ denotes the line integrals along L, a family of lines passing through point (x, y) at various orientations. Provided the data sufficiency condition is met, various algorithms, particularly Filtered Back Projection (FBP), can be employed to reconstruct $\alpha(x, y; E)$ [60].

6.6.3 Polychromatic X-ray Source Consideration

While a monochromatic X-ray source would simplify the equations, current CT systems use a polychromatic X-ray source where the energy of X-ray photons is distributed over a spectrum up to the peak voltage (E_{kVP}) applied to the X-ray tube's anode. This leads to a more complex integral equation:

$$\int_0^{E_{kVP}} S(E)\left\{\int \mu(x,;y,;E)\,dl\right\} dE = \int_0^{E_{kVP}} S(E)\left\{\int\left[\alpha(x,y) f_c(E) + \beta(x,y) f_p(E)\right] dl\right\} \mathrm{dE}$$

Where $S(E)$ is the spectral distribution of the X-ray source [60].

The physical principles and mathematical equations in CT imaging, from the Beer-Lambert Law and X-ray attenuation to advanced reconstruction algorithms, enable the creation of detailed and accurate diagnostic images. These principles ensure the efficient use of X-rays, accurate attenuation mapping, and the effective differentiation of various tissues, enhancing the diagnostic capabilities of CT technology. The reconstructed images can be displayed in various planes (axial, sagittal, coronal) and even rendered in three dimensions, providing comprehensive views of the anatomy. Modern CT scanners are capable of performing this entire process rapidly, often completing scans in just a few seconds, which is crucial for imaging dynamic organs such as the heart or for use in emergency settings. Technological advancements continues to expand the applications and effectiveness of CT imaging in medical diagnostics.

6.7 Windowing in CT Imaging

We discussed the concept of CT Numbers in the previous section. In CT imaging, the image is composed of CT numbers or Hounsfield Units (HU) that range typically from +1000 to −1000, and it represents the various shades of gray. This range of numbers forms a continuous grayscale, with each number corresponding to a specific shade.

Window Width (WW) and Window Level (WL)
The range of CT numbers displayed on the image is referred to as the window width (WW). The window width determines the contrast of the image by defining the range of CT numbers that will be displayed as shades of gray. A narrow window width increases image contrast by displaying a smaller range of CT numbers, which is useful for distinguishing between tissues with similar densities. Conversely, a wide window width reduces contrast, displaying a larger range of CT numbers, which is useful for viewing structures with a wide range of densities.

The window level (WL), also known as the window center (C), sets the midpoint of the range of CT numbers that will be displayed. It essentially shifts the center of the window width range along the CT number scale. By adjusting the window level, one can change the image's brightness, making the image appear lighter or darker.

Mechanism of Windowing
Both the WW and WL are controlled from the console, allowing for adjustments to image contrast and brightness. When a WW of 2000 and a WL of 0 are used, the entire grayscale spectrum is displayed, which can make it difficult for the human eye to perceive small differences in soft tissue attenuation because it can discern only about 40 shades of gray. This process of modifying the grayscale of the CT image is called *windowing*. The WW controls the image contrast, while the WL or C controls the image brightness. As the WL or C increases, the image transitions from white (bright) to dark (less bright), altering the image contrast based on different WW values. Optimizing image contrast for specific anatomy requires setting appropriate values for WW and WL or C during the initial scanning of the patient. However, it's important to note that the image displayed during initial scanning is typically a default setting, and further windowing adjustments are made during image review to optimize visualization of specific tissues or pathologies.

Box 6.1

- **Window Width (WW):** Controls the contrast of the image.
  - **Narrow WW:** Enhances contrast, useful for differentiating between tissues with similar densities (e.g., soft tissues).
  - **Wide WW:** Reduces contrast, useful for visualizing areas with a broad range of densities (e.g., lung tissues).
- **Window Level (WL):** Controls the brightness of the image.
  - **Low WL:** Shifts the grayscale to display more low-density structures, making the image appear brighter.
  - **High WL:** Shifts the grayscale to display more high-density structures, making the image appear darker.

Practical Application of Windowing
During the initial scanning, the appropriate WW and WL settings are chosen based on the anatomical region being examined. This is crucial for optimizing image quality and ensuring accurate diagnosis. For example:

- **Bone Window:** Optimized for imaging bone, with a high WL and a relatively wide WW to enhance the visibility of bone structures.
- **Mediastinal Window:** Optimized for imaging mediastinal structures, with a moderate WL and WW to visualize soft tissues in the chest.
- **Lung Window:** Optimized for imaging the lungs, with a low WL and wide WW to highlight the air-filled structures of the lungs (Fig. 6.13 and Table 6.4).

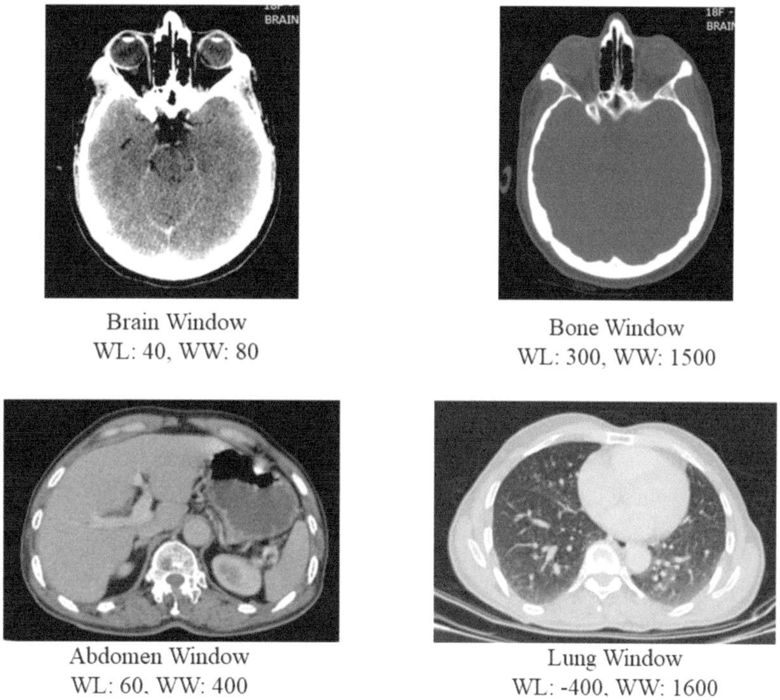

Fig. 6.13 Windowing and window level in CT imaging

Table 6.4 Table summarizing typical window width and level values for various CT imaging applications

Anatomical region	Window width (W)	Window level (L)
Head and neck		
Brain	80	40
Subdural	130–300	50–100
Stroke	30 or 40	30 or 40
Temporal bones	–2800 or 4000	–600 or 700
Soft tissues	350–400	20–60
Chest		
Lungs	~1500	~–600
Mediastinum	~350 to 400	~40 to 50
Abdomen		
Soft tissues	400	50
Liver	~150 to 160	~60 to 88
Spine		
Soft tissues	250	50
Bone	1800	400

This table provides a general reference, but specific values might vary depending on the institution or equipment used. Windowing in CT imaging allows radiologists to optimize image contrast and brightness for better visualization of specific anatomical structures. By adjusting the window width and window level, different tissues can be highlighted, enhancing diagnostic accuracy and providing clearer, more detailed images. This flexibility in image manipulation is one of the key advantages of CT imaging over conventional radiography, enabling more precise and comprehensive diagnostic evaluations.

6.8 CT Instrumentation and Detector Technology

The CT machine integrates complex hardware and sophisticated software systems to provide high resolution images of the human body. The scanning part includes the gantry and patient table, which facilitate the acquisition of raw data. This data is then processed and reconstructed into readable images by the computer system, and finally, the console and workstation manage the storage, display, and advanced processing of these images. Each component plays a critical role in ensuring accurate and efficient diagnostic imaging. The key components of a CT machine and its associated electronics can be broadly categorized into three main parts (Fig. 6.14):

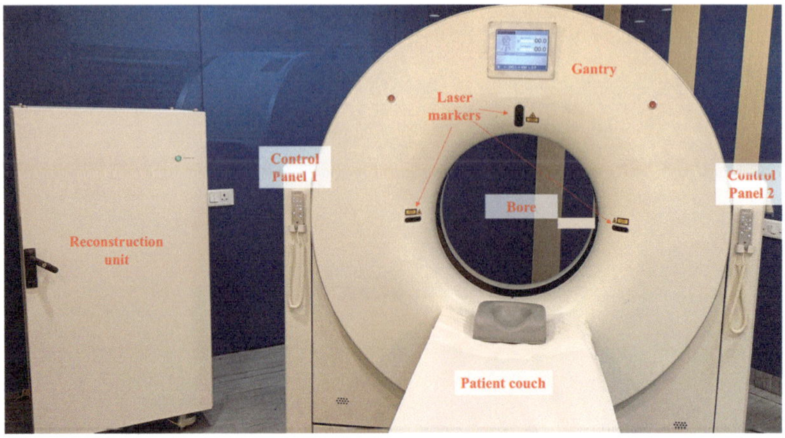

Fig. 6.14 CT instrumentation consist of gantry, patient couch, reconstruction unit and other components

1. The Scanning Part: Gantry and the Patient Table
2. The Computer System for Data Processing and Image Reconstruction
3. The Console and Workstation for Image Storage, Display, and Further Processing

6.8.1 The Scanning Part: Gantry and the Patient Table

The scanning component is primarily composed of the gantry and the patient table. The gantry, which is large ring-like structure, houses several essential elements. It includes the X-ray tube, high-voltage generators, pre-patient collimator, post-patient collimator, detectors, and the data acquisition system (DAS), along with the necessary associated electronics (Fig. 6.15). The size of the patient bore varies depending on the type and design of the machine, tailored to different clinical needs and patient requirements. Standard CT scanners typically have a bore diameter of around 70–80 cm (27.5–31.5 inches), suitable for a wide range of diagnostic imaging needs. Wide-bore CT scanners, with diameters approximately 80–85 cm (31.5–33.5 inches), are designed to accommodate larger patients or those with claustrophobia, providing enhanced comfort and ease of positioning. Ultra-wide bore CT scanners, which can be as large as 90 cm (35.5 inches) or more, are often used in radiation therapy planning and for bariatric patients, where precise positioning and larger bore sizes are necessary.

Portable or mobile CT scanners typically have smaller bores, around 60–70 cm (23.5–27.5 inches), to meet the demands of field settings, emergency situations, or intensive care units where mobility and space constraints are critical. Cardiac CT scanners generally have bore diameters similar to standard scanners, around 70–80 cm (27.5–31.5 inches), but are specialized for cardiac imaging with a focus on high-speed imaging and enhanced temporal resolution. Paediatric CT scanners, often with similar bore sizes as standard scanners, are designed with paediatric protocols and lower radiation doses to ensure safety for children. Additionally, some CT scanners feature extended bore designs that provide a longer scanning area, beneficial for procedures requiring continuous imaging over a longer length of the patient. Interventional CT scanners may have variable bore sizes depending on specific needs, often similar to standard or wide-bore scanners but equipped with additional features for real-time imaging guidance during procedures. The bore size influences patient comfort, positioning accuracy, and the range of possible diagnostic applications, with larger bore sizes offering greater flexibility and comfort, especially for larger or claustrophobic patients, though they may require increased physical space and higher equipment costs.

The patient table also called as patient couch is designed to ensure precise positioning, comfort,

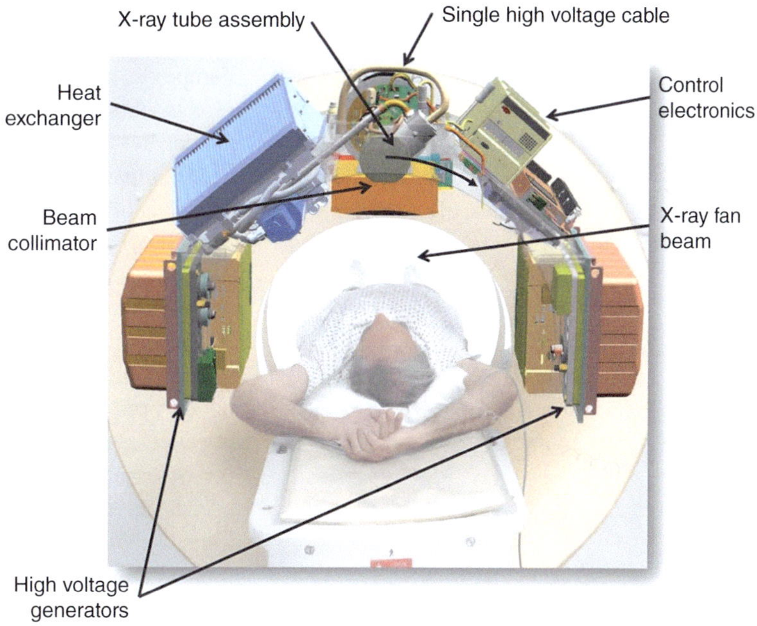

Fig. 6.15 Illustration of a modern high-power X-ray module. Positioned at the top, the X-ray tube receives power from two high-voltage generator blocks, allowing cathode voltages ranging from 80 to 140 kV. The water/glycol-to-air heat exchanger, including pumps, fans, and safety switches, facilitates heat dissipation. A collimator shapes the X-ray beam and incorporates additional X-ray filtering. (Image copyright: Taylor & Francis Group [61]. Reprinted with permission)

and stability during the scanning process. Constructed from carbon fiber or other radiolucent materials, the table minimizes interference with X-ray beams, ensuring high-quality imaging without artifacts. It features motorized controls for precise movements in multiple directions, enabling technologists to position patients accurately within the gantry. Modern CT tables can support a wide range of body weights, typically up to 450 pounds (204 kilograms) or more, with some specialized tables accommodating even higher limits for bariatric patients. The table often includes padding, straps, adjustable headrests, and arm supports to enhance patient comfort and stability. Automated positioning protocols help guide the table to the correct location for specific scans, reducing setup time and increasing accuracy. For pediatric patients, specialized accessories and cushions ensure safety and comfort, securing smaller patients to minimize movement during the scan. Some tables feature extended lengths and tilting capabilities for tall patients and angled views. Integrated with the CT system's software, the patient table ensures seamless communication and coordination during the scanning process, synchronizing movements with imaging sequences for optimal results.

Components Within the CT Gantry

As discussed above, within the gantry, there are several key components work together to facilitate imaging. The X-ray tube, powered by high-voltage generators, produces the X-rays needed for scanning. Pre-patient and post-patient collimators shape and refine the X-ray beam to reduce scatter and improve image quality. Filters are designed to address the issue of beam hardening, where the X-ray beam becomes more intense as it passes through denser tissue, leading to overexposure in certain areas of the image. Detectors capture X-ray photons that pass through the patient and convert them into electrical signals, which the Data Acquisition System (DAS) then digitizes for image reconstruction. The gantry's motor and rotational mechanism allow it to rotate around the patient, acquiring images from multiple angles. Slip rings provide continuous electrical connections, while a cooling system prevents overheating of critical components.

A laser positioning system helps accurately align the patient, and control electronics coordinate the operation of all these components. Together, these elements ensure the production of high-resolution images essential for accurate diagnosis and treatment planning. Let's discuss them one by one in more detail. Though the X-ray tube has been discussed in detail in Chap. 2, we will see a brief outline here again.

Box 6.2 Components within the CT Gantry

X-ray Tube	Data Acquisition System (DAS)
High-Voltage Generators	Slip rings
Pre-patient and post-patient collimators	Motor for rotational mechanism
Filters	Heat Exchanger
Detectors	Laser alignment system

6.8.1.1 X-ray Tubes

X-ray tubes have undergone significant advancements to improve their performance, reliability, and versatility. The production of X-rays involves several key components within an X-ray tube, which can be broadly divided into the X-ray tube insert assembly and the X-ray tube housing assembly.

(a) **X-ray Tube Insert Assembly**

The X-ray tube insert assembly includes the cathode and anode assemblies. The cathode assembly, consisting of a tungsten filament and a focusing cup, serves as the electron source. Through thermionic emission, the heated filament (1900–2500 °C) emits electrons that are accelerated towards the anode by a high voltage (20–150 kV). This electron flow, known as the tube current, interacts with the anode, producing X-rays in all directions, which are then collimated into a beam.

The number of electrons liberated from the cathode depends on the filament temperature, which is regulated by the supply current. Modern X-ray tubes use a heating current of 3–5 amperes, reaching up to 10 amperes in high-performance applications. Without a voltage difference, electrons form a cloud around the cathode, moving towards the anode only under a high electrical potential (kV). This electron flow forms an electric current, typically between 25 and 1000 milliamperes (mA). The cathode's focusing cup directs electrons to a specific location on the anode, known as the focal spot, which significantly impacts image quality and sharpness.

The anode assembly, which is the most expensive component of the X-ray tube, includes the anode target, focal spot, disk, and stem, and it converts the electrons' kinetic energy into X-rays. There are two main types of anodes: stationary and rotating. In CT, rotating anodes are predominantly used, with modern variants such as rotating envelope X-ray tubes and Cathode Innovation for Spectral CT. Rotating anodes, spinning at speeds up to 10,000–15,000 rpm, manage the immense heat generated during X-ray production, enhancing the tube's capacity for higher currents and shorter exposure times.

The tube voltage (kV) determines the X-ray energy, ranging from 0 keV to the peak applied voltage (kVp). X-rays below 20 keV are filtered out using an aluminum filter at the tube window to reduce unnecessary radiation. The product of the tube current (mA) and exposure time (seconds) is called milliampere-seconds (mAs), indicating the total X-ray emission.

Tungsten is preferred for cathodes due to its high melting point (3370 °C), high atomic number (Z = 74), and excellent heat and electrical conductivity. These properties ensure efficient X-ray production and heat dissipation, which is essential since most of the electron energy converts to heat. The anode and cathode assembly is housed within a glass or ceramic tube, maintaining a vacuum to prevent electron interaction with gas molecules, ensuring efficient X-ray generation and tube longevity. Bearings, lubrication, and heat dissipation systems are crucial for maintaining the anode's performance and longevity.

(b) **X-ray Tube Housing Assembly**

The X-ray tube housing assembly plays multiple roles in ensuring effective, safe, and reliable operation. It includes lead shielding to confine emitted X-rays to the intended beam path, high-tension voltage cable sockets for power delivery, and stator electromagnetic coils for anode rotation. Beam pre-collimation shapes the X-ray beam, while the X-ray radiation port and window facilitate controlled X-ray emission. Additional components include a radiation control timer circuit, bellows for accommodating thermal expansion, and heat exchanger parts to dissipate heat. The housing provides mechanical support, protecting the delicate internal components, and incorporates cooling systems, such as fans, oil, or water circulation, to maintain optimal operating temperatures and prevent overheating, thereby extending the tube's lifespan.

6.8.1.2 High-Voltage Generators

High-voltage generators provide the necessary power to produce X-rays by the CT tube. They convert standard electrical power into the high voltages required for X-ray production, ensuring efficient and reliable performance of the CT tubes. The primary function of a high-voltage generator in a CT system is to create the electric field needed to accelerate electrons from the cathode to the anode within the X-ray tube. This acceleration is essential for producing X-rays, as the kinetic energy of the electrons, when they strike the anode, is converted into X-ray radiation. The quality and consistency of this high-voltage supply directly affect the quality of the X-ray images produced, making the generator a vital part of the imaging process.

Components and Operation

High-voltage generators in CT systems consist of several key components that work together to produce the required high voltage. A step-up transformer increases the standard input voltage (typically 110–240 volts AC) to the high kilovoltage levels needed (20–150 kV) for X-ray production. This high voltage is then converted from alternating current (AC) to direct current (DC) using silicon-based rectifiers, as X-ray tubes operate on DC. To ensure precise control of the voltage and current supplied to the X-ray tube, the generator includes advanced regulation systems. A filament transformer supplies low-voltage, high-current power to the cathode filament, heating it to produce electrons via thermionic emission. Modern CT systems use Automatic Exposure Control (AEC) to dynamically adjust the voltage and current, optimizing the radiation dose and image quality based on the patient's size and the area being imaged. Feedback mechanisms within the generator continuously monitor and adjust the output voltage and current, ensuring stable operation and consistent image quality.

Safety and Protection Mechanisms

High-voltage generators are equipped with various safety and protection mechanisms to prevent damage from overcurrent or overvoltage conditions. These include fuses, circuit breakers, and electronic protection systems. Efficient cooling systems, such as forced air, oil, or water cooling, are essential to dissipate the heat generated by the high-voltage components, maintaining optimal operating temperatures and ensuring reliable performance.

Integration with CT Systems

High-voltage generators are integrated into the overall CT system architecture to ensure seamless operation. This integration involves both hardware and software components. The generators are often designed as modular units, making them easier to replace and maintain. Special insulated cables connect the generator to the X-ray tube, and cable management systems help avoid electrical interference and ensure safety. The control software of the CT system interfaces with the high-voltage generator, managing voltage and current settings, exposure timing, and safety protocols. Advanced diagnostic tools are incorporated to monitor the generator's performance, predict maintenance needs, and troubleshoot issues, helping to ensure the generator operates within optimal parameters.

Impact on Image Quality and Patient Safety

The quality of the high-voltage generator directly impacts the quality of the CT images. A stable and precise high-voltage supply ensures that the X-ray tube operates optimally, producing high-resolution images with minimal noise. This is particularly important for detecting fine details in medical imaging, such as small lesions or subtle anatomical structures. Additionally, precise control of the high-voltage generator contributes to patient safety by optimizing the radiation dose. Automatic Exposure Control (AEC) systems adjust the radiation dose based on the patient's anatomy and the diagnostic requirements, minimizing exposure while ensuring diagnostic quality.

Advances and Innovations

Recent advancements in high-voltage generator technology have focused on improving efficiency, reducing size, and enhancing control capabilities. Digital generators incorporate digital control systems for more precise voltage and current regulation, improving image quality and dose control. Some modern generators use energy storage components, such as capacitors, to deliver more consistent power and reduce load on the electrical supply. Integration of IoT (Internet of Things) technologies allows for remote monitoring and diagnostics, improving maintenance and reducing downtime. Continuous innovations in this field aim to enhance the efficiency, reliability, and functionality of these critical components, ensuring that CT systems can provide the highest level of diagnostic capability.

6.8.1.3 Collimators

Collimators in CT significantly enhance image quality, reducing patient radiation dose, and improving overall imaging efficiency. Two main types of collimators are employed: pre-patient collimators and post-patient collimators.

(a) *Pre-patient Collimators*

Pre-patient collimators are located between the X-ray source and the patient (Fig. 6.16). Their primary function is to shape and narrow the X-ray beam before it reaches the patient. This precise shaping ensures that only the region of interest is irradiated, minimizing the exposure to surrounding tissues and thereby reducing the patient's overall radiation dose. These collimators are typically made of lead or other high-density materials capable of effectively blocking X-rays. They consist of adjustable lead shutters that can be positioned to form the desired beam shape and size. In modern CT systems, these collimators are often motorized and computer-controlled, allowing for precise and dynamic adjustments during the scanning process. By accurately controlling the beam width, pre-patient collimators help obtain thin slices, crucial for high-resolution imaging, while also reducing scatter radiation, which can degrade image quality and increase noise.

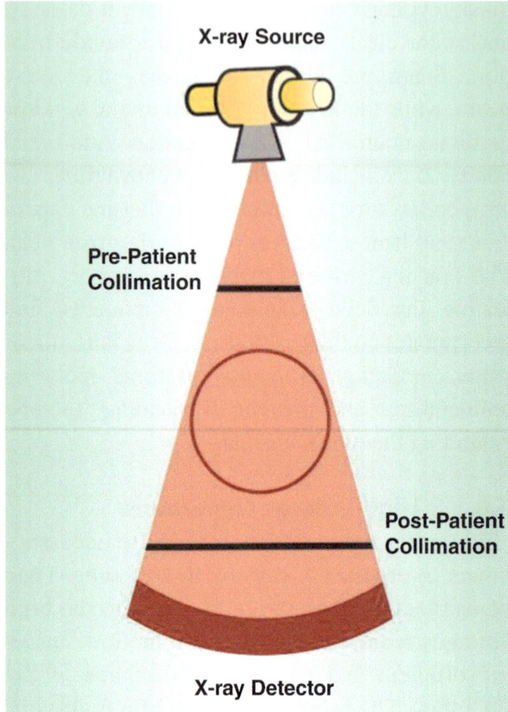

Fig. 6.16 Pre-and post-patient collimation

(b) *Post-patient Collimators*

Post-patient collimators are positioned between the patient and the X-ray detectors. Their main role is to further refine the X-ray beam after it has passed through the patient, ensuring that the detected signal is as accurate and clear as possible. These collimators help eliminate scatter radiation produced when X-rays interact with the patient's body. Scatter radiation can cause artifacts and reduce the contrast and clarity of the final image. Post-patient collimators are designed to ensure that only X-rays that have passed directly through the patient's body in the intended path reach the detectors, improving the signal-to-noise ratio and leading to better image quality.

(c) *Integration and Control*

Both pre-patient and post-patient collimators are integrated into the CT system's overall design and controlled by the system's software. This software allows for precise adjustments of the collimators during scanning, optimizing the beam shape and size for different types of examinations and patient anatomies. Advanced CT systems use real-time feedback mechanisms to adjust collimator settings dynamically, ensuring optimal imaging conditions throughout the scan.

(d) *Advances and Innovations*

Modern CT systems have seen significant advancements in collimator technology, contributing to improved imaging efficiency and patient safety. Innovations include motorized and computer-controlled collimators that enable precise and automated adjustments, enhancing the flexibility and efficiency of the scanning process. These advanced collimators are integrated with the system's software, allowing for fine-tuning during scanning to optimize the beam shape and size for different types of examinations and patient anatomies. Dynamic collimation features have been introduced, which enable real-time adjustments based on the specific requirements of each scan. This capability ensures optimal imaging conditions throughout the scan, improving image quality and reducing the radiation dose to the patient. Adaptive collimation techniques further enhance these benefits by adjusting the collimator settings based on the patient's size, shape, and the specific area being imaged. This optimization helps to achieve the best possible image quality while minimizing the radiation exposure.

The combination of these innovations allows for a more tailored approach to CT imaging, ensuring that each scan is as effective and safe as possible. The integration of motorized, computer-controlled, and adaptive collimation technologies represents a significant leap forward in CT imaging, providing radiologists with more precise tools to capture high-quality images and improve diagnostic outcomes.

6.8.1.4 Filters

Within the CT gantry, filters are designed to shape the beam, improve image quality, and reduce patient radiation dose. The primary types of filters are bow tie filters and spectral filters.

- **Bow Tie Filters (Beam-Shaping Filters):** Bow tie filters are designed to improve dose distribution and image quality by compensating for variations in patient anatomy. These filters are typically placed in the X-ray beam path and are thicker at the edges and thinner in the center. By attenuating the X-ray beam more at the periphery, where less tissue is present, and less at the center where the body is thicker, bow tie filters help achieve a more uniform intensity across the field of view. This results in improved image quality and more consistent radiation dose distribution. Although their primary role is beam-shaping and dose optimization, they also indirectly help minimize artifacts related to beam hardening.
- **Spectral Filters:** Spectral filters are designed to split the X-ray beam into two or more distinct energy spectra, allowing for the differentiation of materials based on their energy-dependent attenuation properties. Spectral filters may employ various materials or techniques to achieve this spectral separation, such as using different thicknesses of materials or incorporating specialized structures into the filter design. By acquiring multiple energy datasets simultaneously, spectral imaging provides additional information about tissue composition and enables applications such as material decomposition and virtual non-contrast imaging.

6.8.1.5 Detectors

Computed tomography (CT) detectors capture the X-ray photons that have passed through the patient and convert them into electrical signals.

Unlike scintillation detection mechanisms used in nuclear medicine, which typically operate in pulse mode, Conventional CT scintillation detection always operates in current mode. While pulse mode preserves individual events' energy and temporal information, current mode in CT provides a stable current, particularly beneficial when event rates are very high. However, in photon counting CTs, each incoming X-ray photon generates a distinct pulse, which is counted and analyzed individually. This allows the system to record the energy and timing of each photon. By preserving the energy information of individual photons, photon counting CT can differentiate materials more precisely. This leads to improved contrast resolution and the ability to perform spectral imaging.

The radiation flux in CT is exceptionally high, approximately on the order of 10^9 quanta per second per mm^2 at the detector level [62]. The CT detectors often utilize inorganic crystals or transparent ceramic scintillators chosen for their good light output, absence of long afterglow, and resistance to radiation damage over prolonged use. Common scintillators include Cesium Iodide thallium activated (CsI(Tl)), Cadmium Tungstate ($CdWO_4$), Gadolinium Oxysulfide (Gd_2O_2S), and Yttria and Gadolinia with Eu activated $(Y, Gd)_2O_3$ or $Y_{1.34}Gd_{0.60}Eu_{0.06}O_3$ (see Table 6.5). General Electric (GE) has used $(YGd)_2O_3$ in over 8000 CT scanners since 1988 and recently introduced Gemstone detectors, while Siemens has utilized proprietary Ultra-fast ceramics (UFC) and Stellar detectors [62].

Table 6.5 Detector properties used in CT imaging

Material	Density (g/cm^3)	Thickness to stop 99% of 140 keV X-rays (mm)	Emission wavelength (nm)	Light yield (ph/MeV)	Temperature coefficient (%/°C)	Primary decay time (μs)	Afterglow (% at 3 ms)
CsI (Tl)	4.52	6.1	550	54,000	0.02	1	0.5
$CdWO_4$ (CWO)	7.9	2.6	495	28,000	−0.3	2, 15	0.05
Gd_2O_3:Eu^{+3}	7.55	2.6	610	–	–	–	–
$Y_{1.34}Gd_{0.6}O_3$, Pr, Tb (YGO)	5.9	6.1	610	42,000	0.04	1000	5
Gd_2O_2S: Pr, Ce, F (GOS)	7.34	2.9	520	50,000	−0.6	2.4	<0.1
Gd_2O_2S: Tb (Ce) (GOS)	7.34	2.9	550	50,000	−0.6	600	0.6
La_2HfO_7:Ti	7.9	2.8	475	13,000	–	10	–
$Gd_3Ga_5O_{12}$, Ce	7.09	4.5	730	39,000	–	150	<0.1

Abbreviations:
CsI (Tl) - Cesium Iodide (Thallium activated) - CsI (Tl)
$CdWO_4$ (CWO) - Cadmium Tungstate
Gd_2O_3:Eu^{+3} - Gadolinium Oxide (Europium activated)
$Y_{1.34}Gd_{0.6}O_3$, Pr, Tb (YGO) - Yttrium Gadolinium Oxide (Europium, Praseodymium, Terbium activated)
Gd_2O_2S: Pr, Ce, F (GOS) - Gadolinium Oxysulfide (Praseodymium, Cerium, Fluorine activated)
Gd_2O_2S: Tb (Ce) (GOS) - Gadolinium Oxysulfide (Terbium activated)
La_2HfO_7:Ti - Lanthanum Hafnate (Titanium activated)
$Gd_3Ga_5O_{12}$, Ce - Gadolinium Gallium Garnet (Chromium, Cerium activated)

Explanation of Parameters:
Density (g/cm^3): Indicates the density of the material.
Thickness to stop 99% of 140 keV X-rays (mm): The thickness required for the material to stop 99% of X-rays at 140 keV energy.
Emission Wavelength (nm): The wavelength at which the material emits light after interacting with X-rays.
Light Yield (ph/MeV): The number of photons emitted per unit of absorbed energy (Mega electron Volt).
Temperature Coefficient (%/°C): The change in light yield per degree Celsius.
Primary Decay Time (μs): The time it takes for the scintillation light to decay to a fraction of its initial intensity.
Afterglow (% at 3 ms): The percentage of remaining light output 3 milliseconds after the initial pulse.

CT detectors can consist of millions of individual detector elements arranged in pixelated arrays. When X-rays interact with the detectors, scintillation light is produced and converted into electrical signals by photodiodes. These signals are then processed by additional circuitry, with many detector channels sharing common electronics. In CT imaging, a spatial resolution of 1 mm at the detector is often required; however, rapid gantry rotation and numerous projections necessitate a high temporal resolution of less than 100 milliseconds.

The scintillation photons generated by the detectors are converted into electrical signals by photodiodes, semiconductor devices that function similarly to photomultiplier tubes (PMTs) by converting light photons into current. The detector elements are positioned in a circular arc, often referred to as the "detector banana," with each detector pixel consisting of a scintillator crystal and an attached photodiode. These photodiodes are connected to electronics channels, including amplifiers and analog-to-digital converters (ADCs), configured for CT detector operation.

An another technology called "Dual-layer detectors" employ two stacked scintillator layers to simultaneously capture low- and high-energy X-ray data during standard CT protocols [63]. This dual-energy capability enhances material discrimination and contrast resolution without needing separate X-ray sources. The top layer absorbs low-energy photons, while the bottom layer captures high-energy photons, enabling the generation of multiple spectral images through projection-space decomposition. These spectral images include material decomposition (iodine-only, virtual non-contrast, effective atomic number) and virtual monoenergetic images, which can be produced on-demand based on clinical requirements [63]. This technology improves vascular contrast, lesion conspicuity, and material characterization while reducing artifacts and radiation dose [63].

Photon-counting detectors (PCDs) now enable spectral imaging by counting individual photons and measuring their energy, offering improved image quality and lower radiation doses. New scintillator materials like enhanced Gadolinium Oxysulfide (GOS) and Yttrium-based compounds offer higher light output and stability. High-density detectors, including ceramic scintillators and those with smaller pixel sizes, provide superior spatial resolution and handle higher photon fluxes. Improvements in electronics and signal processing have increased the dynamic range and sensitivity of modern detectors. Integration with advanced imaging software and AI allows for real-time adjustments and enhanced image reconstruction, further optimizing image quality. Collectively, these innovations have made CT imaging more efficient, accurate, and safer for patients.

6.8.1.6 Data Acquisition System (DAS)

The Data Acquisition System (DAS) involves sampling electrical signals and converting these samples into digital numeric values that can be processed by a computer. The primary functions include measuring the transmitted radiation beam, encoding the measurements into binary data, and transmitting this binary data to a computer for further processing. Following are the functions of DAS:

- **Signal Amplification:** The electrical signals generated by photodiodes in the detector array are initially weak and require amplification. The DAS includes preamplifiers that boost these signals to a level suitable for further processing while minimizing noise introduction.
- **Analog-to-Digital Conversion (ADC):** After amplification, the analog signals are converted into digital form by ADCs within the DAS. This conversion translates the continuous analog signals into discrete digital values, representing the intensity of the detected X-rays.
- **Noise Reduction:** The DAS incorporates techniques to minimize noise from electronic components and external sources. Effective noise reduction ensures the integrity and clarity of the acquired data.
- **Data Synchronization:** Synchronization is vital for collecting and processing data from different detector elements accurately, especially during rapid gantry rotation and high-

speed scans. The DAS ensures precise timing and coordination across the entire detector array.

- **Data Formatting and Transmission:** Once digitized, the data needs to be formatted and transmitted efficiently to the central processing unit (CPU) of the CT scanner. The DAS organizes the data into a suitable structure for transmission to the image reconstruction system.

Components of the DAS

- **Preamplifiers:** Located close to the detector array, preamplifiers boost the initial signals with minimal noise introduction, preparing them for further amplification and processing.
- **Amplifiers:** Additional amplification stages increase the signal strength to levels appropriate for ADC. These stages are carefully designed to maintain signal integrity.
- **Analog-to-Digital Converters (ADCs):** High-speed, high-resolution ADCs convert analog signals into digital form, ensuring precise and rapid data conversion.
- **Multiplexers:** Multiplexers manage the numerous detector channels, allowing multiple signals to be processed through fewer ADCs. They switch between channels at high speed to ensure continuous data acquisition.
- **Data Buffers:** Buffers temporarily store the digitized data before transmission to the CPU, managing data flow and preventing data loss during transmission.
- **Synchronization Circuits:** These circuits ensure that data from different detector elements are collected and processed simultaneously, maintaining temporal alignment across the entire detector array.
- **Transmission Interfaces:** High-speed data transmission interfaces connect the DAS to the central processing unit, enabling rapid and efficient data transfer for image reconstruction.

For Photon-counting detectors, DAS is designed to handle individual photon events, preserving energy and temporal information for each photon, enabling spectral imaging and improved material differentiation. Advances in electronics have allowed for the miniaturization of DAS components, resulting in more compact and integrated designs. This reduces power consumption and enhances overall system reliability.

By efficiently amplifying, converting, and transmitting signals from the detector array, the DAS directly impacts the clarity, resolution, and diagnostic value of the CT images. Ongoing advancements in DAS technology continue to enhance the performance and capabilities of modern CT scanners, supporting more accurate and efficient diagnostic imaging.

6.8.1.7 Gantry Motor and Rotational Mechanism

The gantry rotational mechanism enables the precise movement of the X-ray tube and detector array around the patient, typically powered by a high-torque, variable-speed electric motor. This motor delivers the necessary power to rotate the heavy gantry assembly smoothly and accurately. By facilitating the rotation of the gantry during the scan, it allows for the acquisition of images from multiple angles, producing detailed cross-sectional images. The motor's speed and torque are finely controlled to ensure consistent and precise rotation, which is crucial for maintaining image quality and ensuring patient safety.

6.8.1.8 Slip Rings

Slip rings allow for the transmission of power and data signals without the need for cumbersome wiring that could limit the gantry's rotational capabilities. They enable the gantry to rotate continuously around the patient while maintaining electrical connections. This continuous rotation is the basic principle of CT data acquisition from different angles, which are then reconstructed into cross-sectional images by the CT scanner's computer.

Slip rings were invented by Arthur Hood, West Long Branch, N.J., Morris from New York in 1945 and granted patent in 1949 [64]. They were initially used in electrical motors and generators to allow the transmission of current through rotating parts. Their application in medical imaging, particularly in CT scanners, marked a significant technological advancement in 1987 which prior to 1987, relied mostly on cables to power the X-ray tubes and transmit detector signals [9]. Though the Varian System introduced slip ring in 1976 with third generation CT scanners which supported continuous gantry rotation and transferred high-voltage power, but they had small diameter of slip ring and transferred high power unlike modern CT scanner slip rings that transfer power at low voltage and have a compact high voltage power supply on the gantry [6].

Design and Components

The slip ring assembly typically consists of a rotating ring (or rings) attached to the rotating part of the gantry and stationary brushes or contacts that remain fixed in place. As the gantry rotates, the brushes maintain contact with the rotating rings, allowing for the transfer of electrical signals. The rings are made from conductive materials, such as copper or gold-plated metals, which ensure efficient electrical conductivity. The stationary brushes are usually composed of conductive carbon or metal alloys designed to minimize wear and ensure a reliable connection.

The slip ring assembly is housed in a protective casing that provides insulation and shields the components from dust, debris, and other contaminants. This casing is crucial for maintaining the integrity and longevity of the slip ring assembly. High-speed CT scanners generate significant heat, so slip rings often include cooling mechanisms to prevent overheating. This can involve air or liquid cooling systems integrated into the slip ring assembly.

Advances in materials science have led to the development of more durable and conductive materials for both rings and brushes, enhancing the longevity and performance of slip rings. Modern slip ring assemblies are becoming more compact, allowing for smaller and more efficient gantry designs. This miniaturization helps reduce the overall size and weight of the CT scanner, making it more versatile and easier to install in various clinical settings. Innovations in data transfer technology have increased the bandwidth and speed at which data can be transmitted through slip rings. This capability is particularly important for advanced imaging techniques that require high-resolution and high-speed data acquisition.

6.8.1.9 Heat Exchanger Unit

The heat exchanger unit plays a crucial role in maintaining the optimal performance of the CT scanner, particularly by regulating the temperature of the CT gantry's internal components. The primary function of this system is to manage the substantial heat generated by the X-ray tube during operation. This heat, if left unchecked, can induce thermal stress, cause component failure, and degrade image quality. By ensuring a stable operating temperature, the heat exchanger extends the lifespan of the X-ray tube and other sensitive electronics, thereby reducing the frequency of maintenance and replacement. Consistent thermal regulation is vital to prevent thermal drift, which can otherwise lead to artifacts and noise in the images produced by the CT scanner.

Components of the Heat Exchanger System

(a) **Cooling Medium**: The heat exchanger utilizes a cooling medium—typically a liquid coolant such as water or an oil-based fluid—to absorb and transport heat away from the heated components.
(b) **Pumps**: These devices circulate the cooling medium throughout the heat exchanger system. Pumps ensure a continuous flow of coolant from the hot components to the heat exchanger unit and back.
(c) **Radiators and Fans**: Radiators and fans work together to dissipate the absorbed heat from the cooling medium into the surrounding environment. Heat is transferred from the coolant to the air, with fans often aiding in enhancing airflow and cooling efficiency.
(d) **Heat Exchanger Unit**: The heart of the system, the heat exchanger unit, facilitates the transfer of heat from the coolant to the air. It typically comprises a network of tubes or plates designed to maximize the surface area available for heat exchange.

(e) **Temperature Sensors and Controllers**: These components monitor the temperature of both the coolant and the key components of the CT gantry. Sensors relay temperature data to controllers, which adjust the operation of the pumps and fans to maintain the desired temperature range.

Function

(a) **Heat Absorption**: As the CT scanner operates, the heat generated by the X-ray tube and other electronics is absorbed by the coolant circulating through the system.
(b) **Circulation of Coolant**: The now-heated coolant is transported away from the hot components to the heat exchanger unit by the pumps.
(c) **Heat Dissipation**: At the heat exchanger unit, heat is transferred from the coolant to the air. Radiators and fans facilitate this process, enhancing the efficiency of heat dissipation.
(d) **Cooled Coolant Return**: The cooled coolant is circulated back to the hot components, ready to absorb more heat, thus completing the thermal management cycle.
(e) **Continuous Operation**: Effective thermal management enables the CT scanner to function continuously without the risk of overheating, which is essential during extended or high-throughput scanning sessions.

Efficient thermal management minimizes downtime caused by overheating and eliminating the need for cooling-off periods. This not only enhances the overall efficiency and throughput of the CT scanning process but also ensures the reliability of the CT scanner. By maintaining optimal temperatures, improving image quality, and extending the equipment's lifespan, thermal management significantly contributes to the performance and dependability of modern CT imaging systems.

6.8.1.10 Laser Positioning System

The laser positioning system within a CT gantry is designed to ensure the precise alignment and positioning of the patient and quality assurance tools. This ensures that the anatomical region of interest is accurately centered and aligned with the CT scanner's imaging plane, enabling precise and efficient image acquisition.

The system comprises lateral, sagittal, and coronal lasers. Lateral lasers project horizontal lines along the sides of the patient, helping to center the desired anatomical region within the scanner's field of view (Fig. 6.17). Sagittal lasers project vertical lines along the midline of the patient, ensuring proper alignment in the head-to-foot direction and aiding in positioning the exact slice plane to be scanned. Coronal lasers, projecting lines from above, intersect with the lateral and sagittal lines to align the patient in the anterior-posterior direction, ensuring proper depth positioning within the scanner.

The lasers create visible reference lines on the patient's body, which technologists use to adjust the patient's position on the CT table. By align-

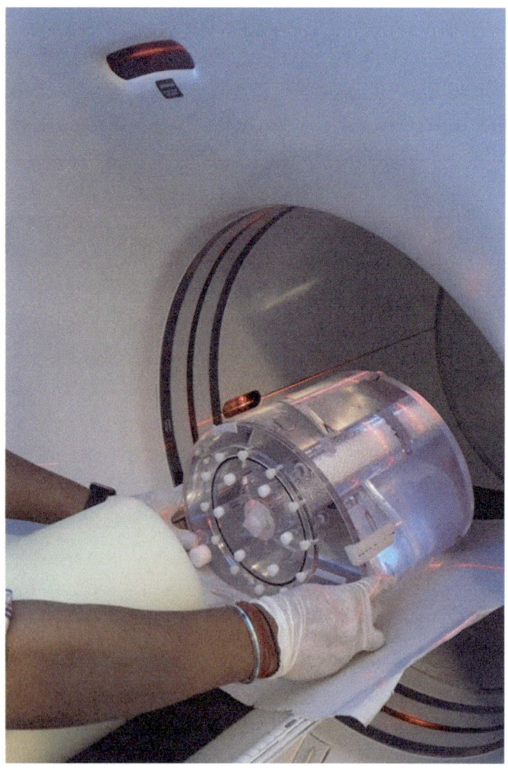

Fig. 6.17 Positioning of phantom using laser lights in a PET-CT machine

ing these lines with anatomical landmarks or external markers, the patient can be positioned precisely. Before the scan begins, the laser lines are used to verify the patient's alignment, ensuring that the scan covers the exact area of interest and that the slices are taken consistently along the desired planes. This coordinated use of lateral, sagittal, and coronal lasers ensures that the cross-sectional images obtained during the scan are accurate and correspond precisely to the anatomical regions being studied, which is vital for diagnostic accuracy and image quality.

When a scan is initiated, the laser positioning system activates, projecting lines of light onto the patient's body, usually in red for high visibility. Technologists then use these projected laser lines to adjust the patient's position. The CT table can be moved up, down, laterally, and longitudinally to align the patient's body with the lasers. Adjustments are made until the laser lines intersect at the desired anatomical landmarks. In some advanced CT systems, the laser positioning can be part of an automated patient positioning system, which uses cameras and software to detect the laser lines and adjust the table position automatically, ensuring precise alignment with minimal manual intervention.

The lateral, sagittal, and coronal lasers work in unison to create a three-dimensional reference framework around the patient. This coordinated operation ensures that the patient's position is adjusted correctly in all three planes (axial, sagittal, and coronal). Once the patient is positioned, the technologists perform a final verification using the laser lines to ensure that the alignment is correct. This step is crucial for preventing misalignment and ensuring that the scan data will be accurate.

6.8.1.11 Control Electronics

Control electronics within the CT gantry ensures the precise control and coordination of the gantry's functions, including the movement of the X-ray tube, detector array, and patient table, as well as the acquisition and processing of imaging data. At the core of the control electronics are microprocessors and controllers that manage the overall operation of the CT scanner. These central processing units execute software instructions to control the gantry's movement, timing the execution of the X-ray tube, and synchronizing data acquisition from the detectors. Motor control circuits are responsible for the high-torque, variable-speed electric motors that rotate the gantry and move the patient table, ensuring smooth and precise movements that are critical for maintaining consistent operation and optimal image quality.

Additionally, diagnostic and safety systems continuously monitor the operation of the CT scanner, detecting any anomalies or malfunctions. These systems provide real-time feedback and alerts to the operator, initiate automatic shutdown procedures if necessary, and ensure the safety of both the patient and the equipment.

6.8.2 The Computer System for Data Processing and Image Reconstruction

The second part of the CT machine is the computer system responsible for processing the data collected by the scanning components. This system, usually housed in a box structure near the gantry, called the "reconstruction unit" or "recon unit," which handles data processing and image reconstruction. Transferring data from the Data Acquisition System (DAS) to the computer system involves a multi-step procedure designed to ensure data integrity and high-quality image production. The DAS captures analog signals from the detectors and converts them into digital signals using an Analog-to-Digital Converter (ADC) located within the DAS, positioned close to the detectors. This digital data is then transmitted to the recon unit for further processing and image reconstruction, ensuring efficient data conversion and minimizing potential signal degradation.

Once preprocessed, the data is transmitted from the DAS to the computer system via high-speed communication channels, often using fiber-optic cables for rapid and reliable transfer. Upon reaching the computer system, the data is temporarily stored in high-speed memory buffers or RAM, allowing efficient access during processing. The data is then organized into a format suitable for image reconstruction, such as sinograms, which represent the intensity of detected signals in relation to the X-ray source's position and angle. The organized data undergoes mathematical transformations, such as the Fourier transform, converting spatial frequency domain data into the spatial domain, and filtering techniques to enhance image quality by reducing artifacts.

Image reconstruction involves algorithms like filtered back projection (FBP), iterative reconstruction (IR), and advanced algorithms like deep learning-based (DL based) methods to create images from the raw data. Each algorithm has its own advantages and disadvantages in terms of speed, image quality, and computational requirements. These algorithms transform the data into cross-sectional images by computing attenuation values for each pixel in the image matrix. The reconstructed images may undergo further post-processing to enhance quality, including image enhancement, contrast adjustment (windowing), noise reduction, enlargement, and quantitative measurements. Advanced features include multi-planar reconstruction (creating images in different planes) and 3D imaging, providing detailed anatomical views for better diagnosis and planning.

Finally, the processed images are stored in a permanent storage system, such as a Picture Archiving and Communication System (PACS), for long-term archival and easy retrieval. The images are then sent to calibrated display monitors for review by radiologists and clinicians, ensuring accurate representation of diagnostic information. This comprehensive process, from data acquisition to image display, is fundamental to the effective use of CT technology in medical imaging.

Let's discuss each step in a detailed manner:

6.8.2.1 Data Preprocessing

Preprocessing steps are performed before the data reconstruction process. These steps clean and correct the raw projection data, making it suitable for reconstruction. The reconstruction algorithms (FBP, IR, or DL based methods) then use this preprocessed data to generate accurate and high-quality cross-sectional images. Preprocessing ensures that the input to the reconstruction process is as accurate and artifact-free as possible, thereby enhancing the final image quality. The data preprocessing involves several steps such as detector calibration, normalization, logarithmic transformation, beam hardening correction, scatter correction, noise reduction, geometric calibration, flat-field correction, motion correction, bad pixel correction, gain and offset correction, and ring artifact correction.

6.8.2.1.1 Detector Calibration

Detector calibration adjusts the detector readings to correct for sensitivity and gain variations, ensuring a consistent and uniform detector response. This step addresses sensitivity variations and gain variations among the detectors. By calibrating the detectors, we ensure that each detector in the array responds uniformly to the same amount of incident X-ray photons. This uniformity is critical for accurate image reconstruction and diagnostic quality. The following steps are involved in detector calibration:

1. **Reference Measurements (Air Scans)**: Reference measurements, also known as air scans, are taken without any object in the path of the X-ray beam. This measurement captures the baseline response of the detectors to the X-ray beam. This measurement provides a baseline reference for each detector. Let $I_{\text{raw}}(x)$ be the intensity measured by the detector at position "x" when no object is in the path (air scan).
2. **Dark Field Measurements and Correction**: Dark field measurements also called "Offset Correction" are taken when the X-ray beam is off, capturing the detector's response to ambient conditions or inherent electronic noise. This basically accounts for the electronic noise or dark current that is present when no X-ray photons are incident on the detectors. This correction ensures that the baseline signal is adjusted to zero when there is no X-ray exposure. Let $D(x)$ be the dark field measurement for the detector at position

x. Then, the dark corrected field measurement:

$$I_{\text{dark corrected}}(x) = I_{\text{raw}}(x) - D(x)$$

3. **Determine the Gain Factor and Its Correction**: Gain correction adjusts the signal amplification to account for differences in detector sensitivity. This step ensures that each detector's response is proportional to the incident X-ray intensity. Let $G(x)$ be the gain factor for the detector at position x. The gain-corrected signal $I_{\text{gain corrected}}(x)$ is given by:

$$I_{\text{gain corrected}}(x) = \frac{I_{\text{dark corrected}}(x)}{G(x)}$$

Thus, the calibrated intensity is:

$$I_{\text{calibrated}}(x) = \frac{I_{\text{raw}}(x) - D(x)}{G(x)}$$

After calibration, the detector readings should be consistent and uniform across the array. This consistency is crucial for accurate projection data and high-quality image reconstruction. The calibrated data is then normalized and logarithmically transformed during subsequent preprocessing steps, ensuring it is ready for the reconstruction algorithms.

6.8.2.1.2 Normalization

Normalization adjusts the projection data to account for variations in detector sensitivity and X-ray source intensity, ensuring consistency across the data. The process involves scaling the raw detector readings so that they reflect only the attenuation properties of the tissues being scanned. Let $I_{\text{raw}}(x, \theta)$ be the raw intensity measured by the detector at position x and projection angle θ.

- **Reference Measurement** I_0: This is the intensity measured without any object in the path, often referred to as the air scan or reference scan.
- **Normalized Intensity** $I(x, \theta)$: This is obtained by dividing the raw intensity by the reference measurement.

$$I(x,\theta) = \frac{I_{\text{raw}}(x,\theta)}{I_0(x,\theta)}$$

Normalization ensures that the measured intensity is scaled relative to the reference measurement, making the data more consistent and comparable across different detectors and projection angles by compensating for variations in source intensity and detector sensitivity.

6.8.2.1.3 Logarithmic Transformation

Logarithmic transformation converts the normalized intensity values into attenuation coefficients, which are more directly related to the tissue properties being imaged. This step transforms the multiplicative attenuation process into an additive form, facilitating the reconstruction process. Using Beer's law, the relationship between the transmitted intensity and the attenuation coefficient can be expressed as:

$$I(x,\theta) = I_0.e^{-\int_{\text{path}} \mu(t)dt}$$

Where $\mu(t)$ is the linear attenuation coefficient along the path t.

Taking the natural logarithm on both sides gives:

$$\ln(I(x,\theta) = \ln(I_0) - \int_{\text{path}} \mu(t)dt$$

Rearranging this, we get:

$$\int_{\text{path}} \mu(t)dt = \ln(I_0) - \ln(I(x,\theta))$$

Since I_0 is constant for a given scan, we can denote $\ln(I_0)$ as a constant C:

$$\int_{\text{path}} \mu(t)dt = C - \ln(I(x,\theta))$$

For practical purposes, this can be simplified as:

$$\int_{\text{path}} \mu(t)dt \approx -\ln(I(x,\theta))$$

Here, the negative sign is important because the intensity decreases as it passes through the object.

The overall process combining normalization and logarithmic transformation can be described mathematically as:

$$P(x,\theta) = -\ln\left(\frac{I_{\text{raw}}(x,\theta)}{I_0(x,\theta)}\right)$$

where $P(x,\theta)$ is the final processed projection data (often referred to as line integrals or sinogram data), suitable for reconstruction.

6.8.2.1.4 Beam Hardening Correction

Beam hardening occurs because lower-energy X-ray photons are absorbed more easily than higher-energy photons as they pass through an object, causing the X-ray beam to become "harder" (having a higher average energy) as it travels through the object. This leads to artifacts in CT images, such as cupping artifacts and streaks. To correct for beam hardening, the process begins by acknowledging the polychromatic nature of the X-ray source, which emits a spectrum of photon energies. Calibration phantoms with known materials are used to model the beam hardening effect, and a correction curve is created to represent how different materials attenuate the X-ray beam at various thicknesses. The initial image reconstruction is performed using the raw projection data, and areas with beam hardening artifacts are identified. These artifacts typically appear as cupping artifacts, where the center of the object appears darker, or as streak artifacts between dense structures. Correction algorithms, often polynomial or iterative in nature, adjust the attenuation values based on the beam hardening model. The projection data is adjusted according to these corrections, and the image reconstruction is repeated iteratively to refine the correction. The mathematics behind this involves using a polynomial model to correct the raw projection data, represented as:

$$P_{\text{corrected}}(x) = P_{\text{raw}}(x) + a_1 P_{\text{raw}}(x)^2 + a_2 P_{\text{raw}}(x)^3 + \ldots\ldots\ldots\ldots\ldots$$

where a_1, a_2, a_3, …… are coefficients derived from calibration.

6.8.2.1.5 Scatter Correction

Scatter radiation results from X-ray photons being deflected from their original path due to interactions within the object, causing additional, unwanted photons to reach the detector and leading to a loss of contrast and artifacts in the images. The first step in scatter correction involves measuring the scatter radiation using detectors positioned outside the primary beam path or using Monte Carlo simulations or physical scatter models to estimate the scatter distribution. A scatter model is then developed based on these measurements or simulations, incorporating parameters such as object size, shape, and composition. The estimated scatter is subtracted from the detected signal to correct the projection data. This involves using the scatter model to calculate the scatter contribution for each detector reading. Similar to beam hardening correction, iterative methods can be employed to refine the scatter correction. Initial scatter estimates are refined by re-measuring the scatter after preliminary correction. The mathematics of scatter correction involves the raw detected signal being the sum of the primary and scatter signals:

$$I_{\text{detected}}(x) = I_{\text{primary}}(x) + I_{\text{scatter}}(x)$$

The scatter model $S(x)$ estimates the scatter as:

$$I_{\text{scatter}}(x) = S(x)$$

The detected signal is corrected by subtracting the scatter estimate:

$$I_{\text{corrected}}(x) = I_{\text{detected}}(x) + S(x)$$

The corrected signal is then transformed using a log transformation for further processing:

$$P_{\text{corrected}}(x) = \ln\left(\frac{I_0}{I_{\text{corrected}}(x)}\right)$$

6.8.2.1.6 Noise Reduction

Noise reduction filters out random noise and improves the image quality. Specifically, noise reduction aims to enhance the signal-to-noise ratio (SNR) of the projection data, which is essential for producing clear and accurate images. One common technique used is Gaussian filtering, which smooths out high-frequency noise components while preserving important image details. By applying such filters to the raw projection data, random noise is effectively reduced, leading to more reliable and consistent data for the subsequent reconstruction process. This preprocessing step ensures that the images reconstructed from the filtered data have reduced noise levels, resulting in improved clarity and diagnostic quality.

6.8.2.1.7 Geometric Calibration

Geometric calibration ensures the accuracy and consistency of the spatial relationships within CT images. This involves aligning the imaging system components and correcting for any geometric distortions caused by misalignments or mechanical imperfections. Initially, system alignment is performed to ensure that the X-ray source, detectors, and gantry are correctly positioned. Calibration phantoms with known geometrical properties are then scanned to assess and correct geometric distortions. The data from these phantoms reveal any deviations from the expected geometry, allowing for the generation of correction factors. Geometric distortion correction is applied to the raw projection data, adjusting it to account for these deviations and ensuring that the reconstructed image accurately reflects the true spatial relationships within the scanned object. Additionally, gantry rotation calibration ensures that each projection's angular position is precise, preventing artifacts such as streaking or blurring. Detector calibration ensures consistent sensitivity and accurate spatial positioning of each detector element. These preprocessing steps are essential for minimizing artifacts and ensuring that the data used in the reconstruction process is accurate and reliable.

6.8.2.1.8 Flat-Field Correction

Flat-field correction ensures uniformity in the detector's response, thereby improving image quality and accuracy. This correction addresses variations in detector sensitivity and gain, which can cause inconsistencies and artifacts in the final image. The process involves capturing images of a uniform, homogenous object, often referred to as a flat field or flood field, which ideally should produce a uniform signal across all detectors. By comparing these flat-field images to the raw projection data, correction factors are determined for each detector element. These factors adjust the raw data to account for any deviations in detector response, ensuring that each detector contributes uniformly to the image reconstruction. Mathematically, this involves normalizing the raw detector readings $I_{raw}(x)$ by the flat-field measurements $F(x)$, resulting in corrected values $I_{corrected}(x) = \frac{I_{raw}(x)}{F(x)}$. This correction step is crucial for eliminating artifacts caused by detector inhomogeneities, leading to more accurate and consistent CT images.

6.8.2.1.9 Motion Correction

Motion correction compensates for patient movement during the scan. Motion artifacts can significantly degrade image quality, leading to blurred images and inaccurate anatomical representation. The process of motion correction involves detecting and correcting for any movements that occur during the data acquisition phase. This can be done using several methods, such as tracking fiducial markers placed on the patient's body, using motion sensors, or employing image-based techniques that detect inconsistencies in the projection data. Once motion is detected, algorithms are applied to adjust the projection data accordingly. These algorithms may involve rigid or non-rigid registration techniques, aligning the projection data to a common reference frame. The corrected data is then used in the reconstruction process, resulting in clearer and more accurate images. Motion correction is particularly important in dynamic imaging scenarios, such as cardiac CT, where the beating heart can cause significant motion artifacts. By effectively addressing these artifacts, motion correction ensures that the reconstructed images accurately reflect the true anatomical structures, enhancing the diagnostic utility of the CT scan.

6.8.2.1.10 Bad Pixel Correction

Bad pixel correction addresses the issue of malfunctioning or non-responsive detector elements, known as bad pixels. These defective pixels can result from various factors, including manufacturing defects, radiation damage, or wear and tear over time. Bad pixels fail to accurately record the X-ray signal, leading to artifacts and inaccuracies in the final reconstructed image. The correction process begins with the identification of bad pixels, which can be achieved through regular calibration scans using uniform phantoms or through continuous monitoring during routine operation. Once identified, the values of these bad pixels are corrected by interpolating the data from neighboring pixels that are functioning correctly. This interpolation can be performed using simple linear methods or more sophisticated algorithms, depending on the extent and distribution of the bad pixels. Mathematically, if $P(x)$ is a bad pixel, its corrected value $P_{\text{corrected}}(x)$ might be computed as the average of adjacent pixel values. This ensures that the final dataset is free from anomalies caused by defective detectors, leading to higher quality and more accurate CT images.

6.8.2.1.11 Ring Artifact Correction

Ring artifact correction aims at eliminating ring artifacts that appear as concentric rings centered around the rotation axis of the scanner. These artifacts are typically caused by inconsistencies in the response of individual detector elements or groups of elements, often due to calibration errors, detector defects, or variations in detector gain. The presence of ring artifacts can significantly degrade image quality and obscure important anatomical details. The correction process involves several steps. First, the raw projection data is analyzed to detect the presence and severity of ring artifacts. Techniques such as Fourier transform methods can be used to identify periodic patterns in the data that correspond to ring artifacts. Once detected, various correction algorithms are applied. One common approach is to normalize the detector readings, adjusting the gain and offset values to ensure consistent response across all detectors. Another method involves applying correction filters that specifically target the periodic nature of ring artifacts in the frequency domain. By addressing these inconsistencies, ring artifact correction ensures that the reconstructed images are free from circular artifacts, resulting in clearer and more diagnostically useful CT images.

6.8.2.2 Reconstruction Process

Once the preprocessing steps are complete, the cleaned and corrected projection data is transferred to the reconstruction algorithms. The main reconstruction methods, filtered back projection and Iterative Reconstruction, along with newly introduced Deep Learning Reconstruction [65], then take over to create the final cross-sectional images.

The foundational concept of image reconstruction is attributed to Johann Karl August Radon or Johann Radon, who presented the mathematical theory behind it in 1917. Radon's work laid the groundwork for later developments in medical imaging, including CT. Johann Radon was an Austrian mathematician and formulated the Radon transform, which is a mathematical technique for reconstructing a function from its projections. His 1917, his original publication, titled "Über die Bestimmung von Funktionen durch ihre Integralwerte längs gewisser Mannigfaltigkeiten," appeared in the journal "Berichte der Sachsischen Akadamie der Wissenschaft, vol. 69, pp. 262–277, 1917 [66]," which provided the theoretical basis for tomographic imaging. His paper was translated into the English by P. C. Parks in 1986 with name "On the Determination of Functions from Their Integral Values Along Certain Manifolds" [67] (Fig. 6.18).

To create a cross-sectional image of the body, the absorption profile is processed using reconstruction techniques such as Filtered Back Projection (FBP), iterative reconstruction algorithms or deep learning reconstruction methods. FBP involves applying mathematical filters to the projection data to enhance image quality and reduce noise. The filtered projections are then back projected onto an image matrix, reconstructing the original attenuation values of the tissues. Iterative reconstruction, on the other hand, refines the image by comparing measured projection data with simulated projections from an initial image estimate, making adjustments until the simulated and actual projections closely match.

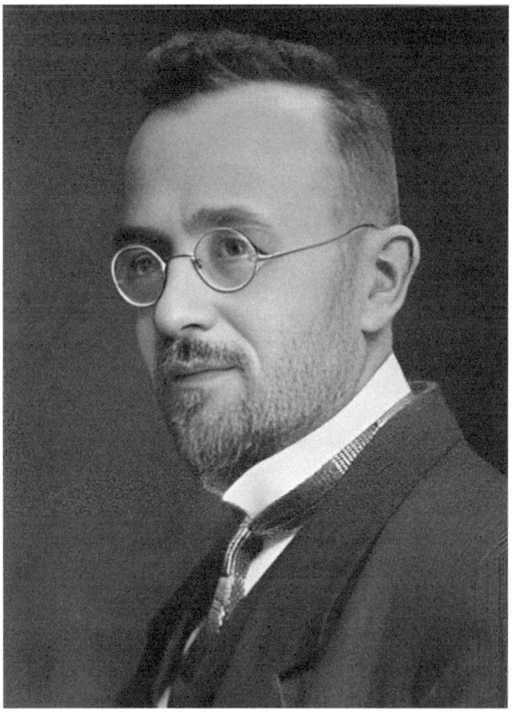

Johann Karl August Radon
(16 December 1887 – 25 May 1956)

Fig. 6.18 Person who gave foundation concept of image reconstruction. (Image courtesy: Wikipedia by unknown author. Reprinted under Creative Commons CC0 License)

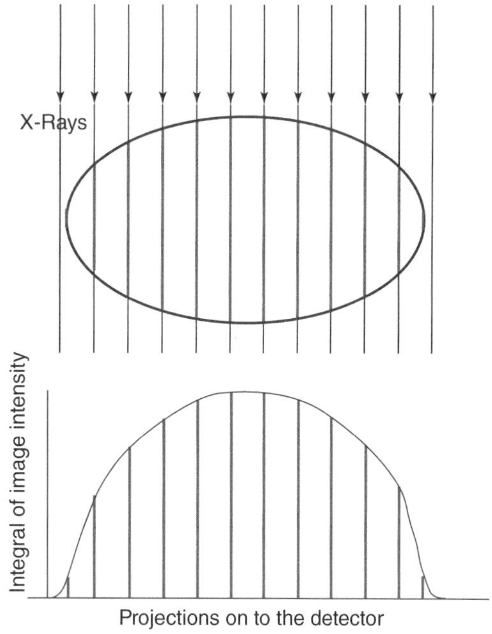

Fig. 6.19 Integral of projections on to the detector

This method produces high-quality images with reduced artifacts.

Several steps are involved during the image reconstruction process, involving multiple mathematical transformations and algorithmic steps. A brief description of each step follows:

6.8.2.2.1 Object

The object is the subject being scanned, typically a patient. The goal is to capture detailed images of internal structures, including bones, organs, and tissues. The varying densities and compositions of these structures affect how X-rays are absorbed, creating contrast in the final image. This contrast is essential for accurate visualization and diagnosis.

6.8.2.2.2 Projections

Projections are the raw data collected by the CT scanner as it rotates around the object. Each projection represents the intensity of X-rays that have passed through the object along a specific path. By acquiring projections from multiple angles (usually 360 degrees around the object), the CT scanner gathers comprehensive data about the object's internal structure. This data forms the basis for the subsequent reconstruction steps. Figure 6.19 shows integral of projections on to the detector, which forms the basis for further image reconstruction.

6.8.2.2.3 Attenuation Map or Absorption Profile

The attenuation map represents how much the X-rays are reduced in intensity due to the tissues they pass through. This reduction is quantified by the attenuation coefficient μ, which varies for different types of tissues. Dense tissues like bone have high attenuation coefficients, while less dense tissues like muscle or fat have lower coefficients. Detectors positioned opposite the X-ray source measure the intensity of the transmitted X-rays after they pass through the body, recording the reduction in beam intensity as projection data. This data represents the cumulative attenuation along the path of each beam and forms the absorption profile of the scanned region.

To illustrate this concept, consider an object placed within the field of view of the X-ray source and detector. The positioning of this object can be described using Cartesian coordinates (x, y), represented by the function $f(x, y)$. The absorption profile created at the detector depends on this function. The projection at an angle θ and location s on the detector represents the conversion of the two-dimensional structure into a one-dimensional absorption profile (Fig. 6.20):

$$R_\theta\left(x\right)=\int_{-\infty}^{\infty} f\left(x,y\right)dy$$

As the X-ray source and detector moves changing the angle θ and at a location s, then $R_\theta(x')$ absorption profile will be generates by projection $p\ (s, \theta)$:

$$R_\theta\left(x'\right)=\int_{-\infty}^{\infty} f\left(x',y'\right)dy'$$

Where $R_\theta(x')$ provides the absorption coefficient, where x' is constant and y' varies from $-\infty$ to ∞. We will find out how (x, y) would be related to (x', y') as understanding the transformation between (x, y) and (x', y') is important in the projection process. Hypothetically, how the coordinates for the same object will change, with respect to the axes, is shown in Fig. 6.21 just for understanding.

6.8.2.2.4 Beer-Lambert's Law, Logarithmic and Radon Transformations

The relationship between the initial and detected X-ray intensities is exponential. To linearize this relationship, a logarithmic transformation is applied to convert the raw projection data into attenuation coefficients.

Consider an experimental setup where the scanned object is represented by the function $f(x, y)$, generates a projection $p\ (s, \theta)$ at an angle θ and at a location s on the detector when X-rays of initial intensity I_0 travel through it. The transmitted X-ray intensity I follows Beer-Lambert's law:

$$I = I_0 e^{-\mu s}$$

When we integrate this along a path, the above equation can be written as:

$$I = I_0 e^{-\int \mu \, ds}$$

Here, μ is the linear attenuation coefficient at each point (x, y) in the object, and the integral is taken along the path ds of the X-ray through the object. This relationship is exponential because the attenuation depends on the cumulative effect of the material through which the X-ray passes.

To linearize this relationship, a logarithmic transformation is applied to the measured intensi-

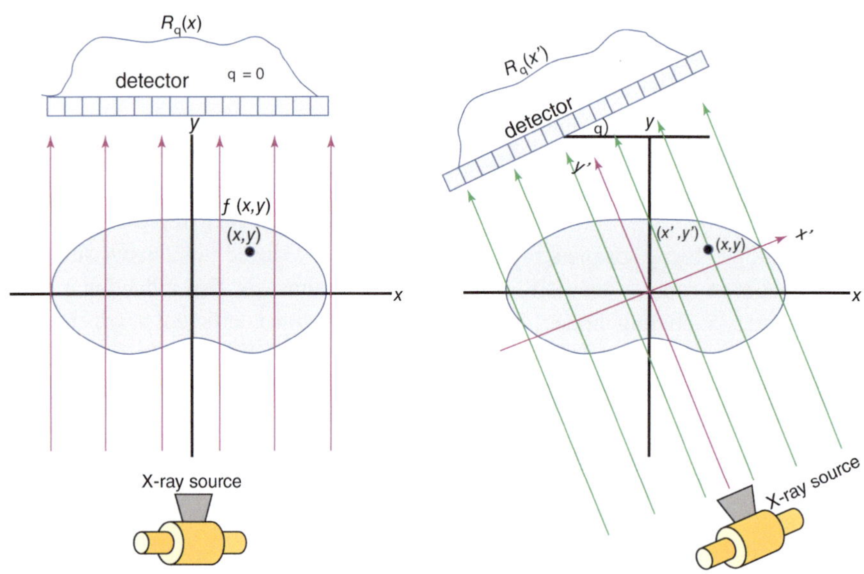

Fig. 6.20 Projections generated from various angles by the source and detector assembly. Here, (x, y) represents the position of any point within the object, while $f(x, y)$ denotes the function that defines the object coordinates

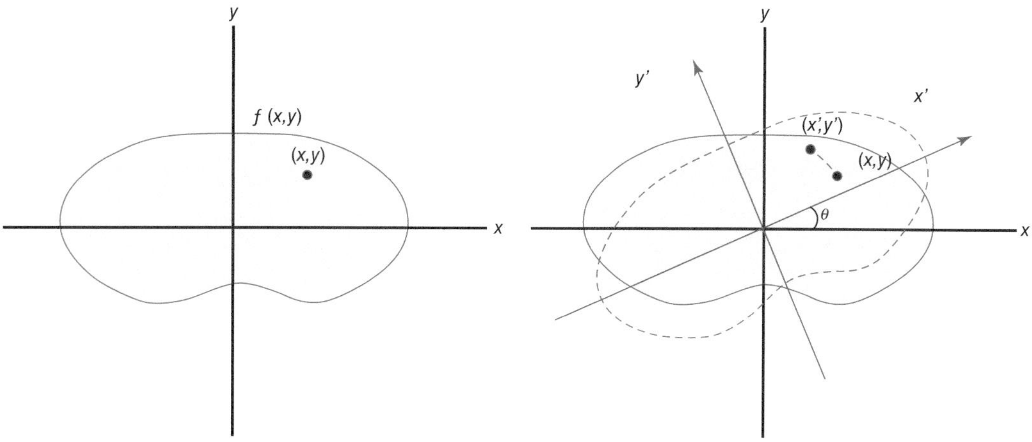

Fig. 6.21 Positional shift in coordinates of object with respect to axis XY and $\theta = 0$. For illustrative purposes, the object is depicted as rotating. In reality, however, the object remains stationary while the assembly of the detector and X-ray source rotates around it

ties. This transformation converts the raw projection data into attenuation coefficients. The projection data $p(s, \theta)$ is given by:

$$p(s,\theta) = -\log \frac{I(s,\theta)}{I_0}$$

Where $I(s, \theta)$ is the detected intensity at position s and angle θ, and I_0 is the initial intensity. This logarithmic transformation linearizes the exponential relationship, making the data suitable for further processing.

Once the projection data has been linearized, the next step is the Radon transformation. The Radon transform converts spatial image data into a set of projections by integrating the attenuation coefficients along straight lines through the object. For a fixed angle θ, the projection $R_\theta(x')$ is given by:

$$R_\theta(x') = \int_{y'=-\infty}^{\infty} f\begin{Bmatrix}(x'\cos\theta - y'\sin\theta), \\ (x'\sin\theta + y'\cos\theta)\end{Bmatrix} dy'$$

This equation integrates the attenuation coefficient along the line perpendicular to the angle θ for each position x', producing a one-dimensional projection for each angle. Proof of this equation is as follows (Fig. 6.22).

During the CT scan, the object remains stationary while the assembly of the detector and X-ray source rotates around it. This movement creates a sinogram, a comprehensive dataset representing all projections at various angles. In this context, the transformation between coordinates (x, y) and (x', y') can be described as follows:

$$x = x'\cos\theta - y'\sin\theta$$

$$y = x'\sin\theta + y'\cos\theta$$

$$\begin{bmatrix} x \\ y \end{bmatrix} = \begin{bmatrix} \cos\theta & -\sin\theta \\ \sin\theta & \cos\theta \end{bmatrix} \begin{bmatrix} x' \\ y' \end{bmatrix}$$

$$X = A.X'$$

$$X' = A^{-1}.X$$

$$A^{-1} = \begin{bmatrix} \cos\theta & \sin\theta \\ -\sin\theta & \cos\theta \end{bmatrix}$$

By applying inverse matrix, we can find,

$$\therefore x' = x\cos\theta + y\sin\theta$$

$$\& y' = -x\sin\theta + y\cos\theta$$

$$\therefore f(x,y) = f\begin{Bmatrix}(x'\cos\theta - y'\sin\theta), \\ (x'\sin\theta + y'\cos\theta)\end{Bmatrix}$$

Therefore, Eq. (6.2)

$$R_\theta(x') = \int_{-\infty}^{\infty} f(x', y')\, dy'$$

Can be written as,

$$R_\theta(x') = \int_{y'=-\infty}^{\infty} f\begin{Bmatrix}(x'\cos\theta - y'\sin\theta), \\ (x'\sin\theta + y'\cos\theta)\end{Bmatrix} dy'$$

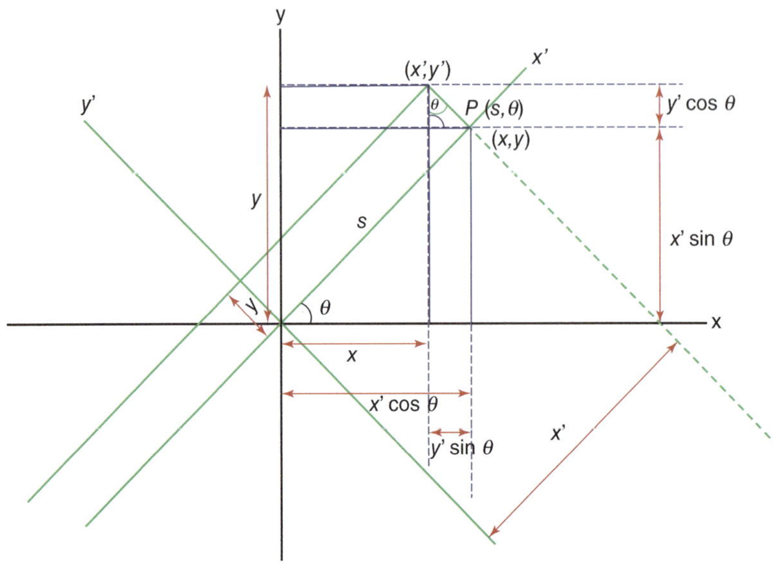

Fig. 6.22 Coordinate change and its new position with respect to old

The above equation is called the *Radon Transformation*. It is a fundamental mathematical tool used to convert spatial image data into a set of projections, facilitating image reconstruction. Named after the Austrian mathematician Johann Radon, this transform provides detailed projections by integrating the attenuation coefficients along straight lines through the object, generating a comprehensive dataset of line integrals for various angles.

Combining these concepts, the projection $p(s, \theta)$ can also be expressed in terms of the attenuation coefficient μ:

$$p(s,\theta) = -\log\frac{I(s,\theta)}{I_0} = \int_{-\infty}^{\infty} \mu \begin{Bmatrix} (x'\cos\theta - y'\sin\theta), \\ (x'\sin\theta + y'\cos\theta) \end{Bmatrix} ds$$

This equation shows that a projection provides an integration of the attenuation coefficient along the object's axis s as a function of the projection angle θ at the location s on the detector. By using multiple projections at different angles, we can determine the distribution of the attenuation coefficient within the scanned object.

The Beer-Lambert law, logarithmic transformation, and Radon transformation work in conjunction to facilitate CT image reconstruction. The Beer-Lambert law describes the exponential attenuation of X-rays, the logarithmic transformation linearizes this relationship, and the Radon transformation converts the spatial image data into a set of projections. Together, these transformations enable the accurate reconstruction of the internal structure of the object from the collected projection data.

6.8.2.2.5 Sinogram Creation

A sinogram is a graphical representation of the Radon transform. It visually encapsulates all the projection data acquired at various angles, serving as an intermediary step in the CT reconstruction process. The term "sinogram" comes from the sinusoidal patterns that projections form when plotted. The structure of the sonogram contains rows and columns which represent some data (Fig. 6.23).

- **Rows and Columns**: Each row in the sinogram corresponds to the projection data acquired at a specific angle θ. Each column corresponds to a specific detector position t.
- **Data Representation**: The intensity of each point in the sinogram represents the degree of X-ray attenuation along a particular path through the object at a specific angle (Fig. 6.23).

Building the Sinogram

1. **Data Collection**: As the X-ray tube rotates around the patient, projections are collected at multiple angles. At each angle θ, the detectors measure the transmitted X-ray intensities after passing through the object.

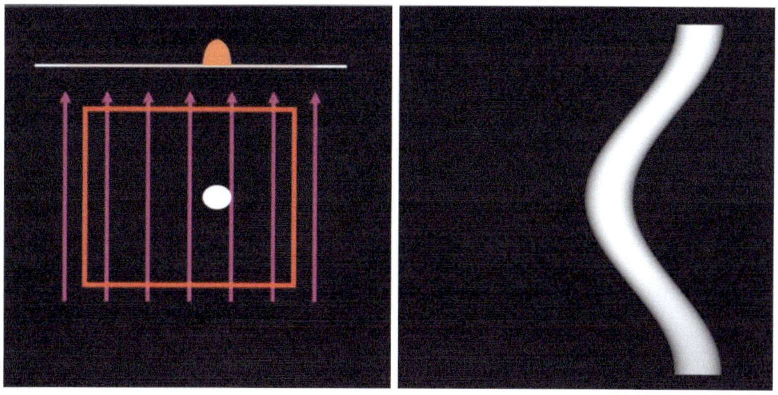

Fig. 6.23 Graphical representation of the Radon transform in the form of sinogram

2. **Projection Data**: For each angle θ, the projection data $p(s,\theta)$ is recorded. Here, $p(s,\theta)$ represents the integral of the attenuation coefficients along the X-ray path at angle θ and detector position s.
3. **Sinogram Plotting**: Each projection $p(s,\theta)$ is plotted as a row in the sinogram. As the angle θ changes from 0 to 180 degrees (or 0 to 360 degrees in some scanners), the corresponding projections fill in the sinogram.

The sinogram thus provides a comprehensive dataset encapsulating all the projection information needed to reconstruct the original two-dimensional image of the scanned object. Each sine wave pattern in the sinogram represents the way different structures in the object attenuate X-rays from different angles, highlighting how these structures contribute to the overall attenuation profile.

6.8.2.2.6 Fourier Transformation

The Fourier transform, developed by mathematician Baron Jean-Baptiste-Joseph Fourier in 1807, converts the projection data from the spatial domain to the frequency domain [1]. This step is critical for applying filters that enhance image quality. By transforming the data into the frequency domain, it becomes easier to manipulate and filter specific frequency components, which correspond to different details in the image.

The Fourier Transform decomposes a function into its constituent frequencies. For a two-dimensional function $f(x,y)$, the 2D Fourier Transform $F(u,v)$ is given by:

$$F(u,v) = \int_{-\infty}^{\infty} \int_{-\infty}^{\infty} f(x,y) e^{-2\pi i(ux+vy)} dxdy$$

The inverse Fourier Transform, which reconstructs the original function from its frequency components, is:

$$f(x,y) = \int_{-\infty}^{\infty} \int_{-\infty}^{\infty} F(u,v) e^{2\pi i(ux+vy)} du\, dv$$

6.8.2.2.7 Fourier Slice Theorem

The Fourier Slice Theorem states that the 1D Fourier Transform of a projection of a 2D object is equal to a slice of the 2D Fourier Transform of the object along a line through the origin.

For a projection $p(s,\theta)$ at angle θ, its 1D Fourier Transform $P(\omega,\theta)$ is:

$$P(\omega,\theta) = \int_{-\infty}^{\infty} p(s,\theta) e^{-2\pi i\omega s} ds$$

According to the Fourier Slice Theorem:

$$P(\omega,\theta) = F(\omega\cos\theta, \omega\sin\theta)$$

This means that $P(\omega,\theta)$ is a slice of the 2D Fourier Transform of the object $f(x,y)$ along the line at angle θ from the origin.

6.8.2.2.8 Relationship Between Radon Transform and Fourier Transform

The Radon Transform of the object, $R_\theta(x')$, is the integral of the object's attenuation coefficient along a line at angle θ. In the frequency domain, the Radon Transform and Fourier Transform are related by the Fourier Slice Theorem.

Given the Radon Transform $R_\theta(x')$:

$$R_\theta\left(x'\right)=\int_{y'=-\infty}^{\infty} f\left\{\begin{matrix}\left(x'\cos\theta-y'\sin\theta\right),\\ \left(x'\sin\theta+y'\cos\theta\right)\end{matrix}\right\}dy'$$

The 1D Fourier Transform of $R_\theta(x')$is:

$$F\left[R_\theta\left(x'\right)\right](\omega)=\int_{-\infty}^{\infty} R_\theta\left(x'\right)e^{-2\pi i\omega x'}dx'$$

By the Fourier Slice Theorem, this is equal to a slice of the 2D Fourier Transform of $f(x, y)$:

$$F\left[R_\theta\left(x'\right)\right](\omega)=F\left(\omega\cos\theta,\omega\sin\theta\right)$$

6.8.2.2.9 Image Reconstruction Using Fourier Transform

To reconstruct the image, we need to invert the process:

1. **Fourier Transform of Projections**: Compute the 1D Fourier Transform of each projection $p(s, \theta)$ to get $P(\omega, \theta)$.
2. **Back-Projection in Frequency Domain**: Map each $P(\omega, \theta)$ to its corresponding location in the 2D Fourier Transform space $F(u, v)$.
3. **Inverse Fourier Transform**: Perform a 2D inverse Fourier Transform on $F(u, v)$ to obtain the reconstructed image $f(x, y)$.

Mathematically, the process involves the following steps:

- Compute the 1D Fourier Transform of the projection data $p(s, \theta)$:

$$P\left(\omega,\theta\right)=\int_{-\infty}^{\infty} p\left(s,\theta\right)e^{-2\pi i\omega s}\,ds$$

- Use the Fourier Slice Theorem to place $P(\omega, \theta)$ into the 2D Fourier space $F(u, v)$:
- $F(u, v)$ is populated using $P(\omega, \theta)$
- Perform the 2D inverse Fourier Transform to reconstruct the image:

$$f\left(x,y\right)=\int_{-\infty}^{\infty}\int_{-\infty}^{\infty} F\left(u,v\right)e^{2\pi i\left(ux+vy\right)}\,du\,dv$$

6.8.2.2.10 Filtered Back Projection (FBP)

The filtered projections are back-projected to reconstruct the image, providing a direct method for image reconstruction. FBP is efficient and widely used due to its computational simplicity and effectiveness in generating high-quality images from the projection data. As CT technology advanced, FBP-based algorithms were improved and extended to match hardware progress, exemplified by Feldkamp et al.'s 1984 solution for reconstructing data from large area detectors [68]. It combines the Fourier Transform with filtering to improve image quality.

- **Filtering**: Ramp filtering, also known as the Shepp-Logan filter, is applied to the frequency-domain data to enhance the high-frequency components, which correspond to edges and fine details in the image. This filter helps to correct the blurring introduced during the back-projection process. Mathematically, it multiplies the Fourier-transformed projections by a ramp function (increasing linearly with frequency) before converting them back to the spatial domain. Apply a filter $|\omega|$ in the frequency domain to enhance high-frequency components:

$$\hat{P}\left(\omega,\theta\right)=\omega P\left(\omega,\theta\right)$$

- **Back-Projection**: Back-projection is a technique used to reconstruct the image from the filtered projection data. It involves smearing each filtered projection back across the image space along the same paths that the X-rays originally took. The projections from different angles are summed to form the final image. However, simple back-projection results in a blurry image, which is why ramp filtering is applied first to sharpen the result (Figs. 6.24 and 6.25).

Perform the inverse Fourier Transform of the filtered data and sum the contributions from all angles:

$$f\left(x,y\right)=\int_{-\infty}^{\pi}\int_{-\infty}^{\infty}\hat{P}\left(\omega,\theta\right)e^{2\pi i\omega\left(x\cos\theta+y\sin\theta\right)}\mathrm{d}\omega\mathrm{d}\theta$$

The Fourier Transform, along with the Fourier Slice Theorem and Radon Transform, provides a powerful framework for CT image reconstruction. By transforming projection data into the frequency domain, the entire reconstruction process is made more efficient and mathematically tractable. The use of Filtered Back Projection further

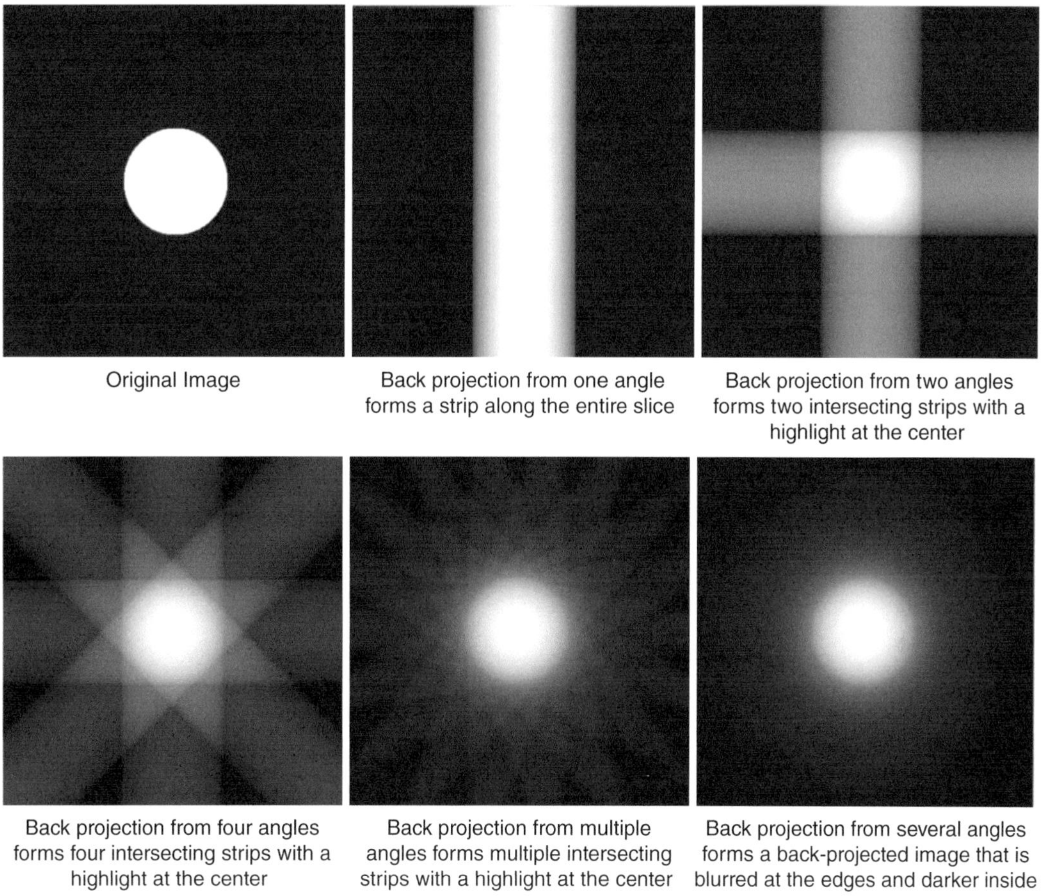

Fig. 6.24 Back projection from multiple angles forms a blurred image without filtering

refines this process, yielding high-quality images that are crucial for accurate diagnosis and treatment planning.

6.8.2.2.11 Iterative Reconstruction (IR)

Iterative reconstruction is an alternative to filtered back-projection that iteratively refines the image estimate to improve quality and reduce artifacts. Developed in 1970 by Gordan et al. and named Algebraic Reconstruction Techniques (ART), Hounsfield initially used ART for the first image reconstructions [69]. However, due to the lack of computational power, ART was not utilized in CT image reconstruction until 2009, when Siemens Healthineers' IR algorithm received FDA approval for commercial use. Until then, simple analytic methods like FBP had been the standard for decades [68]. Within 2 years, four advanced IR algorithms received FDA clearance: ASIR (adaptive statistical iterative reconstruction, GE Healthcare), SAFIRE (sinogram-affirmed iterative reconstruction, Siemens Healthineers), iDose4 (Philips Healthcare), and Veo (GE Healthcare), with the first three being hybrid IR algorithms that, like FBP and IRIS, utilize a single backward projection step [68].

By 2014, major CT manufacturers had introduced iterative reconstruction (IR) algorithms to overcome the limitations of the FBP algorithm, such as image noise and streak artifacts [1]. IR algorithms aim primarily to reduce image noise and lower the higher radiation dose associated with FBP. These algorithms typically utilize FBP-generated CT data, referred to as measured projections, to generate simulated projections. These simulated projections are then compared with the initial measured projections to identify discrepancies in image noise. The observed dif-

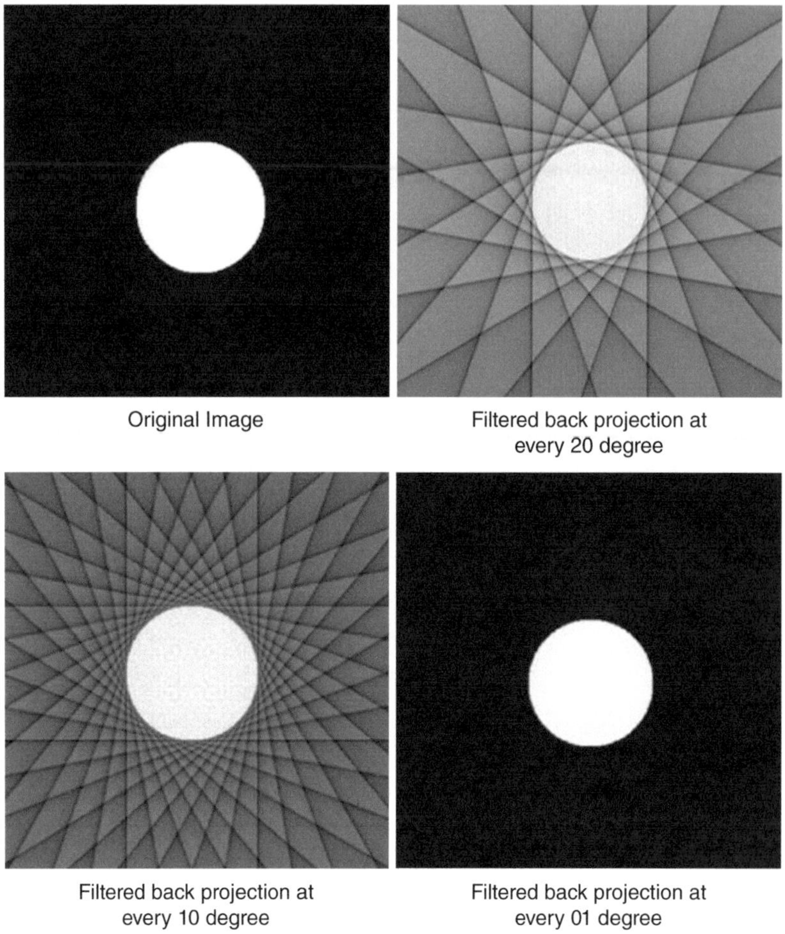

Fig. 6.25 Filtered back projection

ferences are used to correct inconsistencies in the simulated data. The system then reconstructs a new image, and this iterative process repeats until the disparity between the measured and simulated data is minimized to an acceptable level. This iterative approach yields images that faithfully represent the scanned object with significantly reduced noise and artifacts. Iterative reconstruction diverges from FBP by iteratively refining the image estimate to enhance quality and diminish artifacts. This methodology involves several sequential steps:

1. **Initial Estimate:** The initial estimate serves as the starting point for iterative reconstruction. It may be a rudimentary image derived from a basic reconstruction method like FBP or a minimally processed image. This estimate acts as the baseline that undergoes iterative refinement.
2. **Forward Projection:** Forward projection entails generating synthetic projections from the current image estimate. This step simulates the acquisition of projection data by calculating how projections would appear if the estimated image were the true representation. The synthetic projections are compared against actual measured projections to evaluate the accuracy of the estimate.
3. **Comparison:** During this phase, the synthetic projections are compared with the actual measured projections. The disparity between these sets of projections (the error) is computed. This error quantifies how much the current image estimate diverges from the true image.
4. **Error Correction:** Error correction utilizes the computed error to update the image estimate. Various algorithms, such as gradient descent or other optimization techniques, are employed to adjust the image estimate and

minimize errors in the projections. This iterative refinement aims to achieve a more precise reconstruction.

5. **Iteration:** The iterative process involves repeating the steps of forward projection, comparison, and error correction. Each iteration refines the image estimate further, progressively reducing errors and improving overall image quality. Iterations continue until the error reaches an acceptable threshold or the image converges to a stable, accurate solution.

This methodical iterative reconstruction approach contrasts with the traditional FBP method, offering enhanced image quality and reduced artifacts in CT imaging.

> **Box: 6.3**
> **Reconstruction Process**
> 1. **Filtered Back-Projection (FBP)**
>   - **Projection Data Collection**: Uses Radon transform to collect projection data.
>   - **Fourier Transform**: Converts spatial domain data to frequency domain.
>   - **Filtering (Convolution)**: Applies filter function (e.g., ramp filter) to enhance high-frequency components.
>   - **Inverse Fourier Transform**: Transforms filtered data back to spatial domain.
>   - **Back-Projection**: Spreads filtered data onto image matrix and sums contributions from all angles.
> 2. **Iterative Reconstruction (IR)**
>   - **Initial Guess**: Starts with an initial image guess.
>   - **Forward Projection**: Simulates projections from the initial guess.
>   - **Comparison and Correction**: Compares simulated projections to actual projections and updates image based on the error.
>   - **Fourier Transform and Filtering**: Utilizes transforms and filtering within each iteration for noise reduction.
>   - **Reiteration**: Repeats process until convergence and error minimization.

Iterative reconstruction can incorporate models for noise reduction, edge preservation, and artifact correction, leading to higher-quality images, especially in low-dose CT scans. Notable iterative reconstruction algorithms include ASIR (adaptive statistical iterative reconstruction), SAFIRE (sinogram-affirmed iterative reconstruction), iDose4, and Veo. These algorithms, particularly hybrid IR algorithms, use a single backward projection step similar to FBP.

6.8.2.2.12 Deep Learning Reconstruction

Deep learning reconstruction (DLR) harnesses the power of artificial intelligence and neural networks to significantly enhance image reconstruction from raw projection data. This modern approach offers substantial improvements over traditional methods such as filtered back projection (FBP) and iterative reconstruction (IR). By training deep learning models on extensive datasets of paired raw projection data and high-quality images, these models learn to reconstruct new images with remarkable accuracy, even from noisy or sparse inputs. The advanced capabilities of deep learning enable it to uncover complex patterns and features in the data, resulting in superior image quality and robustness compared to conventional techniques. Consequently, DLR is increasingly favored in modern CT imaging for its ability to reduce artifacts and improve image resolution.

Principles of Deep Learning in Image Reconstruction

The foundation of deep learning in image reconstruction involves several key principles, including feature engineering, convolutional neural networks (CNNs), nodes and layers, and the processes of forward and backward propagation, along with weight adjustment and the phases of training, validation, and testing. These concepts are crucial for understanding how deep learning enhances CT image reconstruction, particularly in addressing noise, radiation, and artifact reduction.

Feature Engineering

In traditional CT image reconstruction, feature engineering involves manually crafting filters and techniques to emphasize critical image aspects. Deep learning automates this process by

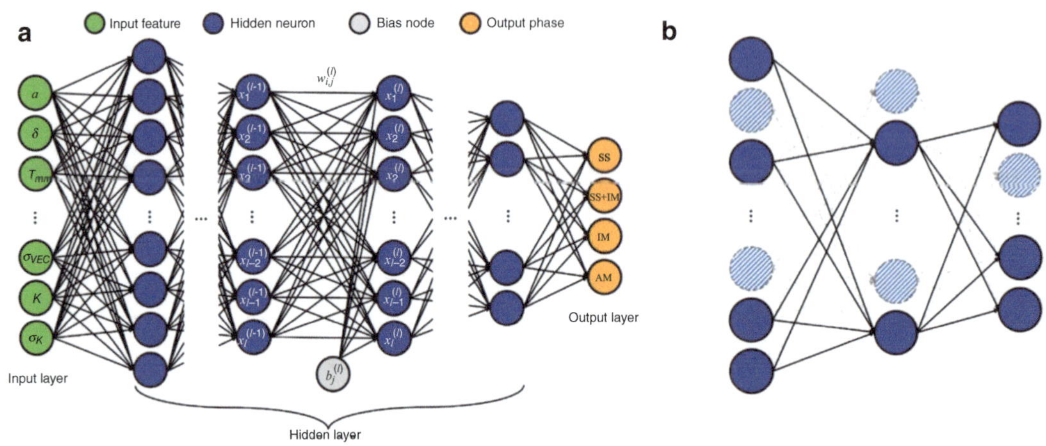

Fig. 6.26 Schematic diagram of the deep neural network: (**a**) illustrates the architecture of the DNN model, which consists of input, hidden, and output layers; (**b**) depicts the dropout regularization technique, which manages the connections between neurons in the hidden layers. (Figure originally published by Lee et al. [70]. Republished under CCNY 4.0 license)

enabling the network to learn and extract relevant features directly from raw CT data. This automation improves both the efficiency and accuracy of image reconstruction, as the network adapts to complex data patterns and structures (Fig. 6.26).

Convolutional Neural Networks (CNNs)
CNNs are central to deep learning applications in CT image reconstruction. They consist of multiple layers, including convolutional layers that apply filters to the input image to generate feature maps. These layers can detect edges, textures, and complex patterns through successive processing stages. The hierarchical learning capabilities of CNNs make them particularly effective at enhancing image quality by reducing noise and artifacts, which is especially beneficial in low-dose CT scans.

Nodes and Layers
A deep learning network designed for CT image reconstruction typically includes an input layer, multiple hidden layers, and an output layer. Each layer contains nodes (neurons) that process information. Nodes in one layer connect to those in the next layer, with each connection assigned a weight. This architecture refines image quality progressively as data passes through the layers, enabling the network to produce high-resolution reconstructed images.

Forward and Backward Propagation

- **Forward Propagation**: During forward propagation, the input CT data moves through the network. Each node processes inputs from the previous layer, applies weights and biases, and passes the result through an activation function. This process continues until the final reconstructed image is produced. Forward propagation is essential for assessing how well the current weights and biases contribute to achieving the desired image quality.
- **Backward Propagation**: In backward propagation, the network adjusts weights and biases to minimize the discrepancy between the reconstructed image and the ground truth. The error is propagated back through the network, and gradients of the loss function with respect to each weight are calculated. Optimization algorithms, such as gradient descent, are used to update the weights, enhancing the network's accuracy in image reconstruction.

Weight Adjustment
Weights in a deep learning network are crucial as they determine the influence of connections between nodes. During training, these weights are iteratively adjusted to minimize the loss function, which measures the difference between the reconstructed and actual images. Proper weight

adjustment ensures that the network reconstructs images with high fidelity, effectively reducing noise and artifacts.

Phases of Training, Validation, and Testing

- **Training Phase**: The network undergoes training on a large dataset of CT images, learning to reconstruct images by adjusting weights through forward and backward propagation. The goal of this phase is to minimize the loss function and enhance the network's ability to produce clear and accurate images from potentially noisy or low-dose inputs.
- **Validation Phase**: The model's performance is assessed on a separate validation set during training. This phase is crucial for tuning hyperparameters and preventing overfitting. Validating the model on unseen data ensures it generalizes well to various CT images beyond the training set.
- **Testing Phase**: The model is evaluated on an independent test set to gauge its overall performance and generalizability. This phase provides a final assessment of the network's capability to reconstruct high-quality CT images, offering insights into its practical applicability.

Deep learning, especially through CNNs, has revolutionized CT image reconstruction by mitigating noise, reducing radiation doses, and minimizing artifacts. By leveraging extensive datasets, deep learning models can reconstruct high-quality images from low-dose scans, thus decreasing patient exposure to radiation while maintaining diagnostic accuracy. The enhanced image quality supports radiologists in making more precise diagnoses, ultimately improving patient outcomes (Fig. 6.27).

CT Image Reconstruction Using Deep Learning

The introduction of deep learning to CT image reconstruction has revolutionized the field by developing two primary frameworks: indirect and direct deep learning-based reconstruction (DLR) frameworks. These frameworks differ in their integration with traditional reconstruction methods such as filtered back projection (FBP) or iterative reconstruction (IR).

Indirect DLR Frameworks

Indirect DLR frameworks incorporate traditional reconstruction methods at some stage in the reconstruction process and are classified into three main types: sinogram-based, image-based, and hybrid frameworks.

- *Sinogram-Based Frameworks*: These frameworks optimize the sinogram data using deep learning techniques before applying FBP or IR. The pre-processing step aims to enhance the quality of the sinogram, thereby improving the final reconstructed image.
- *Image-Based Frameworks*: In this approach, initial reconstruction is performed using FBP or IR, and the resulting image is then refined by a deep learning network. This post-

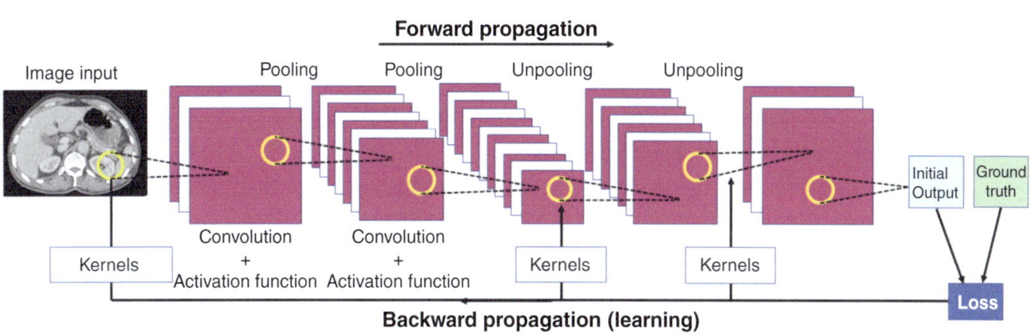

Fig. 6.27 An illustration of the forward and backward propagation process in a convolutional neural network (CNN). The forward pass involves applying convolutions, pooling, and activation functions to extract features from the input image, while the backward pass (learning phase) updates the network's parameters to minimize the loss function

processing step aims to reduce noise and artifacts, resulting in a clearer final image.

- *Hybrid Frameworks*: Hybrid frameworks combine sinogram and image optimization. Deep learning networks process both the sinogram data and the initial reconstructed image, leveraging the advantages of both approaches to produce high-quality images.

Commonly used models in these frameworks include convolutional neural networks (CNNs) such as wavelet transform-based U-Net and residual encoder-decoder CNNs. Additionally, non-CNN approaches like transformer-based neural networks and generative adversarial networks (GANs) are utilized to further enhance reconstruction quality.

Direct DLR Frameworks

Direct DLR algorithms reconstruct images directly from sinogram data without employing traditional methods like FBP or IR. This approach can potentially eliminate artifacts associated with traditional methods, leading to clearer images. Notable examples of direct algorithms include AUTOMAP and iRadonMAP, which use advanced deep learning techniques to map sinogram data directly to reconstructed images.

Building and Tuning a DLR Model

Developing an effective deep learning-based reconstruction model involves several critical steps:

- *Training Phase*: The model is trained on a dataset of low-dose CT images paired with high-dose or routine-dose images as ground truth. This supervised learning process allows the model to learn how to mitigate noise and artifacts.
- *Validation Phase*: The model's performance is evaluated on a separate validation set to fine-tune hyperparameters and prevent overfitting. This phase ensures that the model generalizes well to new, unseen data.
- *Testing Phase*: Finally, the model is tested on an independent test set to assess its real-world applicability and overall performance in reconstructing high-quality CT images.

Meticulous tuning of the model and the use of extensive datasets significantly improve image quality, enhance diagnostic accuracy, and reduce patient radiation exposure.

Current DLR Algorithms

Several CT vendors and independent software companies have developed FDA-approved DLR algorithms:

- *TrueFidelity (GE Healthcare)*: Utilizes CNNs trained on lower-dose sinograms to produce images with FBP-like noise texture, sharpness, and artifact properties.
- *AiCE (Canon Medical Systems):* An indirect, image-based DLR algorithm trained on lower-dose HIR images, offering benefits in noise and artifact reduction.
- *Precise Image (Philips Healthcare)*: A direct DLR algorithm employing CNNs trained on lower-dose sinograms, providing optimized workflows and shorter reconstruction times compared to MBIR.

Independent software companies have also developed DLR-based denoising algorithms, such as ClariCT.AI and PixelShine, which further enhance image quality by reducing noise and artifacts [65].

Image Quality and Artifact Reduction

DLR algorithms improve image quality by reducing noise and artifacts compared to traditional methods. Key metrics used to assess improvements include noise magnitude, signal-to-noise ratio (SNR), and contrast-to-noise ratio (CNR). Radiologists often find that DLR images offer superior noise texture, reduced artifacts, and sharper features compared to traditional methods [65].

Advantages of Deep Learning Reconstruction

DLR algorithms offer several advantages:

1. *Noise Reduction and Image Quality*: DLR effectively reduces image noise, enhancing clarity and diagnostic accuracy, particularly in low-dose imaging protocols where maintaining quality is challenging.

2. *Radiation Dose Reduction*: DLR can reduce radiation doses by up to 71% compared to traditional methods without compromising image quality, making it a safer option for patients, especially in repeated imaging scenarios [65].
3. *Artifact Reduction*: DLR minimizes artifacts such as beam hardening and streak artifacts, which are common in conventional techniques, improving image interpretation accuracy.
4. *Improved Spatial Resolution*: DLR maintains high spatial resolution even in low-dose conditions, crucial for detecting small lesions and anatomical details.

Clinical Applications of DLR

DLR has been tested in various imaging subdomains:

1. *Brain Imaging*: DLR improves image noise, reduces artifacts, and enhances differentiation between gray and white matter, which is critical for detecting hemorrhages and other brain abnormalities [71].
2. *Chest and Cardiac Imaging*: In chest imaging, DLR enhances image quality metrics such as SNR, CNR, and sharpness [72]. For cardiac applications, DLR enables significant dose reduction while preserving or enhancing image quality, suitable for cardiac CT angiography and stenosis assessment [73–75].
3. *Abdominal Imaging*: DLR improves image quality and lesion detectability in abdominal CT imaging, particularly in low-contrast tissue interfaces [76]. However, further evaluation is needed to address concerns about blurring small lesions and vessels [77].
4. *Pediatric Imaging*: Reducing radiation dose is crucial for pediatric imaging. Studies demonstrate that DLR improves image quality and reduces noise in lower-dose protocols, making it ideal for pediatric patients [78, 79].

Challenges and Prospects of DLR

Despite its benefits, DLR faces several challenges [65]:

1. *Quality Assessment*: Comprehensive evaluation of image quality and diagnostic performance is necessary before adopting new techniques. Clinical superiority in lesion detection and other factors should guide the transition to new methods.
2. *Training Data Quality*: The effectiveness of DLR algorithms depends on the quality and diversity of training data. Collecting large, diverse datasets is essential but challenging due to associated costs and time.
3. *Artifact and Blurring Concerns*: DLR may introduce artifacts or blur small structures. Accurate training data and robust testing are crucial to mitigate these issues.
4. *Standardization and Vendor Partnerships*: Variations in DLR algorithms complicate cross-vendor comparisons of CT examinations. Enhanced partnerships and standardization in training data and pathology are needed.

Future Prospects

Photon-counting CT, which offers images with reduced noise and higher spatial resolution, holds promise for further enhancing DLR performance. By improving ground truth image quality, photon-counting CT can refine DLR algorithms for better noise reduction and artifact handling. DLR also has potential for processing raw CT data, which contains all necessary diagnostic information. This capability could be especially useful in emergency settings where timely assessment is critical. Preliminary studies suggest that deep learning can analyze CT sinograms to detect intracranial hemorrhage and cranial abnormalities without full image reconstruction.

With ongoing advancements and increased standardization, DLR is set to become a cornerstone in clinical CT imaging, providing safer and more accurate diagnostic tools. The continuous development of diverse training datasets and the integration of emerging technologies like photon-counting CT will further enhance DLR's capabilities, cementing its role as a transformative technology in medical imaging [65].

6.8.3 The Console and Workstation for Image Storage, Display, and Further Processing

Parameters Control and Image Storage

The console acts as the central control hub for the CT scanner, enabling radiologists or technologists to configure scanning parameters such as slice thickness, rotation speed, and X-ray dosage. It provides real-time image display during the scan, ensuring proper patient positioning and scan progression. Images and raw data are initially stored on the console's local storage for immediate review and quality assessment before being transferred to a more permanent storage system connected to the hospital's network. Typically, images are saved in a digital format compliant with medical standards like DICOM (Digital Imaging and Communications in Medicine).

The workstation, in contrast, is equipped for advanced image processing and analysis. It offers tools for generating 3D reconstructions, performing multiplanar reformats (MPR), and volume rendering. Diagnostic tools available at the workstation allow for detailed measurement of structures, annotation of findings, and comparison of different image sets. Post-processing adjustments such as window level modifications, filters, and image enhancements are applied to improve the visualization of anatomical features and pathologies. Workstations are generally connected to a Picture Archiving and Communication System (PACS), which ensures secure storage, retrieval, and distribution of medical images. PACS manages a database of patient images and metadata, including patient information, scan parameters, and diagnostic reports, facilitating efficient image organization, search, and retrieval.

Data Flow from Console to Workstation

Data flow begins with raw data acquisition by the CT scanner's detectors, which is sent to the console. The console performs initial processing to create preliminary images, followed by quality checks by technologists. Once images pass quality assessment, they are securely transferred to the workstation over a network. The workstation then conducts advanced processing and analysis, with the final images and associated patient and scan information being stored in the PACS for long-term management and access.

Security and Accessibility

Advanced storage systems ensure patient data protection through encryption, access controls, and regular backups, adhering to healthcare regulations such as HIPAA (Health Insurance Portability and Accountability Act). The secure storage system allows access by authorized healthcare providers for collaborative diagnosis and treatment planning. Additionally, archived images support medical research and the training of healthcare professionals. The seamless integration of the console and workstation within the CT imaging workflow guarantees the production, secure storage, and accessibility of high-quality images for clinical use.

Software Processing in CT Imaging

After initial processing, advanced software tools on the workstation refine and analyze CT data to enhance image quality and extract diagnostic information. Radiologists can adjust image parameters such as brightness, contrast, and sharpness to improve the visibility of anatomical structures. Techniques like windowing and leveling highlight various tissues by modifying grayscale values, while filters reduce noise and artifacts to enhance clarity. The software also includes tools for precise measurements of anatomical structures, including lengths, angles, and areas, which are vital for assessing abnormalities like tumors. Annotation tools enable radiologists to mark areas of interest, add notes, and highlight features, facilitating communication and supporting clinical decision-making.

Sophisticated analytical tools perform complex evaluations, such as detecting abnormalities, quantifying tissue densities, and calculating volumes. For example, software can automatically measure tumor size, monitor growth, and compare characteristics with a pathology database.

Modern workstation software supports 3D modeling from CT data, providing a comprehensive spatial view of scanned areas. Volume rendering and surface rendering techniques create realistic 3D images that can be rotated, zoomed, and sliced, aiding in surgical planning, treatment evaluation, and patient education. Some advanced workstations offer functional imaging techniques, such as perfusion imaging, to assess tissue blood flow and physiological status. Quantification tools measure parameters like blood flow and perfusion rates, which are critical for diagnosing conditions such as stroke, tumors, and vascular diseases.

The integration of artificial intelligence (AI) and machine learning enhances CT workstations with automated detection and diagnosis capabilities. AI algorithms analyze CT images to identify patterns and anomalies, offering preliminary diagnoses, prioritizing urgent cases, and highlighting areas of concern, thereby improving diagnostic efficiency and accuracy. Additionally, the workstation software can integrate CT images with other modalities, such as MRI or PET, and include data from electronic health records (EHR). This multi-modal approach provides a holistic view of the patient's condition, facilitating more informed diagnoses and personalized treatment plans. The correlation of CT findings with clinical history, lab results, and other imaging studies enhances diagnostic accuracy and supports comprehensive patient care.

6.9 Artefacts in CT Imaging

CT image artifacts are distortions or errors in the reconstructed images that do not represent the actual anatomical structures. These artifacts can arise due to various factors, including limitations in imaging hardware, patient movement, and computational methods used in image reconstruction. Some of the corrections are discussed in image pre-processing section. Below is a detailed explanation of various types of CT image artifacts, their causes, and their impact on image quality. Artifacts can be broadly classified into 2D and 3D categories based on how they manifest in the images.

6.9.1 2D Artifacts

2D artifacts are distortions that are typically observed in individual CT slices or planes.

6.9.1.1 Beam Hardening Artifacts

Beam hardening artifacts arise from the polychromatic nature of X-ray beams used in electron-impact sources. These sources generate X-rays when fast electrons collide with a solid metal anode, producing a spectrum that includes both continuous bremsstrahlung radiation and characteristic emission lines unique to the anode material. As an X-ray beam passes through an object, its spectrum changes because lower-energy (soft) X-rays are more readily absorbed than higher-energy (hard) X-rays, leading to an overall hardening of the beam.

This phenomenon results in artifacts because the X-ray attenuation is dependent not only on the path length but also on the energy of the photons [80]. The basic mathematical model for X-ray attenuation, represented by Lambert-Beer's law, assumes a monoenergetic beam and linear attenuation, which does not hold true for polychromatic X-ray sources. When considering the energy dependence of attenuation, the model becomes more complex, and the simple logarithmic ratio of incident to transmitted intensity fails to account for the spectral changes.

Beam hardening artifacts manifest as dark streaks or "cupping" effects in CT images, particularly around dense objects like bone or metal implants (Fig. 6.28) [80]. These artifacts occur because the reconstruction algorithm, typically filtered back projection (FBP), interprets the varying attenuation coefficients incorrectly, leading to inconsistencies in the measured projections. In practice, the detectors measure the integral intensity over all wavelengths, unable to distinguish between different photon energies, exacerbating the artifact.

To mitigate beam hardening artifacts, several techniques are employed:

- **Pre-filtering**: Placing materials like aluminum or copper filters near the X-ray source to absorb soft X-rays before they reach the patient.

- **Computational Corrections**: Applying corrections during image reconstruction, often using the attenuation properties of water as a reference for soft tissues.
- **Dual-Energy CT**: Using different tube voltages to acquire images, which allows for better modeling of the energy dependence of attenuation and improved correction of beam hardening effects.

Despite these corrections, some residual artifacts may persist, especially in areas with a mix of materials with different attenuation properties. The development of new reconstruction algorithms and improvements in CT technology continue to enhance the ability to minimize and correct beam hardening artifacts, leading to clearer and more accurate diagnostic images.

6.9.1.2 Partial Volume Artifacts

Partial volume artifacts arise from the limited resolution of the detector system when imaging objects with sharp boundaries. When a boundary falls within the width of a detector element, the intensity of the X-ray signal is averaged over that detector width ($\Delta\xi$), leading to a blurring effect. This averaging causes problems during the reconstruction process, especially when the object's structure partially overlaps multiple detector elements [80].

For instance, consider an axial abdomen slice containing a highly absorbing vertebra. The transition from the vertebral body to the surrounding tissue creates a sharp boundary. If the detector

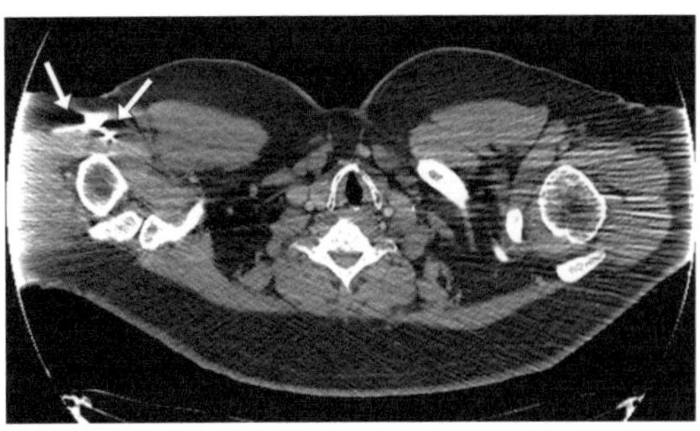

Fig. 6.28 Beam hardening artifacts shown with arrows

elements cannot resolve this boundary due to their finite width, the resulting projection signal is averaged over $\Delta\xi$, causing a blurred image. This effect shows that reducing the detector width mitigates the blurring at the object boundary.

The mathematical basis for the partial volume effect lies in the logarithmic relationship used in CT reconstruction. The intensity $I(\xi)$ of the X-ray passing through the object is given by:

$$I(\xi) = I_0(\xi)e^{-\int \mu(\xi,\eta)d\eta}$$

$I_0(\xi)$ is the initial intensity and $\mu(\xi,\eta)$ is the attenuation coefficient. The projection value $p(\xi)$, used in reconstruction methods, is:

$$p(\xi) = \int \mu(\xi,\eta)d\eta$$

The logarithmic relationship introduces non-linearity. Specifically, the logarithm of the linearly averaged intensities does not equal the sum of the logarithms of the individual intensities. Mathematically, this is expressed as:

$$\ln\left(\alpha I(\xi_1) + (1-\alpha)I(\xi_2)\right) \neq \alpha \ln\left(I(\xi_1)\right) + (1-\alpha)\ln\left(I(\xi_2)\right)$$

Here, $\alpha \in (0,1)$ represents the fraction of the detector element covered by the high-contrast object boundary. This non-linearity means that the effective attenuation coefficient calculated from the averaged intensities is inaccurately low, resulting in a smoothed edge and incorrect mean attenuation.

This inconsistency leads to artifacts in the reconstructed image, visible as streaks extending from the point of inconsistency along the back-projection path. When back-projections from multiple directions are superimposed, the erroneous values cannot be consistently corrected, leading to partial volume artifacts. These artifacts often appear as ghost lines along sharp object boundaries, as the back-projections from different directions fail to accurately represent the true attenuation profile.

6.9.1.3 Motion Artifacts

Motion artifacts result from inconsistencies caused by movement during data acquisition. It arises when there is movement within the slice being reconstructed during data acquisition

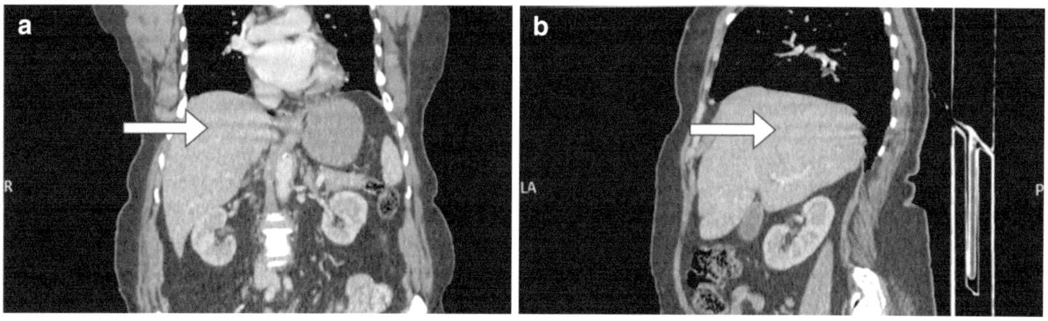

Fig. 6.29 Motion artifact due breathing. (**a**) Coronal image. (**b**) Sagittal image

(Fig. 6.29). Various methods, including interpolation and data-driven approaches, have been developed to address these artifacts. However, the ultimate solution lies in enhancing the speed of data acquisition while overcoming the associated technical limitations.

The assumption of a static morphology is violated when the attenuation coefficient, $\mu = \mu(\xi, \eta, E, t)$, varies over time, resulting in inconsistent data. This inconsistency occurs because the continuously moving table ensures that no single measured projection profile perfectly matches the others.

One approach to mitigate this issue is using spiral CT data interpolation, which leverages the known speed of table movement to interpolate missing data within certain limits, defined by the pitch factor. However, this method is limited by the accuracy of the pitch factor and the degree of motion.

Schumacher and Fischer [81] proposed, data-driven method which addresses motion artifacts. This method involves learning motion parameters directly from the raw data. It integrates reconstruction and motion correction into a single step, formulated as a regularized optimization problem:

$$(f,\omega)_{\min} = \min_f \sum_{i=1}^{K} A_i T(\omega_i) f - p_i 2 + \alpha R(f)$$

In this equation,

- K denotes the number of projection sets where the object is at rest.
- A_i is the system matrix modeling the projection geometry.
- p_i is the projection data, ω represents the motion parameters.
- $T(\omega_i)$ describes the transformation.
- $R(f)$ is a regularization term.

Since this system is over-determined, least squares minimization can be used to estimate both the image f and the motion parameters ω.

Despite these advancements, a fundamental goal for engineers is to accelerate the data acquisition process to reduce motion artifacts, particularly those caused by anatomical and physiological movements. Modern CT scanners, such as multi-slice sub-second CTs, attempt to achieve this, but they still struggle to produce clear images of rapidly moving organs, like the heart, without ECG triggering.

The speed of data acquisition cannot be increased indefinitely due to technical limitations. For instance, mechanical constraints limit the angular velocity and angular momentum of the gantry, which can weigh up to 1000 kg [80]. Additionally, data transmission from the rotating sampling unit to the fixed gantry poses a bottleneck, restricting the data rate and thus the potential for faster imaging.

6.9.1.4 Ring Artifacts

Ring artifacts are prominent circular distortions in reconstructed CT images caused by the failure of a detector channel or its corresponding processing channel. The geometry of the CT scanner explains their formation. The X-ray source and detector array are fixed together and move as a unit during scanning. When a detector element fails, it produces erroneous readings that propagate through the reconstruction process.

During filtered backprojection, the virtual lines connecting the defective detector element and the X-ray source create tangents of a circle in the image plane. This configuration results in inconsistencies in the measured values across different projection directions, which affect every point along these lines. Consequently, this causes significant distortions outside the circle formed by these tangents.

In image reconstruction, the defective channel manifests as a straight line in the overview along the table feed direction due to the fixed orientation of the X-ray tube and detector array. Despite the 360-degree rotation of the sampling unit with around 1000 angular steps, the defective channel remains visible as a straight line. The ring artifact arises from the accumulation of these tangents, which are backprojected over the entire image, creating a circular distortion. Within the circle formed by these tangents, the image is relatively free from artifacts, although smaller waves may appear near the artifact. These waves are due to reconstruction artifacts from the convolution of the projection signal before backprojection, which broadens the error in the filtered projection compared to the raw projection. This error diminishes with distance from the circle, leading to a cleaner image within the circle.

The severity of ring artifacts varies depending on the consistency of the detector failure across the array. Different Moiré patterns may emerge during reconstruction, which vary with the number of measured projection angles (N_p). These patterns can further complicate the image outside the defective circle, making ring artifacts a significant challenge for high-quality CT imaging.

6.9.1.5 Noise

Noise in CT imaging arises from two primary sources: quantum noise and detector noise.

Quantum Noise: This noise results from stochastic fluctuations during the scattering and absorption of X-ray quanta as they pass through the object being imaged. The number of quanta reaching the detector varies due to these random processes, even under identical radiographic conditions. Quantum noise is modeled as additive noise, with the noise level increasing linearly with X-ray exposure. It reflects the fact that X-ray energy is delivered in discrete packets, leading to statistical fluctuations in the detected signal.

Detector Noise: This type of noise is associated with the electronic properties of the detector, primarily arising from thermal effects. It is produced by the random motion of electrons within the detector material and is independent of X-ray exposure. Detector noise can be measured even without radiation.

The final reconstructed images are a combination of both the primary sources of noise. Consequently, noise present in the raw projection data propagates through the reconstruction process, potentially degrading image quality.

The noise can be minimized through several techniques. Increasing the X-ray dose improves signal-to-noise ratio, but this must be balanced with patient safety (Fig. 6.30). Advanced reconstruction algorithms, such as iterative reconstruction and model-based techniques, effectively reduce noise by incorporating statistical and physical models into the reconstruction process. Filtering methods applied during post-processing can also help diminish noise. Additionally, using high-quality detectors and optimizing scan parameters, such as exposure time and imaging protocol, further contributes to noise reduction and enhances image clarity.

6.9.1.6 Aliasing Artifacts

Aliasing artifacts in CT imaging occur due to under-sampling, which means the data collected does not capture the full detail of the object being scanned. This inadequacy can lead to misrepresentations in the reconstructed image. When the sampling rate is below the Nyquist rate, which is twice the highest frequency present in the object, high-frequency components are incorrectly interpreted as lower frequencies. This phenomenon, known as aliasing, can cause false patterns or structures to appear in the image, distorting the actual anatomical details.

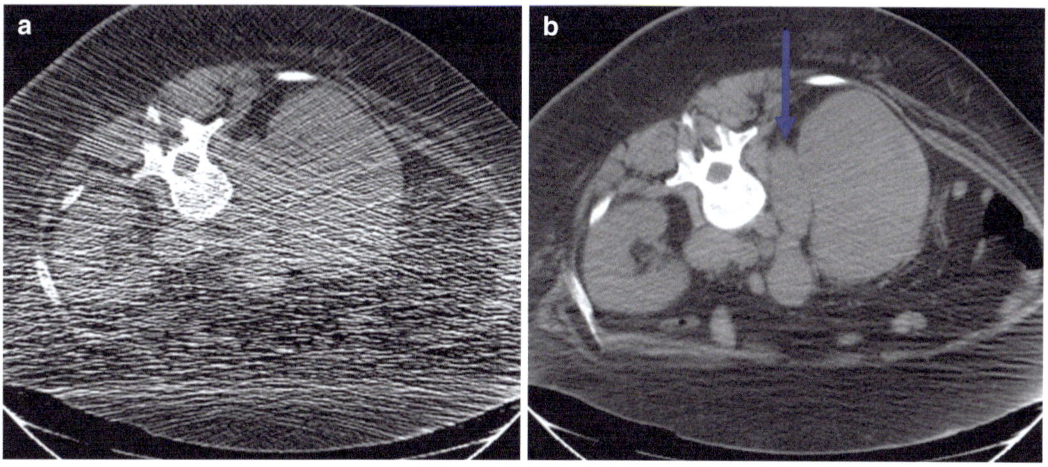

Fig. 6.30 Effect of mA on Poisson noise. (**a**) A low-dose CT image taken during a CT-guided biopsy displays extensive Poisson noise. These streaks persist regardless of whether the abdomen or arms are partially outside the field of view. (**b**) A post-biopsy image taken at 7.3 times the initial dose exhibits $\sqrt{7.3} = 2.7$ times less noise. The images reveal an enlarged retroperitoneal lymph node (arrow) and infiltration of the right kidney in a patient with Hodgkin's lymphoma [82]. (Image Courtesy: F Edward Boas and Dominik Fleischmann. Republished under conditions of open access)

The root cause of aliasing artifacts lies in the limited resolution of the detector system. If the spatial sampling interval is too large, the detector fails to accurately capture sharp edges and fine details. As a result, high-frequency information, such as abrupt changes in density or small structures within the scanned object, is not properly recorded. This missing information is then misrepresented during the reconstruction process, leading to visible artifacts.

One common manifestation of aliasing artifacts is the appearance of streaks or bands in the reconstructed image, particularly around areas with high contrast, such as the edges of bones or metallic implants. These artifacts can significantly impair the diagnostic quality of the images by introducing misleading visual information.

To mitigate aliasing artifacts, it is crucial to ensure an adequate sampling rate during the data acquisition process. This can be achieved by increasing the number of projections or detector elements, thereby capturing more detailed information about the scanned object. Additionally, advanced reconstruction algorithms that incorporate anti-aliasing techniques can help reduce the impact of these artifacts, leading to clearer and more accurate images.

6.9.2 3D Artifacts

3D artifacts affect the volume-rendered images or 3D reconstructions generated from multiple 2D slices.

6.9.2.1 Metal Artifacts

Metal artifacts can severely degrade CT image quality and obscure anatomical details, arising from metal objects like dental fillings, implants, or surgical hardware. The high density and atomic number of metals cause them to attenuate X-rays more strongly than surrounding tissues, leading to several issues during data acquisition and image reconstruction (Figs. 6.31 and 6.32).

As X-rays pass through metal, they are significantly absorbed, creating areas with little to no transmitted signal and causing inconsistencies in the measured projections. This often results in streaks radiating from the metal object, which can obscure surrounding structures and complicate diagnosis. Additionally, metals cause beam hardening—where lower-energy X-rays are absorbed more than higher-energy ones—skewing the reconstruction algorithms. They can also introduce scatter and photon starvation, reducing

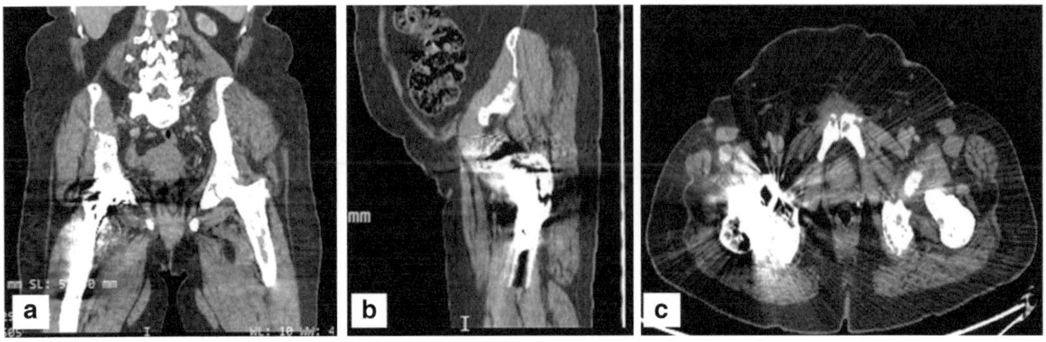

Fig. 6.31 Metal artifact due to metal implant in hip joint. (**a**) Coronal view. (**b**) Saggital view. (**c**) Axial view

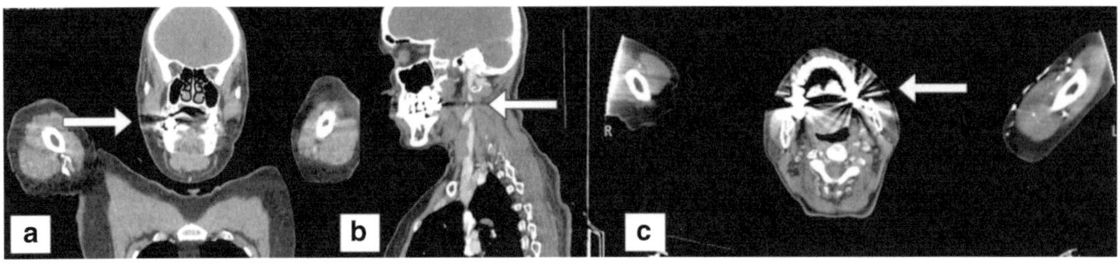

Fig. 6.32 Artifact due to dentures

the X-rays' intensity reaching the detector and further complicating reconstruction.

When slices containing metal artifacts are used to create 3D reconstructions, these artifacts can propagate through the volume, compounding the distortion. For instance, in jaw tomography, metal fillings can produce strong radial streak artifacts that degrade the entire image, affecting both coronal and sagittal reformatted slices.

To address these issues, metal artifact reduction (MAR) algorithms and dual-energy CT techniques are employed. MAR algorithms correct inconsistencies by modifying affected projections, while dual-energy CT differentiates between metal and soft tissues to reduce artifact severity. Despite these strategies, metal artifacts remain a persistent challenge, with ongoing development aimed at enhancing image accuracy and quality in the presence of metal objects. Accurate correction is crucial for reliable diagnosis and treatment planning, especially for patients with metallic implants or dental work.

6.9.2.2 Spiral CT Artifacts

While spiral or helical CT reduces motion artifacts and staircasing through continuous data acquisition, it introduces new challenges. One significant artifact is the scalloping artifact, which arises from interpolation inaccuracies and is influenced by the pitch factor.

Scalloping artifacts become noticeable due to increased slice sensitivity in spiral CT, making partial volume artifacts more pronounced in areas with rapid anatomical changes along the axial direction. For instance, in skull tomography, where the skull's diameter changes quickly, scalloping appears at slice positions with significant curvature variations. This results in reconstructed slices with apparent thickness differences, despite consistent nominal slice thickness. Scalloping manifests as thin fringes or ripples around structures, particularly where the surface normal vectors vary sharply between slices. These irregularities lead to visual distortions along the edges of structures.

The severity of scalloping can increase with excessively high pitch factors. A high pitch factor results in larger gaps between data points as the table moves rapidly through the gantry. This leads to interpolation inaccuracies, especially in areas with rapid anatomical changes, enlarging and shifting the fringe artifacts.

Minimizing scalloping artifacts requires careful pitch factor selection based on imaging requirements and anatomical characteristics. By choosing an appropriate pitch factor, gaps between data points can be reduced, decreasing the need for interpolation and mitigating scalloping in clinical practice.

6.9.2.3 Cone Beam Artifacts

Similar to spiral CT artefact, the cone-beam reconstruction method also generates a variety of artifacts, although some image errors, such as motion artifacts, may be reduced due to the increased acquisition speed. However, artefacts emerge with this method, particularly those related to the shadow zones in Radon space caused by incomplete data sets [80].

Reconstruction using data from a 4-line detector with 1 mm slice thickness and a feed rate of 12 mm/s remains acceptable for clinical applications with standard reconstruction, even without considering the cone aperture angle [80]. However, the standard reconstruction's mathematical approximations regarding the actual inclination of the reconstruction plane in three-dimensional space become invalid with larger cone aperture angles. Consequently, using a 16-line detector with 1 mm slice thickness and a feed rate of 48 mm/s results in significant artifacts, as the standard reconstruction method fails to account for the cone beam's geometry [80].

6.9.2.4 Zebra Artifacts

Zebra artifacts, also known as zebra stripes or zebra noise, appear as alternating dark and light bands parallel to the detector rows in CT images (Fig. 6.33). They are particularly noticeable in uniform density areas, like large water-filled structures or regions with consistent attenuation. These artifacts arise from imperfections or inconsistencies within the detector elements or their readout electronics, causing variations in recorded signal intensities across adjacent detectors. During image reconstruction, these variations manifest as periodic patterns or stripes that do not reflect actual anatomical structures. The severity of zebra artifacts can vary with the type of CT scanner, detector quality, and imaging parameters. They are more pronounced in older or lower-quality scanners with less precise detector uniformity and calibration. High X-ray tube currents or scanning protocols involving rapid movements or changes in contrast media can exacerbate the artifacts.

Mitigation strategies include regular calibration and maintenance of CT scanners to ensure detector uniformity, along with advanced reconstruction algorithms and post-processing techniques. Noise reduction filters and iterative reconstruction algorithms can smooth out zebra artifacts, improving image quality and diagnostic accuracy. Radiologists are trained to recognize and differentiate zebra artifacts from true anatomical features to avoid misinterpretation. Despite efforts to minimize these artifacts, they remain a challenge, particularly in older equipment or under suboptimal conditions, underscoring the need for ongoing technological advancements and quality assurance in medical imaging.

6.9.2.5 Staircase Artifacts

Staircase artifacts arise during three-dimensional reconstruction of objects with rapidly changing boundaries along the table feed direction, manifesting as step-like features in the image. These artifacts occur because the discrete nature of CT slices averages boundary information, leading to an inaccurate representation of continuous surfaces. This is particularly noticeable in high-contrast areas like the skull, where rapid changes along the z-axis create visible steps between adjacent slices.

The severity of staircase artifacts is pronounced in high-resolution areas where precise detail is crucial. To mitigate this, using very small, collimated slices that overlap can help smooth transitions between slices. A more effective solution is spiral (or helical) CT scanning, which provides continuous data acquisition and enables the reconstruction of densely stacked

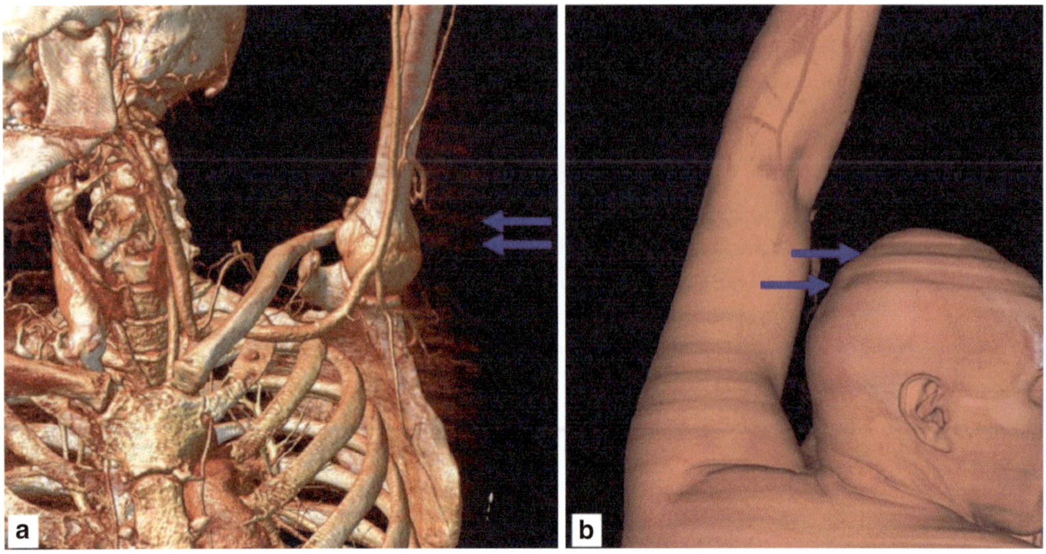

Fig. 6.33 (**a**) Zebra artifacts, resulting from helical interpolation, are more noticeable at the periphery of the field of view. (**b**) Stair-step artifacts, observed in both helical and multidetector row CT, are also more prominent near the field's periphery. Hence, it is crucial to position the object of interest near the center of the field of view [82]. (Image Courtesy: F Edward Boas and Dominik Fleischmann. Republished under conditions of open access)

slices, reducing staircase artifacts by offering more consistent data across the scanned volume.

The pitch factor, the ratio of table feed per rotation to slice thickness, is critical in controlling these artifacts. A pitch factor of less than 1 is recommended for rapid changes in high-contrast structures to ensure sufficient slice overlap and capture more detail, reducing step-like artifacts. Conventional CT with thicker slices, like 6 mm, exacerbates the staircase effect due to coarse inter-slice resolution [80]. Advanced techniques such as volume or cone-beam CT, with isotropic resolutions down to 140 μm, provide higher spatial resolution and improve detail and accuracy in reconstructed images, enhancing tumor detection and quantitative measurements [80].

6.9.2.6 Out-of-Field Artifacts

Out-of-field artifacts in CT imaging occur when parts of the patient's body extend beyond the scan field of view (SFOV). These artifacts typically manifest as bright pixels or streaks at the edge of the image, significantly degrading the overall image quality and potentially obscuring important diagnostic details (Fig. 6.34). The primary cause of these artifacts is the incomplete data acquisition from areas outside the SFOV, which leads to inconsistencies in the reconstructed images. The attenuation effects of out-of-field structures, combined with beam hardening and scatter radiation, contribute to

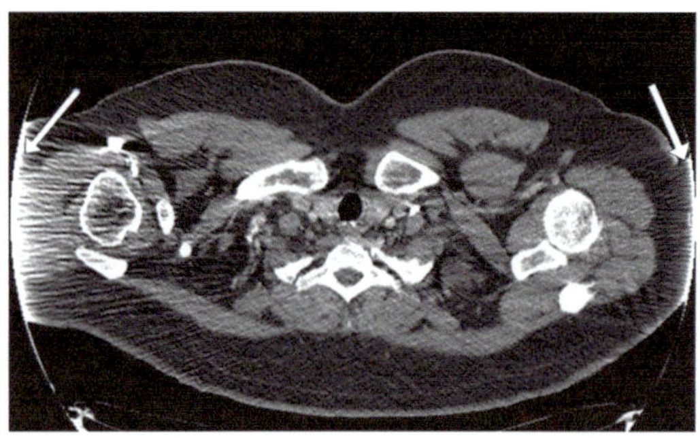

Fig. 6.34 Out-of-field artifacts as shown by arrows

these artifacts. Fortunately, modern CT scanners equipped with advanced reconstruction algorithms can mitigate out-of-field artifacts by accurately extrapolating missing data and correcting for these inconsistencies. Proper patient positioning, ensuring that the entire area of interest remains within the SFOV, also plays a crucial role in reducing the occurrence of these artifacts. Improved reconstruction techniques and careful patient management are essential for maintaining high-quality diagnostic images and minimizing the impact of out-of-field artifacts.

6.10 Quality Control in CT

Developing a comprehensive Quality Assurance (QA) and Quality Control (QC) program for CT systems is essential for ensuring the safety, accuracy, and reliability of imaging. The program encompasses several critical aspects, including basic system performance, acceptance testing, routine QC, and follow-up evaluations. The framework for such a program is established by various leading organizations and should be implemented under the supervision of a Qualified Medical Physicist (QMP). Key components include evaluating geometric accuracy, radiation output, and imaging output both at the commissioning stage (prior to first clinical use) and throughout the life of the CT system.

Several resources provide well-established methods for these evaluations. The American Association of Physicists in Medicine (AAPM) offers detailed procedures in Report 233 [83] for assessing CT system performance, including geometric accuracy, radiation dose measurements, and image quality assessments. The American College of Radiology (ACR) QC Manual for the CT Accreditation Program (CTAP) [84, 85] provides comprehensive guidelines for acceptance testing and routine performance evaluations. The European Commission's Report 162 [86] offers guidelines on CT quality assurance within the European context. The National Electrical Manufacturers Association (NEMA) XR-29 Standard (MITA Smart Dose) [87] outlines requirements for features like automatic exposure control and DICOM-compliant radiation dose reporting. The International Atomic Energy Agency (IAEA) [88] and the International Electrotechnical Commission (IEC) [89] also provide key guidelines and standards. Additionally, manufacturer-specific QC protocols are essential for maintaining performance and warranty compliance, aligning with each CT system's unique hardware and software specifications. Country-specific guidelines also regulate the quality control of imaging devices; however, they mainly follow the guidelines and procedures mentioned by the above-mentioned guidelines.

The Quality Control in CT involves a series of procedures designed to detect and correct defects or imperfections in CT equipment and imaging processes. By identifying and addressing these issues, QC helps maintain the high standards of image quality and patient safety. The QC process can be divided into two primary steps:

1. **Acceptance Testing:** Acceptance testing is conducted on newly installed CT equipment or the equipment that has undergone major repairs. The goal is to detect any defects or imperfections that might compromise the equipment's performance. Major repairs that necessitate acceptance testing include the replacement or repair of significant components such as x-ray tubes or detector assemblies. This step ensures that the equipment is functioning correctly before it is used for patient imaging. It also serves to establish baseline performance parameters for the CT equipment. By measuring and documenting these parameters, medical physicists can create a reference point for future comparisons.
2. **Routine QC for Performance Monitoring:** Routine QC involves regular monitoring and evaluation of the CT equipment's performance to detect and diagnose changes before they become apparent in clinical images. This proactive approach allows for early intervention and correction of any issues, thereby preventing potential degradation in image quality and ensuring consistent, reliable imaging results. When a defect or deterioration in equipment performance is detected, follow-up

measurements are performed to verify that the corrective actions have been successful. This step ensures that the equipment has been restored to its optimal performance level and is safe for clinical use.

6.10.1 QC Tests and Their Frequencies

QC involves systematic tests and inspections conducted at various intervals—daily, weekly, monthly, quarterly, and annually. Table 6.6 names the test, their frequency and purpose of those test.

6.10.2 Quality Control Procedures [84]

6.10.2.1 Daily Quality Control

Frequency Before the first clinical scan of the day

Components

1. **Water CT Number and Standard Deviation (Noise)**
   - **Warm-Up:** Prepare the X-ray tube as per manufacturer's recommendations.
   - **Calibration Scans:** Perform air-calibration scans to calibrate the system.
   - **Position QC Phantom:** Place and align the QC phantom accurately at the scanner isocenter.
   - **Set Up Scan:** Configure daily QC scan parameters for water mean and standard deviation. Follow manufacturer's recommendations or use pre-programmed settings provided by the Qualified Medical Physicist (QMP).
   - **Limits:** Water mean should be 0 ± 5 HU (or 0 ± 7 HU with ACR CT phantom); noise levels depend on scan technique (Fig. 6.35).

1. **Artifact Evaluation**
   - **Obtain Images:** Use axial mode or same images from water CT number and noise analysis.
   - **Reconstructed Images:** Ensure they are thin and span the *z*-axis.
   - **Visual Assessment:** Check for rings, streaks, or other artifacts. Set window width to 100 HU and center to 0 HU.
   - **Data Interpretation:**
     - **Ring Artifacts:** May indicate detector issues. Follow manufacturer's recommendations or repeat calibration.
     - **Other Artifacts:** Could be due to spilled contrast. Clean the gantry and retest.
     - **Subtle Artifacts:** Document but consider impact on patient scans. Avoid overreacting to minor issues.

Notes

- Automatic QC procedures can be used but should not replace artifact analysis.
- Maintain and review a library of artifact images for reference (Fig. 6.36).

6.10.2.2 Weekly Test

The weekly QC procedures include a single test:

1. **Wet Laser Printer Quality Control:**
   - This test ensures that the images printed on film match the quality of those displayed on the scanner's monitors.

Equipment Needed

1. Calibrated Densitometer
2. Laser Film QC Chart
3. SMPTE Test Pattern

Procedure

1. **Wet Laser Film Quality Control:**
   - Display the SMPTE test pattern on the filming console, setting the display window width/level to manufacturer-specified values.
   - Film the SMPTE pattern using a 6-on-1 format.
   - Measure the optical density of the 0, 10%, 40%, and 90% gray level patches using a film densitometer.
   - Plot these optical densities on the Laser Film QC Chart, circling any points outside control limits.

Table 6.6 CT quality assurance program schedule as per the ACR guideline 2017 [84], and revision in 2022 [85]

QC test	Frequency	Purpose
Acceptance Testing	Upon Installation	Verify system performance against manufacturer's specifications.
Annual Medical Physicist Survey	Annually (up to 14 months)	Ensure compliance with ACR QC requirements.
Participation in Review of Clinical Protocols	Acceptance and then Annually	Ensure protocols are up-to-date and optimized for safety and quality.
Scout Prescription and Alignment Light Accuracy	Acceptance and then Annually	Verify accuracy of patient positioning and alignment.
Table Travel Accuracy	Acceptance and then Annually	Ensure precise movement of the patient table.
Radiation Beam Width	Acceptance and then Annually	Measure beam width for correct collimation and dose distribution.
Low-Contrast Performance	Acceptance and then Annually	Assess ability to differentiate between tissues with minor differences.
Spatial Resolution	Acceptance and then Annually	Evaluate ability to distinguish small structures.
CT Number Accuracy	Acceptance and then Annually	Check accuracy of Hounsfield units for various tissues.
Artifact Evaluation	Acceptance and then Annually	Identify and mitigate artifacts affecting image quality.
CT Number Uniformity	Acceptance and then Annually	Ensure uniformity of CT numbers across the imaging field.
Dosimetry	Acceptance and then Annually	Measure and verify the radiation dose delivered.
CT Scanner Display Calibration	Acceptance and then Annually	Ensure display monitors accurately represent scanned images.
Other Tests as Required by State or Local Regulations	Acceptance and then Annually	Compliance with regional regulatory requirements.
Daily Tests		
Water CT Number and Standard Deviation[a]	Daily	Verify consistency of CT numbers in water to ensure scanner stability.
Artifact Evaluation	Daily	Monitor for new artifacts affecting clinical images.
Weekly Tests		
Wet Laser Printer Quality Control (if applicable)	Weekly	Ensure quality and accuracy of printed images.
Monthly Tests		
Visual Checklist	Monthly	Check physical condition of the scanner and its components.
Dry Laser Printer Quality Control (if applicable)	Monthly	Ensure quality and accuracy of printed images.
Display Monitor Quality Control	Monthly	Assess display accuracy for proper image visualization.

[a]It is recommended that the Water CT Number and Standard Deviation test be performed in both axial and helical scan modes

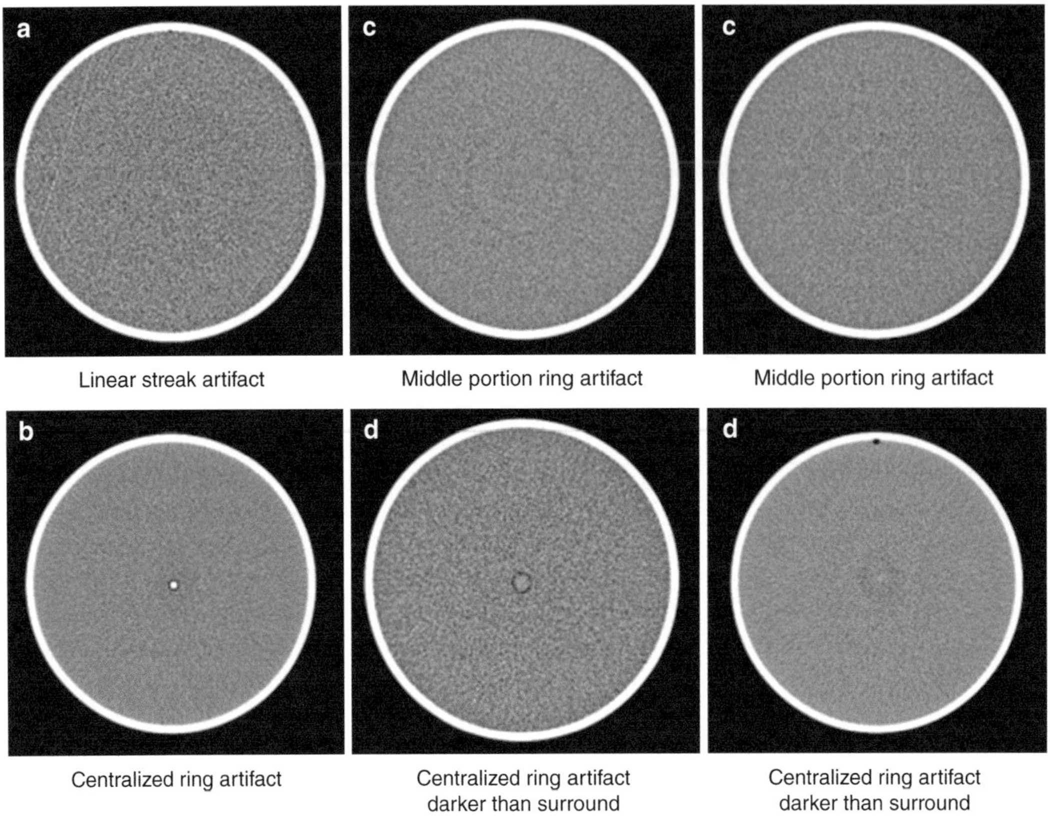

Fig. 6.35 Artifacts from Water Phantoms. (Image Courtesy: Dillon et al. [84]. Reprinted with permission)

- Inspect the film on a light box for streaks, uneven densities, and other artifacts.

SMPTE Pattern Performance Criteria
- **0% Patch:** 3.00 ± 0.15
- **10% Patch:** 2.20 ± 0.15
- **40% Patch:** 1.15 ± 0.15
- **90% Patch:** 0.30 ± 0.15

Corrective Actions
1. **If Optical Densities or Artifacts Are Outside Control Limits:**
   - Repeat the QC procedure to confirm the issue
   - Check for common issues:
     - Light leaks in the darkroom
     - Correct type and orientation of the film
     - Establish new action limits if the film type has changed
     - Clean processor rollers if streaking is present
     - Ensure correct water temperature and replenishment rates
   - Inform the QMP for assistance
- Consult the supervising radiologist to decide if filming can continue while resolving the issue

6.10.2.3 Monthly Quality Control Procedures

(i) **Visual Checklist**

Purpose: Verify CT system components for operational integrity and safety.
Frequency: Monthly
Inspection Points:

- **Gantry:**
  - Table height, position, angulation indicators
  - Laser localization light
  - Table motion and X-ray on indicators

Fig. 6.36 Common artifacts visible only in a larger uniform phantom. (Image Courtesy: Dillon et al. [84]. Reprinted with permission)

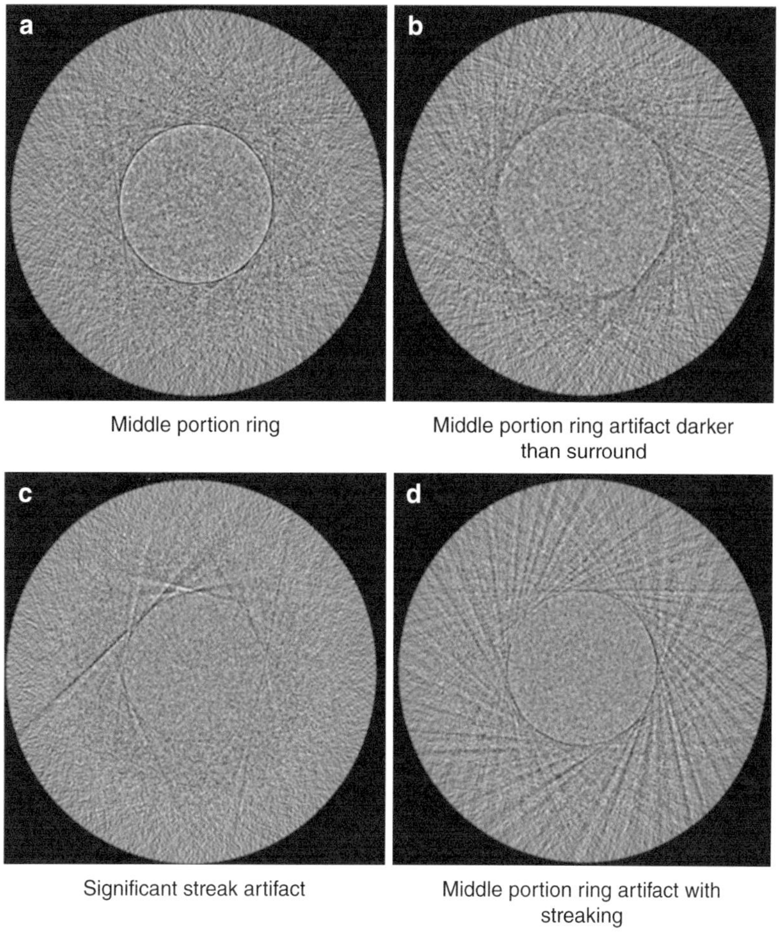

- **Control Console:**
  - Exposure switch, panel switches, lights, meters
  - X-ray on indicator and intercom functionality
  - Warning labels and postings
- **Other:**
  - Service records maintenance and accessibility

(ii) **Hard Copy Image Quality Control of Dry Laser Printers**

Purpose: Ensure diagnostic-quality film images match CT scanner monitor displays.

Frequency: Monthly; for backup printers, test before use and after changes.

Equipment Needed:

- Calibrated densitometer
- Laser Film QC Chart
- SMPTE test pattern

Procedure:

1. **Establish Operating Levels:**
   - Set by Qualified Medical Physicist (QMP) and verified monthly
2. **Dry Laser Film QC:**
   - Film SMPTE pattern on a 6-on-1 format
   - Measure optical densities of 0%, 10%, 40%, and 90% gray patches
   - Plot densities on the Laser Film QC Chart

SMPTE Pattern Criteria:

- 0% Patch: 3.00 ± 0.15
- 10% Patch: 2.20 ± 0.15
- 40% Patch: 1.15 ± 0.15
- 90% Patch: 0.30 ± 0.15

Corrective Actions:

1. Verify measurements and check common issues (e.g., light leaks, film type).
2. Consult QMP and radiologist if unresolved.

(iii) **Gray Level Performance of CT Scanner Acquisition Display Monitors**

Purpose: Confirm monitors display the full range of gray shades.

Frequency: Monthly, at QC program initiation, and after significant changes.

Equipment Needed:

- SMPTE Test Pattern or equivalent

Procedure:

1. Display the test pattern using manufacturer-specified settings.
2. Verify even gray level progression:
   - Distinguish 5% and 95% patches
   - Ensure all gray level steps are distinct

Corrective Actions:

1. Adjust monitor position to avoid glare.
2. Perform annual maintenance checks.
3. Address common issues (e.g., brightness/contrast adjustment, ambient lighting).
4. Follow manufacturer's adjustment procedures or consult QMP/service engineer.

6.10.2.4 Annual Quality Control

The Qualified Medical Physicist should include the following assessments in the annual testing program:

6.10.2.4.1 Clinical Protocol Review

- **Scanner Features Utilization:** Verify that clinical protocols effectively use scanner features such as kV, mAs, detector configuration, scan width, pitch, and dose reduction options (e.g., automatic exposure controls, iterative reconstruction). Ensure protocols provide necessary diagnostic image quality while minimizing patient radiation exposure.
- **Guideline Consistency:** Review protocols in line with AAPM Medical Physics Practice Guideline 1.a. on CT protocol management.

6.10.2.4.2 Scout Prescription and Alignment Light Accuracy

- **Purpose:** Confirm that alignment lights and scout images accurately reflect the scan position.
- **Required Equipment:** Phantom with radiopaque fiducial markers (e.g., ACR CTAP Phantom Module 1).
- **Test Procedure:** Align the phantom using lights, zero the table location, perform an axial scan, and check the alignment of scout images with fiducial markers. Repeat the process for verification.
- **Data Interpretation:** Assess alignment light and scout prescription accuracy by comparing the visibility of markers in images. Follow manufacturer's protocols if available.
- **Performance Criteria:** Ensure accuracy within 2 mm. If deviations exceed this threshold, contact service.

6.10.2.4.3 Table Travel Accuracy

- **Objective:** Verify table movement consistency.
- **Required Equipment:** Phantom with external fiducial markers (e.g., ACR CTAP Phantom Modules 1 and 4).
- **Test Procedure:** Position the phantom, zero the table, move it between fiducial markers, and record positions.

- **Data Interpretation:** Compare measured distances to known values and initial versus final positions.
- **Performance Criteria:** Table translation should be accurate within 2 mm. Consult specifications or contact service if inaccuracies exceed this limit.

6.10.2.4.4 Radiation Beam Width

- **Objective:** Measure and compare the radiation beam width to the nominal collimated beam width.
- **Required Equipment:** External radiation detector (e.g., CR plate, OSL strip), flat radiation attenuator (e.g., lead or acrylic).
- **Test Procedure:** Place the detector on the attenuator, adjust for isocenter, and measure beam width for each N × T product.
- **Data Interpretation:** Assess the actual beam width and compare it to the nominal width, ensuring it is accurate within 3 mm or 30% of the nominal width.
- **Performance Criteria:** The measured beam width should not be less than the nominal width. Contact service if discrepancies are found.

6.10.2.4.5 Low-Contrast Performance

- **Objective:** Ensure clinical protocols provide adequate low-contrast performance for diagnosis.
- **Required Equipment:** Phantom with low-contrast targets (e.g., ACR CTAP Phantom Module 2).
- **Test Procedure:** Scan the phantom with Auto mA disabled in various protocols (Adult Head, Pediatric Head, Adult Abdomen, Pediatric Abdomen).
- **Data Interpretation:** Measure and calculate Contrast-Noise Ratio (CNR) for each protocol.
- **Performance Criteria:** Achieve CNR standards: Adult Head: 1.0, Pediatric Head: 0.7, Adult Abdomen: 1.0, Pediatric Abdomen: 0.4. Adjust mAs or pitch if standards are not met.

6.10.2.4.6 Spatial Resolution

- **Objective:** Verify spatial resolution performance.
- **Required Equipment:** Phantom with high-contrast targets (e.g., ACR CTAP Phantom Module 4).
- **Test Procedure:** Scan the phantom with Auto mA disabled and measure the highest visible frequency.
- **Data Interpretation:** Compare results to standards for spatial resolution.
- **Performance Criteria:** Meet ACR CTAP Phantom standards: Adult Abdomen: 6 lp/cm, High-Resolution Chest: 8 lp/cm. Address discrepancies by evaluating equipment or reconstruction algorithms.

6.10.2.4.7 CT Number Accuracy

- **Objective:** Confirm CT number accuracy.
- **Required Equipment:** Phantom with known CT numbers (e.g., ACR CTAP Phantom Module 1).
- **Test Procedure:** Perform scans with Auto mA disabled for different protocols and measure CT numbers.
- **Data Interpretation:** Compare measured CT numbers to ACR Phantom standards.
- **Performance Criteria:** Meet standard ranges for water, air, Teflon, polyethylene, and acrylic. Recalibrate the scanner or consult service if values are outside ranges.

6.10.2.4.8 Artifact Evaluation

- **Objective:** Detect and address artifacts in uniform test phantom images.
- **Required Equipment:** Water phantom (ACR CT Phantom Module 3) or a larger phantom.
- **Test Procedure:** Scan the phantom using typical settings, reconstruct images, and inspect for artifacts.
- **Data Interpretation:** Identify and record artifacts such as rings or streaks.
- **Performance Criteria:** Correct artifacts like ring imbalances and address any issues that affect clinical interpretation.

6.10.2.4.9 CT Number Uniformity

- **Objective:** Identify non-uniformities in CT numbers.
- **Required Equipment:** Water phantom (ACR CT Phantom Module 3).
- **Test Procedure:** Scan the phantom and place ROI at various positions to measure and compare CT numbers.
- **Data Interpretation:** Ensure the difference between peripheral and central ROI values does not exceed 5 HU.
- **Performance Criteria:** Correct non-uniformities within 30 days or before they impact clinical use.

6.10.2.4.10 Dosimetry

- **Objective:** Measure doses for verifying scanner performance and patient dose estimates.
- **Required Equipment:** Calibrated electrometer, CTDI pencil ionization chamber, Head and Body CTDI phantoms.
- **Test Procedure:** Scan using various protocols, record CTDI values, and calculate CTDI_vol.
- **Data Interpretation:** Compare results to scanner-reported values and ACR standards.
- **Performance Criteria:** Ensure differences are within 5% year-to-year and 20% of scanner-reported values.

6.10.2.4.11 CT Scanner Display Calibration

- **Objective:** Ensure the monitor displays the full range of gray shades.
- **Required Equipment:** SMPTE Test Pattern, calibrated photometer.
- **Test Procedure:** Display the pattern, check gray levels, brightness, and contrast.
- **Data Interpretation:** Ensure distinct gray levels and check brightness non-uniformity.
- **Performance Criteria:** Maintain display non-uniformity within specified limits for CRTs and flat-panel displays. Consult with the QMP or service engineer if issues persist.

This streamlined approach to annual quality control covers essential assessments, procedures, and performance criteria to ensure accurate and reliable CT imaging.

6.11 Contrast Enhancement in Computed Tomography

Contrast media are used to enhance the visibility of internal structures within the body, thereby facilitating the differentiation between various tissues and organs. These agents, commonly iodine-based dyes, play a pivotal role in improving the clarity and detail of imaging studies, making it easier for radiologists and physicians to identify and evaluate abnormalities. By increasing the contrast between different tissues, these media help in accurately diagnosing a wide range of conditions, including tumors, vascular diseases, and inflammatory processes.

Administered via different routes such as orally, intravenously, or rectally, contrast media cater to specific diagnostic needs and target different parts of the body. Oral administration is often used to highlight the gastrointestinal tract, providing clear images of the stomach, intestines, and related structures. Intravenous injection is widely utilized for enhancing the visibility of blood vessels and soft tissues, aiding in the assessment of organs like the brain, liver, kidneys, and heart. Rectal administration, on the other hand, is primarily used to visualize the lower gastrointestinal tract, including the rectum and colon.

6.11.1 Physics of Contrast Media

The physics of contrast media involves the differential attenuation of X-rays by various tissues. Contrast agents, such as iodine or barium, contain elements with high atomic numbers that absorb X-rays more effectively than surrounding tissues. When introduced into the body, these agents create a stark contrast between areas where they accumulate and the surrounding tissues. This increased absorption leads to a notable difference in X-ray intensity detected by CT scanners, measured in

Hounsfield Units (HU). By elevating the HU values in regions like blood vessels or tumors, contrast agents enhance the visibility of these structures on CT images, improving the differentiation between tissues and revealing fine details such as tumors, blood vessel abnormalities, or inflammatory regions.

6.11.2 Types of Contrast Media

Contrast media can be broadly classified into two categories: iodinated and non-iodinated contrast media, each with its specific applications, properties, and considerations.

6.11.2.1 Iodinated Contrast Media

Iodinated contrast media are the most commonly used agents in CT imaging due to their high effectiveness in absorbing X-rays. They can be further divided into non-ionic and ionic types.

1. **Non-ionic Iodinated Contrast Media**:
   - **Chemical Structure, Properties, and Advantages**: Non-ionic contrast agents do not dissociate into charged particles (ions) in solution. They are composed of molecules that remain whole when dissolved in water, resulting in lower osmolality compared to ionic agents. Osmolality refers to the concentration of particles in a solution and is a critical factor in determining the safety and comfort of contrast media. The lower osmolality of non-ionic iodinated contrast media reduces the risk of adverse reactions, such as discomfort, pain, or allergic responses. Patients receiving non-ionic contrast agents generally experience fewer side effects, making these agents the preferred choice in clinical practice.
   - **Clinical Applications**: Non-ionic iodinated contrast media are widely used in various CT examinations, including imaging of the brain, chest, abdomen, and pelvis. Their safety profile makes them suitable for use in patients with a higher risk of contrast-induced reactions.
2. **Ionic Iodinated Contrast Media**:
   - **Chemical Structure and Properties**: Ionic contrast agents dissociate into charged particles when dissolved in water, resulting in higher osmolality. This higher osmolality can increase the likelihood of side effects and adverse reactions such as nausea, vomiting, and allergic reactions. Due to these potential issues, their use has decreased in favor of non-ionic agents.
   - **Clinical Applications**: Despite their drawbacks, ionic contrast media remain valuable in specific clinical situations due to their unique properties. They are commonly utilized in certain vascular studies where their characteristics are advantageous. While intravenous administration is the most frequent route for contrast studies, ionic iodinated contrast media can also be administered through various other routes, including gastrointestinal (oral, rectal), cystourethral, vaginal, and intraosseous methods. One notable advantage of ionic contrast media is their lower cost compared to non-ionic contrast media, making them a more economical choice in certain applications.

6.11.2.2 Non-iodinated Contrast Media

Non-iodinated contrast media are less commonly used in CT imaging but can be valuable in specific situations, especially when iodine-based agents are contraindicated. These contrast agents include gadolinium-based agents and other specialized compounds.

1. **Barium-based Contrast Agents**:

   Barium-based contrast agents are primarily used for gastrointestinal (GI) studies. These agents, containing barium sulfate, are highly radiopaque and enhances the visualization of the GI tract. They are commonly employed in CT enterography to assess the small intestine for conditions such as Crohn's disease, in CT colonography (virtual colonoscopy) to examine the colon and rectum for polyps or tumors. Additionally, barium-based agents are used in CT upper GI series to investigate abnormalities in the esophagus, stomach, and duodenum.

2. **Gadolinium-based Contrast Agents**:

   Gadolinium-based contrast agents are primarily used in magnetic resonance imaging rather than in computed tomography (CT) imaging. Gadolinium enhances the quality of MRI images by improving contrast in various tissues, making it particularly useful for imaging the brain, spinal cord, blood vessels, and joints. It works by altering the magnetic properties of tissues, thereby enhancing the contrast between different structures and improving the visualization of pathological conditions.

6.11.3 Usage and Considerations

The choice of contrast media and administration route depends on the clinical scenario, the area being examined, and the patient's health status. Before administering contrast media, patients are `typically screened for allergies, kidney function, and other risk factors to minimize potential adverse reactions. Common side effects of contrast media include a feeling of warmth or flushing during injection, nausea, and a metallic taste in the mouth. Serious allergic reactions are rare but can occur. The appropriate selection and administration of contrast media are essential for obtaining high-quality diagnostic images while minimizing potential risks to patients.

6.12 Applications of Volume Scanning

Volume scanning, unlike traditional slice-by-slice CT scanning, acquires continuous volumetric data, allowing for comprehensive imaging of anatomical structures. This increases the speed and efficiency of scans along with enhanced resolution and accuracy of the images produced. By capturing large datasets in a single, continuous sweep, volume scanning enables a variety of sophisticated imaging techniques, including real-time imaging, three-dimensional reconstructions, detailed vascular studies, and even virtual reality-based visualizations. Volume scanning, whether achieved through single-slice spiral/helical or multislice spiral/helical CT, produces significantly more data compared to traditional slice-by-slice CT scanning. This extensive data acquisition has led to the development of several innovative applications that provide radiologists and other physicians with enhanced diagnostic tools.

6.12.1 CT Fluoroscopy

CT fluoroscopy, or continuous imaging, relies on spiral/helical data acquisition, high-speed processing, and advanced image reconstruction algorithms. Unlike conventional CT, which has a time lag between data acquisition and image reconstruction, CT fluoroscopy enables real-time image reconstruction and display at variable frame rates. Approved by the U.S. FDA in 1996, this technique is based on three technological advancements [90]:

1. **Fast, Continuous Scanning:** Enabled by spiral/helical scanning principles.
2. **Rapid Image Reconstruction:** Achieved through specialized hardware and new algorithms.
3. **Continuous Image Display:** Utilizing cine mode at frame rates of two to eight images per second.

CT fluoroscopy is further supported by tools such as the Fluoro Assisted Computed Tomography System, which integrates a flat-panel amorphous silicon digital detector with an X-ray tube on a C-arm as part of the CT gantry.

Three-Dimensional Imaging and Volume Visualization

Three-dimensional (3D) imaging is widely used in various fields, including radiation treatment planning, craniofacial imaging, surgical planning, and orthopedics. 3D images can be created through hardware-based or software-based approaches, both of which involve transforming trans-axial CT data into simulated 3D images using rendering techniques. These techniques generally include three steps:

1. **Volume Formation:** Stacking images to create a volume with preprocessing.
2. **Classification:** Determining tissue types in the slices.
3. **Image Projection:** Projecting classified volume data to form a 2D representation of the 3D volume.

Advancements in computer graphics have played a significant role in the evolution of 3D imaging, allowing for more sophisticated and refined images. Volume visualization tools, ranging from simple windowing tools to advanced interactive and cine visualization tools, aid diagnosticians in interpreting these images.

6.12.2 CT Angiography

CT angiography involves imaging blood vessels opacified by contrast media. The entire area of interest is scanned using spiral/helical CT during contrast injection, capturing images when the vessels are fully opacified to show arterial or venous phases of enhancement. This technique employs 3D imaging principles to visualize the vasculature through intravenous contrast media injection. Key elements include:

1. **Patient Preparation:** Ensuring optimal imaging conditions.
2. **Acquisition Parameters:** Optimizing scan time, slice thickness, and table speed.
3. **Contrast Media Injection:** Enhancing vessel visibility.
4. **Postprocessing Techniques:** Utilizing algorithms for 3D image display in interactive cine modes, multiplanar reconstruction, maximum intensity projection, shaded surface display, and volume rendering.

6.12.3 CT Endoscopy: Virtual Reality Imaging

Virtual reality in CT imaging has led to the development of virtual endoscopy, which creates inner views of tubular structures using volume CT data. This technique immerses users in a computer-generated environment, allowing for interaction with 3D scenes with virtual endoscopy.

6.12.4 Cardiac CT Imaging

Imaging the beating heart requires reducing motion artifacts and preserving spatial and contrast resolution. The synchronization with electrocardiograms (ECGs) with latest multislice CT (MSCT) or dual-source CT (DSCT) scanners offer excellent image quality by meeting technical requirements like low-contrast resolution, high-contrast resolution, and temporal resolution. These scanners enable fast data acquisition and use dedicated reconstruction algorithms to merge synchronized transmission data from multiple heart cycles, improving temporal resolution. Applications include coronary artery calcification assessment, ventricular function assessment, and coronary angiography.

6.13 Digital Image Processing

Digital image processing in CT imaging begins with acquiring X-ray attenuation data from multiple angles. This data is reconstructed into cross-sectional images using algorithms such as filtered back projection or iterative reconstruction. Post-processing techniques, including edge detection algorithms like Sobel and Canny, and segmentation methods such as thresholding and region-growing, further refine image quality. These techniques enhance diagnostic accuracy by highlighting anatomical structures and lesions.

6.13.1 Matrix Size in CT

Matrix size in CT imaging plays a crucial role in determining image resolution and detail. Initially, clinical CT images were produced with an 80 × 80 matrix of 3 mm × 3 mm × 13 mm voxels. Today, standard matrix sizes have evolved to 512 × 512 or 1024 × 1024 pixels. The choice of matrix size depends on the anatomy under study and the desired resolution. The Field of View (FOV) or reconstruction circle is the circular area from which transmission measurements are recorded. The scan FOV, covered by the matrix, creates the image slice, while the display FOV can be equal to or less than the scan FOV, affecting image detail and zoom. The matrix size, selected before the CT examination, influences pixel size and image resolution. Larger matrices provide finer detail but require more data storage and processing power. For example, with a 25 cm (250 mm) FOV and a 512 × 512 matrix, the pixel size is approximately 0.49 mm. Pixel sizes in clinical CT scans typically range from 0.5 mm to 2 mm, though older systems may have pixel sizes up to 10 mm. Each pixel represents a small square area, while each voxel (volume element) represents a 3D space volume. Isotropic imaging occurs when voxel dimensions are equal in length, width, and height.

6.13.2 Image Formation, Resolution, and Bit Depth

Each pixel in a CT image can display various shades of gray, representing different tissue densities. CT images can have bit depths of 8, 9, 10, 11, or 12 bits per pixel, impacting the grayscale range. For instance, a 12-bit CT image can display 4096 (2^12) shades of gray, ranging from −1000 to 3095 Hounsfield units. Higher matrix sizes, such as 1024 × 1024, capture more detailed information, beneficial for diagnosing small abnormalities, though they generate larger data volumes and require more processing time. Standard matrix sizes, like 512 × 512, offer a balance between detail and data management, making them suitable for general diagnostic purposes. The ability to choose appropriate matrix sizes and FOV allows technologists to tailor CT scans to the specific needs of the examination, optimizing image quality and diagnostic value.

Digital imaging represents images as pixel matrices, facilitating extensive post-processing, and easy storage, retrieval, and sharing. Resolution is defined by pixel count, while bit depth determines the range of grayscale values or colors. In 3D imaging, voxels represent volumetric units, affecting spatial resolution. The digitization process involves scanning, sampling, and quantization to convert analog images into digital format, with Analog-to-Digital Conversion (ADC) translating signals into digital values. This process simplifies storage, manipulation, transmission, and integration with electronic health records. Various processing techniques, including point, local, and global operations, and geometric transformations, enhance image quality.

6.13.3 Image Compression and Its Effects

Image compression is used to reduce file size while preserving visual content. Lossless compression maintains data integrity, making it suitable for medical imaging, while lossy compression reduces file size by discarding some data, which is more appropriate for multimedia. Lossy compression can introduce artifacts and reduce detail, necessitating a balance between compression benefits and image quality needs. Overall, advancements in digital image processing have significantly enhanced diagnostic accuracy and image quality.

6.14 CT Dose and Dosimetry

The assessment and management of radiation dose in Computed Tomography (CT) ensures patient safety while maintaining diagnostic image quality. Dosimetry for CT involves the measurement and calculation of the radiation dose absorbed by the patient's body. This field has seen significant advancements, with comprehensive guidelines provided by the International Commission on Radiation Units and Measurements (ICRU) [91], the American Association of Physicists in Medicine [92], and the International Atomic Energy Agency (IAEA) [93]. These guidelines introduce various dosimetric indices essential for optimizing CT examinations and safeguarding patient health.

6.14.1 Standard Terms Used in CT Dose Assessment

6.14.1.1 Computed Tomography Dose Index (CTDI)

The term Computed Tomography Dose Index (CTDI) was proposed by Shope et al. [94] in 1981 to quantify the radiation output from a CT scanner during a single 360-degree rotation of the X-ray tube with no table motion. CTDI measures the radiation dose from a CT tube when it completes a full rotation, providing a standardized metric for comparing the radiation output of different CT systems. It is calculated by integrating the axial dose profile along the z-axis for a single CT slice and dividing by the beam width (Fig. 6.37). The formula is expressed as:

$$\mathrm{CTDI}_{\infty} = \frac{1}{nT}\int_{-\infty}^{\infty} K(z)\,\mathrm{d}z$$

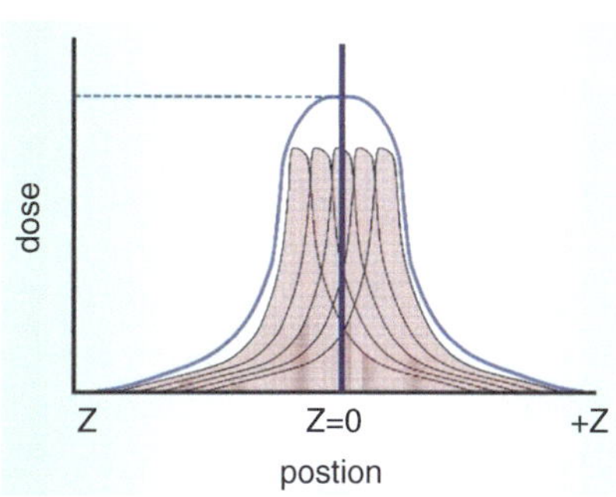

Fig. 6.37 A CT dose profile distribution of radiation dose along the path of an X-ray beam during a scan

Where:

- n is the number of data channels used in a particular scan.
- T is the nominal width of the tomographic section along the z-axis imaged by one data channel.
- $K(z)$ is the air kerma as a function of position on the z-axis.

The product nT, known as the nominal beam width, is an important measure in CT acquisition protocols and dosimetry. Historically, the air kerma $K(z)$ was referred to as $D(z)$ [95], but since it represents the absorbed dose to air in the ionization chamber rather than to the phantom material, the notation was updated to $K(z)$ [92] .

CTDI values are measured in milli-Gray (mGy). These values predict the dose resulting from a series of contiguous scans. When measured at the scanner isocenter without any patient or phantom, it is termed $\mathrm{CTDI}_{\mathrm{air}}$. In multi-detector CT (MDCT) machines, the number of detector rows and data channels is more relevant than the number of slices. Detector rows refer to the arrangement of discrete elements across the detector, while data channels are the electronics converting analogue signals from the detector into digital values for image reconstruction.

6.14.1.2 CTDI_{100}

CTDI_{100} represents a specific measurement of CTDI, utilizing a 100 mm long pencil-shaped ionization chamber to integrate the CT axial dose profile over a single full 360-degree rotation of the CT tube within a 15 cm long polymethyl methacrylate (PMMA) cylindrical phantom. This method is designed to measure the radiation dose within a standardized length of the phantom.

Standard Phantoms For adult CT exams, standard 16 cm (head) and 32 cm (body) PMMA phantoms are used. Custom-made phantoms for pediatric studies, with varying diameters corresponding to different ages, are also utilized. These phantoms are placed concentrically with the isocenter of the CT scanner, ensuring accurate and consistent dose measurements.

Calculation and Formula The formula for $CTDI_{100}$ is:

$$CTDI_{100} = \frac{1}{nT}\int_{-50}^{+50} K(z)\,dz$$

This formula integrates the air kerma over a 100 mm length along the *z*-axis, providing an accumulated dose measure within this specific range. While $CTDI_{100}$ offers a practical dose estimate for a defined scan length, it tends to underestimate the accumulated air kerma for longer scan lengths, as noted in ICRU Report 87.

$CTDI_{100}$ measurements are taken by placing the ionization chamber in central and peripheral holes within the phantoms. For more comprehensive assessments, head and body phantoms may include multiple peripheral holes at various angles, with values typically averaged to obtain a more accurate dose distribution.

6.14.1.3 Weighted Computed Tomography Dose Index ($CTDI_w$)

$CTDI_w$, or weighted CTDI, is a metric used to approximate the average radiation dose within a CT dosimetry phantom. It accounts for the variation in absorbed doses between the center and periphery of the scanned volume. In a 32-cm body phantom, which simulates the adult body, surface doses at the periphery can be twice as high as those at the center (Fig. 6.38). Conversely, in a head phantom, doses are more uniform between the central and peripheral regions.

It is calculated using measurements from both the center and periphery of the phantom, integrating these to provide an averaged dose value. The formula is:

$$CTDI_w = \frac{2}{3}CTDI_p + \frac{1}{3}CTDI_c$$

Where:

- $CTDI_p$ is the CTDI measured at the periphery of the phantom.
- $CTDI_c$ is the CTDI measured at the center of the phantom.

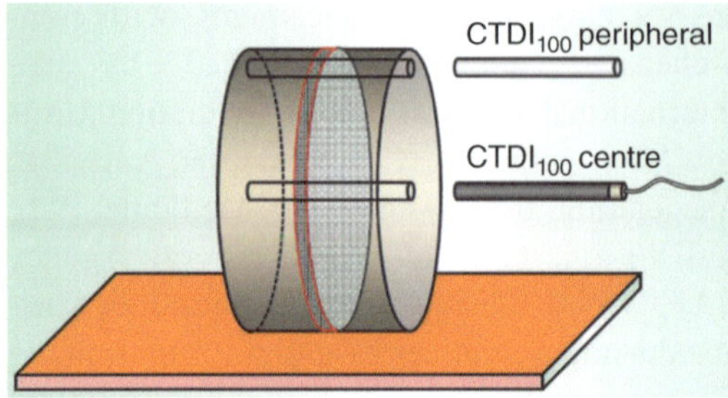

Fig. 6.38 CT Dose Index

This weighted calculation reflects the dose distribution more accurately, considering that in a single full rotation of the CT tube, half of the energy is deposited directly in the irradiation volume, while the other half is deposited in scattered tails adjacent to the directly irradiated volume. The intensity of scattered radiation diminishes rapidly according to the inverse square law, but tissues beyond the directly irradiated region are still exposed to this scattered radiation.

6.14.1.4 Volume Computed Tomography Dose Index ($CTDI_{vol}$)

$CTDI_{vol}$, or volume CTDI, is used in helical or spiral scanning modes where the CT gantry rotates continuously with concurrent patient table movement. It accounts for gaps or overlaps in the scanned volume by adjusting for the pitch, which is the ratio of the distance traveled by the table in one gantry rotation to the beam width or beam collimation. The formula for $CTDI_{vol}$ is:

$$CTDI_{vol} = \frac{CTDI_w}{\text{pitch}}$$

where the pitch is the table movement per rotation divided by the beam width. $CTDI_{vol}$ is independent of the total scan length and provides a measure of radiation intensity incident on the patient. If the pitch is 1.0, $CTDI_{vol}$ equals $CTDI_w$. If pitch <1.0, dose increases due to overlapping scans, and if pitch >1.0, dose decreases.

$CTDI_{vol}$ is a universal metric indicating the intensity of radiation incident on patients but does not represent the patient dose directly. It depends on various factors including X-ray tube voltage (kV), tube current (mA), tube rotation time (sec), CT pitch (P), and phantom size.

6.14.1.5 Dose-Length Product (DLP)

The dose-length product (DLP) quantifies the total radiation dose incident on a patient by considering both the intensity and length of the scan. It provides a cumulative measure of the radiation exposure over the entire scanned volume. The formula for DLP is:

$$\text{DLP} = \text{CTDI}_{\text{vol}} \times \text{Scan length}\left(L\right)$$

DLP is measured in milliGray-centimeters (mGy·cm) and is proportional to the total energy imparted to the patient. It serves as a good indicator of the overall radiation exposure and is directly related to the patient's stochastic risk, which includes the potential for radiation-induced effects. DLP can be used to establish reference values for different types of CT examinations, adhering to the ALARA (As Low As Reasonably Achievable) principle to minimize radiation exposure while achieving necessary diagnostic outcomes.

6.14.1.6 Size-Specific Dose Estimate (SSDE)

Since 2002, CT scanners have been mandated to display CTDI_{vol} (Computed Tomography Dose Index volume) and DLP (Dose-Length Product) before and after the scan as part of a "dose report." However, these values are determined using only 16-cm and 32-cm PMMA head and body reference phantoms, which means the dose estimates generated by the system pertain to the phantoms, not the actual patients. This poses a significant challenge in accurately assessing patient doses due to wide variations in patient sizes, particularly among pediatric patients, where the absorbed doses can differ by a factor of 2–3 times compared to the phantoms. To address this discrepancy and improve dose estimation accuracy, the American Association of Physicists in Medicine (AAPM) provided detailed guidelines on "Size-Specific Dose Estimate (SSDE)" in its Report 204 (2011) [96].

The SSDE is a more accurate "patient dose estimate" that incorporates corrections based on the patient's size. It uses linear dimensions measured directly on the patient or from patient images. The AAPM Report 204 provides tables related to 32-cm and 16-cm diameter PMMA phantoms, respectively. These tables include correction factors that are used to adjust the CTDI_{vol} reported by CT scanners. The formula for calculating SSDE is:

$$\text{SSDE} = \text{CTDI}_{\text{vol}} \times \text{size specific conversion factor}$$

Measuring Patient Dimensions

To obtain the necessary size-specific conversion factor, "Anterior-Posterior (AP)" and/or "Lateral" dimensions must be measured. These measurements can be taken using electronic calipers. The AAPM tables provide data within four sub-tables that offer conversion factors based on these dimensions.

- **AP Dimension:** This is the thickness of the body part from anterior to posterior or vice versa.
- **Lateral Dimension:** This is the measurement from left to right or vice versa.

Using these dimensions, an effective diameter can be calculated. The effective diameter is defined as the diameter of a circle whose area is the same as that of the patient's cross-section.

6.14.1.7 Estimating Effective Diameter by Age

In cases where the AP and lateral dimensions are not available, the AAPM Report 204 offers a table that estimates the effective diameter based on the patient's age. This table is useful when only the patient's age is available. The estimated effective diameter from this table can then be matched with the conversion factors to calculate the SSDE. However, it is important to note that this method should only be used when patient-specific dimensions are not available, as there can be significant size variation among patients of the same age.

Patient Absorbed Dose Calculation

To estimate the patient dose from the $CTDI_{vol}$, the following formula is used:

$$\text{Patient absorbed dose} = CTDI_{vol} \times \text{Patient size factor} \times \text{Scan length}$$

This formula takes into account the volume CT dose index ($CTDI_{vol}$), a patient size-specific factor, and the length of the scan. These elements together provide a comprehensive estimation of the radiation dose absorbed by a patient during a CT scan.

6.14.2 CT Dosimetry Phantoms

6.14.2.1 AAPM Report 31 (1990) Phantoms

The Association of American Physicists in Medicine (AAPM) Report 31 (1990) [97] describes two essential phantoms used for obtaining $CTDI_{100}$ measurements. These phantoms include:

1. A 16-cm diameter adult head phantom, which also serves as a pediatric body phantom equivalent to the cross-sectional area of a typical 2-year-old child.
2. A 32-cm diameter adult body phantom.

Both phantoms are 15 cm in length and constructed from Polymethyl methacrylate (PMMA), a clear plastic also known under trade names such as Lucite, Perspex, and Plexiglass. PMMA has a chemical formula of $(C_5H_8O_2)_n$ and a density of 1.185 g/cm^3. These phantoms feature ~12 mm diameter holes at the center and periphery to allow for the insertion of an ionization chamber.

These PMMA phantoms have been widely used and proven to be very useful in CT dosimetry. In addition to these standard phantoms, several custom-made PMMA phantoms are designed specifically for pediatric studies. These phantoms, also 15 cm in length, have diameters tailored to approximate average body sizes at different ages: 10 cm for newborns, 13 cm for 1-year-olds, 16 cm for 5-year-olds, 20 cm for 10-year-olds, and 25 cm for 15-year-olds (Fig. 6.39). These pediatric phantoms enable accurate dosimetric measurements for various patient sizes, ensuring that CT imaging protocols are appropriately adjusted for different age groups. However, they have certain limitations, including:

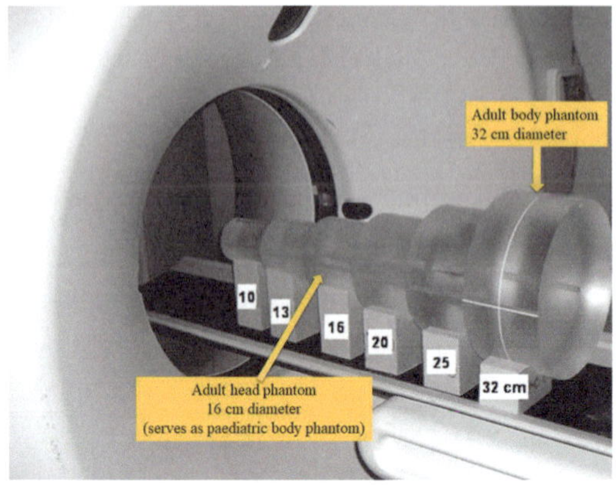

Fig. 6.39 Cylindrical PMMA phantoms used for CT dose assessment, with varying diameters for adult head, adult body, and pediatric body simulations. (Image copyright John Wiley and Sons; Brisse et al. [98], reprinted with permission)

- Exclusion of dose accumulation for longer scans
- Unsuitability for newer scanners with very wide beams exceeding 100 mm

6.14.2.2 AAPM Report 111 Recommendations and ICRU/AAPM Phantom

Recognizing the limitations of the older phantoms, AAPM Report 111 [99] offered several recommendations for new measurement methodologies and suggested new phantom designs. Subsequently, the AAPM and The International Committee on Radiation Units and Measurements (ICRU) jointly developed a new phantom suitable for a wide range of CT scanner designs and scanning conditions, discussed in AAPM Report 200 (2020) [92].

6.14.2.3 ICRU/AAPM Phantom

This new phantom is cylindrical, made of polyethylene with a density of 0.97 g/cm^3, chosen to closely mimic the absorption properties of human adipose tissue. Key characteristics include:

- Diameter: 30 cm
- Length: 60 cm
- Lightweight, readily available, and relatively expensive

To enhance manageability, the phantom can be divided into three sections:

- Each section is 20 cm long and has a mass of approximately 13.7 kg.
- The total weight of the fully assembled phantom is 41.1 kg, similar to the fully assembled 32-cm CTDI phantom.

Advantages and Future Adoption The ICRU/AAPM phantom has shown good correlation with radiation absorption properties and can be adopted as future standards (as cited in AAPM Report 200 and ICRU Report 87). This phantom design addresses the limitations of previous models and accommodates the needs of modern CT scanners, providing a more accurate representation of dose distribution and absorption in human tissues.

6.14.3 Estimating Effective Doses

Definition and Purpose

The effective dose, as defined in ICRP 60 (1991) [100] and modified in ICRP 103 (2007) [101], is a measure used to compare the radiation detriments of various radiological and nuclear medicine procedures. It is a generic quantity based on weighting factors derived from radiobiological considerations and reflects the overall risk of any radiation exposure to a reference person. This dose is not intended to assess an individual patient's radiation dose, as it is averaged over all ages and both sexes.

Methods for Calculating Effective Doses in CT Scans

There are two common methods to calculate effective doses in CT scans:

1. **Organ Dose Estimates Method (Gold Standard):** This method uses tissue-weighting factors specified by the ICRP to estimate organ doses. It is considered the gold standard for calculating effective doses.
2. **Dose-Length Product (DLP) Method:** This simpler method uses the DLP and a dose conversion coefficient (k) determined for different anatomical regions. The conversion coefficients are provided in Table 6.7, which lists values for various age groups and body regions based on 16-cm and 32-cm diameter phantoms. The effective dose (E) can be calculated using the formula:

$$E \approx k \times \text{DLP}$$

Table 6.7 Conversion factors for effective dose calculation (ICRP 103)

Region of the body	16-cm diameter phantom	32-cm diameter phantom	References
Head	0.0024	0.0049	[102]
Neck	0.0053	0.0107	[102]
Head and neck	0.0045	0.0090	[102]
Chest	0.0102	0.0204	[102]
Abdomen	0.0082	0.0163	[102]
Pelvis	0.0071	0.0143	[102]
Abdomen + pelvis	0.0086	0.0171	[102]
Chest + abdomen + pelvis (trunk)	0.0093	0.0186	[102]
Whole body (head + torso)	0.0077	0.0154	[102]
Lower extremities (male)	–	0.0060	[103]
Lower extremities (female)	–	0.0073	[103]

Table originally published in Pankaj Tandon, Dibya Prakash et al. [104]. Republished with permission

where E is the effective dose in mSv, DLP has units of mGy.cm, and k has units of mSv/(mGy.cm).

Conversion Coefficients for Effective Dose Calculation

To estimate the effective dose from CT scans, conversion coefficients are used based on the Dose-Length Product (DLP). The coefficients vary by age and the region of the body being scanned. The tables below summarizc thcsc coefficients.

- **Conversion Factors**: The values listed under each phantom size represent the conversion factors used to calculate the effective dose from the Dose-Length Product (DLP) for specific body regions.
- **16-cm Diameter Phantom**: Typically used for head scans.
- **32-cm Diameter Phantom**: Typically used for body scans.

6.14.4 Software and Tools for Effective Dose Calculation

Effective dose estimation, which incorporates organ dose estimates and tissue weighting factors, is based on Monte Carlo data sets from the National Radiological Protection Board (NRPB), UK. This process is facilitated by the ImPACT Excel spreadsheet and other specialized software. The ImPACT spreadsheet, available for download from the impactscan.org website, calculates effective doses in accordance with ICRP 103 and ICRP 60 guidelines. Additionally, code data sets can be requested for free from the UK government via email at medicalradiationdoses@phe.gov.uk.

The NRPB data sets comprise 23 series of Monte Carlo calculations that simulate exposure conditions for various CT scanner models. Each data file includes 208 sets of normalized dose data for 27 organs of a mathematical phantom, segmented into 5 mm thick transverse slabs. This extensive data allows for precise modeling and effective dose estimation across different CT scanner types and configurations.

ImPACT Excel Spreadsheet

- This tool uses organ dose estimates and tissue weighting factors based on NRPB Monte Carlo data sets.
- Available for download at impactscan.org.
- Contains data for 27 organs and models exposure conditions for various CT scanners.
- Calculates effective doses according to ICRP 103 and ICRP 60.

6.14.5 Calculation of Effective Dose Using Dose Reports

Here is an example which show the process of calculating the effective dose from a patient dose report obtained from a PET-CT scanner using the DLP (Dose-Length Product) method. We will use the conversion coefficients from Table 6.7 (based on ICRP 103) for the corresponding anatomic regions and assume SSDE (Size-Specific Dose Estimate) factor as 1 (Fig. 6.40).

1. **Calculate the Effective Dose from HRCT Thorax**:
   - DLP (Dose-Length Product) for HRCT Thorax: 248.24 mGy-cm
   - Conversion Coefficient: 0.0204 mSv/(mGy-cm)
   - Effective Dose: 248.24 × 0.0204 = 5.06 mSv
2. **Calculate the Effective Dose from Whole-Body CT**:
   - DLP (Dose-Length Product): 879.08 mGy-cm
   - Conversion Coefficient: 0.0154 mSv/(mGy-cm)

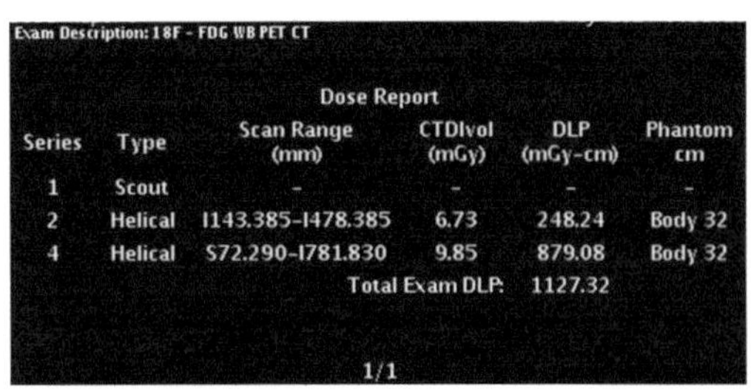

Exam Description: 18F - FDG WB PET CT

Dose Report

Series	Type	Scan Range (mm)	CTDIvol (mGy)	DLP (mGy-cm)	Phantom cm
1	Scout	-	-	-	-
2	Helical	I143.385-I478.385	6.73	248.24	Body 32
4	Helical	S72.290-I781.830	9.85	879.08	Body 32
			Total Exam DLP:	1127.32	

1/1

Fig. 6.40 CT dose report for whole-body CT exam as part of 18F-FDG Whole-body exam, showing CT dose parameters including $CTDI_{vol}$, DLP, and the phantom size

- Effective Dose: 879.08 × 0.0154 = 13.54 mSv

3. **Calculate the Total Effective Dose**:
   - Sum of Effective Doses: 5.06 mSv (HRCT Thorax) + 13.54 mSv (Whole-Body CT) = 18.6 mSv

6.14.6 Factors Influencing CT Doses

1. **Tube Current (mA) and Scan Rotation Time:** CT doses are directly proportional to the milliampere (mA) and the scan rotation time. An increase in either parameter results in a higher radiation dose.
2. **Tube Voltage (kV):** Increasing the tube voltage significantly increases the dose. The relationship between $CTDI_{vol}$ and the tube voltage is expressed as:

$$CTDI_{vol} \alpha \left(kV\right)^{2.6}$$

   For example, increasing the kVp from 80 to 140 kVp results in approximately a five-fold increase in $CTDI_{vol}$. This exponential relationship highlights the sensitivity of the dose to changes in tube voltage.
3. **Tube Current Modulation:** Modern CT scanners often include software-assisted tube current modulation, which adjusts the tube current around the patient to minimize the dose while maintaining image quality. This modulation helps reduce the overall radiation dose without compromising diagnostic effectiveness.
4. **Pitch:** The pitch, defined as the ratio of the table movement per gantry rotation to the beam width, inversely affects the dose. A lower pitch results in a higher dose, whereas a higher pitch reduces the dose. Specifically:
   - A pitch of 0.5 doubles the dose.
   - A pitch of 2 halves the dose.
5. **Dose Distribution:** The dose profile along the patient's axis is not uniform. Surface doses tend to be higher than central doses. The ratio of surface to central doses varies:
   - In head scans, the ratio is approximately 1:1.
   - In body scans, the ratio is approximately 2:1.
6. **Slice Thickness and Number of Slices:** The patient dose is directly proportional to the product of the acquired slice thickness and the total number of slices. Thus, thicker slices and more slices lead to higher doses.
7. **Multiphase Studies:** Multiphase studies, which involve multiple scans of the same region, significantly increase the patient dose. In some cases, the dose can be up to four times higher than a single-phase study.

Box 6.4

CTDI provides a broader measure of the radiation dose output from a CT scanner for a single rotation, integrating the dose profile along the entire *z*-axis.

$CTDI_{100}$ focuses on a specific 100 mm length of the scan, offering a more practical and standardized measure for routine clinical assessments, particularly in standard dosimetry phantoms.

$CTDI_w$ provides an average dose measure by combining central and peripheral dose values within a dosimetry phantom, offering a more comprehensive representation of dose distribution.

$CTDI_{vol}$ adjusts the weighted dose index for helical or spiral scans by considering the pitch, thus accounting for non-contiguous scanning.

DLP integrates the $CTDI_{vol}$ over the scan length, representing the total radiation dose incident on the patient, useful for assessing overall radiation exposure and associated risks.

SSDE Developed by AAPM to provide a more accurate patient dose estimate by incorporating corrections based on patient size. It is calculated by multiplying $CTDI_{vol}$ by a size-specific conversion factor derived from patient dimensions or age. AP and lateral dimensions are measured using electronic calipers. Effective diameter is calculated from these measurements to find the appropriate conversion factor. When

(continued)

Box 6.4 (continued)

patient dimensions are not available, an effective diameter can be estimated based on age, though this method should be used with caution due to potential size variations among patients of the same age.

AAPM Report 31 *Phantoms* includes a 16-cm diameter head phantom and a 32-cm diameter body phantom, both made of PMMA. They are widely used but have limitations with longer scans and wide beam scanners.

ICRU/AAPM Phantom: A newer design made of polyethylene, with a 30 cm diameter and 60 cm length, divisible into three sections for manageability. It is designed to mimic human adipose tissue and is suitable for a wide range of CT scanner designs and conditions, potentially becoming the new standard in CT dosimetry.

6.15 Clinical Applications of CT

Computed tomography is an indispensable diagnostic tool in modern medicine, which offers detailed cross-sectional views of the body and assist in diagnosing a wide array of conditions across various clinical domains. In head and brain imaging, it identifies injuries, strokes, tumors, and neurological disorders. Chest CT imaging evaluates lung diseases, heart conditions, and thoracic structures. Abdominal and pelvic CT imaging aids in diagnosing organ abnormalities, gastrointestinal issues, and reproductive system disorders. Musculoskeletal CT scans provide information on bone fractures, joint diseases, and soft tissue injuries. Cardiac CT angiography evaluates coronary artery disease and other heart conditions. CT guidance is instrumental in invasive procedures, ensuring precise needle placement for biopsies and interventions. Dental and maxillofacial CT imaging assists in dental implant planning and diagnosing oral pathologies. Gastrointestinal CT imaging visualizes the GI tract for various digestive conditions, while urological CT scans assess the urinary system. Similarly, orthopedic imaging evaluates complex fractures, joint conditions, and sports injuries, making CT imaging an indispensable asset in comprehensive patient care. A detailed overview of major imaging areas are as follows:

6.15.1 Head and Brain CT Imaging

CT imaging rapidly assesses head injuries, including fractures, hemorrhages, and brain contusions. It helps in diagnosing strokes, tumors, vascular anomalies, infections, and inflammatory conditions within the brain. Additionally, CT scans are highly effective in identifying skull and facial bone fractures, evaluating sinus and ear conditions, and investigating various neurological disorders. These scans provide detailed images that assist surgeons in planning brain surgeries and determining the safest approach. Post-treatment, CT scans monitor brain changes, assess the effectiveness of interventions, and detect any recurrence of conditions. It is crucial in diagnosing acute neurological dysfunctions, often presenting as paralysis or transient ischemic attacks (TIA), caused by factors such as cerebral infarction, spontaneous brain hemorrhage, infections, or tumors. Hemorrhages in the brain can result from vascular anomalies, such as tumors or arteriovenous malformations (AVMs), or weakened capillary vessel walls due to hypertension. Hemorrhages can also occur in the subarachnoid space or between the brain and its meninges, leading to bloody cerebrospinal fluid or blood accumulation in the epidural and subdural spaces. On CT scans, acutely extravasated blood appears white, with the degree of brainstem compression determining the mass effect and impacting the patient's level of consciousness, often measured using the Glasgow Coma Scale. It is vital to avoid delays in scanning patients with scores below 13 or 14 after head injuries, as these scores can change rapidly in the presence of expanding intracranial hematomas.

6.15.2 Chest CT Imaging

CT chest helps to assess the lungs for conditions such as pneumonia, lung nodules, tumors, and other pulmonary abnormalities. It also visualizes the heart, major blood vessels, esophagus, trachea, bronchi, and other thoracic structures, offering insights into their size, shape, and potential abnormalities. The mediastinum, containing the heart, great vessels, and other structures, is thoroughly evaluated for masses, lymph node enlargement, or other abnormalities. Additionally, CT chest imaging assesses the chest wall, ribs, and bony structures for fractures, tumors, or other issues. Pleural conditions, including effusions or pneumothorax, are also identifiable through CT scans. CT angiography of the chest is particularly useful for visualizing thoracic blood vessels, aiding in diagnosing conditions like aortic aneurysms or dissections. It can reveal signs of infectious diseases affecting the chest, such as abscesses or fungal infections. Prior to chest surgeries, CT scans provide detailed anatomical information for surgical planning. They also assess airways, including the trachea and bronchi, for conditions such as bronchiectasis, bronchial wall thickening, or obstruction. Post-treatment, CT scans monitor chest changes following surgeries, chemotherapy, or radiation therapy.

6.15.3 Abdominal and Pelvic Imaging

Abdominal and pelvic CT imaging reveals insights into the organs, blood vessels, and structures of the abdominal and pelvic regions. It enables the examination of organs such as the liver, spleen, pancreas, kidneys, and adrenal glands, identifying abnormalities like tumors, cysts, or inflammation. The stomach, intestines, and colon are visualized to detect conditions such as bowel obstructions, inflammatory bowel disease, or colorectal cancer. CT scans also identify kidney stones, tumors, infections, and other abnormalities, and evaluate the bladder and ureters for conditions like urinary tract obstruction. In females, the uterus and ovaries, and in males, the reproductive organs, can be examined for tumors or cysts. CT angiography of abdominal and pelvic vessels provides detailed images of blood vessels, aiding in diagnosing aneurysms, stenosis, or thrombosis. The scans can reveal enlarged or abnormal lymph nodes, helping diagnose various diseases, including cancer. Abnormalities in the abdominal wall, muscles, and soft tissues, such as hernias or tumors, are also detectable. CT imaging also diagnoses appendicitis by assessing the appendix's size and inflammation. The liver and biliary system are examined for conditions like cirrhosis, gallstones, or bile duct obstruction. After abdominal or pelvic surgeries, CT scans help monitor postoperative changes.

6.15.4 Musculoskeletal Imaging

Musculoskeletal CT excels in detecting and characterizing bone fractures, offering detailed images for assessing fracture location, extent, and alignment. CT scans evaluate joints, such as the hip, knee, shoulder, and wrist, for arthritis, ligament injuries, or dislocations. They identify bone tumors and soft tissue masses within the musculoskeletal system. Orthopedic surgeons rely heavily on CT for surgical planning, especially for complex fractures or joint reconstructions. It also offers detailed soft tissue images, including muscles, tendons, and ligaments, aiding in assessing soft tissue injuries or abnormalities. CT scans detect calcifications in joints or soft tissues, aiding in diagnosing arthropathies. They are vital in trauma cases for assessing injuries from accidents or falls, providing decision-making information for treatment planning. Athletes undergo musculoskeletal CT to evaluate sports-related injuries, such as stress fractures, ligament tears, or muscle injuries. Additionally, CT assesses the position and condition of joint prosthetics or orthopedic implants, determining their effectiveness and identifying issues.

6.15.5 Cardiac Imaging

Cardiac CT angiography (CTA) helps to identify blockages, stenosis, or plaques in the coronary arteries, determining the severity and extent of arterial blockages. Cardiac CTA also detects coronary anomalies, enhancing understanding of cardiac health. It provides detailed images of cardiac anatomy, including chambers, valves, and surrounding structures, aiding preoperative planning for cardiac surgeries and interventions. Cardiac CTA evaluates diseases of the aorta, such as aneurysms, dissections, or vascular abnormalities, extending its utility beyond coronary arteries. It assesses cardiac function and wall motion, enhancing diagnostic capabilities. In clinical practice, cardiac CTA is crucial for ruling out or confirming coronary artery disease in chest pain cases, aiding in diagnosing and managing cardiac masses or tumors. Post-interventional assessments, like stent placement or bypass surgery, use cardiac CTA to evaluate procedural success and detect complications, ensuring optimal patient outcomes.

6.15.6 Guided Biopsies for Tissue Characterization in Oncological Treatment Planning

CT-guided biopsies and interventions help oncological treatment planning by utilizing CT imaging for real-time guidance during needle insertion and other procedures. This technique is crucial for accurately locating and visualizing lesions, tumors, or abnormalities, facilitating precise sampling or treatment. Biopsies involve inserting a needle to obtain tissue samples, which are essential for diagnosing and characterizing tumors. Additionally, CT guidance supports tumor ablation procedures, such as radiofrequency ablation (RFA) or cryoablation, which employ extreme temperatures to shrink or destroy tumors. For abscesses or fluid collections, CT guidance is used to place drainage catheters or perform aspirations, thereby alleviating symptoms. This guidance is also vital for pain management interventions, including nerve blocks or joint injections. Furthermore, CT guidance is indispensable for spinal procedures, including biopsies, facet joint injections, and epidural injections, as well as for lung procedures like lung biopsies or abscess drainage. Similarly, liver procedures such as biopsies, tumor ablations, or abscess drainage are effectively guided by CT. It also aids in renal procedures, such as biopsies or cyst drainage, ensuring precise needle placement while avoiding critical structures. This meticulous approach enhances the accuracy and efficacy of oncological treatments, contributing significantly to patient care.

6.15.7 Dental and Maxillofacial Imaging

Dental and maxillofacial CT imaging, or cone-beam computed tomography (CBCT), captures three-dimensional images of teeth, jaws, and surrounding structures. It assists in planning dental implant placement by providing details on bone density, volume, and adjacent structures. It diagnoses dental and maxillofacial pathologies, such as impacted teeth, cysts, tumors, and infections. CBCT is invaluable in orthodontic treatment planning, offering detailed views of teeth, jaw bones, and soft tissues. It evaluates the temporomandibular joint, aiding in diagnosing TMJ disorders, and captures images of the paranasal sinuses for sinus pathology evaluation or sinus lifts in dental implants. It assesses fractures and dislocations in facial trauma, aiding treatment planning, and evaluates the upper airway for dimensions and obstructions. In endodontics, CBCT assesses root canal anatomy and complex configurations. It is essential for preoperative planning in oral and maxillofacial surgeries, including wisdom tooth extractions, jaw surgeries, and reconstructions, ensuring detailed preoperative information.

6.15.8 Gastrointestinal Imaging

Gastrointestinal CT imaging visualizes the gastrointestinal (GI) tract, including the esophagus, stomach, small intestine, large intestine, and associated organs, aiding in diagnosing abdominal pain, bowel obstructions, inflammatory bowel diseases, tumors, Crohn's disease, and postoperative changes. It identifies conditions like liver cirrhosis, hepatic lesions, pancreatic tumors, and locates sources of gastrointestinal bleeding. CT colonography offers a non-invasive alternative to traditional colonoscopy for colorectal cancer screening.

6.15.9 Urological Imaging

Urological CT imaging visualizes the urinary tract and reproductive organs, providing detailed images of the kidneys, ureters, bladder, and surrounding structures. It diagnoses kidney stones, urinary tract obstructions, renal masses, tumors, and infections. CT scans investigate urological trauma, identify hematuria sources, characterize renal cysts, detect ureteral strictures, and evaluate bladder conditions. While not primarily used for prostate assessment, CT is employed for prostate cancer evaluation and aids in preoperative planning for urological surgeries.

6.16 CT Room Design and Layout

Designing a CT room involves a multifaceted approach that prioritizes safety, functionality, patient comfort, and regulatory compliance. By addressing these considerations, healthcare facilities can create CT rooms that provide a safe, efficient, and comfortable environment for both patients and healthcare providers, ultimately enhancing the quality of care and operational efficiency. The following key considerations should be taken into account:

6.16.1 Room Size and Dimensions

The room size and dimensions are critical for accommodating the CT scanner, associated equipment, and ensuring the comfort and safety of patients and healthcare providers. Typically, a CT room should be at least 500–600 square feet to provide sufficient space for the CT scanner and patient table, while also allowing for the movement of staff and equipment. The ceiling height should be a minimum of 9 feet to ensure enough space for the CT gantry, ventilation, and proper lighting. Adequate space is necessary to ensure that all components of the CT system are easily accessible for operation and maintenance, and to provide a comfortable environment for patients during scanning procedures (Fig. 6.41).

6.16.2 Room Layout

The layout of the CT room should be designed for maximum efficiency and safety. The CT scanner should be centrally positioned to allow easy access from all sides, minimizing the need for patient repositioning and facilitating the smooth transfer of patients onto the scanner table. Adjacent to the CT room, a shielded control room with large windows should be provided for radiologists and technologists to operate the CT scanner and monitor patients. This control room should offer a clear view of the CT scanner to ensure proper patient oversight. A patient preparation area, including changing rooms and waiting areas, should be conveniently located near the CT room to ensure patient privacy and comfort. Additionally, ample storage space for consumables, contrast media, and emergency equipment should be provided to keep the room organized and functional.

6.16.3 Radiation Shielding

Radiation protection is a paramount consideration in CT room design. All walls, doors, and windows should be lined with lead or other appropriate shielding materials to protect staff and patients from radiation exposure. The thickness of the shielding will depend on the CT scanner's specifications and the frequency of its use. The control room, where operators spend a significant amount of time, must have adequate shielding to protect against scatter radiation. This includes using leaded glass windows to maintain visibility while ensuring radiation protection. Proper radiation shielding ensures compliance with safety standards and protects the health of both patients and staff.

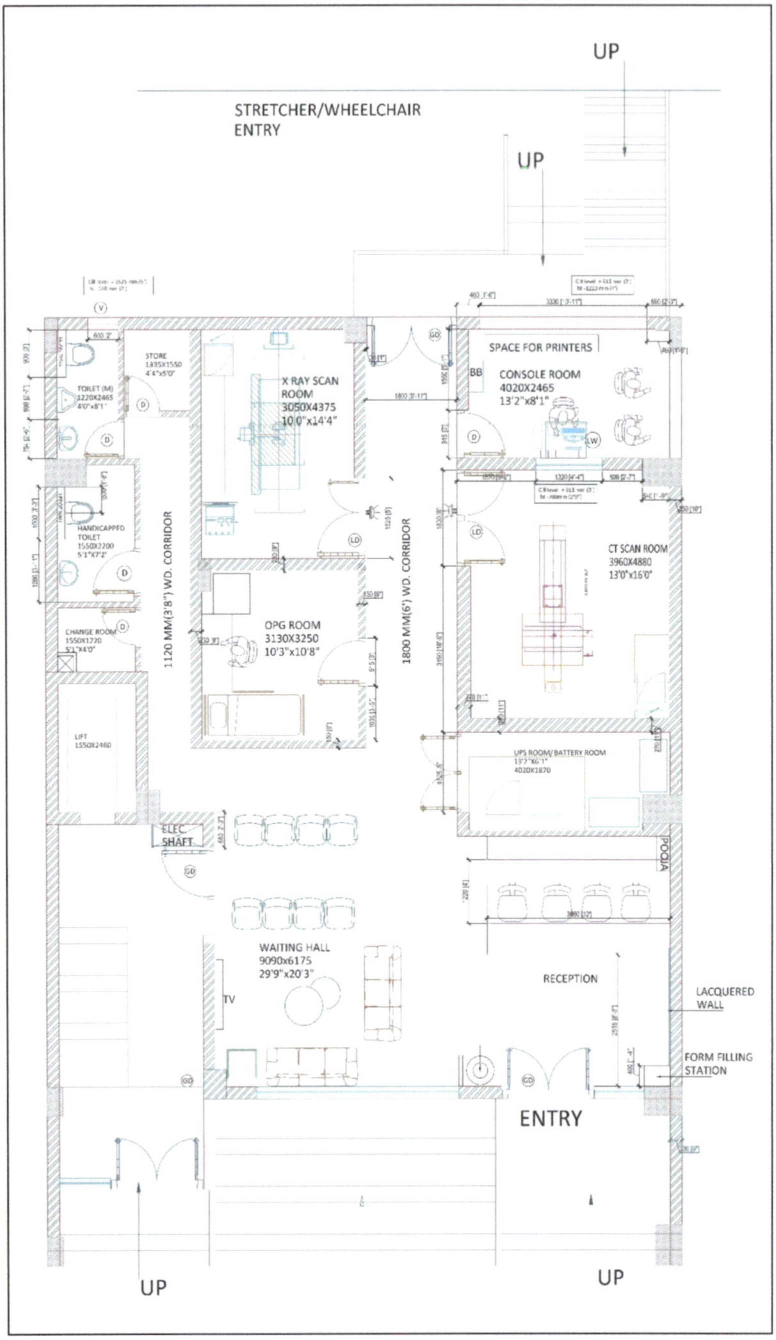

Fig. 6.41 Typical layout of radiology department including CT

6.16.4 Electrical and Mechanical Considerations

The CT scanner requires a stable and reliable power supply, necessitating dedicated electrical circuits and backup power systems, such as uninterruptible power supplies (UPS), to prevent interruptions during scanning. The room must also be equipped with an efficient heating, ventilation, and air conditioning (HVAC) system to maintain a stable temperature and humidity level, as CT scanners generate significant heat during operation. Adequate cooling is essential to ensure the equipment operates within optimal temperature ranges. Proper cable management is also crucial, with cables being routed and organized to prevent tripping hazards and interference, thereby maintaining a safe and efficient workspace.

6.16.5 Safety and Accessibility

Safety and accessibility are vital components of CT room design. Emergency power-off switches should be strategically placed and easily accessible in case of an emergency. Clear signage and protocols for emergencies, such as fires or equipment failures, must be prominently displayed. The design should comply with standards to ensure accessibility for patients with disabilities, which includes wide doorways, ramps, and accessible restrooms. Ensuring that all patients can comfortably and safely access the CT room is essential for providing equitable healthcare services.

6.16.6 Patient Comfort and Experience

Enhancing patient comfort and experience plays an important role in patient care. The interior design should feature calming colors, adequate lighting, and soundproofing to reduce patient anxiety. Soft, adjustable lighting can create a more relaxing environment, while comfortable furniture in the waiting area can improve the overall patient experience. Noise control measures, such as soundproofing, help minimize the operational noise of the CT scanner, further enhancing patient comfort. Privacy considerations, such as separate changing areas and privacy screens, ensure that patients feel secure and respected during their visit.

6.16.7 Workflow Efficiency

The CT room layout should facilitate efficient workflow to optimize the productivity of the healthcare team. Ergonomic design principles should be applied to minimize the distance staff need to travel between the CT scanner, control room, and patient preparation areas. Streamlined workflow processes help reduce the time required for each scan, increase the number of patients that can be seen, and improve the overall efficiency of the department. Integration of digital systems, such as Picture Archiving and Communication System (PACS) and Hospital Information System (HIS), enables seamless data transfer and image storage, enhancing workflow and reducing administrative burdens.

6.16.8 Regulatory Compliance

Compliance with local, state, and regulatory bodies is mandatory in the design of a CT room and ensure adherence to guidelines set forth by them. Ensuring that the design meets all safety and operational standards is essential to avoid legal issues and ensure the health and safety of patients and staff. Regular inspections and certifications are necessary to maintain compliance and ensure that the CT room operates within the required safety parameters. These measures ensure that the facility meets the highest standards of safety and performance.

6.16.9 Environmental Considerations

Incorporating environmental considerations into the CT room design promotes sustainability and reduces the environmental impact of the facility. Using environmentally friendly materials and energy-efficient systems can significantly reduce energy consumption and environmental footprint. Proper waste management systems must be in place for the disposal of medical and radiological waste, ensuring hygiene and safety. Sustainable design practices not only benefit the environment but can also reduce operational costs and enhance the reputation of the healthcare facility as an environmentally conscious institution.

6.17 Safety Aspects in CT

Ensuring safety in CT imaging involves optimizing radiation dose, maintaining equipment, conducting quality assurance, and adhering to regulatory standards. Key areas include:

6.17.1 Dose Reduction Techniques

- **Protocol Optimization:** Customize imaging protocols based on the patient's size and clinical needs. Adjust scan parameters such as tube current (mA) and tube voltage (kVp) to balance dose and image quality. Use the largest practical collimation to enhance dose efficiency; for example, 4 × 5 mm collimation can be more dose-efficient compared to 2 × 5 mm.
- **Technical Adjustments:** For pediatric scans, reduce mA and kVp settings to decrease radiation. Limit scan length to cover only the region of interest and adjust the Field of View (SFOV) to avoid unnecessary radiation to surrounding tissues.
- **Advanced Techniques:** Utilize iterative reconstruction methods to reduce image noise and allow for lower doses without compromising diagnostic quality. Implement automatic dose modulation to dynamically adjust radiation based on the patient's size and the scan area.

6.17.2 Pediatric-Specific Considerations

- **Size-Based Adjustments:** Adapt protocols specifically for pediatric patients, taking size into account rather than age alone. Use appropriate phantoms to simulate different sizes and ensure precise dose measurement.
- **Communication:** Clearly explain the imaging procedure to parents and guardians to reduce anxiety and improve cooperation. Ensure proper positioning and immobilization of the patient to minimize motion artifacts and reduce the need for repeat scans.
- **Training and Education:** Provide specialized training for radiologic technologists on pediatric imaging and dose reduction techniques. Offer ongoing education to keep staff informed about the latest best practices and guidelines for pediatric CT imaging.

6.17.3 Regulatory and Best Practice Guidelines

- **ACR Guidelines:** Follow guidelines for image thickness and protocol specifications. For standard scans, the reconstructed image thickness should be ≤5 mm. Consult manufacturer manuals and AAPM guidelines for detailed protocol recommendations for various clinical scenarios.
- **Image Gently Principles:** Design imaging protocols to minimize radiation while maintaining diagnostic quality. For example, use high-resolution reconstruction kernels for chest scans and thin axial images for high-resolution chest protocols. Monitor $CTDI_{vol}$ values to ensure they meet ACR pass/fail levels and develop dose thresholds for new protocols.

6.17.4 Quality Assurance and Monitoring

- **Regular QA Procedures:** Perform routine quality assurance checks on CT equipment to ensure compliance with safety standards and dose reduction protocols. Implement systems to monitor and track patient doses, comparing them with reference and pass/fail values.
- **Data Collection and Review:** Regularly audit imaging practices and review dose reports to ensure adherence to safety guidelines. Identify areas for improvement and implement necessary changes.
- **Incident Reporting:** Establish protocols for reporting and investigating deviations or incidents. Ensure corrective actions are taken promptly to address any issues.

By following these comprehensive practices, healthcare providers can achieve safe and effective CT imaging, minimizing radiation exposure while ensuring high diagnostic quality.

Exercise

Multiple-Choice Questions

1. What does CT stand for in the context of medical imaging?
   A. Computerized Tomography
   B. Computed Axial Tomography
   C. Computer-Assisted Tomography
   D. Computed Tomography
2. Which algorithm is used for edge detection in CT image processing?
   A. K-means Clustering
   B. Sobel
   C. Region-Growing
   D. Fourier Transform
3. What is the primary material used in the construction of CT dosimetric phantoms mentioned in the text?
   A. Polycarbonate
   B. Polyethylene
   C. Polymethyl methacrylate (PMMA)
   D. Polyvinyl chloride
4. Which technology allows CT scanners to capture multiple slices simultaneously?
   A. Dual-Energy CT
   B. Cone-Beam CT
   C. Multi-slice CT (MDCT)
   D. Photon Counting CT
5. Who were awarded the Nobel Prize in Physiology or Medicine in 1979 for their work on CT imaging?
   A. Godfrey Hounsfield and James Ambrose
   B. Allan Cormack and James Ambrose
   C. Allan Cormack and Godfrey Hounsfield
   D. Godfrey Hounsfield and Rayleigh Hounsfield
6. Which of the following describes the mechanism used by first-generation CT scanners?
   A. Fan-beam X-ray with stationary detectors
   B. Translate-and-rotate with multiple detectors
   C. Translate-and-rotate with a single X-ray tube and detector
   D. Rotational X-ray with multiple detector rows
7. When were second-generation CT scanners introduced, and what was their primary improvement over the first generation?
   A. 1971, with increased detector sensitivity
   B. 1974, with increased number of detectors and faster acquisition time
   C. 1976, with reduced patient exposure time
   D. 1981, with improved image resolution
8. What was a significant limitation of third-generation CT scanners?
   A. Lack of rotational motion capability
   B. High image artifacts due to detector misalignment
   C. Restricted scan speed due to gantry acceleration and deceleration
   D. Poor spatial resolution and image quality
9. Which generation of CT scanners introduced slip-ring technology?
   A. First Generation
   B. Second Generation
   C. Third Generation
   D. Fourth Generation
10. What was a key advancement provided by the fourth generation of CT scanners?
   A. No moving parts and high-speed scanning
   B. Enclosed stationary detector ring with rotating X-ray tube
   C. Improved image quality through reduced scan time
   D. Enhanced image reconstruction algorithms
11. In which generation did Electron Beam CT (EBCT) scanners become prominent, and what was their key feature?
   A. Second Generation, with faster data acquisition
   B. Third Generation, with slip-ring technology
   C. Fourth Generation, with high-speed scanning and no moving parts
   D. Fifth Generation, with improved spatial resolution

12. What does the “pitch” value in helical CT scanning determine?
    A. The thickness of each slice being imaged
    B. The distance the table moves during one 360° gantry rotation relative to the slice thickness
    C. The speed of data acquisition and processing
    D. The number of slices acquired per rotation
13. Which of the following is NOT a primary advantage of CT over conventional radiography?
    A. Detailed Cross-Sectional Imaging
    B. Superior Contrast Resolution
    C. Limited Depth Information
    D. Reduced Artefacts
14. What does the window width (WW) in CT imaging determine?
    A. The amount of X-ray exposure
    B. The range of CT numbers displayed as shades of gray
    C. The thickness of the CT slices
    D. The speed of the CT scan
15. In CT imaging, what is the primary use of Hounsfield Units (HU)?
    A. To measure the speed of the CT scanner
    B. To calculate the thickness of the body slices
    C. To differentiate between tissues based on radiodensity
    D. To adjust the window level
16. Which of the following is true about the Beer-Lambert Law in the context of CT imaging?
    A. It describes how X-rays are produced in the CT scanner.
    B. It is used to calculate the contrast resolution of CT images.
    C. It relates to the attenuation of X-rays as they pass through materials.
    D. It measures the time required for a CT scan.
17. How does window level (WL) affect CT imaging?
    A. It changes the width of the grayscale spectrum displayed.
    B. It sets the midpoint of the CT number range displayed on the image.
    C. It adjusts the speed of the image acquisition.
    D. It alters the thickness of the CT slices.
18. What is the primary purpose of the pre-patient collimator in a CT scanner?
    A. To shape and narrow the X-ray beam before it reaches the patient
    B. To filter out low-energy X-rays after they have passed through the patient
    C. To capture X-ray photons and convert them into electrical signals
    D. To regulate the voltage supplied to the X-ray tube
19. Which component within the CT gantry is responsible for converting X-ray photons into electrical signals?
    A. High-voltage generator
    B. Data Acquisition System (DAS)
    C. Detectors
    D. Laser positioning system
20. What is the role of the slip rings in a CT scanner?
    A. To transmit power and data signals while allowing continuous gantry rotation
    B. To regulate the temperature of the X-ray tube
    C. To focus the X-ray beam onto the patient
    D. To amplify electrical signals from the detectors
21. What is a key feature of photon-counting detectors compared to conventional CT detectors?
    A. They operate in pulse mode and preserve energy and temporal information of each photon
    B. They use scintillation materials to capture X-ray photons
    C. They require high-voltage generators for operation
    D. They rely on analog-to-digital converters for data processing
22. Which type of filter in a CT scanner is designed to address beam hardening?
    A. Bow tie filter
    B. Spectral filter
    C. Pre-patient collimator
    D. Post-patient collimator

23. What is the main function of the high-voltage generator in a CT system?
    A. To convert standard electrical power into high voltages required for X-ray production
    B. To amplify the electrical signals from the detectors
    C. To regulate the temperature of the CT gantry
    D. To shape and refine the X-ray beam before it reaches the patient
24. Which component of the CT scanner's gantry helps in reducing scatter radiation and improving image quality?
    A. Data Acquisition System (DAS)
    B. Pre-patient collimator
    C. Heat exchanger unit
    D. Laser positioning system
25. How does the heat exchanger unit contribute to the performance of a CT scanner?
    A. By regulating the temperature of the CT gantry's internal components
    B. By capturing X-ray photons and converting them into electrical signals
    C. By allowing continuous rotation of the gantry
    D. By shaping and refining the X-ray beam
26. What is the primary function of the computer system in a CT machine?
    A. X-ray emission
    B. Data preprocessing
    C. Image reconstruction
    D. Detector calibration
27. Which of the following algorithms is used in the CT image reconstruction process?
    A. Principal Component Analysis (PCA)
    B. Filtered Back Projection (FBP)
    C. Fast Fourier Transform (FFT)
    D. Singular Value Decomposition (SVD)
28. What does beam hardening correction address in CT imaging?
    A. Variations in detector sensitivity
    B. Electronic noise in detectors
    C. Artifacts caused by the differential absorption of X-ray photons
    D. Motion artifacts due to patient movement
29. What is the purpose of normalization in CT data preprocessing?
    A. To convert raw data into attenuation coefficients
    B. To correct for variations in detector sensitivity and X-ray source intensity
    C. To adjust for patient movement during the scan
    D. To filter out high-frequency noise
30. In the context of CT imaging, what does the Radon Transform facilitate?
    A. Conversion of spatial data into projections
    B. Correction of scatter radiation
    C. Enhancement of image quality through noise reduction
    D. Calibration of detector sensitivity
31. Which of the following best describes the primary advantage of deep learning reconstruction (DLR) over traditional methods like filtered back projection (FBP) and iterative reconstruction (IR)?
    A. Faster processing times
    B. Reduced patient exposure to radiation
    C. Enhanced image quality and artifact reduction
    D. Lower cost of implementation
32. In convolutional neural networks (CNNs) used for image reconstruction, what is the primary function of the convolutional layers?
    A. To adjust weights and biases
    B. To detect edges, textures, and complex patterns
    C. To handle forward and backward propagation
    D. To preprocess the sinogram data
33. Which phase of deep learning model development focuses on assessing the model's performance on an independent dataset to determine its generalizability?
    A. Training Phase
    B. Validation Phase
    C. Testing Phase
    D. Optimization Phase

34. What is the main benefit of using direct DLR frameworks compared to indirect DLR frameworks?
    A. They incorporate traditional methods like FBP or IR
    B. They can potentially eliminate artifacts associated with traditional methods
    C. They require less training data
    D. They are more computationally efficient
35. What is the primary cause of beam hardening artifacts in CT imaging?
    A. Detector noise
    B. Polychromatic nature of X-ray beams
    C. Patient movement
    D. Inadequate sampling rate
36. Which artifact is characterized by dark streaks or "cupping" effects around dense objects like bone or metal implants?
    A. Partial volume artifact
    B. Ring artifact
    C. Metal artifact
    D. Beam hardening artifact
37. How can partial volume artifacts be mitigated in CT imaging?
    A. Increasing the X-ray dose
    B. Using high-quality detectors
    C. Reducing the detector width
    D. Employing dual-energy CT
38. What method is commonly used to address motion artifacts in CT imaging?
    A. Using pre-filters
    B. Spiral CT data interpolation
    C. Applying metal artifact reduction (MAR) algorithms
    D. Increasing the pitch factor
39. Which of the following organizations provides detailed procedures for assessing CT system performance?
    A. European Commission
    B. National Electrical Manufacturers Association
    C. American Association of Physicists in Medicine
    D. International Atomic Energy Agency
40. What is the primary objective of Acceptance Testing in CT Quality Control?
    A. To verify daily imaging consistency
    B. To assess equipment performance prior to clinical use
    C. To monitor routine QC tests
    D. To review clinical protocols
41. Which test is performed daily to ensure scanner stability?
    A. Wet Laser Printer Quality Control
    B. Artifact Evaluation
    C. Water CT Number and Standard Deviation
    D. Visual Checklist
42. What is the purpose of the Annual Medical Physicist Survey in the CT Quality Assurance program?
    A. To verify daily QC results
    B. To ensure compliance with ACR QC requirements
    C. To assess patient positioning accuracy
    D. To evaluate the quality of printed images
43. What does the Computed Tomography Dose Index (CTDI) primarily measure?
    A. The total radiation dose absorbed by the patient
    B. The radiation output from a CT scanner during a single 360-degree rotation
    C. The intensity of radiation incident on the patient during helical scanning
    D. The cumulative radiation exposure over the length of the scan
44. Which CT dose metric accounts for variations in absorbed doses between the center and periphery of a scanned volume?
    A. $CTDI_{vol}$
    B. Dose-Length Product (DLP)
    C. Weighted Computed Tomography Dose Index ($CTDI_w$)
    D. Size-Specific Dose Estimate (SSDE)
45. How is the Dose-Length Product (DLP) calculated?
    A. $CTDI_w$ multiplied by the pitch
    B. $CTDI_{vol}$multiplied by the scan length
    C. $CTDI_{100}$ divided by the pitch
    D. $CTDI_{vol}$multiplied by the beam width
46. Which of the following factors does NOT influence CT dose?
    A. Tube Current (mA)
    B. Tube Voltage (kV)
    C. Slice Thickness
    D. Patient Age

47. Which of the following conditions is NOT typically assessed using chest CT imaging?
    A. Lung tumors
    B. Bone fractures
    C. Pleural effusions
    D. Mediastinal masses
48. In CT imaging of the head and brain, which of the following is a primary application of the technology?
    A. Evaluating abdominal aortic aneurysms
    B. Diagnosing lung infections
    C. Identifying brain tumors and hemorrhages
    D. Planning dental implants
49. What is the main purpose of CT-guided biopsies in oncological treatment planning?
    A. To assess lung function
    B. To plan orthopedic surgeries
    C. To provide real-time guidance for precise tissue sampling
    D. To evaluate the digestive system
50. Which design consideration is crucial for maintaining a safe CT room environment?
    A. The color of the walls
    B. The thickness of radiation shielding
    C. The layout of the patient waiting area
    D. The type of furniture in the control room

Short Answer Questions

1. What is the significance of contrast agents in CT imaging?
2. What were the early limitations of CT technology before the advancements made by Hounsfield and Cormack?
3. How does the matrix size in CT imaging affect the image resolution?
4. Describe the major technological improvement introduced by the second-generation CT scanners.
5. Explain the role of slip-ring technology in modern CT scanners.
6. What were the advantages of fourth-generation CT scanners over earlier generations?
7. What is the significance of the "pitch" value in spiral CT scanning?
8. What is the principle behind CT imaging that allows it to produce detailed cross-sectional images?
9. What is the significance of Hounsfield Units (HU) in CT imaging?
10. Describe one advantage of using CT over conventional radiography in emergency settings.
11. Describe the function of the Data Acquisition System (DAS) in a CT scanner.
12. Explain the purpose of the laser positioning system in a CT gantry.
13. What are the advantages of using a rotating anode in X-ray tubes used in CT scanners?
14. Explain the role of detector calibration in CT imaging.
15. Describe the process of logarithmic transformation in CT data preprocessing.
16. Explain the role of forward propagation in deep learning-based image reconstruction.
17. Describe the primary difference between indirect and direct DLR frameworks in CT image reconstruction.
18. Explain the primary difference between 2D and 3D CT image artifacts.
19. Describe how ring artifacts occur and mention one method used to correct them.
20. Describe the main goal of Routine Quality Control (QC) in CT imaging.
21. What are the recommended corrective actions if optical densities or artifacts are outside control limits during Wet Laser Printer Quality Control?
22. Define the formula for Weighted Computed Tomography Dose Index (CTDI_w) and explain its components.
23. What is the purpose of the Size-Specific Dose Estimate (SSDE), and how is it calculated?
24. Describe how CT imaging aids in diagnosing neurological disorders in the brain.
25. What are the key considerations for designing a CT room to ensure patient comfort?

Long Answer Question

1. Discuss the historical development of CT technology, highlighting the contributions of key figures and the evolution of the technology.
2. Discuss the evolution of CT technology from first-generation to multi-slice CT scanners. Include key technological advancements, their impacts on imaging speed, resolution, and clinical applications.
3. Analyze the benefits and limitations of wide cone beam CT compared to traditional multi-slice CT scanners. Address issues related to image quality, scan speed, and technical challenges.
4. Explain how CT imaging overcomes the limitations of conventional radiography related to structural superimposition and depth information.
5. Discuss the role of window width (WW) and window level (WL) in optimizing CT images for different anatomical regions. Provide examples of how these settings might be adjusted for specific imaging scenarios.
6. Discuss the role and importance of collimators in CT imaging. Include descriptions of both pre-patient and post-patient collimators, and explain how their integration and control contribute to image quality and patient safety.
7. Explain the advancements in detector technology in CT imaging, focusing on photon-counting detectors and dual-layer detectors. How do these technologies improve image quality and diagnostic capabilities compared to traditional detectors?
8. Discuss the significance of the Radon Transform in CT image reconstruction. Include its mathematical basis and its role in converting spatial image data into a set of projections.
9. Discuss the key principles of deep learning in image reconstruction and how they contribute to improving CT image quality.
10. Discuss the impact of metal artifacts on CT imaging and describe at least two techniques used to mitigate these artifacts.
11. Explain the key components and procedures involved in the annual Quality Control for a CT system. Include details about the types of tests performed, their objectives, and the acceptable performance criteria for each.
12. Discuss the limitations of the traditional PMMA phantoms used in CT dosimetry and explain how the ICRU/AAPM phantom addresses these limitations.

Answers to MCQs

Answers

1. D. Computed Tomography
2. B. Sobel
3. C. Polymethyl methacrylate (PMMA)
4. C. Multislice CT (MDCT)
5. C. Allan Cormack and Godfrey Hounsfield
6. C. Translate-and-rotate with a single X-ray tube and detector
7. B. 1974, with increased number of detectors and faster acquisition time
8. C. Restricted scan speed due to gantry acceleration and deceleration
9. C. Third Generation
10. B. Enclosed stationary detector ring with rotating X-ray tube
11. C. Fourth Generation, with high-speed scanning and no moving parts
12. B. The distance the table moves during one 360° gantry rotation relative to the slice thickness
13. C. Limited Depth Information
14. B. The range of CT numbers displayed as shades of gray
15. C. To differentiate between tissues based on radiodensity
16. C. It relates to the attenuation of X-rays as they pass through materials.
17. B. It sets the midpoint of the CT number range displayed on the image
18. A. To shape and narrow the X-ray beam before it reaches the patient
19. C. Detectors
20. A. To transmit power and data signals while allowing continuous gantry rotation

21. A. They operate in pulse mode and preserve energy and temporal information of each photon
22. A. Bow tie filter
23. A. To convert standard electrical power into high voltages required for X-ray production
24. B. Pre-patient collimator
25. A. By regulating the temperature of the CT gantry's internal components
26. C. Image reconstruction
27. B. Filtered Back Projection (FBP)
28. C. Artifacts caused by the differential absorption of X-ray photons
29. B. To correct for variations in detector sensitivity and X-ray source intensity
30. A. Conversion of spatial data into projections
31. C. Enhanced image quality and artifact reduction
32. B. To detect edges, textures, and complex patterns
33. C. Testing Phase
34. B. They can potentially eliminate artifacts associated with traditional methods
35. B. Polychromatic nature of X-ray beams
36. D. Beam hardening artifact
37. C. Reducing the detector width
38. B. Spiral CT data interpolation
39. C. American Association of Physicists in Medicine
40. B. To assess equipment performance prior to clinical use
41. C. Water CT Number and Standard Deviation
42. B. To ensure compliance with ACR QC requirements
43. B. The radiation output from a CT scanner during a single 360-degree rotation
44. C. Weighted Computed Tomography Dose Index ($CTDI_w$).
45. B. $CTDI_{vol}$ multiplied by the scan length
46. D. Patient Age
47. B. Bone fractures
48. C. Identifying brain tumors and hemorrhages
49. C. To provide real-time guidance for precise tissue sampling
50. B. The thickness of radiation shielding

References

1. Euclid S. Computed tomography: physical principles, clinical applications, and quality control, 2016. [Online]. Available: http://evolve.elsevier.com/Seeram/YOU'VEJUSTPURCHASED
2. Hounsfield GN. Computerized transverse axial scanning (tomography): Part I. Description of system, 1973.
3. Professor Torgny Greitz. The Nobel Prize in Physiology or Medicine 1979 | Allan M. Cormack Godfrey N. Hounsfield | Award ceremony speech. https://www.nobelprize.org/prizes/medicine/1979/ceremony-speech/.
4. Wells PNT. Sir Godfrey Newbold Hounsfield KT CBE. 28 August 1919–12 August 2004, 2005, https://doi.org/10.1098/rsbm.2005.XXXX.
5. Beckmann EC. CT scanning the early days. Br J Radiol. 2006;79(937):5–8. https://doi.org/10.1259/bjr/29444122.
6. Schulz RA, Stein JA, Pelc NJ. How CT happened: the early development of medical computed tomography. J Med Imaging. 2021;8(05) https://doi.org/10.1117/1.JMI.8.5.052110.
7. Hounsfield GN. Computed medical imaging, 1979.
8. McCollough C, Orton C. AAPM virtual museum of Medical Physics on CT, https://museum.aapm.org/exhibit/07-ct/.
9. Goldman LW. Principles of CT and CT technology. J Nucl Med Technol. 2007;35(3):115–28; quiz 129–30. https://doi.org/10.2967/jnmt.107.042978.
10. Cormack AM. Representation of a function by its line integrals, with some radiological applications. J Appl Phys. 1963;34(9):2722–7. https://doi.org/10.1063/1.1729798.
11. Ledley RS, Di Chiro G, Luessenhop AJ, Twigg HL. Computerized transaxial X-ray tomography of the human body. Science (1979). 1974;186(4160):207–12. https://doi.org/10.1126/science.186.4160.207.
12. Simpson RG, Chen CT, Grubbs EA, Swindell W. A 4-MV CT scanner for radiation therapy: the prototype system. Med Phys. 1982;9(4):574–9. https://doi.org/10.1118/1.595102.
13. Napel S, et al. CT angiography with spiral CT and maximum intensity projection. Radiology. 1992;185(2):607–10. https://doi.org/10.1148/radiology.185.2.1410382.
14. Mozzo P, Procacci C, Tacconi A, Tinazzi Martini P, Bergamo Andreis IA. A new volumetric CT machine for dental imaging based on the cone-beam technique: preliminary results. Eur Radiol. 1998;8(9):1558–64. https://doi.org/10.1007/s003300050586.
15. Ltd. Canon Electron Tubes & Devices Co., Company History - Canon.
16. Robert IK, Kim H. Thin rotating plate target for X-ray tube US6560315, US - Patents, 2002.

17. Schardt P, et al. New x-ray tube performance in computed tomography by introducing the rotating envelope tube technology. Med Phys. 2004;31(9):2699–706. https://doi.org/10.1118/1.1783552.
18. Paolo R. Handbook of X-ray imaging. York CRC Press, the Taylor & Francis Group; 2018.
19. Koninklijke Philips NV. Philips introduces IQon Spectral CT system at RSNA 2013, RSNA 2013: imaging innovations from Philips, 2013.
20. Padole A, Khawaja RDA, Kalra MK, Singh S. CT radiation dose and iterative reconstruction techniques. Am J Roentgenol. 2015;204(4):W384–92. https://doi.org/10.2214/AJR.14.13241.
21. Behling R. X-ray sources: 125 years of developments of this intriguing technology. Phys Med. 2020;79:162–87. https://doi.org/10.1016/j.ejmp.2020.07.021.
22. Zhang Z, Seeram E. The use of artificial intelligence in computed tomography image reconstruction - a literature review. Elsevier Inc; 2020. https://doi.org/10.1016/j.jmir.2020.09.001.
23. Dillon WP. 50th anniversary of computed tomography: past and future applications in clinical neuroscience. J Med Imaging. 2021;8(05) https://doi.org/10.1117/1.JMI.8.5.052112.
24. Boyd DP, Gould RG, Quinn JR, Sparks R, Stanley JH, Herrmmannsfeldt WB. A proposed dynamic cardiac 3-D densitometer for early detection and evaluation of heart disease. IEEE Trans Nucl Sci. 1979;26(2):2724–7. https://doi.org/10.1109/TNS.1979.4330523.
25. Casian R, Velasco R. Crest ® + Oral-B ® at dentalcare.com | the trusted resource for dental professionals. [Online]. Available: www.dentalcare.com/en-us/professional-education/ce-courses/ce531
26. Esquivel A, et al. Photon-counting detector CT: key points radiologists should know. Korean J Radiol. 2022;23(9):854. https://doi.org/10.3348/kjr.2022.0377.
27. Yu Z, et al. Noise performance of low-dose CT: comparison between an energy integrating detector and a photon counting detector using a whole-body research photon counting CT scanner. J Med Imaging. 2016;3(4):043503. https://doi.org/10.1117/1.JMI.3.4.043503.
28. Cormode DP, et al. Atherosclerotic plaque composition: analysis with multicolor CT and targeted gold nanoparticles. Radiology. 2010;256(3):774–82. https://doi.org/10.1148/radiol.10092473.
29. Sartoretti T, et al. Photon-counting multienergy computed tomography with spectrally optimized contrast media for Plaque removal and Stenosis assessment. Investig Radiol. 2021;56(9):563–70. https://doi.org/10.1097/RLI.0000000000000773.
30. Muenzel D, et al. Simultaneous dual-contrast multi-phase liver imaging using spectral photon-counting computed tomography: a proof-of-concept study. Eur Radiol Exp. 2017;1(1):25. https://doi.org/10.1186/s41747-017-0030-5.
31. Pourmorteza A, Symons R, Henning A, Ulzheimer S, Bluemke DA. Dose efficiency of quarter-millimeter photon-counting computed tomography. Investig Radiol. 2018;53(6):365–72. https://doi.org/10.1097/RLI.0000000000000463.
32. Leng S, et al. 150-μm spatial resolution using photon-counting detector computed tomography technology. Investig Radiol. 2018;53(11):655–62. https://doi.org/10.1097/RLI.0000000000000488.
33. Rajendran K, et al. Dose reduction for sinus and temporal bone imaging using photon-counting detector CT with an additional tin filter. Investig Radiol. 2020;55(2):91–100. https://doi.org/10.1097/RLI.0000000000000614.
34. Klein L, et al. Effects of detector sampling on noise reduction in clinical photon-counting whole-body computed tomography. Investig Radiol. 2020;55(2):111–9. https://doi.org/10.1097/RLI.0000000000000616.
35. Gutjahr R, et al. Human imaging with photon counting–based computed tomography at clinical dose levels. Investig Radiol. 2016;51(7):421–9. https://doi.org/10.1097/RLI.0000000000000251.
36. Goldman LW. Principles of CT: multislice CT. J Nucl Med Technol. 2008;36(2):57–68. https://doi.org/10.2967/jnmt.107.044826.
37. Tan Z, et al. The primary study of low-dose pancreas perfusion by 640- slice helical CT: a whole-organ perfusion. Springerplus. 2015;4(1):192. https://doi.org/10.1186/s40064-015-0950-6.
38. Commandeur F, Goeller M, Dey D. Cardiac CT: technological advances in hardware, software, and machine learning applications. Curr Cardiovasc Imaging Rep. 2018;11(8):19. https://doi.org/10.1007/s12410-018-9459-z.
39. Hsieh J, Flohr T. Computed tomography recent history and future perspectives. J Med Imaging. 2021;8(05) https://doi.org/10.1117/1.jmi.8.5.052109.
40. Standring S. Gray's anatomy the anatomical basis of clinical practice. 42nd ed. Elsevier; 2021.
41. Flohr T, Schmidt B. Technical basics and clinical benefits of photon-counting CT. Lippincott Williams and Wilkins; 2023. https://doi.org/10.1097/RLI.0000000000000980.
42. Grunz J-P, et al. Spectral shaping via tin Prefiltration in ultra-high-resolution photon-counting and energy-integrating detector CT of the temporal bone. Investig Radiol. 2022;57(12):819–25. https://doi.org/10.1097/RLI.0000000000000901.
43. Woeltjen MM, et al. Low-dose high-resolution photon-counting CT of the lung: radiation dose and image quality in the clinical routine. Diagnostics. 2022;12(6):1441. https://doi.org/10.3390/diagnostics12061441.
44. Zsarnoczay E, et al. Ultra-high resolution photon-counting coronary CT angiography improves coronary stenosis quantification over a wide range of heart rates – A dynamic phantom study. Eur J

Radiol. 2023;161:110746. https://doi.org/10.1016/j.ejrad.2023.110746.
45. Schwartz FR, Samei E, Marin D. Exploiting the potential of photon-counting CT in abdominal imaging. Investig Radiol. 2023;58(7):488–98. https://doi.org/10.1097/RLI.0000000000000949.
46. Bette S, et al. Optimal Conspicuity of liver metastases in virtual monochromatic imaging reconstructions on a novel photon-counting detector CT—effect of keV settings and BMI. Diagnostics. 2022;12(5):1231. https://doi.org/10.3390/diagnostics12051231.
47. Emrich T, et al. Reduced iodinated contrast media administration in coronary CT angiography on a clinical photon-counting detector CT system. Investig Radiol. 2023;58(2):148–55. https://doi.org/10.1097/RLI.0000000000000911.
48. Rajiah PS, et al. High-pitch multienergy coronary CT angiography in dual-source photon-counting detector CT scanner at low iodinated contrast dose. Investig Radiol. 2023;58(9):681–90. https://doi.org/10.1097/RLI.0000000000000961.
49. Wildberger JE, Alkadhi H. New horizons in vascular imaging with photon-counting detector CT. Investig Radiol. 2023;58(7):499–504. https://doi.org/10.1097/RLI.0000000000000957.
50. Emrich T, et al. Coronary computed tomography angiography-based calcium scoring. Investig Radiol. 2022;57(8):536–43. https://doi.org/10.1097/RLI.0000000000000868.
51. Symons R, et al. Low-dose lung cancer screening with photon-counting CT: a feasibility study. Phys Med Biol. 2017;62(1):202–13. https://doi.org/10.1088/1361-6560/62/1/202.
52. Jungblut L, et al. Potential of photon-counting detector CT for radiation dose reduction for the assessment of interstitial lung disease in patients with systemic sclerosis. Investig Radiol. 2022;57(12):773–9. https://doi.org/10.1097/RLI.0000000000000895.
53. Hagen F, et al. Image quality and dose exposure of contrast-enhanced abdominal CT on a 1st generation clinical dual-source photon-counting detector CT in obese patients vs. a 2nd generation dual-source dual energy integrating detector CT. Eur J Radiol. 2022;151:110325. https://doi.org/10.1016/j.ejrad.2022.110325.
54. Tsiflikas I, et al. Low dose pediatric chest computed tomography on a photon counting detector system—initial clinical experience. Pediatr Radiol. 2023;53(6):1057–62. https://doi.org/10.1007/s00247-022-05584-4.
55. Kappler S, et al. In: Pelc NJ, Nishikawa RM, Whiting BR, editors. First results from a hybrid prototype CT scanner for exploring benefits of quantum-counting in clinical CT; 2012. p. 83130X. https://doi.org/10.1117/12.911295.
56. Wrazidlo R, et al. Radiation dose reduction in contrast-enhanced abdominal CT: comparison of photon-counting detector CT with 2nd generation dual-source dual-energy CT in an oncologic cohort. Acad Radiol. 2023;30(5):855–62. https://doi.org/10.1016/j.acra.2022.05.021.
57. Hagen F, et al. Image quality and radiation dose of contrast-enhanced chest-CT acquired on a clinical photon-counting detector CT vs. second-generation dual-source CT in an oncologic cohort: preliminary results. Tomography. 2022;8(3):1466–76. https://doi.org/10.3390/tomography8030119.
58. Van der Bie J, et al. Photon-counting CT: review of initial clinical results. Elsevier Ireland Ltd; 2023. https://doi.org/10.1016/j.ejrad.2023.110829.
59. Jun Choi H, Jung Lee H, Kang SG. The Clinical significance of Hounsfield number of metallic and non-metallic foreign bodies in the soft tissue, 2010.
60. Tang X, Xie H. X-ray computed tomography for diagnostic imaging—from single-slice to multi-slice, ch. 32. In: Paolo R, editor. Handbook of X-ray imaging physics and technology. CRC Press Taylor & Francis Group; 2018.
61. Behling R. Modern diagnostic X-ray sources; technology, manufacturing, reliability. 2nd ed; 2021.
62. Tandon P, Prakash D, Kheruka SC, Bhat NN. Working mechanism of radiation detectors used in nuclear medicine, ch. 15. In: Radiation safety guide for nuclear medicine professionals. Singapore: Springer Nature Singapore; 2022. p. 153–75. https://doi.org/10.1007/978-981-19-4518-2_15.
63. Rassouli N, Etesami M, Dhanantwari A, Rajiah P. Detector-based spectral CT with a novel dual-layer technology: principles and applications. Springer Verlag; 2017. https://doi.org/10.1007/s13244-017-0571-4.
64. Hood A, Branch WL, Sobel M, York N, Terhune EA, Bank R. Slip Ring.
65. Koetzier LR, et al. Deep learning image reconstruction for CT: technical principles and clinical prospects. Radiology. 2023;306(3) https://doi.org/10.1148/radiol.221257.
66. Radon JKA. Über die Bestimmung von Funktionen durch ihre Integralwerte längs gewisser Mannigfaltigkeiten. Berichte der Sachsischen Akadamie der Wissenschaft. 1917;69:262–77.
67. Radon J. On the determination of functions from their integral values along certain manifolds, 1986.
68. Willemink MJ, Noël PB. The evolution of image reconstruction for CT—from filtered back projection to artificial intelligence. Eur Radiol. 2019;29(5):2185–95. https://doi.org/10.1007/s00330-018-5810-7.
69. Gordon R, Bender R, Herman GT. Algebraic Reconstruction Techniques (ART) for three-dimensional electron microscopy and X-ray photography, 1970.
70. Lee SY, Byeon S, Kim HS, Jin H, Lee S. Deep learning-based phase prediction of high-entropy alloys: optimization, generation, and explanation. Mater Des. 2021;197 https://doi.org/10.1016/j.matdes.2020.109260.
71. Kim I, Kang H, Yoon HJ, Chung BM, Shin N-Y. Deep learning–based image reconstruction

for brain CT: improved image quality compared with adaptive statistical iterative reconstruction-Veo (ASIR-V). Neuroradiology. 2021;63(6):905–12. https://doi.org/10.1007/s00234-020-02574-x.
72. Hata A, et al. The image quality of deep-learning image reconstruction of chest CT images on a mediastinal window setting. Clin Radiol. 2021;76(2):155.e15–23. https://doi.org/10.1016/j.crad.2020.10.011.
73. Nam JG, et al. Image quality of ultralow-dose chest CT using deep learning techniques: potential superiority of vendor-agnostic post-processing over vendor-specific techniques. Eur Radiol. 2021;31(7):5139–47. https://doi.org/10.1007/s00330-020-07537-7.
74. Franck C, Zhang G, Deak P, Zanca F. Preserving image texture while reducing radiation dose with a deep learning image reconstruction algorithm in chest CT: a phantom study. Phys Med. 2021;81:86–93. https://doi.org/10.1016/j.ejmp.2020.12.005.
75. Kim JH, Yoon HJ, Lee E, Kim I, Cha YK, Bak SH. Validation of deep-learning image reconstruction for low-dose chest computed tomography scan: emphasis on image quality and noise. Korean J Radiol. 2021;22(1):131. https://doi.org/10.3348/kjr.2020.0116.
76. Yang S, et al. Impact of novel deep learning image reconstruction algorithm on diagnosis of contrast-enhanced liver computed tomography imaging: comparing to adaptive statistical iterative reconstruction algorithm. J Xray Sci Technol. 2021;29(6):1009–18. https://doi.org/10.3233/XST-210953.
77. Jensen CT, et al. Image quality assessment of abdominal CT by use of new deep learning image reconstruction: initial experience. Am J Roentgenol. 2020;215(1):50–7. https://doi.org/10.2214/AJR.19.22332.
78. Brady SL, Trout AT, Somasundaram E, Anton CG, Li Y, Dillman JR. Improving image quality and reducing radiation dose for Pediatric CT by using deep learning reconstruction. Radiology. 2021;298(1):180–8. https://doi.org/10.1148/radiol.2020202317.
79. Sun J, et al. Improving the image quality of pediatric chest CT angiography with low radiation dose and contrast volume using deep learning image reconstruction. Quant Imaging Med Surg. 2021;11(7):3051–8. https://doi.org/10.21037/qims-20-1158.
80. Buzug TM. Computed tomography: from photon statistics to modern cone-beam CT, 2008.
81. Schumacher H, Fischer B. A new approach for motion correction in SPECT imaging. In: Bildverarbeitung für die Medizin. Berlin/Heidelberg: Springer Berlin Heidelberg; 2007. p. 51–5. https://doi.org/10.1007/978-3-540-71091-2_11.
82. Boas FE, Fleischmann D, CT artifacts: causes and reduction techniques, 2012.
83. Samei E, Bakalyar D, Boedeker KL, Brady S, Fan J, Leng S, Myers KJ, Popescu LM, Ramirez Giraldo JC, Ranallo F, Solomon J, Vaishnav J, Wang J. Performance evaluation of computed tomography systems: Summary of AAPM Task Group 233. Med Phys. 2019;46(11):E735–E756. https://doi.org/10.1002/mp.13763.
84. Dillon C, et al. Computed tomography radiologist's section radiologic technologist's section qualified medical physicist's section - Quality Control Manual, 2017.
85. Katie A. Quality Control_ CT (Revised 11-9-2022) _ Accreditation Support, 2022.
86. European Commission. European Commission Radiation Protection Report 162 - criteria for acceptability of medical radiological equipment used in diagnostic radiology, nuclear medicine and radiotherapy, 2012, https://doi.org/10.2768/22561.
87. NEMA. Standard attributes on CT equipment related to dose optimization and management, 2013. [Online]. Available: www.nema.org
88. IAEA. Quality Assurance Programme for computed tomography: diagnostic and therapy applications IAEA HUMAN HEALTH SERIES, 2012. [Online]. Available: http://www.iaea.org/Publications/index.html
89. IEC. INTERNATIONAL STANDARD NORME INTERNATIONALE Evaluation and routine testing in medical imaging departments-Part 3–5: Acceptance and constancy tests-Imaging performance of computed tomography X-ray equipment, 2019.
90. Katada K, et al. Guidance with real-time CT fluoroscopy: early clinical experience. Radiology. 1996;200(3):851–6. https://doi.org/10.1148/radiology.200.3.8756943.
91. ICRU. Radiation dose and image-quality assessment in computed tomography the International Commission on Radiation Units and Measurements downloaded from, 2012. [Online]. Available: http://jicru.oxfordjournals.org/
92. A. Task Group. The design and use of the ICRU/AAPM CT radiation dosimetry phantom: an implementation of AAPM report 111 the report of AAPM Task Group 200, 2020.
93. IAEA. Dosimetry in diagnostic radiology: an international code of practice, technical reports series No. 457, 2007.
94. Shope TB, Gagne RM, Johnson GC. A method for describing the doses delivered by transmission x-ray computed tomography. Med Phys. 1981;8(4):488–95. https://doi.org/10.1118/1.594995.
95. Boone JM, et al. Report 87. J ICRU. 2012;12(1):NP-NP. https://doi.org/10.1093/jicru/ndt006.
96. Task Group 204. AAPM RPT 204: Size-specific Dose Estimate (SSDE) in paediatric and adult CT examination, 2011.
97. Chu RYL, American Institute of Physics., and American Association of Physicists in Medicine. Standardized methods for measuring diagnostic x-ray exposures. American Institute of Physics for the American Association of Physicists in Medicine; 1990.

98. Brisse HJ, et al. Automatic exposure control in multichannel CT with tube current modulation to achieve a constant level of image noise: experimental assessment on pediatric phantoms. Med Phys. 2007;34(7):3018–33. https://doi.org/10.1118/1.2746492.
99. A. Task Group, Comprehensive methodology for the evaluation of radiation dose in X-Ray computed tomography report of AAPM task Group 111: the future of CT dosimetry a new measurement paradigm based on a Unified Theory for axial, helical, fan-beam, and cone-beam scanning with or without longitudinal translation of the patient table, 2010.
100. Clarke RH, et al. Annals of the ICRP published on behalf of the international commission on radiological protection members of the main commission of the ICRP, 1991.
101. Icrp 103. Annals of the ICRP Published on behalf of the International Commission on Radiological Protection, 2007.
102. Huda W, Magill D, He W. CT effective dose per dose length product using ICRP 103 weighting fac tors. Med Phys. 2011;38(3):1261–5. https://doi.org/10.1118/1.3544350.
103. Saltybaeva N, Jafari ME, Hupfer M, Kalender WA. Estimates of effective dose for CT scans of the lower extremities. Radiology. 2014;273(1):153–9. https://doi.org/10.1148/radiol.14132903.
104. Tandon P, Prakash D, Kheruka SC, Bhat NN. Computed tomography dose assessment. In: Radiation safety guide for nuclear medicine professionals. Singapore: Springer Nature Singapore; 2022. p. 299–315. https://doi.org/10.1007/978-981-19-4518-2_20.

7 Hybrid Imaging: Physics, Principle of Operation, and Quality Control

Learning Objectives

Introduction to hybrid imaging
The need for hybrid imaging
Advantages of hybrid imaging
Radiation detectors and their properties and mechanism of detection used in SPECT, PET, and CT
Positron emission tomography (PET) and how it works
- Historical developments of positron emission tomography (PET) and PET-CT
- Development of positron-emitting radiopharmaceuticals
- Coincidence detection and construction of first PET scanner
- The positron physics
- Working of PET
- PET-CT data acquisition
- PET-CT instrumentation
- Detector, detector block, sizes, and shape
- 2D versus 3D PET
- Axial-paired (3D) detector ring
- Time-of-flight (TOF) detection
- Total body PET scanners with whole-body coverage

Performance characteristics and quality control in PET-CT
- Spatial resolution
- Sensitivity
- Scatter fraction, count losses, and randoms
- Image quality, accuracy of attenuation, and scatter correction and accuracy of radioactivity quantitation
- Coincidence timing resolution or time-of-flight resolution and energy resolution
- PET-CT co-registration accuracy
- Uniformity check of the reconstructed image test
- Normalization and well counter corrections

The gamma camera, the single photon emission computed tomography (SPECT) and how do they work
- Collimator
- Scintillation crystal and photomultiplier tubes
- Preamplifier and amplifier
- Analogue-to-digital converter (ADC)
- Pulse height analyzer (PHA)
- *X*, *Y* positioning circuit and the energy signals (*Z*)
- Uniformity, linearity, and energy resolution correction
- Image display
- Single photon emission computed tomography (SPECT) imaging

Quality control in gamma camera/SPECT imaging
(A) Intrinsic (collimator removed) gamma camera performance
- (a) Centering of pulse height analyzer (PHA) window
- (b) Intrinsic flood field uniformity
- (c) Intrinsic flood field uniformity through narrowed and asymmetric (off-centered) PHA windows
- (d) Intrinsic spatial resolution and linearity
- (e) Energy resolution
- (f) Multiple window spatial registration
- (g) Intrinsic count rate performance and dead time with and without scatter medium
- (h) Maximum count rate performance in air
- (i) Intrinsic flood field uniformity and spatial resolution at 75 kcps

(B) Extrinsic (with collimator) gamma camera performance
- (a) Extrinsic flood field uniformity
- (b) Extrinsic spatial resolution (FWHM and FWTM) at 0, 10, and 20 cm distance from the detector surface
- (c) System spatial linearity
- (d) System planar sensitivity at 10 cm from the detector surface
- (e) Collimator hole angulation
- (f) Detector head shielding leakage
- (g) Scan speed for the whole-body scan

(C) Tomographic (SPECT) characteristics
- (a) Pixel size (*X* and *Y* direction)
- (b) Integral tomographic uniformity, RMS noise with flood correction, and contrast resolution
- (c) Tomographic resolution in the air (*X* and *Y* direction)
- (d) Multiple head registration (MHR), center of rotation offset, and alignment of axes
- (e) Slice thickness at the center of the field of view
- (f) Variations of sensitivity with angle

(D) Co-registration of SPECT and CT modalities
- Alignment (registration) calibration

Image reconstruction algorithms
- Filtered back projection (FBP)
- Iterative reconstruction
- Newer techniques used for reconstruction of SPECT, PET, and fusion images

Clinical applications of hybrid imaging
- Clinical applications of PET-CT
- Clinical applications of PET-MRI
- Clinical applications of SPECT-CT
- Clinical applications of PET-CT-MRI

D. Prakash, R. P. Kotian, *Fundamentals of X-ray Imaging*,
https://doi.org/10.1007/978-981-96-7328-5_7

7.1 Introduction to the Hybrid Imaging

Hybrid imaging, also known as multimodal imaging or fusion imaging, refers to the combination of two or more imaging modalities to obtain a more comprehensive and detailed assessment of a particular area or condition in the human body. This approach combines the strengths of different imaging techniques, providing complementary information and improving diagnostic accuracy. The most common types of hybrid imaging involve the fusion of anatomical and functional imaging modalities. Here are some examples:

- **PET-CT (positron emission tomography-computed tomography)**
  PET provides functional information by identifying the distribution of a radiotracer injected into the body. It is used to visualize metabolic or other molecular activities, such as the uptake of glucose or specific molecules. The CT component of the scanner uses X-rays to produce high-resolution, detailed anatomical images and provides information about the structure and density of tissues, allowing for precise localization and characterization of abnormalities detected by PET. Combining PET and CT images makes it possible to precisely localize and correlate areas of abnormal metabolic activity with anatomical structures.
- **SPECT-CT (single photon emission computed tomography-computed tomography)**
  SPECT uses radioactive tracers and gamma cameras to create functional images. It is commonly used in nuclear medicine to study organ function. By combining SPECT with CT, anatomical localization and characterization of functional abnormalities can be improved.
- **PET-MRI (positron emission tomography-magnetic resonance imaging)**
  PET-MRI combines the functional information obtained from PET with the excellent soft tissue contrast and anatomical detail of MRI. The MRI component of the scanner utilizes a strong magnetic field and radio waves to generate detailed images of the body's soft tissues, organs, and structures. The MRI can provide detailed information about various tissues' morphology, composition, and function.
- **PET-CT-MRI equipment**
  It is also known as PET-CT-MRI scanners or trimodality scanners and is an advanced imaging system that combines the capabilities of positron emission tomography (PET), computed tomography (CT), and magnetic resonance imaging (MRI) into a single device. These hybrid scanners offer a comprehensive imaging solution by providing functional, anatomical, and detailed soft tissue information in a single examination. By combining PET, CT, and MRI capabilities, these scanners offer several advantages, including comprehensive information, precise localization, and multi-parametric imaging with reduced imaging time.

This hybrid imaging modality is particularly useful in oncology for tumor detection, staging, and monitoring treatment response. The benefits of hybrid imaging include improved sensitivity, specificity, and accuracy compared to individual imaging modalities alone. By integrating the strengths of different techniques, clinicians can better visualize and understand the underlying physiological processes, leading to more precise diagnosis, treatment planning, and patient management.

7.2 The Need for Hybrid Imaging

Each modality of imaging has its own merits and demerits, and therefore none is complete. PET and SPECT are functional imaging modalities that provide information about physiological processes, whereas CT (computed tomography) and MRI (magnetic resonance imaging) primarily provide detailed anatomical information about tissues and structures in the body. Combining both modalities can give an excellent view of physiological and anatomical details. The following are some of the limitations of each modality, which necessitates the need for hybrid imaging.

7.2.1 Limitation of PET Imaging

While positron emission tomography (PET) imaging is a powerful diagnostic tool, it does have certain limitations, such as:

- *Limited Spatial Resolution*: PET scanners have lower spatial resolution than other imaging modalities like computed tomography (CT) or magnetic resonance imaging (MRI). The resolution is typically a few millimeters, which can limit the ability to visualize small structures or detect very small lesions. The spatial resolution of positron emission tomography (PET) scanners can vary depending on several factors, including the specific scanner technology, reconstruction algorithms, and acquisition parameters. However, in general, the typical spatial resolution of PET imaging is in the range of 4–7 millimeters (mm).
- *Limited Availability of Radiotracers*: PET imaging relies on the availability of specific radiotracers that can bind to or interact with certain molecules or receptors in the body and mimic certain pathophysiology of the human body, which can be detected being a radiotracer. The production and availability of radiotracers can be limited, and not all molecular targets or diseases have suitable radiotracers available. Though many radiotracers are under research and in routine use, PET imaging is an important modality in patient care, especially in oncology, neurology, cardiology, and infection imaging.
- *Long Scan Times*: PET imaging requires a certain amount of time for the radiotracer to distribute and accumulate in the body. Also, the acquisition time is longer than other modalities. Thanks to hybrid imaging, where CT is used for attenuation correction; otherwise, in the early days when only PET was used for attenuation correction, the scans were going up to around 30–60 min for a single patient depending upon case to case. However, the advancements in PET technology, such as time-of-flight PET, improved reconstruction techniques, and the use of CT for attenuation correction, have helped to reduce scan times by around 10–20 min.
- *Lack of Anatomical Detail*: PET images provide functional information but lack detailed anatomical information. This can make it challenging to localize abnormalities detected by PET alone precisely. To overcome this limitation, PET is often performed with CT or MRI (PET-CT or PET-MRI) to provide functional and anatomical information.
- *False-Positive and False-Negative Results*: PET imaging can produce false-positive or false-negative results. False-positive results may occur due to uptake of the radiotracer in noncancerous tissues with increased metabolic activity. False-negative results can occur when the disease or abnormality has not significantly increased metabolic activity or the radiotracer is not specific to the target of interest.
- *Radiation Exposure*: PET imaging involves the administration of a radiotracer, which emits positrons. The radioactive material decays and releases positrons that annihilate electrons, producing gamma rays detected by the PET scanner. This exposure to radiation poses a small risk although it is typically considered safe when used appropriately. However, it may concern certain patient populations, such as pregnant women and children.
- *Cost*: PET imaging is generally more expensive than other imaging modalities due to the cost of radiotracers, specialized equipment, and maintenance requirements. The availability of PET scanners may be limited in some regions or healthcare settings due to cost considerations.

Despite these limitations, PET imaging remains valuable in various clinical applications, particularly oncology, neurology, and cardiology. Ongoing research and technological advancements continue to address these limitations and enhance the capabilities of PET imaging.

7.2.2 Limitations of SPECT Imaging

Despite several advantages of single photon emission computed tomography (SPECT) imaging, SPECT has several limitations, including:

- *Lower Spatial Resolution*: SPECT scanners generally have lower spatial resolution than imaging modalities such as CT, MRI, and PET. The resolution of SPECT images is typically in the range of several millimeters to centimeters (for typical conventional clinical SPECT systems range is 6–12 mm), which may limit the ability to visualize small structures or detect very small lesions accurately. However, organ-specific SPECT cameras, such as cardiac SPECT can achieve improved spatial resolution, often in the range of 4–8 mm, and dedicated brain SPECT systems with specialized collimators can achieve even higher spatial resolutions, ranging from 3 to 7 mm.
- *Limited Quantification*: The quantification accuracy in SPECT can vary depending on the specific radiotracer, imaging protocol, reconstruction techniques, and calibration methods used. Therefore, when comparing SPECT images quantitatively or tracking changes in radiotracer uptake, it is crucial to account for these limitations and utilize appropriate calibration methods to obtain reliable and meaningful results.
- *Longer Acquisition Time*: SPECT imaging requires longer acquisition than other imaging modalities. This is because the gamma camera used in SPECT rotates around the patient to acquire multiple projections from different angles or even the planar gamma camera studies are longer. The longer acquisition times can increase patient discomfort and, typically in SPECT, limit the feasibility of performing dynamic imaging or capturing rapidly changing processes.
- *Limited Spatial Resolution with Attenuation Correction*: Attenuation correction is a technique used to compensate for the attenuation of photons as they pass through the body's tissues. However, the attenuation correction in SPECT is often based on a simple model and does not account for tissue inhomogeneity or scatter, resulting in limited accuracy. This can affect the overall image quality and quantitative accuracy of SPECT images. Artificial intelligence may solve this challenge in the future.
- *Limited Availability of Radiotracers*: Similar to PET imaging, SPECT imaging relies on specific radiotracers that can bind to or interact with target molecules or receptors in the body and follow certain pathophysiology to mimic human physiology. The availability of radiotracers can be limited, and not all molecular targets or diseases have suitable radiotracers available for SPECT imaging or planar gamma camera imaging.
- *Lower Sensitivity*: SPECT imaging has lower sensitivity than positron emission tomography (PET) imaging. This means that SPECT may require higher doses of radiotracer or longer acquisition times to achieve adequate image quality, which can increase radiation exposure to the patient.
- *Limited Anatomical Details*: SPECT images lack detailed anatomical information similar to PET imaging. While SPECT can be performed with CT (SPECT-CT) to provide functional and anatomical information, the spatial registration between SPECT and CT images can be challenging and may introduce inaccuracies.

Despite these limitations, SPECT imaging remains valuable in various clinical applications, particularly cardiology, neurology, and oncology. Ongoing research and technological advancements continue to address these limitations and improve the capabilities of SPECT imaging.

7.2.3 Limitations of CT Imaging

Computed tomography (CT) imaging is a widely used diagnostic tool in medical imaging. However, it does have certain limitations. Here are some of the limitations associated with CT imaging:

- *Lack of Physiological Information:* CT (computed tomography) imaging primarily provides detailed anatomical information rather than direct physiological insights. It creates cross-sectional images of the body, valuable for visualizing tissues and organs' structure, shape, and density. CT does not directly capture physiological processes or provide information about metabolic activity or cellular function. It focuses more on the structural aspects of the body. Though it can reveal abnormalities, lesions, or structural changes, it may not comprehensively understand the underlying physiological mechanisms or functional status. This limitation becomes apparent when evaluating conditions that involve altered cellular metabolism or specific molecular targets.
- *Limited Soft Tissue Differentiation*: While CT imaging excels in visualizing bones and dense structures, it has limitations in differentiating soft tissues, especially when compared to magnetic resonance imaging (MRI). Soft tissues with similar densities can be challenging to distinguish, potentially leading to limited sensitivity in detecting certain pathologies.
- *Motion Artifacts*: CT scans require the patient to lie still during the examination to avoid motion artifacts. However, patients who cannot remain still, such as young children, critically ill individuals, or those with certain medical conditions, may experience motion artifacts that can affect image quality and interpretation.
- *Contrast Agents*: Contrast agents are sometimes used in CT imaging to enhance certain structures' visibility or highlight abnormalities. While generally safe, contrast agents carry a small risk of adverse reactions, such as allergic reactions or kidney damage, particularly in individuals with preexisting renal conditions or allergies to contrast agents.
- *Ionizing Radiation*: CT imaging involves X-rays exposing patients to ionizing radiation. Although CT scanners are designed to minimize radiation exposure, repeated or unnecessary CT scans may increase the cumulative radiation dose over time. This is particularly important for pediatric patients and individuals who require multiple imaging studies.
- *Spatial Resolution*: CT scanners have improved significantly in terms of spatial resolution, allowing for detailed visualization of anatomical structures. However, CT still has limitations in capturing extremely fine details, such as small blood vessels or tiny lesions. In some cases, additional imaging modalities like MRI may be required for more precise characterization.
- *Cost and Accessibility*: CT scanners are complex and expensive equipment, and the cost of performing CT scans can be relatively high. This can limit accessibility to CT imaging in some healthcare settings or regions, potentially impacting patient access to this diagnostic tool.

Despite these limitations, CT imaging remains valuable for various diagnostic purposes, including trauma evaluation, detection of certain cancers, and visualization of anatomical structures. Ongoing advancements in CT technology continue to address these limitations and improve the capabilities of CT imaging.

7.2.4 Limitations of MR Imaging

Magnetic resonance imaging (MRI) is a powerful, versatile modality that provides detailed anatomical and functional information, including bony ones. It provides excellent soft tissue contrast and is particularly well suited for imaging the brain, muscles, joints, organs, bone marrow abnormalities, bone tumors, and joint diseases and assessing soft tissue structures around bones, such as ligaments and tendons. MRI can offer various techniques to assess physiological processes; for example, functional MRI (fMRI) is commonly used to map brain activity by detecting changes in blood oxygenation levels, allowing for the identification of active brain regions during specific tasks or stimuli. Additionally, MRI can be utilized for diffusion-weighted imaging (DWI) to assess the movement of water molecules in tissues, providing information about tissue microstructure. Furthermore, MRI can offer perfusion imaging techniques to assess blood flow and tissue perfusion. Dynamic contrast-enhanced MRI (DCE-MRI) involves the injection of a contrast agent to track its distribution through tissues, providing information about blood flow and tissue vascularization. Arterial spin labeling (ASL) is a non-contrast-based perfusion imaging technique that measures blood flow using magnetically labeled arterial blood water as an endogenous contrast agent. Despite so many advantages mentioned above, MRI does have certain limitations. Here are some of the limitations associated with MRI imaging:

- *Patient Discomfort*: The small-bore size of some MRI scanners can cause discomfort for certain patients. Individuals who are larger or who experience physical discomfort when confined in small spaces may find the tight enclosure of the MRI scanner uncomfortable. This discomfort can affect patient cooperation and lead to difficulty in obtaining high-quality images.
- *Noise*: MRI scanners produce loud knocking, thumping, and buzzing noises during imaging. These noises result from the magnetic field gradients and radiofrequency pulses that generate the images. The loud and repetitive nature of these sounds can cause anxiety and discomfort for patients. However, modern MRI scanners are equipped with noise-reducing technology, and patients are typically provided with earplugs or headphones to mitigate the noise levels.
- *Claustrophobia*: Claustrophobia, the fear of enclosed spaces, is a common concern for patients undergoing MRI scans. The small-bore size of some MRI scanners can exacerbate feelings of claustrophobia, making it challenging for some individuals to tolerate the procedure. The enclosed environment and the need to remain still for an extended period inside the scanner can trigger anxiety and discomfort. Open-bore or wide-bore MRI scanners are designed to address this limitation by offering a larger, more open space, reducing feelings of confinement and claustrophobia.
- *Sensitivity to Motion*: MRI is highly sensitive to patient motion; even small movements during the scan can result in motion artifacts, compromising image quality and interpretation. Patient cooperation and remaining still during imaging are crucial for obtaining clear and accurate MRI images.
- *Cost*: MRI scanners are complex and expensive equipment, making MRI examinations more expensive than other imaging modalities such as X-rays or ultrasound. The high cost of equipment, maintenance, and specialized personnel required for MRI can limit its availability in some healthcare settings.
- *Time-consuming*: MRI scans can be time-consuming, often requiring the patient to remain in the scanner for an extended period. The duration of an MRI examination varies depending on the specific imaging protocol and the body area being scanned. Longer scan times can be challenging for patients who are claustrophobic or have difficulty remaining still, including young children and individuals with certain medical conditions.
- *Patient Limitations*: Certain patient populations may have limitations with MR imaging. For example, individuals with metallic implants or devices, such as pacemakers, cochlear implants, or some types of aneurysm clips, may not be eligible for MRI due to safety concerns. Additionally, patients who experience claustrophobia may find it challenging to undergo MRI scans although open-bore or wide-bore MRI scanners are available to address this limitation to some extent.
- *Limited Accessibility for Emergency Situations*: In emergencies, such as trauma or acute stroke, MRI may not be the first-line imaging modality due to its time-consuming nature. Other modalities like computed tomography (CT) are often preferred due to their faster acquisition times and wider availability in emergencies.
- *Contraindications with Certain Conditions*: MRI may have contraindications in patients with specific conditions. For instance, patients with certain metallic implants or foreign bodies that are not MRI compatible may not be

suitable for MRI scanning due to safety concerns. Patients with severe renal impairment may require special considerations when using contrast agents.

- *Limited Availability of Contrast Agents*: While contrast agents can enhance the visibility of certain structures or pathologies in MRI, not all areas or pathologies can be adequately visualized with contrast-enhanced MRI. Additionally, some patients may have contraindications or adverse reactions to contrast agents, such as those with impaired renal function or allergies.

Despite these limitations, MRI remains a valuable imaging modality in various clinical applications, providing detailed anatomical and functional information without ionizing radiation. Ongoing advancements in technology and techniques continue to address these limitations and improve the capabilities of MRI imaging.

7.3 Advantages of Hybrid Imaging

Hybrid imaging offers several advantages over a single imaging modality. Which combines two or more imaging modalities offers several advantages over stand-alone imaging techniques. Here are some key benefits of hybrid imaging:

- *Comprehensive Information*: By integrating different imaging modalities, hybrid imaging provides a more comprehensive assessment of the human body. It combines functional and anatomical information, allowing a more complete understanding of disease processes. This comprehensive data can enhance diagnostic accuracy and improve treatment planning.
- *Improved Localization*: Hybrid imaging enables precise localization of abnormalities by overlaying functional information onto detailed anatomical images. This helps to pinpoint the exact location of diseases or abnormalities, aiding in surgical planning, biopsy guidance, and targeted therapy.
- *Synergistic Effect*: The combination of multiple imaging modalities can have a synergistic effect, where the strengths of each modality complement each other. For example, combining functional information from positron emission tomography (PET) or single photon emission computed tomography (SPECT) with the anatomical detail provided by computed tomography (CT) or magnetic resonance imaging (MRI) can enhance the interpretation and diagnostic confidence of the results.
- *Improved Sensitivity and Specificity*: Hybrid imaging can improve the sensitivity and specificity of diagnostic examinations. Combining the strengths of different modalities can help differentiate between benign and malignant lesions, detect subtle abnormalities, and reduce false-positive or false-negative findings.
- *Treatment Monitoring*: Hybrid imaging techniques effectively monitor treatment response. By comparing pre- and posttreatment scans, clinicians can evaluate changes in functional and anatomical characteristics, helping to assess the effectiveness of therapies and make informed decisions regarding treatment adjustments.
- *Reduced Examination Time and Radiation Dose*: In some cases, hybrid imaging can reduce the need for separate imaging examinations, saving time and reducing patient discomfort. For instance, a single PET-CT or PET-MRI scan can provide functional and anatomical information. Additionally, combining imaging modalities can optimize imaging protocols to minimize radiation dose while maintaining diagnostic quality.
- *Research and Advancements*: Hybrid imaging techniques have opened new avenues for research and advancements in various fields, including oncology, neurology, cardiology, and more. They provide opportunities to study complex diseases, understand physiological processes, and develop novel diagnostic and therapeutic approaches.

The advantages of hybrid imaging may vary depending on the specific modalities being combined, the clinical scenario, and the expertise of the interpreting physician. Nonetheless, hybrid imaging has proven to be a valuable tool in modern medicine, offering enhanced diagnostic capabilities and contributing to improved patient care.

7.4 Radiation Detectors and Their Properties and Mechanism of Detection Used in SPECT, PET, and CT

In Chap. 1, Sect. 1.5.2, we discussed the interaction of radiation with matter. In imaging, mainly photons are used in detection and image formation. The properties of two main interactions, photoelectric effect and Compton scattering, are utilized for imaging as other kinds of interactions mentioned in Chap. 1 are unsuitable for imaging because of lower or higher energies. In imaging, scintillation and semiconductor detectors are typically used in SPECT or PET imaging.

7.4.1 Scintillation Detectors

Sir William Crookes (1832–1919), a British chemist and physicist, was the first to observe scintillation with alpha particles striking on a ZnS screen in 1902. Certain materials, from solids, liquids, or gases, emit light while interacting with radiation. This process of emitting light is called scintillation (Fig. 7.1). It is a rapid and intermittent light emission, often in discrete flashes or scintillations. Scintillation occurs when the energy from incident radiation excites electrons within a scintillator material, causing them to emit light photons as they return to lower energy states. The emission of light photons can be proportional to the amount of radiation absorbed; hence, these materials can be used as radiation detectors. The emitted light photons are converted into electrical pulses with the help of electronics and used for radiation detection.

These detectors are of three types: inorganic, organic, and gaseous scintillators. The choice among these detectors depends on properties such as detector efficiency, decay time, dead time, wavelength of emission, ability to grow in different sizes, transparency to its wavelength of emissions, etc. The meaning of detector efficiency is that the detector material should be able to convert the kinetic energy of radiation to detectable light with high scintillation efficiency and proportional to deposited energy over a wide range. The decay time of the produced scintillation should be short so that fast signals can be processed and dead time is minimum. The dead time of a scintillation detector refers to the period

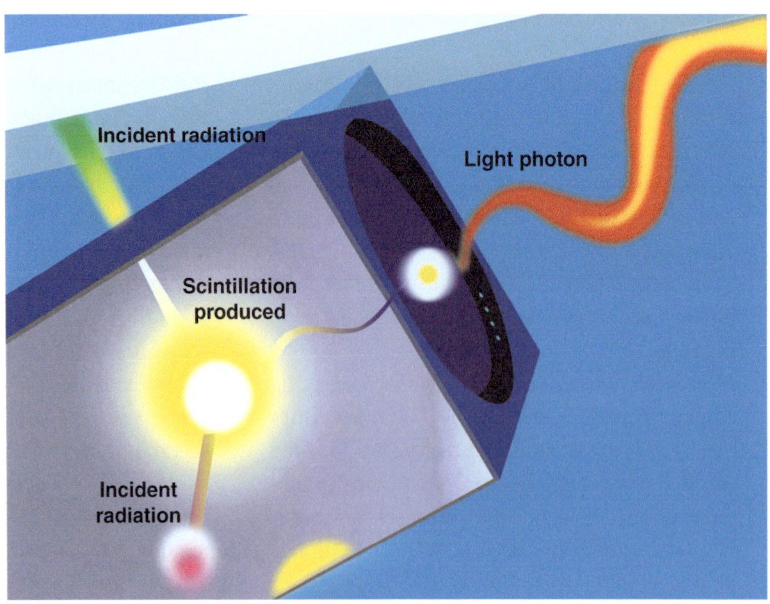

Fig. 7.1 Scintillation produced in a crystal

during which the detector cannot register subsequent radiation events immediately after detecting an initial event. It is a temporary insensitivity or "dead time" during which the detector recovers from the initial event and resets itself to detect subsequent events.

Commonly used scintillator detectors are inorganic crystals, for example, sodium iodide thallium activated (NaI(Tl)), cesium iodide thallium activated (CsI(Tl)), bismuth germanate (bismuth germanium oxide, BGO), and lutetium oxyorthosilicate cerium activated (LSO(ce)) (Fig. 7.2). Although the inorganic materials offer good linearity and light output, their response times are generally slow. Organic scintillators, on the other hand, produce less light but are typically faster. Inorganic crystals with high Z and density are employed in gamma-ray spectroscopy, but organic crystals with high hydrogen content are chosen for beta spectroscopy and fast neutron detection.

In nuclear medicine, scintillator detectors are used in PET, SPECT, or gamma cameras, thyroid probes, well counters, organ-specific such as cardiac or breast imaging gamma cameras, gamma probes for sentinel node detection, and as CT detectors in PET-CT machines.

7.4.2 Mechanism of Scintillation Detection

Inorganic materials, the crystalline lattice's energy levels, affect its scintillation mechanism. The outermost electrons in an atom are known as valence electrons, and they orbit the nucleus at various energy levels. When given enough energy, valence electrons can break out from their orbit and move freely within the crystal lattice. These free electrons, which aid in conduction, always have more energy than the valence electrons. A valence band refers to the energy range of valence electrons, whereas a conduction band refers to the energy range of conduction electrons. A forbidden band is an area between these two bands in a crystalline crystal where electrons are absent. In a diagrammatic representation, the lower band can be shown as the valence band, whereas the upper band can be the conduc-

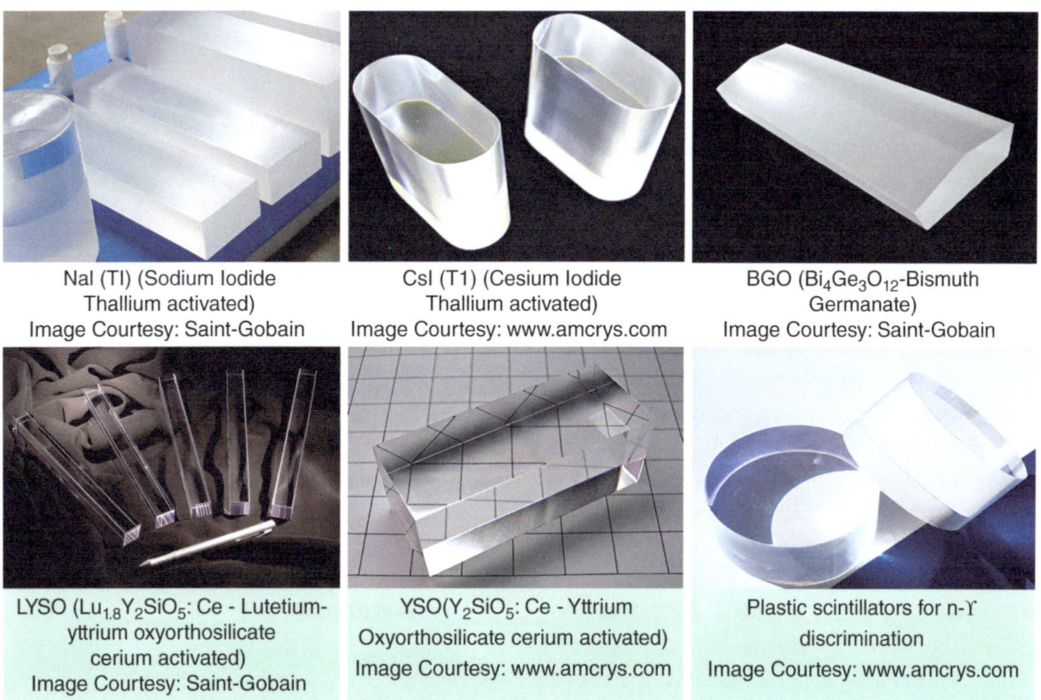

Fig. 7.2 Scintillator crystals. (Image originally published in Tandon et al. [1]. Republished with permission)

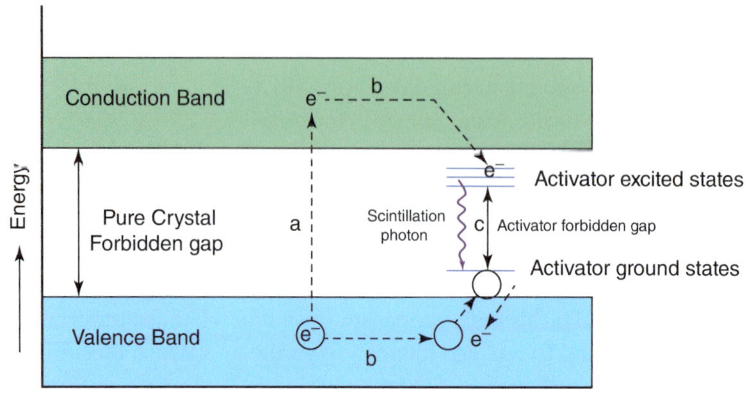

Fig. 7.3 Energy levels of activated crystalline scintillator

tion band. The gap between these two bands is called the forbidden band.

On receiving energy from radiation, electrons from the valence band move to the conduction band and leave a gap in the valence band. Upon returning to the valence band, they create light photons. In pure crystals, the difference in energy between the two bands is usually significant, which means that photon emission is inefficient and visible light is unlikely. To enhance the chances of visible light emission, trace amounts of activator contaminants are added intentionally. These impurities create unique energy locations in the crystal lattice's energy band that are lower than the full forbidden gap of a pure crystal (see Fig. 7.3). These transitions can now give photons of visible light. This is a basic principle of the scintillation process, where activator-forbidden gaps determine the emission spectrum.

The activators are chosen wisely depending on their emissions of visible energy range. Typical lifetimes for such excited states are of the order of 30–500 ns [2]. Tables 7.1 and 7.2 provide various characteristics of scintillation crystals suitable for gamma and PET cameras, respectively.

To convert the scintillation light into electric pulses and amplify these pulses enough to be read by further electronics, the scintillator detectors are always connected to photomultiplier (PM) tubes or photodiodes. Internal reflections are reduced by using a clear optical "coupling grease" between the crystal and the PM tube (Fig. 7.4). Each light pulse is converted into an electron by the photocathode material inside the PM tube, which is then significantly amplified to create a voltage pulse that can be read and interpreted. The quantity of these pulses is determined by counting them over time, while the size of each generated pulse allows for detecting the radiation's specific energy.

Table 7.1 Properties of common crystals used in gamma camera [1]

Principle properties	NaI (Tl)	CsI (Tl)	CsI (Na)
Effective atomic number	50	54	54
Density (g/cm^3)	3.67	4.51	4.51
Hygroscopic	Yes	Slightly	Yes
Wavelength of emission max (nm)	415	550	420
Decay time (ns)	250	1000	630
Light yield (photon/keV)	38	54	41
Comments	General purpose Good energy resolution	High Z, rugged, good match to photodiodes	High Z, rugged

7.4.3 Computed Tomography (CT) Detectors

As discussed above, the scintillation detection method used in CT scans differs from that used in nuclear medicine. PET and gamma cameras work

Table 7.2 Properties of common crystals used in PET detectors [1]

Principle properties	BGO $Bi_4Ge_3O_{12}$	LSO $Lu_2SiO_5(Ce)$	LYSO $Lu_{1.8}Y_{0.2}SiO_5(Ce)$
Effective atomic number	73	66	66
Density (g/cm^3)	7.1	7.4	7.1
Hygroscopic	No	No	No
Attenuation length for 511 keV (cm)	1.0	1.15	1.2
Energy resolution (%) @662 keV	12	9	8
Wavelength of emission max (nm)	480	420	420
Decay time (ns)	300	40	36
Light yield (photon/keV)	9	26	33
Comments	High Z, compact detector, low afterglow	Bright, high Z, fast, dense background from ^{176}Lu activity	Bright, high Z, fast, dense background from ^{176}Lu activity, better energy resolution, and decay time

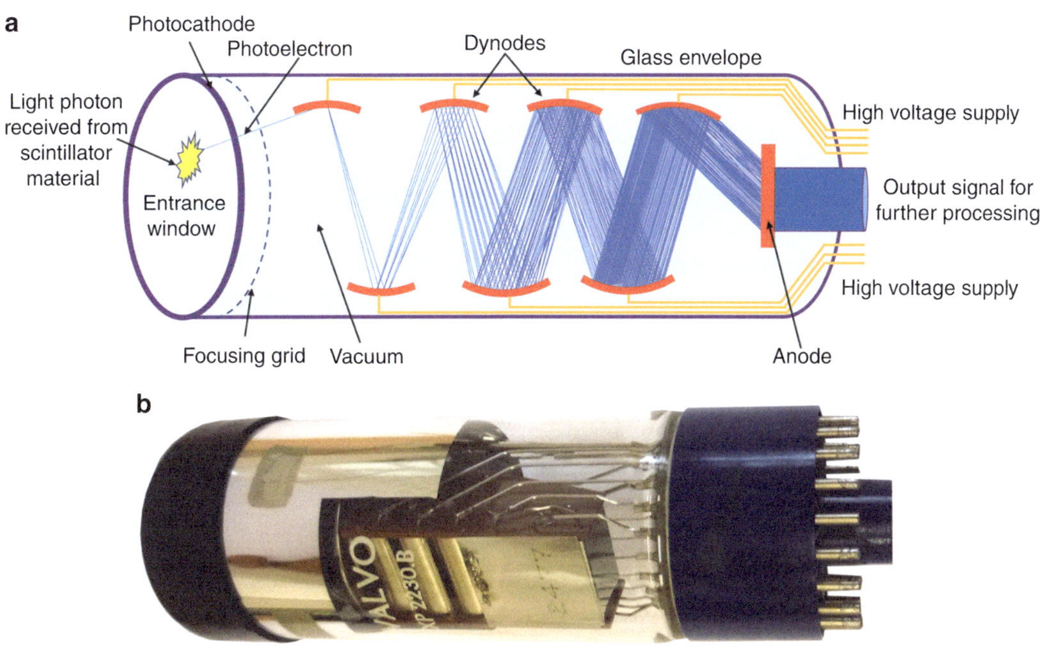

Fig. 7.4 Photomultiplier tube assembly. (**a**) Cross-sectional diagram of PMT. (**b**) Original PM tube. (Image courtesy: Philipp Bielefeldt, published under Creative Commons license 4.0. Published with modifications)

in pulse mode, whereas CT operates in the current mode. When event rates are very high, the current mode can be employed to provide a stable current, whereas in pulse mode, the information about the energy and time of individual events is retained. In PET and gamma cameras, the radiation flux is much lower (1–100 quanta/s/mm^2 for a gamma camera and 100 quanta/s/mm^2 for a typical PET application), whereas CT has very high radiation flux (i.e., in the order of 10^8 to 10^9 quanta/s/mm^2 at the detector, and individual counting in CT is therefore impractical) [1].

X-rays and computed tomography have utilized inorganic crystals or clear ceramic scintillators for radiation detection. The selection of the detectors is based on their high light output, lack of long afterglow, and resistance to radiation damage over time. Scintillators like yttria and gadolinium with Eu activated $(Y, Gd)_2O_3$:Eu or $Y_{1.34}Gd_{0.60}Eu_{0.06}O_3$ or self-activated cadmium tungstate ($CdWO_4$), gadolinium oxysulfide (Gd_2O_2S), and others have been utilized. General Electric (GE) has been using $(YGd)_2O_3$ in thousands of CT scanners; however, recently, they have used complicated rare earth-based oxide gemstone detectors, whereas Siemens has employed proprietary detectors like Ultra Fast Ceramics (UFC) and Stellar Infinity detectors [1]. The characteristics of several detectors used in X-ray imaging applications are shown in Table 7.3.

CT detectors can be found in countless millions, each one configured in a separate channel array in pixelated form. Like nuclear medicine, radiation (X-rays) strikes the detectors, scintillation light is generated, and photodiodes transform the light into electrical signals. The additional circuitry, shared by many or all detector channels, is then connected to the pixel electronics. Figure 7.5 presents a general illustration of the CT detecting system, whereas Fig. 7.6 presents X-ray flat panel detector.

In CT imaging, a spatial resolution of 0.5–1 mm is often needed at the detector, but due to quick gantry rotation and a large number of projections, a very high temporal resolution of 50–100 μs is needed. Gadolinium oxysulfide has a light output of 35–60 photons/keV compared to cadmium tungstate's 20 photons/keV. To prevent lateral crosstalk of the scintillation light between the individual crystals, the scintillator crystals are made into small pieces of around 2–5 mm^3 and put next to each other with reflective material between them. The detector components are arranged in a circular shape with an arc of 1 m, sometimes called the "detector banana." A scintillator crystal and a matched photodiode make up each detector pixel. The electronics channel, which normally consists of an amplifier and an analogue-to-digital converter (ADC) optimized for the operation of the CT detector, is then connected to the photodiode.

In X-ray flat panel detectors, the readout integrated circuits (ROICs) and gate drivers that are part of the electronic circuitry comprise an array of sensing components known as pixels. The relative strength of the signals collected by the pixel array estimates the body area's composition in the scanner because soft tissue, bone, and blood have varied X-ray attenuation properties. The ROICs transform the electrical impulses into digital outputs sent to a back-end computing system. The output of the digital signal from the computer is rendered as an image that can be printed or viewed on a monitor.

Table 7.3 Important characteristics of X-ray scintillators used in imaging

Material	Density (g/cm^3)	Thickness to stop 99% of 140 keV X-rays (mm)	Emission (nm)	Light yield (photon/MeV)/temperature coefficient (%/°C)	Primary decay time (μs)	Afterglow (% at 3 ms)
CsI (Tl)	4.52	6.1	550	54,000/0.02	1	0.5
$CdWO_4$ (CWO)	7.9	2.6	495	28,000/−0.3	2, 15	0.05
$Gd_2O_3:Eu^{+3}$	7.55	2.6	610	–	–	–
$Y_{1.34}Gd_{0.6}O_3$:Eu, Pr, Tb (YGO)	5.9	6.1	610	42,000/0.04	1000	5
Gd_2O_2S:Pr, Ce, F (GOS)	7.34	2.9	520	50,000/−0.6	2.4	<0.1
Gd_2O_2S:Tb (Ce) (GOS)	7.34	2.9	550	50,000/−0.6	600	0.6
La_2HfO_7:Ti	7.9	2.8	475	13,000/–	10	–
$Gd_3Ga_5O_{12}$:Cr, Ce	7.09	4.5	730	39,000/–	150	<0.1

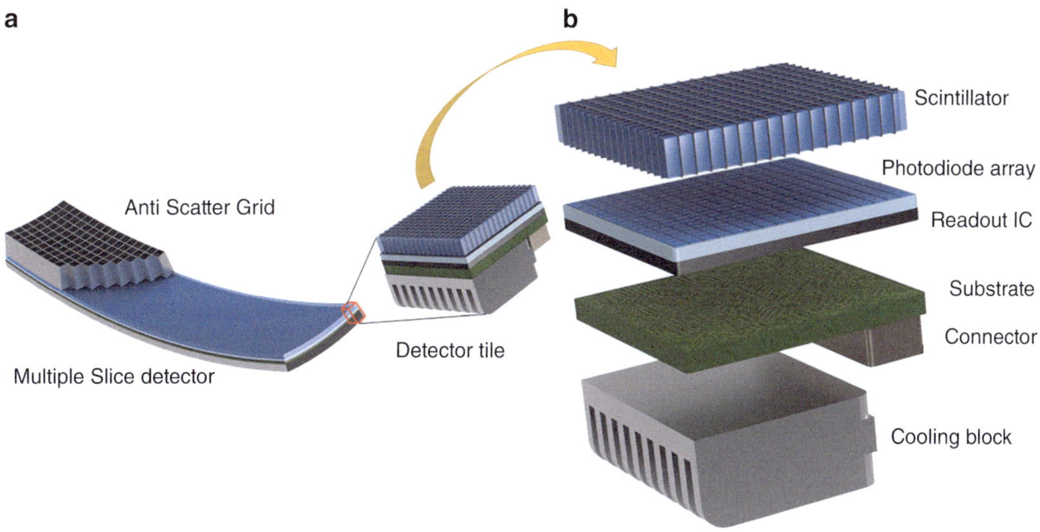

Fig. 7.5 CT detection system. (**a**) Multiple slice CT detector array with anti-scatter grid, showing arrangement of detector tiles. (**b**) Exploded view of a single CT detector tile illustrating key components: scintillator, photodiode array, readout integrated circuit (IC), substrate, connector, and cooling block. (Image courtesy: AMS OSRAM. Printed with permission)

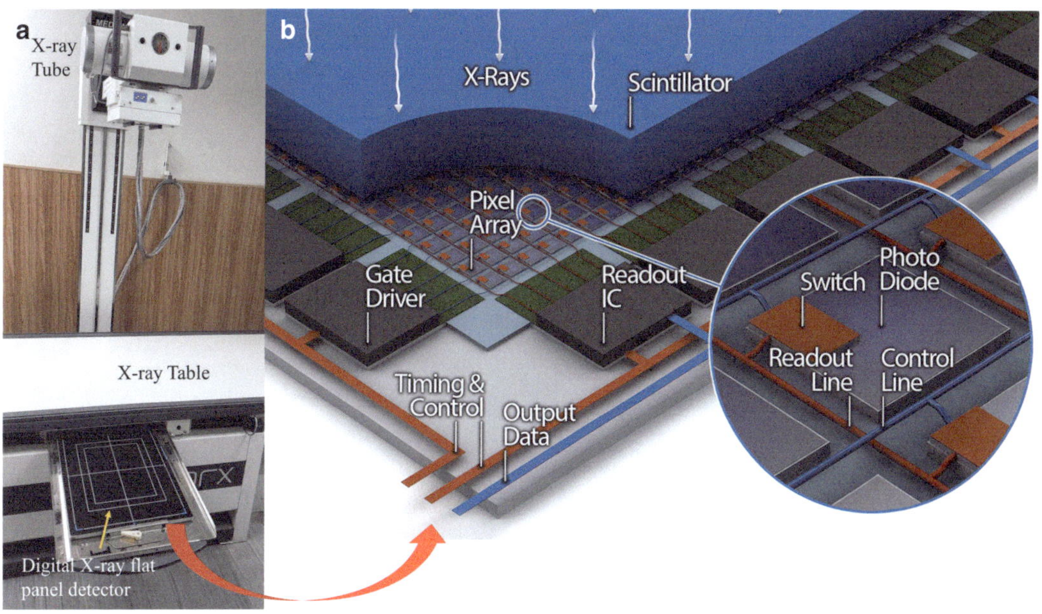

Fig. 7.6 X-ray flat panel detectors; (**a**) X-ray machine with flat panel detector; (**b**) X-ray flat panel detector with readout integrated ICs. (Image courtesy: AMS OSRAM, printed with permission)

7.5 Positron Emission Tomography (PET) and How It Works

7.5.1 Historical Developments of Positron Emission Tomography (PET) and PET-CT

Discovery of Positron

The discovery of positrons is a significant development in particle physics and fundamental understanding of matter. Positrons, also known as antielectrons, are positively charged particles with the same mass as electrons but with opposite charge. The discovery of positrons played a crucial role in developing positron emission tomography (PET) imaging.

In 1928, Paul Dirac proposed the concept of positive electrons and given an equation [4] that combined quantum mechanics and special relativity, known as the Dirac equation (Fig. 7.7). The Dirac equation predicted the existence of particles with both positive and negative energies. Dirac interpreted the negative energy solutions as antimatter particles, which he called positrons.

Experimental confirmation of Dirac's theory came in 1932 when American physicist Carl D. Anderson observed the tracks of particles in a cloud chamber [5]. Anderson was studying cosmic rays, high-energy particles originating from outer space. He noticed a peculiar track that curved in the opposite direction to the expected path of an electron. Through further experiments, Anderson identified these particles as positrons. The tracks were caused by the positrons colliding with electrons, resulting in mutual annihilation and the production of gamma rays. This discovery marked the first experimental evidence of antimatter.

Paul Dirac was awarded the Nobel Prize in 1933, whereas Anderson was awarded in 1936, for advancing our understanding of particle physics. The discovery of positrons provided crucial evidence supporting the concept of antimatter and contributed to the development of quantum field theory.

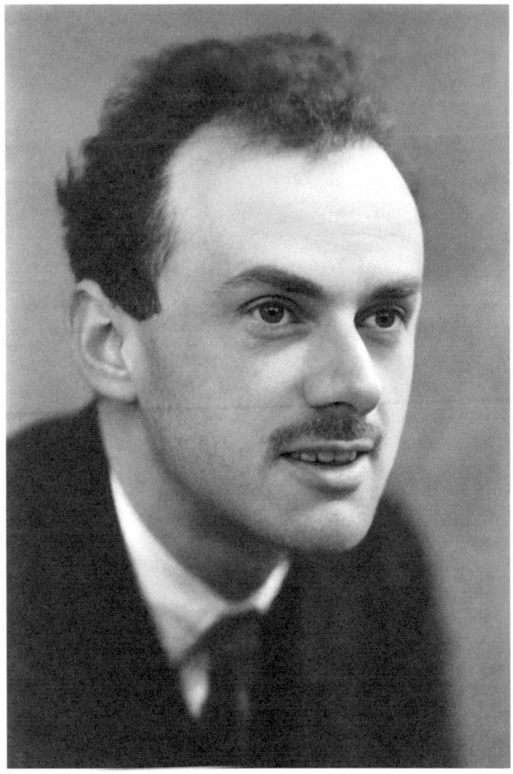
Paul Dirac (1902-1984)

Fig. 7.7 Paul Dirac, proposer of positive electrons. (Image courtesy: Wikimedia. Published under Creative Commons license)

7.5.2 Development of Positron-Emitting Radiopharmaceuticals

In the 1940s and 1950s, researchers began experimenting with positron-emitting isotopes for medical imaging. Carbon-11 (^{11}C) and nitrogen-13 (^{13}N) were the first isotopes used. They were incorporated into small molecules like carbon monoxide and ammonia to study regional cerebral blood flow and brain metabolism.

One of the most significant breakthroughs was the introduction of fluorodeoxyglucose (FDG) as a radiopharmaceutical. In the 1970s, researchers recognized the similarity between FDG and glucose and explored its potential for imaging glucose metabolism. The positron-emitting isotope fluorine-18 (^{18}F) labeled the glucose molecule, resulting in ^{18}F-FDG. FDG rapidly became the most widely used radiopharmaceutical in PET imaging.

7.5.3 Coincidence Detection and Construction of First PET Scanner

In the 1950s, scientists recognized the importance of coincidence detection in PET imaging. Coincidence detection involves detecting two photons emitted in opposite directions simultaneously, indicating the annihilation of a positron and electron (discussed in detail in Sect. 7.5.4). Michael E. Phelps (Fig. 7.8) and his team at Washington University in St. Louis made a notable contribution to the development of PET technology. They built one of the earliest PET scanners, the "Positron Emission Transaxial Tomograph III (PETT III)" scanner, operational by 1973 [6]. Here the III signifies that it was the third iteration of the PET scanner developed by Michael Phelps, Edward Hoffman, and colleagues at Washington University in St. Louis in the early 1970s. The team had already built two earlier versions of prototypes with limitations, and PETT III was the first widely recognized and used system. This scanner utilized a ring of detectors to detect the coincident gamma rays resulting from positron annihilation.

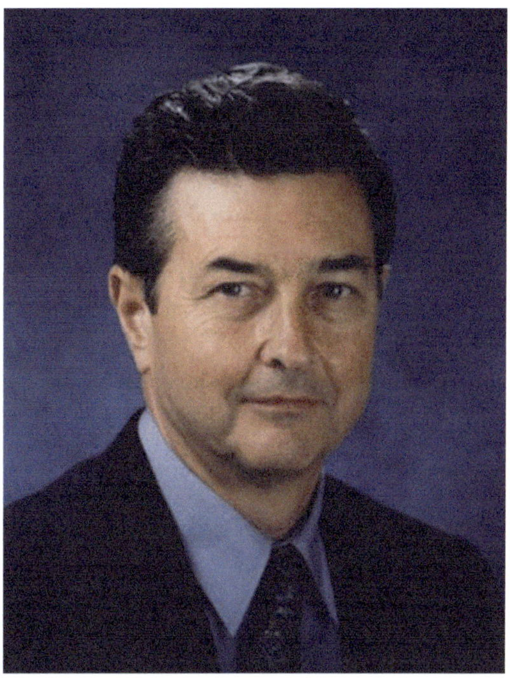

Michael E. Phelps (Born 1939)

Fig. 7.8 Michael E. Phelps—built one of the earliest PET scanners. (Copyright: Springer Nature. Republished with permission)

In the 1980s, advancements in computer technology facilitated the development of 2D and 3D reconstruction algorithms. These algorithms allowed for more accurate and detailed images, improving the diagnostic capabilities of PET.

In the late 1990s, the concept of combining PET with computed tomography (CT) was introduced, leading to the development of PET-CT scanners with the working prototype of the first PET/CT scanner developed in 1998 [7]. The first commercial PET-CT was available in 2001 [8] with a single-slice CT system [9], but now the PET-CT scanners are available with up to 256-slice CT. The hybrid imaging technology provided anatomical and functional information in a single examination, enhancing PET's diagnostic accuracy and clinical utility. But to understand the concept in detail, we need to see it from the basics of positron physics and then build up the knowledge of PET scanners.

7.5.4 The Positron Physics

Nuclides with excess protons tend to undergo positron decay or electron capture. This occurs to reduce the proton-to-neutron ratio and achieve a more stable configuration. Positron decay occurs in lighter nuclides, whereas electron capture is more common in heavier elements, particularly those with a higher atomic number (Z). Some nuclides undergo a competitive decay of both; for example, F-18 undergoes approximately 97% positron decay and 3% electron capture.

During positron decay, which is also known as beta-plus decay, a proton decays down into a neutron, a positron, and a neutrino. The nucleus emits the positron ($\beta+$) and neutrino (ν), while the neutron stays within the nucleus. The atomic number of the nucleus is changed since a proton has been converted into a neutron, and it typically moves the nucleus toward a more stable configuration. This process reduces the atomic number of the nucleus by one while leaving the mass number unchanged. The following equation represents the decay:

$$ {}_{Z}^{A}X \rightarrow {}_{Z-1}^{A}Y + {}_{1}^{0}\beta + \nu \tag{7.1} $$

Example:

$$ {}_{9}^{18}F \xrightarrow{\beta+} {}_{8}^{18}O + {}_{1}^{0}\beta + \nu $$

When a positron is emitted from a nucleus, it collides with atoms of the surrounding matter, loses its kinetic energy, and comes to rest. Within a few millimeters (different for different isotopes, and it is called a range) from the location of its origin to the point where its kinetic energy becomes zero, it temporarily forms an atom called "positronium" (Fig. 7.9). Positronium is a short-lived atom-like particle consisting of an electron in "orbits" and a positron as its "nucleus." It can exist in two forms: ortho-positronium (o-Ps) and para-positronium (p-Ps), depending on the relative spin orientations of the electron and positron. The average lifetime of ortho-positronium is approximately 140 nanoseconds (ns), while para-positronium has a shorter average lifetime of about 125 picoseconds (ps). These lifetimes refer to the average time it takes for the positronium to decay.

The electron (or positron) has a mass-energy equivalence of 511 keV (kilo electron volt). Both electron and positron combinedly provide rest mass-energy equivalence to 1.022 MeV (million electron volt), which is ejected out in the form of two gamma photons of 511 keV each in opposite directions. The reason gamma-ray photons are emitted approximately 180 degrees apart in the annihilation of positron-electron pairs is related to the conservation of momentum. To conserve momentum, the total momentum before annihilation must equal the total momentum after annihilation. To achieve this, the two gamma-ray photons are emitted in opposite directions, essentially back to back, with a total momentum of zero. This configuration ensures that the net momentum of the system is conserved, as the momenta of the photons cancel each other out.

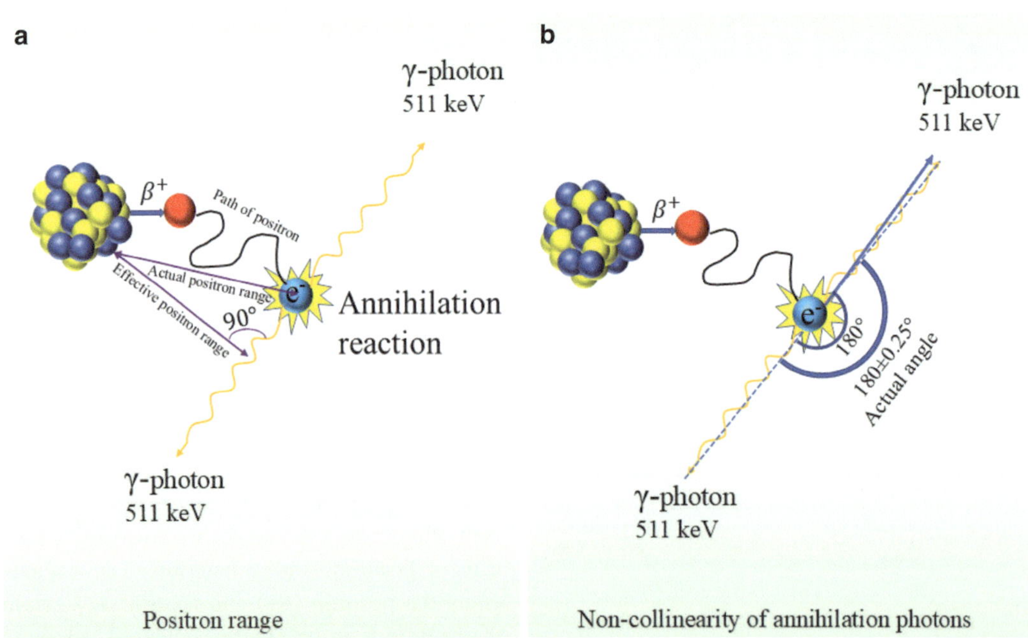

Fig. 7.9 Annihilation reaction between a positron ($\beta+$) and an electron ($e-$). (**a**) Positron range responsible for image blurring. (**b**) Noncollinearity causes positioning error

It's important to note that the 180-degree emission angle is an idealized scenario. In practice, due to various factors such as the finite size of the positronium atom and interactions with surrounding matter, the emitted gamma-ray photons may deviate slightly from the exact 180-degree angle (180 ± 0.25°). However, the overall emission pattern remains predominantly back to back, ensuring momentum conservation.

7.5.5 Working of PET

Positron emission tomography utilizes the physics of positron annihilation to generate images of biological processes in the body. Here's a step-by-step explanation of how PET works:

Radiotracer Injection

A small amount of a radiotracer, a radioactive substance, is injected into the patient's body. The radiotracer contains a positron-emitting isotope, such as fluorine-18 (F-18). 18F-fluorodeoxyglucose (FDG) is the most widely used radiotracer in PET imaging. It is a glucose analogue that accumulates in tissues with high glucose metabolism, such as cancer cells. FDG-PET is commonly used for cancer diagnosis, staging, restaging, and treatment response monitoring. Other commonly used radiotracers are 68Ga-DOTA, 68Ga-PSMA, 11C-Methionine (MET), 18F-Fluorothymidine (FLT), 18F-Sodium Fluoride (NaF), 18F-Florbetapir, 18F-Flutemetamol, 18F-FDOPA, and 68Ga-FAPI (Gallium-68-labeled Fibroblast Activation Protein Inhibitors), among others.

Positron Decay and Gamma Emission

The radiotracers mentioned above contain short-lived isotopes that undergo radioactive decay, emitting a positron from their nucleus. The positron is a positively charged particle with the same mass as an electron but opposite charge. The emitted positron travels a short distance within the body until it encounters an electron. Positrons have a relatively short range due to their interactions with electrons. When a positron interacts with an electron, both particles annihilate each other. This annihilation process results in the complete conversion of their masses into energy through two gamma photons. The annihilation produces two gamma photons, each with an energy of 511-kilo electron volts (keV). These gamma photons are emitted in nearly opposite directions, typically approximately 180 ± 0.25° degrees from each other.

Detection

The PET scanners, a specialized detector, surround the patient and detect the gamma photons emitted during annihilation. The detectors record the timing and location of each detected photon. PET scanners consist of a ring or a series of detector modules surrounding the patient. These detectors are typically made of scintillation crystals, such as Bismuth Germanate (BGO), lutetium oxyorthosilicate (LSO), or lutetium-yttrium oxyorthosilicate (LYSO), coupled with photodetectors (such as photomultiplier tubes or silicon photomultipliers). When the annihilation photons interact with the scintillation crystals, they deposit energy, causing the crystals to emit light flashes (scintillation). The photodetectors detect this light. The scintillation light is converted into an electrical signal by the photodetectors. The amplitude of the electrical signal is proportional to the energy deposited by the annihilation photons in the scintillation crystals. Electronic circuits within the PET scanner amplify and process the electrical signal. This includes amplification, filtering, and digitization of the signal.

Some modern PET scanners incorporate time-of-flight measurement, which involves measuring the time it takes for the annihilation photons to travel from their emission point to the detectors. This information helps improve the spatial resolution and image quality of the PET system. PET event detection relies on detecting coincident events, which are pairs of photons detected almost simultaneously in different detector elements of the PET scanner. This indicates that the photons likely originated from the same annihilation event.

Data Acquisition and Image Reconstruction

The coincidence events, along with the corresponding timing and energy information, are recorded by the PET scanner's data acquisition system (DAS). This data forms the basis for image reconstruction and analysis. The recorded data is processed and reconstructed to create a three-dimensional image representing the radiotracer distribution in the body. Advanced algorithms, such as iterative reconstruction techniques, Ordered Subset Expectation Maximization (OSEM), Maximum Likelihood Expectation Maximization (MLEM), Time-of-Flight (TOF) Reconstruction, Model-Based Iterative Reconstruction (MBIR), etc., are used to estimate the activity distribution accurately.

PET event detection plays a crucial role in PET imaging as it allows for the localization of positron annihilation events and the reconstruction of images that reflect the distribution of radiotracer uptake in the body. The information obtained from PET event detection provides valuable insights into metabolic processes, organ function, and the presence of abnormal tissue, contributing to the diagnosis, staging, and monitoring of various diseases, including cancer, cardiovascular disorders, and neurological conditions.

7.5.6 PET-CT Data Acquisition

The data acquisition system (DAS) in a PET (positron emission tomography) scanner is responsible for capturing, digitizing, and processing the signals generated by the detectors during a PET imaging study. It is critical to acquire the necessary data for image reconstruction and analysis. Following are the components and functions of a typical PET DAS system:

- *Analog Front End*: The DAS begins with the analogue front end, which receives the electrical signals from the photodetectors or detector modules. This front end typically includes preamplifiers, amplifiers, and filters to amplify and condition the signals. It helps to boost the weak electrical signals and remove unwanted noise.
- *Analog-to-Digital Conversion*: The conditioned analogue signals from the front end are converted into digital signals by analogue-to-digital converters (ADCs). ADCs assign discrete digital values to the continuous analogue signals, allowing for further digital processing and storage of the data.
- *Time-to-Digital Conversion*: In PET scanners with time-of-flight (TOF) capability, time-to-digital converters (TDCs) measure the time difference between coincident photons arriving at different detectors. This information is crucial for improving spatial resolution and image quality.
- *Coincidence Detection*: The DAS detects coincident events, which are pairs of photons detected nearly simultaneously in different detector elements. This process involves comparing the timing information from different detector channels to identify coincidences. Coincident events indicate that the photons likely originated from the same positron annihilation event.
- *Coincidence Sorting*: The DAS sorts the detected coincidence events based on their timing and energy information. It identifies true coincidences (valid pairs of photons) and rejects random coincidences (accidental pairings of photons).
- *Data Buffering*: The DAS uses data buffers to temporarily store the detected event information before transferring it to the data processing and storage components. The buffer allows for efficient handling of the large amount of data generated by the PET scanner.
- *Data Transfer*: The DAS transfers the acquired event data to the computer system for further processing. This can be done through Ethernet, USB, or dedicated high-speed data transfer protocols.
- *Real-Time Monitoring and Quality Control*: The DAS provides real-time monitoring and quality control functionalities to ensure the proper functioning of the PET scanner. It continuously checks for system errors, detector malfunctions, and other issues that could affect data acquisition and image quality.
- *Triggering and Synchronization*: The DAS coordinates the timing and synchronization of various components within the PET scanner, including the detectors, data acquisition mod-

ules, and other subsystems. It ensures precise timing measurements and synchronization of events for accurate image reconstruction.

The data acquisition system is a crucial component of a PET scanner, responsible for collecting the raw data needed for image reconstruction and analysis. It requires high-speed processing capabilities, efficient data handling, and accurate event detection to produce reliable and high-quality PET images. Continuous advancements in DAS technology have led to improved imaging performance, faster acquisition times, and enhanced diagnostic capabilities in PET imaging.

7.5.7 PET-CT Instrumentation

The PET-CT (positron emission tomography-computed tomography) machine is housed with two components, viz., PET and the CT. The CT component has been discussed in detail in Chap. 6. Here, we will focus on PET components. The images are obtained sequentially from PET and CT parts and fused to give excellent images full of anatomical and physiological information. The fusion of PET and CT images allows for better localization and interpretation of abnormalities, improves diagnostic accuracy, and aids in treatment planning.

7.5.7.1 PET Scanner

The PET component of the instrumentation consists of a ring of detector modules surrounding the patient. Each module contains multiple scintillation crystals coupled to photomultiplier tubes (PMTs) or silicon photomultipliers (SiPMs). These detectors detect the gamma photons emitted from the radiotracer during positron decay, and a line of response (LOR) is generated within a coincidence timing window of usually 2–6 ns [10]. The timing and position information of the detected photons are recorded for image reconstruction. The scintillation detectors are discussed in Sect. 7.4.1. These detectors are crucial in determining the imaging performance, including spatial resolution, sensitivity, and image quality.

7.5.7.2 Coincidence Detection

PET relies on detecting two annihilation photons emitted in opposite directions during positron decay. To achieve this, PET detectors are arranged in pairs, each pair of detectors positioned on opposite sides of the patient. When a pair of detectors simultaneously detect the annihilation photons, it is called a coincidence event. PET can reconstruct the radiotracer distribution in the body by analyzing these coincidence events. While detecting coincidence, there can be scatter and random events apart from true events, which must be eliminated while reconstructing the final image.

7.5.7.3 Events in PET

The line of responses represents the imaginary line connecting the two detectors that detected the coincident photons. It does not directly provide information about the location of annihilation photon generation within the patient's body. Instead, collecting many lines of response from different detector pairs forms a projection dataset, which, combined with sophisticated reconstruction algorithms, generates the final PET image. While generating a line of responses, different types of events are detected and recorded during the imaging process. The main types of events in PET technology are:

True Coincidence Events

True coincidence occurs when both annihilation photons produced by the positron-electron annihilation are detected almost simultaneously in two different detectors of the PET system.

These events represent the desired signals that provide information about the radiotracer distribution within the patient's body. True coincidence events are used for image reconstruction and quantifying radiotracer uptake in specific regions of interest.

Random Coincidence Events

Random coincidence occurs when two unrelated photons from different annihilation events are detected within a certain time window (Fig. 7.10). These events do not correspond to true positron annihilation and can introduce

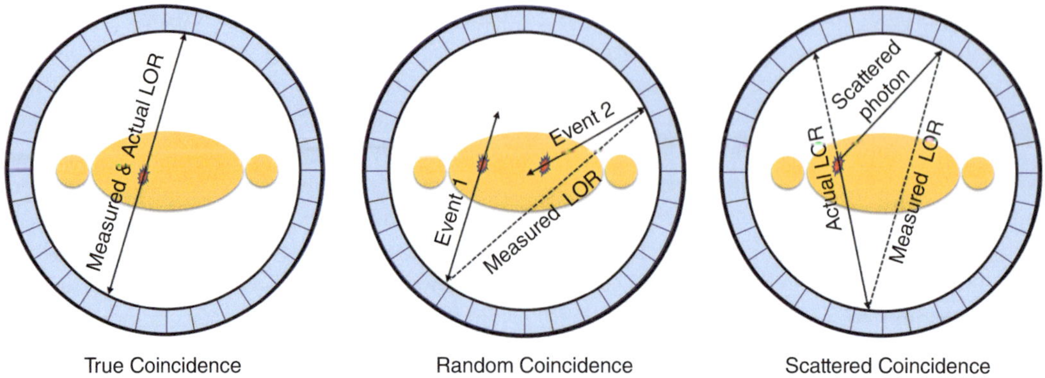

Fig. 7.10 Scatter, random, and true events measured during the PET scan

noise and degrade image quality if not properly accounted for. Random coincidence events are caused by the random arrival times of the annihilation photons and are more likely to occur in areas with high activity levels. Various techniques, such as time-of-flight (TOF) information and random event subtraction algorithms, are employed to reduce the impact of random coincidences on image quality.

Scatter Events

Scatter events occur when one or both annihilation photons undergo Compton scattering within the patient's body before being detected. Scatter events can introduce inaccuracies and distortions in the reconstructed PET image as they result in erroneous information about the location of the radiotracer distribution. Sophisticated correction algorithms compensate for scatter events and improve image accuracy.

Single Events

Single events occur when only one annihilation photon is detected by a PET detector without a corresponding detection in another detector. Single events can arise due to incomplete photon detection or the escape of one annihilation photon from the field of view. Single events are generally not used in image reconstruction and are usually discarded or accounted for in the data analysis.

Accurate identification and characterization of these event types are essential for proper image reconstruction, image artifact correction, and quantifying radiotracer uptake in PET imaging. Various algorithms and techniques are employed to optimize image quality and minimize the impact of random coincidences and other events on the final PET image.

7.5.8 Detector, Detector Block, Sizes, and Shape

A detector refers to the individual unit or crystal responsible for detecting and measuring the annihilation photons emitted during PET imaging, whereas a detector block, also known as a module or panel, is a combination of multiple individual detectors arranged in a specific configuration. PET technology utilizes various size detector elements and blocks depending on the specific PET system design and application. The crystals used in PET detectors are typically cuboid or rectangular. The overall shape of a PET detector can be a circular ring (or rings) made up of detector blocks, and detector blocks are a combination of various crystals (Fig. 7.11). However, organ-specific PET cameras can have different shapes depending on the need. The precise sizes of crystals and blocks can differ among different PET systems, manufacturers, and research advancements. Table 7.4 provides various scintillation crystals, sizes, and other performance parameters of various PET-CT machines.

Detector Blocks

Detector blocks are composed of multiple detector elements arranged in a specific configuration. These blocks are used to capture and measure the

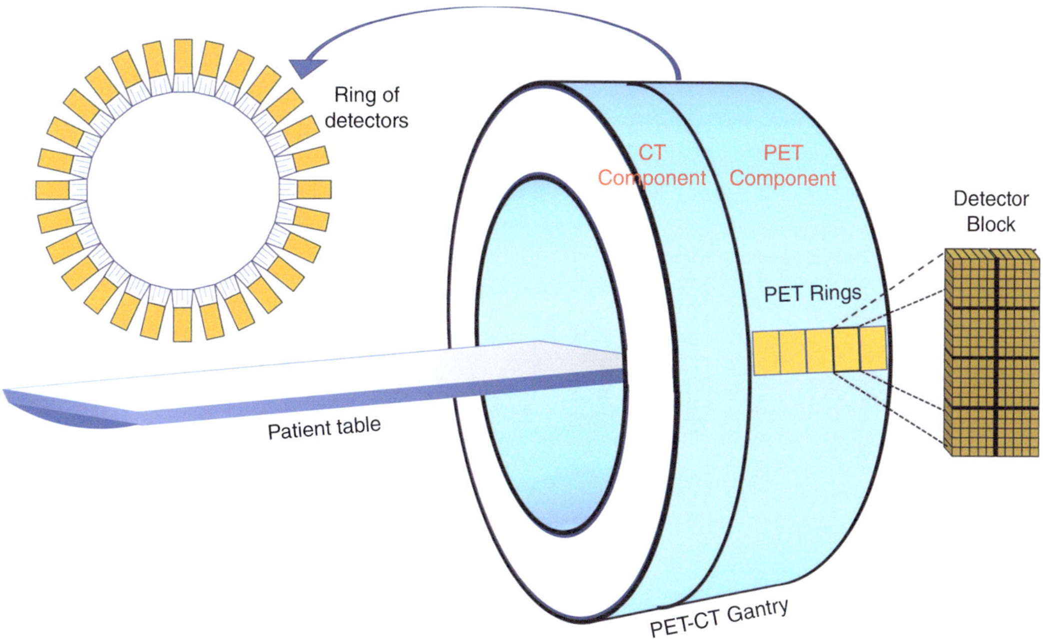

Fig. 7.11 PET-CT gantry, ring of detectors, and detector block

annihilation photons more efficiently. The dimensions of detector blocks can vary, but they are typically a few centimeters in width, length, and height. The block size may depend on the specific PET system and the desired balance between sensitivity, spatial resolution, and timing resolution. They can be arranged in different configurations, such as rectangular, square, or hexagonal, to optimize the overall system performance. The selection of specific sizes depends on factors such as the desired spatial resolution, sensitivity, cost considerations, and the specific application of the PET system (e.g., whole-body imaging, dedicated organ imaging, or preclinical research). Advancements in detector technology, such as small pixel sizes, improved crystal materials, and high-resolution photodetectors, continue to push the limits of PET imaging capabilities, enabling higher spatial resolution and improved image quality.

7.5.9 2D Versus 3D PET

Most scanners made before the early 1990s, with a few exceptions, had lead septa between the detector rings that limited the contributions of random coincidences and scattered photons (within the object), but it caused low geometric sensitivity and long scan times since only true coincidence events detected within a series of 2D slices could be detected [17]. Operating in 3D mode by removing septa increases the sensitivity of true coincidences by five to ten times (Fig. 7.12). However, this significantly increases random and scattered events, requiring careful correction [17]. All PET-CT systems operate in 3D mode, with no septa between the detectors.

7.5.10 Axial-Paired (3D) Detector Ring

In this arrangement, PET detectors are positioned in a continuous ring around the patient, similar to the axial arrangement. However, each detector module in the ring consists of multiple detector elements or crystal elements. The crystal elements are arranged axially in a segmented fashion. This 3D arrangement allows for more precise localization of the annihilation events along the axial direction, improving sensitivity and image quality.

Table 7.4 Specifications of various make and models of PET-CT machines

PET-CT make and model	GE discovery IQ	GE discovery MI	Siemens biograph vision	Phillips ingenuity TF	United uMI550
Crystal	BGO	LYSO	LSO	LYSO	LYSO
Crystal size (mm^2)	6.3 × 6.3	3.95 × 5.3	3.2 × 3.2	4 × 4	2.76 × 2.76
Crystal depth	30 mm	25 mm	20 mm	22 mm	16.3 mm
Number of crystals	19,200	40,352 (3 rings), 48,672 (4 rings) [11]	32,448	28,336	34,560
Patient port size (cm)	70	70 [12]	78	70	70
Coincidence window (ns)	9.5	4.9	3.9	4.5	4.0
Detector type	PMT	SiPM	SiPM	PMT	SiPM
No. of PMTs	720	–	–	420	–
Physical axial field of view (cm)	26 cm (5 rings)	20 cm (3 rings), 26 cm (5 rings)	21.8 cm	19.7 cm	24 cm
Spatial resolution Tangential/radial/axial (1 cm offset from the FOV center)	4.7/4.2/4.8 mm [13]	4.3/4.3/5 mm [13]	3.7/3.5/3.6 mm [13]	4.8/4.8/4.9 mm [14]	2.9/3/3 mm [13]
Timing resolution (ps)	Non-TOF	381.7	178 [15]	495 [16]	372

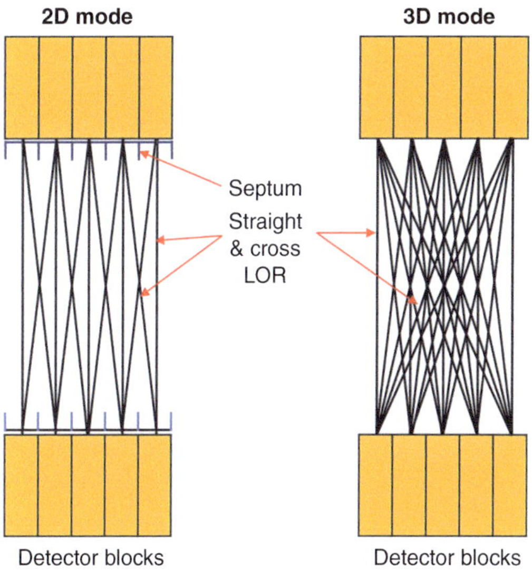

Fig. 7.12 2D and 3D modes of acquisition

7.5.11 Time-of-Flight (TOF) Detection

TOF PET systems incorporate additional timing information to improve image quality and resolution. In this arrangement, the PET detectors are equipped with timing electronics that measure the time difference between detecting the two annihilation photons. By knowing the time-of-flight of the photons, the location of the annihilation event can be determined more accurately, resulting in improved spatial resolution and image quality.

7.5.12 Total Body PET Scanners with Whole-Body Coverage

PET systems are designed to provide whole-body coverage, enabling imaging of the entire patient from head to toe. Conventionally, PET acquisition is carried out by moving bed positions. Each bed position is equal to the axial field of view of the PET system. This is between 16 cm and 26 cm coverage in many PET systems. This allows 8–10 bed position movements for an average-height patient in the vertex to mid-thigh scan range. Nowadays, "*total-body PET scanners*," also known as whole-body PET scanners, are designed by vendors to capture images of the entire body in a single scan. They have a long axial field of view (AFOV) that allows for the coverage of a large portion of the patient's body. This extended AFOV enables imaging from the top of the head to the feet without needing multiple scans or repositioning the patient. The AFOVs are between 1 and 2 m, showing a tremendous increase in system sensitivity and allowing short-term, low-dose, and dynamic total body imaging and new examination methods in almost all areas of imaging [18] (Fig. 7.13).

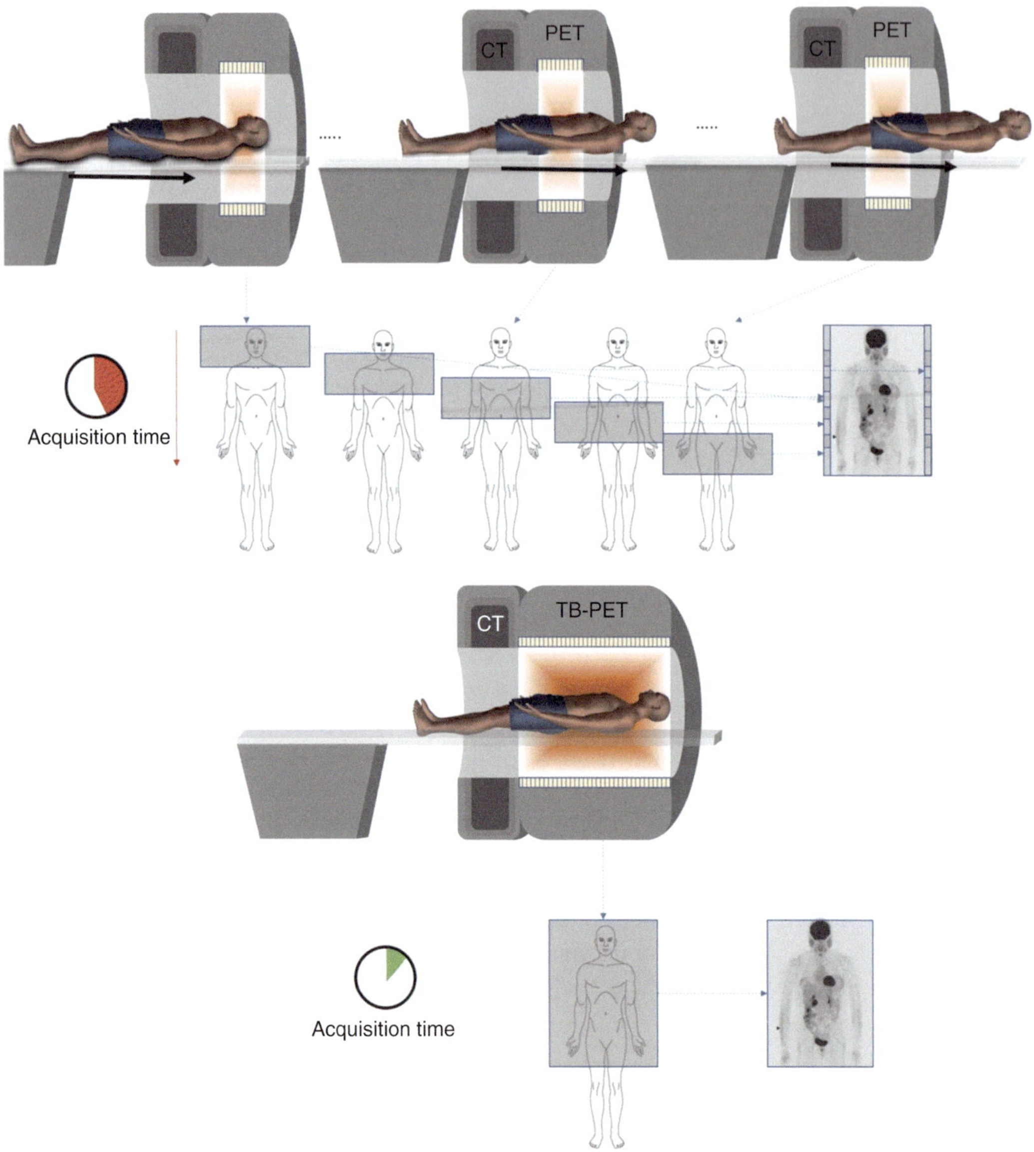

Fig. 7.13 Comparing a current PET-CT to a total body PET-CT (top and bottom figures). It is no longer necessary to scan the body in various bed positions. The broader solid angle coverage (shown by the shading) inside the total body PET FOV results in increased sensitivity for all areas in the FOV. Due to the greater sensitivity, the overall acquisition time can be drastically decreased for the same activity injected into the patient [19]. (Image copyright: Vandenberghe et al. [19]. Reprinted under Creative Commons CC BY license)

7.6 Performance Characteristics and Quality Control in PET-CT

Performance characteristics of PET-CT are performed annually, half-yearly, quarterly, weekly, and daily, depending upon the manufacturer's recommendation. A baseline performance is set at the time of the acceptance test, and after that, periodic assessment gives any deviation from its initial assessment. The NEMA (National Electrical Manufacturers Association), which develops and publishes standards, guidelines, and technical documents to promote standardization and ensure the safety, reliability, and compatibility of various electrical and imaging products, provides guidelines and criteria to assess the performance characteristics of PET systems.

The first NEMA standard addressing PET systems was NEMA NU 2-1994, titled "Performance Measurements of Scanners for Positron Emission Tomography." It was published in 1994 and served as a foundational document for evaluating the performance characteristics of PET scanners. Subsequently, this guideline was revised to keep pace with recent advancements in PET technologies. The revised documents were published in documents NU 2-2001, NU 2-2007, and NU 2-2012, and the recent recommendations were published in NU 2-2018. These standards help ensure consistency and comparability between different PET scanners.

The NEMA standards cover various aspects of PET system performance, including spatial resolution, sensitivity, count rate performance, image quality, and accuracy. Here are some key NEMA characteristics of PET.

7.6.1 Spatial Resolution

The term "spatial resolution" says resolution in "space." It refers to the ability of an imaging system to distinguish and resolve small structures or details in space. It measures the system's ability to differentiate between two closely spaced objects or detect the smallest discernible feature size. It is particularly important for accurately visualizing and distinguishing small anatomical structures or lesions.

The spatial resolution of PET is affected by several factors and primarily by the physical size of the detector element although other factors, including acollinearity, positron range, penetration into the detector ring, and decoding errors in the detector modules, play an important role in determining overall system resolution. Statistical noise and sampling geometry also reduce the effective resolution even more [20].

Table 7.5 describes the detector sizes of different PET scanners available these days, which plays a major limiting role in determining system spatial resolution. However, any system cannot achieve better spatial resolution than the positron range of a particular radionuclide as this much blurring will always be present in PET images. The ejected positron from the nucleus possesses kinetic energy and travels some distance before combining with an electron, forming positronium, which decays to a pair of annihilation photons of 511 keV. The detection is carried out for the annihilation of photons, whereas the origin of the positron is somewhere else, probably a distance away mentioned in Table 7.5.

The NEMA standards for spatial resolution in PET (positron emission tomography) primarily involve point sources. This standard defines the minimum detectable size of sources and provides metrics such as full width at half maximum (FWHM) to quantify the spatial resolution. It is a simplified measure of spatial resolution and provides a useful summary of system performance. While FWHM is a commonly used metric, it may not fully capture all aspects of spatial resolution.

A point source is a small radioactive source that emits radiation, for example, positrons (in the case of PET) or other form of radiation. It is used to simulate a single point of emission within the imaging field. In an ideal imaging system, a point source would produce a perfectly sharp and localized image representing a true point in space. However, due to various factors such as

Table 7.5 Properties of commonly used PET isotopes

Isotope	Half-life	Branching (β^+) in %	E_{max} (MeV)	E_{mean} (MeV)	Range$_{max}$ (mm)	Range$_{mean}$ (mm)
^{11}C	20.4 min	99.8	0.960	0.386	4.2	1.2
^{13}N	10.0 min	99.8	1.199	0.492	5.5	1.8
^{15}O	2 min	99.9	1.732	0.735	8.4	3.0
^{18}F	110 min	96.9	0.634	0.250	2.4	0.6
^{64}Cu	12.7 h	17.5	0.653	0.278	2.5	0.7
^{89}Zr	78.4 h	22.7	0.902	0.396	3.8	1.3

Table originally printed in Springer Nature by Maurizio Conti et al. [21]. Reprinted under Creative Commons CC BY license

detector size and efficiency, depth of interaction on the detector with photon, limitation of electronics, positron range, scattering, reconstruction algorithms, or other system imperfections, the detected events are not confined to a single point but are spread out or blurred to some extent.

The blurred image of the point source is called the point spread function, and it represents the spreading or blurring of the detected events originating from the point source in the PET image. The point spread function characterizes the shape and extent of the response to a point source. It explains how the system detects and localizes the emitted photons and how the reconstructed PET image represents the spatial information.

By analyzing the point spread function, one can understand the system's ability to resolve small structures, quantify the blurring effect, and assess the overall spatial resolution of the PET system. The width of the point spread function, often measured as the full width at half maximum (FWHM) and full width at tenth maximum (FWTM), is an important parameter used to characterize the system's spatial resolution. Both parameters are important as the same FWHM can have different FWTM (Fig. 7.14). A smaller FWHM indicates better spatial resolution, implying that the blurring effect is minimal and the details in the image are more distinct.

The spatial resolution is expressed in length units (e.g., millimeters) and represents the minimum discernible separation between two objects in the image. A smaller FWHM or FWTM corresponds to higher spatial resolution and the ability to distinguish smaller details in the image.

The FWHM and FWTM are measured for all three directions, for example, axial, radial, and tangential (Fig. 7.14). The axial direction is typically aligned with the *z*-axis of the imaging system. The radial direction is perpendicular to the imaging plane and extends from the center of the field of view toward the periphery, whereas the tangential direction is parallel to the imaging plane and lies within the plane itself. Three-point sources are prepared, and point sources must be less than 1 mm in axial length. If the source is longer than 1 mm, it will give falsely larger FWHM, reducing spatial resolution. 185 mega becquerels (MBq) of 18F-FDG are taken in 1 mL, and multiple 1 mm droplets on created on the plastic surface. Droplets are picked up in capillary tubes with the open end sealed with sealing clay (Fig. 7.15). Three similar-sized capillary tubes are picked and fixed gently in the holder and then on the patient's couch (Fig. 7.15).

Using the laser positioning system, locate the isocenter of the scanner (0, 0) cm by using a capillary tube positioning device to place the three-point sources at either location at (0, 1), (0, 10), and (10, 0) cm (NEMA NU 2-2007) or (0, 1), (0, 10), and (0, 20) cm (NEMA NU 2-2012) (Fig. 7.18). The variance in positioning of point sources in *X–Y–Z* values should be below ±1.0 mm (Fig. 7.17). Acquire the scan and analyze the spatial

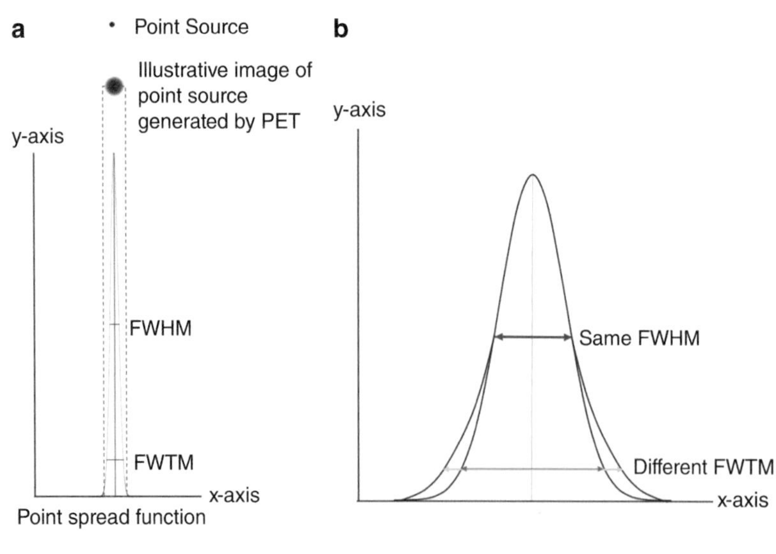

Fig. 7.14 An illustrative depiction of point spread function, FWHM, and FWTM. Image (**a**) shows the point spread function of the point source generated by an imaging device (imaginary—to make the reader understand the concept). Image (**b**) shows same FWHM can have different FWTM and describes why both measurements are important

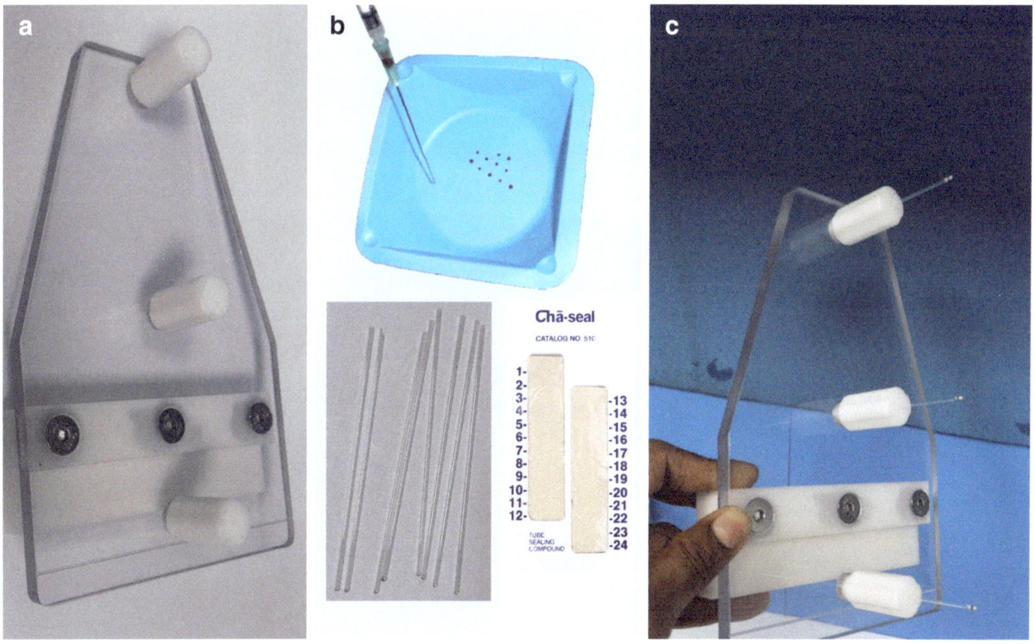

Fig. 7.15 Point source holder and source preparation. (**a**) Custom-designed acrylic point source holder with three mounting positions for source alignment, (**b**) Materials used for source preparation, such as capillary tubes, sealing compound for radioactive source containment and dripping to radioactivity to pick in capillary tube, (**c**) Assembled point source holder with prepared sources mounted in position, ready for experimental use

resolution scans with a minimum of 500K counts. A typical spatial resolution report generated by a PET system is shown in Fig. 7.16. For more detailed information, NEMA NU2-2018-Performance Measurements of Positron Emission Tomography [22], The American Association of Physicists in Medicine (AAPM) report 126 (2019)-PET/CT Acceptance Testing and Quality Assurance [23], and the manufacturer manual may be referred.

7.6.2 Sensitivity

Sensitivity measures the ability of the PET system to detect and accurately quantify the radiotracer activity in the patient. Higher sensitivity allows for detecting lower levels of radioactivity, which is particularly important for imaging small lesions or areas of low tracer uptake. Sensitivity is typically measured using a uniform cylindrical phantom containing a known activity of a radioactive source. The NEMA standard specifies the acquisition parameters and provides guidelines for calculating sensitivity in counts per second per unit activity.

Several factors, including the design of the detectors, the efficiency of the scintillation crystals, the distance between the detectors and the patient, and the use of appropriate collimation or shielding, can influence the sensitivity of a PET-CT system. Advances in detector technology, such as using lutetium-based scintillators, can enhance sensitivity.

The sensitivity of PET scanners is typically measured using a uniform cylindrical aluminum sleeve of varying diameter that contains a known activity of a radioactive source placed inside those sleeves as a line source (five different-sized metal tubes and a fillable line source) (Fig. 7.17). The phantom is positioned centered in the scanner's field of view, and data is acquired starting with a thinner sleeve (inner diameter 3.9 mm, outer diameter 6.4 mm, length 700 mm). Specifications of each aluminum sleeve and tubing placed inside these sleeves are mentioned in Table 7.6. Subsequently, each sleeve is added one

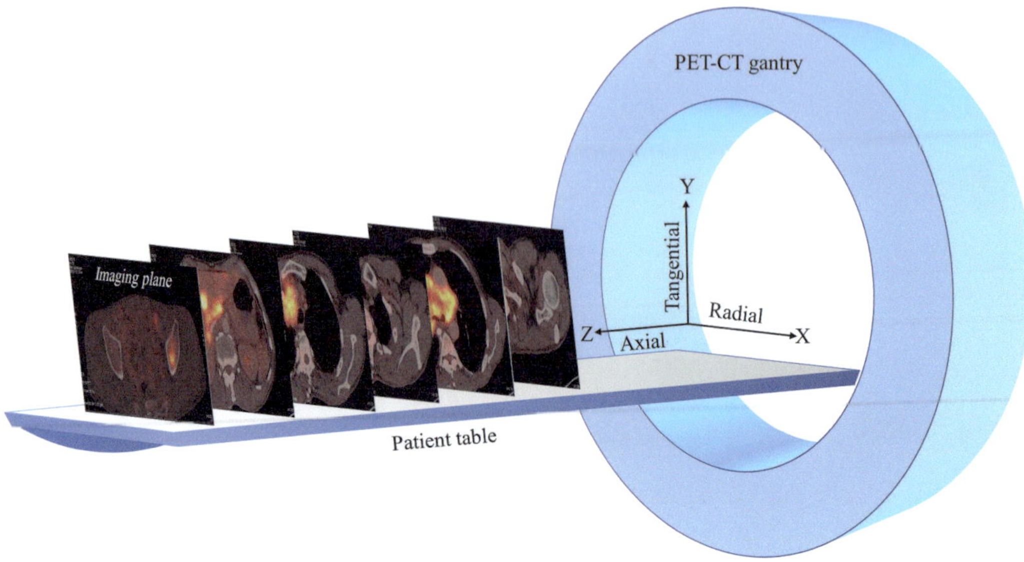

Fig. 7.16 Axial, radial, and tangential directions in PET-CT machine

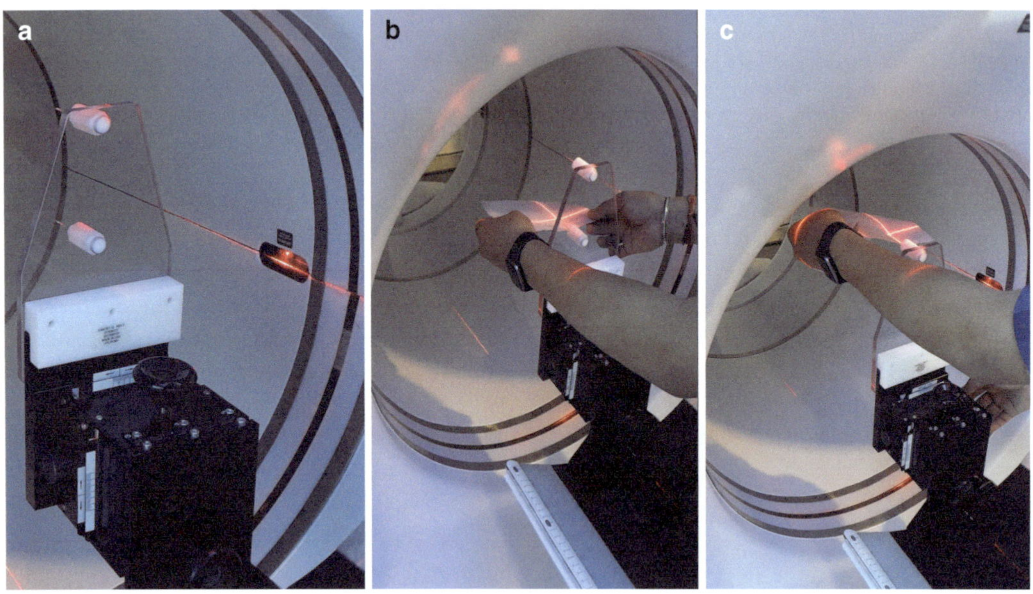

Fig. 7.17 Positioning of point sources for spatial resolution test. (**a**) Point source holder mounted on the scanner bed and aligned with the scanner's laser positioning system. (**b**) Manual adjustment of the point source position along the axial direction for precise alignment. (**c**) Final verification of point source placement using laser cross-hairs before initiating the scan

by one, with all five sleeves on top of each other, and counts are recorded with varying thickness of attenuating material.

The test is conducted at such low activity levels that count losses are negligible, i.e., dead time loss and random coincidence rate is less than 5% of total prompts (total detected coincidence events) [23]. The scanner's sensitivity is calculated using extrapolation to give the scanner sensitivity having no attenuation material. The randoms are subtracted from the prompts to generate results that reflect true sensitivity alone.

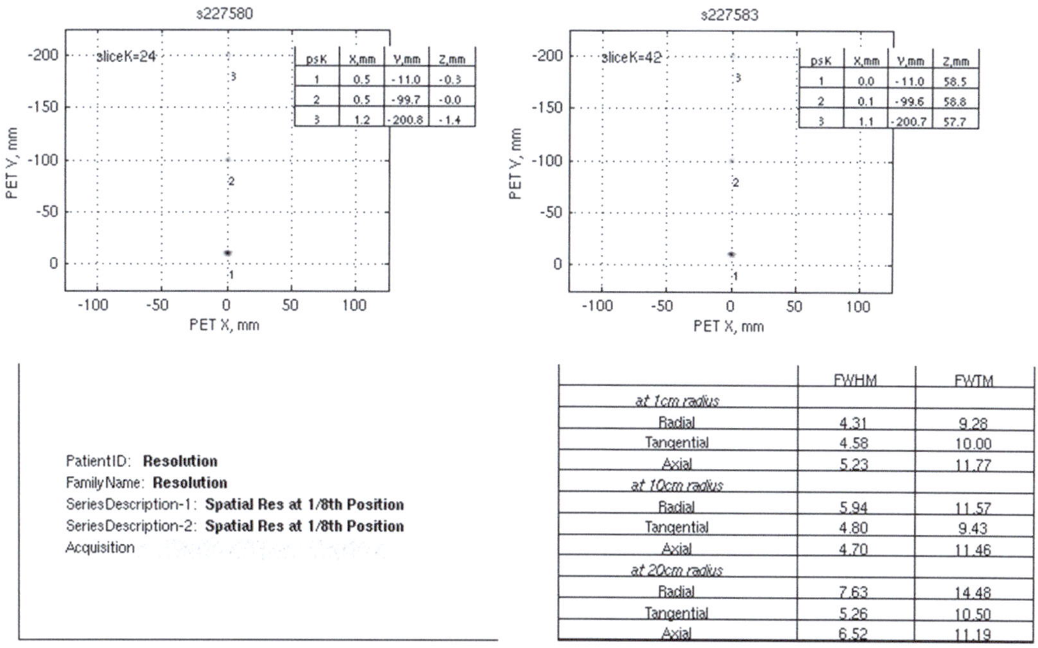

	FWHM	FWTM
at 1cm radius		
Radial	4.31	9.28
Tangential	4.58	10.00
Axial	5.23	11.77
at 10cm radius		
Radial	5.94	11.57
Tangential	4.80	9.43
Axial	4.70	11.46
at 20cm radius		
Radial	7.63	14.48
Tangential	5.26	10.50
Axial	6.52	11.19

Fig. 7.18 Typical spatial resolution report generated by a PET system

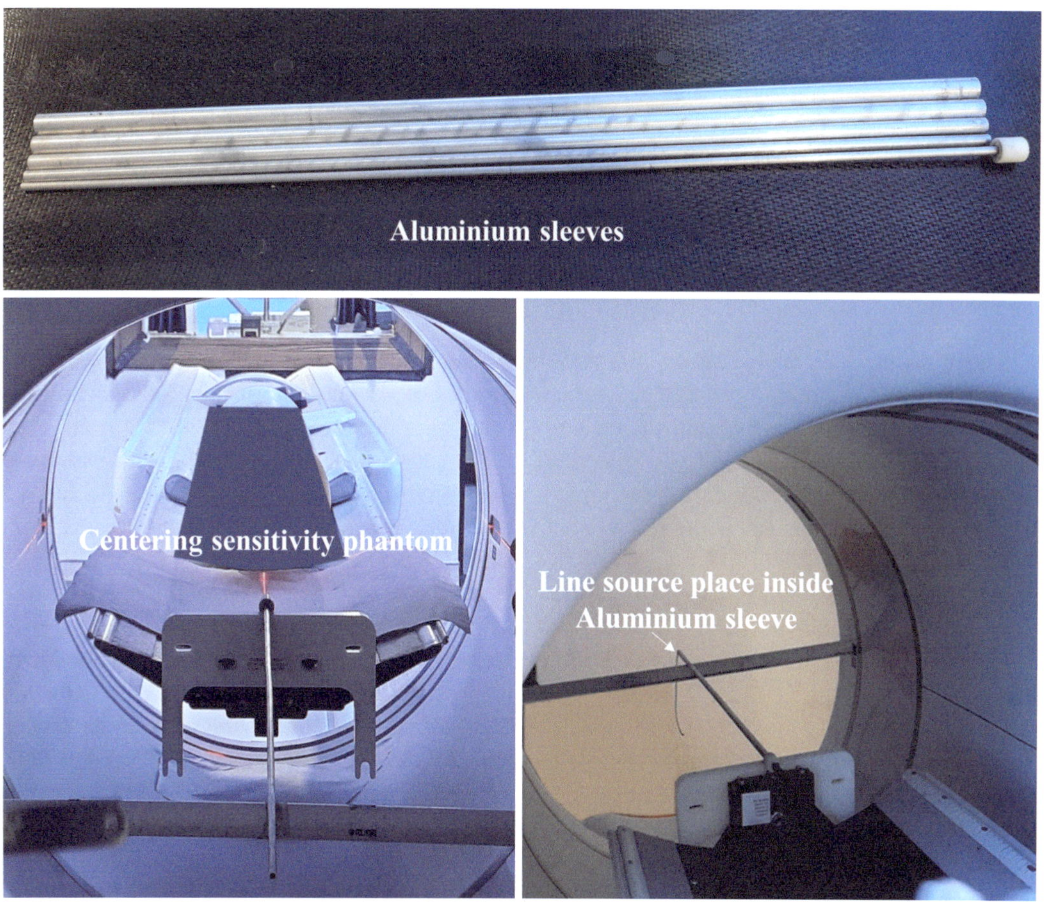

Fig. 7.19 Sensitivity measurement

Table 7.6 Specifications of each aluminum sleeve and tubing inside these sleeves

Sleeve number (all with length 700 mm)	Inner diameter (mm)	Outer diameter (mm)
1st	3.9	6.4
2nd	7.0	9.5
3rd	10.2	12.7
4th	13.4	15.9
5th tube	16.6	19.1
The innermost tube, a fillable polyethene tubing	1	3

The sensitivity measurements are made with differing amounts of attenuating material, with the results extrapolated to give the scanner sensitivity with no attenuating material. The randoms are subtracted from prompts to obtain true-only sensitivity results. The activity should be between 1 and 4 MBq to produce no more than 5% randoms but sufficient to produce measurable results. Manufacturers recommend starting with a higher activity (e.g., 20 MBq) and waiting until the activity decays to below 4 MBq as most dose calibrators have a larger error at the lower line to decay.

The unit of sensitivity is typically expressed as counts per second per unit activity (cps/kBq) .

In Fig. 7.20, the graph shows (a) acquired counts with the thinnest sleeve on and, subsequently, a linear fall in counts by adding more attenuating material (adding more sleeves) and (b) shows the sensitivity measurement in axial profile width at fine axial intervals.

Sensitivity can vary depending on the scanner design, detector technology, energy resolution, system geometry, and image reconstruction algorithms. Additionally, sensitivity can be influenced by acquisition parameters such as the energy window settings, coincidence timing window, and acquisition duration. Therefore, sensitivity measurements are usually performed periodically as part of quality control procedures to ensure the scanner performs optimally.

7.6.3 Scatter Fraction, Count Losses, and Randoms

Scatter Fraction and Count Losses: Scatter fraction refers to the fraction of scattered events in the acquired PET data, which can degrade image quality. Count losses are the loss of true coincidence events due to random coincidences, dead time, and detector inefficiencies. These factors contribute to reduced count statistics and affect image quality.

Random coincidences occur when two unrelated gamma photons are detected as a coincidence event. Randoms contribute to noise in PET data and can lead to image degradation. Randoms can be estimated and corrected for during image reconstruction.

The PET scanner's scatter fraction and count rate performance are measured using the scatter phantom, which is 70 cm long and 20 cm in diameter, made of polyethene and cylindrical shape (Fig. 7.21). The scatter phantom is filled with a polyethene plastic tube filled with 800–900 MBq (~25 mCi) FDG that was 70 cm long in ~5 mL volume, and this line is thicker than the one used for NEMA sensitivity (3 mL). The line source insert was parallel to the phantom's central axis and 45 mm radially displaced from the center of the phantom. Additionally, the phantom is turned so that the line source is closest to the patient's bed.

The scatter phantom is positioned in the patient's bed in the center of the field of view (FOV) and aligned with laser light at the center of the FOV. Enter the pre- and post-injection details with the source volume as 22,000 mL. The acquisition protocol is designed to contain the appropriate number of frames for the total scan time. There is a total of 34-time frames in PET scan methodology with 20 frames of 15 min each, 11 frames of 25 min but 25 min pause before the start of acquisition, and the final 3 frames are 25 min each (this protocol is set in GE Discovery IQ systems, may vary with other manufacturers). The total duration of the study is 15 h 25 min (Fig. 7.22). During the initial 20 frames of 15 min each, the count rate is high, and scatter and true coincidences are detected. The count rate decreases significantly during the subsequent frames due to radioactive decay. This reduction in count rate leads to a decrease in scatter events, making their contribution negligible. The scatter fraction can be accurately calculated by comparing the scatter-free data with the scatter-inclusive data acquired under similar conditions but with reduced scatter events (Fig. 7.23).

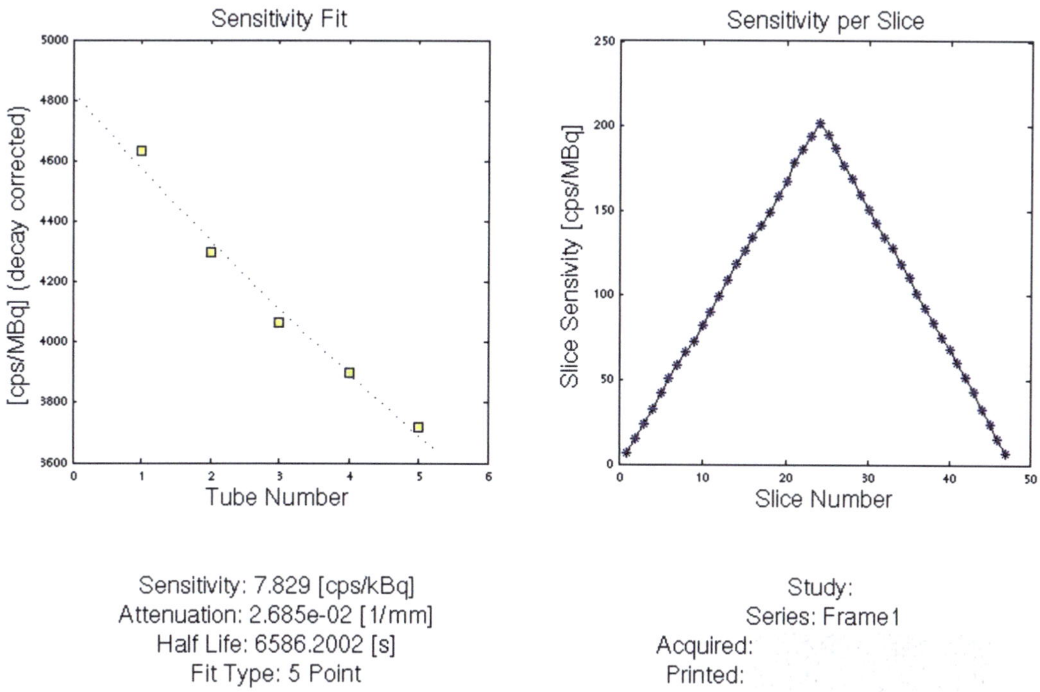

Fig. 7.20 Sensitivity measurement of a typical PET scanner at the center

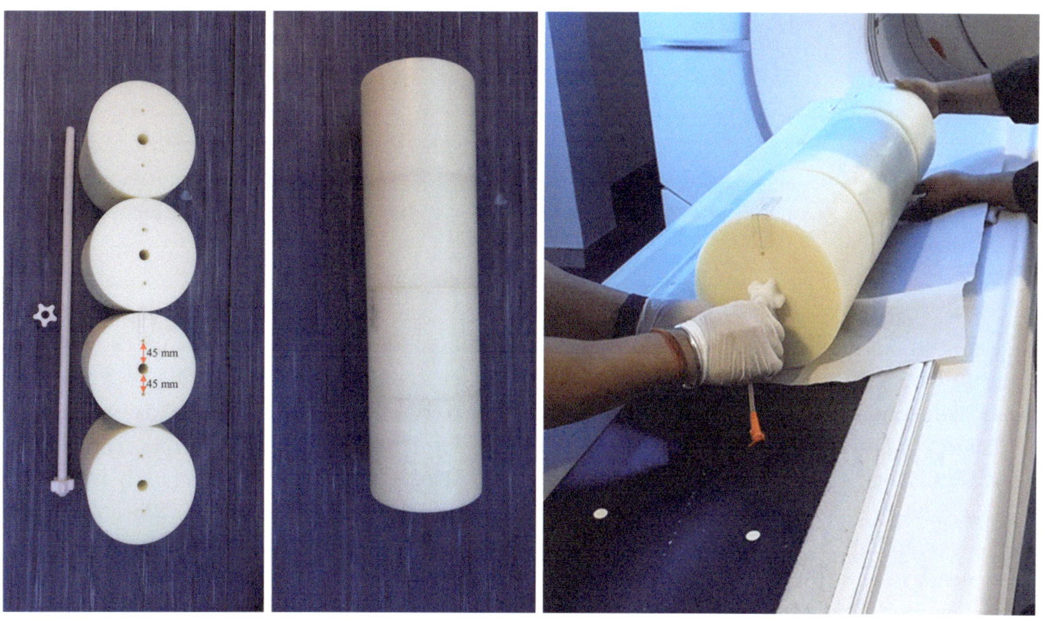

Fig. 7.21 Scatter phantom polyethene phantom with line source insertion

The list mode data is obtained during each time frame and histogrammed into prompt and delayed sinograms using SSRB (single-slice rebinning), and the noise equivalent count (NEC) rates (total, true, random, scatter, and so forth) are calculated [12]. Single-slice rebinning is a data processing technique used in PET imaging to reduce data storage requirements and process-

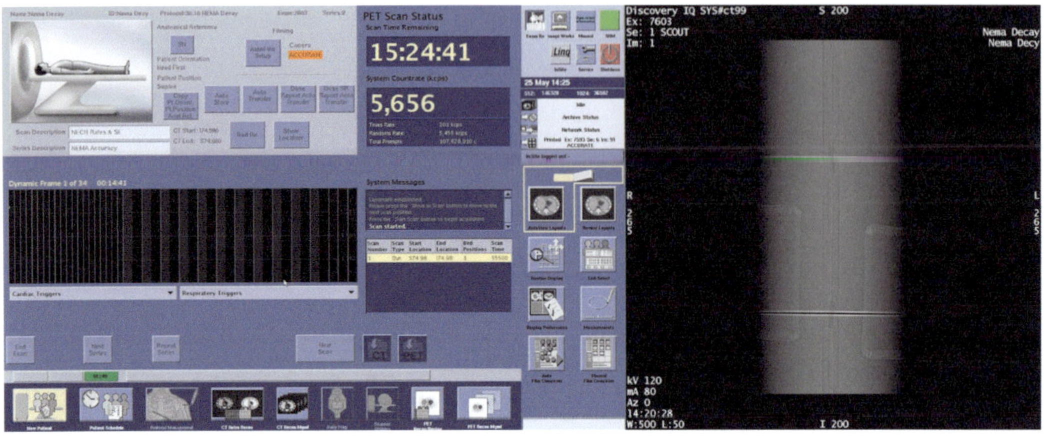

Fig. 7.22 Scatter fraction and count rate performance acquisition

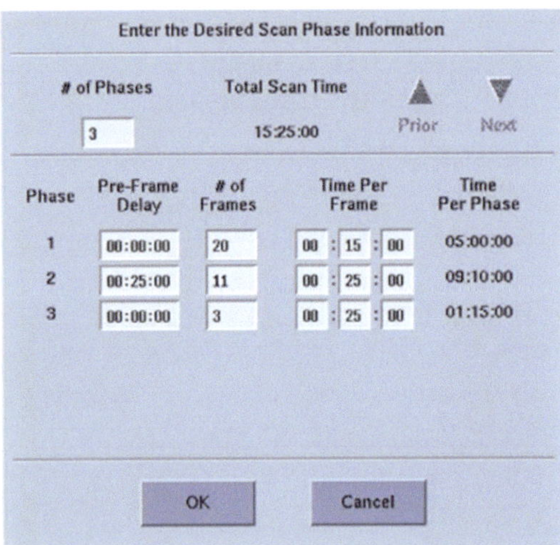

Fig. 7.23 Scan protocol of scatter fraction

ing time while preserving image quality. It combines the data from multiple detector elements in the axial direction to create a single virtual slice.

The report provides various values, including Noise Equivalent Count Rate (NECR), scatter fraction, and peak true count rate. It plots the graph containing the total Prompts, Noise Equivalent Counts (NECs), Trues, Randoms, and Scatter events. The *Noise Equivalent Counts (NECs)* refer to the counts equivalent to the noise level in the acquired data. It represents the statistical fluctuations in the data and depends on true, scatter, and random count rates (kcps), the fraction of the FOV subtended by the phantom, and the k factor that depends on the random counts correction technique ($k = 1$ for noiseless random counts estimate, such as estimating random counts from single photon rates; $k = 2$ for noisy random counts estimate) (AAPM report 126) [23]. Most new PET scanners have $k = 1$ value, but checking with the vendor for the appropriate k-value will be more helpful.

$$\mathrm{NEC} = \frac{R_T^2}{R_T + R_S + \left(k \times f \times R_R\right)} \tag{7.2}$$

where R_T, R_S, and R_R are true, scatter, and random counts, k is the random counts correction factor, and f is the fraction of FOV subtended by the phantom (Fig. 7.24).

The graph typically shows the count rates or counts per unit time on the *Y*-axis and the activity concentration or count rate on the *X*-axis. The scatter fraction and NECR (Noise Equivalent Count Rate) are typically plotted as functions of activity concentration or count rate. The specific axis labels and data representation may vary depending on the test setup and reporting format, but here is a general explanation:

7.6.3.1 Scatter Fraction

The *X-axis* shows activity concentration or count rate (e.g., in kilo becquerels per milliliter or counts per second), whereas the *Y-axis* plots the scatter fraction (expressed as a percentage). The scatter fraction is calculated as the ratio of scatter coincidences to total true coincidences. The plot

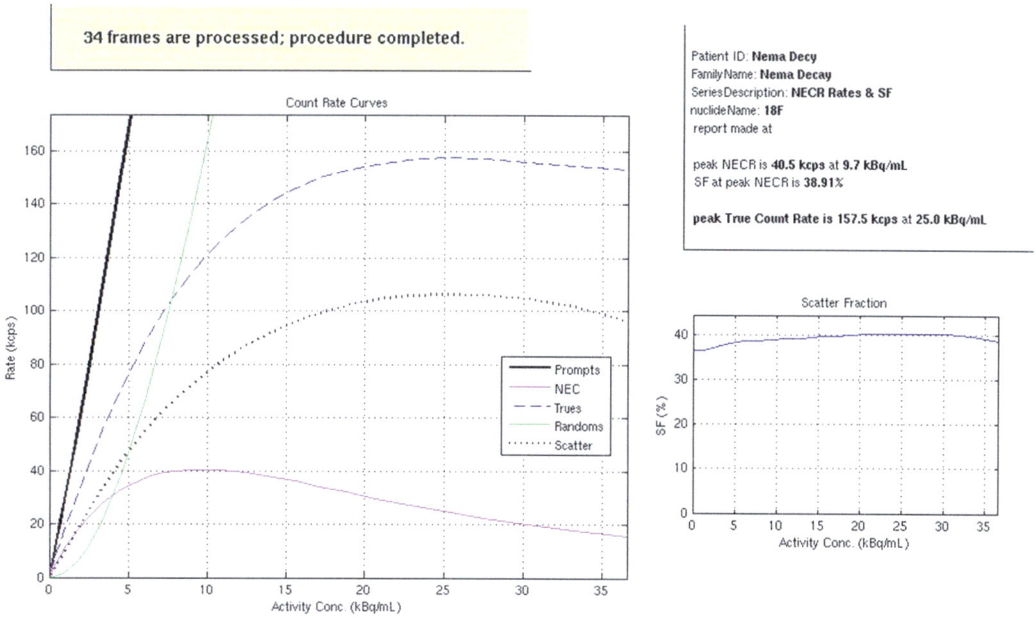

Fig. 7.24 Scatter fraction results

Table 7.7 Scatter fraction

Description	Measured	Reference	Tolerance
Scatter fraction (3D mode) in %	38.91	≤44	≤1.05 of reference

Table 7.8 Noise Equivalent Count Rate

Description	Measured	Reference	Tolerance
Peak NECR (kcps) in 3D mode	40.5	≥32.8	≥0.95 of reference
Activity (MBq) at which peak NECR is achieved in 3D mode	9.7	≤11	≥0.95 of reference

shows how the scatter fraction varies with activity concentrations or count rates. It helps evaluate the impact of scatter on image quality and quantification, with lower scatter fractions indicating better image quality.

7.6.3.2 NECR (Noise Equivalent Count Rate)

The *X*-axis describes activity concentration or count rate (e.g., in kilo becquerels per milliliter or counts per second), whereas the *Y*-axis shows NECR (expressed in counts per second or minute). The NECR represents the maximum count rate at which the signal-to-noise ratio remains acceptable. The plot shows the relationship between the count rate and the corresponding NECR values. The goal is to achieve a high NECR, indicating a high count rate capability while maintaining acceptable image quality.

The NECR should be greater than or equal to the manufacturer's specification, while the scatter fraction should be lower. Tables 7.7 and 7.8 describes the typical result of the PET system for scatter fraction and Noise Equivalent Count Rate.

> ? The scatter fraction phantom is 70 cm long, and the sensitivity phantom is again 70 cm long. What is the significance of 70 cm in PET quality control?

The 70 cm-long phantom approximates the activity distribution in whole-body imaging because the effects of out-of-field activity (OFA) are included in the performance measurement [24]. While the actual length of patients may vary, using a standardized length of 70 cm allows for consistent measurements and comparisons across different PET scanners. It serves as a reference for evaluating system performance and optimizing imaging protocols. These measurements aim not to precisely mimic every patient but to provide a standardized approach for assessing and comparing system performance.

Notably, the 70 cm length specifically refers to the axial dimension (*z* direction) of the phantoms used in these measurements, not the *xy*-plane. This choice is a result of consensus and standardization efforts within the field. The specific value of 70 cm was likely determined through practical considerations and agreement among researchers, manufacturers, and regulatory bodies involved in developing the NEMA standards.

7.6.4 Image Quality, Accuracy of Attenuation and Scatter Correction, and Accuracy of Radioactivity Quantitation

An image-simulating phantom, called image quality phantom, which includes hot and cold lesions with nonuniform attenuation, is used to assess the actual image quality in clinical conditions. However, the NEMA NU 2-2018 rules out the cold spheres, and as per new recommendations, all six spheres will be hotter [25]. The image quality is assessed by calculating image contrast and background variability ratios for hot and cold spheres [26]. This test also assesses the accuracy of the absolute quantification of radioactivity concentration in the uniform volume of interest inside the phantom. Three replicates of this test should be performed to improve the reliability of the results.

The image quality phantom mimics internal structures, contains three rods and six spheres, and comprises poly (methyl methacrylate) or PMMA material. It has an exterior length of ~217 mm, interior length of ~193 mm, and 18 cm in interior length to cover the whole axial field of view of PET. The six hollow spheres have internal diameters of 10 mm, 13 mm, 17 mm, 22 mm, 28 mm, and 37 cm, and the wall thickness is ~1 mm (Fig. 7.25). At the center, a cylindrical insert with a 5.0 ± 0.2 cm outer diameter is filled with low atomic number material to mimic lung attenuation with an average density of 0.3 ± 0.1 g/mL and extends axially through the entire phantom.

This test necessitates the employment of a second phantom in addition to the image quality phantom to simulate out-of-field radiation. The 70 cm-long scatter phantom with the off-center line source, previously used to calculate the scatter fraction, count losses, and randoms, is also used to simulate background activity as in the human body (Fig. 7.26).

The phantom is prepared by filling an F-18 solution of 5.3 ± 0.27 kBq/mL radioactivity concentration. The 5.3 kBq/mL radioactivity concentration corresponds to a total injected radioactivity of 5.3 kBq/mL × 70,000 mL = 371 MBq (~10 mCi), a typical injected dose for whole-body PET studies. If the manufacturer recommends a lower dose for whole-body scans, a lower radio-

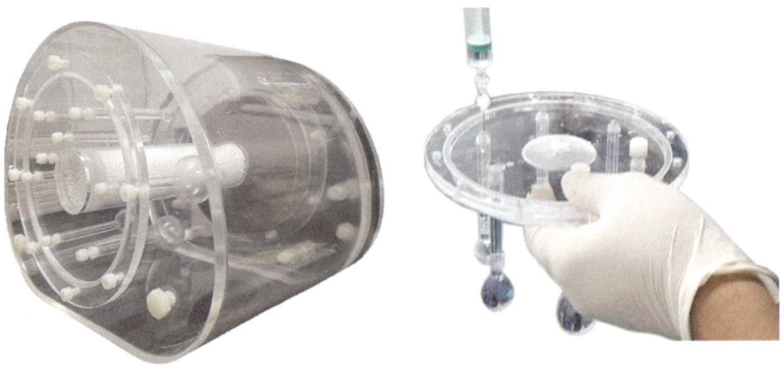

Fig. 7.25 NEMA/IEC image quality phantom

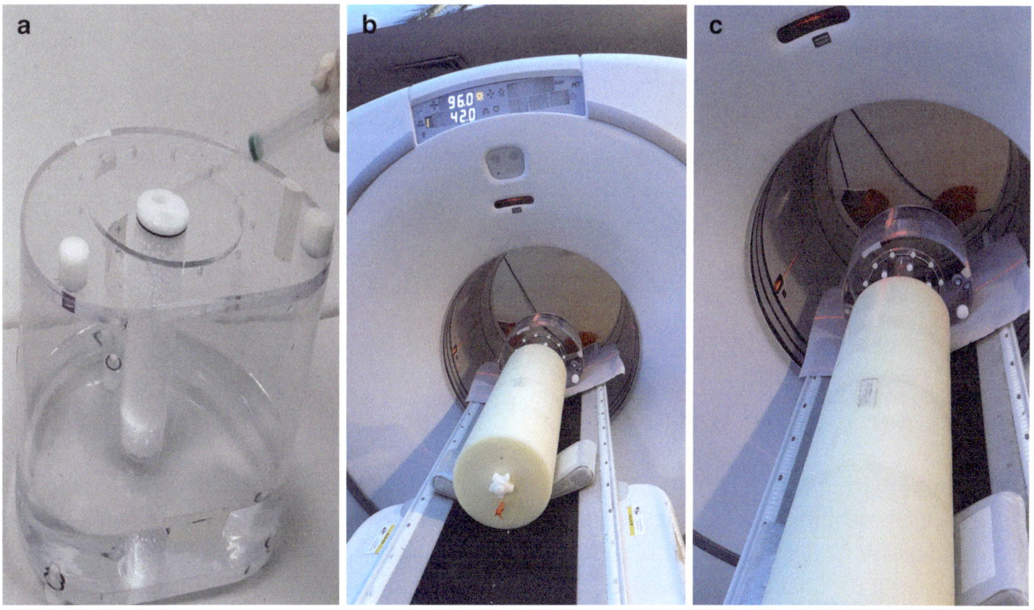

Fig. 7.26 Source preparation and positioning of image quality phantom and scatter phantom. (a) Filling of image quality phantom with the prepared radioactive solution. (b) Placement of the image quality phantom and the scatter phantom on the PET/CT scanner bed. (c) Final alignment of the combined phantom setup using the scanner's laser positioning system prior to acquisition

Table 7.9 Source activities at the time of scan

Phantom	Typical volume	Activity	Activity concentration
Background filling	9792 mL	52 MBq (1.5 mCi)	5.3 kBq/mL
Hot spheres	~ 60 mL (all six spheres) as per NEMA NU 2-2018	NA	21 kBq/mL
Tubing inserted in scatter phantom	5 mL	120 MBq (3 mCi)	NA

activity concentration than 5.3 kBq/mL could be used and reported for this test.

A typical image quality phantom background volume is 9792 mL, and the sphere volume is approximately 20 mL. At scan time, the activity concentration should be 21 kBq/mL (0.6 μCi/cc) in spheres and 5.3 kBq/mL (0.15 μCi/cc) in the background (Fig. 7.25). A typical time may be 45 min to prepare the sources for the scan. We need to fill higher activities at the time of fill so they can take care of decay to the correct activities by the time of the scan (Table 7.9).

A practical approach to accurately achieve a 4:1 sphere-to-background ratio without spills is to fill the body compartment with a quarter of its total volume, add the radioactivity intended for the background compartment, use this solution to fill the spheres, and then fill the body compartment with water and cover the phantom with the lid to which the spheres are attached [26].

This test evaluates several parameters to assess the imaging system's performance. Here's what these parameters mean:

Contrast Recovery

Contrast recovery refers to the ability of the imaging system to detect and measure differences in radioactivity concentration accurately. It is typically evaluated using small spherical objects of known radioactivity concentration placed within a background medium (Fig. 7.27). The contrast recovery coefficient (CRC) is calculated as the ratio of the measured radioactivity concentration in the sphere to the true radioactivity concentration. It indicates the system's ability to distinguish small variations in radioactivity concentration.

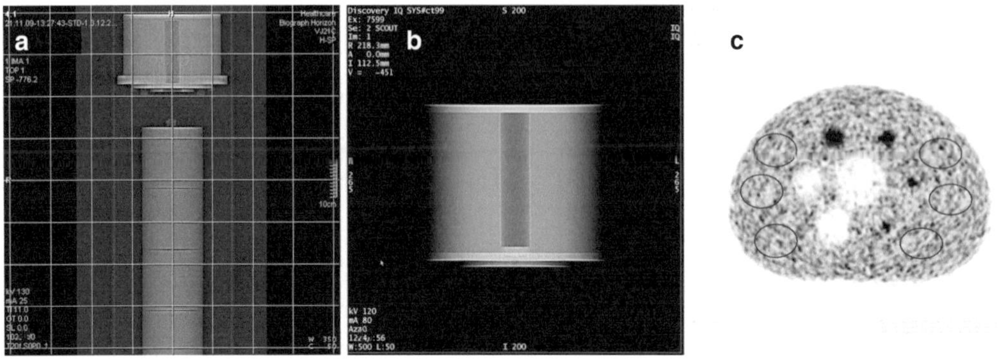

Fig. 7.27 Scout and ROI drawing. (**a**) Scout obtained in Siemens Biograph system. (**b**) Scout obtained in GE Discovery IQ system. (**c**) ROIs drew in the GE Discovery system

Background Variability
Background variability measures the uniformity of the radioactivity distribution in the surrounding background medium. It is assessed by calculating the coefficient of variation (COV) of the radioactivity concentration in the background region. A lower COV indicates a more uniform background distribution, which is desirable for accurate quantitative analysis.

Lung Residual Mean
The lung residual mean evaluates the system's accuracy in measuring radioactivity concentration in lung regions. It is calculated by comparing the measured radioactivity concentration in a simulated lung region to the known true concentration. A lower residual mean indicates better accuracy in quantifying radioactivity in lung tissue.

These parameters collectively provide insights into the image quality, accuracy of radioactivity quantification, and ability to detect and measure small differences in radioactivity concentration (Fig. 7.28). They help assess the performance of the PET imaging system and ensure its suitability for clinical applications.

7.6.5 Coincidence Timing Resolution or Time-of-Flight Resolution and Energy Resolution

Time-of-flight (TOF) resolution or coincidence timing resolution refers to the measurement of the system's ability to accurately determine the time difference between detecting two annihilation photons during a positron emission event. PET imaging uses TOF information to improve image quality and spatial resolution.

TOF resolution can be assessed using the data acquired for the scatter fraction test in PET NEMA imaging or by aligning a line source with the system axial center and acquiring coincidence data after system calibration. The time difference between the detected photons from multiple point sources in the phantom is measured, and this information is utilized both for calculating the scatter fraction and determining the TOF resolution. During the acquisition, the PET system records the timing information for each detected photon, which allows for calculating the time difference between pairs of photons originating from different point sources. This information evaluates the TOF resolution, representing the system's ability to measure these time differences accurately (Fig. 7.29).

The TOF resolution is calculated as the full width at half maximum (FWHM) of the distribution of time differences. A smaller TOF resolution indicates a higher precision in determining the arrival time of annihilation photons. This information can be used to improve image reconstruction algorithms and reduce image artifacts, leading to better spatial resolution and overall image quality in PET imaging.

The energy resolution of a PET system is typically determined by measuring the full width at half maximum (FWHM) of the photopeak in the energy spectrum of a radioactive source. The energy spec-

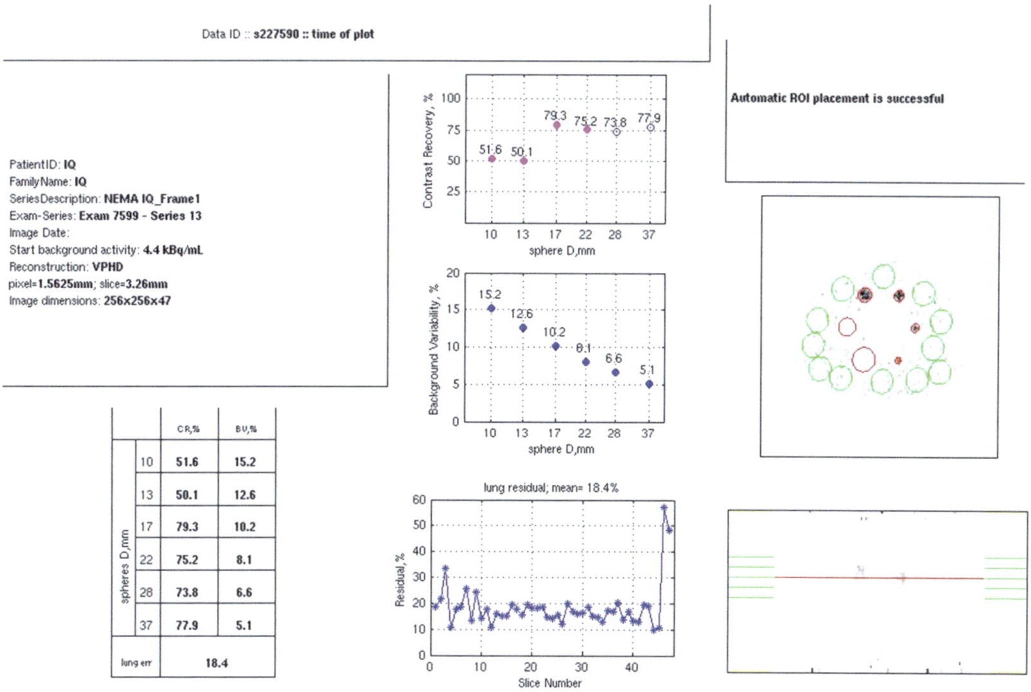

Fig. 7.28 Results obtained for image quality test in GE Discovery IQ PET system as per NEMA NU 2-2012

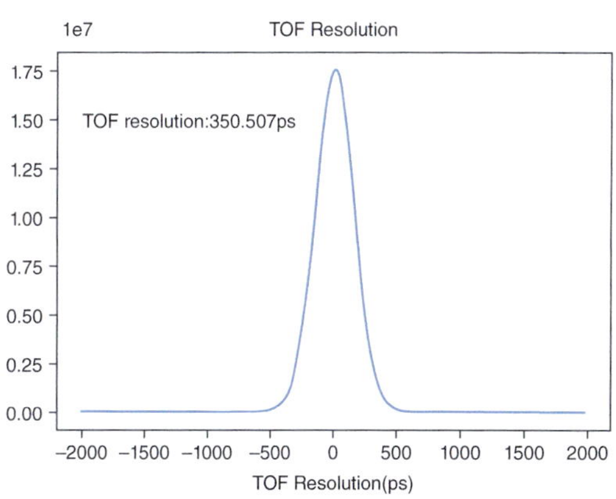

Fig. 7.29 Time-of-flight resolution graph of a typical PET system

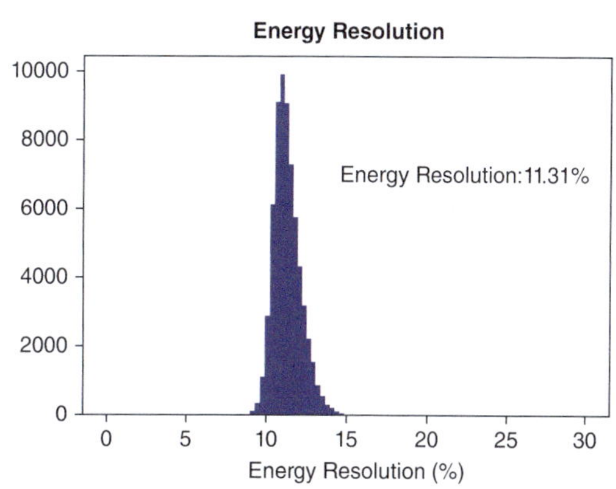

Fig. 7.30 Energy resolution graph of a typical PET system

trum is obtained by acquiring data from the PET system while imaging a source with known energy (e.g., a standard radioactive material).

The energy resolution provides information about the system's ability to distinguish between different photon energies and is an important parameter for quantifying the image quality and accuracy of PET measurements. A lower energy resolution indicates better energy discrimination and improved image quality (Fig. 7.30).

7.6.6 PET-CT Co-registration Accuracy

PET-CT co-registration accuracy is a test to assess the co-registration accuracy between PET and CT images in a PET-CT system. This test evaluates the alignment and spatial correspondence between the PET and CT images, which is crucial for accurate anatomical localization and fusion of functional and anatomical information.

The test typically involves using a specialized phantom containing PET and CT features. The phantom may have inserts or structures that mimic anatomical structures, such as bones or lesions. The phantom is positioned and scanned using the PET-CT system, acquiring PET and CT images.

General Electric (GE) PET-CTs, such as Discovery IQ and some other models of GE PET-CTs, use the VQC (Volumetric Quality Control) phantom for PET-CT alignment tests. It is a cylindrical phantom that contains multiple inserts and contrasts to simulate various anatomical structures. A typical VQC phantom may consist of five spheres with Ge-68 radioactivity and different Hounsfield Unit (HU) values, though this can vary depending on the specific manufacturer and model of the phantom (Fig. 7.31). It evaluates the co-registration accuracy between the PET and CT images. The phantom allows for the assessment of alignment and registration between the PET emission and CT transmission data, providing information about the accuracy of anatomical localization in the combined PET-CT images.

Specific regions or landmarks in the PET and CT images are identified and marked to evaluate the co-registration accuracy. These regions can be reference points, fiducial markers, or anatomical structures with known spatial coordinates. The co-registration accuracy is then assessed by measuring the spatial deviation or discrepancy between the corresponding landmarks or structures in the PET and CT images.

Various metrics, such as distance measurements or overlap indices, can be used to quantify the co-registration accuracy. The test results provide information about the spatial alignment and accuracy of co-registration between PET and CT images, indicating the system's ability to align functional and anatomical information precisely (Figs. 7.32 and 7.33).

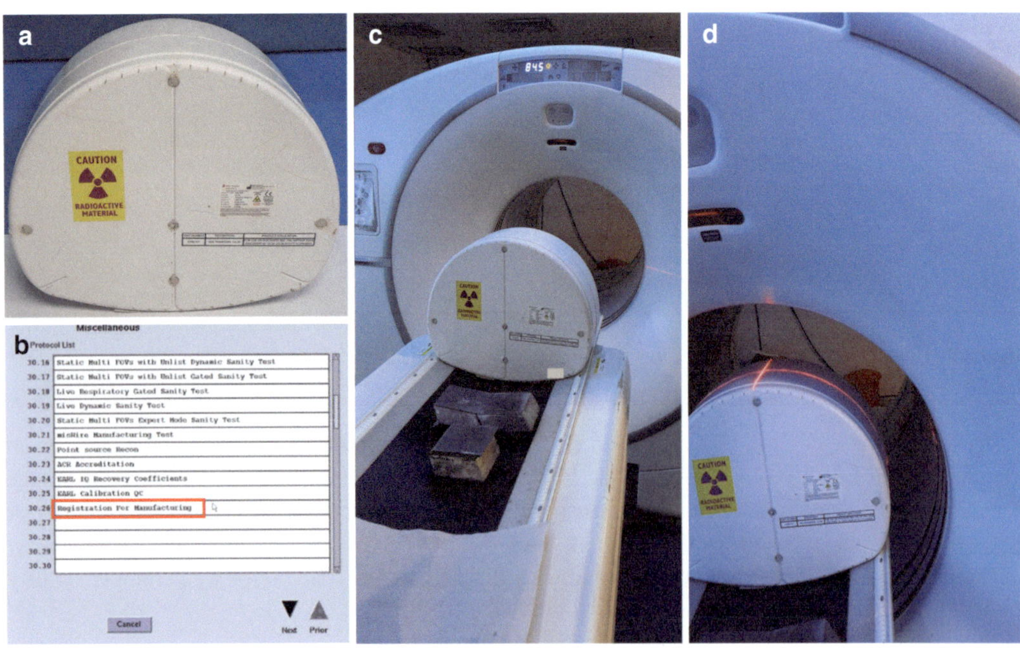

Fig. 7.31 VQC phantom and its placement. (**a**) VQC phantom. (**b**) Protocol selection. (**c**) Placement on patient table. (**d**) Positioning and alignment with the help of laser light

Measurement Items

Direction	ReferenceRange	Current Value	Measurement Result
X Direction(mm)	-1.5~1.5	-0.21	Qualified
Y Direction(mm)	-1.5~1.5	-0.20	Qualified
Z Direction(mm)	-1.5~1.5	0.27	Qualified

Measurement Analysis

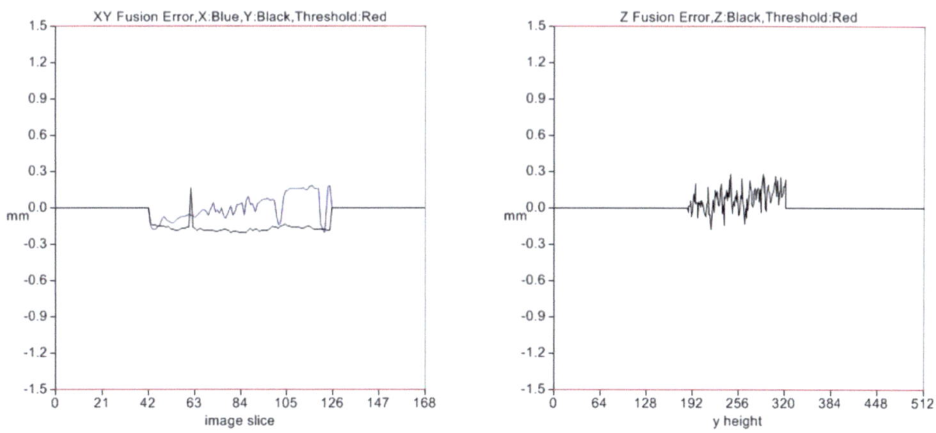

Fig. 7.32 PET-CT registration image of United MI 550 PET-CT

Fig. 7.33 PET-CT registration data of GE Discovery IQ PET-CT

Sphere	Axis	Img 1	Img 2	Diff
1	x (L)	8.48	9.19	**-0.71**
	y (P)	98.92	98.31	**0.61**
	z (S)	-55.14	-55.35	**0.21**
Distance Magnitude = 0.97 mm				
2	x (L)	5.96	6.39	**-0.43**
	y (P)	-190.08	-187.89	**-2.19**
	z (S)	-54.00	-54.67	**0.66**
Distance Magnitude = 2.33 mm				
3	x (L)	7.27	8.03	**-0.76**
	y (P)	9.69	9.83	**-0.14**
	z (S)	-4.97	-5.29	**0.33**
Distance Magnitude = 0.84 mm				
4	x (L)	-191.87	-188.98	**-2.89**
	y (P)	10.16	10.50	**-0.34**
	z (S)	44.96	44.51	**0.44**
Distance Magnitude = 2.95 mm				
5	x (L)	205.13	203.94	**1.18**
	y (P)	7.10	7.26	**-0.16**
	z (S)	46.62	45.88	**0.74**
Distance Magnitude = 1.41 mm				

The PET-CT co-registration accuracy test ensures the reliability and accuracy of PET-CT image fusion, which is essential for proper interpretation and clinical use of PET-CT imaging data. It helps identify potential issues or misalignments in the co-registration process, allowing for adjustments or corrections to improve the accuracy of image fusion and localization in clinical practice.

7.6.7 Uniformity Check of the Reconstructed Image Test

The uniformity test for the reconstructed PET images is assessed to evaluate the scanner's ability to produce images with consistent and accurate activity values across the field of view.

This test scans a phantom with known activity concentrations using the PET scanner. The phantom may contain regions of varying activity concentrations or specific patterns designed to challenge the scanner's ability to reconstruct the activity distribution accurately.

After acquiring the PET images, regions of interest (ROIs) are defined within the phantom (Fig. 7.34). The activity concentrations within these ROIs are measured, and the nonuniformity of the reconstructed image is quantified using metrics such as the coefficient of variation (CV) or percent standard deviation (%SD). In GE Discovery IQ, the images are used from 3D WCC data (discussed in the next section) with retro-reconfiguration by changing parameters to 256 × 256 pixels instead of the default 128 × 128 and a few more changes as suggested by manufacturers.

The nonuniformity is a measure of the variability or inconsistency in activity values across the field of view. A high nonuniformity value indicates significant deviations from the expected activity distribution, which can indicate issues such as image artifacts, reconstruction errors, or calibration problems.

The test results are compared against predefined acceptance criteria or manufacturer specifications to determine if the PET system meets the required nonuniformity standards. This test helps evaluate the accuracy and reliability of the reconstructed PET images, ensuring that the scanner produces consistent and valid quantitative measurements.

7.6.8 Normalization and Well Counter Corrections

Normalization and well counter correction are two important processes in positron emission tomography (PET) imaging. Let's explore each of them in detail:

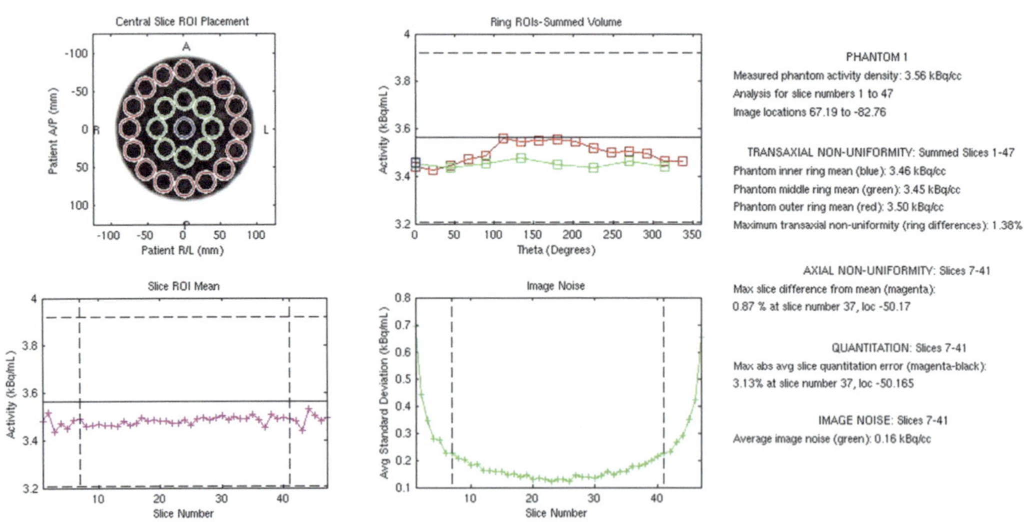

Fig. 7.34 Uniformity for the reconstructed image in the GE Discovery IQ machine

Normalization in PET

Normalization aims to correct for nonuniformities in the scanner's response across the field of view (FOV). These nonuniformities can be caused by various factors such as detector inhomogeneities, differences in crystal efficiencies, or variations in electronic response. It ensures that the measured PET data accurately represent the true distribution of the radiotracer within the patient's body. It involves acquiring data using a uniform radioactive source that emits gamma rays. This source is typically a cylindrical phantom filled with a radioactive material. The phantom is positioned within the PET scanner's FOV, and the scanner acquires data from it. The acquired data are then processed to generate a normalization map or correction factors that can be applied to the patient data during image reconstruction. The normalization correction factors account for the nonuniformities in the scanner's response and are used to normalize the acquired PET data. This correction helps to produce images with more accurate quantification and uniformity across the FOV.

Well Counter Correction in PET

The well counter correction (WCC) calibration involves matching a known amount of activity concentration to the pixel values displayed in the PET image. The goal is to establish a conversion factor that allows the true count rate measured by the PET scanner to be converted into activity concentration, typically expressed in kilo becquerels per milliliter (kBq/mL). In simpler terms, it converts PET true count rate into activity concentration, i.e., kBq/mL, which is required to calculate standard uptake values (SUVs) (Fig. 7.35).

The calibration begins with a radioactive source containing a known activity concentration, usually in the form of a calibration phantom. The activity concentration is typically determined through a separate measurement method, such as a well counter or a dose calibrator. The calibration phantom is positioned within the field of view of the PET scanner, and the scanner acquires data. The acquired data represent the true count rate corresponding to the known activity concentration in the phantom (Fig. 7.36).

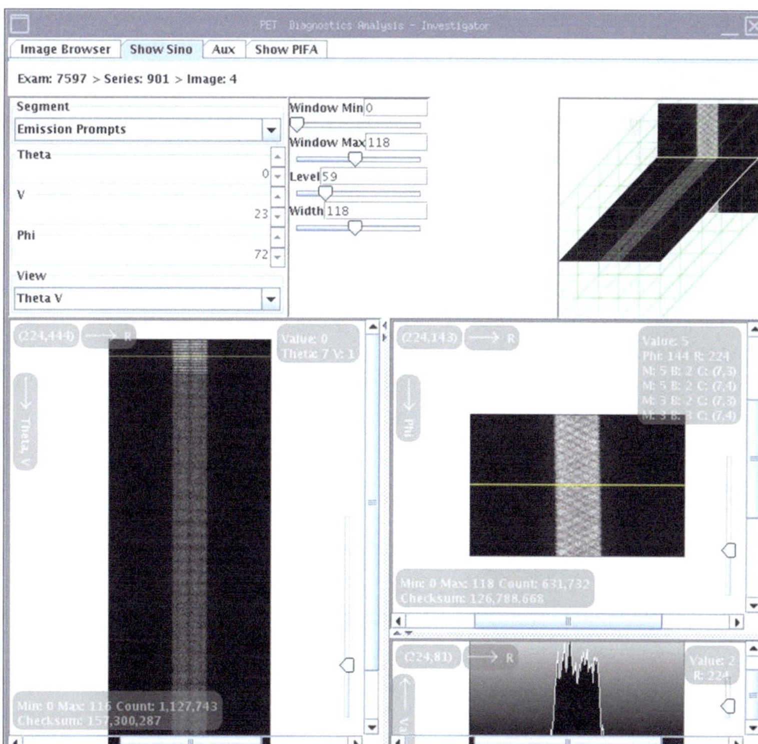

Fig. 7.35 Sinogram image of PET GE Discovery IQ

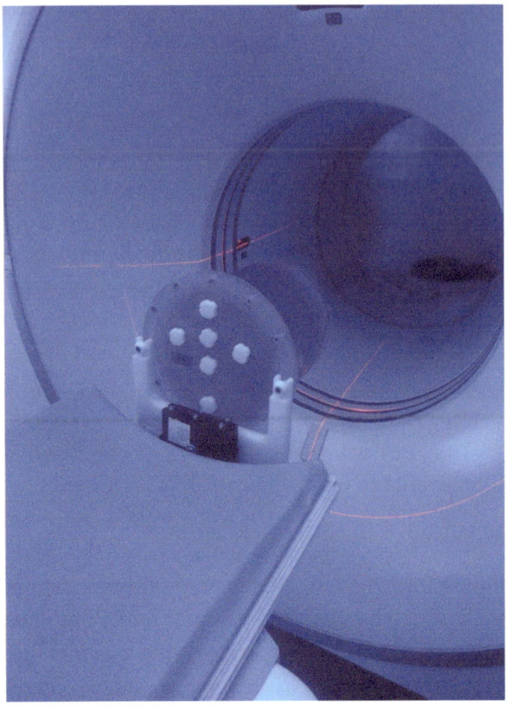

Fig. 7.36 Well counter correction phantom placement

The acquired PET data are then reconstructed to generate a PET image. The pixel values in the image represent the measured count rates. The acquired count rates in the PET image are compared to the known activity concentration in the phantom. A conversion factor or calibration curve is determined by correlating the measured count rates with the known concentration. The derived conversion factor or calibration curve is used to convert the measured count rates in the PET image to activity concentration units (kBq/mL). This conversion allows the image's pixel values to represent the radiotracer concentration in the imaged tissue or region.

The resulting PET image with calibrated activity concentration can be used for quantitative analysis, such as determining the uptake of a radiotracer in specific tissues, assessing treatment response, or evaluating metabolic activity.

The well counter correction (WCC) calibration process is crucial for accurately quantifying and interpreting PET images. It ensures that the pixel values in the image correspond to the true activity concentration in the imaged tissue, enabling meaningful and quantitative analysis in PET imaging studies.

It's important to note that the specific details of the WCC calibration process may vary depending on the PET scanner, reconstruction algorithms, and calibration methods used by the imaging facility or research institution.

7.7 The Gamma Camera, the Single Photon Emission Computed Tomography (SPECT), and How Do They Work

A gamma camera, also known as a scintillation camera or Anger camera, is a specialized imaging device used in nuclear medicine for diagnostic purposes. It detects and measures the gamma rays emitted by radiopharmaceuticals, allowing the visualization of functional processes and the distribution of radiotracers within the body. The rotating gamma camera is called single photon emission computed tomography (SPECT). The gamma camera rotates around the patient in SPECT imaging, capturing data from various angles. The rotation allows the camera to acquire multiple views of the emitted gamma rays, providing information about the distribution and intensity of the radiotracer in different regions of interest. The acquired data are subsequently processed and reconstructed to generate cross-sectional or volumetric images, allowing for the visualization and analysis of functional processes in the body.

In 1957, Hal Anger introduced a scintillation camera that utilized a large sodium iodide crystal coupled with an array of photomultiplier tubes (PMTs) (Fig. 7.37). This groundbreaking design was known as the Anger camera, gamma camera, or scintillation camera. The crystal was the gamma-ray detector, while the PMTs converted the scintillation light into electrical signals.

The gamma camera consists of several essential components:

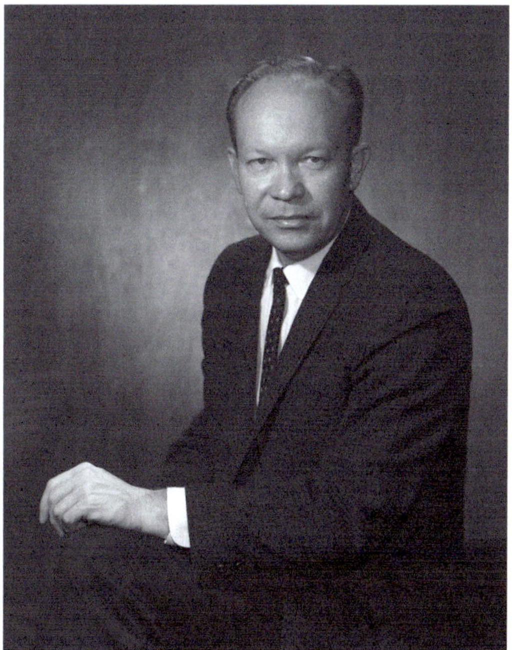

Hal Anger (1920 - 2005)

Fig. 7.37 Hal Anger. (Image © The Regents of the University of California, Lawrence Berkeley National Laboratory. Printed with permission)

7.7.1 Collimator

The collimator is a lead or tungsten sheet with a pattern of small holes or channels. Its purpose is to shape and direct the incoming gamma rays. The collimator acts as a filter, allowing only gamma rays from specific angles to pass through to the detector. There are five basic designs of collimators such as parallel hole collimators, slant-hole collimators, converging and diverging collimators, fan-beam collimators, and pinhole collimators. They are used for different purposes. The parallel hole collimators can be of different types, such as "low energy high resolution (LEHR)," "low energy all purpose (LEAP)," and medium- and high-energy collimators. They all can be used with the same gamma camera to optimize imaging for different clinical applications. The most commonly used collimators are LEAP, LEHR, and high-resolution collimators. LEAP and LEHR collimators are used in routine Techenitium-99m studies, where high-energy collimator is used for I-131 studies (Fig. 7.38).

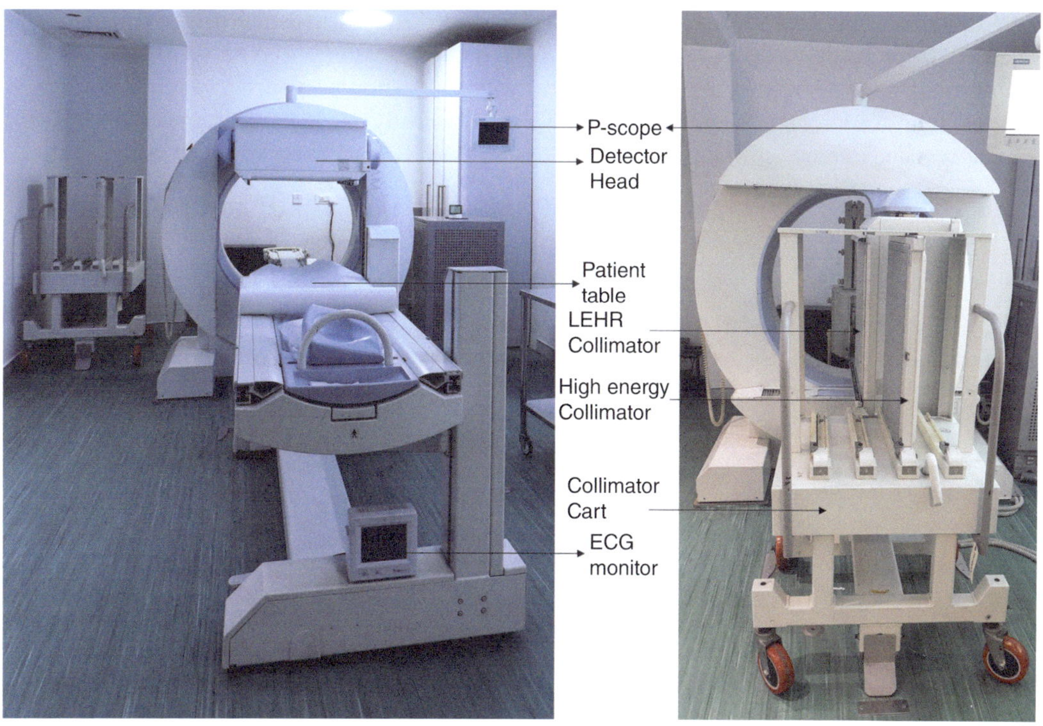

Fig. 7.38 Gamma camera and its parts

Difference in Low Energy All Purpose (LEAP) and Low Energy High Resolution (LEHR)

The difference between low-energy all-purpose and low-energy high-resolution collimators lies primarily in their construction and design, influencing their imaging characteristics.

The LEAP collimators typically have larger and wider holes than the LEHR collimators. The larger holes allow for higher sensitivity, enabling a higher detection efficiency for gamma rays. In contrast, LEHR collimators have smaller and narrower holes to enhance spatial resolution by reducing the acceptance of scattered and off-axis gamma rays (Fig. 7.39).

The LEAP collimators usually have longer holes compared to LEHR collimators. The longer holes allow for a wider angular acceptance of gamma rays, including those emitted from off-axis locations. This broader acceptance improves the overall sensitivity of the collimator but sacrifices spatial resolution. The density of the collimator material can also differ between the two types. The LEAP collimators often use materials with lower density, such as lead or tungsten, which provides good sensitivity, whereas LEHR collimators, on the other hand, use denser materials like tungsten to enhance the collimation of gamma rays and improve spatial resolution.

The septal thickness, which refers to the thickness of the material between adjacent holes, can also vary between the two collimator types. Low-energy high-resolution collimators tend to have thinner septa, allowing for better spatial resolution by minimizing the interaction of gamma rays with neighboring holes, whereas low-energy all-purpose collimators may have thicker septa to increase structural integrity and provide better collimation of gamma rays emitted from a wider range of angles.

These construction differences between low-energy all-purpose and low-energy high-resolution collimators impact their imaging performance, balancing sensitivity, and spatial resolution. Low-energy all-purpose collimators are designed for general imaging purposes, providing good sensitivity but sacrificing spatial resolution, whereas low-energy high-resolution collimators, on the other hand, prioritize spatial resolution at the expense of sensitivity by minimizing scatter and off-axis gamma rays.

7.7.2 Scintillation Crystal and Photomultiplier Tubes

The collimator is coupled to a scintillation crystal, typically made of sodium iodide thallium activated (NaI(Tl)) or cesium iodide thallium

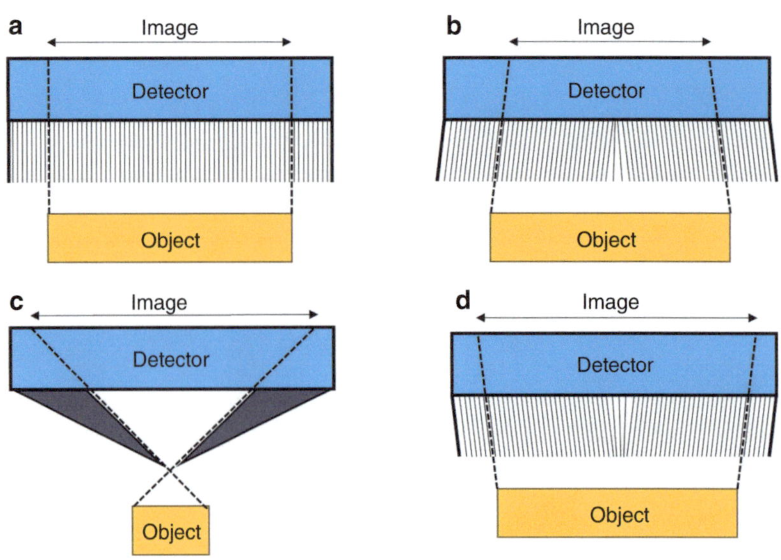

Fig. 7.39 Collimators used in gamma camera. (**a**) Parallel hole collimator. (**b**) Diverging hole collimator. (**c**) Pinhole collimator. (**d**) Converging hole collimator

activated (CsI(Tl)). In recent years, cadmium zinc telluride (CZT) semiconductor-based new gamma cameras equipped with wide-field detectors have been introduced into routine nuclear medicine practice [27]. The scintillation detectors and PMTs have been discussed in detail in Sects. 7.4.1 and 7.4.2. Sodium iodide (NaI) crystals are gamma cameras' most commonly used scintillation crystals. NaI crystals have been widely utilized in gamma cameras due to their favorable scintillation properties and relatively high light output. NaI crystals have high density, high light yield, and good energy resolution, making them suitable for gamma-ray detection in nuclear medicine applications. However, it's important to note that other scintillation crystals, for example, cesium iodide (CsI) or semiconductor-based detectors, are also used. "The CZT cameras offer better sensitivity, higher energy resolution, and improved image contrast compared to the traditional SPECT camera, while maintaining similar spatial resolution. The adoption of this new technology could potentially lead to changes in current nuclear medicine practices, such as reduced acquisition time and lower injection of radioactive material into patients [27]."

When a gamma ray passes through the collimator and enters the crystal, it interacts with the crystal's atoms, causing the emission of light photons. The detectors are coupled with photomultiplier tubes (PMTs) or photodiodes to convert light photons into electrical signals. PMTs are light-sensitive detectors that convert the emitted light photons into electrical signals. Each PMT corresponds to a specific region or pixel of the gamma camera (Fig. 7.40).

7.7.3 Preamplifier and Amplifier

The preamplifier and amplifier work to amplify the weak electrical signals generated by the PMTs in response to scintillation photons. The preamplifier amplifies the signals immediately

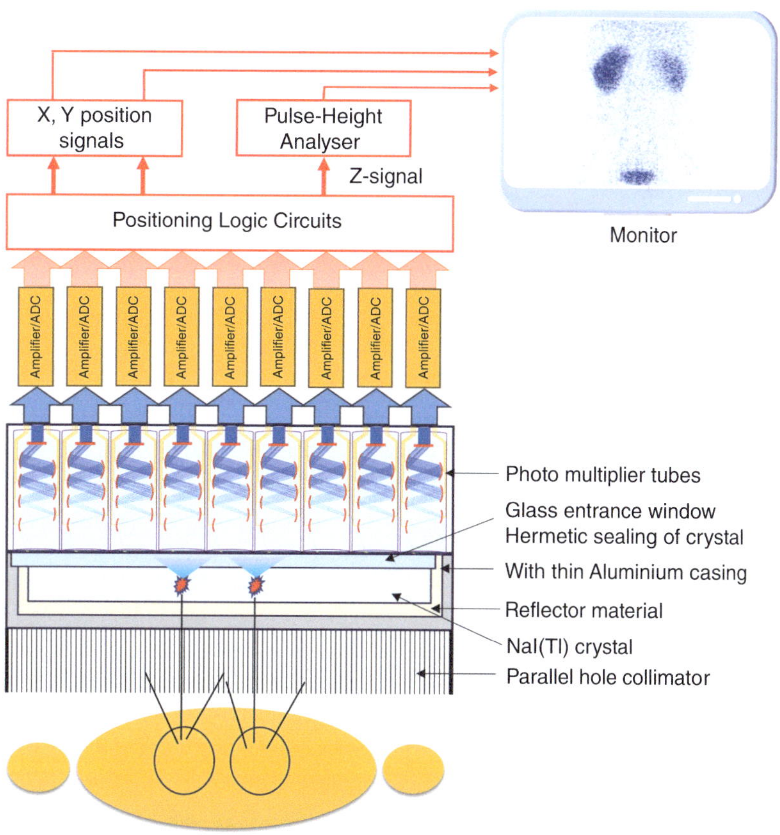

Fig. 7.40 The working principles of gamma camera

after generation by the PMTs, while the amplifier further amplifies the signals to an optimal level for subsequent processing and analysis in the gamma camera system.

The first stage of signal processing in the gamma camera system is preamplifier. Its primary function is to amplify the weak electrical signals generated by the PMTs in response to scintillation photons. The preamplifier is typically placed close to the PMTs to minimize signal degradation. The preamplifier performed the following functions:

- Signal Amplification: The preamplifier amplifies the weak electrical signals from the PMTs to a level suitable for further processing.
- Noise Reduction: It helps reduce the impact of external noise and interference on the signals by amplifying the signal-to-noise ratio.
- Signal Shaping: The preamplifier can shape the signals' waveform to improve their compatibility with downstream processing stages.

The amplifier is responsible for further amplifying the signals from the preamplifier to an optimal level for subsequent processing and analysis. It strengthens the electrical signals to ensure they are within the appropriate voltage range and can be effectively digitized. The functions of the amplifier are as follows:

- Signal Amplification: The primary role of the amplifier is to amplify the electrical signals from the preamplifier to a level suitable for further processing.
- Gain Adjustment: The amplifier may have adjustable gain settings to accommodate different signal strengths and optimize the amplification level.
- Filtering: The amplifier may incorporate filters to eliminate unwanted noise and interference that could affect the quality of the signals.
- Signal Conditioning: The amplifier may perform additional signal conditioning, such as impedance matching or equalization, to ensure optimal signal integrity.

The preamplifiers and amplifiers are important components that work together to process and amplify the electrical signals generated by the photomultiplier tubes (PMTs).

7.7.4 Analogue-to-Digital Converter (ADC)

The ADC in a gamma camera plays a critical role in converting the continuous analogue signals from the PMTs into discrete digital values that digital systems can process and analyze. The digital signals can be used for energy analysis, pulse height discrimination, positioning calculations, and subsequent image reconstruction.

- Amplification and Shaping: The electrical signals from the PMTs, which represent the scintillation photons detected by the crystal, are initially weak and in analogue form. Before being sent to the ADC, the signals typically undergo amplification and shaping processes to enhance their amplitude and optimize their waveform.
- Sampling: The ADC samples the analogue signal regularly to capture discrete values. The sampling rate determines how frequently the signal is measured and is typically determined by the Nyquist-Shannon sampling theorem, ensuring an accurate representation of the original analogue signal.
- Quantization: The ADC quantizes the sampled analogue signal by assigning digital values to each sample. The quantization process involves dividing the signal's amplitude range into a finite number of discrete levels or bins. The number of bits used to represent each sample determines the resolution of the ADC.
- Binary Encoding: After quantization, the ADC assigns a binary code to each discrete level, representing the digital value of the sample. This binary encoding allows for efficient storage and processing of the digital signal.
- Digital Output: The ADC provides a digital representation of the analogue signal as its output. This digital signal is a stream of binary values, typically a digital waveform or a series of numerical values, which digital systems such as computers can further process, analyze, and store.

The specific design, resolution, and sampling rate of the ADC can vary between different gamma camera systems and manufacturers. The choice of ADC parameters depends on the desired signal accuracy, system requirements, and available technology at the design time.

7.7.5 Pulse Height Analyzer (PHA)

The pulse height analyzer plays a crucial role in energy discrimination, allowing the gamma camera to differentiate between gamma rays of different energies. It is responsible for analyzing the amplitude (energy) of electrical signals generated by the photomultiplier tubes (PMTs) in response to scintillation photons. Setting appropriate energy windows helps filter out background noise and unwanted events, ensuring that only relevant gamma-ray events are included in the subsequent image reconstruction process. The pulse height analyzer works in a gamma camera for:

- Voltage Amplitude Representation: The amplified electrical signals from the PMTs, after passing through the preamplifier and amplifier, are sent to the pulse height analyzer. The PHA converts the analogue signals into digital representations using an analogue-to-digital converter (ADC).
- Energy Window Setting: The PHA allows the operator to set specific energy windows or bins. Each window represents a range of energy levels that are interesting for imaging. Setting energy windows aims to discriminate against noise and unwanted events while retaining gamma-ray events within the desired energy range.
- Pulse Height Discrimination: The PHA compares the voltage amplitude of each digitized signal to the energy windows set by the operator. If the signal falls within one of the energy windows, it is accepted as a valid event for further processing and image reconstruction. Signals outside the set energy windows are rejected.
- Energy Spectrum: The PHA records the number of events falling within each energy window, creating an energy spectrum. This spectrum represents the distribution of gamma rays based on their energy levels, providing valuable information about the radiotracer and its uptake in different regions of the patient's body.

7.7.6 *X–Y* Positioning Circuit and the Energy Signals (*Z*)

The combination of the *X–Y* positioning circuit and the energy signals (*Z*) in a gamma camera enables the precise localization of gamma-ray interactions within the detector crystal and provides information about the energy levels of the detected gamma rays. *X–Y* positioning circuit processes the signals from multiple PMTs to determine the *X* and *Y* coordinates of the gamma-ray interaction within the detector crystal. Various algorithms, such as centroid calculation or Anger logic, can calculate the position.

Centroid Calculation

Centroid calculation is a straightforward algorithm used to determine the center of gravity or centroid of the distribution of signals from multiple photomultiplier tubes (PMTs). The gamma camera's data acquisition system acquires electrical signals from the PMTs, representing the gamma-ray interactions. Each PMT signal is multiplied by a weighting factor, which depends on the distance between the PMT and the calculated position. The weighted signals from all the PMTs are summed. The summed signal is divided by the total signal amplitude to normalize the result. The centroid position is calculated based on the normalized summed signal. The centroid's *X* and *Y* coordinates represent the gamma-ray interaction's estimated spatial coordinates.

The centroid calculation algorithm provides a simple and computationally efficient method to estimate the position of the gamma-ray interaction based on the signal distribution across multiple PMTs. However, it may be susceptible to noise and variations in signal intensity.

Anger Logic

Anger logic, also known as Anger positioning, is a more sophisticated algorithm developed by Hal O. Anger, a pioneer in nuclear medicine imaging. It uses the timing and amplitude information from multiple PMTs to determine the position of the gamma-ray interaction. The electrical signals from the PMTs are acquired and processed by the gamma camera's data acquisition system. The algorithm identifies the PMTs that register signals within a specified time window, indicating a coincidence event. The algorithm further filters the signals based on their energy level, ensuring they fall within the desired energy window. The position calculation involves comparing the timing and amplitude of the coincident signals from the PMTs to determine the *X* and *Y* coordinates of the gamma-ray interaction. The algorithm uses a weighted summation of the signals to estimate the position accurately.

The Anger logic algorithm provides more precise positioning than centroid calculation as it considers both timing and amplitude information from multiple PMTs. It improves the spatial resolution and reduces the impact of noise and background events.

Both centroid calculation and Anger logic are widely used in gamma cameras for position calculation. The choice of algorithm depends on factors such as the desired spatial resolution, computational requirements, and system design considerations. Manufacturers may implement variations or enhancements to these algorithms based on their specific gamma camera designs and technologies.

7.7.7 Uniformity, Linearity, and Energy Resolution Correction

Both linearity and uniformity corrections are crucial for accurately quantifying and interpreting the gamma camera images. By applying these corrections, the acquired image data can be adjusted to account for nonlinearities in the system's response and nonuniformities in detector sensitivity. This helps to improve the overall image quality, enhance diagnostic accuracy, and ensure consistency in the interpretation of images over time.

Linearity Correction

Linearity correction addresses nonlinearities in the gamma camera system's response to different levels of gamma-ray energies. Nonlinearities can occur due to various factors, including detector nonuniformity and variations in the amplification and signal processing components. A calibration process is carried out using known radioactive sources to correct these nonlinearities. The calibration data is used to create a correction curve or lookup table, which is then applied to the acquired image data to linearize the response across the energy spectrum. This correction ensures that the intensity of the acquired image is directly proportional to the actual radioactivity present in the imaged object.

Uniformity Correction

Uniformity correction addresses nonuniformities in the gamma camera's response across the field of view. Nonuniformities can arise due to variations in detector sensitivity, PMT gain, or other factors. To perform uniformity correction, a flood source containing a known radioisotope (such as Technitium-99m or Cobalt-57) is used to irradiate the entire field of view of the gamma camera. This flood acquisition data provides information about the inherent nonuniformities. By analyzing this data, correction factors are derived and applied to the acquired image to compensate for nonuniformities, resulting in a more uniform representation of the radioactivity distribution.

Energy Resolution Correction

The energy resolution of a gamma camera refers to its ability to distinguish between different energy levels of detected gamma rays. Energy resolution corrections are usually applied during the data processing stage, where the acquired raw data from the gamma camera is reconstructed into images and analyzed. The corrections mentioned, such as energy window settings, energy calibration, energy resolution smearing correction, and energy peak shift correction, are part of the post-processing and analysis steps performed on the acquired data. These corrections are typically carried out using specialized software and algorithms that account for the energy response characteristics of the gamma camera system.

In gamma camera imaging, linearity, uniformity, and energy resolution corrections are important to ensure accurate and reliable image quality before the final display.

7.7.8 Image Display

After performing uniformity and linearity corrections in gamma camera imaging, the processed image data is ready for display on a monitor. The image display visually represents the radioactivity distribution within the imaged object. The gamma camera system typically provides a dedicated workstation or software interface for image viewing and analysis. The processed image is visualized on a high-resolution monitor, allowing nuclear medicine physicians or technologists to examine the radioactivity distribution in different regions of interest.

The image display software often provides tools for image manipulation and analysis. Users can adjust the display settings, such as windowing, zooming, panning, and image orientation, to optimize the visualization of specific areas of interest. Quantitative analysis tools may also be available to measure the radioactivity concentration in specific regions or perform comparison studies.

7.7.9 Single Photon Emission Computed Tomography (SPECT) Imaging

When the gamma camera rotates around the patient and acquires images from various directions, it is called SPECT. During a SPECT scan, the gamma camera acquires projection images from different angles around the patient. Each projection image represents the detected gamma-ray counts for a specific projection angle. The data from each projection is processed and rearranged to form a sinogram. The sinogram is a two-dimensional representation of the acquired projection data and is generated by arranging the projection data based on the angle of projection.

The sinogram has dimensions corresponding to the number of projection angles and detector elements or bins along the projection lines. The *x*-axis of the sinogram represents the projection angles, typically ranging from 0 to 180 degrees. The *y*-axis of the sinogram represents the position along the projection line or the number of detector elements (bins) along the line (Fig. 7.41).

Each element or pixel in the sinogram represents the measured gamma-ray counts for a specific angle and position. The values in the sinogram reflect the intensity of the detected

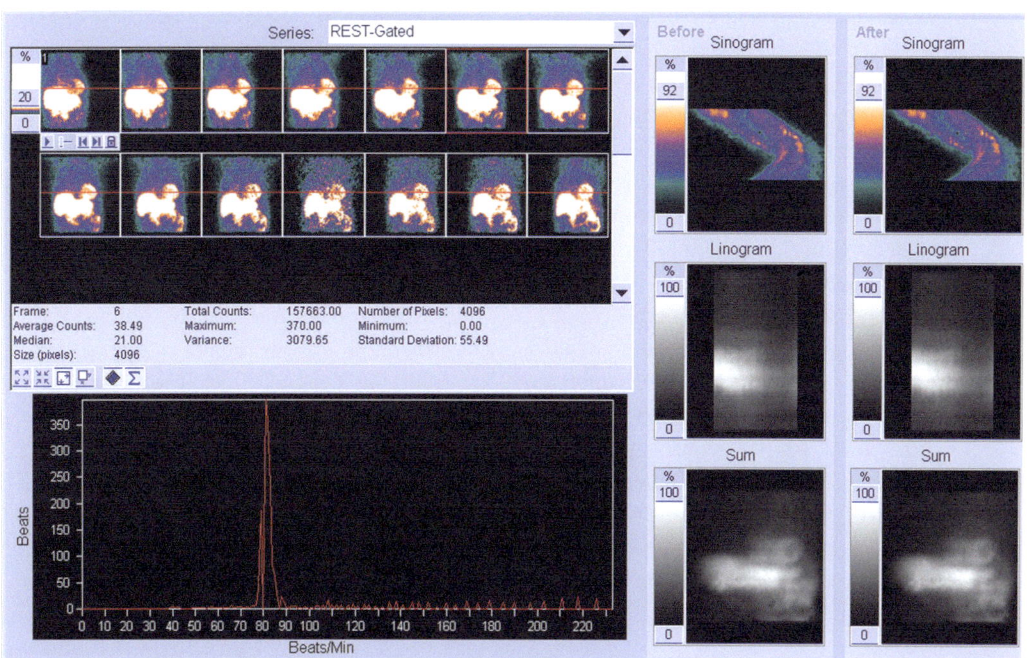

Fig. 7.41 Sinogram in SPECT imaging

radiation along each projection line. It serves as the input data for the image reconstruction algorithm in SPECT. Reconstruction techniques, such as filtered back projection or iterative methods, use the sinogram data to generate a three-dimensional image representation of the radiotracer distribution within the imaged object.

Box 7.1 Summary of Working Principles of Gamma Camera

A radioactive substance is administered to the patients, which emits gamma rays. These gamma rays interact with a scintillation crystal, typically made of sodium iodide thallium-activated crystals (NaI(Tl)) or cesium iodide thallium-activated crystals (CsI(Tl)) or newly introduced cadmium zinc telluride (CZT) semiconductor detectors. This interaction produces scintillation photons (flashes of light) in the crystal. But before interacting with crystals, they pass through the collimators.

The collimation: The collimator consists of parallel holes of lead or tungsten. It allows only gamma rays traveling along specific paths to pass through while rejecting scattered and off-axis radiation.

Scintillation Process: The gamma rays that successfully pass through the collimator interact with the scintillation crystal. The interaction of the gamma rays with the detector crystal generates scintillation photons. The crystal is coupled to several photomultiplier tubes (PMTs), covering almost the entire crystal area, detecting these scintillations, and converting them into electrical signals.

Preamplifier and Amplifier: The preamplifier and amplifier work to amplify the weak electrical signals generated by the PMTs in response to scintillation photons. The preamplifier amplifies the signals immediately after generation by the PMTs, while the amplifier further amplifies the signals to an optimal level for subsequent processing and analysis in the gamma camera system.

Analogue-to-Digital Converter (ADC): The ADC in a gamma camera plays a critical role in converting the continuous analogue signals from the PMTs into discrete digital values that digital systems can process and analyze. The digital signals can be used for energy analysis, pulse height discrimination, positioning calculations, and subsequent image reconstruction.

Pulse Height Analyzer (PHA): The electrical signals from the PMTs are fed into a pulse height analyzer. The PHA analyzes the amplitude (energy) of the electrical signals, sorting them into energy windows or bins corresponding to different energy levels. This allows for energy discrimination and the creation of an energy spectrum.

Anticoincidence Circuit: The anticoincidence circuit consists of additional detectors or scintillation crystals around the primary detector. It helps identify and reject events where gamma rays are detected simultaneously in both the primary and anticoincidence detectors, reducing background or scattered radiation.

Data Acquisition System: The processed electrical signals, including their energies and positions, are sent to the data acquisition system. The data acquisition system collects, processes, and stores the information needed for image reconstruction.

***X–Y* Positioning Circuit and the Energy Signals (*E*):** The combination of the *X–Y* positioning circuit and the energy signals (*E*) in a gamma camera enables the precise localization of gamma-ray interactions within the detector crystal and provides information about the energy levels of the detected gamma rays. *X–Y* positioning circuit processes the signals from multiple PMTs to determine the *X* and *Y* coordinates of the gamma-ray interaction within the detector crystal.

(continued)

Box 7.1 (continued)

Image Corrections: Various corrections are applied to the acquired data to improve image quality. Some common corrections include:

- Uniformity Correction: This correction accounts for nonuniform response across the detector crystal, ensuring consistent sensitivity throughout the field of view.
- Linearity Correction: Linearity correction compensates for any nonlinear response in the gamma camera's detection system, ensuring accurate measurement of gamma-ray energy.
- Energy Resolution Correction: This correction helps optimize the energy resolution of the gamma camera, ensuring accurate energy discrimination and better image quality.

Reconstruction: The acquired data, including the *X–Y* positions and energy information, are processed using reconstruction algorithms. These algorithms convert the data into two-dimensional or three-dimensional images, representing the radiotracer distribution within the patient's body.

Filters: Filters can be applied to the reconstructed images to enhance image quality, reduce noise, or emphasize specific features of interest.

Display: The final reconstructed and filtered images are displayed, providing visual information about the distribution and functional processes being studied.

7.8 Quality Control in Gamma Camera/SPECT Imaging

Quality control in gamma camera/SPECT imaging ensures accurate and reliable results. It involves a series of tests and procedures to assess the performance and functionality of the gamma camera system, detect potential issues or deviations, and maintain optimal imaging quality. The NEMA (National Electrical Manufacturers Association) and national regulatory bodies provide guidelines for quality control of gamma cameras, and they have been developed over several decades to establish standardized procedures and recommendations for ensuring the performance and reliability of gamma camera systems. The first guideline by NEMA was published in 1994 and NU 1-1994, which was revised and expanded in 1997 with new guidelines named NU 1-1997. Subsequently, revised guidelines, viz., NU 1-2001, NU 1-2007, NU-2012, and a recent guideline on this is NU 1-2018. These editions provide comprehensive recommendations and procedures for assessing the performance of gamma camera systems, covering areas such as spatial resolution, uniformity, energy resolution, and count rate performance.

The NEMA guidelines have evolved to reflect advancements in technology, changes in imaging practices, and the need for standardized quality control procedures. These guidelines aim to ensure consistency, accuracy, and reliability in gamma camera imaging by providing standardized procedures for quality control testing. Imaging facilities need to adhere to these guidelines to maintain the performance and reliability of their gamma camera systems.

Several performance characteristics of gamma cameras are evaluated during quality control tests, for example, intrinsic characteristics or detector and electronics characteristics *without collimator*; extrinsic characteristics, i.e., performance of detector and electronics *with collimator* in planar imaging, SPECT, or three-dimensional imaging parameters; and if CT is integrated with the camera, the CT performance as well as co-registration of both modalities. The summarized below characteristics demand several tests and include a recommendation from NEMA, AAPM, and country-specific requirements:

A. *Intrinsic (collimator removed) gamma camera performance*
   (a) Centering of pulse height analyzer (PHA) window
   (b) Intrinsic flood field uniformity
   (c) Intrinsic flood field uniformity through narrowed and asymmetric (off-centered) PHA windows
   (d) Intrinsic spatial resolution and linearity
   (e) Energy resolution
   (f) Multiple window spatial registration
   (g) Intrinsic count rate performance and dead time with and without scatter medium
   (h) Maximum count rate performance in air
   (i) Intrinsic flood field uniformity and spatial resolution at 75 kcps
B. *Extrinsic (with collimator) gamma camera performance*
   (a) Extrinsic flood field uniformity
   (b) Extrinsic spatial resolution (FWHM and FWTM) at 0, 10, and 20 cm distance from the detector surface
   (c) System spatial linearity
   (d) System planar sensitivity at 10 cm from the detector surface
   (e) Collimator hole angulation
   (f) Detector head shielding leakage
   (g) Scan speed for the whole-body scan
C. *Tomographic (SPECT) characteristics*
   (a) Pixel size (*X* and *Y* direction)
   (b) Integral tomographic uniformity, RMS noise with flood correction and contrast resolution
   (c) Tomographic resolution in the air (*X* and *Y* direction)
   (d) Multiple head registration (MHR) and center of rotation offset and alignment of axes
   (e) Slice thickness at the center of the field of view
   (f) Variations of sensitivity with angle
D. *Co-registration of SPECT and CT modalities*—alignment (registration) calibration

English and Zimmerman [28] suggest the gamma camera shall meet or exceed certain specifications at 140 keV energy in the central field of view (CFOV), as mentioned in Table 7.10.

Let us discuss these parameters in detail:

7.8.1 Tests of Intrinsic Gamma Camera Detector Characteristics

The intrinsic characteristics of a gamma camera detector refer to its inherent properties that affect image quality and performance. The term "intrinsic" specifically refers to the detector properties without the influence of the collimator. These characteristics determine the uniformity, sensitivity, resolution, linearity, energy response, etc. Let's discuss these characteristics:

7.8.1.1 Centering of Pulse Height Analyzer Window

The test for centering of PHA (pulse height analyzer) assesses the accuracy of the energy window settings in the gamma camera's PHA system. The PHA window refers to a specific energy range within which the gamma camera detects and counts gamma rays. The centering of the PHA window ensures that it is aligned with the desired energy range for optimal image acquisition and quantification.

A radioactive source with known energy emission is used during the centering of the PHA window test. The source is positioned in the gamma camera's field of view, and an energy spectrum is obtained. The goal is to determine the PHA window settings that align with the expected energy range of the radioactive source. The acquired spectrum is verified if it is centered correctly on the expected energy peak. Any deviations from the desired energy range may indicate misalignment or calibration issues in the PHA system,

Table 7.10 Gamma camera standard performance specifications

Parameter	Sub-parameter	Minimum requirement
Intrinsic uniformity	Integral	±3.0%
	Differential	±4.0%
Intrinsic resolution	FWHM	4.0 mm
	FWTM	8.0 mm
Intrinsic energy resolution		11.0%
Intrinsic spatial linearity	Absolute	1.0 mm
	Differential	0.4 mm
Intrinsic count rate performance	20% loss (normal mode)	75 kcps
	20% loss (high count rate mode)	110 kcps
	Maximum count rate	200 kcps
Intrinsic spatial resolution at 75 kcps (FWHM)		5.0 mm
Multiple window spatial registration		2.0 mm
Intrinsic flood field uniformity	Integral at 75 kcps	±7.0%
Point source sensitivity		±4.0%
Extrinsic spatial resolution (low-energy collimator)	FWHM (air)	10.5 mm
	FWTM (air)	17.8 mm
	FWHM (10 cm H_2O)	11.2 mm
	FWTM (10 cm H_2O)	22.9 mm
System sensitivity		330 cpm

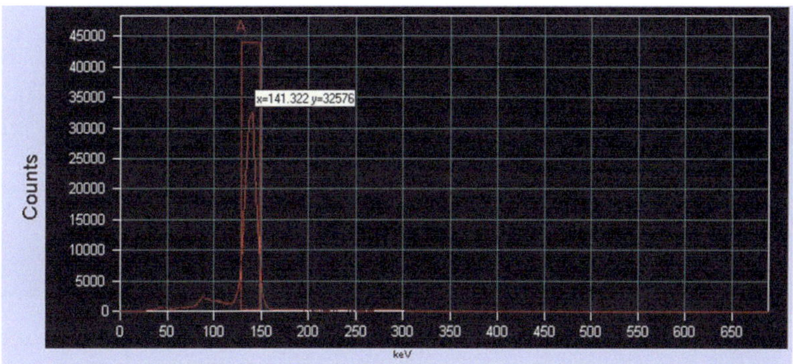

Fig. 7.42 Energy spectrum of ^{99m}Tc obtained from gamma camera

affecting the accuracy and reliability of subsequent image quantification.

By performing the PHA window's centering test, gamma camera operators can ensure that the energy window settings are properly calibrated, allowing for accurate detection and quantification of gamma rays within the desired energy range. This quality control measure helps maintain the performance and reliability of the gamma camera system for optimal imaging results (Fig. 7.42).

7.8.1.2 Intrinsic Flood Field Uniformity

The intrinsic flood field uniformity test evaluates the uniformity of the detector response across the field of view when exposed to a flood source of radiation. Four terms are used in this test: central FOV (CFOV), useful FOV (UFOV), and integral and differential uniformities. The terms UFOV (useful field of view) and CFOV (central field of view) describe regions of the detector's field of view. The UFOV represents 95% of the entire FOV, whereas the CFOV represents 75% of the UFOV. This test assesses two aspects of uniformity: integral and differential.

Prepare a point source of ^{99m}Tc with 25 μCi (925 kBq) activity for Siemens systems or 10–20 MBq (0.3–0.5 mCi) activity for GE and other systems, which the manufacturer recommends. In Siemens ecam systems, the point source is kept at 20 cm away from detectors, and for other systems, the point source is kept at five

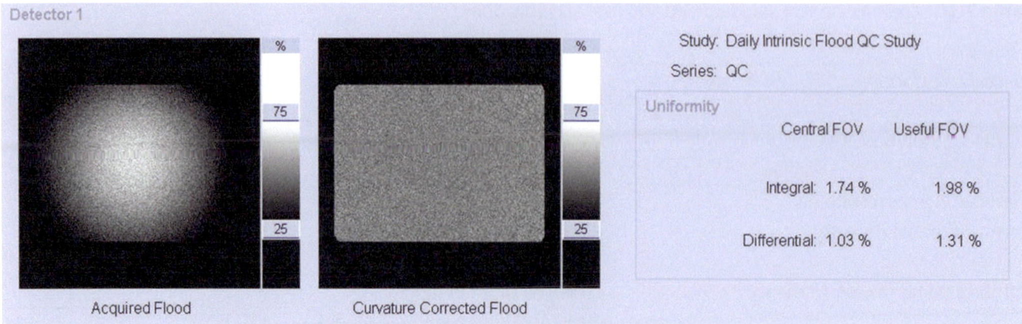

Fig. 7.43 Intrinsic uniformity report generated by single-head gamma camera

times of largest UFOV dimension and 30K counts/s with the manufacturer's default PHA window is acquired (Fig. 7.43). A similar way can be done for the other radioisotopes intended to be used on the camera.

Integral Uniformity

Integral uniformity evaluates the overall uniformity of the detector response across the entire field of view and is based on the image's maximum and minimum pixel count. It can be calculated using the following formula:

$$\text{Integral uniformity}\,(\text{in}\%) = \frac{\text{Pixel}_{\max} - \text{Pixel}_{\min}}{\text{Pixel}_{\max} + \text{Pixel}_{\min}} \times 100 \qquad (7.3)$$

where $\text{Pixel}_{\max}$ and $\text{Pixel}_{\min}$ are maximum and minimum pixel counts within the image.

Differential Uniformity

Differential uniformity assesses the local variations or differences in the detector response in five consecutive pixels vertically or horizontally in the image. Mathematically, it can be calculated with the following formula:

$$\text{Differential uniformity}\,(\text{in}\%) = \frac{\text{Pixel}_{\text{high}} - \text{Pixel}_{\text{low}}}{\text{Pixel}_{\text{high}} + \text{Pixel}_{\text{low}}} \times 100 \qquad (7.4)$$

$\text{Pixel}_{\text{high}}$ and $\text{Pixel}_{\text{low}}$ are maximum and minimum count differences for any five consecutive pixels (horizontally or vertically) in the image.

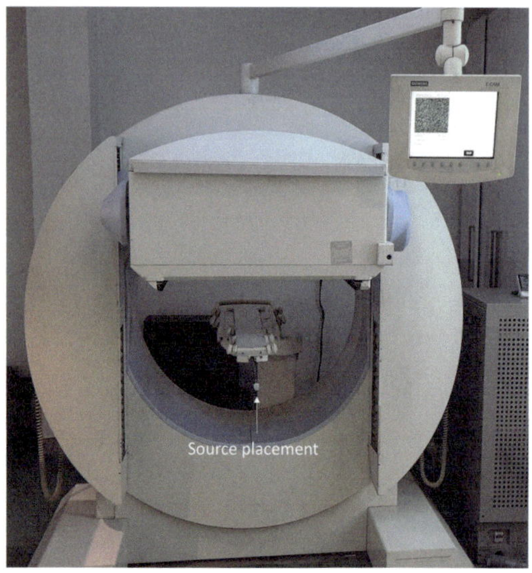

Fig. 7.44 Flood source placement for intrinsic uniformity

Both parameters, i.e., integral and differential uniformities, are evaluated within the center field of view (CFOV) and the useful field of view (UFOV).

During the intrinsic flood field uniformity test, the flood phantom uniformly irradiates the detector surface, and the gamma camera acquires the image. The acquired data is then analyzed to calculate integral and differential uniformity in UFOV and CFOV (Fig. 7.44).

7.8.1.3 Test of Intrinsic Flood Field Uniformity Through Narrowed and Asymmetric (Off-Centered) PHA Windows

Asymmetric energy windows are used to assess the hydration of crystals, sometimes known as the measles effect, tuning of PM tubes, and identify any electronic issues. Even when the same amount of asymmetric shift is applied, some scintillation cameras are more sensitive to off-peak windows than others [29]. The hydrated areas appear more obviously as hotspots on the asymmetric low image and cold spots on the asymmetric high image in the corresponding positions [29] (Fig. 7.45).

The source for the intrinsic uniformity test (previous test) can also be used. 30,000K counts each are acquired in three energy window settings, viz., 140 keV (15% window), 10% window at energies centered at 130 and 150 keV for lower and higher asymmetric windows and observed for any hydration of the crystal and uniformity in all three images to verify all PMTs are well tuned.

7.8.1.4 Test of Intrinsic Spatial Resolution and Linearity

The intrinsic spatial resolution of a gamma camera refers to its ability to accurately determine a radioactive source's spatial location. It is a measure of the smallest distance between two-point sources that the gamma camera can distinguish. The spatial resolution is typically measured in full-width half resolution (FWHM) and full-width tenth value resolution (FWTM). For more details on FWHM and FWTM, please refer to Sect. 7.6.1 in PET spatial resolution (Fig. 7.46).

In its recommendations, the International Atomic Energy Agency (IAEA) describes two methods to test intrinsic spatial resolution [29]. The first method is called the "visual image method," which can be used if only "quadrant bar phantom" is available, and this method does not even need any software to process the data. The second method is called the "quantitative method," which uses "intrinsic spatial resolution and linearity (ISRL) phantom" and software to process the data. The ISRL phantom is constructed of a lead sheet at least 3 mm in thickness

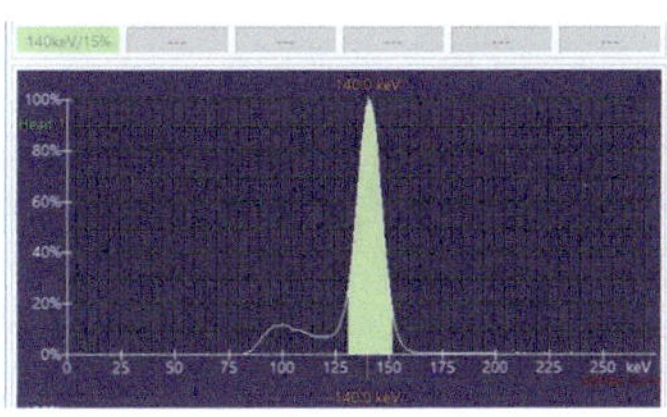

15% symmetric narrowed window

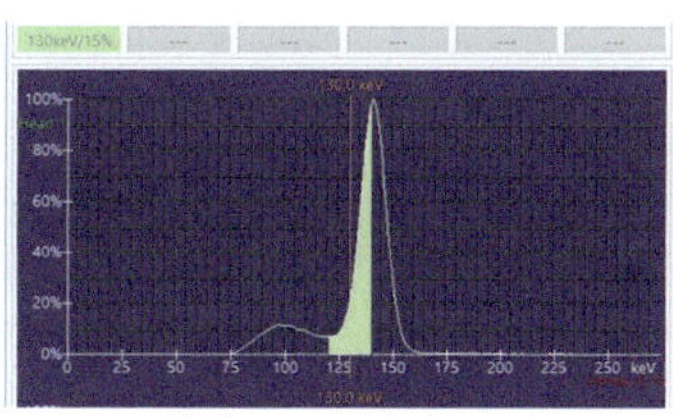

10% energy window set asymmetrically over the lower half of the photopeak

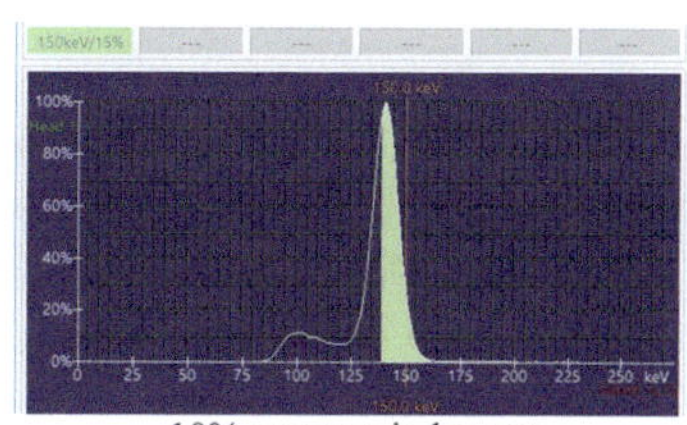

10% energy window set asymmetrically over the upper half of the photopeak

Camera response at 15% symmetric narrowed window

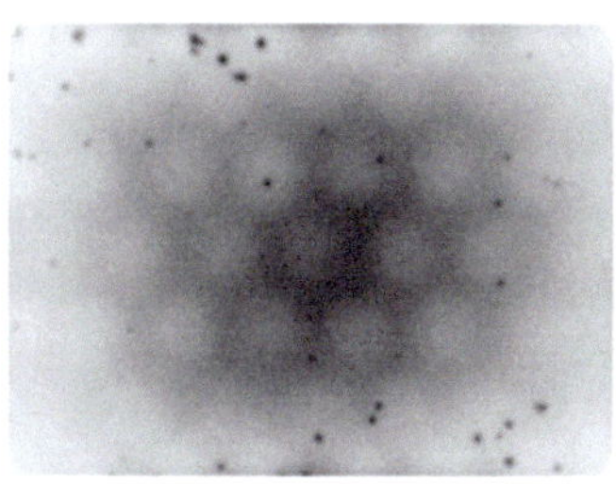

The hydrated areas appears as hotspots on the asymmetric low image

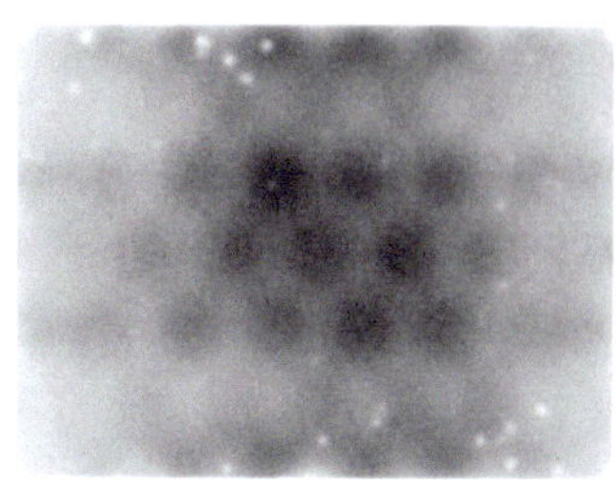

The hydrated areas appears as cold spots on the asymmetric high image

Fig. 7.45 Intrinsic flood field uniformity through narrowed and asymmetric PHA windows

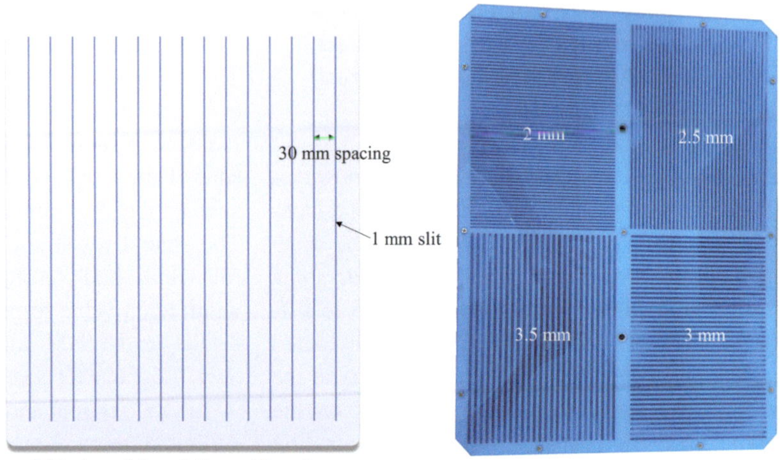

Intrinsic spatial resolution and linearity phantom (IRSL)

Quadrant bar phantom

Fig. 7.46 Spatial resolution phantoms—intrinsic spatial resolution and linearity phantom (ISRL phantom) and quadrant bar phantom

with 1 mm slits at 30 mm spacing. These phantoms are kept on the surface of the detector without a collimator and exposed to a point source containing activity of 20–40 MBq (0.5–1 mCi) kept at a distance of ≥5 times of UFOV for the uniform flood of radiation [29].

The visual image method keeps the quadrant bar phantom as close as possible to the detector. The bars are carefully aligned to the *X* and *Y* axes of the detector, and 60K counts are acquired using the largest available matrix size. The phantom is rotated for 90°, and the procedure is repeated a couple more times. The phantom is inverted, and the procedure is repeated for each quarter. A total of eight images are acquired, and the smallest resolved bar width is noted down in both *X* and *Y* directions. The FWHM is calculated using the formula:

$$\mathrm{FWHM} = 1.75B \tag{7.5}$$

where *B* is the width of the smallest resolve bar. The spatial linearity can be noted by observing whether lines are straight, indicating a good spatial linearity.

The quantitative method uses two ISRL phantoms for *X* and *Y* directions per manufacturer recommendation. A point source containing 40 MBq (1 mCi) of ^{99m}Tc is kept at a distance of ≥5 times UFOV, and the first phantom is mounted. Counts are acquired as per manufacturer recommendations. The second phantom with slits parallel to the other direction is placed once the first phantom test is over. A second image using the parameters for the total count as instructed by the manufacturer is also acquired. A special analysis software provided by the manufacturer analyzes FWHM and the FWTM in the UFOV and CFOV. This is done in the *X* and *Y* directions (Figs. 7.47 and 7.48). The software also reports the intrinsic spatial linearity.

7.8.1.5 Test of Energy Resolution

The energy resolution in a gamma camera refers to its ability to distinguish between different energy levels of gamma rays. It measures the camera's capability to resolve small differences in the energy spectrum of detected gamma rays. The energy resolution is affected by various factors, including the properties of the scintillation crystal, the PMT characteristics, the electronic noise, and the energy calibration procedures (Fig. 7.49).

A lower energy resolution indicates a higher ability to differentiate between gamma rays of slightly different energies. This is important for accurately identifying specific radionuclides and distinguishing between different energy peaks in the acquired gamma-ray spectrum.

The energy resolution is typically expressed as a percentage of the full width at half maximum (FWHM) of the energy peak in the energy spectrum. For example, an intrinsic energy resolution of 10% at 140 keV means that the FWHM of the energy peak at 140 keV is 10%

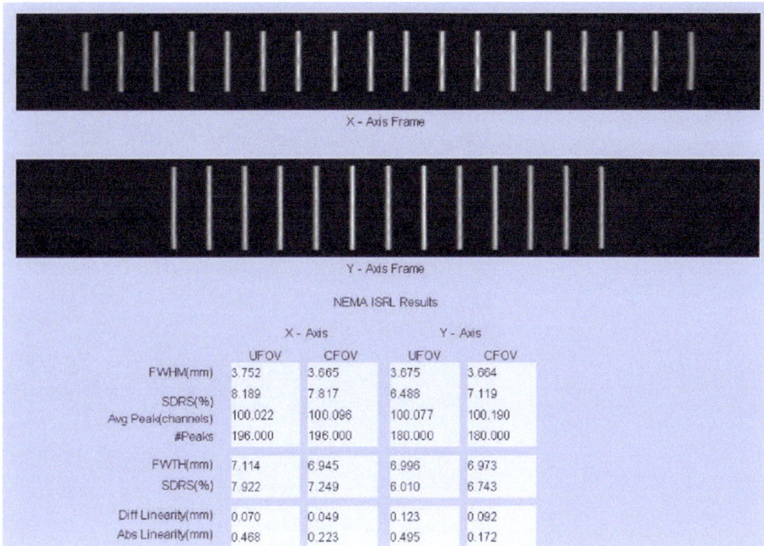

Fig. 7.47 Siemens ecam single-head gamma camera intrinsic spatial resolution calculation using quantitative method

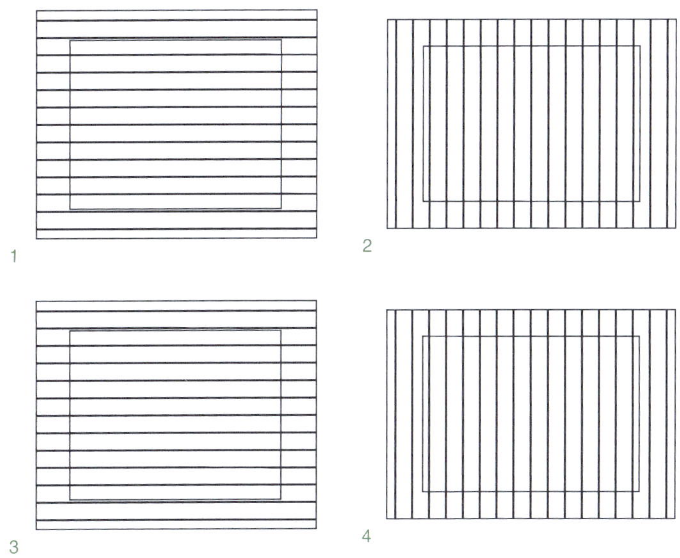

		UFOV	CFOV
1	FWHM [mm]	4.26	4.25
	FWTM [mm]	8.09	8.05
2	FWHM [mm]	4.43	4.34
	FWTM [mm]	8.36	8.19
3	FWHM [mm]	4.52	4.55
	FWTM [mm]	8.57	8.61
4	FWHM [mm]	4.54	4.50
	FWTM [mm]	8.62	8.54

No.	Angle[°]	Head / No	Lines	Orientation	kcps	Max.	mm/Pixel	Line Distance
1	0.000	rectang. 1	13	horizontal	3.631	1000	1.20 (1.20)	25.1Pixel/30mm
2	–0.335	rectang. 1	17	vertical	3.432	1000	1.19 (1.20)	25.1Pixel/30mm
3	0.000	rectang. 2	13	horizontal	3.704	892	1.20 (1.20)	25.1Pixel/30mm
4	0.000	rectang. 2	17	vertical	3.352	939	1.19 (1.20)	25.1Pixel/30mm

Fig. 7.48 MI ecam dual-head gamma camera intrinsic spatial resolution calculation using quantitative method

of the peak energy or 14 keV. Achieving high energy resolution is desirable in gamma cameras to enhance the accuracy and reliability of nuclear medicine imaging studies.

While running the energy spectrum graph, some systems display FWHM (Fig. 7.50); for others, a manual calculation can be done using Eq. (7.6). and obtain a graph.

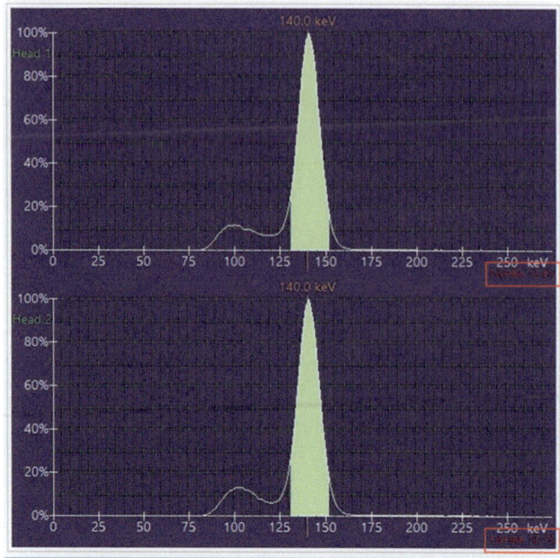

Fig. 7.49 Energy resolution in MI ecam dual-head gamma camera

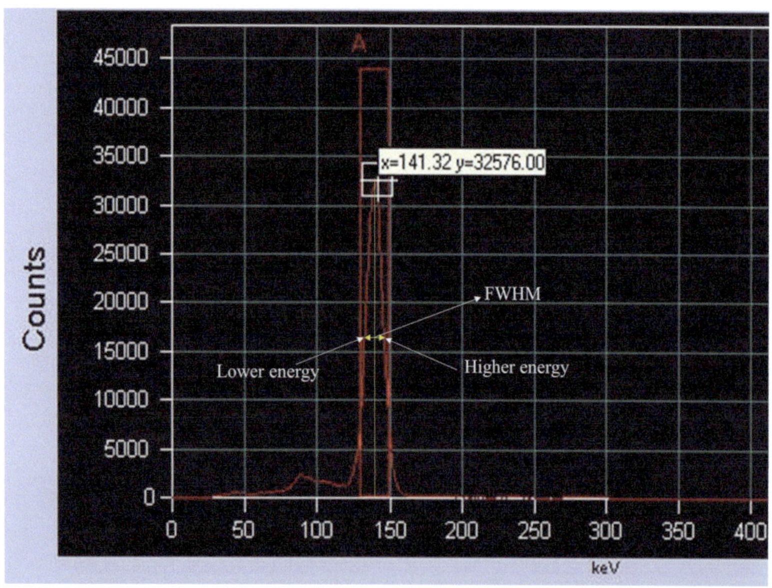

Fig. 7.50 Manual energy resolution

$$\text{Energy resolution} = \frac{\text{Higher energy} - \text{lower energy}}{\text{Energy peak}} \times 100 \quad (7.6)$$

$$\text{Energy resolution} = \frac{146 - 133}{141} \times 100 = 9.2\%$$

7.8.1.6 Multiple Window Spatial Registration

The multiple window spatial registration (MWSR) tests is a method used to evaluate the gamma camera positional response or spatial registration of objects across different energies of gamma photons. The gallium-67 isotope is used for this test as it has gamma photon energies of 93 keV (39%), 184 keV (21%), and 300 keV (17%) or for approximation in remembering it has energies at around 100, 200, and 300 keV. Without moving a source, the counts can be acquired in all three energy ranges, i.e., low, medium, and high. Some gamma camera allows only two energy windows counting; in that case, low and high energies, i.e., energy window centering at 93 and 300 keV can be taken.

The MWSR accuracy is measured at multiple locations along the *x*- and *y*-axis of the gamma camera.

A nine-point source holder MWSR phantom is used for this test in which source holding points are placed along the *x*- and *y*-axis of the gamma camera and contains four sources on the *x*-axis, four sources on the *y*-axis, and one source at the center. The two sources on either side of the central hole are situated at 40% and 80% of UFOV. The lead-lined source holder collimates the gallium-67 source on the detector through the cylindrical lead tunnel. This tunnel is 5 mm in diameter and 25 mm in depth; the other specifications are shown in Fig. 7.51.

Approximately 7–11 MBq (200–300 mCi) of Ga-67 is placed on each holder, and 1K counts are acquired in the peak pixel of each photo peak image with pixel size not more than 2.5 mm [30], and a composite image is obtained in the software-generated report (Fig. 7.52). The software calculates each image's centroid and compares the displacement between the point source at different energy windows. The maximum displacement between the centroids indicates the performance parameter in the MWSR test.

Many companies provide a tolerance of ≤0.6 mm in their product specifications; however, regulatory authorities may allow a tolerance of ≤1.10 mm of reference.

7.8.1.7 Test of Intrinsic Count Rate Performance and Dead Time With and Without Scatter Medium

The test of intrinsic count rate performance and dead time for a gamma camera is used to assess the camera's ability to handle high count rates and measure the system's dead time characteristics. Dead time is when the gamma camera cannot detect additional radiation events because it is still processing a previous event. NEMA NU-1-2012 [31] and 2018 [32] suggest the decaying source method and copper plates method; however, AAPM report no. 6 [33] and report no. 9 [34] suggest two-source method with specific conditions of scatter and count rates. This method is easy and fast and requires scatter phantom. However, instead of scatter phantom, a beaker filled with rice can also be used as scatter media. The country-specific regulatory authorities demand the test for count rate performance and dead time with and without scatter medium having two source methods or the manufacturer's method [35]. The count rate performance with scatter media is simulated using a gamma camera in clinical conditions [36].

In two source methods, two sources of similar activities, i.e., 1.85 MBq (50 μCi), are prepared which each can produce ~20,000 counts per second (cps) (±10%) (R_1 and R_2) at a 1-m distance and 34,000–36,000 cps (R_{12}) when kept together at 1-m distance. "In the

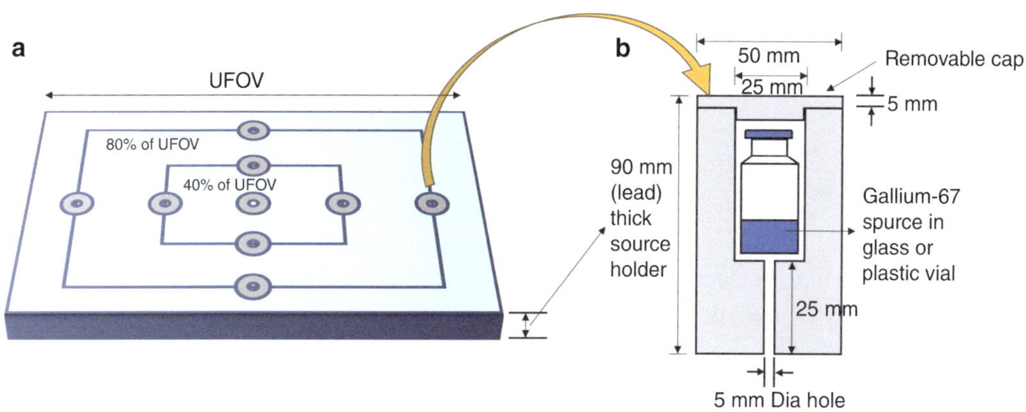

Fig. 7.51 Multiple windows spatial registration phantom with lead-lined point sources holder. (**a**) MWSR phantom with nine source holders. (**b**) Cross-section of source holder and source via

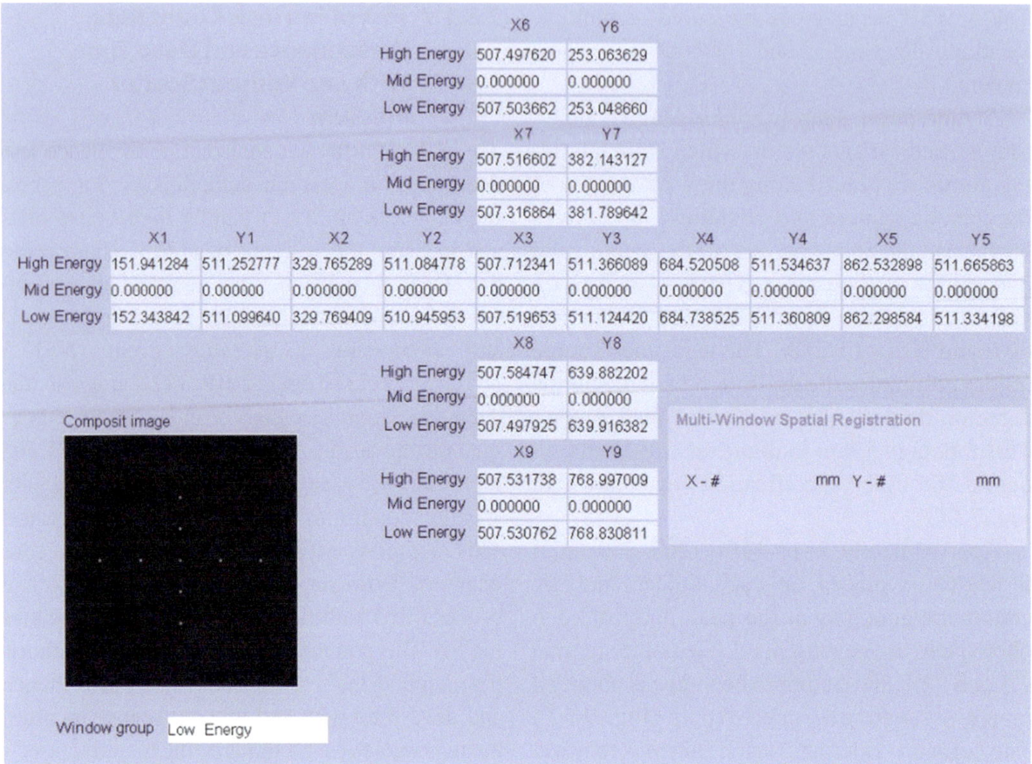

Fig. 7.52 A software-generated nine-point centroid readings

20,000–36,000 cps range, the deadtime (τ) does not vary more than 5%, and these counting rates are of critical concern for most deadtime corrections. At lower counting rates, the correction factors are small, and a slight under-correction or over-correction is usually not significant, but at higher counting rates, the deadtime losses may be excessive" [36]. The formula for the calculation of dead time for the gamma camera is:

$$\text{Dead time}(\tau) = \left[\frac{2 \times R_{12}}{(R_1 + R_2)^2}\right] \ln\left(\frac{R_1 + R_2}{R_{12}}\right) \tag{7.7}$$

Once the dead time is calculated, the input count rate at 20% counting losses ($R_{-20\%}$) is calculated using the formula:

$$R_{-20\%} = \frac{1}{\tau} \times \ln\left(\frac{10}{8}\right) \tag{7.8}$$

or

$$R_{-20\%} = \frac{0.2331}{\tau(\text{in s})} \tag{7.9}$$

The input or true count rate refers to the rate at which radiation events (such as gamma-ray detections) enter the detection system or gamma camera. It represents the actual count rate of radiation events before any effects of dead time or other system limitations come into play. It helps provide a baseline reference for comparison with the observed count rate (which may be affected by dead time, system limitations, or other factors). By comparing the observed count rate to the input count rate, one can assess the impact of dead time or other system characteristics on the accuracy and reliability of the count rate measurement.

Procedure

Articles needed

- Two-point sources of 50 μCi each
- One small beaker filled with rice

Two-point sources are prepared with the activity of 50 μCi each, and then one of the two sources is kept at a distance of 1 m from the detector surface. The system is set to acquire counts for 100 s. The second point source is also positioned alongside the first source without moving it, and counts for both the sources are acquired for 100 s. In the third reading, the first source is removed and counts for only the second source is observed again for 100 s.

A similar procedure is repeated for "with scatter" measurements. The point sources are kept inside a small beaker filled with rice. The readings are obtained first with one source, then with both sources, and then by removing the first source from the beaker (Fig. 7.53).

Calculation Data

Figure 7.53 shows the counts obtained in 100 s. They are converted to counts per second by dividing 100.

Without scatter

R_1 = 21,730 counts/s (for the first source at 1 m)

R_{12} = 41,350 counts/s (for both sources together at 1 m)

R_2 = 21,580 counts/s (for the second source at 1 m)

With scatter

R_1 = 17,800 counts/s

R_{12} = 34,800 counts/s

R_2 = 18,650 counts/s

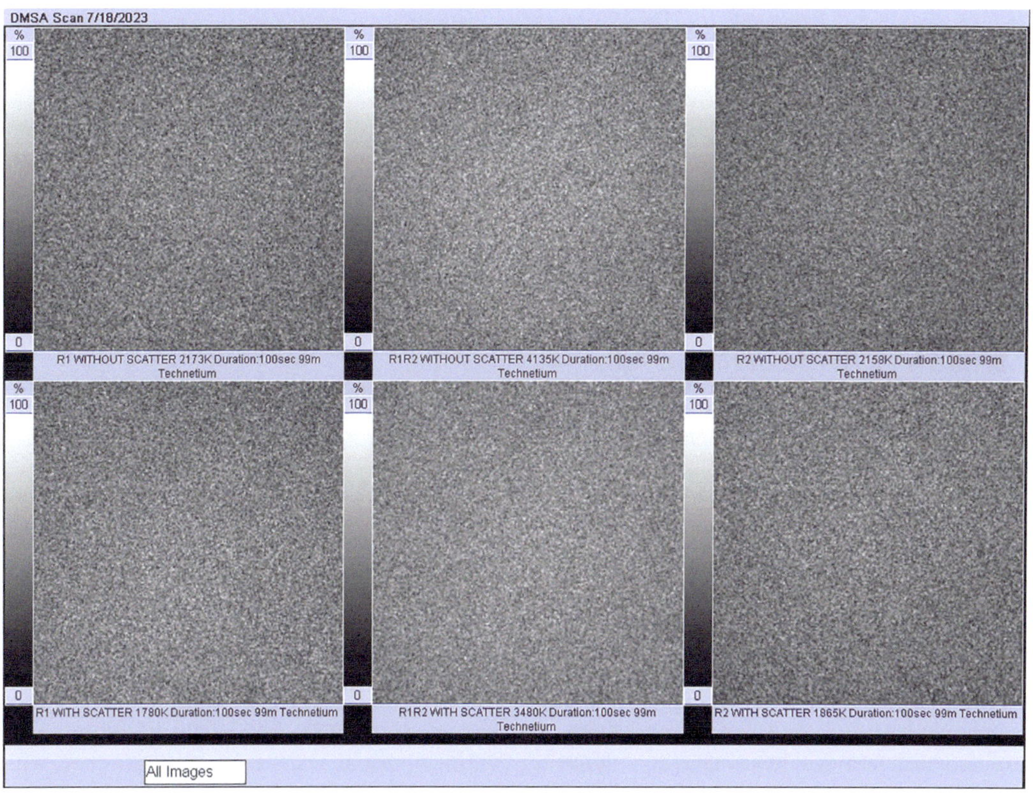

Fig. 7.53 Raw data for calculation of dead time with and without scatter using the two-source method

Dead Time Calculation

$$\text{The formula for dead time }(\tau)=\left[\frac{2\times R_{12}}{(R_1+R_2)^2}\right]\ln\left(\frac{R_1+R_2}{R_{12.}}\right)$$

Dead time without scatter, i.e.,

$$\text{Dead time in air}(\tau_{\text{air}})=\left(\frac{2\times 41{,}350}{(21{,}730+21{,}580)^2}\right)\ln\left(\frac{21{,}730+21{,}580}{41{,}350}\right)$$

$$=\frac{82{,}700}{1{,}875{,}756{,}100}\ln(1.047)$$

$$=4.41\times 10^{-5}\times 0.046$$

$$(\tau_{\text{air}})=2.02\,\mu s$$

Similarly, dead time in scatter media (τ_{scatter}) = 2.43 µs

$$\text{Now, the Input count rate for 20\% data loss}(R_{-20\%})\text{ in air}=\frac{1}{\tau_{\text{air}}}\times\ln\left(\frac{10}{8}\right)=\frac{0.2331}{\tau_{\text{air}}(\text{in s})}$$

$$=\frac{0.2331}{2.02\times 10^{-6}}=115.4\text{K}$$

$$\text{And Input count rate for 20\% data loss}(R_{-20\%})\text{ in scatter}=\frac{1}{\tau_{\text{scatter}}}\times\ln\left(\frac{10}{8}\right)=\frac{0.2331}{\tau_{\text{scatter}}(\text{in s})}$$

$$=\frac{0.2331}{2.43\times 10^{-6}}=95.9\text{K}$$

Then compare with the manufacturer's specifications. Reporting can be done in the following Table 7.11.

7.8.1.8 Test of Maximum Count Rate in Air

The test of the maximum count rate in the air for a gamma camera is performed to determine the highest count rate the gamma camera can handle without saturating or exceeding its counting capabilities. This test is essential to understand the camera's maximum count rate limit and to ensure its proper functioning during high-activity imaging studies.

NEMA again suggests a decaying source and copper plate method; however, this measurement can also be determined by using a set of dynamic images acquired from a source, slowly moving toward the crystal surface of the detector without a collimator. A 100 µCi ^{99m}Tc point source is taken and suspended in a trolley at about a 2-m distance and slowly moved toward the camera, and dynamic acquisition per second is acquired. A graph of distance versus count rate was plotted (Fig. 7.54, Table 7.12).

7.8.1.9 Intrinsic Flood Field Uniformity and Spatial Resolution at 75 kcps

If the gamma camera is used with high count rates, some tests, such as flood field uniformity and spatial resolution, can be repeated at 75 kcps. Though clinical static acquisitions do not reach such a count rate, cardiac first-pass studies using a 30-mCi bolus of activity may reach such count rates.

This test is supplementary to the test performed as intrinsic flood field uniformity and intrinsic spatial resolution and performed with the same method but with a high count rate, i.e., 75,000 counts per second count rate, and results are reported along with manufacturer specifications for comparison.

Table 7.11 Table for reporting dead time and input count rate at 20% count loss with and without scatter

	With scatter			Without scatter (in air)		
Description	Measured	Reference	Tolerance	Measured	Reference	Tolerance
Dead time	2.43 μs	As specified by the manufacturer	±10% of reference	2.02 μs	As specified by the manufacturer	±10% of reference
Input count rate	95.9K	As specified by the manufacturer	±10% of reference	115.4K	As specified by the manufacturer	±10% of reference

Table 7.12 The reporting of the maximum count rate in the air can be made in the following table

Description	Measured	Reference	Tolerance
Maximum count rate	243 kcps	As specified by the manufacturer	±20% of the reference value

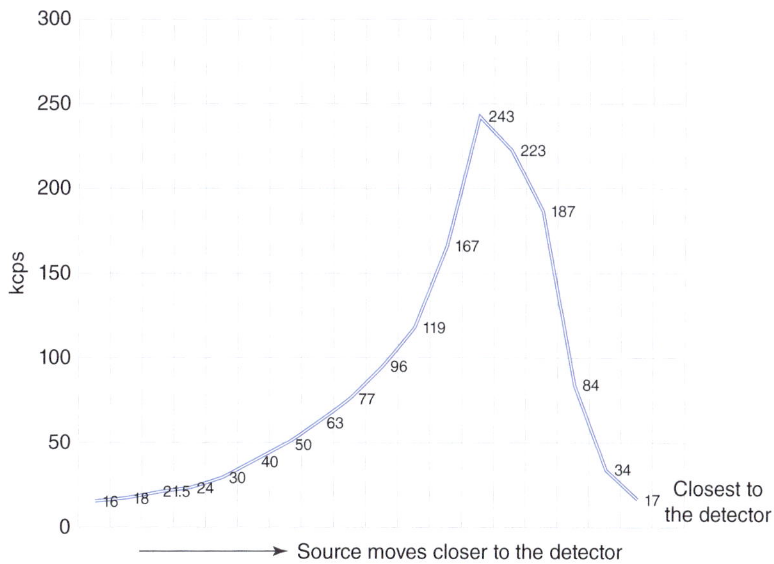

Fig. 7.54 Graph for maximum count rate performance

7.8.2 Extrinsic (with Collimator) Gamma Camera Performance Parameters

7.8.2.1 Extrinsic Flood Field Uniformity

Extrinsic flood field uniformity assesses the uniformity of gamma camera response across the field of view when collimators are placed on top of the detector. In clinical conditions, the gamma camera is used with collimators on; this test gives uniformity response of the system as a whole. This test is not mentioned in NEMA recommendations [32]; however, the AAPM [33, 37], the IAEA [38], and country-specific regulatory bodies [35] recommend this test to be performed. The IAEA recommends frequency for this test as a reference test and half yearly after that. Most manufacturers supply water-fillable phantoms for performing this test as routine when they supply machine as part of their accessories. However, the Co-57 sheet source can be used instead of the water-fillable phantom with ^{99m}Tc. The Co-57 sheet source is easy and ready to use but is expensive and requires frequent replacements as Co-57 has a half-life of 270 days, and these sources have a shelf life of 2 years (Fig. 7.55).

LEHR (low-energy high-resolution) collimator is mounted on the detector head. ^{99m}Tc flood or ^{57}Co sheet source containing 5–7 mCi is taken with uniform filling. The count rate should be below 30 kcps with the collimator on the camera. By selecting the appropriate protocol, this test is done by an Auto-Run procedure available in the software. The detector will undergo acquisition

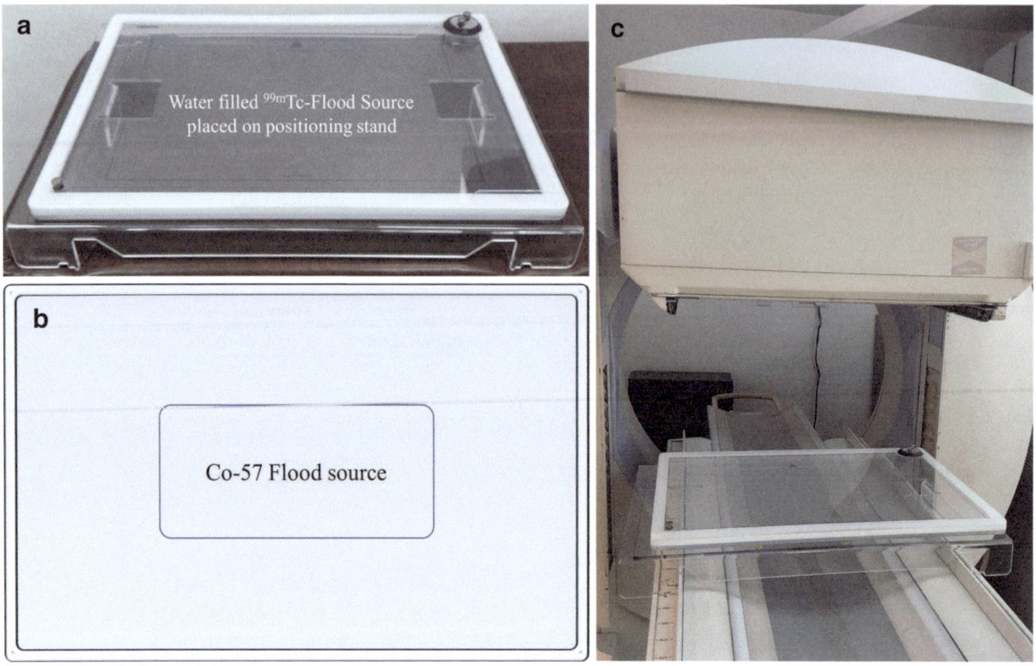

Fig. 7.55 Extrinsic flood field uniformity test. (**a**) Water-filled ^{99m}Tc flood phantom placed on positioning stand. (**b**) Schematic diagram of Co-57 flood source. (**c**) Water-filled phantom kept on the table before readings

one by one in an automated manner, with ten million counts acquired for each detector head.

Using the same source (phantom), the procedure is repeated for the HE (high-energy) collimator.

7.8.2.2 Extrinsic Spatial Resolution (FWHM and FWTM) at 0, 10, and 20 cm Distance from the Detector Surface and Test of System Spatial Linearity

The NEMA recommended spatial resolution with and without scatter and performed at a distance of 10 cm from the collimator [32]. Two capillary tubes with inner diameters less than or equal to 1 mm and at least a length greater than 30 mm, along with two acrylic scattering blocks of sizes 10 cm and 5 cm thickness, are used to perform this test. The method is mentioned in the standards. The IAEA suggests two methods, viz., *visual and quantitative methods*, and recommends to be performed at 0, 10, and 20 cm with scatter media [38]. In the visual method, the flood phantom is used for extrinsic uniformity, and the bar phantom has spacings of about 4, 6, 8, and 10 mm. The bar phantom is kept on the detector, flood phantom is kept on top of that, and a total of 6×10^6 counts is acquired. The quadrant bar phantom is rotated through 90°, and counts are acquired again. The same procedure is repeated twice, and then the phantom acquires a similar set of four images so that each quadrant in each direction images the smallest bars. The visual inspection of this image gives *system spatial linearity*.

The same procedure is repeated but with the quadrant bar phantom and flood phantom at a distance of 10 cm from the face of the collimator. The phantom should be supported with non-scattering material such as Styrofoam cups or other materials. At the same distance, the procedure is repeated with a scattering phantom to get system spatial resolution at 10 cm with scatter.

The widths of the smallest bars are determined visually by which scintillation camera can resolve in the X and Y directions at 0 and 10 cm positions. The system spatial resolution is estimated in the

X and *Y* directions in terms of the FWHM of the line spread function using the formula:

$$\mathrm{FWHM} = 1.75B \tag{7.10}$$

where B is the width of the smallest bars that the camera can resolve.

The procedure is repeated for each direction and averaged to get system spatial resolution at 0, 10, and 20 cm with scatter.

The quantitative method accurately assesses system spatial resolution regarding FWHM and FWTM. To perform this test, four microcapillaries having an internal diameter of 0.5 mm, minimum 30 mm in length, each filled with 1.5–2 mCi of ^{99m}Tc solution and sealed with sealing clay or wax are mounted on the edge of 10 cm square drawn on rigid plastic or cardboard. Static acquisitions for 60K counts at 0, 10, and 20 cm are obtained per country-specific requirements and may be acquired at 0 and 10 cm with and without scatter counts. If the gamma camera software permits its evaluation, it can be done there, or IAEA software can be used to know the FWHM and FWTM (Fig. 7.56).

7.8.2.3 System Planar Sensitivity at 10 cm from the Detector Surface

System planar sensitivity measures the gamma camera's ability to detect and register gamma rays emitted from a radioactive source outside the camera. The count rate response of the gamma camera is measured from a known source of radioactivity measured in a dose calibrator. Count per minute/μCi unit is typically used to denote system planar sensitivity.

Approximately 1 mCi of the source is measured in a dose calibrator in a syringe, and activ-

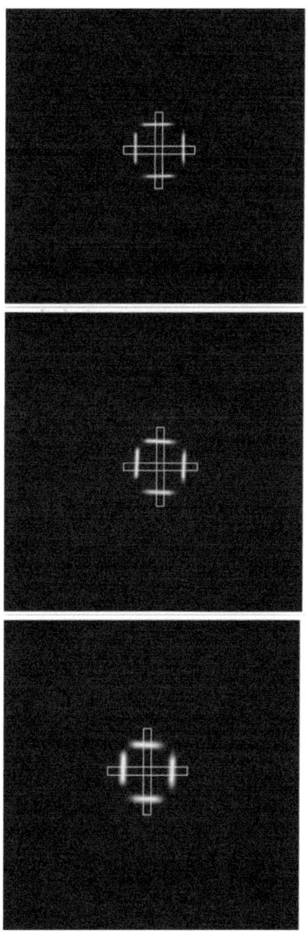

At 0 cm

Test	X (mm)	Y (mm)	Difference (%)
FWHM (mm)	3.1298	3.2212	2.8758
FWTM (mm)	5.7045	5.8709	2.8758

At 10 cm

Test	X (mm)	Y (mm)	Difference (%)
FWHM (mm)	4.8999	5.0383	2.7849
FWTM (mm)	8.9307	9.1829	2.7849

At 20 cm

Test	X (mm)	Y (mm)	Difference (%)
FWHM (mm)	7.3651	7.5417	2.3691
FWTM (mm)	13.4238	13.7456	2.3691

Fig. 7.56 Spatial resolution at 0, 10, and 20 cm of typical gamma camera

ity is noted down. The same source is measured at 10 cm from the surface of the gamma camera. The counts are recorded for 100 s, and sensitivity can be calculated as shown in Fig. 7.57.

7.8.2.4 Collimator Hole Angulation

In gamma cameras, collimator hole angulation or septal angulation refers to the orientation of the collimator holes relative to the detector face. Parallel hole collimators are commonly used in gamma cameras for planar imaging and single photon emission computed tomography (SPECT) imaging. And they consist of multiple holes, and the angulation of these holes affects the imaging characteristics. Any angulation in collimator design is critical and can influence the spatial resolution and sensitivity of the gamma camera. The collimator holes are designed to be perfectly parallel and perpendicular to the detector face for optimal spatial resolution. This configuration ensures that gamma rays travel straight through the collimator without undergoing any scattering or additional blurring effects.

There are many methods explained in various literatures [37–40] to perform this test, and they can give angulation in a measured form. However, the IAEA technique mentioned in reference [37] seems the easiest and does not require any additional phantom or article. But it has the limitation of only visual inspection, and reporting can be as done as "the collimator hole appears to be parallel." Many machine vendors do not provide any reference limit in their technical specifications. As per this method, a point source containing 200–320 MBq (5–8 mCi) of ^{99m}Tc is placed at least 2.5 m away from the detector face and in the line of center of the field of view. The same procedure is repeated at four additional locations on the collimator, and each location should be almost halfway to the edge of the FOV. Acquire the images of 5000K counts with largest available matrix size.

The obtained images are visually inspected and displayed with maximum matrix size. The central image should appear round, and other images should be symmetrical. Hole angulation or collimator defects should appear as streaks (Fig. 7.58) or distorted shapes.

7.8.2.5 Detector Head Shielding Leakage

The detector head shielding in a gamma camera is designed to prevent the gamma camera's detector from receiving radiation from directions other than the intended imaging field of view. The shielding is essential to minimize background radiation and ensure that the detected gamma rays are primarily from the patient or the imaging target. The shielding material, typically made of lead or other dense materials, is strategically

Measured activity in dose calibrator excluding post injection = 0.9 mCi

Counts obtained in 100 seconds in Gamma Camera at 10 cm = 307982

$$\text{Counts in 100 seconds per } \mu\text{Ci} = \frac{307982}{0.9 \times 1000}$$

$$\therefore \text{Counts in 100 seconds per } \mu\text{Ci} = 342 \text{ counts}$$

$$\therefore \text{Counts per minute per } \mu\text{Ci} = \frac{342 \times 60}{100} \approx 205 \text{ counts}$$

$$\therefore \text{Sensitivity} \approx 205 \text{ counts}/\mu\text{Ci}/\text{minute}$$

Fig. 7.57 System planar sensitivity at 10 cm

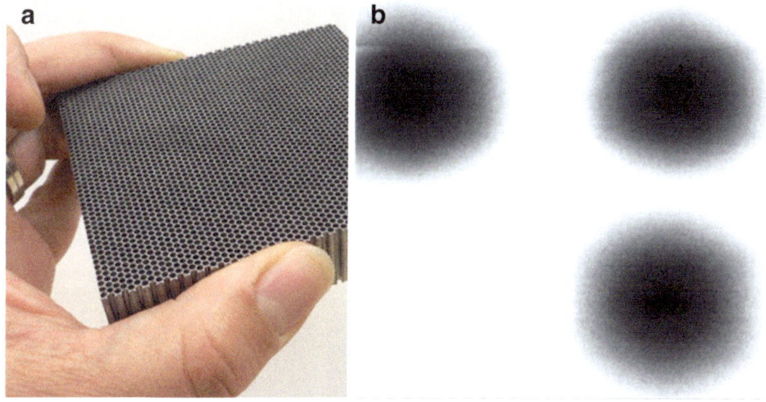

Fig. 7.58 Collimator hole angulation test. (**a**) A piece of hexagonal parallel hole collimator. (Image courtesy: www.nuclearfields.com, accessed on 22.07.2023, printed with permission). (**b**) The alignment of collimator septa and holes was evaluated using a distant point source, with the discontinuity lines in the top two images indicating misalignment, rendering the collimator unacceptable and in need of replacement. (Image courtesy: IAEA [38], reprinted with permission)

placed around the detector head to absorb and attenuate radiation that could otherwise reach the detector from unintended directions. This helps improve image quality by reducing background noise and improving the signal-to-noise ratio.

The testing indicates the gamma camera only responds to the radiation incident upon the crystal which passes through the collimator. A point source of 100 μCi is pasted over the detector head in different positions around the detector, i.e., on the front, back, both sides, up, and backside, and the counts are observed for 60 s for each position. Finally, one reading will be obtained without any source for the same duration to check for background counts (B). Calculate the standard deviation of background counts, i.e., $\sqrt{B}$. And check for whether any side count is more than $B+3\sqrt{B}$. All side counts should have counts below $B+3\sqrt{B}$ [41] (Fig. 7.59).

7.8.2.6 Scan Speed for the Whole-Body Scan

The test for scan speed in whole-body scans using a gamma camera ensures that the camera's movement speed is accurate and consistent. A proper scan speed is crucial for obtaining high-quality whole-body images with accurate tracer distribution and precise localization of abnormalities.

The IAEA has recommended two methods [38] in the first method; a flood source or line source is used to see the entire field of view, and in the second method, 10 points sources each of 20 MBq (0.5 mCi) distributed over entire scan length are imaged.

Alternatively, seven-point sources placed at a distance of 30 cm in the entire field of view, i.e., 200 cm, can be imaged at a speed of 30 cm/min. The 30 cm/min scan speed is the maximum speed used in clinical conditions [42] and the maximum standard speed offered by manufacturers [43] is also 30 cm/min. However, they offer maximum scan speed up to 200 cm/min. In this test, the time taken for the gamma camera to complete the entire scan, starting from the first acquisition position until the last position, is measured. The expected scan speed is calculated based on the distance covered during the scan and the time taken. The measured scan speed, the expected scan speed, and the manufacturer's specifications are compared. Ensure that the actual scan speed falls within an acceptable range. If the measured scan speed is outside the acceptable range or deviates significantly from the expected scan speed, the cause of the deviation is to be ascertained; corrective action will be initiated as necessary (Fig. 7.60).

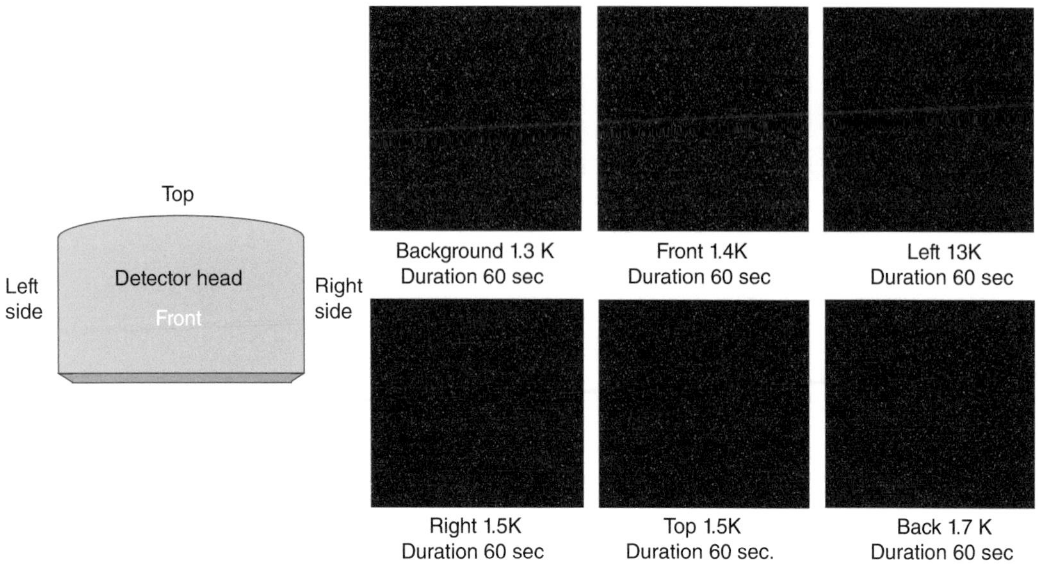

Fig. 7.59 Counts obtained during detector head shielding test

7.8.3 Tomographic (SPECT) Characteristics

7.8.3.1 Pixel Size (*X* and *Y* Direction)

A picture element, which stores a value in digital memory, is called a pixel. It represents an area defined by dimensions in *X* and *Y* directions at a known position defined by *X* and *Y* coordinates. While using a gamma camera, it is important that *X* and *Y* axes are being reconstructed correctly. Accurate pixel size calibration is required for estimating the size volume or depth of organs, attenuation correction in SPECT reconstruction, etc. The pixel size can be calibrated with point or line sources placed at known distances or slit or grid phantoms [44]. Then their centroid and the separation between these sources are calculated. The pixel size in the *X* and *Y* directions is then determined by dividing the distance between the point sources by the number of pixels [45].

This test is performed using one-point or two-point sources. The point source is placed on the camera face approximately 5 cm from the field of view's edge along the *X*-axis. Obtain a single planar image with 50K counts using a matrix size of 256 × 256 or 512 × 512 without zoom. The point source is now moved horizontally to a position within 1 mm of the known distance and approximately 5 cm from the opposite edge of the field of vision. Repeat the same procedure of obtaining counts. Repeat for each of the clinically applicable tomographic zoom conditions. The difference between the *X* and *Y* values should be less than 5% of the manufacturer's specification.

7.8.3.2 Tomographic Uniformity, RMS Noise with Flood Correction, and Contrast Resolution

In single photon emission computed tomography (SPECT), tomographic uniformity refers to the degree of uniformity of the gamma camera's detector system across the entire field of view and throughout the different slices or planes of the tomographic reconstruction in the imaging volume. The nonuniformities can lead to image artifacts and inaccuracies, affecting the quantitative accuracy and diagnostic quality of SPECT images.

The RMS noise refers to the Root Mean Square Noise, which is a measure of the statistical variability or fluctuations in the pixel intensity values of the SPECT images. It is a quantitative parameter used to assess the level of noise present in the reconstructed images. The noise can arise from various sources, such as statistical fluctuations in the detected counts, elec-

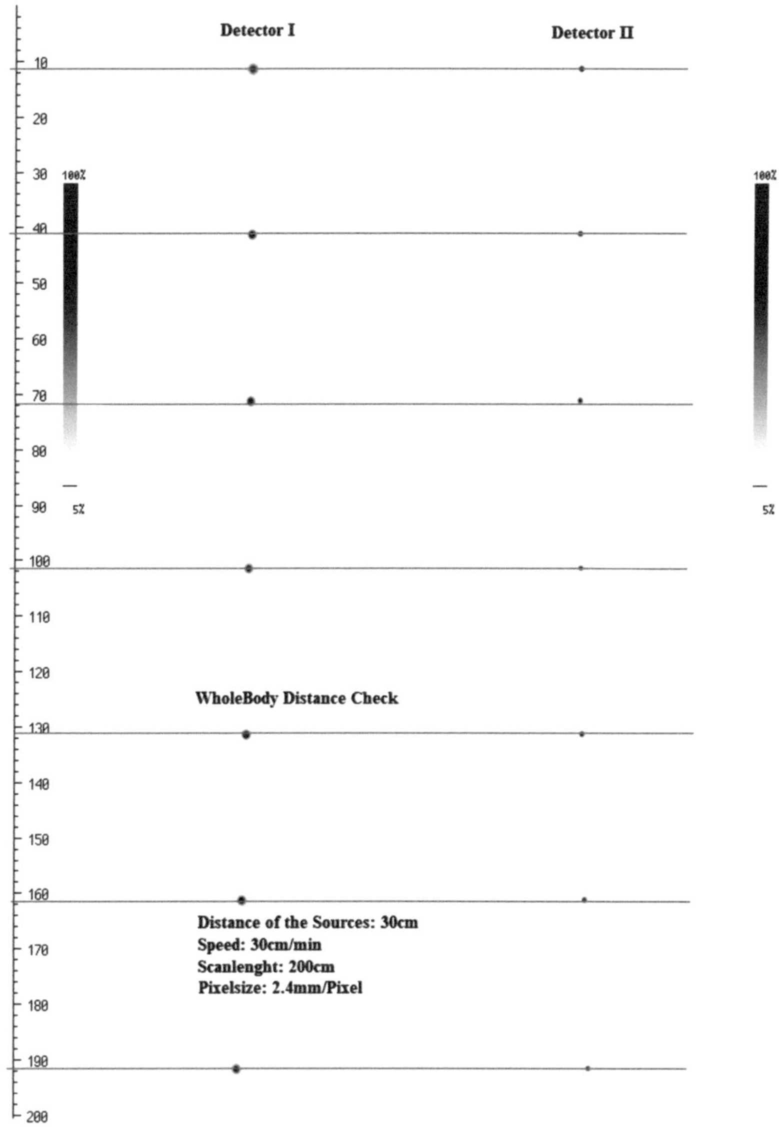

Fig. 7.60 Whole-body scan speed test from a typical gamma camera

tronic noise, and background noise. Higher noise levels can degrade image quality, reduce contrast, and affect the accuracy of quantitative measurements. It can be calculated by choosing a region of interest (ROI) which covers the area with uniform or constant pixel intensity values. Pixel intensity values within the selected ROI and Root Mean Square Noise are calculated using the pixel intensity values within the ROI. The RMS noise represents the standard deviation of the pixel intensity values, which indicates the degree of image noise. A lower RMS noise value indicates that the image has less noise and better image quality. High-quality SPECT images with low noise are important for accurate diagnosis and improved visualization of structures and features of interest.

Contrast resolution is the ability of the imaging system to distinguish small differences in radiotracer uptake or activity concentrations between different tissues, such as tumors, lesions, or areas of altered physiological function or structures within the imaged region. It measures the system's sensitivity to detect subtle changes in the radiotracer distribution and is crucial for visualizing and accurately characterizing various physiological and pathological features. To evaluate contrast resolution in SPECT, phantoms with known activity distributions or hot and cold regions of varying sizes can be imaged, and the ability to differentiate the hot and cold regions and resolve small features is then assessed.

These tests are conducted using a phantom called Jaszczak phantom, SPECT phantom, or Data Spectrum ECT phantom. It is a versatile tool that assesses various aspects of the SPECT system's performance and image quality, such as tomographic uniformity, RMS noise, contrast resolution, SPECT spatial resolution, attenuation, and scatter correction or alignment tasks. It comprises a core, acrylic plastic cylinder or tank and several inserts. Six sets of "cold" rods and six solid spheres are present in every Jaszczak phantom. The sizes of the spheres in different models may vary. Since different models of the phantom have rods of various diameters, the number of rods in each set depends on the size of the rod in that set. The deluxe variant has rod sizes of 4.8, 6.4, 7.9, 9.5, 11.1, and 12.7 mm, while the sphere diameters are 9.5, 12.7, 15.9, 19.1, 25.4, and 31.8 mm (Fig. 7.61).

The AAPM report 177 [46] explains this test in detail and an extract of the procedure mentioned here to carry out the test. In SPECT phantom, tap water can be used, and to mix the activity properly, 30–40 mL of air bubble is left and used for mixing. A 400–1000 MBq (10–27 mCi) of ^{99m}Tc is added through fill port, recapped, and mixed thoroughly. To completely mix the radionuclide, the phantom must undergo several inversions. Add more water to get the air bubble down to under 5 mL. The phantom activity should be added to keep the detector count rate under 30,000 cps.

The phantom is placed on the patient table with its center at least within 2 cm of the axis of rotation, as close as possible to the center of rotation. Use a 128 × 128 matrix and a magnification factor that results in 2.5–3.5 mm pixels. Obtain 120 or 128 360-degree views. A dual-headed

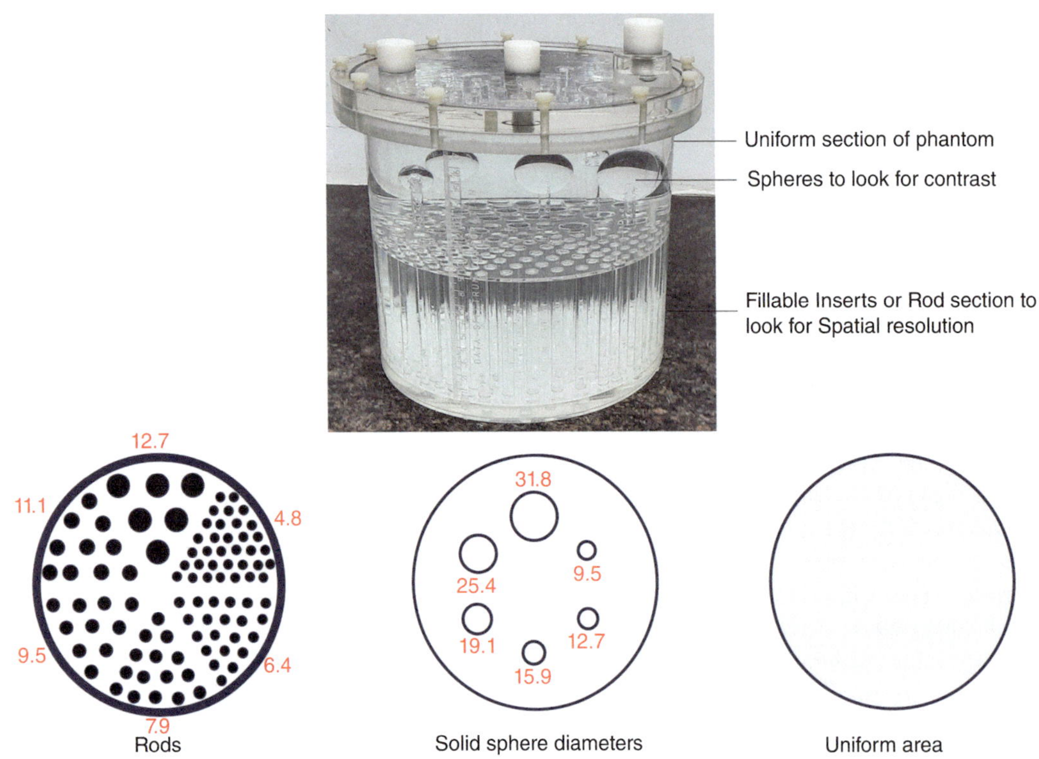

Fig. 7.61 Jaszczak phantom and its parts

camera acquires two views simultaneously, so for instance, 64 stops (or angles) will result in 128 views. There should be 32 million counts in total for the acquisition. The time per view is computed by multiplying 32 million by the sum of the count rate and the number of views (120 or 128).

$$\text{Time per projection} = \frac{32{,}000{,}000}{28{,}000\left(\text{count rate,e.g.}\right)\times 128\left(\text{number of projections}\right)} \quad (7.11)$$

Reconstruct the slices using filtered back projection and a Butterworth low-pass frequency filter with a clinical study-appropriate order and cutoff frequency. The cutoff frequency may be adjusted to obtain the desired outcome of images with the maximum resolution and contrast with a midrange of noise level. The smoothing of the images should be avoided. Utilize the vendor-provided software to apply Chang's method for attenuation correction to the trans-axial slices. The attenuation is calculated by specifying the phantom boundaries in the image slices and allocating a linear attenuation coefficient (0.11 or 0.12/cm for ^{99m}Tc). This value may be adjusted so that the count density is the same at the center and periphery.

The spatial resolution, contrast, and uniformity are visually inspected on reconstructed slices. The smallest visualized sector, of which more than half of the rods can be visualized, gives the spatial resolution of the SPECT system. The smallest sphere that can be visualized for contrast detectability calculation is identified, and the corresponding sphere diameter is recorded. Additionally, the contrast of each sphere is calculated using the following formula:

$$\text{Sphere contrast} = \frac{\text{Mean pixel count from uniform section} - \text{minimum sphere pixel count}}{\text{Mean pixel count from the uniform section}} \quad (7.12)$$

As per AAPM, the uniformity index is not calculated but inspected for artifacts such as attenuation, focal, and ring artifacts. However, using the IAEA tool NMQC, it can be calculated. The noise analysis, i.e., root-mean-squared (RMS) noise, is calculated by drawing a large ROI (>100 cm^2) in a SPECT slice within the central portion of the uniform section and measuring the mean pixel count and standard deviation. The RMS noise is calculated with the following formula:

$$\text{RMS noise}\left(\%\right) = \frac{100\times \text{standard deviation}}{\text{Mean pixel counts}} \quad (7.13)$$

7.8.3.3 Tomographic Spatial Resolution in Air

Many factors affect the reconstructed tomographic spatial resolution, including planar spatial resolution with certain collimators, the radius of rotation, detector orientation, multiple head registration (MHR), the electronic center of rotation (COR), axial head tilt, and the reconstruction algorithm.

The test is performed using a line source positioned at the center of the axis of rotation with detectors set to a 20 cm radius of rotation. A minimum of 60 images having 128 × 128 matrix size are acquired over 360 degrees of rotation with 2000–3000 counts in the first image [46]. The images are reconstructed using filtered back projection and ramp filter. The reconstructed image of the line source appears as a point source axially. The FWHM of the point spread function is determined.

The earlier source is used for planar imaging having the same distance from the detector to the source, and at least 100,000 counts are acquired. The FWHM of line spread function is also determined.

The planar spatial resolution and SPECT spatial resolution are compared, and SPECT-reconstructed spatial resolution should not exceed 10%.

7.8.3.4 Center of Rotation (COR), Multiple Head Registration (MHR), and Alignment of Axes

The COR represents the point or axis around which the gamma camera rotates during the SPECT acquisition process. It is a critical parameter that needs to be accurately calibrated to ensure proper alignment and registration of the acquired data during image reconstruction. During the COR calibration process, specialized phantoms or point sources are used to determine the true center of rotation of the gamma camera system. The goal is to ensure that the true center of rotation coincides with the known physical center of rotation of the gamma camera. Any misalignment between the true center of rotation and the physical center can lead to image artifacts and distortions in the reconstructed SPECT images. By calibrating the COR correctly, nuclear medicine facilities can achieve accurate spatial registration, improve image quality, and provide reliable diagnostic information for patient care. Regular COR calibration is typically part of the routine quality assurance program to maintain optimal performance in SPECT imaging.

Multiple head registration (MHR) is an important step in multiheaded gamma cameras as each detector head acquires data from a specific angle, and the data from all detector heads are combined to create a unified and coherent image. It is necessary to estimate each detector head sample to the same volume. MHR involves the calibration of the relative positions of the detector heads and compensating for any mechanical or positional variations between them. The SPECT system can optimize image quality, achieve accurate spatial registration, and enhance diagnostic capabilities by calibrating and aligning the data from all detector heads.

The calibration of both COR and MHR is generally combined into one measurement. However, separate measurements are required for all the available detector configurations, such as 76-, 90-, and 180-degree. To conduct these tests, 1-point, 3-point, and 5-point sources are used per the manufacturer's recommendation. The SPECT acquisition for point sources is obtained for the full 360-degree rotation of each detector. The tomographic reconstruction is not performed, and images are tracked as a function of detector angle by manufacturer-provided software. The MHR-COR is calculated from the projected source positions itself (Figs. 7.62 and 7.63).

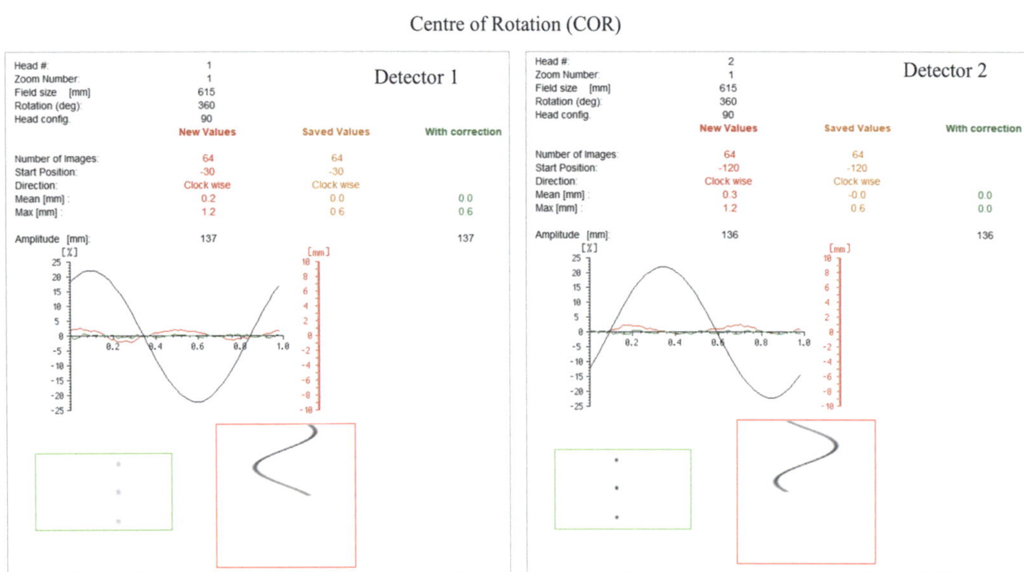

Fig. 7.62 Center of rotation results of a typical dual-head gamma camera

Multiple Head Registration (MHR)

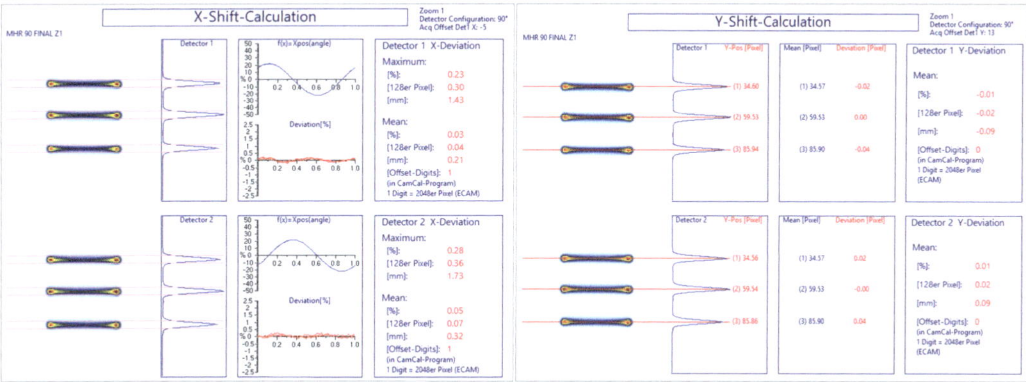

Fig. 7.63 Multiple head registration results of a typical dual-head gamma camera

7.8.3.5 Slice Thickness at the Center of the Field of View

The "Slice Thickness Test" in SPECT (single photon emission computed tomography) is a quality assurance procedure used to measure and verify the actual thickness of the reconstructed image slices at the center of the field of view (FOV) in a SPECT system. During a SPECT scan, the gamma camera rotates around the patient to acquire data from multiple angles, resulting in projection images. These projection images are then reconstructed to form tomographic slices representing the radiotracer distribution within the patient. The "Slice Thickness Test" specifically focuses on the accuracy of the slice thickness in the reconstructed images at the center of the FOV.

The data collected in previous tests also act as raw data for this test; however, the analysis is different. The slice showing the point source clearly is located and then the pixel containing the maximum number of counts is observed. The (X, Y) coordinates and the maximum value of this pixel are noted. All adjacent slices which contain maximum counts for the same (X, Y) pixel position are recorded, and a profile of the point source is generated along the Z-axis using these values. The FWHM of this profile is calculated and converted into millimeters using the pixel size.

7.8.3.6 Variations of Sensitivity with Angle

The "variations of sensitivity with angle" test in SPECT (single photon emission computed tomography) assesses the sensitivity of the gamma camera system at different rotation angles during a SPECT scan. The sensitivity of the gamma camera system can vary at different angles due to mechanical and geometric factors. The variation in sensitivity should be > ±1% of the mean value.

This test was important for detectors made before 1990, but magnetic shielding for PMTs has gotten significant attention since then [38]. This test can be important for the gamma camera, which is close to the magnetic resonance imaging scanner.

This test can be performed using a flood source of about 200 MBq (5 mCi) of ^{99m}Tc, which can safely be attached to the collimator face, and the system can be rotated. ^{57}Co sources are more suitable for this test. Perform a 360-degree SPECT rotation with at least 10^6 counts per image. The process is repeated for fast and slow rotations. NEMA integral uniformity for each angular position is calculated. The mean, standard deviation, and maximum deviation from the mean are calculated.

7.8.3.7 Co-registration of SPECT and CT Modalities—Alignment (Registration) Calibration SPECT/CT

Co registration of SPECT and CT modalities is a crucial quality assurance test in SPECT-CT imaging systems. SPECT-CT combines the functional information from SPECT (single photon emission computed tomography) with the anatomical information from CT (computed tomography) to provide fused images that offer functional and anatomical details in a single examination. The co-registration test aims to ensure that the SPECT and CT images are aligned and fused, enabling precise localization and correlation of functional abnormalities with anatomical structures.

The SPECT phantom used before can again be used to perform this test; just the iodinated CT contrast should be added to the ^{99m}Tc solution to more clearly identify the source location on the CT images. The procedure can be repeated the same way, and co-registration between SPECT and CT can be evaluated using fusion software provided by the manufacturer.

7.9 Image Reconstruction Algorithms

7.9.1 Filtered Back Projection (FBP)

Filtered back projection (FBP) is a widely used reconstruction algorithm in single photon emission computed tomography (SPECT) imaging. A deterministic, analytical algorithm aims to reconstruct a three-dimensional image from the acquired projection data. The following steps take place in the FBP algorithm:

- *Projection of data*: During a SPECT scan, a gamma camera acquires a set of two-dimensional projection images from different angles around the patient. Each projection image represents the attenuated and detected gamma rays from various directions as the camera rotates around the patient.
- *Filtering*: The acquired projection data is preprocessed before reconstruction using a Fourier-based frequency domain filter. The filter's purpose is to suppress high-frequency noise and artifacts in the projection data while preserving the low-frequency information. Commonly used filters include the ramp filter, Hanning window filter, Shepp-Logan filter, and Butterworth filter. Filter choice depends on factors such as noise characteristics and desired image characteristics.
- *Back projection*: The back projection step begins once the projection data is filtered. It involves converting the filtered projection data back into the three-dimensional reconstruction space. The filtered projections are back projected onto a reconstruction grid or voxel array. For each pixel in the projection image, the corresponding line of response (LOR) is determined and contributes to reconstructing the corresponding voxels along that LOR. This process is repeated for all projection images, accumulating the contributions from each angle to form the final reconstructed image.
- *Pixel weighting*: During back projection, pixel weighting can be applied to account for nonuniform detector response, collimator response, and other system-specific factors. The weighting factors help to compensate for nonideal characteristics and improve the uniformity and accuracy of the reconstructed image.

Filtered back projection is a computationally efficient and widely used reconstruction algorithm in SPECT imaging. It provides relatively fast image reconstruction, but it may introduce some artifacts and have limitations in terms of resolution and noise suppression compared to iterative methods. The choice of reconstruction algorithm depends on various factors, including image quality requirements, computational resources, and specific clinical applications.

7.9.2 Iterative Reconstruction

Iterative reconstruction is an advanced technique used in medical imaging, including single photon emission computed tomography (SPECT), to generate high-quality images by iteratively refining an initial estimate of the reconstructed image. Unlike the deterministic filtered back projection (FBP) algorithm, iterative reconstruction incorporates statistical modeling and optimization techniques to iteratively update the image estimate based on the acquired projection data. The following steps take place in iterative reconstruction:

- Initial Image Estimate: The iterative reconstruction process starts with an initial estimate of the reconstructed image. The initial image can be a uniform, low resolution, or even an image obtained from a previous reconstruction.
- Forward Projection: The initial image estimate is forward projected to simulate the acquisition of projection data compared to the actual acquired projection data. The forward projection calculates the expected projection data based on the estimated image, incorporating the imaging system geometry, attenuation correction, collimator response, and other factors.
- Comparison and Update: The forward projected image is compared to the acquired projection data, and the differences (residuals) between the two are calculated. Based on the residuals, an update is made to the current image estimate to improve its agreement with the acquired data.
- The update can be performed using various mathematical techniques, such as Maximum Likelihood Estimation (MLE), Maximum Posteriori (MAP) estimation, or other optimization algorithms. The update step minimizes the differences between the acquired and estimated data by iteratively adjusting the image estimate.
- Iterative Process: The forward projection, comparison, and update process are repeated iteratively to refine the image estimate. Each iteration incorporates new information from the acquired data to improve the accuracy and quality of the reconstructed image. The number of iterations can vary depending on image quality requirements, convergence criteria, and computational resources.
- Regularization and Constraints: Regularization techniques are often applied to prevent overfitting and improve the stability of the iterative reconstruction. Regularization adds constraints to the update step, encouraging smoother or more realistic solutions that align with prior knowledge about the imaged object. Common regularization techniques include Tikhonov regularization, total variation regularization, or anatomical priors.
- Convergence and Final Image: The iterative process continues until a convergence criterion is met, such as reaching a maximum number of iterations or achieving a desired level of image quality. The final image estimate represents the reconstructed image that best fits the acquired data and incorporates statistical properties and regularization constraints.

Iterative reconstruction methods, such as Ordered Subset Expectation Maximization (OSEM), Maximum Likelihood Expectation Maximization (MLEM), or other variants, offer advantages over FBP in terms of noise reduction, improved resolution, and the ability to handle complex imaging scenarios. However, they are computationally more demanding and may require longer processing than FBP. The choice of the iterative reconstruction algorithm depends on factors such as image quality requirements, computational resources, and specific clinical applications.

7.9.3 Newer Techniques Used for Reconstruction of SPECT, PET, and Fusion Images

Several newer techniques and advancements have been developed to reconstruct single photon emission computed tomography (SPECT) and positron emission tomography (PET) images. These techniques aim to improve image quality, resolution, noise reduction, and quantitative accuracy. Here are some notable techniques:

7.9.3.1 Based on Iterative Reconstruction Algorithms

- **Time-of-Flight (TOF) PET Reconstruction**
  Time-of-flight (TOF) PET reconstruction is an advanced reconstruction technology used in positron emission tomography (PET) imaging, which leverages the time difference between the detection of annihilation photons to improve spatial resolution and image quality. In PET imaging, positron-emitting radiotracers are administered to the patient, which undergo annihilation when they encounter an electron. Annihilation results in the emission of two photons traveling in approximately opposite directions. TOF PET takes advantage of the time it takes for the photons to travel from the annihilation point to the detectors.
  TOF PET scanners have detectors with excellent timing resolution, capable of accurately measuring the time difference between the detection of the two photons. The detectors record the arrival times of the photons, allowing for precise timing measurements. The TOF information provides an estimate of the distance traveled by the photons based on the speed of light. The distance between the annihilation event and the detector can be estimated by knowing the time difference and assuming constant speed. This information helps to localize the origin of the photons more accurately.
  The TOF information is incorporated into the image reconstruction algorithm during the reconstruction process. The TOF information constrains the possible locations of the annihilation event, resulting in improved spatial resolution. The reconstruction algorithm uses the TOF data to generate a high-resolution image that better represents the actual distribution of the radiotracer in the imaged object.
- **Advantages of TOF PET**
  - Improved Spatial Resolution: TOF PET allows for better localization of the annihilation event, resulting in improved spatial resolution.
  - Enhanced Signal-to-Noise Ratio: The TOF information helps to differentiate true coincidences from random events, leading to an improved signal-to-noise ratio.
  - Reduced Image Artifacts: TOF PET can mitigate certain image artifacts, such as those caused by scattered or attenuated photons, by providing more accurate localization information.
  - Improved Quantitative Accuracy: TOF PET improves the accuracy of quantitative measurements by reducing partial volume effects and improving image quality.

  TOF PET reconstruction technology has revolutionized PET imaging by providing higher resolution and improved image quality. It allows for more accurate localization and quantification of radiotracer uptake in tissues, enhancing diagnostic capabilities. The incorporation of TOF information in PET scanners has significantly advanced the field and contributed to the clinical success of PET imaging.
- **Resolution Modeling**
  This technique models the inherent blurring effects in the imaging system, such as the point spread function (PSF) or system response function (SRF). Incorporating the system response into the reconstruction process helps restore resolution lost due to physical limitations and improves image quality.
- **Bayesian Methods**
  Bayesian reconstruction methods utilize Bayesian statistics to estimate the most probable distribution of radioactivity given the acquired projection data. These methods incorporate prior knowledge about the imaged object and incorporate regularization to achieve high-quality images with reduced noise and improved quantitative accuracy.
- **Maximum Likelihood Expectation Maximization (MLEM) Variants**
  MLEM is an iterative reconstruction algorithm commonly used in PET and SPECT. Variants of MLEM, such as the Ordered Subset Expectation Maximization (OSEM) algorithm, have been developed to improve convergence speed and noise handling while maintaining good image quality.

7.9.3.2 Statistical Reconstruction-BBased Techniques

- **Penalized Likelihood (PL) Reconstruction**
  PL reconstruction incorporates regularization techniques based on penalizing image variations. It balances the trade-off between noise reduction and preserving image details, improving image quality and quantitative accuracy.
- **Total Variation Regularization**
  This technique promotes images with piecewise smooth regions and sharp edges by minimizing the total variation of the image. It helps to reduce noise and enhance the visualization of structures with distinct boundaries.
- **Compressed Sensing (CS)**
  CS exploits the sparsity or compressibility of the imaged object to reconstruct high-quality images from highly under-sampled data. It enables faster acquisition times and reduced radiation exposure while maintaining image quality.

7.9.4 Hybrid Imaging Reconstructions

7.9.4.1 SPECT/CT and PET/CT Fusion

The fusion of SPECT or PET with computed tomography (CT) images allows for combining functional and anatomical information. Hybrid imaging techniques facilitate accurate localization and correlation of metabolic or functional abnormalities with anatomical structures, enhancing diagnostic capabilities.

7.9.4.2 CT Image Reconstruction

CT (computed tomography) image reconstruction converts acquired raw X-ray attenuation measurements into a three-dimensional image representing the imaged object's anatomical structures. The steps involved in CT image reconstruction, including iterative reconstruction, are as follows:

- Raw Data Acquisition: During a CT scan, an X-ray source emits a fan-shaped or cone-shaped X-ray beam that passes through the patient's body. The X-ray beam is detected by an array of detectors positioned on the opposite side of the patient. The detectors measure the intensity of the X-ray beam after it has passed through the patient, producing raw X-ray attenuation measurements.
- Preprocessing: Before reconstruction, the raw X-ray data may undergo preprocessing steps, such as calibration, normalization, and correction for artifacts like detector malfunctions or noise.
- Reconstruction Algorithms:
  - Filtered Back Projection (FBP): FBP is a common reconstruction algorithm used in CT imaging. It involves filtering the raw data in the spatial domain using techniques like the Ram-Lak filter, followed by back projection to generate the reconstructed image slices.
  - Iterative Reconstruction: Iterative reconstruction is an alternative to FBP that has recently gained popularity. It employs an iterative process to refine the reconstructed image by updating the image estimate based on a mathematical model and the acquired raw data. The iterative reconstruction algorithm starts with an initial estimate of the image and iteratively adjusts the image estimate based on the mismatch between the estimated projection data and the acquired raw data.

Various algorithms are used in iterative reconstruction, such as the Maximum Likelihood Expectation Maximization (MLEM) algorithm, Ordered Subset Expectation Maximization (OSEM), or statistical-based algorithms. The iterative process continues until convergence is reached, improving the quality and accuracy of the reconstructed image.

- Voxel Reconstruction: Whether using FBP or iterative algorithms, the reconstruction process generates a stack of two-dimensional image slices. These image slices are combined to form a three-dimensional volume of image data called a voxel volume. Each voxel represents a three-dimensional pixel in the reconstructed image and contains information about the X-ray attenuation properties at that location.

- Post-processing: After the CT image reconstruction, post-processing steps can be applied to enhance the quality and visualization of the reconstructed images. Post-processing techniques may include noise reduction, contrast enhancement, image filtering, or other methods to improve image quality or highlight specific structures.

The resulting CT image provides detailed cross-sectional views of the imaged anatomy, enabling the detection, diagnosis, and evaluation of various conditions or diseases. Both filtered back projection (FBP) and iterative reconstruction algorithms are crucial in generating accurate and high-quality CT images. The choice between the two depends on factors such as image quality requirements, reconstruction time, and available computational resources.

7.9.4.3 Co-registration of SPECT with CT Images and PET with CT Images

The SPECT and CT images are co-registered to accurately align the functional SPECT data with the anatomical CT data. Image registration techniques such as rigid or deformable registration align the corresponding structures in both images. Rigid registration is a technique used to align images by applying rigid transformations such as translation, rotation, and scaling, whereas deformable registration is a technique used to align images by allowing local deformations or nonrigid transformations. Both rigid and deformable registration techniques have advantages and applications in medical image analysis. Rigid registration is faster and more suitable when there are minimal deformations or when aligning images with similar anatomy. Deformable registration, on the other hand, offers more flexibility and is better suited for aligning images with varying anatomy or when capturing local deformations is essential. Registration may involve manual or automated methods to ensure spatial correspondence between the SPECT and CT data or PET and CT data.

Fusion

The co-registered SPECT and CT images are fused to create a hybrid image. Various fusion methods, such as overlaying the SPECT data onto the CT data or PET data onto the CT data, combine the functional and anatomical information. This fusion allows for better localization and correlation between the functional SPECT information and the anatomical CT structures (Figs. 7.64 and 7.65).

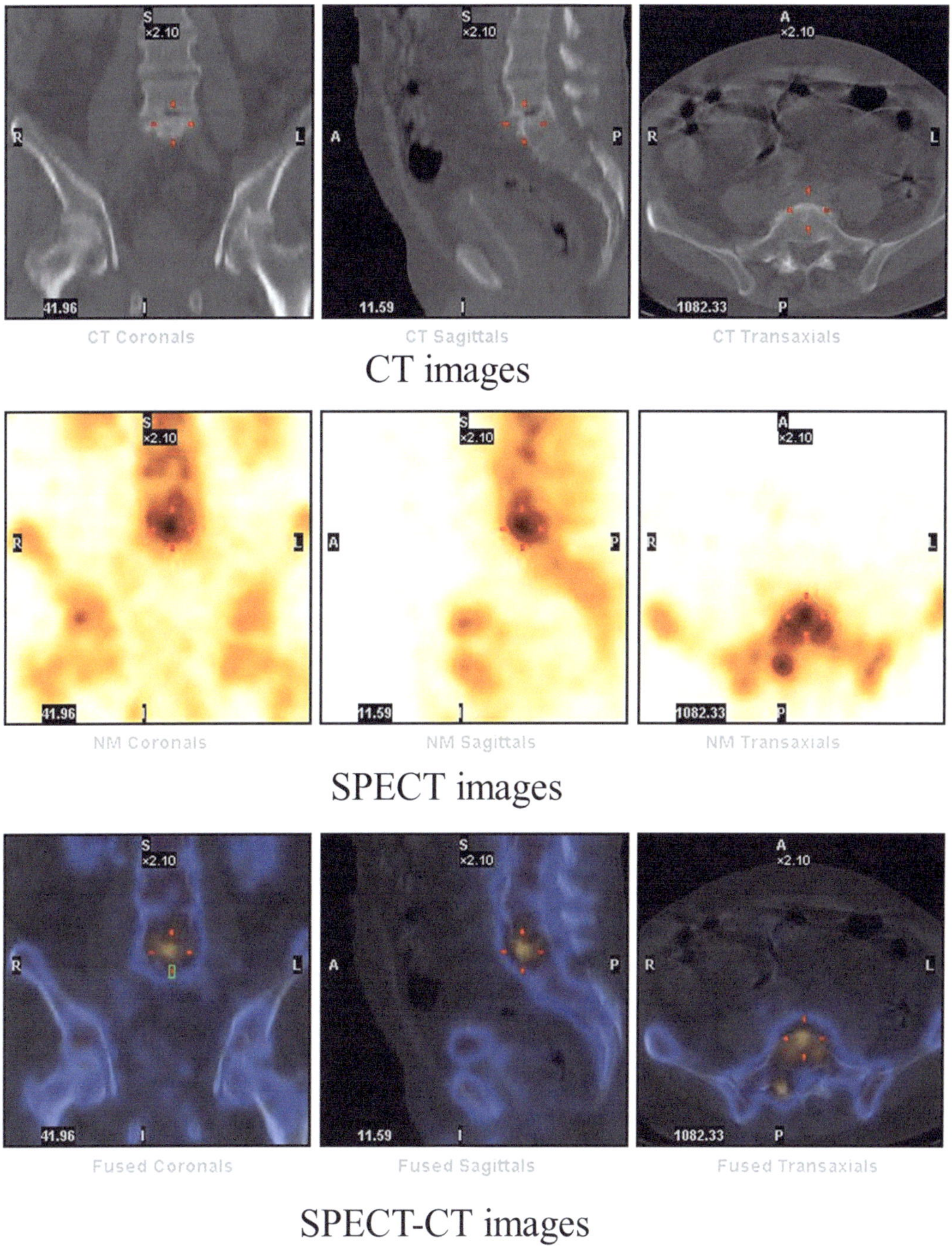

Fig. 7.64 CT, SPECT, and SPECT-CT image

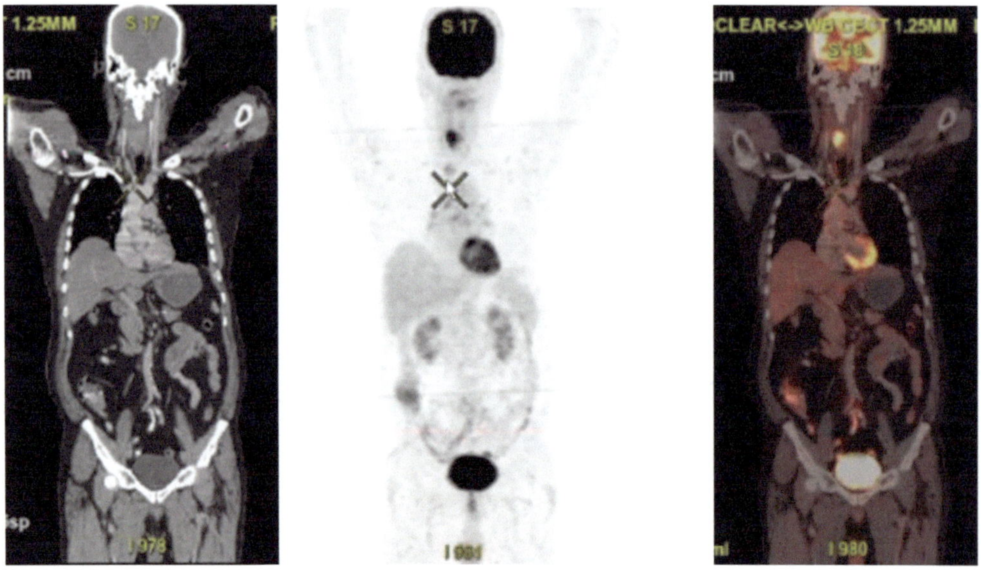

Whole Body CT image Whole Body PET image Whole Body PET-CT Fusion image

Fig. 7.65 CT, PET, and PET-CT fusion images

7.10 Clinical Applications of Hybrid Imaging

The integration of PET with CT, MRI, and their combinations offers a range of clinical applications across oncology, neurology, cardiology, musculoskeletal disorders, and infection management. These advanced imaging modalities provide complementary information, enhancing the precision of diagnosis, staging, treatment planning, and monitoring in various medical specialties.

7.10.1 PET-CT Applications

Oncology

PET-CT, a fusion imaging technique that combines positron emission tomography (PET) and computed tomography (CT), is extensively utilized in oncology. This modality is instrumental in cancer detection, staging, and treatment planning. PET's ability to identify abnormal metabolic activity complements CT's detailed anatomical imaging, providing a comprehensive assessment of primary tumors, cancer spread (metastasis), and treatment response.

Radiation Therapy Planning

In radiation therapy, PET-CT is crucial for accurately delineating tumor volumes and identifying areas of high metabolic activity. This precision enables radiation oncologists to deliver targeted radiation therapy while minimizing damage to surrounding healthy tissues.

Neurology

PET-CT is valuable in neurology for diagnosing and evaluating neurological disorders. It helps differentiate between benign and malignant brain tumors, localize epileptic foci, and assess neurodegenerative diseases such as Alzheimer's disease and Parkinson's disease.

Cardiology

In cardiology, PET-CT assesses myocardial viability and perfusion. It evaluates the extent of coronary artery disease, identifies viable myocardium in patients with impaired cardiac function, and monitors the response to cardiac interventions.

Infection and Inflammation

PET-CT is employed in cases of suspected infections or inflammation. It identifies the presence and extent of infectious or inflammatory processes, guides biopsy or aspiration procedures, and monitors treatment response.

Pulmonary Disorders
PET-CT aids in evaluating lung nodules to determine their malignant or benign nature. It is also useful in assessing pulmonary diseases, such as lung cancer staging, identifying infection sites, and evaluating lung function and ventilation/perfusion matching.

Bone Metastases
PET-CT detects and assesses skeletal metastases from various primary cancers. The combination of PET's metabolic activity detection with CT's high-resolution anatomical information provides accurate localization and characterization of bone metastases.

7.10.2 PET-MRI Applications

Oncology
PET-MRI merges positron emission tomography (PET) with magnetic resonance imaging (MRI) to enhance cancer imaging, staging, and treatment planning. PET provides functional information on abnormal metabolic activity, while MRI offers detailed anatomical and soft tissue characterization, aiding in precise tumor localization, extent assessment, and treatment response evaluation.

Neurology
In neurology, PET-MRI assists in diagnosing and evaluating neurological disorders. It helps assess brain tumors, identify epileptic foci, evaluate neurodegenerative diseases, and map brain function and connectivity using functional MRI (fMRI) and PET.

Cardiology
PET-MRI evaluates myocardial perfusion, viability, and function. It assesses myocardial blood flow, detects ischemia or scar tissue, and provides insights into cardiac function and myocardial metabolism.

Inflammation and Infection
PET-MRI is useful in assessing inflammatory and infectious conditions by localizing and characterizing areas of increased metabolic activity associated with these processes, guiding treatment planning, and monitoring therapy response.

Musculoskeletal Disorders
PET-MRI aids in evaluating bone and joint diseases, assessing tumor activity, and characterizing inflammatory conditions like arthritis. It provides functional and anatomical information for diagnosis, treatment planning, and disease progression monitoring.

Pediatric Imaging
PET-MRI is particularly advantageous in pediatric imaging due to its ability to combine functional and anatomical assessments without ionizing radiation exposure. It is used in oncology, neurology, and other areas requiring simultaneous functional and structural evaluation.

Research Applications
PET-MRI is extensively used in research to explore various aspects of human physiology and disease. It facilitates comprehensive multimodal imaging for investigations into brain function, tumor biology, metabolic pathways, and treatment responses.

> ? What are the distinctions in clinical conditions in PET-CT and PET-MRI cases?

While there are overlaps in their applications, the choice between PET-CT and PET-MRI depends on factors such as the specific clinical question, availability of equipment, patient factors, and institutional preferences. Both modalities have their strengths and limitations. PET-CT is superior in anatomical localization and is widely available, while PET-MRI provides simultaneous functional and anatomical information without radiation exposure. Different studies show clinical conditions, such as patients with NSCLC and melanoma, may benefit from PET/MRI, which detects brain and liver metastases that go undetected on PET/CT [47].

Ming et al. (2020) suggest, "In cases of primary breast cancer, PET/MRI had comparable results to MRI, but outperformed PET/CT. Both PET/CT and PET/MRI have higher sensitivity than MRI for detecting nodal metastases within and outside the axilla, but when it comes to detecting lung metastases, PET/CT is more effective, while PET/MRI is better for detecting liver and bone metastases. Furthermore, PET/CT is superior in tracking local recurrence [48]."

Al-Nabhani et al. (2014) concluded that the PET data on both modalities were similar; however, PET-MR can be superior in soft tissue-based malignancies of head and neck, pelvis, and colorectal cancers, whereas PET-CT in lung and mediastinal nodal disease points [49]. Ehman et al. (2017) enquired about PET-CT versus PET-MRI and concluded that "the higher cost, the complexity of operating and interpreting the studies obtained on a PET/MRI system, make it less common. PET/MRI has advantages such as lower radiation dose, better motion correction, and convenient combined exams. However, PET/CT remains dominant due to its established access, cost, speed, and familiarity. The imaging community needs to determine where PET/MRI will add the most value, and its future role is yet to be determined [50]."

7.10.3 SPECT-CT Applications

Oncology

SPECT-CT, which combines single photon emission computed tomography (SPECT) with computed tomography (CT), is employed in oncology for cancer diagnosis, staging, and treatment planning. It provides functional information on tumor metabolism or receptor expression (SPECT) along with precise anatomical localization (CT), aiding in accurate tumor characterization, evaluation of metastatic spread, and guiding targeted therapies.

Bone Disorders

SPECT-CT is valuable in assessing bone disorders such as osteomyelitis, infections, and metastases. SPECT provides functional information on blood flow or tracer uptake in bones, while CT offers detailed anatomical information, helping localize and characterize abnormalities.

Cardiology

In cardiology, SPECT-CT evaluates myocardial perfusion and function, assessing blood flow to the heart muscle, identifying ischemic or scarred regions, and aiding in the diagnosis and management of coronary artery disease.

Orthopedics

SPECT-CT is used in orthopedics to evaluate joint diseases like osteoarthritis or inflammatory arthritis. It helps localize and characterize areas of increased tracer uptake, assisting in diagnosis, treatment planning, and monitoring disease progression.

Endocrinology

SPECT-CT assesses the functional status of various endocrine glands. It is useful in evaluating conditions like hyperparathyroidism, detecting parathyroid adenomas, and guiding surgical interventions.

Infection and Inflammation

SPECT-CT identifies and localizes infection or inflammation areas, assisting in diagnosing and managing conditions such as abscesses, osteomyelitis, vasculitis, and soft tissue infections.

Neurology

In neurology, SPECT-CT is used to assess brain perfusion, identify seizure foci, and locate areas of abnormal brain activity. It aids in evaluating epilepsy, dementia, brain tumors, and other neurological disorders.

7.10.4 PET-CT-MRI Applications

Oncology
The combined use of PET-CT-MRI enhances comprehensive cancer evaluation by providing simultaneous assessments of tumor metabolism (PET), precise anatomical localization (CT), and detailed soft tissue characterization (MRI). This integration supports tumor detection, staging, treatment planning, and monitoring treatment response.

Neurology
PET-CT-MRI is valuable in neurology for evaluating brain tumors, neurodegenerative disorders, and epilepsy. It integrates functional information on cerebral metabolism and blood flow (PET), precise anatomical localization (CT), and detailed soft tissue visualization (MRI) to aid in tumor characterization, localization of epileptic foci, and assessment of neurodegenerative diseases.

Cardiology
PET-CT-MRI facilitates comprehensive cardiac assessment by combining the evaluation of myocardial perfusion and viability (PET) with detailed anatomical information (CT) and assessment of myocardial function and tissue characterization (MRI). This approach aids in diagnosing and managing coronary artery disease, myocardial infarction, and cardiac sarcoidosis.

Musculoskeletal Imaging
PET-CT-MRI is effective in evaluating musculoskeletal conditions such as bone and soft tissue tumors, arthritis, and sports injuries. It combines tumor metabolism assessment (PET), anatomical localization (CT), and detailed soft tissue and bone evaluation (MRI) to support accurate tumor staging, joint inflammation characterization, and musculoskeletal pathology assessment.

Infection and Inflammation
PET-CT-MRI provides valuable insights into infectious and inflammatory conditions. It combines functional PET imaging, anatomical localization (CT), and detailed soft tissue characterization (MRI) to aid in the localization, characterization, and monitoring of infections and inflammation and to guide treatment response.

Exercise

Multiple Choice Questions

1. Which hybrid imaging modality combines positron emission tomography (PET) with computed tomography (CT)?
   A. PET-MRI
   B. SPECT-CT
   C. PET-CT
   D. PET-CT-MRI
2. What is a significant limitation of PET imaging?
   A. High spatial resolution
   B. Excessive anatomical detail
   C. Limited spatial resolution
   D. Rapid scan times
3. Which of the following hybrid imaging techniques combines single photon emission computed tomography (SPECT) with computed tomography (CT)?
   A. PET-CT
   B. PET-MRI
   C. SPECT-CT
   D. PET-CT-MRI
4. What is a primary advantage of hybrid imaging?
   A. Reduced imaging time and radiation dose
   B. Increased cost of equipment
   C. Lack of detailed anatomical information
   D. Longer scan times
5. Which hybrid imaging modality provides excellent soft tissue contrast and anatomical detail combined with functional information?
   A. PET-CT
   B. SPECT-CT
   C. PET-MRI
   D. PET-CT-MRI

6. Which type of radiation detector uses scintillation to convert radiation into light photons, which are then converted into electrical signals?
   A. Photomultiplier tube (PMT)
   B. Semiconductor detector
   C. Scintillation detector
   D. Ionization chamber
7. What property of scintillation detectors affects their ability to detect high-energy radiation effectively?
   A. Scintillation efficiency
   B. Dead time
   C. Decay time
   D. Wavelength of emission
8. Which scintillator material is commonly used in PET imaging for its high light yield and fast decay time?
   A. Sodium iodide (NaI)
   B. Cesium iodide (CsI)
   C. Lutetium oxyorthosilicate (LSO)
   D. Bismuth germanate (BGO)
9. In computed tomography (CT) detectors, what is a key characteristic of the scintillator material used?
   A. High afterglow
   B. High light yield and resistance to radiation damage
   C. High sensitivity to visible light
   D. Slow decay time
10. Which method is employed by CT scanners to handle the high radiation flux efficiently?
    A. Pulse mode
    B. Current mode
    C. Digital mode
    D. Analog mode
11. What was the primary contribution of Paul Dirac to the discovery of positrons?
    A. Observation of positron tracks in a cloud chamber
    B. Proposal of the Dirac equation predicting antimatter
    C. Identification of positron decay
    D. Development of the first PET scanner
12. Which radiopharmaceutical is most widely used in PET imaging due to its role in imaging glucose metabolism?
    A. 11C-Methionine
    B. 18F-FDG
    C. 68Ga-PSMA
    D. 18F-Fluorothymidine
13. In PET imaging, what is the purpose of coincidence detection?
    A. To measure the time-of-flight of photons
    B. To detect photons emitted in opposite directions from positron-electron annihilation
    C. To enhance spatial resolution through detector arrangements
    D. To correct for scatter events in the data
14. How does positron emission tomography (PET) typically improve diagnostic accuracy when combined with computed tomography (CT)?
    A. By providing higher resolution images
    B. By fusing anatomical and functional information into a single examination
    C. By increasing the scanning speed
    D. By reducing the patient's radiation exposure
15. What is the role of time-of-flight (TOF) technology in PET imaging?
    A. To increase the field of view
    B. To improve spatial resolution by measuring the time difference between detecting two annihilation photons
    C. To reduce the incidence of random coincidences
    D. To extend the life of the scintillation crystals
16. Which of the following NEMA standards was the first to address PET systems?
    A. NEMA NU 2-2001
    B. NEMA NU 2-2007
    C. NEMA NU 2-1994
    D. NEMA NU 2-2012
17. What is primarily used to measure the sensitivity of a PET scanner according to NEMA standards?
    A. Uniform cylindrical phantom
    B. Scatter phantom
    C. Image quality phantom
    D. Time-of-flight phantom
18. In PET imaging, what does a higher Noise Equivalent Count Rate (NECR) indicate?
    A. Increased scatter fraction
    B. Decreased count rate capability
    C. Improved signal-to-noise ratio
    D. Lower sensitivity

19. Which measurement technique involves assessing the ability to determine the time difference between detecting two annihilation photons?
    A. Spatial resolution
    B. Energy resolution
    C. Time-of-flight (TOF) resolution
    D. Sensitivity measurement
20. What does the uniformity check of the reconstructed image test assess in PET imaging?
    A. Co-registration accuracy between PET and CT images
    B. Consistency of activity values across the field of view
    C. Sensitivity and count rate performance
    D. Scatter fraction and count losses
21. What is the primary purpose of a collimator in a gamma camera?
    A. To convert scintillation light into electrical signals
    B. To direct and shape incoming gamma rays
    C. To amplify electrical signals from photomultiplier tubes
    D. To reconstruct images from projection data
22. What distinguishes a low-energy all-purpose (LEAP) collimator from a low-energy high-resolution (LEHR) collimator?
    A. LEAP collimators have thinner septa compared to LEHR collimators.
    B. LEAP collimators are used for high-energy studies, while LEHR are used for low-energy studies.
    C. LEAP collimators have larger and wider holes compared to LEHR collimators.
    D. LEAP collimators provide better spatial resolution than LEHR collimators.
23. How does the Anger logic algorithm improve the positioning of gamma-ray interactions compared to centroid calculation?
    A. By using a simpler computational method
    B. By incorporating timing and amplitude information from multiple PMTs
    C. By reducing the number of PMTs used in the calculation
    D. By increasing the distance between PMTs
24. Which component of the gamma camera system converts analogue signals into discrete digital values?
    A. Pre-amplifier
    B. Pulse-height analyzer
    C. Analogue-to-digital converter (ADC)
    D. Scintillation crystal
25. What is the purpose of uniformity correction in gamma camera imaging?
    A. To enhance the spatial resolution of the images
    B. To correct for nonuniformities in the detector's response across the field of view
    C. To amplify weak electrical signals from the PMTs
    D. To set energy windows for pulse height analysis
26. What is the primary purpose of quality control in gamma camera/SPECT imaging?
    A. To increase the imaging speed
    B. To ensure accurate and reliable imaging results
    C. To reduce the cost of imaging procedures
    D. To expand the field of view of the gamma camera
27. Which edition of the NEMA guidelines is the most recent as of 2018?
    A. NU 1-1997
    B. NU 1-2001
    C. NU 1-2012
    D. NU 1-2018
28. Which parameter is assessed during the test of intrinsic flood field uniformity?
    A. Collimator hole angulation
    B. Integral and differential uniformities
    C. Scan speed for the whole-body scan
    D. Maximum count rate performance in air
29. The energy resolution of a gamma camera is measured as a percentage of which of the following?
    A. Full width at half maximum (FWHM) of the energy peak
    B. Full width at tenth maximum (FWTM) of the energy peak
    C. The average energy of detected gamma rays
    D. The total number of detected gamma rays

30. What is evaluated in the multiple window spatial registration (MWSR) test?
    A. Detector head shielding leakage
    B. Spatial registration of objects across different gamma photon energies
    C. System planar sensitivity at 10 cm from the detector surface
    D. Variations of sensitivity with angle
31. Which method is recommended for testing intrinsic count rate performance and dead time of a gamma camera?
    A. Visual inspection method
    B. Two-source method
    C. Single-source method
    D. Gamma-ray emission method
32. What is the purpose of using a scatter medium in the intrinsic count rate performance test?
    A. To increase the gamma camera's sensitivity
    B. To simulate clinical conditions and measure count rate performance with scatter
    C. To improve image resolution
    D. To reduce the effect of background radiation
33. What is the recommended procedure for testing the maximum count rate in the air for a gamma camera according to NEMA?
    A. Using a set of dynamic images acquired from a slowly moving source
    B. Using a static source at a fixed distance
    C. Performing a calibration with a known radioactive source
    D. Measuring the count rate with a scatter phantom
34. What is the formula for calculating the dead time (τ) for a gamma camera?
    A. $\tau = \left[\frac{2 \times R_{12}}{(R_1 + R_2)^2}\right] \ln\left(\frac{R_1 + R_2}{R_{12}}\right)$
    B. $\tau = \left[\frac{2 \times R_{12}}{(R_1 + R_2)^2}\right] \ln\left(\frac{R_1 + R_2}{R_{12}}\right)$
    C. $\tau = \left[\frac{2 \times R_{12}}{(R_1 + R_2)^2}\right] \ln\left(\frac{R_1 + R_2}{R_{12}}\right)$
    D. $\tau = \left[\frac{2 \times R_{12}}{(R_1 + R_2)^2}\right] \ln\left(\frac{R_1 + R_2}{R_{12}}\right)$
35. For assessing the system planar sensitivity of a gamma camera, which measurement unit is commonly used?
    A. Counts per minute (cpm)
    B. Counts per second (cps)
    C. Counts per μCi (cpm/μCi)
    D. Counts per Bq (cps/Bq)
36. What is the primary purpose of filtering in the filtered back projection (FBP) algorithm for SPECT imaging?
    A. To enhance high-frequency noise
    B. To suppress high-frequency noise and artifacts
    C. To increase image resolution
    D. To decrease image acquisition time
37. Which technique is commonly used in iterative reconstruction for improving the accuracy and quality of the reconstructed image?
    A. Time-of-flight (TOF) PET
    B. Bayesian methods
    C. Filtered back projection (FBP)
    D. Compressed sensing (CS)
38. In time-of-flight (TOF) PET reconstruction, what is the role of measuring the time difference between the detection of annihilation photons?
    A. To increase the energy of the photons
    B. To localize the origin of the photons more accurately
    C. To enhance the color contrast of the image
    D. To reduce the number of detectors required
39. What advantage does the iterative reconstruction technique have over filtered back projection (FBP) in PET imaging?
    A. Faster processing time
    B. Increased computational simplicity
    C. Improved noise reduction and spatial resolution
    D. Reduced requirement for regularization
40. Which newer technique utilizes prior knowledge about the imaged object to improve image quality and quantitative accuracy?
    A. Penalized likelihood (PL) reconstruction
    B. Time-of-flight (TOF) PET
    C. Filtered back projection (FBP)
    D. Resolution modeling

Short Questions

1. Describe how PET-CT hybrid imaging enhances diagnostic accuracy compared to PET or CT alone.
2. Explain the role of hybrid imaging in oncology.
3. Explain the significance of decay time in scintillation detectors and its impact on the detector's performance.
4. Describe the role of scintillator crystals in PET imaging and how they contribute to the image quality.
5. Describe the significance of the discovery of positrons in the context of positron emission tomography (PET).
6. Explain the basic principle of how PET imaging generates images of biological processes in the body.
7. Explain the significance of using a 70 cm long phantom in PET quality control.
8. Describe how normalization in PET imaging helps to correct for nonuniformities across the field of view.
9. Explain the role of the scintillation crystal in a gamma camera system.
10. Describe how SPECT imaging improves upon conventional gamma camera imaging techniques.
11. Describe the significance of centering the pulse height analyzer (PHA) window in gamma camera quality control.
12. Explain the purpose of using asymmetric energy windows during the intrinsic flood field uniformity test.
13. Describe the procedure for testing extrinsic flood field uniformity of a gamma camera.
14. Explain the importance of calibrating the center of rotation (COR) in SPECT imaging.
15. Describe the role of pixel weighting in the filtered back projection (FBP) algorithm for SPECT imaging.
16. What are the benefits of combining SPECT or PET with CT imaging through fusion techniques?

Long Questions

1. Discuss the limitations of MRI imaging and how these limitations compare to the advantages of hybrid imaging modalities. Include considerations such as patient comfort, scan duration, and the ability to provide both anatomical and functional information.
2. Discuss the advantages and limitations of scintillation detectors compared to semiconductor detectors in radiation imaging. Include aspects such as sensitivity, response time, and suitability for different types of radiation.
3. Discuss the evolution of PET imaging from its early development to the introduction of PET-CT scanners. Include details about historical milestones, technological advancements, and how the integration of PET with CT has enhanced diagnostic capabilities.
4. Discuss the impact of spatial resolution on PET imaging and how factors such as detector size and positron range affect this characteristic. Include details on how spatial resolution is measured and its importance for visualizing small anatomical structures or lesions.
5. Discuss the processes and significance of image reconstruction in SPECT imaging. Include an explanation of how the sinogram is used in image reconstruction and the common techniques employed for this purpose.
6. Discuss the evolution of the NEMA guidelines for gamma camera quality control from the first edition to the most recent one. How have these guidelines adapted to advancements in technology and changes in imaging practices? Include details on the types of tests covered in these guidelines and their importance in maintaining gamma camera performance.
7. Discuss the various methods available for testing tomographic spatial resolution in SPECT imaging, including the use of line sources, phantoms, and the comparison between planar and tomographic spatial resolutions. Include the impact of factors such as collimator design, detector orientation, and reconstruction algorithms on spatial resolution.

8. Compare and contrast filtered back projection (FBP) and iterative reconstruction techniques in SPECT and PET imaging. Discuss their respective advantages and disadvantages, including their impact on image quality, computational requirements, and clinical applications.

Answers to MCQs

1. C. PET-CT
2. C. Limited spatial resolution
3. C. SPECT-CT
4. A. Reduced imaging time and radiation dose
5. C. PET-MRI
6. C. Scintillation detector
7. A. Scintillation efficiency
8. C. Lutetium oxyorthosilicate (LSO)
9. B. High light yield and resistance to radiation damage
10. B. Current mode
11. B. Proposal of the Dirac equation predicting antimatter
12. B. 18F-FDG
13. B. To detect photons emitted in opposite directions from positron-electron annihilation
14. B. By fusing anatomical and functional information into a single examination
15. B. To improve spatial resolution by measuring the time difference between detecting two annihilation photons
16. C. NEMA NU 2-1994
17. A. Uniform cylindrical phantom
18. C. Improved signal-to-noise ratio
19. C. Time-of-flight (TOF) resolution
20. B. Consistency of activity values across the field of view
21. B. To direct and shape incoming gamma rays
22. C. LEAP collimators have larger and wider holes compared to LEHR collimators
23. B. By incorporating timing and amplitude information from multiple PMTs
24. C. Analogue-to-digital converter (ADC)
25. B. To correct for nonuniformities in the detector's response across the field of view
26. B. To ensure accurate and reliable imaging results
27. D. NU 1-2018
28. B. Integral and differential uniformities
29. A. Full width at half maximum (FWHM) of the energy peak
30. B. Spatial registration of objects across different gamma photon energies
31. B. Two-source method
32. B. To simulate clinical conditions and measure count rate performance with scatter
33. A. Using a set of dynamic images acquired from a slowly moving source
34. A. $\tau = \left[\frac{2 \times R_{12}}{\left(R_1 + R_2\right)^2}\right] \ln\left(\frac{R_1 + R_2}{R_{12}}\right)$
35. C. Counts per μCi (cpm/μCi)
36. B. To suppress high-frequency noise and artifacts
37. B. Bayesian methods
38. B. To localize the origin of the photons more accurately
39. C. Improved noise reduction and spatial resolution
40. A. Penalized likelihood (PL) reconstruction

References

1. Tandon P, Prakash D, Kheruka SC, Bhat NN. Working mechanism of radiation detectors used in nuclear medicine. In: Radiation safety guide for nuclear medicine professionals. Singapore: Springer; 2022. p. 153–75. https://doi.org/10.1007/978-981-19-4518-2_15.
2. Knoll GF. Radiation detection and measurement. 4th ed. Hoboken: Wiley; 2010.
3. Lecoq P. Development of new scintillators for medical applications. Nucl Instrum Methods Phys Res A. 2016;809:130–9. https://doi.org/10.1016/j.nima.2015.08.041.
4. Dirac PAM, John S. The quantum theory of the electron. Roy Soc Proc A. 1927;43:227.
5. Andhrson CD. The positive electron. Phys Rev. 1933;43:491. [Online]. Available: https://journals.aps.org/pr/pdf/10.1103/PhysRev.43.491. Accessed 5 July 2023.
6. Steiner MA. PET—the history behind the technology. [Online]. Available: https://trace.tennessee.edu/utk_interstp2. Accessed 5 July 2023.
7. Townsend DW, Beyer T, Blodgett TM. PET/CT scanners: a hardware approach to image fusion.

Semin Nucl Med. 2003;33(3):193–204. https://doi.org/10.1053/snuc.2003.127314.
8. Townsend DW, Carney JPJ, Yap JT, Hall NC. PET/CT today and tomorrow. J Nucl Med. 2004;45(Suppl 1):4S–14S.
9. Townsend DW, Beyer T. A combined PET/CT scanner: the path to true image fusion. Br J Radiol. 2002;75 Spec No:S24–30. https://doi.org/10.1259/bjr.75.suppl_9.750024.
10. Aide N, Lasnon C, Desmonts C, Armstrong IS, Walker MD, McGowan DR. Advances in PET/CT technology: an update. Semin Nucl Med. 2022;52(3):286–301. https://doi.org/10.1053/j.semnuclmed.2021.10.005.
11. Chicheportiche A, Marciano R, Orevi M. Comparison of NEMA characterizations for Discovery MI and Discovery MI-DR TOF PET/CT systems at different sites and with other commercial PET/CT systems. EJNMMI Phys. 2020;7(1):4. https://doi.org/10.1186/s40658-020-0271-x.
12. Chen S, Hu P, Gu Y, Yu H, Shi H. Performance characteristics of the digital uMI550 PET/CT system according to the NEMA NU2-2018 standard. EJNMMI Phys. 2020;7(1):43. https://doi.org/10.1186/s40658-020-00315-w.
13. Singh MK, Mohan P, Mahajan H, Kaushik C. Technical and clinical assessment of latest technology SiPM integrated digital PETCT scanner. Radiography. 2023;29(4):705–11. https://doi.org/10.1016/j.radi.2023.04.020.
14. Zorz A, et al. Performance evaluation of a new time of flight PET/CT scanner: results of a multicenter study. Phys Med. 2019;68:146–54. https://doi.org/10.1016/j.ejmp.2019.11.017.
15. van Sluis J, et al. Performance characteristics of the digital biograph vision PET/CT system. J Nucl Med. 2019;60(7):1031–6. https://doi.org/10.2967/jnumed.118.215418.
16. https://www.usa.philips.com/healthcare/product/HC882456/ingenuity-tf-petct-system.
17. Daube-Witherspoon ME, Cherry SR. Scanner design considerations for long axial field-of-view PET systems. PET Clin. 2021;16(1):25–39. https://doi.org/10.1016/j.cpet.2020.09.003.
18. Nadig V, Herrmann K, Mottaghy FM, Schulz V. Hybrid total-body pet scanners—current status and future perspectives. Eur J Nucl Med Mol Imaging. 2022;49(2):445–59. https://doi.org/10.1007/s00259-021-05536-4.
19. Vandenberghe S, Moskal P, Karp JS. State of the art in total body PET. EJNMMI Phys. 2020;7(1):35. https://doi.org/10.1186/s40658-020-00290-2.
20. Moses WW. Fundamental limits of spatial resolution in PET. Nucl Instrum Methods Phys Res A. 2011;648:S236–40. https://doi.org/10.1016/j.nima.2010.11.092.
21. Conti M, Eriksson L. Physics of pure and non-pure positron emitters for PET: a review and a discussion. EJNMMI Phys. 2016;3(1):8. https://doi.org/10.1186/s40658-016-0144-5.
22. NEMA. Performance measurements of positron emission tomographs (PET). 2018. [Online]. Available: https://www.nema.org/standards/view/Performance-Measurements-of-Positron-Emission-Tomographs. Accessed 15 June 2023.
23. AAPM Task Group. AAPM report no. 126: PET/CT acceptance testing and quality assurance. The report of AAPM Task Group 126. Alexandria: AAPM; 2019.
24. Daube-Witherspoon ME, et al. PET performance measurements using the NEMA NU 2-2001 standard. J Nucl Med. 2002;43(10):1398–409. [Online]. Available: http://www.nema.org/.
25. NEMA. NEMA standards publication NU 2-2018: performance measurements of positron emission tomographs (PETS). Rosslyn: NEMA; 2018. [Online]. Available: http://www.nema.org/.
26. IAEA. IAEA human health series no. 1. Quality assurance for PET and PET/CT systems. Vienna: IAEA; 2009.
27. Desmonts C, Bouthiba MA, Enilorac B, Nganoa C, Agostini D, Aide N. Evaluation of a new multipurpose whole-body CzT-based camera: comparison with a dual-head Anger camera and first clinical images. EJNMMI Phys. 2020;7(1):18. https://doi.org/10.1186/s40658-020-0284-5.
28. English RJ, Zimmerman RE. Performance and acceptance testing of scintillation cameras for SPECT. J Nucl Med Technol. 1988;16(3):132–8.
29. IAEA. IAEA quality control atlas for scintillation camera systems. Vienna: IAEA; 2003.
30. NEMA Standards Publication NU 1-2007. 2007.
31. NEMA Standards Publication NU 1-2012. Performance measurements of gamma cameras. 2013. [Online]. Available: www.medicalimaging.org.
32. Performance measurements of gamma cameras. 2019. [Online]. Available: www.medicalimaging.org.
33. AAPM Task Group. Scintillation camera acceptance testing and performance evaluation. AAPM; 1980.
34. AAPM Task Group. Computer-aided scintillation camera acceptance testing. New York: AAPM; 1982.
35. AERB. Quality assurance tests for SPECT-CT/SPECT/gamma camera imaging equipment. Mumbai: Radiological Safety Division, Atomic Energy Regulatory Board; 2021.
36. Adams R, Hine GJ, Zimmerman CD. Deadtime measurements in scintillation cameras under scatter conditions simulating quantitative nuclear cardiography. J Nucl Med. 1978;19:538–44. [Online]. Available: https://jnm.snmjournals.org/content/jnumed/19/5/538.full.pdf. Accessed 18 July 2023.
37. AAPM report 22 SPECT QC.
38. IAEA. IAEA human health series no. 6. Quality assurance for SPECT systems. Vienna: IAEA; 2009. [Online]. Available: http://www.iaea.org/Publications/index.html.
39. Zeinali HZ, Ataee M, Ravanbakhsh H, Goodarzi EM, Ghoreishi S, Raisali G. The precise methods for the measurement of collimator hole angulation and center of rotation of SPECT by adaptive quality control phan-

tom. World J Nucl Sci Technol. 2014;4(4):208–15. https://doi.org/10.4236/wjnst.2014.44026.
40. Busemann-Sokole E. Measurement of collimator hole angulation and camera head tilt for slant and parallel hole collimators used in SPECT. J Nucl Med. 1987;28:1592–8.
41. IAEA-TECDOC-317. Quality control of nuclear medicine instruments. 1984. [Online]. Available: https://www-pub.iaea.org/MTCD/Publications/PDF/te_317_prn.pdf. Accessed 22 July 2023.
42. Van den Wyngaert T, et al. The EANM practice guidelines for bone scintigraphy. Eur J Nucl Med Mol Imaging. 2016;43(9):1723–38. https://doi.org/10.1007/s00259-016-3415-4.
43. GE HealthCare. Discovery NM/CT 670 CZT A DIGITAL SPECT/CT.
44. Rhoe D. Minimum quality control requirement for nuclear medicine equipment. 2007. [Online]. Available: www.anzsnm.org.au.
45. IAEA. IAEA human health series no. 35. SPECT-CT atlas of quality control and image artefacts. Vienna: IAEA; 2019. [Online]. Available: www.iaea.org/books.
46. AAPM Task Group. Acceptance testing and annual physics survey recommendations for gamma camera, SPECT, and SPECT/CT systems. The report of AAPM Task Group 177. Alexandria: AAPM; 2019.
47. Mayerhoefer ME, et al. PET/MRI versus PET/CT in oncology: a prospective single-center study of 330 examinations focusing on implications for patient management and cost considerations. Eur J Nucl Med Mol Imaging. 2020;47(1):51–60. https://doi.org/10.1007/s00259-019-04452-y.
48. Ming Y, et al. Progress and future trends in PET/CT and PET/MRI molecular imaging approaches for breast cancer. Front Oncol. 2020;10:1301. https://doi.org/10.3389/fonc.2020.01301.
49. Al-Nabhani KZ, et al. Qualitative and quantitative comparison of PET/CT and PET/MR imaging in clinical practice. J Nucl Med. 2014;55(1):88–94. https://doi.org/10.2967/jnumed.113.123547.
50. Ehman EC, et al. PET/MRI: where might it replace PET/CT? J Magn Reson Imaging. 2017;46(5):1247–62. https://doi.org/10.1002/jmri.25711.

8 Dental Radiography: Physics, Principle of Operation, Quality Control, and Safety

Learning Objectives

8.1 Introduction

Dental imaging plays a pivotal role in modern dentistry, providing essential diagnostic information that aids in the identification, treatment planning, and monitoring of various dental and oral health conditions. These imaging techniques allow dental professionals to look for the internal structures of the teeth, jaws, and surrounding tissues, enabling accurate diagnosis and effective treatment delivery. These structures include:

D. Prakash, R. P. Kotian, *Fundamentals of X-ray Imaging*,
https://doi.org/10.1007/978-981-96-7328-5_8

- **Teeth**: Caries (cavities), cracks, fractures, and root morphology (shape)
- **Bone**: Bone loss, jawbone structure, and potential for implant placement
- **Soft tissues**: Abscesses, cysts, and tumors

Dental imaging helps in treatment planning for various dental procedures, including restorative dentistry, endodontic therapy, orthodontic treatment, oral surgery, and dental implant placement. By providing detailed information about tooth anatomy, bone morphology, and soft tissue structures, dental images help dentists develop precise treatment plans tailored to each patient's needs. Sequential radiographs taken during orthodontic treatment, endodontic therapy, or dental implant placement allow dentists to evaluate changes in tooth alignment, root canal morphology, bone healing, and implant integration, ensuring optimal treatment outcomes.

By visualizing subtle changes in tooth structure, bone density, and soft tissue morphology, dental images facilitate the early detection of conditions such as dental caries, periodontal disease, oral cancer, and temporomandibular joint disorders (TMJ). It also serves as a valuable tool for research and education in dentistry. Researchers use imaging techniques to investigate the etiology, progression, and treatment outcomes of various dental conditions, contributing to advancements in the field. Dental schools utilize imaging technology to educate dental students and trainees, allowing them to develop proficiency in interpreting and utilizing dental images in clinical practice.

Various imaging modalities are used in dental imaging to visualize internal structures and diagnose dental problems effectively, such as intraoral radiography, panoramic radiography, cephalometric radiography, and cone-beam computed tomography (CBCT). Each technique offers strengths and weaknesses, and the choice depends on the specific information needed. An overview of each modality, highlighting their respective advantages and limitations, is mentioned below:

8.1.1 Intraoral Radiographs (X-Rays)

Intraoral radiographs capture images of structures inside the mouth, such as teeth, surrounding bone, and supporting tissues. These radiographs are taken with the film or sensor placed inside the patient's mouth, allowing for a detailed examination of individual teeth and their surrounding structures.

There are several types of intraoral radiographs commonly used in dental practice:

- **Periapical Radiographs**: These images show the entire tooth, from the crown to the root tip and surrounding bone. They are used to diagnose conditions such as tooth decay, infections, and bone loss.
- **Bitewing Radiographs**: These images capture the crowns of the upper and lower teeth in a single view. They are particularly useful for detecting cavities between teeth, assessing the fit of dental restorations, and monitoring changes in bone levels.
- **Occlusal Radiographs**: These provide a broader view of the entire arch of teeth and surrounding bone. They help assess the development of teeth, detect abnormalities, and identify foreign objects in the mouth.

Intraoral radiographs offer numerous benefits in dental diagnosis and treatment planning as they provide detailed information about the condition of teeth and surrounding structures, aiding in detecting dental caries, periodontal disease, developmental anomalies, and other oral pathologies. Additionally, they help dentists visualize the anatomy of teeth before performing procedures such as extractions, root canal therapy, or dental implant placement. The benefits and limitations for intraoral radiographs are as follows:

- **Benefits**:
  - High resolution for visualizing details like caries (cavities), cracks, fractures, and root morphology
  - Relatively low radiation dose compared to other techniques

- **Limitations**:
  - Limited field of view, showing only a few teeth at a time
  - Two-dimensional (2D) images can lead to overlapping structures and difficulty assessing spatial relationships.

8.1.2 Panoramic Radiograph (OPG)

A panoramic radiograph, also known as an orthopantomogram (OPG), provides detailed view of the entire mouth, including the teeth, jaws, temporomandibular joints (TMJ), and surrounding structures. This radiographic technique captures a single image of the entire oral and maxillofacial region, offering a broad overview that is particularly useful for assessing dental and skeletal relationships. Key aspects of panoramic radiographs are as follows:

Image Acquisition
During a panoramic radiograph, the patient sits or stands in front of the X-ray machine while the film or digital sensor rotates around the head in a semicircular motion. This movement captures a detailed image of the oral and facial structures, including the upper and lower dental arches, jawbones, sinuses, and surrounding tissues.

Diagnostic Applications
- Assessing the overall dental and skeletal development in pediatric patients
- Detecting dental caries, periodontal disease, and other dental pathology
- Evaluating unerupted or impacted teeth's presence, position, and eruption status
- Examining the condition of the temporomandibular joints (TMJ) and detecting signs of temporomandibular joint disorder (TMD)
- Planning for orthodontic treatment, dental implants, extractions, and other dental procedures
- Assessing the presence of tumors, cysts, or other abnormalities in the oral and maxillofacial region

Advantages
- Convenience: A single panoramic image captures the entire mouth, eliminating the need for multiple intraoral X-rays.
- Patient comfort: Patients do not need to bite down on film or sensors, making the procedure more comfortable, especially for individuals with a strong gag reflex.
- Comprehensive view: Panoramic radiographs provide a broad overview of dental and skeletal structures, aiding in comprehensive treatment planning and diagnosis.

Limitations
- *Reduced image detail*: Compared to intraoral radiographs, panoramic images may have lower resolution and less detail, making detecting small dental caries or fractures challenging.
- *Distortion*: The panoramic technique can introduce distortion, particularly in the anterior teeth region, which may affect the accuracy of measurements and assessment of dental relationships.
- *Overlapping structures*: In some cases, anatomical structures may overlap, obscuring certain areas of interest and complicating interpretation.

It provides valuable information about the overall oral and maxillofacial anatomy and offers numerous benefits for comprehensive dental evaluation, treatment planning, and patient care.

8.1.3 Cephalometric Radiograph

A cephalometric radiograph, also known as a cephalogram, provides a two-dimensional image of the side of the face and skull. This radiographic technique is commonly used in orthodontics and oral and maxillofacial surgery to assess the relationship between the teeth, jaws, and facial structures. It captures lateral (side) and sometimes posteroanterior (front-to-back) images of the head to assess facial profile, jaw development, and the relationship between teeth and jaws. The key aspects of cephalometric radiographs are as follows:

Image Acquisition

During a cephalometric radiograph, the patient stands or sits upright while the X-ray machine captures an image of the side of the head. The patient's head is positioned using standardized head-holding devices to ensure consistency and accuracy in imaging. The X-ray beam transmits through the patient's head and is captured on a film or digital sensor on the opposite side.

Anatomical Structures

- The skeletal structures of the face and skull include the maxilla (upper jaw), mandible (lower jaw), and cranial base.
- The teeth and their positions relative to the jaws and facial bones.
- Soft tissues, such as the palate, nose, and lips.
- Diagnostic applications: Cephalometric radiographs are used for a variety of diagnostic purposes in orthodontics and oral and maxillofacial surgery, including:
- Assessing facial growth and development in pediatric patients
- Evaluating the skeletal and dental relationships, including the position of the jaws and teeth relative to each other and the cranial base
- Planning orthodontic treatment, including the placement of braces, orthodontic appliances, and corrective jaw surgery
- Diagnosing and evaluating craniofacial anomalies, such as cleft lip and palate, facial asymmetry, and skeletal deformities
- Monitoring treatment progress and evaluating the outcomes of orthodontic and surgical interventions

Advantages

- Objective assessment: Cephalometric measurements provide quantitative data about the relationship between facial structures, enabling more accurate diagnosis and treatment planning.
- Treatment prediction: Cephalometric analysis helps orthodontists predict how different treatment approaches affect facial growth and development, allowing personalized treatment plans.
- Comprehensive evaluation: Cephalometric radiographs provide a comprehensive view of the patient's facial anatomy, facilitating a thorough assessment of orthodontic and surgical needs.

Limitations

- Two-dimensional representation: Cephalometric radiographs provide a flat, two-dimensional image of the facial structures, which may not fully represent the three-dimensional nature of the face.
- Radiation exposure: Like all X-ray procedures, cephalometric radiographs involve exposure to ionizing radiation. However, modern digital imaging techniques have reduced radiation doses compared to traditional film-based radiography.

Cephalometric radiographs are essential diagnostic tools in orthodontics and oral and maxillofacial surgery, providing valuable information about facial growth and development, skeletal relationships, and treatment planning. While they have some limitations, cephalometric radiographs offer significant benefits for the comprehensive evaluation and management of orthodontic and craniofacial conditions.

8.1.4 Cone-Beam Computed Tomography (CBCT)

Cone-beam computed tomography (CBCT) is used in dentistry and maxillofacial imaging to produce three-dimensional (3D) images of the teeth, jaws, temporomandibular joints (TMJ), and surrounding structures. CBCT technology utilizes a cone-shaped X-ray beam to capture high-resolution images with minimal radiation exposure compared to conventional computed tomography (CT) scans. It creates 3D images of the jaws and surrounding structures using a cone-shaped X-ray beam and computer software reconstruction. Some key aspects of CBCT imaging are as follows:

Image Acquisition

During a CBCT scan, the patient sits upright while the CBCT machine rotates around their head in a complete or partial circle, capturing a series of 2D X-ray images from various angles. Computer software then reconstructs these images to create a detailed 3D representation of the oral and maxillofacial region.

Anatomical Structures

- Teeth: CBCT images accurately depict the size, shape, and position of individual teeth, including roots and surrounding bone.
- Jaws: CBCT scans show the entire maxilla (upper jaw) and mandible (lower jaw), allowing for precise assessment of bone density, morphology, and pathology.
- Temporomandibular joints (TMJ): CBCT imaging enables evaluation of TMJ anatomy, including the articular surfaces, disc position, and presence of degenerative changes or disorders.
- Sinuses and airway: CBCT scans can assess the paranasal sinuses and airway anatomy, aiding in diagnosing sinusitis, airway obstructions, and other respiratory conditions.

Diagnostic Applications

- Dental implant planning: CBCT scans provide detailed information about bone volume, quality, and proximity to vital structures, facilitating precise implant placement.
- Orthodontic treatment planning: CBCT images allow orthodontists to assess tooth and bone relationships in three dimensions, aiding in treatment planning for complex malocclusions and surgical orthodontic procedures.
- Endodontic evaluation: CBCT imaging helps endodontists visualize root canal anatomy, detect root fractures, and assess the extent of periapical pathology.
- Surgical planning: CBCT scans aid oral and maxillofacial surgeons in planning for jaw surgery, orthognathic surgery, tumor resection, and other complex procedures by providing detailed 3D images of the anatomical structures involved.

Advantages

- High image resolution: CBCT scans produce high-quality, detailed images with superior resolution compared to conventional radiographs, allowing for precise diagnosis and treatment planning.
- Three-dimensional visualization: CBCT imaging provides a comprehensive 3D view of the oral and maxillofacial region, enabling a more accurate assessment of anatomical structures and pathology.
- Low radiation dose: While CBCT scans involve exposure to ionizing radiation, modern CBCT machines are designed to minimize radiation dose while still producing diagnostic-quality images.

Limitations

- *Cost*: CBCT scans can be more expensive than conventional radiographs, making them less accessible in some clinical settings.
- *Radiation exposure*: Although CBCT scans use lower radiation doses than conventional CT scans, they still involve exposure to ionizing radiation, particularly in pediatric and young adult patients.
- *Interpretation challenges*: Interpreting CBCT images requires specialized training and expertise due to the complexity of the 3D data sets and the potential for artifacts and image distortion.

By understanding each method's distinct capabilities and limitations, dental professionals can select the most appropriate imaging modality based on the specific diagnostic needs of each patient, ensuring optimal care and minimizing unnecessary radiation exposure.

8.2 Highlights of the Historical Development of Dental X-Ray Equipment

Following Röntgen's groundbreaking discovery in 1895, dental radiography began to gain traction rapidly. However, commercialization and widespread implementation took time. By 1905, the first dental X-ray machines were manufactured in Germany by Siemens [1]. By 1912–1913, dental X-ray units reached the United States although only a few dentists initially adopted them. By 1932, nearly half of newly graduated dentists in the United States had acquired an X-ray unit for their practice.

Early experimentation with X-rays in 1896 was facilitated by the accessibility of tools used by Röntgen and his predecessors. No new equipment was needed; an induction coil coupled with a Crookes-Hittorf tube was sufficient to generate X-rays. The high vacuum in the Crookes-Hittorf tube resulted in a constant electron stream, improving radiographic detail. Early improvements to the tube were made by researchers like König and Harrison. C.E. Kells also explored optimizing X-ray technology, preferring the Crookes-Hittorf tube. However, X-ray quantity and quality consistency remained an issue until Mackee and Remer proposed using a "radiochromometer" and radiometer.

In 1913, William David Coolidge designed the Coolidge-type tube, still in use today, which improved safety and provided better control over X-ray quantity and quality. The adaptation of this tube for dental radiography followed soon after.

Handheld X-ray units for intraoral radiography were first described in 1993, with increasing interest in forensic and clinical dentistry. However, their main limitations include operator exposure to scatter radiation and low tube output, necessitating longer exposure times. They are recommended for specific environments, such as remote areas or facilities with immobile patients where mobile units are unavailable. A timeline illustrating brief history of dental radiology is shown in Table 8.1.

Table 8.1 Highlights in the history of dental radiology

Year	Concept	Persons associated	Additional information
1895	Discovery of X-rays	Wilhelm Conrad Röntgen	Pioneered the use of X-rays, laying the foundation for the field of dental radiography
1896	First dental radiograph	Otto Walkhoff	Took the first dental radiograph, exposing himself to significant radiation, which led to skin damage
1896	First dental radiograph in the US (skull and live)	W.J. Morton and C.E. Kells	Morton produced the first dental radiograph on of a skull in the US. Kells later took the first dental x-ray in America of a living person's mouth.
1901	Dangers of X-radiation	William Herbert Rollins	Advocated for radiation safety after identifying the risks associated with X-ray exposure
1904	Bisecting angle technique	Weston A. Price	Introduced a method to improve image clarity by optimizing the angle between the X-ray beam and the tooth
1913	First dental text and prewrapped films	Howard Riley Raper and Eastman Kodak Company	Raper authored the first dental radiology textbook, and Eastman Kodak developed prewrapped dental X-ray films, enhancing standardization and hygiene.
1913	First X-ray tube with hot cathode	William David Coolidge	Revolutionized X-ray technology by creating more consistent and reliable X-ray generation
1920s	Paralleling technique and machine-made film packets	Franklin W. McCormack and Eastman Kodak Company	Improved the accuracy of dental radiographs and made the process more accessible to dental practitioners
1923	First dedicated dental X-ray machine	Victor X-ray Corporation of Chicago	Developed the first machine specifically designed for dental radiography, enhancing the precision and convenience of dental imaging
1925	Bitewing technique	Howard Riley Raper	Introduced a method crucial for detecting interproximal caries, improving diagnostic capabilities
1933	Rotational panoramic radiography concept	Dr. Hisatugu Numata	Pioneered the concept of panoramic X-rays, which allow for a broad view of the dental arches
1947	Long cone paralleling technique	F. Gordon Fitzgerald	Enhanced the paralleling technique, improving image quality and reducing patient radiation exposure

(continued)

Table 8.1 (continued)

Year	Concept	Persons associated	Additional information
1948	Panoramic radiography	Dr. Yrjö Veli Paatero	Developed the first practical panoramic radiography system, providing a comprehensive view of the jaw and teeth
1950s	D-speed film	Eastman Kodak Company	Introduced faster film that reduced exposure time and improved image quality
1957	First variable kilovoltage dental X-ray machine	General Electric	Developed a machine that allowed for the adjustment of X-ray energy levels, improving image quality and patient safety
1960s	First commercially available panoramic X-ray machine	Marketed by SS White and Co.	Made panoramic radiography widely accessible, leading to its widespread adoption in dental practices
1969	CT scanner prototype	Sir Godfrey Hounsfield	Invented the first CT scanner, which eventually led to the development of CBCT technology for dental and maxillofacial imaging
1970s	Dental xeroradiography		Introduced a technique that offered certain advantages, such as edge enhancement, though it was not widely adopted in dental practice
1980s	E-speed film and intraoral digital radiography	Eastman Kodak Company	Introduced faster film and began the transition to digital imaging, allowing for real-time viewing of X-rays and reducing patient exposure
1987	DentaScan and CBCT technology development		Introduction of DentaScan, the first dedicated dental CT software; early CBCT research also began during this period, laying the foundation for advanced 3D imaging in dentistry and maxillofacial applications
2000s	"F" speed films and CBCT commercialization		Introduced even faster film and saw the widespread commercialization of CBCT, providing high-resolution 3D imaging for diagnostics and treatment planning
2010s and beyond	Digital sensors and advancements in CBCT		Continued advancements in digital sensor technology, with CBCT systems becoming more sophisticated, including features like low-dose imaging and AI integration for improved diagnostic accuracy

8.3 Instrumentation of Dental X-Ray Imaging

As mentioned earlier, dental imaging employs various equipment for different diagnostic purposes, broadly categorized as intraoral, panoramic, cephalometric, and cone-beam computed tomography (CBCT). The instrumentation of each modality is detailed as follows:

8.3.1 Intraoral X-Rays

Intraoral X-rays are integral in dentistry because they provide detailed images of specific teeth and surrounding bone structures. Periapical radiographs offer a comprehensive view of one or two entire teeth, including the crowns and roots, aiding in the detection of infections, bone loss, and developmental abnormalities, Bitewing radiographs capture both upper and lower teeth in a single section, enabling early detection of cavities between teeth and facilitating precise treatment planning.

They offer detailed visualization, allowing dentists to observe intricate dental structures that may not be apparent during a clinical examination. Moreover, their role in early cavity detection, monitoring treatment progress, and delivering relatively low radiation doses compared to other imaging techniques makes them indispensable in routine dental care. Dentists often recommend intraoral X-rays during routine checkups to investigate tooth-related concerns like pain or swelling, assess jawbone health before procedures, and monitor the progress of ongoing treatments, ensuring comprehensive dental care for patients.

8.3.1.1 History of Intraoral Radiography

Just 2 weeks following Röntgen's groundbreaking discovery, German dentist Otto Walkhoff, assisted by Fritz Giesel, obtained a radiograph of his teeth which took an exposure time of 25 minutes [1]. However, the image lacked diagnostic quality. Subsequent efforts by other pioneers rapidly improved radiographic quality. In 1896, Walkhoff and Giesel established the first dental X-ray laboratory [2]. Early X-ray tubes required recalibration before each exposure, a process known as "setting," often done by adjusting tube current based on the operator's hand in front of a fluoroscope. Dentists sometimes held intraoral plates during exposure, leading to health risks.

C.E. Kells, an American dentist, adopted X-rays for dentistry in 1896 [3]. He developed a film holder allowing patients to swallow during exposure and advocated for parallel film placement and minimal object-film distance, pioneering the paralleling technique. He also suggested using holders for proper film positioning and two films simultaneously for recordkeeping. William J. Morton, also in the United States, presented intraoral radiographs of a skull in 1896 and highlighted X-rays' potential in dentistry [1].

In England, Frank Harrison discussed dental radiography's potential applications in 1896 [1]. Physicist Walter König reduced exposure times by adapting X-ray tubes. In the United States, W.H. Rollins advocated for radiation protection principles, including shielding and proper collimation, despite initial disregard. Weston A. Price emphasized accurate labeling and meticulous radiographic recordkeeping.

In 1909, Howard Riley Raper (1887–1978) pioneered a new field, which he named radiodontia and initiated the inaugural dental radiography course for undergraduate dental students at the Indiana Dental College (now recognized as Indiana University School of Dentistry) (Fig. 8.1). By 1913, Raper authored one of the earliest textbooks on dental radiology titled "Elementary and Dental Radiography," followed by another textbook named "Electro-radiographic Diagnosis" in 1921 [4]. Notably, in 1915, Raper became the pioneering specialist in the practice of dental radiology. By 1925, Dr. Raper had introduced the concept of bitewing films and collaborated with George Eastman of the Eastman Kodak Company. The first utilization of paralleling principles in intraoral dental radiography was credited to Franklin W. McCormack, a medical X-ray technician from San Francisco, California.

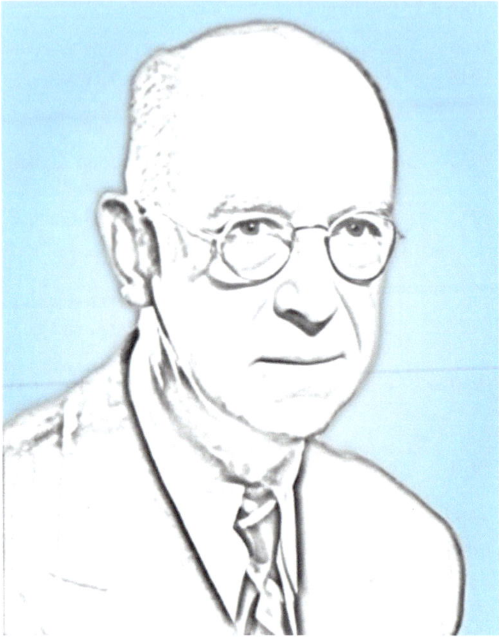

Fig. 8.1 Dr. Howard Riley Raper

In 1940, Dr. Gordon Fitzgerald (1907–1981) developed a long cone for dental X-ray machines, drawing inspiration from McCormack's tabletop long-distance (36-inch FFD) technique and adapting it for dental chair use. In 1949, the American Academy of Oral Roentgenology, now known as the American Academy of Dental Radiology, was established.

While some early adopters faced health issues due to radiation exposure, their pioneering work laid the foundation for modern dental radiography, contributing to its widespread adoption and safer practices.

8.3.1.2 Working Principle of Intraoral Radiography

Intraoral X-rays remain fundamental in dental diagnostics, offering high-resolution, two-dimensional projections of individual teeth and surrounding structures. This section delves into the intricate technical aspects of the intraoral radiography process, encompassing equipment, patient positioning, beam path and film placement, image formation, and interpretation.

Equipment and Setup

- **X-ray source**:
  - Generates a collimated X-ray beam with a narrow field of view (typically 4–8 mm diameter) using a tungsten target and filtration system.
  - The filtration system, often composed of aluminum and copper, removes low-energy photons, optimizing spectral quality for dental applications by reducing patient exposure to unnecessary radiation while ensuring sufficient penetration through dense tissues.
  - Modern units frequently utilize cone-beam collimation or paralleling beam devices to restrict scattered radiation further and enhance image detail by minimizing the geometric blurring effect of the penumbra.
- **Image receptor**:
  - **Film-based systems**:
    - Employ X-ray film cassettes loaded with photosensitive films of varying sizes (sizes 0, 1, 2) based on the desired field of view and targeted tooth.
    - Film selection also considers speed characteristics, balancing image quality with exposure times. Faster films require less radiation exposure but may exhibit lower image quality than slower films.
  - **Digital sensors:**
    - Utilize solid-state technology of amorphous silicon or CMOS (complementary metal-oxide semiconductor) detectors.
    - These detectors convert incident X-ray photons directly into an electrical signal for digital image formation.
    - Sensor selection involves considerations of active area size, pixel resolution, and dynamic range for optimal image capture.

Patient Positioning

- The patient is comfortably positioned supine or semi-supine with their head stabilized using a headrest and bite block.
- The bite block serves a dual purpose:
  - **Positioning**: Ensures proper placement of the film/sensor within the oral cavity, aligning the receptor is parallel to the long axis of the tooth to minimize geometric distortion
  - **Immobilization**: Minimizes patient movement during exposure, reducing image blur

8.3.1.3 Beam Path and Film Placement

- The X-ray source is positioned extraoral at a specific:
  - **Vertical angulation**: Typically ranging from +40° to +90° relative to the targeted tooth
  - **Horizontal angulation**: Mesial, distal, or occlusal, depending on the desired visualization of the tooth and surrounding structures
- This specific angulation ensures the central ray of the X-ray beam traverses the tooth along the desired path, minimizing:
  - Superimposition of anatomical structures, allowing for clearer visualization of specific aspects like the periapical region
  - Geometric distortion
- **Intraoral placement**: To achieve optimal image quality, the film/sensor is positioned within the oral cavity using specific techniques like the bisecting angle or paralleling technique. These techniques ensure proper alignment of the receptor with the long axis of the tooth and minimize geometric distortion.

8.3.1.4 Image Formation and Processing

- **Film-based systems**:
  - When the X-ray beam interacts with the silver halide crystals in the film, it causes a latent image to be formed. The film's degree of exposure (darkness) corresponds to the X-ray photon flux reaching different areas.
  - The exposed film undergoes a multistep chemical processing (developing, fixing,

washing) to convert the latent image into a permanent, visible radiograph.

- **Digital sensors**:
  - X-ray photons interact with the photodiodes within the sensor and generate electrical signals proportional to the incident photon flux. This signal variation across the sensor area corresponds to different tissues' spatial distribution of X-ray attenuation.
  - This signal is converted into a digital image through an analog-to-digital converter (ADC) for electronic display on a monitor or storage. Image processing algorithms may be applied to enhance contrast and visualization.

8.3.1.5 Handheld and Wall-Mounted Scanners

Intraoral scanners can be of two types, for example, handheld and wall mounted. These scanners have undergone significant advancements since inception and offer dentists versatile and efficient tools for comprehensive patient care. Their portability, convenience, and imaging capabilities make them valuable assets in modern dental practices, facilitating accurate diagnosis, treatment planning, and dental health monitoring.

8.3.1.5.1 Handheld Scanners

Handheld scanners are portable devices that allow dentists to capture X-ray images directly in the patient's mouth without cumbersome equipment setups. Their lightweight and ergonomic design facilitates easy maneuvering and accurate positioning to ensure optimal image quality. Handheld scanners are particularly useful when mobility and flexibility are essential, such as in pediatric dentistry or when treating patients with limited mobility (Fig. 8.2).

- **Pros**:
  - **Greater Maneuverability**: Offers more flexibility for capturing data from various intraoral locations and angles.
  - **Portability**: This can be easily moved between operatories or used for chairside consultations.
  - **Generally Lower Cost**: Typically a more affordable option compared to wall-mounted scanners.
- **Cons**:
  - **Requires Operator Skill**: Requires good hand-eye coordination and technique for efficient scanning.
  - **Potential for Patient Discomfort**: The scanner wand might cause discomfort in patients with limited mouth opening.

8.3.1.5.2 Wall-Mounted Scanners

Wall-mounted scanners are fixed imaging units installed within the dental operatory. They are designed to be mounted on the wall or ceiling, offering a stable and permanent imaging solution for dental practices. Wall-mounted scanners typically feature adjustable arms or articulating mounts, allowing for precise positioning and alignment with the patient's oral anatomy. These scanners are ideal for practices with high patient volumes and consistent imaging needs, providing reliable and efficient X-ray imaging capabilities (Fig. 8.3).

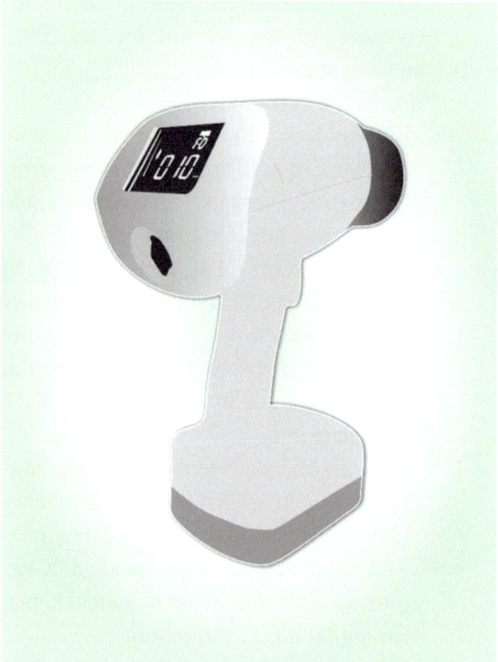

Fig. 8.2 Handheld portable intraoral X-ray machines

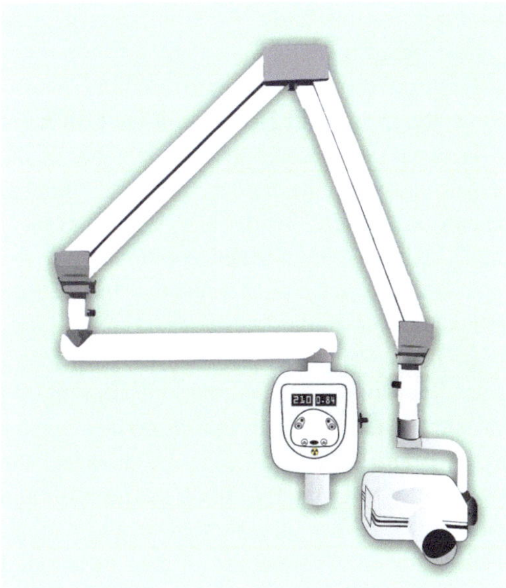

Fig. 8.3 Wall-mounted dental X-ray unit with the head supported on a jointed positioning arm

- **Pros**:
  - **Improved Ergonomics**: Frees up the dentist's hands, potentially reducing fatigue during longer scanning procedures.
  - **Standardized Scanning**: This can potentially lead to more consistent and reproducible scans due to the fixed position of the scanner head.
  - **Potential for Improved Patient Comfort**: Patients with limited mouth opening may be more comfortable as the dentist doesn't need to hold the scanner intraorally.
- **Cons**:
  - **Limited Maneuverability**: The fixed position of the scanner head might limit access to certain areas of the mouth.
  - **Higher Cost**: Typically a more expensive investment compared to handheld scanners.
  - **Less Portable**: Not easily moved between operatories or used for chairside consultations.

Additional Considerations

- **Scanning Speed**: Newer scanner models offer faster scanning times, improving workflow efficiency.
- **Image Quality**: High-resolution cameras and advanced software algorithms contribute to superior image quality and accurate 3D models.
- **Integration with CAD/CAM Systems**: Seamless integration with computer-aided design and computer-aided manufacturing software allows for efficient design and fabrication of dental restorations.

Intraoral handheld and wall-mounted scanners offer valuable tools for capturing digital impressions in dentistry. The choice between these types depends on individual practice needs, workflow preferences, and budget considerations.

8.3.2 Panoramic Radiograph (OPG)

The terms "panoramic radiography" and "OPG" (orthopantomogram) are often used interchangeably due to the widespread adoption of this imaging technique as the standard for capturing comprehensive views of the teeth, jawbone, and surrounding structures on a single film or digital sensor. This method generates a single tomographic image encompassing the entire facial structure, including the upper (maxillary) and lower (mandibular) jaw arches and their supporting structures. Synonyms for this type of radiography include "rotational radiography" and "pantomography." The term "pantomography" is derived from "pan" meaning "wide," "tomo" meaning "slices," and "graphy" meaning "to write." While OPG or panoramic radiographs are commonly used in dentistry alongside bitewing and periapical X-rays, they offer different advantages and limitations.

Unlike projection images (bitewing and periapical) that capture specific areas with high detail, panoramic radiographs provide a broader view of the jaw, encompassing multiple structures. However, this broader view comes at the cost of reduced sharpness and overlapping structures in certain areas. Consequently, their diagnostic value is better suited for identifying general anomalies where fine details are less crucial [5] as it is not useful for detecting small carious lesions, periapical disease, or the fine structure of the marginal periodontium [6].

The primary benefit of panoramic radiographs is their ability to visualize a large area and show the relative positions of various structures. However, they are not routinely used during checkups due to lower resolution and higher radiation exposure compared to individual intraoral images. Studies suggest that panoramic radiographs are less effective than periapical and bitewing radiographs in detecting proximal caries [7].

Panoramic radiographs become more relevant when clinical examination suggests a need for a broader view, particularly for conditions affecting larger areas such as tumors or developmental disorders. In such cases, a panoramic radiograph can be a valuable supplement to individual intraoral images.

8.3.2.1 History of Panoramic Radiography

The panoramic radiography technique is largely attributed to Dr. Yrjö Veli Paatero, a Finnish dentist. However, its origins trace back to earlier contributions. In 1922, Zulauf proposed a narrow-beam scanning technique in the United States and introduced the term "panoramic radiography" [8]. Dr. H Numata in Japan published clinical results of a prototype "parabolic radiography" device in 1933, contributing to the early development of panoramic imaging techniques [9].

During World War II, Paatero took up a position at the Institute of Dentistry of the University of Helsinki and became the sole member of the Department of Radiology. Despite limited resources, Paatero made significant advancements. In 1946, he published a preliminary report on his work, unaware of previous publications and patents on similar techniques [1] (Fig. 8.4).

In 1949, Paatero introduced the "parabalograph," utilizing a long, curved film placed intraorally and exposed with a moving narrow X-ray beam. Later that year, he modified the technique, placing the film extraorally and rotating the X-ray tube relative to the patient, leading to the development of the "orthoradial pantomograph," commonly known as "orthopantomograph" or "OPG" [1].

In the early 1950s, Paatero collaborated with engineer Timo Nieminen via the Finnish company Lääkintäsähkö, leading to the development of a panoramic radiography unit with a triple rotation center. Clinical testing followed, and through collaboration with Siemens, commercialization of the orthopantomograph began in 1960 [11, 12].

Meanwhile, in the United States, after clinical testing of a double eccentric machine by

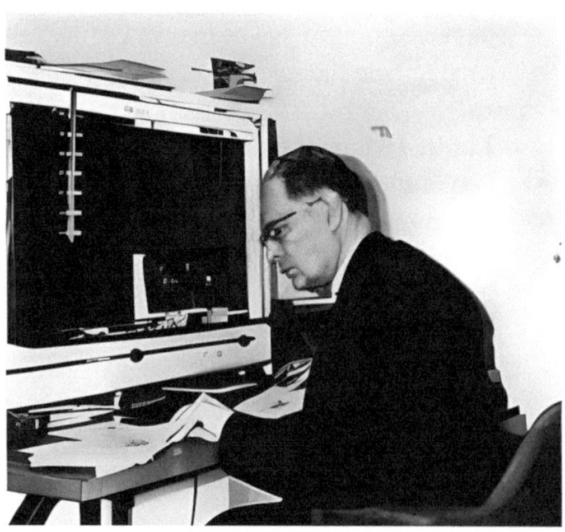

Dr Yrjö Veli Paatero

Fig. 8.4 Dr. Yrjö Veli Paatero, known as the "father of panoramic radiography," pioneered the development of panoramic dental X-rays. (Courtesy: Oxford University Press [10])

Hudson et al., the S.S. White company commenced production of the "Panorex." In the United Kingdom, dentist S. Blackman, inspired by a panoramic radiography unit from Helsinki, collaborated with Watson and Sons to develop the "Rotograph" [1].

These efforts marked the widespread adoption of panoramic radiography worldwide, transforming dental diagnostic imaging and improving patient care. Panoramic radiography underwent further development with its clinical implementation. Early models often used one-pulse AC generators, but hospitals' adoption allowed coupling to 12-pulse generators, enabling rotating anode tubes [11]. In 1978, Soredex introduced DC generators [11]. A 1979 dosimetric study found the energy imparted by panoramic radiography ranging from 0.45 to 4.5 mJ in the head and neck region, similar to conventional radiographs [13].

Mechanical movement was gradually replaced by step motors and electronic control systems, improving device ergonomics and patient positioning. While initially focusing on dental arch visualization, later developments allowed customization and refinement of image layers. Computed panoramic radiography emerged in the 1980s [14], followed by direct digital panoramic radiography in the early 1990s [15, 16]. Some current units feature direct conversion receptors.

Recent dosimetric studies show absorbed doses ranging from 0.62 mGy to 17.6 μSv for different types of panoramic radiography, with effective doses between 14 and 24 μSv reported in earlier studies [17]. However, more recent studies have found effective doses ranging from 5 to 15 μSv for digital panoramic radiography, with dose reductions observed for collimated radiographs [17].

8.3.2.2 Working Mechanism of Orthopantomography (OPG)

The technical aspects of the OPG procedure, including equipment setup, beam path trajectory, image formation principles, and resulting image characteristics, are mentioned below:

Equipment and Setup

- The OPG unit typically comprises an X-ray source (collimator, anode, and generator), a patient positioning system (chair, headrest, and chin support), and an image receptor (film cassette or digital sensor) mounted on a movable arm.
- The patient is positioned in a seating or standing upright posture with their chin resting on the chin support and head stabilized against the headrest, ensuring minimal movement during the acquisition process (Fig. 8.5).
- The X-ray source and the image receptor are positioned on opposite sides of the head of the patient, maintaining a specific geometric relationship defined by the chosen unit's configuration and desired field of view.

8.3.2.3 Beam Path Trajectory and Synchronization

- The core principle of OPG lies in the synchronized movement of the source and the image receptor along complementary paths.
- The X-ray source executes a curvilinear path around the patient's head, following an arc that approximates the shape of the dental arches. This trajectory ensures that the X-ray beam traverses the maxillofacial region at varying angles, capturing different anatomical structures within the desired field of view.

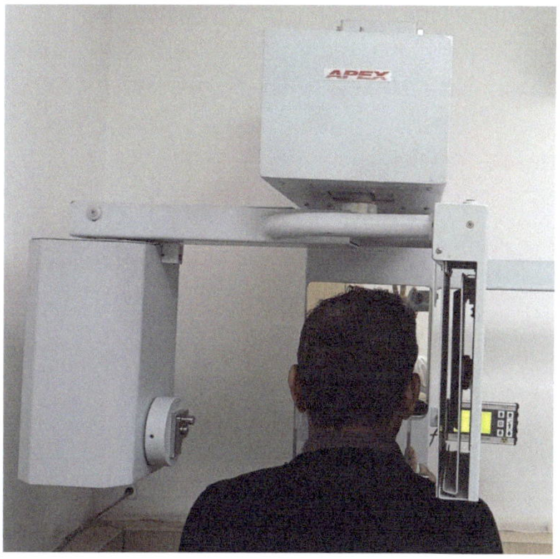

Fig. 8.5 Acquiring OPG images

- Simultaneously, the image receptor undergoes a reciprocal, synchronized movement along a curved path on the opposite side of the patient's head. This movement ensures that a specific "slice" of the maxillofacial region remains aligned with the central axis of the X-ray beam throughout the acquisition process.

8.3.2.4 Image Formation and Blurring

- The synchronized movement of the X-ray source and the image receptor allows for the targeted acquisition of a specific "slice" of the maxillofacial region.
- Structures within this designated "slice" are consistently projected onto the same location of the image receptor throughout the movement, resulting in a sharp and clear depiction.
- Conversely, structures positioned outside the intended "slice" are projected onto different locations on the image receptor during the movement. This intentional misalignment leads to the blurring of these structures, effectively minimizing their visual interference with the structures of interest within the chosen slice.

8.3.2.5 Resulting Image and Applications

- The final OPG image provides a flattened, panoramic representation of the entire maxillofacial region, encompassing the upper and lower jaws, surrounding bony structures, and various anatomical landmarks (Fig. 8.6).
- The distinct advantage of OPG over periapical radiography lies in its broad field of view, enabling the comprehensive assessment of multiple teeth, jaws, and surrounding structures in a single image. This makes OPG a valuable tool for various dental diagnostic applications, including:
  - Evaluation of jaw development and abnormalities
  - Assessment of dental impactions, unerupted teeth, and supernumerary teeth
  - Diagnosis of fractures, cysts, and other pathological conditions affecting the jaws
  - Preoperative planning for surgical procedures and dental implant placement

OPG combines synchronized movement, targeted beam path, and intentional blurring to capture a comprehensive image of the maxillofacial region in a single acquisition. This technique offers valuable diagnostic information for various dental applications, making it a cornerstone of contemporary dental imaging.

8.3.3 Cephalometric Dental Units

Cephalometric dental units are specialized X-ray machines used in dentistry and orthodontics to capture a comprehensive view of the patient's facial skeleton, teeth, and jaws (Fig. 8.7). This information is crucial for various dental procedures, such as:

- **Orthodontic treatment planning**: Cephalometric X-rays provide valuable insights for

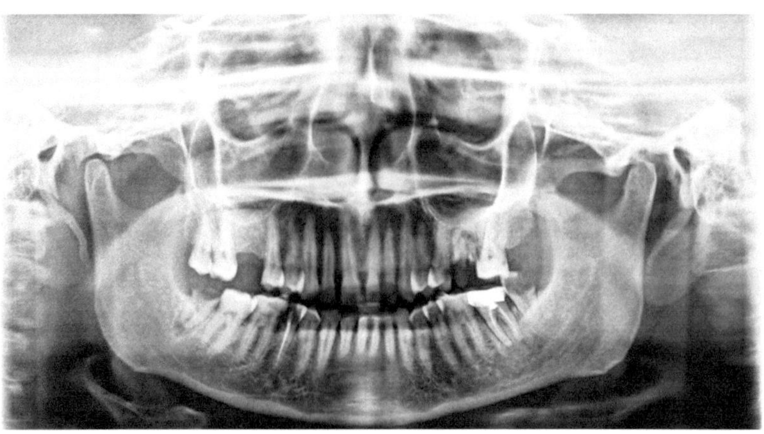

Fig. 8.6 OPG image

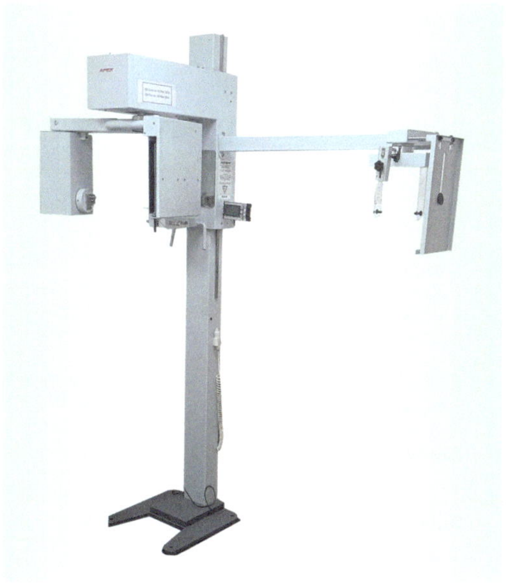

Fig. 8.7 OPG cum cephalometric dental unit

orthodontists when planning treatment for misaligned teeth or bite problems. They help assess jaw growth patterns, tooth position, and potential issues related to bite alignment.

- **Evaluation of facial symmetry**: These X-rays can reveal asymmetries in the jaw or facial structures, which can be helpful for orthodontic treatment and oral surgery planning.
- **Diagnosing jaw abnormalities**: Cephalometry can help identify issues like prognathism (jutting lower jaw) or retrognathia (receded lower jaw).
- **Presurgical planning**: Cephalometric X-rays provide valuable anatomical details for surgeons to plan the surgery precisely for procedures involving the jaws or facial bones.
- **TMJ (temporomandibular joint) assessment**: While not always the primary diagnostic tool, cephalometric X-rays can sometimes be used to evaluate potential issues with the jaw joint.

8.3.3.1 History of Cephalometric Radiography

In 1931, the introduction of cephalometric X-ray by BH Broadbent in the United States [18] and H. Hofrath in Germany [19] marked a significant advancement in diagnostic tools available to orthodontists. Before this innovation, clinicians relied solely on clinical observation and patient study casts. However, cephalometric X-rays provided a deeper insight into facial structure, allowing for a correlation between each patient's malocclusion and their facial skeletal and dental morphology [20]. This facilitated a more detailed study of dentoalveolar components and the development of improved treatment plans tailored to individual patient needs [20].

Initially, cephalometric analysis was primarily used for morphological assessment, describing an individual's facial makeup without significant clinical predictive value for future facial development [20] (Fig. 8.8). While numerous morphological analyses exist today, they often vary based on individual preferences and may lack robust data to support their use across larger patient populations. Furthermore, modern computerized cephalometric analyses often provide excessive data, posing challenges for orthodontic practitioners [20].

In response to these complexities, a simplified cephalometric analysis known as the "Björk Morphological Analysis" has emerged, offering practical applicability for most clinicians [20]. Additionally, the introduction of cone-beam computed tomography (CBCT) several decades ago has revolutionized diagnostic capabilities in orthodontics. CBCT allows for creating high-resolution lateral head films from DICOM files, offering detailed insights into dental and skeletal issues.

8.3.3.2 Working Principle of Cephalometric Dental X-Ray Machines

Cephalometric dental X-ray machines are specialized imaging devices that capture head and facial structures radiographic images. The working principle of these machines involves the following key components and steps:

- **X-Ray Tube**: Like other dental X-ray machines, cephalometric units consist of an X-ray tube that generates X-rays. The X-ray tube produces a focused beam of X-rays directed toward the patient's head and facial region.

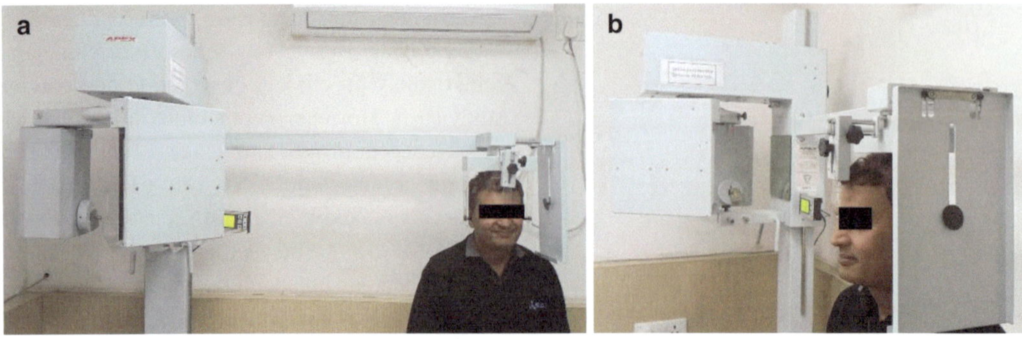

Fig. 8.8 Performing a cephalometric test. (**a**) Front view. (**b**) Sideways view

- **Cephalostat**: The cephalostat is a mechanical device that holds the patient's head in a fixed position during the X-ray exposure. It ensures that the patient's head remains stable and properly aligned for accurate imaging.
- **Head Positioning**: The patient's head is positioned within the cephalogram in a standardized orientation, typically concerning anatomical landmarks such as the ear canal and the corner of the eye. This positioning ensures consistent and reproducible images for accurate analysis.
- **Exposure Parameters**: Before the X-ray exposure, the operator selects the appropriate exposure parameters, such as the X-ray tube voltage (kVp) and current (mA), based on the patient's age, size, and specific imaging requirements. These parameters determine the energy and intensity of the X-ray beam.
- **X-Ray Exposure**: Once the patient is properly positioned, the X-ray is initiated by activating the X-ray tube. The X-ray beam is directed toward the patient's head and passes through the tissues, including the bones and soft tissues of the face and skull.
- **Image Receptor**: The X-ray beam that passes through the patient's head is captured by an image receptor positioned on the opposite side. Digital sensors or phosphor plates are commonly used as image receptors in modern cephalometric units. These receptors convert the X-ray energy into digital signals or latent images for subsequent processing and analysis.
- **Image Processing**: After the X-ray exposure, the captured images are processed using specialized software. The software enhances the image quality, adjusts the contrast and brightness, and applies image corrections to optimize the diagnostic information.
- **Image Analysis**: The processed images are then analyzed by dental professionals, such as orthodontists or maxillofacial surgeons, to assess anatomical structures and diagnose dental and facial abnormalities. Cephalometric images provide valuable information for treatment planning in orthodontics, orthognathic surgery, and other dental specialities (Fig. 8.9).

Overall, the working principle of cephalometric dental X-ray machines involves precise positioning of the patient's head, controlled X-ray exposure, and digital image capture and processing to obtain detailed radiographic images of the craniofacial region for diagnostic and treatment purposes.

8.3.4 Cone-Beam Computed Tomography (CBCT)

Cone-beam computed tomography also called as CBCT is a 3D imaging technique used in dentistry to produce detailed scans of the maxillofacial skeleton. In a CBCT scan, the X-ray source and detector move in a circle around the object being scanned (Fig. 8.10). Depending on the settings, this takes about 10–40 seconds but can be faster

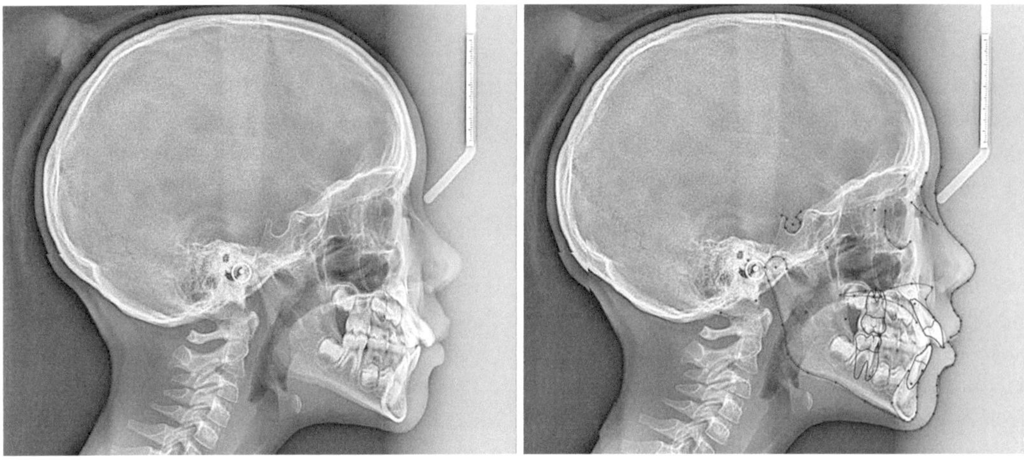

Fig. 8.9 Cephalometric dental X-ray. (Image Source: https://cephx.com/cephalometric-analysis-based-x-ray-scans/. Accessed on 02.02.2024)

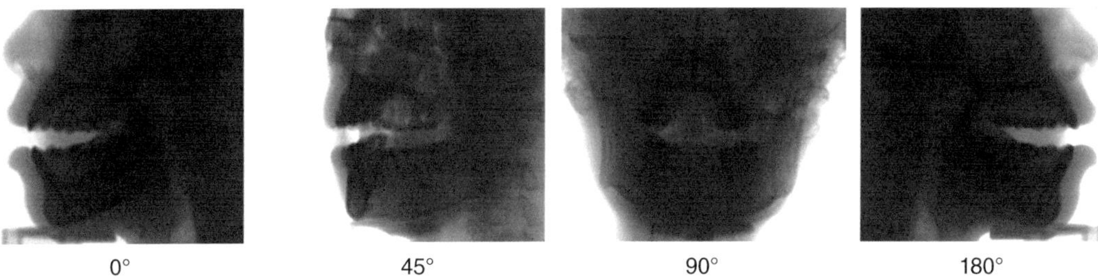

Fig. 8.10 Two-dimensional projections at different angles at 0°, 45°, 90°, and 180°. (Image copyright: Oxford University Press [21], republished with permission)

or slower. During this movement, the X-rays form a cone or pyramid shape, capturing hundreds of individual images from varied angles. These obtained images are combined to create a 3D picture of the scanned object [21].

CBCT machines are compact and cost-effective compared to traditional medical computed tomography (CT) scanners. It uses a cone-shaped beam to capture images of the head and neck, providing horizontal, vertical, and axial views of structures. The machine rotates around the patient's head, capturing imaging data from different angles and then reconstructing it into tomographic images using a computer. CBCT is particularly useful in dental specialities, including implantology, endodontics, orthodontics, and pathology assessment. It allows for accurate measurements, improved localization of impacted teeth, visualization of airway abnormalities, identification of asymmetry, assessment of periodontal structures, and evaluation of temporomandibular joint (TMJ) bony structures. However, it is important to consider the potential risks and limitations of CBCT, such as higher radiation dosages compared to traditional radiographic techniques. Therefore, the usage of CBCT should be restricted to situations where its benefits outweigh the potential risks and where it is justifiable. CBCT was initially applied to other fields such as angiography, musculoskeletal, breast, respiratory, and cardiac applications [22].

The machine used for cone-beam computed tomography is similar in size to the one used for panoramic radiography. While scanning, the x-ray beam is projected toward the object or the parts of the human body. The exact shape of this X-ray beam varies according to the X-ray scanner used, i.e., for MSCT scanners, it is cylindrical, whereas for CBCT scanners, it is cone shaped. Thus, the "cone bean" is the cone-shaped beam used with the CBCT scanner. The cone shape of the X-ray enables good-quality images while significantly reducing the radiation level the patient is exposed to.

Unlike traditional CT scanners that capture thin slices, cone-beam technology scans a larger volume in a single rotation, reducing the need for multiple rotations. This approach efficiently gathers all the required data to reconstruct the region of interest (ROI). By using this method, dentists can generate high-quality 2D images in multiple planes and create detailed 3D reconstructions while minimizing radiation exposure. The scanning process involves an X-ray tube and a 2D sensor rotating around the patient's head, typically covering an arc between 180° and 360°. The collected data is then processed by a computer to produce tomographic images.

8.3.4.1 History of CBCT

The cone-beam CT (CBCT) as a method for 3D imaging was developed in 1982 by Richard A. Robb [23]. Though its widespread adoption in medical fields wasn't realized until 1997 for several reasons, such as these scanners were large and bulky, higher cost of the machines, and exposed patients to high doses of radiation [24], the advent of implant surgeries in dentistry prompted the development of compact CT machines. In the late 1990s, independently, Arai et al. in Japan [25] and Mozzo et al. [26] in Italy pioneered the use of CBCT for oral and maxillofacial applications, offering 3D imaging and improved accuracy compared to 2D techniques, similar to conventional CT scans. Arai and colleagues called this prototype-limited cone-beam CT (CBCT) devicc Ortho-CT [25] whereas Mozzo et al. called it NewTom-9000 [26]. This marked a significant advancement in dental imaging technology. Since then, CBCT has rapidly gained popularity in dentistry due to its ability to produce volumetric images of the jawbone at a reasonable cost and radiation dose. CBCT machines have become more compact, affordable, and widely used in various dental specialities, including implantology, endodontics, orthodontics, and pathology assessment. Key milestones and pioneers of CBCT has been shown in Table 8.2. The utilization of CBCT has revolutionized dental diagnostics and treatment planning, providing accurate measurements, improved localization of impacted teeth, visual-

Table 8.2 Key milestones and pioneers of CBCT

Year	Milestone
1982	Developed the concept of CBCT, marking the beginning of 3D imaging in dental radiography
1996	The first commercial CBCT system for dental use, the Accuitomo, is introduced in Japan by J. Morita.
1998	A. Mozzo et al. in Italy introduce the NewTom-9000, pioneering dental CBCT applications and setting new standards in 3D imaging.
1999	Arai et al. developed a prototype-limited cone-beam CT named Ortho-CT, further refining the technology.
2001	J. Morita in Japan launches the first CBCT specifically designed for maxillofacial imaging, enhancing diagnostic capabilities.
2003	Introduction of flat-panel detectors in CBCT, improving image quality and reducing radiation exposure
2004	Sirona Dental Systems release the Galileos, significantly impacting CBCT's clinical adoption and setting a benchmark for future systems.
2007	Integration of digital imaging and communication in medicine (DICOM) standards, allowing better data management and interoperability
2010s	Several manufacturers join the market, driving innovation and competition, leading to more accessible and diverse CBCT systems.
2015	Introduction of dose reduction technologies, making CBCT safer for patients while maintaining high image quality
2018	Emergence of ultra-low-dose protocols in CBCT, further minimizing radiation exposure while ensuring diagnostic accuracy
Present	AI integration in CBCT systems is gaining traction, promising further advancements in diagnostic accuracy, image processing, and treatment planning efficiency.

ization of airway abnormalities, assessment of periodontal structures, and evaluation of temporomandibular joint (TMJ) bony structures. However, it is important to consider the potential risks and limitations of CBCT, and its usage should be limited to cases where it is justifiable.

8.3.4.2 Working Principle of CBCT Machines

CBCT machines use cone-shaped X-ray beams to capture three-dimensional images of the dental and maxillofacial structures. These machines offer various field of view (FOV) options, ranging from small to large volumes, allowing for targeted imaging of specific areas or capturing the entire maxillofacial region. The resolution of a CBCT machine refers to the level of detail in the captured images. It's typically measured in terms of voxel size, with smaller voxels (Fig. 8.11).

Sizes indicating higher resolution, these include parameters such as tube voltage, tube current, and exposure time, which is adjusted to optimize the image quality and minimize radiation dose to the patient. The time it takes for the CBCT machine to complete a scan varies depending on the selected scan volume and exposure parameters. Scan times typically range from a few seconds to a minute or more.

CBCT machines deliver a relatively low radiation dose compared to conventional CT scanners. However, it's still important to consider radiation

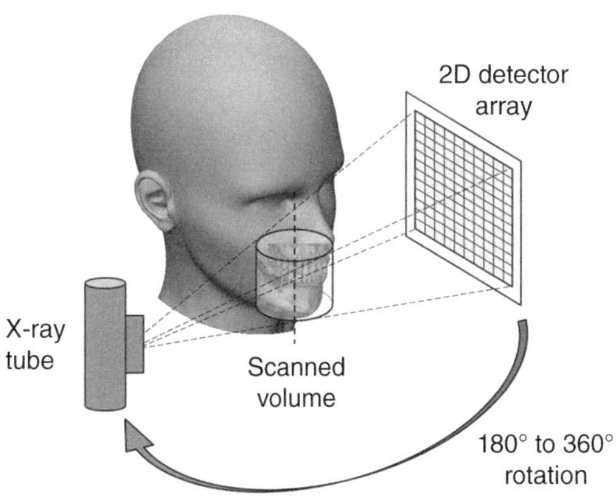

Fig. 8.11 The X-ray tube and detector move concomitantly around the rotation axis. 2D, two-dimensional. (Image copyright: Oxford University Press [21], republished with permission)

safety and dose optimization techniques, especially for pediatric patients and individuals undergoing multiple scans. These machines utilize specialized software algorithms to reconstruct the acquired projection images into a three-dimensional volume, which can be viewed and analyzed from different angles and planes. Advanced CBCT machines may offer features for image enhancement, such as noise reduction algorithms, artifact correction, and dynamic range adjustment, to improve image quality and diagnostic accuracy. Some CBCT machines are designed to integrate seamlessly with computer-aided design (CAD) or computer-aided manufacturing (CAM) systems, allowing for precise treatment planning and fabrication of dental prosthetics and implants. Technical characteristics of some commercially available CBCT devices are shown in Table 8.3. These machines are typically equipped with adjustable positioning devices and ergonomic design features to ensure patient comfort and optimize image acquisition. CBCT machines may have built-in storage capabilities or be network connected for efficient storage and transfer of imaging data to electronic health record (EHR) systems or external storage devices. Some of the key features of CBCT machines are summarized below:

- **X-Ray Source**:
  - Energy levels: 70–120 kVp, optimized for dental applications
  - Flat-panel detectors: Capture high-resolution images with low noise
  - Collimation options: Tailor the beam size to the specific FOV
- **Image Acquisition**:
  - Single or multiple rotations around the head, depending on FOV and desired detail
  - Acquisition time varies with FOV and resolution (typically 5–20 seconds).
- **Image Reconstruction**:
  - Filtered back projection: Standard algorithm for reconstructing 3D volumes
  - Iterative reconstruction: Advanced technique for reducing noise and artifacts
  - Voxel size: Crucial for detail; 0.15–0.3 mm common in dentistry

Table 8.3 Technical characteristics of some commercially available CBCT devices

CBCT machine	Availability of pan and ceph	FOV available (height × diameter in cm)	Voxel size (mm)	Manufacturer	Exposure time (seconds)	Key features and applications
Veraviewepocs 3D R100	Yes	4 × 4, 4 × 8, 8 × 5, 8 × 8, 10 × 5, 10 × 8	0.125	J. Morita, Japan	4–9.4	**Key features**: High-resolution images with minimal distortion, dual scan mode **Applications**: Implant planning, endodontics, and general dental diagnostics
Galileos Comfort Plus	Yes	15.4 cm spherical	0.25/0.125	Sirona Dental Systems, Germany	2–5	**Key features**: Integrated with CAD/CAM, 3D implant planning software **Applications**: Comprehensive maxillofacial imaging, orthodontics, and implantology
i-CAT FLX	Yes	4 × 16, 6 × 16, 8 × 8, 8 × 16, 10 × 16, 11 × 16, 13 × 16, extended FOV: 17 × 23	0.125–0.4	Imaging Sciences Int'l, USA	4.8, 8.9, 14.7, 17.8, or 26.9	**Key features**: QuickScan+ for low-dose imaging, customizable FOVs **Applications**: Orthodontics, implant planning, airway analysis, and oral surgery
KaVo OP 3D Maxio	Yes	5 × 5, 6.1 × 7.8, 7.8 × 7.8, 7.8 × 15, 13 × 15	0.085–0.420	KaVo, Germany	1.2–9	**Key features**: Low-dose imaging protocols, flexible FOVs **Applications**: General dental diagnostics, maxillofacial surgery, endodontics, and TMJ imaging
NewTom 5G	Yes	6 × 6, 8 × 8, 12 × 8, 15 × 5, 15 × 12, 18 × 16	0.075–0.250	QR, Inc., Verona, Italy	18–36	**Key features**: 360° scans, adjustable voxel sizes **Applications**: Implant planning, orthognathic surgery, TMJ assessment, and airway analysis
PreXion3D Eclipse 3D	Yes	8.1 × 7.5, 11.3 × 7.2	0.150	PreXion, Inc., USA	4–7	**Key features**: High-resolution imaging, compact design **Applications**: Implantology, endodontics, periodontal assessment, and general dental diagnostics

(continued)

Table 8.3 (continued)

CBCT machine	Availability of pan and ceph	FOV available (height × diameter in cm)	Voxel size (mm)	Manufacturer	Exposure time (seconds)	Key features and applications
Planmeca ProMax 3D S	Yes	8 × 8, 8 × 5, 5 × 8, 5 × 5, stitched volume: 14 × 10.5 × 8	0.075–0.400	Planmeca OY, Helsinki, Finland	7.5–27	**Key features**: Scalable FOVs, ultra-low-dose protocols **Applications**: Orthodontics, implant planning, oral and maxillofacial surgery, airway analysis
Soredex 3D CBCT	No	5 × 5, 6.1 × 7.8, 7.8 × 7.8, 7.8 × 15, 13 × 15	0.085–0.420	Soredex, Helsinki, Finland	4–9	**Key features**: High image resolution, ease of use **Applications**: Comprehensive diagnostics, including endodontics, implant planning, and general dental imaging
Carestream 9300 3D	Yes	5 × 5, 8 × 8, 10 × 5, 10 × 10, 17 × 6, 17 × 11, 17 × 13.5	0.090–0.500	Carestream Health, Rochester, USA	4–8.9	**Key features**: Wide range of FOVs, user-friendly interface **Applications**: Maxillofacial surgery, orthodontics, implantology, TMJ, and airway analysis
Gendex GXDP-70	Yes	6.1 × 4.1, 6.1 × 7.8	0.085–0.300	Gendex Dental Systems, USA	2.3–12.6	**Key features**: Compact design, fast scanning times **Applications**: General dental diagnostics, including endodontics, implant planning, and orthodontics
Papaya 3D Plus	Yes	4 × 5, 7 × 7, 8 × 8, 14 × 8, 14 × 14	0.075–0.400	Genoray America Inc., USA	4–7	**Key features**: High-resolution imaging, flexible FOVs **Applications**: Implantology, maxillofacial surgery, orthodontics, and TMJ assessment
Hyperion X9	Yes	5 × 5, 8 × 5, 8 × 8, 11 × 5, 11 × 8, 11 × 13	0.075	MyRay, Italy	18	**Key features**: 3D reconstruction, multimodality imaging (3D, panoramic, cephalometric) **Applications**: Comprehensive diagnostics, including implant planning, TMJ, and airway assessment

(continued)

Table 8.3 (continued)

CBCT machine	Availability of pan and ceph	FOV available (height × diameter in cm)	Voxel size (mm)	Manufacturer	Exposure time (seconds)	Key features and applications
PaX-Reve3D	Yes	5 × 5, 8 × 6, 12 × 8, 15 × 15, 15 × 19	0.080–0.250	Vatech Korea	15/24	**Key features**: High-resolution imaging, broad FOV range **Applications**: Implantology, maxillofacial surgery, orthodontics, and airway analysis

- **Advanced Features**:
  - Metal artifact reduction: Algorithms to minimize artifacts from fillings or implants
  - Low-dose protocols: Balance image quality with radiation reduction
  - Multiplanar reformatting: Generate 2D slices for various diagnostic views

8.3.4.3 Differences Between Cone-Beam Computed Tomography Scanners (CBCT) and Medical Computed Tomography Scanners, i.e., Multi-Slice CT Scanners (MSCT)

CBCT and MSCT use fundamentally different approaches to capturing images. MSCT employs a fan-shaped beam, whereas CBCT leverages a cone-shaped beam originating from a single point [21]. The difference between both is schematically explained in Table 8.4 and Fig. 8.12. Basically, in CBCT, the beam originating from an X-ray source is used, whereas in MSCT, the beam is collimated to reach its detectors to create a flat, two-dimensional image across detectors.

- **Spatial Resolution**: Cone-beam computed tomography scanners generally have a better spatial resolution and range from 0.4 mm to as low as 0.125 mm [23] with a relatively lower radiation dose than MSCT [27], whereas the best achievable in-plane spatial voxel dimensions of state-of-the-art clinical MSCTs are 0.23–0.4 mm and 0.3 mm in the z direction [28]. However, the spatial resolution depends upon the physical characteristics of the detector (number and size of unitary elements), geometrical characteristics of the beam (focal spot size, beam collimation), and incremental or helical acquisition mode (number of projections, rotation duration time) [29]. Moreover, reconstruction parameters, such as kernel type, pixel reconstructed size, and reconstruction algorithm, impact image resolution [30, 31].
- **Image Contrast**: In most of the CBCT scanners these days, different types of indirect flat-panel detectors (FPDs) are used, which contain a layer of scintillator material, either gadolinium oxysulfide (Gd_2O_2S: Tb) or cesium iodide (CsI: Tl) coupled with thin-film transistor (TFT) array spread across a flat panel, essentially functioning like millions of tiny pixel sensors [21]. These detectors historically have had lower quantum efficiency and slower response than ceramic detectors used in helical MSCT. Therefore, this nature of the FPD can limits contrast resolution due to the reduction in temporal resolution and dynamic range, compared to standard MSCT detectors [22]. Reduced temporal resolution decreases image quality and impairs low-contrast detectability, causing artifacts such as image ghosting, "afterglow," memory effects, and streak artifacts [32].
- **Gantry Rotation**: The gantry of CBCT machines rotates once around the patient from 180° to 360°, covering the defined anatomical

Table 8.4 Summary of differences between CBCT and MSCT

Feature	CBCT	MSCT
Spatial resolution	0.4–0.125 mm: High spatial resolution suitable for detailed imaging of dental and maxillofacial structures, with customizable voxel sizes	0.23–0.4 mm (in-plane), 0.3 mm (z direction): Offers high spatial resolution for broader medical applications, allowing for precise imaging across multiple planes
Image contrast	Lower due to detector limitations: Adequate for hard tissue imaging but less effective for soft tissues, limiting some diagnostic capabilities	Higher with ceramic detectors: Superior contrast resolution ideal for imaging soft tissues and vascular structures in whole-body scans
Gantry rotation	Single rotation (180–360°): Reduces scan time and radiation exposure but may limit certain complex imaging applications	Multiple rotations: Enables more comprehensive imaging but requires longer scan times and higher radiation exposure
Cost	3–5 times less expensive: More affordable, making it accessible for dental practices and specialized imaging centers	Higher: Significant investment, typically used in hospitals and large medical centers for a wide range of diagnostic purposes
Size and weight	Smaller and lighter: Compact design allows for easier installation in smaller clinics and more flexibility in patient positioning.	Larger and heavier: Bulkier equipment requires more space and robust infrastructure, limiting portability.
Radiation dose	Generally lower compared to MSCT: Beneficial for repeated use in dental and orthodontic practices, especially for pediatric patients	Higher: Often necessary for comprehensive imaging of large body areas or dense tissues
Applications	Dental, maxillofacial, ENT: Primarily used for detailed imaging of dental structures, jaw, sinuses, and airways, with emerging applications in ENT	Whole body, various medical uses: Versatile use across multiple specialties, including cardiology, oncology, and neurology
Strengths	High spatial resolution, lower cost, smaller size: Excels in producing detailed images of hard tissues at a lower cost, ideal for dental and orthodontic use	Excellent contrast resolution, wider applications: Supports a broader range of diagnostic procedures with superior contrast resolution and multi-slice capability
Limitations	Lower contrast resolution, limited applications: Cost-effective and compact, but limited contrast resolution makes it less suitable for soft tissue imaging	Higher cost, larger size, higher radiation dose: Cost, size, and radiation dose are challenges but unmatched diagnostic capabilities for complex cases.

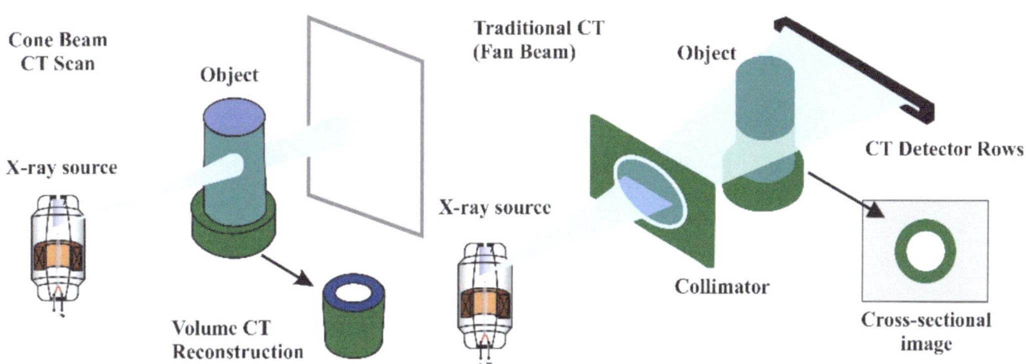

Fig. 8.12 CBCT versus MSCT

volume (complete dental/maxillofacial volume or limited regional area of interest) rather than slice-by-slice imaging having multiple rotations found in conventional CT.

- Cone-beam computed tomography scanners are less expensive than CT scanners. They cost approximately 3–5 times less.
- Cone-beam computed tomography scanner equipment is smaller and lighter.

While CBCT provides several benefits, it is important to recognize its limitations. Compared to conventional radiographic methods like intraoral and panoramic imaging, CBCT may produce lower contrast images and expose patients to higher radiation doses. Specifically, effective doses from CBCT are generally higher than those from intraoral and panoramic radiography, potentially by tens or hundreds of μSv, depending on the technique employed. As a result, its application should be carefully considered and reserved for situations where its advantages clearly outweigh the associated risks. The use of CBCT should be justified based on clinical necessity.

8.3.4.4 Clinical Applications of CBCT

The CBCT has many clinical applications and some are outlined below:

- **Implantology**:
  - Precise assessment of bone volume and density for implant placement
  - Evaluation of nerve proximity and anatomical landmarks
  - Virtual implant planning and surgical guide fabrication
- **Endodontics**:
  - Identification of complex root canal anatomy (curved canals, additional canals)
  - Diagnosis of root fractures and periapical lesions
  - Guided endodontic surgery for inaccessible canals
- **Oral Surgery**:
  - Visualization of jaw fractures, impacted teeth, and unerupted wisdom teeth
  - Preoperative planning for complex surgeries (tumor removal, orthognathic surgery)
  - Assessment of temporomandibular joint (TMJ) disorders
- **Orthodontics**:
  - 3D evaluation of jaw and tooth development
  - Monitoring tooth movement during treatment
  - Diagnosis of impacted teeth and other developmental anomalies

8.4 Quality Control in Dental Radiography

8.4.1 Acceptance Testing and Routine Quality Control (QC) of Dental Equipments

The American Association of Physicists in Medicine (AAPM) provides detailed guidelines on acceptance testing and routine quality control of dental equipment. The AAPM task group reports 175 [33] provides the details of the evaluation of intraoral, panoramic, and cephalometric dental units whereas report 261 [34] provides cone-beam computed tomography (CBCT) systems. The QC test and its procedures are adapted from these two reports.

8.4.1.1 Intraoral Dental Units

The acceptance testing and quality control for intraoral dental units have been divided into the following sections. However, they are not applicable for handheld units, which can be there with general dentists in dental clinics:

(a) Tube head stability and positioning
(b) Leakage radiation and visual inspection
(c) Collimation and minimum source-to-skin distance
(d) Beam quality
(e) Kilovoltage (kVp) accuracy
(f) Timer accuracy
(g) Exposure reproducibility

(h) Milliampere (mA) or milliampere-second (mAs) linearity
(i) Darkroom quality control (if X-ray film is used)
(j) Film processing quality control for intraoral film
(k) Quality control for digital intraoral image receptors (sensors/phosphor plates)
(l) Evaluation of the site's quality control program
(m) Technique factors and entrance skin air kerma
(n) Scattered radiation survey

(a) **Tube Head Stability and Positioning**

This test does not apply to handheld devices. To ensure compliance with the National Council on Radiation Protection and Measurements (NCRP) report no. 185 (2020) [35], the dental X-ray unit's tube head must exhibit minimal movement once the operator releases it. Specifically:

- **Stopping time**: After releasing the tube head, it must stabilize within 1 second.
- **Maximum movement**: Any residual movement (drift) after stabilization should not exceed 0.5 cm.

Regular checks are necessary to verify that the tube head meets these requirements.

(b) **Leakage Radiation and Visual Inspection**

Regularly inspect the X-ray machine's tube housing to ensure the radiation shielding is intact. In case of any suspect of any damage:

- **Measure radiation levels**: Use a special detector to compare readings near the suspected leak and a normal area. Similar readings indicate no problem.
- **Alternatively, use an X-ray film or sensor**: If any light or dark spots appear on the film or sensor after exposure, it suggests a leak.

If a leak is confirmed, stop using the machine immediately and seek professional help.

(c) **Collimation and Minimum Source-to-Skin Distance**

This check ensures the X-ray beam is safe and accurate by limiting its size and ensuring it's at a safe distance from the patient as per regulatory and recommended limits, and it looks for:

1. **Beam size**:
   - **Limit**: The beam size shouldn't be wider than 7 cm for circular beams or 4x5 cm for rectangular beams at the end of the position indicating device (PID). The beam size should be as small as practically possible while still covering the area of interest to minimize patient dose.
   - **Measurement**: An X-ray film or large plate can be used to measure the beam size.
2. **Distance from skin (SSD)**:
   - **Minimum**: The X-ray source must be at least 7 inches (approximately 18 cm) for intraoral radiographs using rectangular collimation. For units with kVp settings below 50 kVp, a longer minimum SSD of 18 cm is generally recommended.
   - **Reason**: Lower voltages (below 60 kVp) are not recommended by the AAPM and require this minimum source-to-skin distance for safety. For dental intraoral radiography, the SSD is critical to minimize dose and maximize image quality. Longer PIDs are preferred to increase the SSD.
3. **Collimator**:
   - **Fixed units**: If the collimator (beam shaper) is fixed, it only needs checking during the initial setup, not yearly. However, regular checks for proper alignment and any potential damage are still prudent.
4. **Rectangular collimation**:
   - **Recommendation**: The beam size in each direction should be almost the same size as the X-ray film or sensor.
   - **Positioning**: A special device is highly recommended to ensure the X-ray beam covers the entire film/sensor. These are called positioning devices, paralleling devices, film holders, or sensor holders.

(d) **Beam Quality**

The beam quality is measured in terms of the power of penetration by the X-ray beam and is measured in the half-value layer for the commonly used kilovoltage. The method of performing the test is as follows:

1. Place the X-ray beam at a detector.
2. Place thin aluminum sheets in front of the beam, one by one.
3. Measure how much the beam weakens with each sheet.
4. Stop adding sheets when the beam weakens by half.

The number of aluminum sheets needed to weaken the beam by half is called the half-value layer (HVL). This test ensures the HVL meets two requirements:

- Matches the manufacturer's specifications
- Meets the standards of the regulatory body

If an X-ray machine has different voltage settings, this test should be repeated for each setting.

(e) **Kilovoltage (kVp) Accuracy**

As the name suggests, the test looks for the accuracy of kilovoltage potential, and it is performed in the following way:

- Position the detector so all its sensors are within the X-ray beam.
- If the machine has different voltage settings, measure the voltage for each setting.
- Measure the voltage after the machine warms up, not during the initial start-up.
- If available, the voltage reading should be within ±10% of the setting chosen or meet the manufacturer's specifications.

The AAPM recommends avoiding voltages below 60 kVp as higher dose rates to the patient's skin may result, and low-energy X-rays have limited diagnostic value.

(f) **Timer Accuracy**

Since most X-ray machines have a warm-up time, measuring the exact exposure time is difficult. Therefore, measuring the exact time is not necessary. However, checking if the timer is accurate is still recommended, especially if the machine shows the exposure time setting. If available, the timer reading should be within ±10% of the chosen setting or meet the manufacturer's specifications.

(g) **Exposure Reproducibility**

This test is performed as follows:

- Position the detector so the entire sensitive volume is directly exposed to the X-ray beam.
- During acceptance testing, measure the radiation output for different settings, such as the strongest, typical (like adult molar bitewing), and weakest exposures.
- For routine quality checks, typically only the typical setting (e.g., molar bitewing) must be measured.
- Take at least three measurements at each setting to calculate the consistency of the radiation output to determine the coefficient of variation (COV) by dividing the standard deviation by the mean value.
- The COV should be within the manufacturer's specifications or a maximum of 0.05 if no specific value is provided.

(h) **Milliampere (mA) or Milliampere-Second (mAs) Linearity**

This text describes a test for X-ray units with variable power settings and only applies to X-ray machines with different power settings at the same voltage level. The following is done for this test:

- Measure the radiation output (air kerma) for each power setting (mA or mAs) at the most commonly used voltage.
- Calculate a value called "X" for each set by dividing the air kerma by the chosen power setting (mAs).
- Compare every pair of neighboring power settings:
  - The difference between their "X" values ($|X1 - X2|$) must be less than 10% of the average of their "X" values ($X1 + X2$).

In simpler terms, this test checks if the X-ray machine delivers a consistent amount of radiation per power unit across different power settings.

(i) **Darkroom Quality Control (If X-Ray Film Is Used)**

This text explains how to test the darkroom and daylight loader for dental film processing to ensure good image quality. Exposure to unwanted light (fog) can reduce the contrast and detail in X-rays, making it harder to see important information.

How often should this test be required to be done?

- Darkroom:
  - Initially for a new darkroom and annually after that
  - Whenever changed:
    - Safelight filter or bulb
    - Door, door sweep, weather stripping, or air baffle
- Daylight loader:
  - Initially, for a new daylight loader
  - Annually after that
  - Whenever the room lighting is changed
  - Whenever the daylight loader modified

What is done for the test?

1. Turn off the darkroom lights and wait for eyes to adjust. Check for light leaks from doors, vents, or the processor. Fix any leaks if found.
2. Partially cover a piece of film with something opaque. Expose it in the darkroom and process it.
3. Look for a difference in darkness between the covered and uncovered parts.
   - No difference: Good!
   - Difference: Investigate the cause.
   - Safelight too bright or close?
   - Is the safelight filter faded, damaged, or wrong?
   - Too many safelights in the room?
   - Is light leaking into the room?

4. **Repeat the test for the daylight loader**, following similar steps with covering the film and checking for light leaks.

One should not worry if a tiny difference is seen right at the edge where the film was covered as this is normal. Look for larger differences across the entire film. Regularly checking for light leaks ensures X-rays are clear and accurate for proper dental care.

(j) **Film Processing Quality Control for Intraoral Film**

Proper processing of X-ray films ensures:

- Clear images with good contrast (ability to see details).
- To minimize radiation exposure for patients and staff. It also minimizes the need for retaking X-rays.
- Regularly checking the film processing ensures everything is working well.

How often to check:

- Daily, before processing any patient films
- Done by on-site staff, then reviewed by a qualified expert (QMP) at least annually

Two methods are available:

1. Crabtree Device (Dental Radiographic Quality Control Device)
   - This tool helps determine the correct exposure for the film.
   - It also allows to check the quality of the processing equipment.

2. Conference of Radiation Control Program Directors (CRCPD) Method
   - This method doesn't require a specific tool.
   - It uses a sensitometer and a densitometer (specialized equipment).
   - If panoramic or cephalometric machines are used, this method is mandatory.

Regularly checking film processing can ensure accurate and reliable X-rays for better dental care.

(k) **Quality Control for Digital Intraoral Image Receptors**

In digital X-rays, quality control is important for good image quality. Here's why:

- **Underexposed images**: These can be too noisy, making it difficult to see important details.
- **Overexposed images** use more radiation, increasing the dose for patients and staff.

Therefore, regular checks are essential to ensure the X-ray system works well and produces clear images with minimal radiation exposure.

Frequency of Test

- Routine QC tests should be performed periodically, often Daily, weekly, monthly, or quarterly, as recommended by manufacturers or regulatory bodies.
- More often, if sensor damage is suspected, replace sensors.
- Reviewed by a qualified expert (QMP) at least annually, or as needed for acceptance testing or major system changes.

There isn't a single standard way to check, but some options include:

- **Special phantoms**: These are objects used specifically for testing X-ray machines.
- **Test patterns**: These are displayed on the screen and help check display quality.

Before checking the phantom image, ensure the screen we use works properly. One can do this by displaying a test pattern and adjusting the brightness/contrast until the image looks good.

The initial evaluation can be done using:

- Check the phantom image for any large issues like blurring or missing information.
- Make sure all the gray levels are visible.
- Adjust the screen brightness/contrast if needed.

Before the initial evaluation, ensure regular X-ray images don't have any strange markings or distortions. Once the initial evaluations are done, the phantom manufacturer's instructions for routine checks will be followed. This might involve:

- *Uniformity (monthly to quarterly)*: Checks how consistent the image is across its entire area
- *Contrast resolution (quarterly to semiannually)*: Checks how well the image shows fine details
- *Spatial resolution (quarterly to semiannually)*: Checks how sharp the image is

Additionally:

- Check the monitor quality and for image distortions regularly.
- If rarely used, erase PSP receptors before use to avoid unwanted background signals.
- Store PSP receptors away from radiation sources.

By regularly checking digital X-ray system, one can ensure it produces clear and safe images for better dental care.

(l) **Evaluation of Quality Control Program**

Once a year, the Qualified Medical Physicist (QMP) should review the quality control (QC) program. This should include:

- **Checking the QC activities performed by the staff**: This ensures the staff follows the proper quality control procedures.

- **Reviewing the service history of the X-ray equipment**: This helps identify any potential problems with the equipment that could affect image quality.

(m) **Technique Factors and Entrance Skin Air Kerma**

Each X-ray machine's radiation output (measured in air kerma or exposure) should be checked for the most common type of X-ray (like a back bitewing). This measurement will compare recommended safe levels (DRLs) and achievable doses. Some important points are as follows:

- The X-ray settings should follow the manufacturer's recommendations for digital sensors (or film).
- Use techniques that minimize radiation exposure while maintaining good image quality.
- A chart showing the recommended settings should be displayed near the X-ray control panel.

Generally, the recommended safe level (DRL) for dental X-rays is 1.6 millisieverts (mGy), regardless of the sensor type.

(n) **Scattered Radiation Survey**

At the time of acceptance testing of the new X-ray unit, it's recommended to check the amount of scattered radiation they produce. Here's how it's done:

- Take a head-shaped object (phantom) or a filled water jug and X-ray it using typical settings.
- Measure the scattered radiation around the machine, especially near where staff usually stands (like by the control panel).
- Since the scattered radiation is weak, use a special meter to detect low amounts (between 9 and 90 nano gray or 1–10 micro roentgen). The unit μR is an older unit for exposure and may not be standard for scattered radiation measurements in newer guidelines.
- Choose a meter that can measure the total scattered radiation over the entire X-ray exposure, not just the rate at which it's emitted.
- Good options for meters include integrating solid-state detectors or integrating ion chambers.

Following these steps ensures that scattered radiation levels are within safe limits for the staff.

8.4.1.2 Panoramic Dental Units

(a) Leakage radiation and visual inspection
(b) X-ray beam slit length and width coincidence
(c) Beam quality
(d) Kilovoltage accuracy
(e) Exposure reproducibility
(f) Darkroom quality control (if X-ray film is used)
(g) Quality control for digital panoramic image receptors
(h) Technique factors
(i) Evaluation of the site's quality control program
(j) Scattered radiation survey

(a) **Leakage Radiation and Visual Inspection**

Checking the X-ray machine's tube housing is important to ensure it's not damaged and protects against radiation leakage. Firstly, we should visually inspect the housing for any signs of damage such as dents or cracks. If any damage is suspected, use a survey meter to measure the radiation levels around the suspected area and nearby. The used survey meter should be sensitive enough to detect low radiation levels (like an integrating detector or ion chamber). The readings from both locations should be similar if the housing is intact. Alternatively, one can place an X-ray film or sensor over the suspected area and take an X-ray. Look for any dark spots on the resulting image, which could indicate a leak. Be aware that the film/sensor size might not perfectly cover the leak so that a larger detector might be preferable. If any evidence of a radiation leak is found, stop using the machine immediately and contact a qualified professional for repair.

(b) **X-Ray Beam Slit Length and Width Coincidence**

This text describes a method to check if the X-ray beam size in a panoramic X-ray machine matches the size of the image receptor. The following items are needed to do this test (Fig. 8.13):

- Paper clips
- Intraoral films, PSP receptors, or radiochromic films (choose two)
- Pencils

Steps

- Attach a paper clip to each of the two films, ensuring the paper clip runs along the long side and is centered.
- Mark the top and bottom edges of the X-ray beam slit (the narrow opening) on the film holder with a pencil.
- Place the films with the paper clips on the holder, lining them up with the slit or the marks made. Make sure the paper clip ends in the center of the film and lines up with the slit marks.
- Take a panoramic X-ray using these films.

Alternative Method

- Instead of films, use a fluorescent screen.
- Set up the screen similar to the films in steps 1–3.
- Use camera to record the screen during the X-ray exposure.

Evaluating the Results

- No universal standards yet exist, so a qualified professional (QMP) will assess the results based on manufacturer guidelines, regulations, or future international standards.
- In ideal situations, the X-ray beam should be of the same size and shape as the image receptor and completely covered by the beam slit (if present). However, it's important to note that the beam should ideally be slightly larger than the image receptor to ensure full coverage, while still being tightly collimated to minimize patient dose.
- In the vertical direction (up and down), the beam should be within 2% of the total error of the source-image distance (SID) when compared to the slit (if present).
- The beam should not be larger than the image receptor in the long direction. According to regulatory standards, the X-ray field should not extend beyond any edge of the image

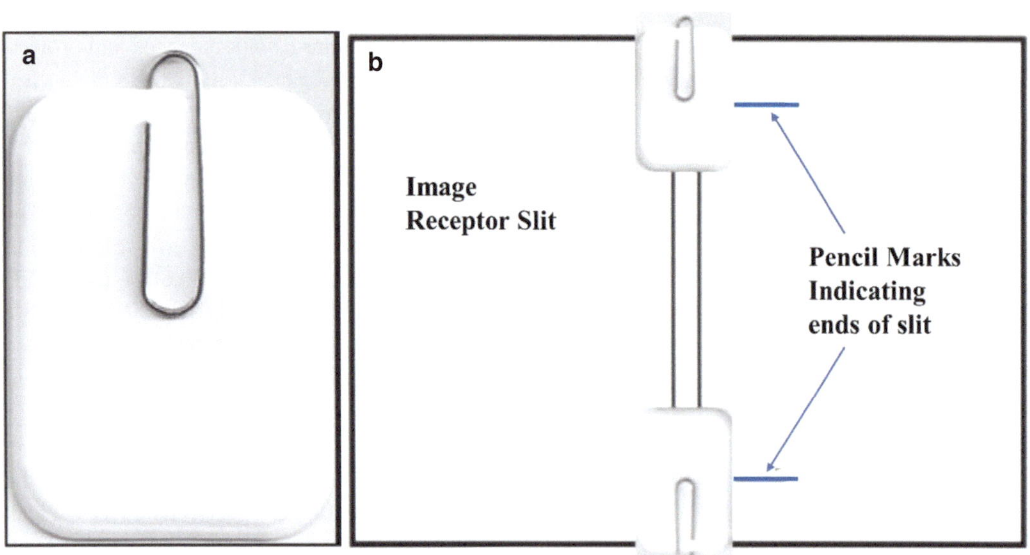

Fig. 8.13 (**a**) Intraoral radiographic film packet secured with a paperclip. (**b**) Intraoral packets with paper clips covered with image receptors. (Image Source: AAPM Report 175 [33]. Reprinted with permission)

receptor when the beam is aligned with the center of the image receptor.

Remember: This is just one possible method; a qualified professional should always interpret the results.

(c) **Beam Quality**

This test is performed by positioning a radiation detector in the X-ray beam, such as near the chin support, and the following steps are performed:

- Measure the half-value layer (HVL) in millimeters of aluminum for the most frequently used kilovoltage setting.
- Place aluminum sheets, as far as possible, directly on the front of the collimator housing in front of the detector.
- Ensure the measured HVL meets the minimum required by:
  - The manufacturer's specifications
  - Regulatory standards

Note: If using a solid-state detector with multiple sensors, ensure all sensors are aligned and exposed to the X-ray beam for accurate measurement.

(d) **Kilovoltage Accuracy**

To perform this test, position a kilovoltage detector (kV detector) along the center of the X-ray beam. Since the panoramic unit uses a moving beam, one might need to attach the kV detector to the moving part to stay in the beam during the X-ray. Make sure the ear and nose positioning devices are not blocking the X-ray beam, and do the following:

- Take X-rays at different voltage settings, including the lowest, highest, and middle settings.
- All units must meet the manufacturer's specifications for voltage accuracy.
- The voltage should be accurate within 10% of the selected setting for older units without manufacturer specifications.

(e) **Exposure Reproducibility**

Position the radiation detector directly in the X-ray beam to do this test. Since the detector might not be fully exposed in every position, ensure it's placed the same way for each measurement to get consistent results. This test can be performed using a pencil chamber, and the following steps are performed:

- Tape a pencil chamber (CT) or other suitable detector before the panoramic unit's slot.
- Make sure the chamber's length aligns with the X-ray beam's height.
- Secure the cable to avoid entanglement with the moving machine and prevent noise in the readings.

Testing

- For initial testing, measure with various technique combinations.
- For routine QC checks, using the typical technique is usually enough.
- Take at least three measurements at each setting to calculate the coefficient of variation (COV). This compares the variation of the readings to their average.
- The unit's air kerma (or exposure) COV must meet the manufacturer's specifications.
- A maximum COV of 0.05 (5%) is recommended if no specification exists.

(f) **Darkroom Quality Control (If X-Ray Film Is Used)**

Checking for the darkroom fog and detecting unwanted light exposure are very important, and this test checks if excessive light leaks in the darkroom are affecting the quality of X-ray images. Light leaks can fog the X-rays, reducing their clarity and contrast, leading to misdiagnosis. This is how it is done:

Darkroom Test:

- Turn on lights in nearby rooms and the film processor.
- Turn off all darkroom lights and safelights. Wait for the eyes to adjust to the darkness (3–5 minutes).
- Look for and fix any light leaks from doors, vents, or the processor.
- Preexpose a panoramic film (needed due to its screen-film setup) to a medium gray density.
- Cover half of the exposed film with opaque material in the darkroom.
- Wait 2 minutes and then process the film.
- Examine the developed film for density differences between the covered and uncovered sides. A difference indicates fog from light leaks.
  - Note: The human eye can detect small density variations, but only a significant difference (around 0.10) indicates a problem.
- Possible causes:
  - Safelights: Too bright, too close, damaged filter, or too many lights
  - Light leaks: From outside the darkroom

Daylight Loader Fog Test:

- Preexpose a panoramic film as in the darkroom test.
- Load the film: In the daylight loader, cover half with opaque material.
- Wait 2 minutes and then process the film.
- Examine for a density difference between covered and uncovered sides. A difference indicates excessive light entering the loader.
- Possible causes:
- Daylight loader filter: Changed, damaged, or incorrect
- Room lights: Too bright
- Loader filter or port material: Cracked, worn, or missing

Remember: Consistent annual tests and tests after specific changes are crucial to ensure optimal image quality in the X-rays. For both darkroom and daylight loader fog tests, if a significant density difference is observed, identify and rectify the source of the light leak or safelight issue before resuming patient film processing.

(g) **Quality Control for Digital Panoramic Image Receptors**

Maintaining optimal X-ray image quality in digital panoramic radiography is very important. Digital X-ray systems offer a wider range of image details compared to traditional methods. However, this also means that improper settings can lead to:

- *Underexposure*: Loss of detail due to excessive noise, making it difficult to see small differences in image density
- *Overexposure*: An excessively dark image with a loss of detail in areas of high density. Overexposure not only increases radiation dose to patients, it but also degrades image quality by making the image appear too dark and obscuring important diagnostic details.

Therefore, regular QC ensures optimal image quality and minimizes radiation exposure.

How often is this QC needed?

- *Uniformity and artifact evaluations*: Monthly to quarterly (as recommended by Ref. [20]) or whenever sensors are replaced or suspected to be damaged
- *Display functionality checks*: Before each uniformity and artifact evaluation

This will be performed by on-site personnel and reviewed by the Qualified Medical Physicist (QMP) during program evaluation. Currently, there's no single standard method. Follow the manufacturer's recommendations if available.

Checking display functionality:

Before evaluating X-ray images, ensure the display is functioning properly using standardized test patterns:

- SMPTE Medical Diagnostic Imaging Test Pattern: Set the window width to encompass all pixel values and adjust the window level accordingly.
- TG18-QC Pattern (DICOM/16-bit TIFF format): Set the window width to 0-4095 and adjust the window level as needed.

Expected results:

- The test image should be free of noticeable artifacts like blurring or bleeding.
- All gray levels should be visible, and specific areas should be distinct.
- Adjust the display brightness and contrast to achieve these conditions.

For detailed information on the TG18-QC pattern, refer to Section 4 of the AAPM Online Report No. 3.

By following these guidelines and performing regular QC, one can ensure digital panoramic X-ray system produces high-quality images while minimizing radiation exposure.

(h) **Technique Factors**

The exposure settings applied must align with the recommendations provided by the equipment or film manufacturer. To ensure this:

- Follow the manufacturer's recommendations for exposure settings to ensure optimal image quality.
- Lower dose techniques are encouraged if they maintain clear and informative images.
- A technique chart summarizing these settings should be readily accessible near the control panel.

Dose Levels:

- NCRP Report No. 172 recommends a diagnostic reference level (DRL) of 100 mGy cm^2 for the air kerma-area product in panoramic radiography.
- This report also suggests an achievable dose-area (AD) product of 76 mGy cm^2.

Newer X-ray systems might display the air kerma-area product directly.

(i) **Evaluation of the Site's Quality Control Program**

Annually, the QMP should assess the site's QC procedures and outcomes. This evaluation should scrutinize the QC tasks conducted by on-site staff and examine the equipment's service record.

(j) **Scattered Radiation Survey**

As part of the acceptance testing for intraoral units, conducting a scattered radiation survey may be advisable. This helps ensure the safety of staff who work near the machine. Here's how to do it:

- Use a head-shaped object (phantom) or a filled water jug.
- Take an X-ray using the typical settings used for patients.
- Measure the scattered radiation around the machine, especially near where staff usually stands. This could be by the control panel, for example.
- Since the scattered radiation is weak, use a special meter to detect low amounts. Look for a meter ranging from 9 to 90 nano gray (nGy) or 1–10 microRoentgen (μR).
- Choose a meter that can measure the total scattered radiation over the entire X-ray exposure, not just the rate at which it's emitted.
- Good options for meters include integrating energy-compensated solid-state detectors or integrating ion chambers.

Following these steps ensures that scattered radiation levels are within safe limits for the staff.

8.4.1.3 Cephalometric Dental Units

(a) Leakage radiation and visual inspection
(b) Collimation
(c) Exposure reproducibility, typical entrance air kerma, and technique factors
(d) Beam quality
(e) Kilovoltage accuracy
(f) Milliampere (mA) or milliampere-second (mAs) linearity (if applicable)
(g) Timer accuracy (if applicable)
(h) Darkroom quality control (if X-ray film is used)
(i) Quality control for digital cephalometric image receptors

(j) Evaluation of the site's quality control program
(k) Scattered radiation survey

(a) **Leakage Radiation and Visual Inspection**

This test is the same as acceptance testing and quality control recommendations for panoramic dental units. Please refer to previous section.

(b) **Collimation**

It's important to note that this test should be conducted individually for both panoramic and cephalometric modes. For broad-beam units, ensure the entire radiation field is within the image receptor. Adjust the field size manually or choose an aperture to achieve this. Set the size precisely to a clear value on the field size indicator, such as 8 × 10 inches.

Checking Light-Radiation Field Coincidence (If Applicable):

- Turn on the light field (if available) and tape five coins onto the image receptor's surface within the illuminated area.
- Place one coin in the center of each side, with its edge exactly touching the light field border.
- Place the fifth coin in a corner to indicate the image orientation.
- Take an X-ray at a low kVp and mAs combination and process the image.
- Measure the distance from each coin's edge to the corresponding exposed area of the X-ray (radiation field edge).
- Add the absolute values (without considering positive or negative signs) of the differences between opposite edges of the light field and the radiation field. This sum must be less than 2% of the SID (source-to-image distance).

Checking Field Size Indicator Accuracy:

- Measure the actual height and width of the exposed area on the X-ray (radiation field).
- Compare each dimension of the radiation field to the corresponding setting on the field size indicator. They should agree within 2% of the SID.

Checking Radiation Field and Image Receptor Alignment:

- Draw diagonal lines on the image, connecting opposite corners of the exposed area (radiation field). Do the same for the entire image receptor (e.g., film).
- Measure the distance between the points where the two diagonal lines intersect. This distance must be no more than 2% of the SID.

(c) **Exposure Reproducibility, Typical Entrance Air Kerma, and Technique Factors**

To measure and evaluate radiation dose in cephalometric X-ray systems, place a radiation detector at the center of the ear positioning device or the head position. Ensure the entire detector volume is exposed by the main X-ray beam for accurate entrance air kerma calculations (explained later).

Measuring Entrance Air Kerma:

- Perform measurements for common adult and pediatric techniques, taking at least three measurements each to calculate the coefficient of variation (COV).
- The COV, calculated by dividing the standard deviation by the mean value of measurements, must not exceed the manufacturer's specification or 0.05 (whichever is lower).

Comparing to Reference Levels:

- NCRP Report No. 172 discusses the importance of DRLs for optimization of patient dose. DRLs for cephalometric radiography in the United States are typically established based on local surveys of patient dose data, and may vary depending on the facility and equipment. The IAEA reports typical DRL values for adult lateral cephalometric radiography range from 41 to 146 mGy·cm^2, and for children from 25 to 121 mGy·cm², expressed in terms of kerma-area product (KAP).

Calculating Entrance Skin Air Kerma:

Using the average air kerma from the air kerma measurement step, calculate the entrance skin air kerma for common adult and pediatric techniques with the formula:

$$\text{ESAK} = K_a \times BSF \times \left[\text{SDD} / (\text{SID} - FSD)\right]^2$$

where,

ESAK: entrance skin air kerma
K_a: averaged air kerma
SDD: source-to-detector distance (cm)
SID: source-to-image distance (cm),
FSD: Focus-to-skin distance (cm), which is the distance to the point on the patient's skin where the entrance dose is being calculated.
17.5 cm: Defined entrance skin location based on Michigan's cephalometric survey.

Utilizing Air Kerma-Area Product (Newer Systems):

If the system displays the air kerma-area product:

- NCRP recommends:
  - 32.6 mGy cm^2 as the DRL for adults
  - 17 mGy cm^2 as the achievable dose
- Children:
  - 26.4 mGy cm^2 as the DRL
  - 14 mGy cm^2 as the achievable dose

Optimizing Exposure Settings:

- Use exposure settings recommended by the sensor/film manufacturer.
- Prioritize lower patient dose techniques while maintaining necessary image quality.
- Display a technique chart near the control panel for easy reference.

(d) **Beam Quality**

Using the same setup as the exposure reproducibility test:

- Measure the half-value layer (HVL) in millimeters of aluminum for the most commonly used kilovoltage (kVp).
- Place aluminum sheets as far as possible from the radiation detector, ideally directly in front of the collimator housing. This minimizes the influence of scattered radiation.
- Aim for a field size at the detector slightly larger than its actual size. This ensures the entire detector is exposed to the beam.

HVL Requirements:

- The measured HVL must be as high as the manufacturer's specifications for the X-ray system.
- It must also comply with federal regulations governing X-ray equipment.

(e) **Kilovoltage Accuracy**

To measure kilovoltage accuracy, position the kilovoltage detector along the central axis of the X-ray beam. For scanning slit systems, attach the sensor to the moving detector to ensure it stays within the beam throughout the exposure. Also, ensure the detector is not obstructed by ear or nasal positioning devices.

Taking Measurements: Take exposures across the usable range of kilovoltages, including:

- Lowest kilovoltage
- Highest kilovoltage
- Central kilovoltage (middle of the range)

Accuracy Requirements:

- All units must meet the manufacturer's specifications for kilovoltage accuracy.
- Units without manufacturer specifications should be accurate to within ±10%.

(f) **Milliampere (mA) or Milliampere-Second (mAs) Linearity (If Applicable)**

This test only applies to X-ray units with multiple milliampere (mA) or milliampere-second (mAs) options at the same kilovoltage setting. For this test, perform the following steps:

- Measure the air kerma (radiation exposure) at each mA/mAs station across the clinical range at the most commonly used kilovoltage.
- For each station, calculate the value X using the formula:

$$X = \text{Air kerma}(\text{mGy}) / \text{Milliampere} - \text{second}(\text{mAs})$$

Compare neighboring mA/mAs stations:

- Calculate the absolute value of the difference between $X1$ (one station) and $X2$ (neighboring station).
- This difference must be less than 10% of the sum of $X1$ and $X2$.

Explanation:

This test ensures consistent X-ray output across different mA/mAs settings at the same kVp. The calculated value "X" represents the radiation emitted per unit of exposure time. By comparing neighboring stations, we ensure they deliver similar radiation output for consistent image quality.

(g) **Timer Accuracy (If Applicable)**

This test applies only to X-ray units with variable exposure time settings. The following steps are followed to do this test:

- Place the radiation detector in the beam.
- Take exposure measurements across the entire usable range of the timer, including:
  - Minimum exposure time
  - Maximum exposure time
  - Central value (middle of the range)

Accuracy Requirements:

- All units: Meet the manufacturer's specifications for timer accuracy.
- Units without specifications: Be accurate to within 10% for settings above 10 milliseconds.
- Pulsed radiation generators: Timer accuracy should be within 1 pulse.

(h) **Darkroom Quality Control (If X-Ray Film Is Used)**

This test assesses if image quality is compromised by excessive darkroom fog (i.e., unintended exposure to light). Since intraoral and cephalometric films have distinct spectral and processing sensitivities, testing the darkroom or daylight loader with the specific film(s) it is intended to process is crucial. This test ensures that excessive light exposure (fog) isn't affecting the quality of the X-ray films. Following are the occasions when this test is to be performed:

Darkroom:

- Initially, for a new darkroom
- Annually after that
- After changing safelight filters or bulbs
- Whenever modifying the darkroom (doors, ventilation, etc.)

Daylight Loader:

- Initially, for a new loader
- Annually after that
- Whenever changing room lights
- After modifying the daylight loader

The following steps are to be taken for the darkroom fog test:

- Turn on adjacent room lights and the film processor.
- Turn off all lights in the darkroom and wait 3–5 minutes for the eyes to adjust.
- Look for and eliminate any light leaks from doors, vents, or the processor (use black tape for small leaks).
- Expose a cephalometric film (preexposed due to its screen-film setup) to an optical density of 1.00.
- Cover half the film with opaque material.
- Look for a density difference between the covered and uncovered parts. This might indicate:
  - High safelight wattage.
  - The safelight is too close to the counter.

- Faded/damaged/incorrect safelight filter.
- Too many safelights.
- Light leaks from outside.

- Repeat the test with safelights off to confirm if the fog is related to the safelights.

Steps (Daylight Loader):

- Preexpose a cephalometric film (same reason as step 4 in darkroom steps).
- Place the film in the loader, remove it, and cover half with opaque material.
- Leave the film for 2 minutes and then process it.
- Look for a density difference between the covered and uncovered parts. This might indicate:
  - Change in daylight loader filter
  - Bright room lights
  - Cracked/faded/damaged/incorrect daylight loader filter
  - Worn/cracked/missing material in loader ports

Note: The human eye can detect small density differences, which are not significant for fog detection. Covering the edge with an object (e.g., pen) helps identify larger differences indicative of fogged film (around 0.10 in optical density).

(i) **Quality Control for Digital Cephalometric Image Receptors**

Digital cephalometry requires quality control to ensure optimal image quality and system functionality. This minimizes the risks of:

- Underexposure: Loss of detail due to excessive noise in low-exposure images
- Overexposure: Increased radiation dose to patients and staff

Frequency:

- Perform QC regularly, typically monthly to quarterly.
- Conduct additional checks if the sensor is suspected to be damaged or replaced.

Responsibility:

- On-site personnel perform the tests.
- The Qualified Medical Physicist (QMP) reviews the results during program evaluation.

Standards:

- Currently, there's no standard method for digital cephalometric QC.
- Follow the manufacturer's recommendations if available.

Display Verification:

Before QC tests, ensure the image evaluation display functions properly. Consider using:

SMPTE Medical Diagnostic Imaging Test Pattern:

- Set window width to display the entire value range.
- Set the window level to the middle or minimum of the window width (system dependent).

DICOM or 16-bit TIFF TG18-QC Pattern:

- Set window width to 0-4095.
- Set the window level to the center or lower end of the window width (system dependent).

Evaluation Criteria:

- Overall image: Inspect for blurring or bleeding artifacts.
- Gray levels: All levels should be visible, separating 0%, 5%, 95%, and 100% areas.
- Brightness and contrast: Adjust to achieve these criteria.

A detailed explanation of the TG18-QC pattern is given in Section 4 of AAPM Online Report No. 3.25.

(j) **Evaluation of the Site's Quality Control Program**

Annually, the QMP should assess the QC procedures and outcomes at the site. This evaluation should encompass a review of the QC tasks conducted by on-site personnel and an examination of the equipment's service history.

(k) **Scattered Radiation Survey**

Consider performing a scattered radiation survey during acceptance testing of the intraoral X-ray unit. This helps assess radiation exposure to personnel in nearby areas.

Method:

- Expose a head phantom or water-filled one-gallon milk jug using typical clinical settings.
- Measure scattered radiation at locations where personnel are likely to be, such as near the control panel.

Meter Requirements:

- Low-level sensitivity: Detect radiation in the 9–90 nGy (1–10 μR) range.
- Integrate mode: Measure scattered radiation during the entire exposure (rate mode is impractical for short exposures).

Instrument Options:

- Integrating energy-compensated solid-state detector
- Integrating ion chamber

Note: This is an optional test and may not be required by all regulations.

8.4.1.4 CBCT Units

Comprehensive quality control procedures and the use of cone-beam computed tomography (CBCT) systems for dental and maxillofacial imaging are guided by the American Association of Medical Physicists Task Group Report 261 (2024) [34]. The extract of this report is mentioned below with an effort to simplify the language and style for better understanding.

Each dental CBCT scanner available on the market is accompanied by an image quality (IQ) testing phantom provided by the vendor. This phantom is tailored to the specific scanner technology and scanning conditions, along with a guidance document outlining setup and testing procedures. The tolerances specified using this phantom delineate the acceptable range of operational IQ specifications for that particular scanner. Moreover, manufacturers have developed automated analysis software suites to aid in the IQ testing process of the scanner. Before conducting further performance testing, it is imperative for the user or QMP to effectively execute and document the tests recommended by the vendor. The following tests are to be performed as part of the acceptance and routine quality control procedures:

(a) Alignment of lasers
(b) Verification of collimation (field-to-receptor size)
(c) Assessment of contrast-to-noise (CNR)
(d) Assessment of image uniformity
(e) Assessment of image artifacts
(f) Assessment of accuracy and linearity of PV numbers
(g) Assessment of low-contrast resolution
(h) Assessment of spatial resolution
(i) Assessment of tube voltage (kV) accuracy and reproducibility
(j) Assessment of beam quality and HVL
(k) Assessment of image display device
(l) Assessment of CBCT dosimetry

(a) **Alignment of Lasers**

Most dental CBCT systems utilize internal lasers for both lateral and longitudinal positioning. Though there is no built-in verification method exists for the *Longitudinal Laser Alignment, Lateral Laser Alignments* can be tested by aligning the lasers with hash marks engraved on the imaging panel cover.

- Tolerance: ±2 mm
- *Recommendation*: Establish a baseline measurement at acceptance testing for future reference.
- *Frequency*: Annual testing with comparison to the baseline measurement

(b) **Verification of Collimation (Field-to-Receptor Size)**

Ensuring proper collimation in Dental CBCT systems is very important. This restricts X-ray exposure to the region of interest (ROI) and minimizes unnecessary patient dose. It contributes significantly to image quality (IQ). The Qualified Medical Physicist (QMP) needs to verify that:

- Optimal scan volumes can be selected for specific anatomical areas.
- The collimation system functions properly and delivers the correct radiation beam size for chosen FOVs.

While ideally all field sizes should be verified, focusing on the most clinically used options is often sufficient due to:

- Practical limitations
- Operational constraints of the scanner

Test Objectives:

- Ensure the irradiated field of view (FOV) matches the nominal FOV (within tolerance).
- Confirm the irradiated field doesn't exceed the detector borders by more than 10% of the source-to-axis rotation distance (SAD). This prevents unnecessary patient exposure.

Challenges and Solutions:

- Nominal field size is defined at the isocenter.
- **Solution**: Apply a magnification correction (distance scaling) to calculate the expected field size at the exit window of the tube housing for comparison with the nominal size.

In theory, collimation verification can be conducted for every available FOV or protocol. One approach involves utilizing self-developing radiochromic-type film, such as XR-QA2 Gafchromic film, attached to the exit window of the tube housing. This location offers:

- Closest proximity to the focal spot
- Small exposure area for film placement
- High exposure levels for adequate film density
  - Use narrow film strips taped together to cover the entire field size at the exit window.
  - Perform full or multiple rotational scans (depending on technique) to achieve appropriate film density.
  - Mark and record films for accurate field size measurements.
  - For practical considerations, test the three most frequently used FOV options to minimize tube overheating.

Recommendations:

- Establish a baseline measurement during acceptance testing.
- Tolerance: The ratio between the field size at the isocenter and the nominal field size should be within 3% of SID in full rotation mode.
- If the system uses offset fields and testing occurs in stationary mode (if accessible), the ratio should be within 10% of SID.
- Frequency: Perform this test annually.

(c) **Assessment of Contrast-to-Noise (CNR)**

Dental CBCT images of a uniform object should have consistent pixel values (PVs) throughout. To verify this, the user or QMP needs to assess image uniformity. The contrast resolution, measured by the contrast-to-noise ratio (CNR), assesses the visibility of different materials (low and high contrast) against a uniform background. The CNR is:

- Easy to assess
- Reproducible
- Useful for constancy tests

Materials and Phantom:

- Focus on intermediate-to-high-density structures relevant to dental imaging, using materials similar to those in the PV accuracy test.
- The phantom insert should contain these materials embedded in a polymethylmethacrylate (PMMA) background.
- The structures should be large enough to accurately measure mean PVs and standard deviations (SDs) in selected regions of interest (ROIs).

Testing Conditions:

- Test CNR with commonly used protocols for small, medium, and large FOVs.
- Maintain consistent:
  - Protocol (beam dimensions, dose settings)
  - Mode of operation
  - Phantom and insert orientation

Calculation and Analysis:

- Measure the material's mean PV (MPV) and background from designated ROIs.
- Calculate CNR: $CNR = |MPV_m - MPV_b|/SD_b$. Here, SD_b is the standard deviation of the background signal.
- Establish a baseline CNR value for each material and protocol.

Considerations:

- For small FOVs or partial rotations (<360°), ensure the insert's position is consistent relative to the rotation center and scan angles.
- Most systems offer automated ROI selection using dedicated QC software.
- Maintain consistent tube voltage, tube current-exposure time product, and exposure parameters resembling those used for adult patients. Consistent phantom positioning is crucial for systems with tube current modulation.

Recommendations:

- Establish a baseline at acceptance testing.
- Tolerance level: CNR value within ±30% of the baseline
- Frequency: Annually

(d) **Assessment of Image Uniformity**

Dental CBCT images of uniform objects should have consistent pixel values (PVs) throughout. This test ensures such uniformity.

Method:

- *Phantom or Water Bottle*:
  - Use the manufacturer's image quality (IQ) test phantom (if available).
  - Alternatively, use a plastic water bottle.
- *Scanning*:
  - Scan the phantom/bottle using a common clinical protocol and high-resolution settings.
  - Monitor tube voltage and tube current during exposure.
- *ROI Selection*:
  - Use the region of interest (ROI) tool in the image analysis software.
  - Create five ROIs of similar size (around 15% of the phantom diameter):
  - One in the center
  - Four peripherally in symmetrical locations (avoiding the image edge)
- *Analysis*:
  - Analyze the mean PVs of the ROIs.
  - Compare the results to the manufacturer's tolerance levels.
- *Additional Notes*:
  - Acceptance Testing: Carefully review images for artifacts during acceptance testing and every time one performs this uniformity test.
  - Baseline and Frequency:
  - Establish a baseline measurement at acceptance testing.
  - Perform the test annually.

Remember: Tolerance levels vary by manufacturer, so consult the specific system's documentation for details.

(e) **Assessment of Image Artifacts**

Dental CBCT images can be affected by various artifacts, decreasing image quality and potentially impacting diagnoses. This section tests if the scanner has the proper software and calibration to minimize these artifacts.

Common Artifacts:

- Ring artifacts: Concentric circles around the image center
  - Causes: Defective detector element, offset scanning geometry
  - Test method: Use a large water or PMMA phantom with the largest FOV and longest acquisition time during acceptance testing.
- Streak artifacts: Streaks or lines in the image
  - Causes: Increased scatter, beam hardening, edge effects, metal objects
  - Test method: Head phantom with metal inserts simulating various implants. This allows qualitative and quantitative assessment:
    - Qualitative: Evaluate the impact of metal inserts visually during acceptance testing.
    - Quantitative: Use dedicated software to measure the standard deviation within a region of interest, excluding the metal inserts. This reflects the impact of streaks.
- Misalignment artifacts: Motion-like artifacts due to misalignment of the X-ray source, rotation center, and detector
  - Cause: Mechanical instability of the scanner
  - Test method: Any dental CBCT phantom scanned with a clinical protocol
- Aliasing artifacts: Moiré patterns caused by undersampling data
  - Cause: Low-dose protocols with reduced projections or pulses
  - Test method: Homogeneous phantom to visualize Moiré patterns at the periphery.

Recommendations:

- Establish a baseline at acceptance testing for future comparisons.
- *Tolerance level*: No clinically relevant artifacts should be present.
- Frequency:
  - An annual investigation is recommended to identify distortions and aliasing.
  - Additional testing may be needed if concerns arise regarding specific artifacts.

Additional Notes:

- Many dental CBCT scanners offer algorithms to reduce metal artifacts. Evaluate their effectiveness during acceptance testing.
- Manufacturers may provide specific phantoms or testing methods for their systems. Consult the user manual for details.

(f) **Assessment of Accuracy and Linearity of PV Numbers**

Dental CBCT pixel values (PVs) represent the X-ray attenuation properties within each image voxel. It is similar to CT Hounsfield Units (HUs) but not directly comparable due to:

- Energy spectrum variations: Different scanners use varying voltage filtration, leading to different energy spectra and affecting PVs.
- Calibration limitations: Dental CBCT systems have limitations in accurately calibrating PVs due to:
  - Scatter radiation contributes to the signal.
  - Partial rotations and offset geometry.

Manufacturer Responsibilities:

- Provide scanner-specific PVs for reference materials:
  - Air, water, PMMA, bone-equivalent materials, and implant material
- Test and provide tolerance values for these reference PVs.

Testing and Evaluation:

- Annually: Compare measured PVs to manufacturer-provided reference values.
  - If data is unavailable, establish baselines and monitor for constancy.
  - Take corrective actions if PVs fall outside acceptable ranges (>20% deviation from baseline).
- For systems claiming conformity between PVs and HUs:
  - Verify a linear relationship between PVs and reference materials' linear attenuation coefficient (μ).
  - Calculate the mean energy of the scanner's spectrum.
  - Plot PVs against μ values and expect a linear trend.
- For systems without HU conformity:
  - Determine the best fit between PVs and $\mu(E)$.
  - Verify the constancy of the fit over time.
  - Consider repeated phantom positioning trials.

Testing Method:

- Use the manufacturer-provided phantom with the recommended protocol.
- Use the scanner's ROI analysis tools to select regions within different materials.
- Compare measured PVs with reference values or established baselines.

Acceptance Testing and Baseline:

- Establish a baseline for reference material PVs during acceptance testing.

Tolerance Levels:

- Meet manufacturer's recommendations or ensure PVs stay within:
  - ±25% of the difference between water and air PVs
- Linearity line with a slope greater than 0.95

Frequency:

- Perform testing annually.

(g) **Assessment of Low-Contrast Resolution**

Low-contrast resolution describes an imaging system's ability to differentiate objects with similar characteristics to their surroundings. This isn't limited by the size of the pixels (spatial limitation) but by inherent noise. It is relevant because, while not central to dental CBCT, advancements may improve the detection of low-contrast structures.

Testing Procedure:

- Follow the manufacturer's recommendations for low-contrast resolution assessment using their test phantom.
- During acceptance testing, scan the provided low-contrast objects with a high-resolution protocol.
- Document the diameter of the smallest visible object.

Recommendations:

- Scan the manufacturer's low-contrast module with their recommended protocol.
- Monitor scanning parameters and ensure they meet the manufacturer's tolerance or the established baseline.

Testing Frequency:

- Perform testing annually.

(h) **Assessment of Spatial Resolution: Resolution Evaluation and Distance Scale Accuracy**

Spatial resolution is crucial in CBCT, determining the smallest visualized object.

Measurement Methods:

- Line Pairs (lp/mm):
  - Simple, visual assessment using vendor-provided phantoms
  - Limitations:
    - Nonuniform for objects at different distances (anisotropic)
  - Recommendation: Use the manufacturer's method and calibrate readings based on facility viewing conditions, not manufacturer recommendations.
- Modulation Transfer Function (MTF):
  - Preferred quantitative method
  - Less common availability in current CBCT systems
  - Recommendation: Encourage more manufacturers to offer MTF measurement tools
- Distance Scale Accuracy:
  - Some phantoms include embedded markers or scales for testing.
  - Tolerance: ±1 mm

Testing Procedure:

- Use the manufacturer's phantom and recommended protocol.
- Apply the analysis filter before reading the results.
- Document the visible line pair resolution.

Recommendations:

- Follow the manufacturer's testing procedures.
- Scan the phantom with a high-resolution protocol.
- Monitor scanning parameters and ensure they meet the following:
  - Manufacturer's tolerance
  - Baseline established at acceptance testing for visible line pairs
- Determine resolution under the facility's viewing conditions.

Testing Frequency:

- Perform testing annually.

Additional Notes:

- Line pairs offer a quick visual assessment but have limitations.
- MTF is a more accurate method but is currently less widely available.
- Distance scale accuracy also needs to be verified.

(i) **Assessment of Tube Voltage (kV) Accuracy and Reproducibility**

Accurate and consistent tube voltage is crucial for X-ray image quality and patient dose optimization.

Testing Method:

- Use a calibrated voltage sensor aligned to the beam. Internal lasers (if available) can aid in alignment.

Data Recording:

- Record initial values during acceptance testing.

Recommendations:

- Tolerance levels:
- Accuracy: ±10% for various kilovoltage settings across a range of voltages
- Reproducibility: ±5%
- Frequency: Annual testing

(j) **Assessment of Beam Quality and HVL**

Half-value layer (HVL) reflects the quality and filtration of the X-ray beam, impacting image quality and patient dose.

Testing Method:

- Use a calibrated ionization chamber or solid-state dosimeter positioned at the center of rotation.
- Mount aluminum filters (99.9% purity) at the tube exit window.

Data Recording:

- Record initial values during acceptance testing.

Tolerance Level:

- Measured HVL values must meet minimum requirements set by FDA or state regulations.

Frequency of testing: Annual

(k) **Assessment of Image Display Device**

A proper image display is crucial for the accurate interpretation of dental CBCT scans.

Testing Method:

- Perform a visual inspection using a test pattern provided by the manufacturer or following guidelines from:
  - AAPM Task Group 18-QC (TG18-QC)
  - AAPM Task Group 270-sQC (TG270-sQC)

Data Recording:

- Record initial values during acceptance testing.

Tolerance Level:

- Measured values must meet the requirements established in the chosen AAPM Task Group standard (TG18-QC or TG270-sQC).

Frequency: Perform testing annually.

(l) **Assessment of CBCT Dosimetry**

Standard CT dose index (CTDI) measures are unsuitable for cone-beam geometry, leading to unclear dosimetry guidelines for dental CBCT.

Limitations:

- European Federation of Organizations for Medical Physics (EFOMP) protocol lacks specific recommendations for dental CBCT testing.
- No dedicated guidance document exists for dental CBCT encompassing comprehensive testing methodologies, tolerances, and frequencies.

Need for Improvement:

- Establishing standardized testing procedures for dental CBCT dosimetry is crucial for the following:
- Ensuring consistent image quality and patient dose optimization
- Providing clear guidance for acceptance testing and periodic QC
- Facilitating comparisons between different CBCT systems

Next Steps:

- Collaboration is essential to develop a dedicated dental CBCT testing guide, addressing:
  - Comprehensive step-by-step testing methodologies using appropriate dosimetry phantoms and protocols
  - Acceptable tolerance levels for various dosimetric parameters relevant to dental CBCT
  - Recommended testing frequencies based on risk factors and clinical practices.

By addressing these needs, we can achieve standardized and consistent quality control practices for dental CBCT, ultimately improving patient safety and care.

Dental CBCT Quality Control Testing Recommendations

Acceptance Testing:

- Prioritize vendor-specific tests, followed by local/state regulations and recommendations from professional organizations (if available).
- Establish baseline values using additional phantoms for future comparisons.
- Ensure the system meets or exceeds performance standards.

Periodic QC Testing:

- Frequency:
  - Follow the manufacturer's recommendations (if available).
  - Standard recommendations: Daily/weekly and annually for optimal performance
- Purpose: Detect changes in:
  - Radiation dose (substantial increase)
  - Image quality (clinically significant degradation)
- Weekly Testing:
- Personnel: Trained dental assistants (following vendor's recommendations, if available)
- QMP responsibilities:
  - Establish baseline values
  - Define action limits
  - Review procedures and results
- Recommended tests (in the absence of vendor recommendations):
  - Uniformity assessment
  - Noise and CNR assessment
  - Artifact evaluation
  - CT number accuracy (water only)
  - Review QC records
- Annual Testing:
- Performed by QMP.
- Includes:
  - Baseline verification and action limit compliance
  - Data collection and reporting
  - Service record review
  - Final report generation
- Recommended tests:
- Laser alignment
  - Radiation field size
  - Noise, CNR, and uniformity
  - Artifact evaluation
  - CT number accuracy and linearity
  - Spatial resolution
  - Geometric distortion
  - Tube voltage and HVL
  - Display monitor
- Radiation dosimetry

8.5 Dose Considerations and Regulatory Requirements in Dental Radiography

8.5.1 Dose Considerations

Dental radiographs, including X-rays and cone-beam CT (CBCT) scans, are valuable tools for dentists to diagnose and treat various dental problems. However, these procedures involve ionizing radiation exposure, and minimizing this exposure is a crucial aspect of dental care. The terms related to dose are explained in detail in Chap. 10. However, few terms which are related to dental radiography are explained below:

- **Diagnostic reference levels (DRLs)** are national or regional benchmarks for typical radiation doses associated with specific X-ray procedures. They help ensure consistency and identify potential overexposure situations.
- **Units of Measurement**:
  - **Entrance Surface Dose**: Measures radiation when the X-ray hits the body (e.g., the patient's cheek). It's expressed in millisieverts (mSv) or mill gray (mGy).
  - **Kerma-Area Product (KAP)** represents the total amount of X-ray energy used during the procedure. It's expressed in milli gray-square centimeters (mGy.cm^2).
  - **Effective Dose**: This reflects the overall radiation risk to the body, considering the type and distribution of radiation exposure. It's expressed in millisieverts (mSv).

8.5.1.1 Typical Doses for Different Procedures

- **Intraoral X-rays**: These provide detailed images of individual teeth and surrounding bone. Their doses are generally low:
  - Entrance surface dose: 0.65–3.7 mGy
  - Kerma-area product: 26–87 mGy.cm^2
  - Effective dose: 1–8 μSv

- **Panoramic X-rays** capture the broad view of upper and lower jaws, teeth, and sinuses. Their doses are slightly higher than intraoral X-rays:
  - Entrance surface dose: 3.3–4.2 mGy
  - Kerma-area product: 84–120 mGy.cm^2
  - Effective dose: 4–30 μSv
- **Lateral cephalometric X-rays**: These provide a side view of the skull, jaws, and teeth, aiding in orthodontic treatment planning. Their doses are comparable to panoramic X-rays:
  - Kerma-area product:
    - Adults: 41–146 mGy.cm^2
    - Children: 25–121 mGy.cm^2
  - Effective dose: 2–3 μSv
- **Cone-beam CT (CBCT) scans**: These create three-dimensional images of the jaws and teeth, offering detailed information for complex cases. However, they involve higher radiation doses:
  - Effective dose: Can vary significantly, ranging from 50 μSv or lower for small scans to potentially up to several hundred μSv for larger scans, and potentially even higher.

Balancing Safety and Information Needs

- Dental professionals prioritize using the least radiation necessary to obtain a clear and diagnostic image. Factors influencing dose include the type of X-ray needed, the size and angulation of the X-ray beam, and the use of digital technology (which generally requires lower doses).
- Justification Principle: X-rays should only be taken when the risk of radiation exposure outweighs the diagnostic benefit.

By working together, patients and dentists can ensure optimal dental care by understanding dose considerations and prioritizing safety.

8.5.2 Regulatory Requirements in Dental Radiography: Ensuring Safety and Quality

To ensure patient safety and diagnostic image quality in dental radiography, regulatory requirements are in place to govern the use of dental X-ray equipment and practices. These regulations vary depending on country to country, but here's a general overview of the key aspects:

- **Institutional Registration**: Dental practices utilizing X-ray equipment must register with a designated regulatory body, often accredited by a national authority. This registration process ensures proper oversight and adherence to safety regulations.
- **Equipment Registration and Quality Assurance (QA)**: All dental X-ray machines require registration with the regulatory body. Periodic quality assurance (QA) testing must be performed on the equipment at specified intervals (typically every 5 years/2 years, depending upon the manufacturer/regulatory requirements) to verify its functionality and ensure it delivers radiation within acceptable limits. Authorized service agencies conduct these tests.
- **Personnel Monitoring**: Personnel who operate dental X-ray equipment may be required to wear dosimeter badges (TLD badges) to monitor their cumulative radiation exposure over time. This helps ensure they stay within safe exposure limits. While not always mandatory, some regulations recommend the use of dosimeter badges for operators in high-volume practices.
- **Machine Operation and Training**: Only trained personnel who are qualified and authorized to operate dental X-ray equipment are permitted to do so. Training programs ensure operators understand proper X-ray techniques, safety protocols, and radiation protection measures for themselves and patients.
- **Patient Protection**: Justification principle: X-rays should only be taken when the diagnostic benefit outweighs the potential risk of radiation exposure. Dentists are expected to use clinical judgment and consider alternative diagnostic methods.
- **Recordkeeping and Decommissioning**: Regulations typically require maintaining records of X-ray procedures performed, equipment maintenance, and QA testing

results for a specified period. When dental X-ray equipment reaches the end of its lifespan, proper decommissioning procedures are mandated to ensure safe disposal and minimize environmental impact.

Importance of Regulatory Compliance: Adherence to regulatory requirements is crucial for:

- **Patient safety**: Minimizing radiation exposure for both patients and staff
- **Image quality**: Ensuring X-ray equipment functions correctly for optimal image acquisition for diagnosis
- **Accountability**: Maintaining proper records for traceability and potential audits

Finding Specific Regulations: Specific regulatory requirements can vary depending on the location. Consult local or national regulatory body for detailed information. Some helpful resources include the following:

- The International Atomic Energy Agency (IAEA) provides general guidance on dental radiology safety: https://www.iaea.org/publications/14720/radiation-protection-in-dental-radiology.
- In the United States, the Food and Drug Administration (FDA) regulates dental X-ray equipment: https://www.fda.gov/regulatory--information/search-fda-guidance-documents/performance-standard-diagnostic-x-ray-systems-and-their-major-components-21cfr-102030-102031-102032.
- Similarly, many countries have their own regulatory bodies which define standards.

By understanding and complying with regulatory requirements, dental practices can ensure the safe and effective use of X-ray technology for optimal patient care.

8.6 Safety in Dental Radiography

Since dental X-rays uses ionizing radiation, the safety becomes paramount before its use. Following roadmap can be used to ensure the well-being of patients, staff, and the public during dental X-ray procedures.

8.6.1 The Three Pillars of Radiation Protection

- **Justification**: X-rays should never be a routine procedure. Dentists must conduct a thorough clinical assessment to determine if an X-ray is necessary for diagnosis and treatment planning.
- **Optimization**: Once necessary, X-ray procedures should be optimized to deliver the least possible radiation dose while acquiring high-quality images. This involves using proper techniques collimators to confine the beam and selecting the most appropriate film or sensor technology.
- **Limitation**: All reasonable steps must be taken to minimize radiation exposure for everyone involved. This includes proper equipment maintenance, optimizing exposure settings, maximizing distance from the X-ray source, and utilizing appropriate shielding.

8.6.2 Protecting Patients: Quality Images with Minimal Dose

- **Clinical Assessment Is Key**: A dentist's expertise is crucial in determining the necessity of an X-ray. A detailed examination and review of existing dental records can often help reduce the need for additional X-rays.

- **Technology Matters**: Modern dental X-ray equipment offers significant advancements. Using digital sensors or F-speed film allows for capturing clear images with minimal radiation compared to traditional film.
- **Retakes Are Costly (and Radiation Heavy)**: Ensuring proper technique from the start, including using image receptor holders and beam-aiming devices for intraoral radiography and patient positioning aids for panoramic radiography, minimizes the need for retakes, and reduces overall radiation exposure.

8.6.3 Lead Aprons for Patients: A Focus on Effectiveness

The use of lead aprons for patients in dental X-rays is a topic of ongoing discussion. Here's a breakdown of current practices:

- **Limited Effectiveness**: Routine use of lead aprons for dental X-rays and cone-beam CT (CBCT) scans may offer some protection from external radiation, but their effectiveness is limited.
- **Targeted Thyroid Protection**: Thyroid collars are only necessary when the thyroid gland is directly in the X-ray beam, such as during specific procedures involving unusual patient positioning.
- **Internal Scattered Radiation**: Lead aprons block external radiation and do not shield against internally scattered radiation within the body, which is the main source of patient exposure during dental X-rays.

8.6.4 Staff Safety: Knowledge, Distance, and Shielding

Dental staff are also at potential risk from radiation exposure. Here's how to safeguard them:

- **Training and Awareness**: All dental staff must be thoroughly trained in radiation safety principles and understand the health risks associated with X-ray exposure.
- **Distance Is the Friend**: Maximizing the distance between staff and the X-ray source during exposure significantly reduces radiation dose. Ideally, the entire X-ray room should be designated as a controlled area, with staff positioned at least 6 feet (1.8) m away.
- **Shielding Matters**: Lead barriers strategically placed around the X-ray unit provide additional protection for staff.
- **Safe Operation Procedures**: Staff should only operate X-ray equipment in accordance with current guidelines and best practices to minimize unnecessary exposures.
- **Personal Monitoring**: Consider implementing personal monitoring for staff in controlled areas to verify that established safety protocols are effective.

8.6.5 Protecting the Public: Keeping Unintended Exposure to a Minimum

The general public in waiting rooms, adjoining areas, or even outdoors near the dental facility should also be considered.

- **Strategic Equipment Placement**: X-ray equipment should be positioned to prevent the primary X-ray beam from reaching occupied areas or outside the building.
- **Proper Wall Shielding**: Walls separating X-ray rooms from public areas must be evaluated and constructed with appropriate materials and thickness to ensure adequate radiation blocking.
- **Consulting a Medical Physicist**: An expert medical physicist can advise on optimal equipment placement, facility design for radiation shielding, and the proper installation of radiation warning signs.

8.6.6 Beyond the Basics: Equipment Considerations

This guide also details specific requirements for the safe installation, operation, and maintenance of dental X-ray equipment, encompassing general X-ray units, panoramic X-ray machines, and image receptor considerations (refer to local regulatory guidelines for specifics).

By adhering to these comprehensive measures, dental professionals can provide a safe environment for stakeholders in dental X-ray procedures. Remember, safe practices protect patients and staff and ensure public safety and responsible use of ionizing radiation in dentistry.

Exercise

Multiple Choice Questions (MCQs)

1. Which of the following imaging techniques is commonly used to evaluate unerupted or impacted teeth?
   A. Intraoral radiographs
   B. Panoramic radiographs
   C. Cephalometric radiographs
   D. Cone-beam computed tomography (CBCT)
2. What is one of the primary benefits of intraoral radiographs?
   A. Provides a comprehensive view of the entire mouth
   B. Offers high-resolution images of individual teeth
   C. Captures the side profile of the face and skull
   D. Allows for three-dimensional visualization of anatomical structures
3. Which of the following is a limitation of panoramic radiographs?
   A. High radiation dose
   B. Difficulty in assessing bone density
   C. Reduced image detail compared to intraoral radiographs
   D. Inability to detect temporomandibular joint disorders
4. Cephalometric radiographs are particularly useful for:
   A. Detecting dental caries
   B. Assessing the condition of the temporomandibular joints
   C. Planning orthodontic treatment and assessing facial growth
   D. Evaluating the presence of tumors in the oral cavity
5. Which imaging technique provides a three-dimensional view of the oral and maxillofacial region?
   A. Intraoral radiographs
   B. Panoramic radiographs
   C. Cephalometric radiographs
   D. Cone-beam computed tomography (CBCT)
6. When were the first dental X-ray machines manufactured in Germany?
   A. 1895
   B. 1905
   C. 1913
   D. 1932
7. Who designed the Coolidge-type tube, which improved the safety and quality control of X-rays?
   A. WC Roentgen
   B. C.E. Kells
   C. William David Coolidge
   D. WH Rollins
8. What significant dental radiography development occurred in 1925?
   A. Discovery of X-rays
   B. Development of the bitewing technique
   C. Introduction of the paralleling technique
   D. First dental text and prewrapped films
9. What is the primary advantage of intraoral X-rays in dentistry?
   A. High radiation dose
   B. Broad view of multiple structures
   C. Detailed images of specific teeth and surrounding bone structures
   D. Low cost compared to other imaging techniques

10. Who pioneered the concept of bitewing films in dental radiography?
    A. C.E. Kells
    B. Howard Riley Raper
    C. Franklin W. McCormack
    D. William J. Morton
11. What was a significant contribution of Yrjö Veli Paatero to dental radiography?
    A. Discovery of X-rays
    B. Development of the first dental X-ray machine
    C. Introduction of panoramic radiography
    D. Invention of digital sensors
12. What technique minimizes geometric distortion in intraoral radiography?
    A. Paralleling technique
    B. Bisecting angle technique
    C. Rotational technique
    D. Cone-beam technique
13. What is a common disadvantage of panoramic radiography compared to intraoral radiography?
    A. Higher radiation exposure
    B. Limited to specific areas
    C. Lack of patient positioning options
    D. Lower resolution and overlapping structures
14. Which of the following is NOT a use of cephalometric X-rays?
    A. Orthodontic treatment planning
    B. Evaluation of facial symmetry
    C. Diagnosing jaw abnormalities
    D. Detection of cavities
15. Who introduced cephalometric X-ray in Germany?
    A. BH Broadbent
    B. H. Hofrath
    C. Richard A. Robb
    D. J. Morita
16. Which of the following is a simplified cephalometric analysis used today?
    A. Mozzo Analysis
    B. Broadbent Analysis
    C. Björk Morphological Analysis
    D. Hofrath Analysis
17. CBCT scans are useful for all of the following EXCEPT:
    A. Visualizing airway abnormalities
    B. Evaluating temporomandibular joint (TMJ) structures
    C. Monitoring heart conditions
    D. Implantology planning
18. What year was the cone-beam CT (CBCT) developed?
    A. 1982
    B. 1998
    C. 2001
    D. 2004
19. Which organization provides detailed guidelines on acceptance testing and routine quality control of dental equipment?
    A. American Dental Association (ADA)
    B. World Health Organization (WHO)
    C. American Association of Physicists in Medicine (AAPM)
    D. National Council on Radiation Protection (NCRP)
20. What is the maximum movement allowed for the tube head after stabilization in intraoral dental units?
    A. 1 cm
    B. 0.5 cm
    C. 2 cm
    D. 1.5 cm
21. What is the minimum source-to-skin distance required for intraoral dental units?
    A. 18 cm
    B. 20 cm
    C. 15 cm
    D. 10 cm
22. What is the diagnostic reference level (DRL) for dental X-rays as per NCRP Report No. 172?
    A. 1.6 mGy
    B. 1.6 mSv
    C. 100 mGy cm^2
    D. 76 mGy cm^2
23. What tool can be used for quality control of digital intraoral image receptors?
    A. Sensitometer
    B. Densitometer

- C. Special phantoms
- D. PSP receptors

24. Which of the following tests involves measuring the distance from coins' edges to the exposed area of the X-ray?
    - A. Leakage radiation and visual inspection
    - B. Collimation
    - C. Exposure reproducibility
    - D. Beam quality
25. What is the maximum allowable sum of differences between opposite edges of the light field and radiation field in the collimation test?
    - A. 1% of the SID
    - B. 2% of the SID
    - C. 3% of the SID
    - D. 4% of the SID
26. What is the diagnostic reference level (DRL) for typical entrance skin dose in cephalometric X-ray systems according to NCRP Report No. 172?
    - A. 0.07 mGy
    - B. 0.09 mGy
    - C. 0.14 mGy
    - D. 0.17 mGy
27. What is used to calculate entrance skin air kerma (ESAK) in the exposure reproducibility test?
    - A. Air kerma and SID
    - B. Air kerma and SDD
    - C. SDD and ESAK
    - D. SID and ESAK
28. Which quality control aspect involves using a phantom with materials similar to dental structures?
    - A. Evaluation of the site's quality control program
    - B. Scattered radiation survey
    - C. Assessment of contrast-to-noise ratio (CNR)
    - D. Quality control for digital cephalometric image receptors
29. What is the unit of measurement used for the entrance surface dose in dental radiography?
    - A. Millisieverts (mSv)
    - B. Mill gray (mGy)
    - C. Microsieverts (μSv)
    - D. Mill gray-square centimeters (mGy.cm^2)
30. Which X-ray procedure typically has the highest range of effective dose?
    - A. Intraoral X-rays
    - B. Panoramic X-rays
    - C. Lateral cephalometric X-rays
    - D. Cone-beam CT (CBCT) scans
31. What does the kerma-area product (KAP) represent in dental radiography?
    - A. The amount of radiation hitting the patient's cheek
    - B. The total amount of X-ray energy used during the procedure
    - C. The overall radiation risk to the body
    - D. The amount of X-ray energy absorbed by the bone
32. What is the principle that states X-rays should only be taken when the diagnostic benefit outweighs the potential risk of radiation exposure?
    - A. Justification principle
    - B. Safety principle
    - C. Quality assurance principle
    - D. Diagnostic principle
33. Which organization provides general guidance on dental radiology safety?
    - A. Food and Drug Administration (FDA)
    - B. International Atomic Energy Agency (IAEA)
    - C. World Health Organization (WHO)
    - D. National Institute of Dental and Craniofacial Research (NIDCR)
34. What is the primary goal of the optimization principle in radiation protection during dental X-rays?
    - A. To minimize the use of lead aprons
    - B. To deliver the least possible radiation dose while acquiring high-quality images
    - C. To maximize the distance from the X-ray source
    - D. To ensure all X-ray procedures are justified
35. How should dental staff minimize their radiation exposure during X-ray procedures?
    - A. By using personal monitoring badges
    - B. By maintaining a close proximity to the X-ray source
    - C. By operating X-ray equipment only during patient exposure

D. By receiving no training in radiation safety principles

Short Questions

1. What are the benefits and limitations of intraoral radiographs in dental imaging?
2. Describe the key applications of cephalometric radiographs in orthodontics and oral and maxillofacial surgery.
3. Describe the contributions of Dr. Yrjö Veli Paatero to the field of dental radiography.
4. Describe the historical development of intraoral radiography and its significance in dental diagnostics.
5. Explain the working principle of intraoral radiography, including the equipment and setup involved.
6. What are the differences between handheld and wall-mounted intraoral scanners, and what are their respective advantages and disadvantages?
7. Describe the key components involved in the working principle of cephalometric dental X-ray machines.
8. What advancements have CBCT machines brought to dental imaging?
9. What are the primary differences between CBCT and MSCT?
10. Describe the purpose and method of the "darkroom quality control" test for intraoral film.
11. What are the steps involved in performing the "beam quality" test for intraoral dental units?
12. Explain the significance of the "exposure reproducibility" test in dental radiography.
13. Describe the steps for checking the alignment of lasers in dental CBCT systems.
14. What factors are considered while evaluating the accuracy of pixel values (PVs) in dental CBCT systems?
15. Explain the significance of low-contrast resolution in dental imaging and how it is assessed.
16. What are diagnostic reference levels (DRLs) in dental radiography?
17. Explain the importance of using dosimeter badges for personnel operating dental X-ray equipment.
18. What are the key aspects of equipment registration and quality assurance in dental radiography?

Long Question

1. Explain the role and advantages of cone-beam computed tomography (CBCT) in dental imaging. Discuss its diagnostic applications, benefits, and limitations.
2. Discuss the development and technological advancements in panoramic radiography, highlighting the contributions of key figures and companies.
3. Compare and contrast the advantages and limitations of intraoral and panoramic radiography in dental diagnostics. Include considerations of patient safety, image quality, and diagnostic applications.
4. Discuss the history and evolution of cephalometric radiography, highlighting significant milestones and contributors.
5. Explain the working principle of CBCT machines, including their key features and applications in dental and maxillofacial imaging.
6. Discuss the quality control procedures for panoramic dental units, including the key tests performed and their significance.
7. Explain the importance of the "evaluation of the site's quality control program" and outline the key components that should be assessed during this evaluation.
8. Discuss the procedure for testing collimation in cephalometric dental units, including the steps for checking light-radiation field coincidence, field size indicator accuracy, and radiation field and image receptor alignment.
9. Explain the quality control measures for digital cephalometric image receptors, including the procedures for display verification and evaluation criteria for image quality.

10. Discuss the dose considerations in dental radiography, including typical doses for different procedures and factors influencing dose.
11. Explain the regulatory requirements in dental radiography, focusing on the importance of regulatory compliance and the role of different regulations in ensuring patient safety and image quality.

Answers to MCQs

1. B. Panoramic radiographs
2. B. Offers high-resolution images of individual teeth
3. C. Reduced image detail compared to intraoral radiographs
4. C. Planning orthodontic treatment and assessing facial growth
5. D. Cone-beam computed tomography (CBCT)
6. B. 1905
7. C. William David Coolidge
8. B. Development of the bitewing technique
9. C. Detailed images of specific teeth and surrounding bone structures
10. B. Howard Riley Raper
11. C. Introduction of panoramic radiography
12. A. Paralleling technique
13. D. Lower resolution and overlapping structures
14. D. Detection of cavities
15. B. H. Hofrath
16. C. Björk Morphological Analysis
17. C. Monitoring heart conditions
18. A. 1982
19. C. American Association of Physicists in Medicine (AAPM)
20. B. 0.5 cm
21. A. 18 cm
22. B. 1.6 mSv
23. C. Special phantoms
24. B. Collimation
25. B. 2% of the SID
26. C. 0.14 mGy
27. B. Air kerma and SDD
28. C. Assessment of contrast-to-noise ratio (CNR)
29. B. Mill gray (mGy)
30. D. Cone-beam CT (CBCT) scans
31. B. The total amount of X-ray energy used during the procedure
32. A. Justification principle
33. B. International Atomic Energy Agency (IAEA)
34. B. To deliver the least possible radiation dose while acquiring high-quality images
35. A. By using personal monitoring badges

References

1. Pauwels R. History of dental radiography: evolution of 2D and 3D imaging modalities. 2020. [Online]. Available: https://www.researchgate.net/publication/340444478.
2. Sansare K, Khanna V, Karjodkar F. Early victims of X-rays: a tribute and current perception. Dentomaxillofac Radiol. 2011;40(2):123–5. https://doi.org/10.1259/dmfr/73488299.
3. Langland OE, Fortier AP. C. Edmund Kells. Oral Surg Oral Med Oral Pathol. 1972;34(4):680–9. https://doi.org/10.1016/0030-4220(72)90353-2.
4. Thunthy KH, Walkhoff FO. Early pioneers of oral and maxillofacial radiology. [Online]. Available: http://www.aaomr.org/?page=AAOMRHistory.
5. van der Stelt PF. Panoramic radiographs in dental diagnostics. Ned Tijdschr Tandheelkd. 2016;123(04):181–7. https://doi.org/10.5177/ntvt.2016.04.15208.
6. White SC, Pharoah MJ. Oral-radiology-principles-and-interpretation. 6th ed. Mosby; 2009.
7. Rushton VE, Horner K. The use of panoramic radiology in dental practice. J Dent. 1996;24(3):185–201. https://doi.org/10.1016/0300-5712(95)00055-0.
8. Zulauf AF. Panoramic X-ray apparatus. 1922.
9. Numatha H. Consideration of the parabolic radiography of the dental arch. J Shimazu Stud. 1933;10:13.
10. Tammisalo EH. Professor Yrjö V. Paatero – the pioneer of panoramic oral tomography. Dentomaxillofac Radiol. 1975;4(1):53–6. https://doi.org/10.1259/dmfr.1975.0010.
11. Hallikainen D. History of panoramic radiography. Acta Radiol. 1996;37:441–86.
12. Dickson G, et al. A panoramic x-ray dental machine. U S Armed Forces Med J. 1957;13:46–55.
13. Wall BF, et al. Doses to patients from pantomographic and conventional dental radiography. Br J Radiol. 1979;52(621):727–34.
14. Kashima I, et al. Computed panoramic tomography with scanning laser-stimulated luminescence. Oral Surg Oral Med Oral Pathol. 1985;60:448–53.

15. Dove SB, et al. Preliminary evaluation of a digital system for rotational panoramic radiography. Oral Surg Oral Med Oral Pathol. 1992;73:623–32.
16. McDavid WD, et al. Electronic system for digital acquisition of rotational panoramic radiographs. Oral Surg Oral Med Oral Pathol. 1991;71:499–502.
17. Gijbels F, Jacobs R, Bogaerts R, Debaveye D, Verlinden S, Sanderink G. Dosimetry of digital panoramic imaging. Part I: patient exposure. Dentomaxillofac Radiol. 2005;34(3):145–9. https://doi.org/10.1259/dmfr/28107460.
18. Broadbent BH. A new X-ray technique and its application to orthodontia. Angle Orthod. 1931;1(2):45–66.
19. Hofrath H. Die Bedeutung der Roentgenfem- und Abstandsaufnahme fur die Diagnostik der Kieferanomalien. Fortschr Orthod. 1931;1:232–58.
20. Nielsen IL. Cephalometric analysis: history and clinical application. Taiwan J Orthod. 2022;34(4). https://doi.org/10.38209/2708-2636.1323.
21. Pauwels R, Araki K, Siewerdsen JH, Thongvigitmanee SS. Technical aspects of dental CBCT: state of the art. British Institute of Radiology; 2015. https://doi.org/10.1259/dmfr.20140224.
22. Izzetti R, Gaeta R, Caramella D, Giuffra V. Cone-beam computed tomography vs. multi-slice computed tomography in paleoimaging: where we stand. Homo. 2020;71(1):63–72. https://doi.org/10.1127/homo/2020/1063.
23. Robb RA. The dynamic spatial reconstructor: an X-ray video-fluoroscopic CT scanner for dynamic volume imaging of moving organs. IEEE Trans Med Imaging. 1982;1(1):22–33. https://doi.org/10.1109/TMI.1982.4307545.
24. Nasseh I, Al-Rawi W. Cone beam computed tomography. Dent Clin N Am. 2018;62(3):361–91. https://doi.org/10.1016/j.cden.2018.03.002.
25. Arai Y, Tammisalo E, Iwai K, Hashimoto K, Shinoda K. Development of a compact computed tomographic apparatus for dental use. Dentomaxillofac Radiol. 1999;28(4):245–8. https://doi.org/10.1038/sj.dmfr.4600448.
26. Mozzo P, Procacci C, Tacconi A, Tinazzi Martini P, Bergamo Andreis IA. A new volumetric CT machine for dental imaging based on the cone-beam technique: preliminary results. Eur Radiol. 1998;8(9):1558–64. https://doi.org/10.1007/s003300050586.
27. Nardi C, et al. Radiation dose in non-dental cone beam CT applications: a systematic review. Springer-Verlag Italia s.r.l; 2018. https://doi.org/10.1007/s11547-018-0910-7.
28. Commandeur F, Goeller M, Dey D. Cardiac CT: technological advances in hardware, software, and machine learning applications. Curr Cardiovasc Imaging Rep. 2018;11(8):19. https://doi.org/10.1007/s12410-018-9459-z.
29. Dillenseger J-P, et al. MSCT versus CBCT: evaluation of high-resolution acquisition modes for dento-maxillary and skull-base imaging. Eur Radiol. 2015;25(2):505–15. https://doi.org/10.1007/s00330-014-3439-8.
30. Pauwels R, et al. Comparison of spatial and contrast resolution for cone-beam computed tomography scanners. Oral Surg Oral Med Oral Pathol Oral Radiol. 2012;114(1):127–35. https://doi.org/10.1016/j.oooo.2012.01.020.
31. Carrino JA, et al. Dedicated cone-beam CT system for extremity imaging. Radiology. 2014;270(3):816–24. https://doi.org/10.1148/radiol.13130225.
32. Schulze R, et al. Artefacts in CBCT: a review. Dentomaxillofac Radiol. 2011;40(5):265–73. https://doi.org/10.1259/dmfr/30642039.
33. Acceptance testing and quality control of dental imaging equipment: the AAPM Report of Task Group 175. 2016.
34. Mihailidis DN, et al. AAPM Task Group Report 261: comprehensive quality control methodology and management of dental and maxillofacial cone beam computed tomography (CBCT) systems. Med Phys. 2024;51:3134. https://doi.org/10.1002/mp.16911.
35. NCRP Report 185.

9 Planning of Radiology Department: A Global Perspective

Learning Objectives

Introduction
General Principles of Installation and Planning
  Regulatory Compliance and Standards
  Site Selection and Facility Design
  Equipment Selection and Installation
  Safety and Quality Assurance
Regulatory Guidelines for:
  X-Ray
  Mammography
  Fluoroscopy
  CT
  Hybrid Imaging
	General Recommendations and Codal Requirements for Layout Planning:
	  X-Ray
	  Mammography
	  Fluoroscopy
	  CT
	  Hybrid Imaging
	Barrier and Shielding Guidelines:
	  X-Ray
	  Mammography
	  Fluoroscopy
	  CT
	  Hybrid Imaging
	Model Layout Plan:
	  X-Ray
	  Mammography
	  Fluoroscopy
	  CT
	  Hybrid Imaging

9.1 Introduction

X-ray imaging is a critical technology in medical diagnostics, providing essential information about the human body's internal architecture. Since Wilhelm Conrad Roentgen discovered X-ray imaging in 1895, the technology and applications have advanced significantly. With the discovery of X-rays, medicine was revolutionized, allowing non-invasive visualization of internal structures and aiding in the diagnosis and treatment of many diseases. Roentgen's pioneering work set the groundwork for the development of X-ray imaging techniques, which are still evolving today.

Radiological imaging plays an important role in precise diagnosis and successful patient treatment; thus, its implementation must be carefully considered considering the local context. The image capability will improve over time, so multiple implementation options should be considered depending on the imaging needs and available resources. Providing a usable result for

D. Prakash, R. P. Kotian, *Fundamentals of X-ray Imaging*,
https://doi.org/10.1007/978-981-96-7328-5_9

a medical imaging project requires a management approach and extensive involvement from all stakeholders. Imaging services vary widely between countries and within countries, regardless of their development level. X-rays and ultrasounds are more commonly used in remote healthcare facilities, while interventional, computed tomography (CT), and magnetic resonance imaging (MRI) technologies are frequently found in urban areas. A successful imaging service depends largely on the type of health care infrastructure [1].

9.2 General Principles of Installation and Planning

When planning and installing radiology equipment, several broad principles must be considered to guarantee that it operates efficiently, safely, and effectively. Here are some crucial principles that guide the process:

1. **Regulatory Compliance and Standards**
   - Local and International Regulations: Comply with all local, national, and international regulations and standards (e.g., American College of Radiology (ACR), International Electrotechnical Commission (IEC), U.S. Food and Drug Administration (FDA), and World Health Organization (WHO) guidelines).
   - Radiation Safety: Follow guidelines for radiation protection to safeguard patients, staff, and the general public. This includes adhering to ALARA (As Low As Reasonably Achievable) principles.
2. **Site Selection and Facility Design**
   - Space Requirements: Ensure adequate space for the equipment, ancillary devices, patient movement, and staff operations. This includes consideration for future expansion.
   - Ergonomics and Workflow: Design the layout to optimize workflow, minimize patient movement, and ensure staff efficiency. The placement of control rooms, imaging rooms, and patient waiting areas should be logical and efficient.
   - Shielding: Install appropriate radiation shielding (lead-lined walls, doors, and windows) as per regulatory requirements to protect staff and the public from radiation exposure.
   - Environmental Conditions: Ensure proper ventilation, temperature control, and humidity levels to maintain optimal operating conditions for the equipment.
3. **Equipment Selection and Installation**
   - Needs Assessment: Evaluate clinical needs, patient volume, and types of procedures to determine the appropriate equipment.
   - Vendor Selection: Choose reputable vendors who provide reliable equipment, service, and support. Consider the total cost of ownership, including maintenance and upgrades.
   - Installation: Ensure proper installation by certified professionals. Follow the manufacturer's guidelines and protocols for installation and calibration.
4. **Safety and Quality Assurance**
   - Radiation Protection Program: Implement a radiation protection program that includes regular training for staff, monitoring of radiation exposure, and maintenance of protective equipment.
   - Quality Control: Establish a quality control program to regularly test and calibrate equipment to maintain image quality and safety. This includes routine checks and preventive maintenance.
   - Emergency Procedures: Develop and train staff on emergency procedures for radiation incidents, equipment failure, and patient emergencies.
5. **Training and Competence**
   - Staff Training: Provide comprehensive training for radiologists, technologists, and support staff on the operation, safety, and maintenance of the equipment.
   - Continuing Education: Encourage ongoing education and certification to keep staff

updated on the latest techniques, safety protocols, and technological advancements.

6. **Patient Care and Comfort**
   - Patient-Centric Design: Ensure that the facility design and equipment setup enhance patient comfort and privacy. Consider patient flow to reduce wait times and stress.
   - Communication: Maintain clear communication with patients regarding procedures, safety measures, and expected outcomes to enhance their experience and compliance.
7. **Technology Integration**
   - Picture Archiving and Communication Systems (PACS) and Radiology Information Systems (RIS) Integration: Integrate PACS and RIS smoothly for efficient data management.
   - Information technology (IT) Infrastructure: Develop a robust IT infrastructure to support the digital needs of modern radiology departments, including cybersecurity measures to protect patient data.
8. **Financial Planning and Budgeting**
   - Cost Analysis: Perform a detailed cost-benefit analysis to justify the investment in new equipment. Consider initial costs, operational costs, and potential revenue generation.
   - Funding and Reimbursement: Explore funding options and understand reimbursement policies for radiological services to ensure financial viability.

By adhering to these principles, radiology departments can ensure that they are equipped to provide high-quality diagnostic imaging services while maintaining safety, efficiency, and patient satisfaction.

9.2.1 Site Planning

Medical imaging requires an infrastructure that is well-maintained, well-trained physicians, and well-equipped equipment. The implementation of a quality assurance (QA) program will also ensure that minimal radiation exposure is incurred during the collection of radiographic data. Furthermore, local infrastructure influences the implementation scenario, such as energy and water supplies, temperature and humidity management, and IT infrastructure. Also, it is important to consider proper equipment maintenance, service contracts, and warranties, as well as necessary software updates. When implementing an imaging service, capital costs are often considered the most important factor.

The need for capacity building must be addressed, however, in order to ensure that there are enough trained personnel ready to carry out their duties in a safe and effective manner. Additionally, it is important to evaluate all expenditures associated with acquiring medical imaging equipment, such as spare parts, maintenance, upgrades, and staffing requirements. Generally, it is more difficult to sustain a site long-term than to purchase and install it initially. Increasingly complex technology makes medical imaging more dependent on a building's utility and quality systems. An example of digital imaging would be the use of a computer server and a network, along with safeguards to protect patient information.

Imaging operations are usually performed in a fixed site, such as a hospital or a standalone institution. Health professionals, architects, engineers, and hospital management work together to design imaging facility layouts. When planning an imaging facility, workload, patient flow, and types of imaging to be performed should be considered.

It is important to consider radiation protection and safety elements at all stages of the design process. Building designs should accommodate future expansions, since imaging departments typically grow over time. Patients should be able to access an imaging facility conveniently, both as inpatients and as outpatients. A larger room is ideal for accommodating patients on bed trolleys, as well as positioning and moving around equipment, depending on the imaging modalities. Whenever designing an imaging facility, you must include areas for changing cubicles, reception areas, reporting areas, server rooms, offices, and consumable storage areas.

Radiation safety precautions should be taken, including the installation of warning lights and signs at the gate entrances of areas that are supervised and regulated. A radiology reading room must control incoming light. In order to make interpretation easier for radiologists, medical images should be exhibited and read in specially constructed rooms. Vendors often provide site planning and installation recommendations. It should also include the final floor layout with the equipment positioned and scaled appropriately, as well as all local building, electrical, and safety requirements. Several factors play a role in site planning, such as the size and character of the project, the local traditions, the climate, and the budget. With regard to department design, including workflow, medical physicists support medical imaging experts, facility managers, planners, and architects. Medical physicists can also observe construction on site to ensure contractors follow architectural specifications [2, 3].

9.2.2 Radiation Shielding

Radiation-shielding frameworks are required for all medical imaging equipment that generates X-rays. It is important to follow applicable legislation and recommendations when designing and shielding facilities. It is the responsibility of a clinically competent medical physicist to offer shielding advice and ensure that shielding calculations follow relevant regulations. During the design phase, shielding estimates should be made. A room's shielding requirements may change if its intended use changes, if the equipment is improved, or if the workload or occupancy of neighboring rooms changes. The shielding of the imaging facility should be adequate before it can be used for clinical purposes. A shielding barrier, including its floors and ceilings, should be built according to applicable regulations, with viewing windows and doors that meet the shielding specifications appropriate to that barrier. Staff members should remain in shielded operator control rooms or areas, not near patients, except during fluoroscopy-guided procedures. It is possible for multiple neighboring imaging rooms to share the operator room. In this situation, ensuring audio and visual communication with patients is equally important.

9.2.3 Equipment Selection

The choice of equipment packages may depend on the imaging requirements and the resources available. As experts in the technical and radiation aspects of medical imaging equipment, medical physicists and medical imaging personnel play a crucial role in the selection, specification, and purchasing processes. Medical physicists must manage the service and repair aspects of equipment life cycles because they are a significant operational cost. In various healthcare settings, there are several types of imaging equipment that should be installed and operational. There is a close functional and operational link between nuclear medicine and diagnostic radiology departments.

Furthermore, local infrastructure, such as electricity and water supplies, temperature control, humidity, and IT infrastructure, is heavily influencing the choice of implementation scenario, in addition to human and financial resources. As previously mentioned, equipment maintenance, service contracts and warranties, and software updates must also be addressed.

Primary health care should meet the majority of patients' imaging needs. A small hospital or health facility uses basic imaging technology such as radiography, X-rays, and ultrasonography. Typically, secondary health care involves more complex imaging techniques. It comprises imaging equipment used in primary health care as well as advanced radiography (including fluoroscopy), Doppler ultrasonography, mammography, angiography, CT, radionuclide scintigraphy, and single-photon emission computed tomography (SPECT)-CT. Finally, tertiary health care includes all the equipment used in the preceding levels of care, as well as MRI, positron emission tomography (PET)-CT, and theranostics. Technical deliverables are connected to clinical quality through functional or performance standards.

It is important that the proposed system be aligned with the radiology departments' aims and the organization's core objectives. This includes objectives such as production, service quality, and efficiency. Among other considerations are workload, image quality, types of radiation monitors, retrieval time for an image or inspection, and so on. Detailed technical specifications for imaging equipment include particular acceptance criteria and are written in terms that can be used to design the equipment and its functions. In order to meet essential technical challenges, technical requirements should be centered on those challenges [2–5].

9.2.4 Staffing Levels

Radiology employs a variety of health professionals, including radiologists, medical imaging technologists, medical physicists, nurses, IT specialists, and service engineers. An imaging facility collaborates with this multidisciplinary team. It is recommended that minimum personnel credentials, education, and training comply with national regulations and international recommendations. It is important that the radiology service has adequate staffing to achieve its goals. A facility's development phase should include resources for staff education and training.

IT expertise is required based on the size of the facility. Smaller facilities may use on-site IT staff during design and installation and then move to off-site support afterward. For larger and more complex facilities, IT staff may be required to ensure the facility's computing technology operates reliably. Using PACS with RIS for managing requests, images, and reports may require a PACS administrator. Providing medical physics services requires clinically qualified medical physicists based on international recommendations and best practices. The Agency created an algorithm to determine how many clinically trained medical physicists are needed in radiology. In order to ensure the method's universal applicability, a variety of field conditions have been tested [6–9].

9.3 Regulatory Guidelines: X-Ray, Mammography, Fluoroscopy, CT, and Hybrid Imaging

Regulatory guidelines for imaging modalities such as X-ray, mammography, fluoroscopy, CT, and hybrid imaging are critical to ensuring patient safety, image quality, and proper technology application. Regulatory guidelines play a crucial role in ensuring the safe and effective use of X-ray imaging modalities across different healthcare settings worldwide. Various regulatory bodies and organizations establish standards and regulations to govern the practice of X-ray imaging, with a focus on optimizing patient care and minimizing radiation risks.

9.3.1 X-Ray Imaging

Regulatory agencies such as the International Atomic Energy Agency (IAEA), the FDA, and the European Commission provide comprehensive guidelines for the use of X-ray imaging equipment in medical diagnosis. These guidelines cover aspects such as equipment specifications, radiation safety measures, QA protocols, and personnel training requirements [10, 11].

X-Ray Imaging

- **IEC:** Establishes standards for X-ray equipment, including safety and performance requirements (IEC 60601).
- **International Commission on Radiological Protection (ICRP):** Provides radiation protection recommendations, such as exposure limits and safety practices.
- **WHO:** Provides tools and guidance for the safe use of X-ray imaging, especially in low-resource situations.

- **European Union (EU):** Implements the Basic Safety Standards (BSS) Directive (2013/59/Euratom), which specifies radiation protection principles and precautions for medical exposures.

9.3.2 Mammography

Mammography, a specialized form of X-ray imaging used for breast cancer screening and diagnosis, is subject to stringent regulatory oversight. Organizations such as the ACR and the European Society of Breast Imaging establish guidelines for mammography equipment performance, image quality standards, and accreditation criteria for mammography facilities [6, 12–18].

Mammography

- ACR: The Mammography Quality Standards Act (MQSA) rules provide high-quality mammographic images and patient safety in the United States.
- **European Reference Organization for Quality Assured Breast Screening and Diagnostic Services:** Determines European standards for mammography screening and QA.
- **IAEA:** Publishes radiation protection and QA recommendations for mammography.

9.3.3 Fluoroscopy

Fluoroscopy involves real-time X-ray imaging for visualizing dynamic anatomical structures during medical procedures. Regulatory agencies such as the FDA and the European Medicines Agency issue guidelines to ensure the safe and appropriate use of fluoroscopic equipment, radiation dose optimization, and quality control measures to minimize patient and staff radiation exposure [19–21].

Fluoroscopy

- **IEC:** The IEC 60601-2-54 specifies standards for fluoroscopic equipment, including safety and performance criteria.
- **ICRP:** Recommends radiation protection principles in fluoroscopy, emphasizing the significance of dose management and minimizing exposure.
- **FDA:** Regulates fluoroscopy equipment and provides manufacturers with rules to assure its safety and efficacy.

9.3.4 CT Imaging

CT imaging utilizes X-ray technology to create cross-sectional images of the body. Regulatory bodies such as the ACR and the ICRP establish guidelines for CT equipment performance, radiation dose management, image QA, and patient-specific dose optimization techniques [10, 22–25].

Computed Tomography

- **American Association of Physicists in Medicine:** Specifies CT imaging guidelines, including advice for dosage optimization and quality control.
- **ICRP:** Provides recommendations on radiation dose management in CT imaging, emphasizing the importance of balancing image quality and patient safety.
- **EU BSS Directive:** Addresses CT imaging-specific standards such as dose reporting and diagnostic reference levels.

9.3.5 Hybrid Imaging

Hybrid imaging modalities, such as PET-CT and SPECT-CT, combine X-ray imaging with other imaging modalities for enhanced diagnostic capabilities. Regulatory guidelines from organizations such as the European Association of Nuclear Medicine and the Society of Nuclear Medicine and Molecular Imaging (SNMMI) address issues related to equipment calibration, image fusion techniques, radiation dose optimization, and QA in hybrid imaging [26–36].

The following is a summary of essential guidelines and standards from major regulatory authorities and professional organizations.

9.3.5.1 Hybrid Imaging (PET/CT, SPECT/CT)

- **IEC:** Standards for hybrid imaging systems include IEC 60601-2-44 for CT components and IEC 60601-2-29 for nuclear medicine components.
- **IAEA:** Provides detailed instructions for safe and reliable use of hybrid imaging technologies, such as radiation protection and QA processes.
- **SNMMI:** Provides clinical guidelines and best practices for hybrid imaging techniques, ensuring accurate diagnosis and patient safety.

9.3.6 General Principles Across Modalities

- **Radiation Protection:** Comply with the ALARA concept, which involves optimizing techniques to reduce radiation exposure as low as reasonably possible while preserving diagnostic quality.
- **QA:** Implement regular quality control procedures to ensure that equipment performance and image quality meet regulatory requirements.
- **Staff Training:** Ensure that all imaging professionals are properly trained to operate imaging equipment, understand radiation safety, and follow emergency protocols.
- **Patient Safety:** Prioritize patient safety by employing proper shielding, positioning strategies, and communication to educate patients about procedures and safety precautions.

9.3.7 Resources Outline

- ICRP Publications: Comprehensive guidelines on radiation protection across various imaging modalities.
- IEC Standards: Technical standards for medical electrical equipment, including imaging devices.
- WHO Radiology Resources: Guidelines and tools for safe and effective imaging, especially in resource-limited settings.
- IAEA Safety Standards: Publications on radiation protection and safety in medical uses of ionizing radiation.
- EU BSS Directive: Legislative framework for radiation protection in medical exposures within the EU.

By adhering to these global regulatory criteria, healthcare providers can assure the safe and effective use of radiological imaging technologies, protecting both patients and employees. In summary, regulatory guidelines play a pivotal role in governing the safe and effective use of X-ray imaging modalities, including X-ray, mammography, fluoroscopy, CT, and hybrid imaging. Adherence to these guidelines is essential for ensuring patient safety, optimizing diagnostic accuracy, and maintaining quality standards in medical imaging practice [18, 37–44].

9.3.8 General Regulatory Requirements for Diagnostic Radiology Departments

1. **Procurement of X-Ray Equipment:** After receiving procurement approval from the Competent Authority, the employer must acquire NOC-validated/type-approved X-ray equipment from authorized vendors.
2. **Operation of X-Ray Equipment:** It is prohibited to use diagnostic X-ray equipment for patient diagnosis without a competent authority's license.
3. **Prerequisites for Obtaining License for Operation of X-Ray Equipment: X-Ray/CT/Interventional Radiology/Mobile Radiography Room Layout and Shielding Requirement.**

There should be an adequate area for staff movement and patient positioning in the room housing X-ray equipment. It is important to provide adequate structural shielding for the walls, doors, ceiling, and floor of the room housing the X-ray equipment to ensure that radiation exposure to workers and the general public is kept to a minimum and that the annual effective dose limit is not exceeded. At joints or discontinuities, shielding materials must overlap appropriately. A separate room outside but adjacent to the CT room should be installed for the control console, along with a place to view the patient directly and communicate with the imaging technologist.

The gantry and couch must be arranged in the control room so that the technologist can see the patient clearly. There must be a nearby control room equipped with adequate shielding, direct viewing, and oral communication capabilities for interventional radiology (IR) equipment. If the radiography equipment is installed in an X-ray room, a chest stand must be installed to prevent significant amounts of radiation from reaching the control console, entry door, and areas that are occupied full-time, as well as to ensure that radiation dosage limits are not exceeded for radiation workers and the general public.

All the same standards apply to mobile X-ray equipment that is operated as fixed X-ray equipment. Registered institutions/hospitals should restrict the movement of mobile X-ray equipment. X-ray installations must have a permanent radiation warning symbol and instructions posted on their entrance doors, indicating that X-ray radiation is produced by the equipment.

4. **Vehicle Mounted X-Ray Equipment:** In order to provide enough protection for anyone present inside and around a mobile truck or vehicle, X-ray equipment must be installed in an enclosure that provides suitable shielding. The equipment must be shielded on all sides up to a height of 2 m from the external ground surface. Both sides of the vehicle must display the radiation warning symbol.
5. **Staffing Requirements:** X-ray installations must have a radiologist/related medical practitioner/X-ray/Imaging technologist with the necessary radiation protection knowledge to operate the X-ray equipment. Employees involved in these operations are considered radiation workers and must follow the duties and obligations outlined in the competent authorities' radiation safety code for the manufacture, supply, and use of medical diagnostic X-ray equipment. The local Competent Authority will establish the minimum qualification and training requirements. All installations that use X-ray equipment with fluoroscopy, CT, or perform special procedures must have the services of a qualified radiologist or related medical practitioner who is knowledgeable about radiation protection and can interpret and report.
6. **Radiological Safety/Protection Officer (RPO/RSO):** The X-ray department must have an RSO/RPO approved by the Competent Authority. The RSO/RPO may be the employer himself/herself or an employee to whom the employer has delegated the obligation for ensuring compliance with the required radiation safety/regulatory standards applicable to his X-ray installation. The Competent Authority will determine the minimum qualification and training requirements.
7. **Radiation Protection Devices:** Radiation protection devices, such as barriers, aprons, goggles, and thyroid shields, should be used when operating X-ray equipment. A periodic verification of their shielding adequacy is required.
8. **Personnel monitoring services:** This will be supplied to all radiation workers. QA requirements. It is the end user's responsibility to ensure that periodic QA is performed on the equipment by local competent authorized entities. It is necessary to perform periodic QA, as well as to conduct radiation-safety repairs, at least once a year.
9. **Servicing:** It is the end user's responsibility to ensure that the X-ray equipment is serviced by authorized agencies.
10. **Periodic Safety Reports:** In accordance with the regulatory body's specifications, utilities must submit periodic safety reports.
11. **Renewal of License:** Licenses issued by the Competent Authority must be renewed before they expire. In order for X-ray equipment to be decommissioned, agencies must notify the competent authority in advance [12, 19, 45–49].

9.4 General Recommendations and Codal Requirements for Layout Planning: X-Ray, Mammography, Fluoroscopy, CT, and Hybrid Imaging

9.4.1 Codal Requirements

- Regulatory Compliance: Ensure that all designs comply with local, national, and international regulations and standards (e.g., National Council on Radiation Protection and Measurements (NCRP), ACR, IEC, and IAEA).
- Radiation Protection: Follow the ALARA principle, implementing necessary shielding and safety measures to minimize exposure.
- QA: Incorporate spaces for routine equipment testing and quality control procedures.
- Emergency Exits: Plan for emergency exits and ensure that they are clearly marked and accessible.
- Environmental Control: Ensure appropriate HVAC systems to control temperature, humidity, and air quality, preventing equipment overheating and ensuring patient comfort.

By adhering to these recommendations and codal requirements, radiology departments can ensure safe, efficient, and compliant operations for various imaging modalities.

When designing radiology department layouts, it is critical to consider both general suggestions and specific codal requirements for various imaging modalities to ensure safety, efficiency, and regulatory compliance. The following are the guidelines for X-ray, mammography, fluoroscopy, CT, and hybrid imaging facilities:

1. **General Layout Recommendations**
   - **Space and Flow:** Optimize patient flow, reduce wait times, and allow for efficient staff movement. Having separate spaces for distinct procedures can help to streamline operations.
   - **Accessibility:** Ensure accessibility for patients, particularly those with disabilities. Consider the positioning of entrances, exits, and waiting spaces.
   - **Ergonomics:** Plan ergonomic workstations to reduce strain on radiologists and technologists, increase productivity, and reduce injury hazards.
   - **Infection Control:** Implement infection control measures, such as clean surfaces, handwashing stations, and adequate ventilation.
2. **X-Ray Imaging**
   - **Room Size:** Ensure that the X-ray room is large enough to accommodate the equipment, patient, and staff, usually at least 15–20 square meters.
   - **Shielding:** Install lead-lined walls, doors, and windows to guard against radiation exposure. The thickness of the lead lining should meet local norms (e.g., 2 mm lead equivalent).
   - **Control Area:** Provide a control booth or area with a lead-glass window so that the imaging technologist may operate the equipment safely.
   - **Ventilation:** Maintain sufficient airflow to prevent heat buildup from the X-ray equipment.
3. **Mammography**
   - **Room Size:** A mammography room should be no less than 10–15 square meters in size.
   - **Shielding:** To safeguard against scattered radiation, use lead-lined walls and doors, just as you would for X-rays.
   - **Privacy:** Design the room to give patients privacy and comfort, including changing areas and secure storage for personal goods.
   - **Control Area:** Create a separate control space for the technologist, preferably with a lead-glass window or sufficient shielding.
4. **Fluoroscopy**
   - **Room Size:** Fluoroscopy rooms should be larger, ranging from 25 to 30 square meters,

to accommodate the equipment and sophisticated procedures.
- **Shielding:** Increased shielding needs due to increased radiation doses; walls, doors, and ceilings should be appropriately shielded (e.g., 3 mm lead equivalent).
- **Control Room:** A specialized control room with appropriate shielding and communication systems is required.
- **Patient Access:** Provide simple access for patients, especially those in stretchers or wheelchairs.

5. **Computed Tomography**
   - **Room Size:** CT rooms should be between 30 and 40 square meters to accommodate the scanner, control equipment, and patient.
   - **Shielding:** Increased radiation exposures necessitate larger shielding requirements, with walls and doors often requiring 2–3 mm of lead equivalent.
   - **Control Room:** A separate, protected control room with clear views of the patient area via lead-glass windows.
   - **Support Areas:** Include areas for patient preparation, recovery, and possible contrast media administration.
6. **Hybrid Imaging (PET/CT, SPECT/CT)**
   - **Room Size:** These rooms must be larger, approximately 40–50 square meters, to accommodate two imaging equipment and allow for patient movement.
   - **Shielding:** The combination of modalities provides enhanced shielding; assess the cumulative radiation exposure and shielding requirement accordingly (e.g., 3 mm lead equivalent or more).
   - **Control Room:** A fully protected control room equipped with sophisticated monitoring and communication equipment.
   - **Patient Preparation:** Include adjacent to facilities for patient preparation and recuperation, as well as spaces for safe radiopharmaceutical handling and administration.

Radiology departments are critical components of modern healthcare institutions, providing vital diagnostic imaging services to aid in the diagnosis, monitoring, and treatment of a wide range of medical disorders. To maintain the safety, efficiency, and efficacy of imaging services, various issues must be carefully considered while establishing and planning radiology departments. The following are the fundamental principles and stages involved in the installation and planning of radiography departments.

1. **Assessment of Needs**
   - **Clinical Requirements:** Recognize the clinical demands of the healthcare facility. This comprises the imaging services needed (such as X-rays, MRIs, CT scans, and ultrasounds) as well as the estimated patient volume.
   - **Technological Needs:** Assess technical requirements based on the present and future needs. This includes selecting the right imaging equipment and software solutions.
2. **Regulatory Compliance**
   - **Radiation Safety Standards:** Comply with national and international radiation safety regulations. This includes following the guidelines established by organizations such as the IAEA and the ACR.
   - **Licensing and Accreditation:** Obtain the required licenses and certificates from the appropriate health authorities and accreditation agencies.
3. **Site Selection and Design**
   - **Location:** Choose a site within the healthcare facility that is convenient for patients and workers while limiting exposure to other areas of the hospital.
   - **Space Planning:** Allow enough space for imaging rooms, control rooms, waiting areas, and administrative offices. Ensure that the arrangement allows for efficient workflow and patient movement.
   - **Shielding:** Use adequate shielding materials (such as lead-lined walls) to safeguard patients and workers from needless radiation exposure.
4. **Infrastructure Requirements**
   - **Power Supply:** Ensure that the power supply is reliable and sufficient to support high-energy imaging equipment.

- **Cooling Systems:** Install effective cooling systems to keep imaging equipment at appropriate working temperatures.
- **Network Connectivity:** Create a strong IT infrastructure to handle digital imaging, data storage, and integration with electronic health record systems.

5. **Equipment Selection and Installation**
   - **Vendor Selection:** Choose a reputable provider for imaging equipment based on quality, service support, and cost-effectiveness.
   - **Installation:** When installing imaging equipment, follow the manufacturer's directions. This includes calibration and testing to ensure precise and consistent performance.
   - **QA:** Implement a QA program to monitor imaging equipment performance and verify compliance with safety regulations.
6. **Staffing and Training**
   - **Qualified Personnel:** Hire qualified radiologists, radiologic technologists, and support personnel to run and administer the radiology department.
   - **Continuous Training:** Provide continuing training and professional development opportunities for employees to stay updated with technological advances and safety regulations.
7. **Workflow Optimization**
   - **Patient Scheduling:** Implement effective patient scheduling systems to reduce wait times and maximize the use of imaging equipment.
   - **Process Standardization:** Standardize imaging processes and procedures to ensure consistent and high-quality imaging services.
   - **Integration With Healthcare Systems:** Integrate seamlessly with hospital information systems and electronic medical records to improve data management and communication.
8. **Patient Safety and Comfort**
   - **Safety Protocols:** Establish and implement safety protocols to keep patients safe from radiation exposure and other hazards.
   - **Patient Comfort:** Design the radiology department with patient comfort in mind, including features such as comfortable waiting spaces, clear signs, and private rooms during imaging procedures.
9. **Maintenance and Upgrades**
   - **Regular Maintenance:** Create a maintenance schedule to ensure the longevity and peak performance of imaging equipment.
   - **Technological Upgrades:** Plan for periodic imaging technology improvements to keep up with advancements and increase diagnostic capabilities.
10. **Evaluation and Continuous Improvement**
    - **Performance Monitoring:** Continuously evaluate the radiology department's performance using key performance indicators such as patient throughput, imaging quality, and patient happiness.
    - **Feedback Mechanism:** Create a feedback process to collect feedback from patients and staff and use it to make necessary modifications.

Installation and design of radiology departments are complex operations that necessitate great attention to detail, adherence to safety regulations, and a dedication to continual development. Following these broad principles can help healthcare facilities assure the successful deployment of radiology services that are safe, efficient, and capable of addressing patients' diagnostic needs [50–59].

9.5 Barrier and Shielding Guidelines: X-Ray, Mammography, Fluoroscopy, CT, and Hybrid Imaging

Barrier and shielding recommendations for X-ray, mammography, fluoroscopy, CT, and hybrid imaging rooms are critical to protecting patients, personnel, and the public from ionizing radiation exposure. The following are specific suggestions for each modality:

1. **X-Ray Imaging**
   - **Primary Barrier:** It protects against direct radiation from the X-ray tube. Built with lead-lined walls, often 1.5–2 mm lead equivalent.
   - **Secondary Barrier:** Protects against scattered radiation. Walls and doors should be 1 mm lead equivalent.
   - **Control Booth:** Includes an observation window made of leaded glass. Walls and doors should be 1.5–2 mm lead equivalent.
2. **Mammography**
   - **Primary Barrier:** Provides shielding against the X-ray source. Walls and doors with a lead equivalent of 0.1–0.2 mm.
   - **Secondary Barrier:** Shields against dispersed radiation. Walls and doors have the same lead equivalent.
   - **Control Area:** Includes a shielded control booth. The leaded glass window has 0.1–0.2 mm lead equivalent.
3. **Fluoroscopy**
   - **Primary Barrier:** Protects against continuous exposure to high-energy radiation. Walls, doors, and ceilings have a lead equivalent of 2–3 mm.
   - **Secondary Barrier:** Protects against scatter and leakage radiation. Walls and doors have 1.5–2 mm lead equivalent.
   - **Control Room:** Fully shielded with leaded glass windows. The glass has 2–3 mm lead equivalent.
4. **Computed Tomography**
   - **Primary Barrier:** Shields against high-energy X-ray beams. Walls, doors, and ceilings with 2–3 mm lead equivalent.
   - **Secondary Barrier:** Protects against scattered radiation. Similar lead equivalent for walls and doors.
   - **Control Room:** Includes a shielded control area. The leaded glass windows have 2–3 mm lead equivalent.
5. **Hybrid Imaging (PET/CT)**
   - **Primary Barrier:** Shields against both X-ray and gamma radiation. Walls, doors, and ceilings have 3 mm lead equivalent or more.
   - **Secondary Barrier:** Provides additional protection against scattered radiation. Similar lead equivalent for walls and doors.
   - **Control Room:** Fully shielded with leaded glass windows. The glass has 3 mm lead equivalent.

General Shielding Guidelines

- **Material Selection:** The common shielding materials are lead-lined gypsum board, concrete, or leaded glass.
- **Lead Equivalent:** Refers to the thickness of lead that provides equivalent attenuation of radiation.
- **Distance:** Increasing distance from the radiation source reduces exposure, but proper shielding is still necessary.
- **Occupancy Factor:** Accounts for time the area is occupied.
- **Use Factor:** Considers the directionality and frequency of use of the X-ray equipment.
- **Workload:** Determines the level of shielding required based on the frequency and types of procedures performed.

Regulatory References

- NCRP
- ICRP
- ACR
- IAEA
- IEC

Adhering to these recommendations ensures that imaging facilities provide adequate radiation protection while also allowing diagnostic imaging equipment to operate safely and effectively.

9.5.1 Options in Shielding Materials

To protect the public from excessive X-ray radiation, X-ray equipment must be installed in appropriately shielded rooms. Shielding effectiveness is determined by its thickness and substance. Material shielding can be achieved in a variety of ways. Bricks and concrete, however, are considered to be the ideal materials because they are readily available and inexpensive and have a high structural strength. A lead shield is appropriate for shielding X-ray energy, but it is weak structurally and prone to loss of homogeneity, so periodic radiation surveys are necessary to keep it effective. Lead is also an environmental threat, and its use is discouraged worldwide. As an alternative to lead, many new materials have been developed for use as shielding materials. Based on the evidence of shielding effectiveness, all international radiation authorities would encourage the use of these materials.

9.5.2 Step-by-Step Guidelines for Submission of Layout Plan in Diagnostic Radiology Facility

- Choose an appropriate room for hosting an X-ray unit to allow for ease of staff movement and patient positioning.
- In the X-ray room, there should be at least one entrance door and a window that is higher than 2 m above the finished floor level.
- For the door to remain closed during the procedure, it should have a hydraulic mechanism, and it should overlap at the joints to prevent streaming.
- Identify the walls as Walls A, B, C, and D (in any order).

Organize each modality's equipment as follows

(a) **Radiography and Fluoroscopy Equipment**: Couch, control console, and chest stand should be arranged so that the chest stand is opposite the entrance door and console. In order to ensure full protection for the operator, the mobile protective barrier should include a lead equivalent glass viewing window. The control console should be as far away from the X-ray tube as possible.

(b) **IR and CT Equipment:** The basic requirements are a gantry/C-arm, a couch, a separate console room, and a viewing window. It is important to position the gantry and couch so that the patient is fully visible from the control panel during the scanning process. From the control console, the gantry room's entrance door must meet the same specifications as the patient's.

(c) **Mammography/ Orthopantomogram (OPG)/ Cone Beam Computed Tomography (CBCT): Control Console, Equipment, and Protective Barrier**

Equipment should be placed as far away from the door and control console as possible.

- The equipment-specific chart can be used to determine the materials and thickness of walls and doors.
- The length between all the walls, doors, and windows should be measured from the center of the couch outward.
- Tabulate the details of layout and shielding as described by the local competent authorities and manufacturer guidelines.
- Shielding materials must be at least 2 m high from the X-ray room's finished floor.
- As part of the commissioning process, the equipment supplier will conduct a radiation survey to evaluate the adequacy of the design and construction of structural shielding. It may be necessary to modify equipment or procedures if the evaluation survey reveals inadequacies.

9.5.3 Shielding Criteria: Mammography, Fluoroscopy, CT, and Hybrid Imaging

Shielding regulations for X-ray, mammography, fluoroscopy, CT, and hybrid imaging installation rooms are vital to maintain radiation safety for patients, workers, and the general public. The following are thorough references and instructions for protecting these various types of imaging facilities.

1. **General Principles of Radiation Shielding**
   - Primary Barriers: Protect against the primary beam from the X-ray source.
   - Secondary Barriers: Protect against scattering and leakage radiation.
   - Shielding Materials: Commonly used materials include lead, concrete, and lead-

equivalent materials. The thickness of these materials depends on the type of imaging, workload, use factor, occupancy factor, and distance.

2. **X-Ray Imaging**
   - Room Size: Minimum 15–20 square meters.
   - Primary Barriers: Lead-lined walls with a thickness of 1.5–2 mm lead equivalent.
   - Secondary Barriers: Typically require 1 mm lead equivalent for walls and doors.
   - Control Booth: Shielding for control booths typically includes leaded glass windows with 1.5–2 mm lead equivalent.
3. **Mammography**
   - Room Size: Minimum 10–15 square meters.
   - Primary Barriers: Usually, 0.1–0.2 mm lead equivalent due to lower energy X-rays used in mammography.
   - Secondary Barriers: 0.1 mm lead equivalent for walls and doors is often sufficient.
   - Control Area: Shielded with 0.1–0.2 mm lead equivalent; leaded glass with 0.1–0.2 mm lead equivalent.
4. **Fluoroscopy**
   - Room Size: Minimum 25–30 square meters.
   - Primary Barriers: 2–3 mm lead equivalent due to the higher energy and continuous exposure.
   - Secondary Barriers: 1.5–2 mm lead equivalent for walls and doors.
   - Control Room: Shielded with 2–3 mm lead equivalent; leaded glass windows with similar lead equivalent.
5. **Computed Tomography**
   - Room Size: Minimum 30–40 square meters.
   - Primary Barriers: 2–3 mm lead equivalent to accommodate higher energy beams.
   - Secondary Barriers: 1.5–2 mm lead equivalent for walls and doors.
   - Control Room: Shielded with 2–3 mm lead equivalent; leaded glass with 2–3 mm lead equivalent.
6. **Hybrid Imaging (PET/CT)**
   - Room Size: Minimum 40–50 square meters.
   - Primary Barriers: 3 mm lead equivalent or more due to the combination of modalities and higher doses.
   - Secondary Barriers: 2–3 mm lead equivalent for walls, doors, and ceilings.
   - Control Room: Shielded with 3 mm lead equivalent; leaded glass windows with similar lead equivalent.
   - Radiopharmaceutical Handling: Additional shielding for areas where radiopharmaceuticals are stored and handled, often involving concrete or lead-lined compartments.
7. **Regulatory and Reference Sources**
   - NCRP Reports:
     - NCRP Report No. 147: Structural Shielding Design for Medical X-ray Imaging Facilities
     - NCRP Report No. 145: Radiation Protection in Dentistry
     - NCRP Report No. 151: Structural Shielding Design and Evaluation for Megavoltage X- and Gamma-Ray Radiotherapy Facilities
   - ACR Guidelines:
     - ACR provides technical standards and guidelines for various imaging modalities, including shielding recommendations.
   - IAEA:
     - Safety Reports Series No. 47: Radiological Protection for Medical Exposure to Ionizing Radiation
     - Technical Reports Series No. 457: Dosimetry in Diagnostic Radiology: An International Code of Practice
   - ICRP Publications:
     - ICRP Publication 60: Recommendations of the International Commission on Radiological Protection
     - ICRP Publication 73: Radiological Protection and Safety in Medicine
   - IEC Standards:
     - IEC 60601-1-3: General Requirements for Radiation Protection in Diagnostic X-Ray Equipment

To ensure compliance and safety in the design of radiology departments, it is crucial to adhere to the above shielding guidelines and consult relevant regulatory documents. These measures protect against excessive radiation exposure and help maintain a safe environment for both patients and healthcare professionals [10, 23, 30, 34–36, 50, 51, 60–71].

9.6 Model Layout Plan: X-Ray, Mammography, Fluoroscopy, CT, and Hybrid Imaging

Radiology model layout and planning involve several key steps to ensure efficient workflow, patient safety, and optimal use of space and resources. Here is a guide to planning a radiology department layout:

1. **Assessment of Requirements**
   - Space Requirements: Determine the number of rooms needed for different imaging modalities (e.g., X-ray, MRI, CT, and ultrasound).
   - Workflow Analysis: Understand the workflow for patient intake, imaging, and reporting to design a layout that minimizes movement and maximizes efficiency.
   - Regulatory Compliance: Ensure compliance with health and safety regulations, including radiation shielding requirements.
2. **Design Principles**
   - Patient-Centered Design: Create a comfortable and accessible environment for patients.
   - Staff Efficiency: Design workspaces that facilitate quick and efficient workflows for radiologists and technicians.
   - Safety: Incorporate features that protect patients and staff from unnecessary exposure to radiation and other hazards.
3. **Key Areas and Their Layouts**
   - Reception and Waiting Area: Comfortable seating, clear signage, and easy access to restrooms
   - Imaging Rooms:
     – X-ray Room: Proper shielding, patient positioning equipment, and control area
     – MRI Room: Shielded from external RF interference, with a control room and patient preparation area
     – CT Room: Similar to the X-ray room with additional space for gantry and control room
     – Ultrasound Room: Comfortable for patient and sonographer, with appropriate space for equipment
   - Reporting and Reading Room: Quiet, well-lit area for radiologists to review images
   - Storage and Maintenance: Space for storing imaging supplies and maintaining equipment
4. **Technology Integration**
   - PACS : Integrate digital imaging storage and retrieval systems.
   - RIS: Efficient patient management and workflow tracking
5. **Future Proofing**
   - Scalability: Design spaces that can be easily modified or expanded as technology and needs evolve.
   - Technological Advancements: Plan for future technology integration and upgrades.
6. **Collaboration with Stakeholders**
   - Medical Staff: Get input from radiologists, technologists, and nurses.
   - Architects and Engineers: Work with professionals to design and construct the facility.
   - Compliance Experts: Ensure that all regulatory and safety standards are met.

Example Layout

1. Entrance:
   - Reception desk
   - Waiting area
   - Patient restrooms
2. Imaging suite:
   - X-ray room
   - CT room
   - MRI room
   - Ultrasound room
3. Support areas:
   - Control rooms adjacent to imaging rooms
   - Equipment storage
   - Staff break room

4. Post-Imaging:
   - Reporting and reading room
   - Consultation room for patient discussions
5. Support services:
   - IT room for PACS/RIS servers
   - Maintenance room for equipment servicing

Effective radiology model layout and planning require a balance of functionality, comfort, and safety. By carefully considering the needs of patients and staff, as well as future technological advancements, a well-designed radiology department can provide high-quality care and efficient services.

Developing a model layout plan for a radiology department, including X-ray, mammography, fluoroscopy, CT, and hybrid imaging capabilities, requires various considerations to assure patient safety, efficiency, and comfort. The following is a detailed plan that outlines the important parts for each type of imaging room, as well as the recommended spatial relationships and architectural aspects [72–75].

General Design Principles

- **Zoning:** Divide the department into distinct zones for each modality to improve patient flow and staff efficiency.
- **Patient Privacy:** Ensure that there are private changing and waiting areas.
- **Accessibility:** Plan for simple access for all patients, including those with disabilities.
- **Safety:** To protect against radiation, incorporate suitable shielding.
- **Workflow Optimization:** Arrange rooms such that patients and personnel have the shortest possible travel lengths.

1. **X-Ray Room**

Designing an X-ray imaging room entails building a space that can house the necessary equipment, assure patient and staff safety, and maximize workflow efficiency. The following is a general layout plan for an X-ray imaging room:

Key Components of an X-Ray Imaging Room

1. X-Ray Equipment:
   - X-Ray Machine: The central piece of equipment often includes a table and an overhead tube crane or a wall-mounted system.
   - Control Panel: Located outside the main imaging area to protect the technician from radiation exposure.
2. Patient Area:
   - X-Ray Table: Adjustable and radiolucent table for patient positioning
   - Standing X-Ray Stand: For upright images, such as chest X-rays
3. Control Room:
   - Adjacent to the X-ray room with leaded glass windows for radiation protection and visual communication
   - Houses control panels and computer systems for operating the X-ray machine and processing images
4. Storage:
   - Cabinets and shelves for storing X-ray cassettes, protective aprons, and other supplies
5. Radiation Protection:
   - Lead-lined walls, doors, and windows to protect staff and patients from radiation exposure
   - Personal protective equipment such as lead aprons, gloves, and thyroid shields
6. Patient Changing Area:
   - A space with privacy for patients to change into gowns before the procedure
7. Utility Areas:
   - Clean Utility: For storing clean and sterile supplies
   - Dirty Utility: For disposing of used instruments and materials
8. Staff Support Areas:
   - Changing rooms, restrooms, and lounges for staff comfort and convenience

Room Size: 15–20 square meters.

Layout Elements as Depicted in Fig. 9.1.

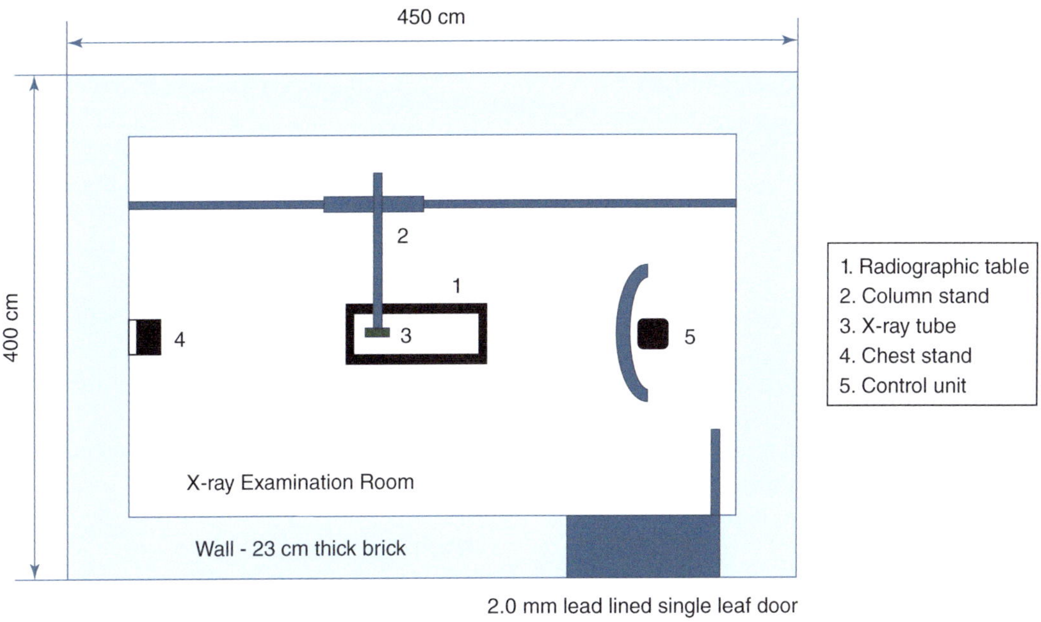

Fig. 9.1 Model X-ray layout

- X-ray equipment is centrally located to facilitate a complete range of motion.
- The control booth is adjacent to the X-ray room and has a lead-glass window for observation.
- Shielding includes lead-lined walls (2 mm lead equivalent), doors, and windows.
- The patient area features a central examination table and clear passageways.

Design:

- The control booth should be accessible from the corridor.
- Enough room surrounding the X-ray machine for patient movement and placement.

2. **Mammography Room**

Designing a mammography room entails establishing an environment that is comfortable for patients, efficient for staff, and meets all technical and safety criteria for mammography imaging. Here is a general reference to the arrangement of a mammography room:

Key Components of a Mammography Room

1. Mammography Equipment:
   - Mammography Machine: The central piece of equipment often includes a dedicated workstation for the technologist.
   - Compression Device: Attached to the mammography machine for positioning and compressing the breast
2. Control Panel:
   - Located outside the main imaging area or in a lead-shielded alcove to protect the technician from radiation exposure
3. Patient Area:
   - Mammography Machine Position: Ensure that there is enough space around the machine for patient and technologist movement.
   - Chair/Stool: For patient comfort if needed during the procedure.
4. Control Room/Area:
   - Adjacent to or within the mammography room with leaded glass windows for radiation protection and visual communication

- Houses control panels and computer systems for operating the mammography machine and processing images

5. Storage:
   - Cabinets and shelves for storing mammography cassettes, protective aprons, and other supplies
6. Radiation Protection:
   - Lead-lined walls, doors, and windows to protect staff and patients from radiation exposure
   - Personal protective equipment such as lead aprons and thyroid shields
7. Patient Changing Area:
   - A space with privacy for patients to change into gowns before the procedure
8. Waiting Area:
   - Comfortable seating for patients waiting for their turn or results
9. Utility Areas:
   - Clean Utility: For storing clean and sterile supplies
   - Dirty Utility: For disposing of used instruments and materials
10. Staff Support Areas:
    - Changing rooms, restrooms, and lounges for staff comfort and convenience

Room Size: 10–15 square meters
Layout Elements as Depicted in Fig. 9.2.

- The mammography unit should be conveniently located for easy access.
- Control Area: A small, shielded area with a lead-glass window.
- Shielding: 0.1–0.2 mm lead equivalent for walls and doors.
- Changing Area: A private space for patients to change.

Design:

- The control area can be a small, shielded corner within the room.
- Separate changing area to enhance patient privacy.

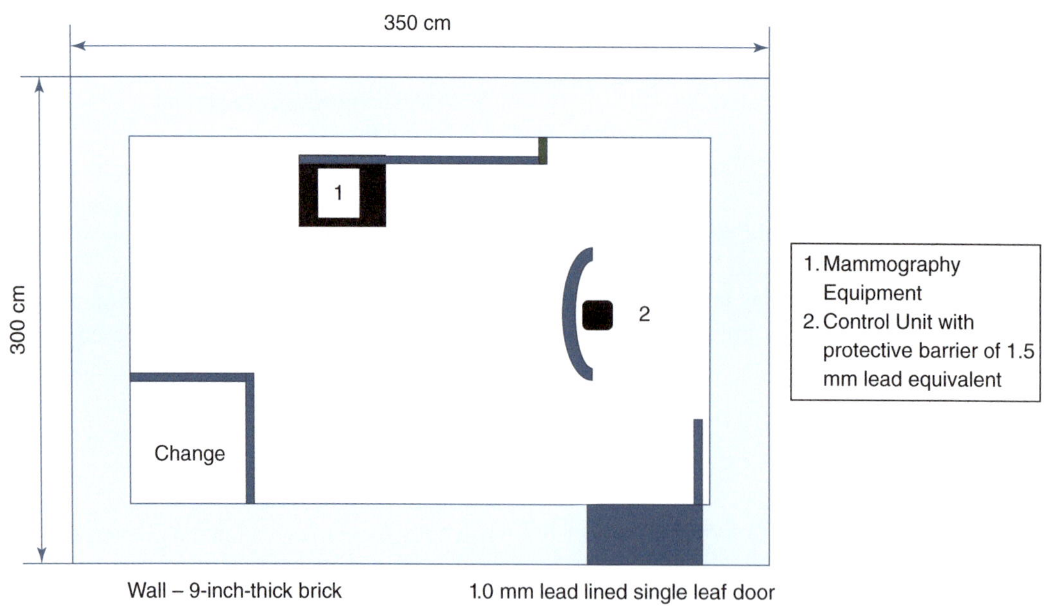

Fig. 9.2 Model layout for mammography

3. **Fluoroscopy Room**

A fluoroscopy room must be carefully designed to accommodate equipment, assure safety, and produce an efficient workflow. Here is a full guide on the layout of a fluoroscopy room:

Key Components of a Fluoroscopy Room

1. Fluoroscopy Equipment:
   - Fluoroscopy Table: Adjustable and radiolucent table for patient positioning
   - C-Arm or Fluoroscopy Unit: The main imaging device, often ceiling-mounted or mobile
   - Monitors: Multiple high-resolution monitors for real-time imaging display
2. Control Room:
   - Adjacent to the fluoroscopy room with leaded glass windows for radiation protection and visual communication
   - Houses control consoles for operating the fluoroscopy unit and viewing images
3. Patient Area:
   - Patient Preparation Area: Space for setting up and preparing patients, including IV administration if necessary
   - Patient Table: Positioned centrally to allow for easy access from both sides
4. Storage:
   - Cabinets and shelves for storing sterile supplies, contrast media, and other necessary equipment
   - Lead-lined storage for any radioactive materials if used
5. Radiation Protection:
   - Lead-lined walls, doors, and windows to protect staff and patients from radiation exposure
   - Personal protective equipment such as lead aprons, thyroid shields, and lead glasses
6. Scrub Area:
   - Dedicated space for staff to scrub in before procedures, ideally located near the entrance to the fluoroscopy room
7. Utility Areas:
   - Clean Utility: For storing clean and sterile supplies
   - Dirty Utility: For disposing of used instruments and materials
8. Staff Support Areas:

- Changing rooms, restrooms, and lounges for staff comfort and convenience

Design Considerations

1. Workflow Efficiency:
   - Ensure smooth movement of staff, patients, and equipment.
   - Minimize the need for staff to leave the room during procedures.
2. Infection Control:
   - Easy-to-clean surfaces and materials
   - Adequate handwashing stations
3. Ergonomics:
   - Adjustable equipment and furniture to reduce staff fatigue
   - Clear line of sight from the control room to the patient area
4. Safety:
   - Proper ventilation to control air quality
   - Backup power supply for critical equipment
5. Patient Comfort:
   - Warm lighting and temperature control
   - Privacy considerations
6. Technical Considerations:
   - Ensure adequate space for the C-arm to move freely around the patient table
   - Shielding for radiation protection, including lead-lined walls, doors, and glass
7. Aesthetics and Ambiance:
   - Soft, calming colors and artwork to reduce patient anxiety
   - Comfortable seating in the patient preparation area

Detailed Room Layout

Control Room:

- Located adjacent to the fluoroscopy room
- Includes computer consoles, monitors, and seating for the technician

Fluoroscopy Room:

- Fluoroscopy Unit (C-arm): Positioned centrally with enough space for full rotation and movement
- Patient Table: Centrally located to allow access from both sides
- Monitors: Positioned for easy viewing by the physician and staff
- Patient Preparation Area: Includes seating, IV setup, and possibly a small sink
- Storage: Shelves or cabinets near the entrance for easy access to supplies

Scrub Area:

- Located near the entrance of the fluoroscopy suite
- Includes sinks and handwashing stations

Utility Areas:

- Clean Utility: For storing clean supplies, located conveniently for staff
- Dirty Utility: For disposing of used materials, located away from clean areas

This layout and these considerations provide a foundation for designing an effective fluoroscopy room. Each facility may have specific requirements that need to be incorporated into the final design.

Room Size: 25–30 square meters
Layout Elements as Depicted in Fig. 9.3.

- The fluoroscopy equipment should be positioned centrally to allow for table movement.
- The control room should be well protected and possess an observation window.
- For walls and doors, shield with 2–3 mm of lead.
- Patient Area: Enough area for patient positioning and staff movement.

Design:

- Direct access from patient preparation areas
- Sufficient space for ancillary equipment (e.g., contrast media injector)

4. **CT Room**

Designing a CT room entails planning for huge equipment, assuring patient and staff safety,

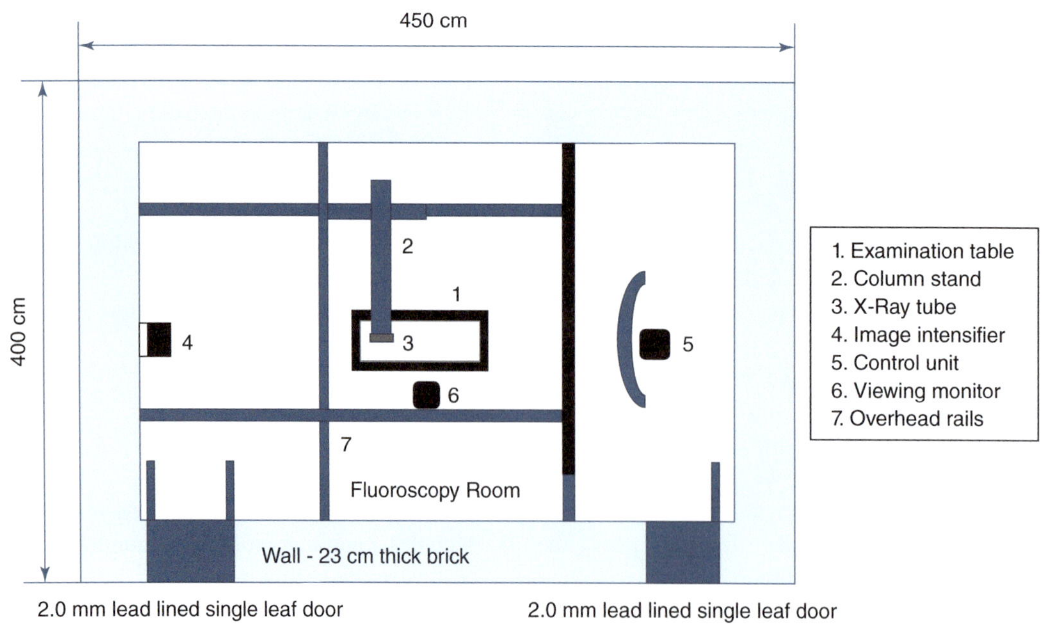

Fig. 9.3 Model layout for fluoroscopy

and maximizing workflow efficiency. Here is a complete guide on the layout of a CT room:

Key Components of a CT Room

1. CT Scanner:
   - Gantry: The main component where the patient lies down for the scan
   - Patient Table: Adjustable table that moves through the gantry
2. Control Room:
   - Adjacent to the CT room with leaded glass windows for radiation protection and visual communication
   - Houses control consoles for operating the CT scanner and monitoring the patient
3. Patient Preparation Area:
   - Space for patients to wait or prepare for the scan, possibly including an IV setup area for contrast administration
4. Storage:
   - Cabinets and shelves for storing supplies, contrast media, and emergency drugs
5. Radiation Protection:
   - Lead-lined walls, doors, and windows to protect staff and patients from radiation exposure
   - Personal protective equipment such as lead aprons and thyroid shields
6. Patient Changing Area:
   - A space with privacy for patients to change into gowns before the procedure
7. Utility Areas:
   - Clean Utility: For storing clean and sterile supplies
   - Dirty Utility: For disposing of used instruments and materials
8. Staff Support Areas:
   - Changing rooms, restrooms, and lounges for staff comfort and convenience

Room Size: 30–40 square meters
Layout Elements as Depicted in Fig. 9.4.

- CT Scanner: Positioned centrally, with ample space around for patient and staff movement
- Control Room: Adjacent, shielded control room with leaded glass window
- Shielding: 2–3 mm lead equivalent for walls, doors, and ceiling
- Patient Preparation Area: Close to the CT room for ease of access

Design:

- Control room with a clear view of the scanner and the patient
- Consider including a separate area for contrast media preparation and administration

5. **Hybrid Imaging Room (PET/CT)**

Designing a PET-CT room entails merging the requirements for PET and CT imaging, guaran-

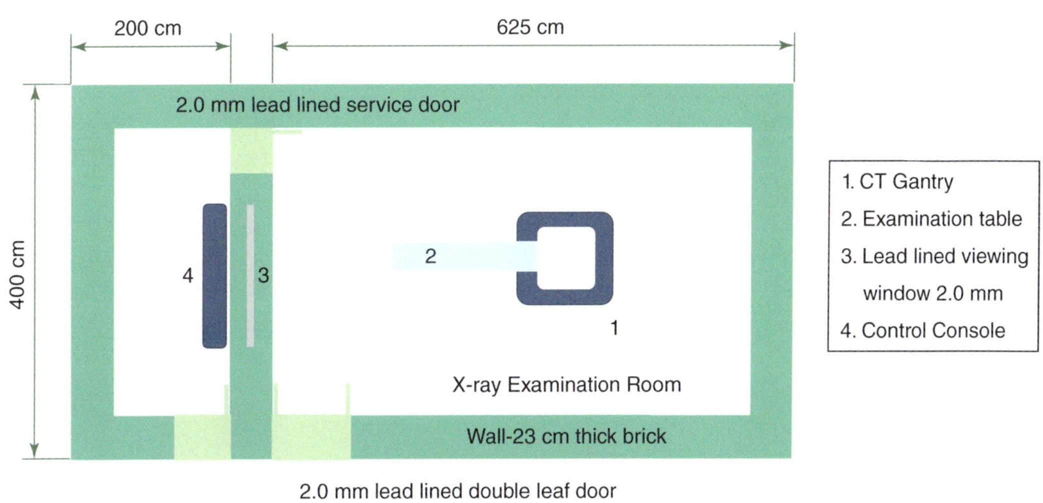

Fig. 9.4 Model CT layout

teeing radiation safety, and establishing an efficient workflow. Here is a detailed guidance on the layout plan for a PET-CT room:

Key Components of a PET-CT Room

1. PET-CT Scanner:
   - Gantry: The main component where the patient lies down for the scan
   - Patient Table: Adjustable table that moves through the gantry
2. Control Room:
   - Adjacent to the PET-CT room with leaded glass windows for radiation protection and visual communication
   - Houses control consoles for operating the PET-CT scanner and monitoring the patient
3. Injection/Preparation Room:
   - Space for administering radioactive tracers to the patient before the scan
   - Seating and IV setup for patient preparation
4. Waiting Area:
   - Comfortable seating for patients waiting for their turn or results
5. Storage:
   - Cabinets and shelves for storing supplies, contrast media, and emergency drugs
6. Radiation Protection:
   - Lead-lined walls, doors, and windows to protect staff and patients from radiation exposure
   - Personal protective equipment such as lead aprons and thyroid shields
7. Patient Changing Area:
   - A space with privacy for patients to change into gowns before the procedure
8. Utility Areas:
   - Clean Utility: For storing clean and sterile supplies
   - Dirty Utility: For disposing of used instruments and materials
9. Staff Support Areas:
   - Changing rooms, restrooms, and lounges for staff comfort and convenience

Design Considerations

1. Workflow Efficiency:
   - Ensure smooth movement of staff, patients, and equipment.
   - Minimize the need for staff to leave the room during procedures.
2. Infection Control:
   - Easy-to-clean surfaces and materials
   - Adequate handwashing stations
3. Ergonomics:
   - Adjustable equipment and furniture to reduce staff fatigue
   - Clear line of sight from the control room to the patient table
4. Safety:
   - Proper ventilation to control air quality
   - Backup power supply for critical equipment
5. Patient Comfort:
   - Warm lighting and temperature control
   - Privacy considerations
6. Technical Considerations:
   - Ensure adequate space for the PET-CT gantry to rotate and for the patient table to move smoothly
   - Shielding for radiation protection, including lead-lined walls, doors, and glass
7. Aesthetics and Ambiance:
   - Soft, calming colors and artwork to reduce patient anxiety
   - Comfortable seating in the patient preparation and waiting areas

Detailed Room Layout as Depicted in Fig. 9.5

Control Room:

- Located adjacent to the PET-CT room
- Includes computer consoles, monitors, and seating for the technician

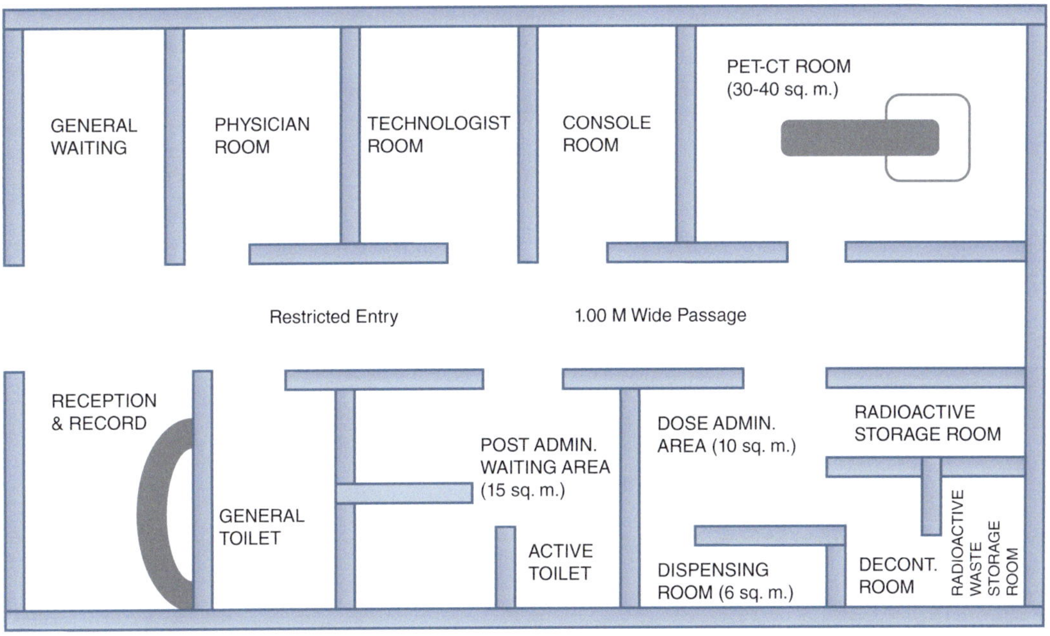

Fig. 9.5 Model PET-CT layout

PET-CT Room:

- PET-CT Scanner: Positioned centrally with enough space for full rotation and movement
- Patient Table: Centrally located to allow access from both sides
- Monitors: Positioned for easy viewing by the physician and staff
- Patient Preparation Area: Includes seating, IV setup, and possibly a small sink
- Storage: Shelves or cabinets near the entrance for easy access to supplies

Injection/Preparation Room:

- Located near the entrance of the PET-CT suite
- Includes seating, IV setup, and possibly a small sink
- Dedicated space for administering radioactive tracers

Waiting Area:

- Comfortable seating for patients waiting for their turn or results

Patient Changing Area:

- Located near the entrance of the PET-CT suite
- Includes lockers or closets for personal belongings

Utility Areas:

- Clean Utility: For storing clean supplies, located conveniently for staff
- Dirty Utility: For disposing of used materials, located away from clean areas

This arrangement and these concepts establish the groundwork for constructing an effective PET-CT room. Each facility may have unique requirements that must be factored into the final design.

Room Size: 40–50 square meters
Layout Elements as Depicted in Fig. 9.6.

- Imaging Equipment: Centrally located to accommodate both modalities
- Control Room: Fully shielded, with lead-glass window for monitoring

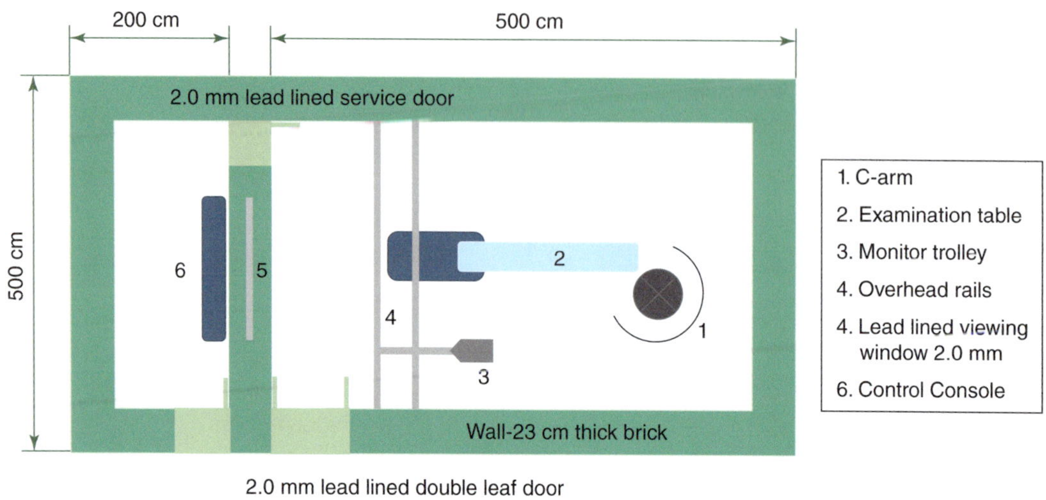

Fig. 9.6 Model layout IR

- Shielding: 3 mm lead equivalent for walls, doors, and ceiling
- Patient Preparation and Recovery Area: Separate spaces for preparing and recovering patients
- Radiopharmaceutical Storage: Secure, shielded storage for radiopharmaceuticals

  Design:

- Control room designed to manage both PET and CT operations
- Close proximity to radiopharmaceutical preparation areas

Spatial Relationships and Workflow

- Reception and Waiting Areas: Centralized to serve all modalities, with clear signage
- Changing Rooms: Strategically located near X-ray, mammography, and CT rooms
- Corridors: Wide enough to accommodate stretchers and wheelchairs
- Staff Areas: Centralized staff workstations for efficient communication and access
- Emergency Exits: Clearly marked and easily accessible from all rooms

6. **Interventional Radiology**

Designing an IR room requires careful consideration to ensure that it fits clinical requirements, safety regulations, and operational efficiency. Here is a general layout plan for an IR room:

Key Components of an IR Room

1. Procedure Room:
   - Size: Typically, around 600–800 square feet to accommodate equipment, staff, and patient movement
   - Ceiling Height: Minimum of 10 feet to accommodate ceiling-mounted equipment
2. Imaging Equipment:
   - Fluoroscopy System: Central piece of equipment, often ceiling-mounted to allow for flexibility
   - Monitors: Multiple high-resolution monitors on movable arms for imaging and data display
3. Patient Area:
   - Procedure Table: Adjustable and radiolucent table for patient positioning
   - Patient Monitoring: Essential for real-time tracking of vitals
4. Control Room:
   - Adjacent to the procedure room with leaded glass windows for radiation protection and visual communication
   - Houses control consoles for imaging equipment and monitors for real-time viewing

5. Scrub Area:
   - Dedicated space for staff to scrub in before procedures, ideally located near the entrance to the procedure room
6. Storage:
   - Cabinets and shelves for storing sterile supplies, instruments, and medications
   - Lead-lined storage for radioactive materials if applicable
7. Anesthesia Workstation:
   - Space for anesthesia equipment and supplies
8. Radiation Protection:
   - Lead-lined walls and doors to protect staff and patients from radiation exposure
   - Personal protective equipment such as lead aprons and thyroid shields
9. Utility Areas:
   - Clean Utility: For storing clean and sterile supplies
   - Dirty Utility: For disposing of used instruments and materials
10. Staff Support Areas:
   - Changing rooms, restrooms, and lounges for staff comfort and convenience

Design Considerations

1. Workflow Efficiency:
   - Ensure smooth movement of staff, patients, and equipment.
   - Minimize the need for staff to leave the room during procedures.

2. Infection Control:
   - Easy-to-clean surfaces and materials
   - Adequate handwashing stations
3. Ergonomics:
   - Adjustable equipment and furniture to reduce staff fatigue
   - Clear line of sight from the control room to the procedure table
4. Safety:
   - Proper ventilation to control air quality
   - Backup power supply for critical equipment
5. Patient Comfort:
   - Warm lighting and temperature control
   - Privacy considerations

This layout and these considerations provide a foundation for designing an effective IR room. Each facility may have specific requirements that need to be incorporated into the final design.

The journey of designing a radiology department is an intricate and dynamic process that demands a careful blend of technical expertise, patient-centered care, and forward-thinking strategies. This book guide has aimed to provide a comprehensive roadmap for planning and executing an efficient and effective radiology model layout [76–84]. As we conclude, it is important to reflect on the key takeaways and the impact of a well-designed radiology department.

Key Takeaways

1. Patient-Centered Design:
   - The layout should prioritize the comfort, privacy, and ease of navigation for patients. This not only enhances patient satisfaction but also contributes to the overall efficiency of the department.
2. Workflow Optimization:
   - Streamlining the workflow for healthcare providers is crucial. A thoughtfully designed layout reduces unnecessary movement, minimizes waiting times, and improves the speed and accuracy of diagnoses.
3. Safety and Compliance:
   - Ensuring compliance with regulatory standards and implementing robust safety measures protects both patients and staff from potential hazards, particularly related to radiation exposure.
4. Technological Integration:
   - The incorporation of advanced technologies such as PACS and RIS enhances the department's functionality, allowing for seamless digital imaging and information management.
5. Future-Proofing:
   - Designing with scalability and technological advancements in mind ensures that the radiology department can adapt to future needs and innovations without significant overhauls.

Impact of an Effective Radiology Department

A well-designed radiology department has far-reaching benefits. It enhances diagnostic accuracy and speed, leading to better patient outcomes. Efficient workflows and a comfortable environment reduce stress for both patients and staff, fostering a positive healthcare experience. Moreover, compliance with safety standards and the integration of cutting-edge technology position the department at the forefront of medical imaging services.

Looking Ahead

The field of radiology is continually evolving, driven by technological advancements and changing healthcare needs. As such, continuous evaluation and adaptation of the radiology department layout are essential. Engaging with stakeholders, including medical staff, patients, and regulatory bodies, ensures that the department remains responsive to new challenges and opportunities.

Final Thoughts

Designing a radiology department is a significant investment in the future of healthcare. By adhering to the principles outlined in this book guide, healthcare providers can create a space that is not only functional and efficient but also compassionate and patient-focused. The ultimate goal is to deliver high-quality imaging services that support the best possible care for patients.

As we conclude this guide, remember that the success of a radiology department lies in the details of its planning and execution. With careful consideration and collaborative effort, the ideal radiology model layout is within reach, promising a brighter future for medical imaging and patient care.

Exercise

Multiple Choice Questions (MCQs)

1. Who discovered X-ray imaging?
   A. Albert Einstein
   B. Wilhelm Conrad Roentgen
   C. Marie Curie
   D. Nikola Tesla
2. What principle ensures minimal radiation exposure to patients, staff, and the public?
   A. PACS
   B. ALARA
   C. RIS
   D. PET
3. What is one of the key considerations when planning and installing radiology equipment?
   A. Color scheme of the room
   B. Type of furniture
   C. Radiation safety
   D. Patient age
4. Which of the following technologies is more commonly used in urban areas for imaging?
   A. Ultrasounds
   B. X-rays
   C. Interventional technologies
   D. Doppler ultrasonography
5. Who is responsible for offering shielding advice and ensuring compliance with regulations?
   A. Radiologists
   B. Medical physicists
   C. Nurses
   D. Engineers
6. Which organization provides guidelines for the safe use of X-ray imaging, especially in low-resource situations?
   A. FDA
   B. IAEA
   C. WHO
   D. IEC
7. What do the MQSA rules ensure in the United States?
   A. Radiation protection in fluoroscopy
   B. High-quality mammographic images and patient safety
   C. Calibration of hybrid imaging systems
   D. General X-ray equipment safety
8. What is the main purpose of regulatory guidelines for X-ray, mammography, fluoroscopy, CT, and hybrid imaging?
   A. To increase the use of imaging equipment
   B. To ensure patient safety and image quality

C. To reduce the cost of medical procedures
D. To promote new imaging technologies

9. Which of the following is a critical aspect of fluoroscopy guidelines?
A. Image fusion techniques
B. Radiation dose optimization
C. Breast cancer screening
D. Calibration of CT equipment

10. Who is responsible for ensuring compliance with radiation safety/regulatory standards in an X-ray department?
A. Radiologist
B. Radiation protection officer (RPO/RSO)
C. Medical physicist
D. Imaging technologist

11. What does the ALARA principle stand for in radiation protection?
A. As Long As Radiation Accumulates
B. As Low As Reasonably Achievable
C. As Low As Radiation Allows
D. As Long As Radiation is Acceptable

12. What is a primary barrier in radiology rooms designed to protect against?
A. Scatter radiation
B. Leakage radiation
C. Direct radiation from the X-ray tube
D. All types of radiation

13. What is the typical lead equivalent for walls and doors in fluoroscopy rooms?
A. 0.1–0.2 mm
B. 1–1.5 mm
C. 2–3 mm
D. 3–4 mm

14. What should be considered in the design of the control area for mammography rooms?
A. It should include a patient waiting area
B. It should have a leaded glass window
C. It should have no shielding requirements
D. It should be outside the imaging facility

15. Which organization provides comprehensive guidelines on radiation protection and safety in imaging?
A. ACR
B. WHO
C. IEC
D. IAEA

16. What are the ideal materials for shielding against X-ray radiation due to their availability, cost, and structural strength?
A. Lead and aluminum
B. Bricks and concrete
C. Steel and copper
D. Titanium and zinc

17. What is a disadvantage of using lead as a shielding material?
A. It is too expensive
B. It is difficult to source
C. It requires periodic radiation surveys
D. It has low shielding effectiveness

18. Which imaging modality requires a minimum room size of 25–30 square meters?
A. X-ray
B. Mammography
C. Fluoroscopy
D. Ultrasound

19. For shielding in a mammography room, what is the typical lead equivalent for primary barriers?
A. 0.1–0.2 mm
B. 1.5–2 mm
C. 2–3 mm
D. 0.5–1 mm

20. Which of the following is not a commonly used material for radiation shielding?
A. Lead
B. Concrete
C. Lead-equivalent materials
D. Aluminum

21. What is the main component of a mammography room used for compressing the breast?
A. Mammography machine
B. Compression device
C. Control panel
D. Lead shield

22. In a fluoroscopy room, where should the control room be located?
A. Adjacent to the fluoroscopy room with leaded glass windows
B. Inside the fluoroscopy room
C. In a separate building
D. In the patient preparation area

23. What is the recommended room size for a CT room?
    A. 10–15 square meters
    B. 25–30 square meters
    C. 30–40 square meters
    D. 40–50 square meters
24. What is the purpose of lead-lined walls, doors, and windows in radiology rooms?
    A. To enhance room aesthetics
    B. To provide insulation
    C. To protect staff and patients from radiation exposure
    D. To improve ventilation
25. Which area in a PET-CT room is dedicated to administering radioactive tracers?
    A. Control room
    B. Injection/preparation room
    C. Patient preparation area
    D. Waiting area

Short Questions

1. Describe the importance of site planning in the installation of medical imaging equipment.
2. What role does a PACS administrator play in a radiology department?
3. Explain the significance of radiation protection devices in X-ray installations.
4. What are the responsibilities of the RPO/RSO in an X-ray department?
5. Describe the general requirements for room size and shielding in a CT imaging facility.
6. What are the primary considerations for infection control in the layout of radiology departments?
7. Describe the general principles of radiation shielding for an X-ray room.
8. What are the key considerations for designing a radiology department layout?
9. Describe the layout considerations for a fluoroscopy room to ensure workflow efficiency.
10. Explain the importance of patient-centered design in the layout of a radiology department.

Long Question

1. Discuss the principles and considerations involved in the selection and installation of radiology equipment, including regulatory compliance, site selection, equipment selection, and safety measures.
2. Discuss the regulatory guidelines and standards for different imaging modalities, focusing on X-ray, mammography, fluoroscopy, CT, and hybrid imaging. Include considerations for radiation safety, quality assurance, and staff training.
3. Discuss the codal requirements and general recommendations for the layout planning of X-ray, mammography, fluoroscopy, CT, and hybrid imaging facilities. Include considerations for space, shielding, and patient safety.
4. Discuss the shielding criteria and layout requirements for a CT room, including the necessary components and considerations for radiation safety, patient and staff comfort, and workflow efficiency.
5. Discuss the key components and design considerations for an IR room. How do these elements contribute to both operational efficiency and patient safety?

Answers for MCQs

1. B. Wilhelm Conrad Roentgen
2. B. ALARA
3. C. Radiation safety
4. C. Interventional technologies
5. B. Medical physicists
6. C. WHO
7. B. High-quality mammographic images and patient safety
8. B. To ensure patient safety and image quality
9. B. Radiation dose optimization
10. B. Radiation protection officer (RPO/RSO)
11. B. As Low As Reasonably Achievable
12. C. Direct radiation from the X-ray tube
13. C. 2–3 mm
14. B. It should have a leaded glass window
15. D. IAEA

16. B. Bricks and concrete
17. C. It requires periodic radiation surveys
18. C. Fluoroscopy
19. A. 0.1–0.2 mm
20. D. Aluminum
21. B. Compression device
22. A. Adjacent to the fluoroscopy room with leaded glass windows
23. C. 30–40 square meters
24. C. To protect staff and patients from radiation exposure
25. B. Injection/preparation room

References

1. Kruskal JB, Reedy A, Pascal L, Rosen MP, Boiselle PM. Quality initiatives: lean approach to improving performance and efficiency in a radiology department. Radiographics. 2012;32(2):573.
2. Krause MO. Atomic radiative and radiationless yields for K and L shells. J Phys Chem Ref Data. 1979;8(2):307.
3. Rankin J, Bedrava J, Covington E, Johnson JL, Pollard-Larkin J, Schipper MJ, et al. Women in the medical physics workforce: insights from membership trends of the American Association of Physicists in Medicine, 1993 to 2023. Int J Radiat Oncol Biol Phys. 2024;119:1336.
4. Mayo CS, Moran JM, Bosch W, Xiao Y, McNutt T, Popple R, et al. American Association of Physicists in Medicine Task Group 263: standardizing nomenclatures in radiation oncology. Int J Radiat Oncol Biol Phys. 2018;100:1057.
5. Skourou C, Sherouse GW, Bahar N, Bauer LA, Fairobent L, Freedman DJ, et al. Code of ethics for the American Association of Physicists in Medicine (revised): report of task group 109. Med Phys. 2019;46(4):e79–93.
6. Amis ES, Butler PF, Applegate KE, Birnbaum SB, Brateman LF, Hevezi JM, et al. American College of Radiology White Paper on radiation dose in medicine. J Am Coll Radiol. 2007;4(5):272.
7. Hendel RC, Patel MR, Kramer CM, Poon M, Hendel RC, Carr JC, et al. Accf/acr/scct/scmr/asnc/nasci/scai/sir 2006 appropriateness criteria for cardiac computed tomography and cardiac magnetic resonance imaging: a report of the american college of cardiology foundation quality strategic directions committee appropriateness criteria working group, american college of radiology, society of cardiovascular computed tomography, society for cardiovascular magnetic resonance, american society of nuclear cardiology, north american society for cardiac imaging, society for ..... J Am Coll Cardiol. 2006;48:1475–1497.
8. European Society of Radiology (ESR), American College of Radiology (ACR). European Society of Radiology (ESR) and American College of Radiology (ACR) report of the 2015 global summit on radiological quality and safety. Insights Imaging. 2016;7(4):481.
9. Mansour Z, Mokhtar A, Sarhan A, Ahmed MT, El-Diasty T. Quality control of CT image using American College of Radiology (ACR) phantom. Egypt J Radiol Nucl Med. 2016;47(4):1665.
10. Geurts MW, Jacqmin DJ, Jones LE, Kry SF, Mihailidis DN, Ohrt JD, et al. AAPM MEDICAL PHYSICS PRACTICE GUIDELINE 5.b: commissioning and QA of treatment planning dose calculations—Megavoltage photon and electron beams. J Appl Clin Med Phys. 2022;23(9):e13641.
11. Vleeming A, Albert HB, Östgaard HC, Sturesson B, Stuge B. European guidelines for the diagnosis and treatment of pelvic girdle pain. Eur Spine J. 2008;17:794.
12. Dance DR, Young KC, Van Engen RE. Estimation of mean glandular dose for breast tomosynthesis: factors for use with the UK, European and IAEA breast dosimetry protocols. Phys Med Biol. 2011;56(2):453.
13. Dance DR, Young KC, Van Engen RE. Further factors for the estimation of mean glandular dose using the United Kingdom, European and IAEA breast dosimetry protocols. Phys Med Biol. 2009;54(14):4361.
14. Kretz T, Mueller KR, Schaeffter T, Elster C. Mammography image quality assurance using deep learning. IEEE Trans Biomed Eng. 2020;67(12):3317.
15. Blum KS, Antoch G, Mohrmann S, Obenauer S. Use of low-energy contrast-enhanced spectral mammography (CESM) as diagnostic mammography-proof of concept. Radiography. 2015;21(4):352.
16. Lalji UC, Jeukens CRLPN, Houben I, Nelemans PJ, van Engen RE, van Wylick E, et al. Evaluation of low-energy contrast-enhanced spectral mammography images by comparing them to full-field digital mammography using EUREF image quality criteria. Eur Radiol. 2015;25(10):2813.
17. Feigin K. Quality assurance in mammography: an overview. Eur J Radiol. 2023;165:110935.
18. Lee CH, Dershaw DD, Kopans D, Evans P, Monsees B, Monticciolo D, et al. Breast cancer screening with imaging: recommendations from the Society of Breast Imaging and the ACR on the use of mammography, breast MRI, breast ultrasound, and other technologies for the detection of clinically occult breast cancer. J Am Coll Radiol. 2010;7:18.
19. Rice JE, Bonoli PT, JsA G, Greenwald MJ, Hutchinson IH, Marmar ES, et al. Central impurity toroidal rotation in ICRF heated Alcator C-mod plasmas. Nucl Fus. 1999;39(9 SPEC. ISS. 1):1175.
20. Markowicz A, Wegrzynek D, Bamford S, Chinea-Cano E. Activities in the IAEA X-ray fluorescence Laboratory at Seibersdorf. X-Ray Spectrom. 2006;35(4):207.

21. Clairand I, Bordy JM, Carinou E, Daures J, Debroas J, Denozire M, et al. Use of active personal dosemeters in interventional radiology and cardiology: tests in laboratory conditions and recommendations ORAMED project. Radiat Meas. 2011;46:1252.
22. Keall PJ, Mageras GS, Balter JM, Emery RS, Forster KM, Jiang SB, et al. The management of respiratory motion in radiation oncology report of AAPM task group 76. Med Phys. 2006;33:3874.
23. Cody DD, Dillon CM, Fisher TS, Liu X, McNitt-Gray MF, Patel V. AAPM medical physics practice guideline 1.b: CT protocol management and review practice guideline. J Appl Clin Med Phys. 2021;22(6):4.
24. Mutic S, Palta JR, Butker EK, Das IJ, Huq MS, Loo LND, et al. Quality assurance for computed-tomography simulators and the computed-tomography-simulation process: report of the AAPM radiation therapy committee task group No. 66. Med Phys. 2003;30:2762.
25. Burton CS, Szczykutowicz TP. Evaluation of AAPM reports 204 and 220: estimation of effective diameter, water-equivalent diameter, and ellipticity ratios for chest, abdomen, pelvis, and head CT scans. J Appl Clin Med Phys. 2018;19(1):228.
26. Harolds JA, Smith GT, Baker SR. Trends and different educational pathways for training physicians in nuclear medicine. Acad Radiol. 2008;15(12):1596.
27. Graham MM, Metter DF. Evolution of nuclear medicine training: past, present, and future. J Nucl Med. 2007;48:257.
28. Zanzonico P, Dauer L, St. Germain J. Operational radiation safety for PET-CT, SPECT-CT, and cyclotron facilities. Health Phys. 2008;95:554.
29. Lopci E, Hicks RJ, Dimitrakopoulou-Strauss A, Dercle L, Iravani A, Seban RD, et al. Joint EANM/SNMMI/ANZSNM practice guidelines/procedure standards on recommended use of [18F]FDG PET/CT imaging during immunomodulatory treatments in patients with solid tumors version 1.0. Eur J Nucl Med Mol Imaging. 2022;49(7):2323.
30. Hossain MN, Mia MS, Biman TA, Hussain R, Kabir MF. Estimating the shielding requirements for a newly planned PET-CT facility. Bangladesh. J Nucl Med. 2019;21(2):102.
31. Elashmawy MM. Design, commissioning and operation of programmable drainage system for PET-CT: an optimized approach to protect personnel and environment in nuclear medicine facilities. Radiat Prot Dosimetry. 2022;198(5):257–64.
32. Fraser L, Parkar N, Adamson K, Fletcher A, Julyan P, Kalirai C, et al. Guidelines & recommendations guidance on medical physics expert support for nuclear medicine. Br J Radiol. 2022;95(1135):20211393.
33. Jacob J, Volpe A, Peng Q, Lechler RI, Smyth LA, Lombardi G, et al. Radiolabelling of polyclonally expanded human regulatory T cells (Treg) with 89Zr-oxine for medium-term in vivo cell tracking. Molecules. 2023;28(3):1482.
34. Tandon P. Regulatory requirements for designing PET-CT facility in India. Indian J Nucl Med. 2010;25:39.
35. Madsen MT, Anderson JA, Halama JR, Kleck J, Simpkin DJ, Votaw JR, et al. AAPM task group 108: PET and PET/CT shielding requirements. Med Phys. 2006;33:4.
36. Uddin MF, Khatun R, Akter S, Jamil HM, Monika AN, Rahaman MA, et al. Radiation shielding analysis and design of tof PET-CT Facility at Institute of nuclear medical physics under Bangladesh atomic energy commission, Bangladesh. Int J Med Phys Clin Eng Radiat Oncol. 2019;08(01):1.
37. Hiratzka LF, Bakris GL, Beckman JA, Bersin RM, Carr VF, Casey DE, et al. 2010 ACCF/AHA/AATS/ACR/ASA/SCA/SCAI/SIR/STS/SVM guidelines for the diagnosis and management of patients with thoracic aortic disease: executive summary: a report of the american college of cardiology foundation/american heart association task force on practice guidelines, american association for thoracic surgery, american college of radiology, american stroke association. Circulation. 2010;121:e16–94.
38. Weinreb JC, Barentsz JO, Choyke PL, Cornud F, Haider MA, Macura KJ, et al. PI-RADS prostate imaging – reporting and data system: 2015, version 2. Eur Urol. 2016;69(1):16.
39. Wang SS, Dibble EH, Gibbs IC, Rubin E, Parikh JR. The 2021 ACR/radiology business management association workforce survey: diversity in radiology. J Am Coll Radiol. 2023;20(12):1269.
40. Lasser EC, Lyon SG, Berry CC. Reports on contrast media reactions: analysis of data from reports to the U.S. Food and Drug Administration. Radiology. 1997;203(3):605.
41. Milam ME, Koo CW. The current status and future of FDA-approved artificial intelligence tools in chest radiology in the United States. Clin Radiol. 2023;78:115.
42. Capote R, Herman M, Obložinský P, Young PG, Goriely S, Belgya T, et al. RIPL – reference input parameter library for calculation of nuclear reactions and nuclear data evaluations. Nucl Data Sheets. 2009;110(12):3107.
43. Brown DA, Chadwick MB, Capote R, Kahler AC, Trkov A, Herman MW, et al. ENDF/B-VIII.0: the 8th major release of the nuclear reaction data library with CIELO-project cross sections, new standards and thermal scattering data. Nucl Data Sheets. 2018;148:1–142.
44. Chadwick MB, Obložinský P, Herman M, Greene NM, McKnight RD, Smith DL, et al. ENDF/B-VII.0: next generation evaluated nuclear data library for nuclear science and technology. Nucl Data Sheets. 2006;107(12):2931.
45. Busch U. Claims of priority – the scientific path to the discovery of X-rays. Zeitschrift fur Medizinische Physik. 2023;33:230.

46. Valentin J. Managing patient dose in multi-detector computed tomography(MDCT). ICRP publication 102. Ann ICRP. 2007;37(1):1.
47. Clarke RH, Valentin J. The history of ICRP and the evolution of its policies. Ann ICRP. 2009;39(1):75.
48. Junda M, Muller H, Friedrich-Nel H. Local diagnostic reference levels for routine chest x-ray examinations at a public sector hospital in Central South Africa. Health SA Gesondheid. 2021;26:1–8.
49. Malone J. X-rays for medical imaging: radiation protection, governance and ethics over 125 years. Phys Med. 2020;79:47.
50. Hechanova A. Technical workforce education and training program at Abu Dhabi polytechnic: integration of academia and industry requirements. In: International Conference on Nuclear Engineering, Proceedings, ICONE; 2018.
51. Vásquez-Maignan X. Nuclear power in The United Arab Emirates: legal framework and regulatory cooperation. NEA News. 2012;30/31(2/1).
52. Alsenaidi M, Mohamed S, AlBlooshi A, Narang M, Bartholomew J. Digital transformation in UAE metrology. In: IMEKO TC6 international conference on metrology and digital transformation; 2022.
53. Kumar R, Kumbharkar P, Vanam S, Sharma S. Medical images classification using deep learning: a survey. Multimed Tools Appl. 2024;83(7):19683.
54. Zhou SK, Greenspan H, Davatzikos C, Duncan JS, Van Ginneken B, Madabhushi A, et al. A review of deep learning in medical imaging: imaging traits, technology trends, case studies with progress highlights, and future promises. Proc IEEE. 2021;109(5):820–38.
55. Sahoo BN, Kandasubramanian B. Recent progress in fabrication and characterisation of hierarchical biomimetic superhydrophobic structures. RSC Adv. 2014;4(42):22053–93.
56. Gopakumar K, Ram Mohan M. Regulatory independence in India: a case of the Atomic Energy Regulatory Board Regulatory Independence in India: a case of the atomic energy regulatory board; 2023.
57. Aggarwa R, George RA, Alam A, Soni BK. E-licensing of radiation applications (eLORA) in armed forces hospitals: 'Nuts and Bolts'. Med J Armed Forces India. 2017;73:80.
58. Ram Mohan MP, Gopakumar KV, Smith T. Nuclear energy safety, regulatory independence, and judicial deference: the case of the atomic energy regulatory Board of India. Adm Soc. 2020;52(7):1009.
59. Anurag L, Gaurav M, Sanjay D, Chandrashekar M. The spectrum of the atomic energy regulatory board under the department of atomic energy with respect to a medical radiation facility. J Datta Meghe Inst Med Sci Univ. 2022;17:766–71.
60. Chen TR, Tyan YS, Chu CH, Wu MC, Tung CJ. Surveyed data for structural shielding calculations of radiographic X-ray installations in Taiwan. Health Phys. 2013;104:S60.
61. Radiation protection in veterinary medicine. NCRP report 2004.
62. Okunade AA. Effective dose as a limiting quantity for the evaluation of primary barriers for diagnostic x-ray facilities. Health Phys. 2005;89(5 SUPPL):S100.
63. Fog LS, Cormack J. Mathematical modeling of the radiation dose received from photons passing over and through shielding walls in a PET/CT suite. Health Phys. 2010;99(6):769.
64. Bibbo G. Shielding of medical imaging X-ray facilities: a simple and practical method. Australas Phys Eng Sci Med. 2017;40(4):925.
65. Judge MA, Keavey E, Phelan N. Scatter radiation intensities around full-field digital mammography units. Br J Radiol. 2013;86(1021):20120130.
66. Ciraj-Bjelac O, Arandjic D, Kosutic D. Comparison of different methods for shielding design in computed tomography. Radiat Prot Dosim. 2011;147(1–2):133–6.
67. Archer BR, Fewell TR, Conway BJ, Quinn PW. Attenuation properties of diagnostic x-ray shielding materials. Med Phys. 1994;21(9):1499.
68. Archer BR, Thornby JI, Bushong SC. Diagnostic x-ray shielding design based on an empirical model of photon attenuation. Health Phys. 1983;44(5):507.
69. United THE, of S. NCRP report no. 49: structural shielding design and evaluation for medical use of X-rays and gamma rays of energies up to 10 MeV. J Nucl Med Technol. 1977;5(2)
70. Jones AK, Heintz P, Geiser W, Goldman L, Jerjian K, Martin M, et al. AAPM no 151: ongoing quality control in digital radiography. Med Phys. 2015;42(11):6658.
71. McCullough SP, Alkhatib H, Antes KJ, Castillo S, Fontenot JD, Jensen AR, et al. AAPM MEDICAL PHYSICS PRACTICE GUIDELINE 2.b.: commissioning and quality assurance of X-ray-based image-guided radiotherapy systems. J Appl Clin Med Phys. 2021;22(9):73.
72. Brittes Benitez G, Sanson Fogliatto F, Bertoglio Cardoso R, Soares Torres F, Sasso Faccin C, Dora JM. Systematic layout planning of a radiology reporting area to optimize radiologists' performance. J Digit Imaging. 2018;31(2):193.
73. Long X, Zhang L, Alwalid O, Lei Z, Liang B, Shi H, et al. Radiology department preventive and control measures and work plan during COVID-19 epidemic-experience from Wuhan. Chin J Acad Radiol. 2021;4:1.
74. Benitez GB, Fogliatto FS, Cardoso RB, Torres FS, Faccin CS, Dora JM. Systematic layout planning of a radiology reporting area to optimize radiologists' performance. J Digit Imaging. 2018;31(2):193.
75. Ileri YY, Çelik A. Hastane Yönetim Etkinliğinde Yerleşim Planının Önemi ve Bir Model Çalışması TT – The importance of layout organization in hospital management efficiency and a model study. Selcuk Üniversitesi Sosyal Bilimler Enstitüsü Dergisi. 2018;39:168–80.
76. Rehani MM, Ciraj-Bjelac O, Vañó E, Miller DL, Walsh S, Giordano BD, et al. Radiological protection in fluoroscopically guided procedures performed outside the imaging department. Ann ICRP. 2010;40(6):1.

77. Vano E, Faulkner K. ICRP special radiation protection issues in interventional radiology, digital and cardiac imaging. Radiat Prot Dosim. 2006;117(1–3):13–7.
78. Vano E. ICRP recommendations on "managing patient dose in digital radiology". Radiat Prot Dosim. 2005;114(1–3):126–30.
79. ICRP. Managing patient dose in digital radiology – ICRP 93. Ann ICRP. 2004;April
80. Howlett DC, Kumi P, Kloeckner R, Bargallo N, Baessler B, Becker M, et al. Clinical audit in European radiology: current status and recommendations for improvement endorsed by the European Society of Radiology (ESR). Insights Imaging. 2023;14(1):71.
81. Rühm W, Yu H, Clement C, Ainsbury EA, Andresz S, Bryant P, et al. ICRP workshop on the review and revision of the system of radiological protection: a focus on research priorities feedback from the international community. J Radiol Prot. 2023;43(4):043001.
82. Rühm W, Cho K, Larsson CM, Wojcik A, Clement C, Applegate K, et al. Vancouver call for action to strengthen expertise in radiological protection worldwide. Radiat Environ Biophys. 2023;62:175.
83. Nyberg NR, McCredden JE, Weller SG, Hardell L. The European Union prioritises economics over health in the rollout of radiofrequency technologies. Rev Environ Health. 2024;39:47.
84. Valentin J. Managing patient dose in digital radiology. Ann ICRP. 2004;34:1–73.

Radiation Safety in Radiology 10

Objectives

- Radiation Protection
- Key Principles or the Framework of Radiation Protection
  - Justification
  - Optimization
  - Dose Limitation
  - Dose Monitoring and Record Keeping
- Fundamental Principles of Radiation Protection
  - Time
  - Distance
  - Shielding
- Terms Related to Radiation Dose and Dose Limit
  - Radiation Absorbed Dose (D)
  - Dose Rate
  - Equivalent Dose
  - Effective Dose
  - Collective Effective Dose or Collective Dose: Assessing Population Exposure
- Dose Limit
  - Dose Limit for Carer and Comforters
  - Dose Limits for Volunteers in Biomedical Research
  - Dose Constraints and Reference Levels
  - Diagnostic Reference Level
  - History and Current Recommendations on Dose Limits
- Principles of Safe Work Practices in Diagnostic Radiology
- Use of Barriers and Techniques for Radiation Protection in Radiology
- Regulatory Bodies
  - International Commission on Radiological Protection
  - International Atomic Energy Agency
  - World Health Organization
  - National Regulatory Authorities
  - Food and Agriculture Organization (FAO)
  - United Nations Scientific Committee on the Effects of Atomic Radiation (UNSCEAR)
  - Health and Medical Organizations
  - Industry-Specific Authorities
- Biological Effects of Radiation
  - Deterministic Effects
  - Stochastic Effects
- Female Patients, Female Radiation Workers, and the Effects of Radiation on the Fetus
  - Conducting Different Diagnostic Procedures During Pregnancy
  - Effects of Radiation on the Fetus During Different Phases of Pregnancy
  - Safety and Handling of Female Patients of Childbearing Age
  - Informed Consent
  - Pregnant Female Radiation Worker
- Radiation Area and Its Classification
  - Controlled Area
  - Supervised Area
  - Unsupervised Area
- Personal Monitoring Devices
  - Thermo-Luminescent Dosimeters
  - $CaSO_4$: Dy TLDs
  - Optically Stimulated Luminescence Dosimeters
  - Pocket Ionization Chambers
  - Digital Pocket Dosimeter
  - Film Badges
  - Extremity Monitors
- Radiation Emergencies
  - Equipment Malfunction
  - Accidental Exposure
  - Terrorism or Sabotage
  - General Preparedness for Radiological Emergencies

D. Prakash, R. P. Kotian, *Fundamentals of X-ray Imaging*,
https://doi.org/10.1007/978-981-96-7328-5_10

10.1 Radiation Protection

Before the discovery of X-rays in 1895 and radioactivity in 1896, people were unaware of the existence of radiation and ionizing substances. On December 12, 1896, the first paper on radiation protection was published, stressing the importance of time, distance, and shielding. However, the concept of protecting from radiation had already been introduced in the early sixteenth century by Georg Bauer, also known as "Agricola" in Latin. He is regarded as the first "Radiation protection officer," since he developed methods to protect mine workers of Erzgebirge, an area on the present-day border between the Czech Republic and Germany, from inhaling the daughter product of radon and falling ill with "Bergsucht" (today known as lung cancer). He encouraged miners' wives to create fine-meshed inhalation filters for their husbands and implemented ventilation systems in the mines [1].

Radiation protection refers to the practice of minimizing the potential risks associated with exposure to ionizing radiation while allowing for its beneficial uses. The ionizing radiation is a type of radiation that has enough energy to remove tightly bound electrons from atoms, creating ions in the process. The common examples of ionizing radiation are X-rays, gamma rays, high-energy ultraviolet radiation, alpha particles, beta particles, neutrons, protons, and heavy ions. The energy carried by ionizing radiation is sufficient to disrupt chemical bonds within molecules and can potentially cause damage to living cells and tissues. This property of ionizing radiation is both beneficial and hazardous. It is typically utilized in medical diagnosis as well as in therapies. Being a double-edged sword, improper exposure to ionizing radiation can lead to health risks, including increased cancer risk, genetic mutations, and acute radiation sickness. Due to its potential dangers, radiation protection measures and regulatory guidelines and standards are established to minimize the risks associated with ionizing radiation exposure.

? Is there any difference between radiation protection and radiation safety, or are they just synonymous?

The concepts of radiation protection and radiation safety are similar and related terms, but they have slightly different meanings in dealing with ionizing radiation.

Radiation Protection

Radiation protection refers to minimizing the potential risks associated with exposure to ionizing radiation while allowing for its beneficial uses. It encompasses a comprehensive approach that involves principles, guidelines, regulations, and practices to ensure that radiation exposure is kept as low as reasonably achievable (ALARA) while still achieving the intended objectives. Radiation protection involves strategies to prevent unnecessary radiation exposure, control exposure pathways, and mitigate ionizing radiation's potential health and environmental impacts.

Example Consider a radiographer performing a fluoroscopy procedure on a patient. Fluoroscopy involves real-time X-ray imaging to visualize the inside of the body. In radiation protection, the radiographer ensures that the equipment is properly calibrated and the patient is positioned correctly to minimize radiation exposure. The principle of ALARA is applied here, where the radiographer adjusts the X-ray settings to obtain clear images while keeping the radiation dose as low as possible. The goal is to achieve the necessary diagnostic information while limiting the patient's radiation exposure.

Radiation Safety
Radiation safety, on the other hand, is a broader term that encompasses protecting individuals from the harmful effects of ionizing radiation and the overall management of radiation-related risks and hazards. It includes measures to ensure the safety of workers, the public, and the environment in areas where ionizing radiation is used or present. Radiation safety programs address exposure to ionizing radiation and issues related to radiation-emitting devices, radioactive materials, and the proper handling, storage, transportation, and disposal of such materials.

Example Let us see radiation safety in a research laboratory working with radioactive isotopes. Researchers are handling and experimenting with radioactive materials for scientific purposes. Regarding radiation safety, the laboratory implements measures to protect researchers, prevent contamination, and ensure that waste materials are properly managed. This involves using protective equipment, shielding materials, proper storage and disposal of radioactive materials, and following protocols to minimize potential exposure and contamination risks.

In these examples, radiation protection focuses on the immediate exposure of the patient during a medical procedure, while radiation safety extends to broader considerations in research settings, such as containment, handling, and proper waste management.

In essence, radiation protection is a key component of radiation safety. Radiation safety encompasses a wider range of considerations, including regulatory compliance, emergency response, and the implementation of best practices to prevent accidents and incidents involving radiation sources. While the terms are related and often used interchangeably, "radiation safety" emphasizes a broader perspective that includes radiation protection and other safety aspects related to ionizing radiation.

The key takeaway is that while these concepts overlap and share common goals, radiation protection often refers to immediate measures taken to reduce individual exposure, while radiation safety encompasses a broader approach to managing radiation-related risks in various contexts.

10.2 Key Principles or the Framework of Radiation Protection

Radiation protection encompasses a set of principles, guidelines, and practices aimed at safeguarding individuals, communities, and the environment from the harmful effects of radiation. The primary goal of radiation protection is to maintain radiation exposures at levels that are ALARA while still achieving the desired outcomes, such as medical diagnosis and treatment, industrial applications, research, and energy production. This field involves implementing safety measures, regulations, and monitoring to prevent excessive radiation exposure and mitigate potential health and environmental impacts. The following key principles guide radiation protection practices.

10.2.1 Justification

The core of justification lies in the *benefit* versus *risk assessment*. Before exposing individuals to ionizing radiation, a thorough analysis is conducted to evaluate whether the potential positive outcomes, such as accurate diagnosis, effective treatment, or valuable research data, outweigh the potential negative effects, such as increased cancer risk or tissue damage. This involves comparing the benefits of the procedure with the possible health risks.

A crucial aspect of justification is the consideration of *alternative methods*. The principle mandates exploring non-radiation alternatives whenever possible. If these alternatives can achieve similar results, they are preferred to minimize radiation exposure. Justification also involves *informed decision-making*. Patients or individuals must be adequately informed about the nature of the radiation procedure, its potential benefits, and the associated risks. This transparency allows them to make an educated decision regarding whether to proceed with the radiation-based activity.

Finally, there is a *professional responsibility* on the part of healthcare practitioners, researchers, and other professionals using ionizing radiation. They must ensure that their actions are justified based on the best available evidence and guidelines. This responsibility includes continuously assessing and re-evaluating the necessity of using radiation.

10.2.2 Optimization

Optimization in radiation protection, often encapsulated by the ALARA principle, is a fundamental concept aimed at minimizing radiation exposure to the lowest reasonable levels while still achieving the intended outcomes of radiation-related activities. This principle is critical across various fields, including medicine, industry, research, and nuclear facilities. The primary goal of optimization is to balance the benefits of using radiation against the potential risks associated with exposure.

This process is not a one-time effort but an ongoing commitment. It involves regularly reviewing and refining procedures, equipment, and practices to identify opportunities for reducing radiation exposure. Advances in technology and techniques play a significant role in achieving lower radiation doses while maintaining the quality of results. Practitioners carefully select the most suitable techniques and equipment to obtain accurate results while minimizing exposure. This selection may involve choosing different imaging modalities, adjusting exposure settings, or employing shielding methods to reduce radiation doses.

Regular monitoring of radiation exposures and the collection of data on doses received by workers, patients, or individuals are integral to the optimization process. This data-driven approach helps identify trends and areas for improvement, enabling practitioners to make informed decisions. The goal is to minimize radiation exposure to levels below regulatory limits and within accepted standards, guided by the ALARA principle. This principle encourages exploring all possible measures for dose reduction without compromising the quality or accuracy of the results.

Optimization reflects an ethical responsibility to prioritize safety while achieving desired outcomes involving ionizing radiation. It underscores a commitment to using radiation effectively and responsibly, contributing to the broader goal of radiation protection.

10.2.3 Dose Limitation

Dose limitation involves establishing and adhering to maximum allowable doses of ionizing radiation exposure for individuals, with the aim of preventing the occurrence of harmful health effects. This principle sets specific dose limits for different categories of people, such as radiation workers, the public, and patients undergoing medical procedures. The limits are based on scientific research and are designed to ensure that radiation exposures remain at levels that are considered safe and acceptable. National and international regulatory bodies, such as the International Commission on Radiological Protection (ICRP) and relevant government agencies, define dose limits and guidelines based on the best available scientific evidence. These standards consider the potential risks associated with different levels of radiation exposure. Dose limits are different for different categories and situations and are discussed in detail in Sect. 10.11.

10.2.4 Dose Monitoring and Record Keeping

Regular radiation exposure monitoring and record keeping are important for individuals working with or around ionizing radiation sources. This helps ensure that exposure remains within acceptable limits and provides data for further optimization. Records of occupational exposure for each worker must be maintained throughout their employment and afterward, at least until the worker reaches or would have reached the age of 75 years, and for a minimum of 30 years after the cessation of work involving occupational exposure [2]. It is generally recommended to keep records of workplace monitoring and instrument calibration for 5 years. However, many records, such as details from specific radiation surveys, are only relevant for a short period and do not need to be kept long term. Other records, like those related to workplace specifications, may need to be retained for the duration of the workplace's existence. For instance, records about the establishment of designated areas should likely be kept for as long as those areas are in use [2].

10.3 Fundamental Principles of Radiation Protection

"Justification," "optimization," and "dose limits" are considered key principles in radiation protection, often encompassing the ethical, regulatory, and scientific aspects of managing radiation exposure. These principles guide decision-making, regulatory frameworks, and ethical considerations in radiation-related activities.

On the other hand, "time," "distance," and "shielding" are fundamental principles often referred to as the "Three Cardinal Principles." These principles are practical strategies individuals can apply to minimize radiation exposure in specific situations. These principles guide the management of radiation exposure to individuals and the environment when working with sources of ionizing radiation. They are simple yet effective strategies to minimize radiation exposure and potential health risks.

10.3.1 Time

The principle of "time" emphasizes reducing the duration of exposure to ionizing radiation. The longer an individual spends near a radiation source, the higher the potential dose they could receive. Minimizing exposure time decreases the overall dose received and is a linear factor.

An example of dose reduction using time techniques in medical imaging is fluoroscopy or X-ray procedures, in which medical professionals aim to limit the patient's exposure to radiation by using short exposure times while still obtaining necessary diagnostic information. When dealing with radiopharmaceuticals, the radiopharmacist minimizes the duration of radiation exposure to reduce the dose, or the technologist who interacts with radioactivity-injected patients minimizes the duration of interaction to decrease their radiation exposure.

10.3.2 Distance

The principle of "distance" highlights the importance of increasing the physical distance between a radiation source and individuals. Radiation intensity decreases with distance according to the inverse square law, so doubling the distance reduces the radiation intensity to one-fourth. This follows an inverse square formula.

Example In some cases, bystanders or family members might be in the radiology room during the procedure. Staff ensure that bystanders are positioned as far away from the X-ray source as possible, reducing their exposure to scattered radiation.

10.3.3 Shielding

The principle of "shielding" involves using physical barriers or materials to absorb or attenuate radiation. Shielding reduces the radiation that can reach individuals and their surroundings, providing additional protection. Shielding materials are selected based on the type and energy of the radiation being used or encountered. Common shielding materials include lead, concrete, steel, and specialized plastics. The choice of material depends on its ability to absorb or scatter radiation effectively.

When radiation passes through a shielding material, its intensity decreases due to attenuation. The interaction between the radiation and the shielding material leads to scattering and absorption, reducing the radiation's energy and intensity. The shielding design involves calculating the appropriate thickness and type of shielding material needed to achieve the desired level of radiation reduction. The design considers factors such as the type of radiation, its energy, the exposure scenario, and the expected radiation dose, and usually, high Z or high-density material is used for shield purposes.

Example Lead aprons are commonly used in medical settings during X-ray procedures to shield sensitive body areas from radiation. In nuclear power plants, thick walls and materials like concrete are used to shield workers from radiation generated by nuclear reactions.

By applying these three cardinal principles, radiation protection professionals can effectively reduce radiation exposure to individuals and minimize the potential risks associated with ionizing radiation. These principles are widely used across various fields, from medical and industrial settings to nuclear facilities and research laboratories.

10.4 Terms Related to Radiation Dose and Dose Limit

There are different terms used when we talk about measuring radiation doses, and sometimes, they, along with their units, can be confusing. However, understanding these terms and units is crucial to know how radiation affects the body and to compare doses from different procedures. The commonly used terms are summarized below:

- Radiation absorbed dose (D)
- Dose rate ($\dot{D}$)
- Equivalent dose (H_T)
- Effective dose (E)
- Collective effective dose or collective dose
- Dose limit

10.4.1 Radiation Absorbed Dose (*D*)

Radiation absorbed dose or simply absorbed dose (D) helps to understand energy deposition by ionizing radiation in a material. Denoted by the symbol D, absorbed dose is a fundamental concept in dosimetry, the field concerned with measuring and quantifying radiation exposure. It essentially tells us how much energy ionizing radiation deposits within a specific mass of material.

It is defined as "Energy deposited per unit mass in a material." The equation for absorbed dose is as follows:

$$D = \frac{E}{m} \tag{10.1}$$

- D: Absorbed dose (in Gray or Joule per kilogram)
- E: Energy deposited by radiation (in Joules)
- m: Mass of the irradiated material (in kilograms)

The SI unit for absorbed dose is Joules per kilogram (J/kg). However, the more commonly used unit in radiation protection is the Gray (Gy), and 1 Gray is equal to 1 Joule of energy deposited per kilogram of material.

Traditional Units (For Reference)

- **Erg per gram (erg/g)**: An older unit, rarely used today
- **Rad (radiation absorbed dose)**: Another historical unit

Conversion Factors

- 1 Gy = 1 Joule/kg = 100 rad
- 1 rad = 100 erg/g

Important Note

It is important to avoid pluralizing units like Gray or rad. They are collective nouns, similar to "staff" or "team." The correct way to refer to them is "one Gray" or "ten rad," not "one Grays" or "ten rads."

Beyond Absorbed Dose
While absorbed dose is a valuable measure, it does not account for the different effects of various radiation types or the varying sensitivities of different tissues. For a more comprehensive understanding of radiation's biological impact, other dose quantities such as equivalent dose and effective dose are derived from absorbed dose.

10.4.2 Dose Rate

Dose rate refers to the rate at which radiation dose is absorbed by a material or living organism. It essentially tells us how much radiation energy is being deposited per unit of time (e.g., per hour and per minute):

$$\dot{D} = \frac{D}{t} \tag{10.2}$$

The unit is gray/time, that is, gray/hour or gray/second.

The dose rate can be an important factor in determining the biological effects of radiation. Here is why understanding dose rate is important:

Biological Effects The biological effects of radiation exposure can depend on the dose rate. High dose rates (intense bursts of radiation) can cause more severe damage compared to low dose rates (spread out over time) for the same total absorbed dose. This is because cells have some ability to repair radiation-induced damage over time.

Acute Versus Chronic Effects High dose rates can lead to acute radiation sickness, characterized by symptoms such as nausea, vomiting, and hair loss. In contrast, chronic exposure to low dose rates may increase the risk of cancer development over time.

Treatment Planning In radiation therapy for cancer, dose rate is a critical factor. Doctors aim to deliver a high enough dose to kill cancer cells while minimizing damage to surrounding healthy tissues. By controlling the dose rate, they can balance these competing effects.

Environmental Monitoring Monitoring radiation levels in the environment after nuclear accidents or other events often involves measuring dose rate to assess potential health risks for exposed populations.

10.4.3 Equivalent Dose

Equivalent dose helps us understand the potential biological impact of radiation exposure by considering both the amount of energy deposited (absorbed dose) and the type of radiation involved, that is, whether it is alpha, beta, gamma, neutron, and so on is interacting with the medium. Different types of radiation have different abilities to cause biological effects based on their linear energy transfer (LET). The LET is the rate at which energy is deposited by ionizing radiation as it travels through matter.

The mean equivalent dose H_T in a target organ or tissue T is given by

$$H_T = \sum_R w_R D_{T,R} \tag{10.3}$$

where $D_{T,R}$ is the mean absorbed dose from radiation R in tissue or organ T, and w_R is the radiation weighting factor.

The unit of equivalent dose is the Sievert (Sv), which is equivalent to 1 Joule per kilogram (J/kg).

Radiation Weight Factor
This accounts for the varying effectiveness of different radiation types in causing biological damage. It essentially reflects the "punch" different radiation types deliver for the same amount of absorbed dose. Higher LET radiation, like alpha

Table 10.1 Radiation weighting factors for different types of radiation

Type of radiation	Weighting factor (wR)	Additional information
X-rays, gamma photons, electrons, positrons, and β-particles	**1**	Standard weighting factor, reflecting the relatively low biological impact of these common types of radiation compared to others
Alpha particles	**20**	Significantly higher due to the dense ionization and greater biological damage caused by alpha particles when interacting with tissues
Protons and charged pions	**2**	Moderate weighting factor, accounting for the greater ionization potential of protons and charged pions relative to X-rays or gamma photons
Neutron	**2.5–20.7**	Continuous function depending on neutron energy, with the factor varying to reflect the differing biological effects of neutrons at various energy levels
Auger electrons	**1–20**	Ranges depending on the specific scenario: **1** when ^{125}**I** is in the cytoplasm, **4** within the nucleus, **7–9** when bound to DNA, and up to **20** based on DNA-bound emitters as per MIRD pamphlet 21

particles or neutrons, typically has a higher w_R due to its ability to cause more localized damage.

It does not have a unit and is a dimensionless factor (Table 10.1).

The concept of equivalent dose is primarily used to estimate the probability of stochastic effects (cancer and genetic effects) from radiation exposure. It is not intended for predicting deterministic effects (tissue damage) that occur at higher radiation doses.

10.4.4 Effective Dose

To account for different organ sensitivity, the tissue weighting factor (w_T) is used. This factor reflects the estimated risk of cancer induction for each tissue. The ICRP has established w_T values based on factors such as sex and the number of organs considered. Here is the formula for calculating effective dose:

$$E = \Sigma\left(H_T \times W_T\right) \quad (10.4)$$

where

E: Effective dose (Sv)
Σ: Summation symbol
H_T: Equivalent dose to a specific organ/tissue (Sv)
w_T: Radiation weighting factor for that organ/tissue

The concept of radiation weighting factors, denoted as w_T, was introduced in Publication 26 by the ICRP in 1977. Initially, these factors served as adjusted nominal risk coefficients for six specific organs/tissues, with the remainder grouped separately. Subsequent revisions, such as Publication 60 in 1991, expanded the number to 12 + 1 (remaining). Further refinement occurred in Publication 103 in 2007, where the salivary gland was included as an additional organ, resulting in a total of 13 + 1 (as detailed in Table 10.2). These coefficients are derived by averaging estimates of radiation-associated lifetime cancer risk across a population with equal representation of males and females. The detriment is modeled based on factors such as life loss, lethality, and reduction in quality of life, as outlined in ICRP 103.

Tissue weighting factors are determined based on the risks of radiation-induced stochastic effects in both males and females, with sex-specific detriments averaged to find the wT values. These factors, along with sex-averaged organ and tissue doses, are then used to calculate the effective dose.

The effective dose (E), measured in Sievert (Sv), provides a single value that represents the

Table 10.2 Tissue weighting factors as per ICRP 103

Tissue	Weighting factor (wT)	No. of tissues	Summation
Red bone marrow, colon, lung, stomach, breast, and remainder tissues	0.12 each: Significant contributors to overall radiation sensitivity, reflecting their importance in radiation protection	06	0.72
Gonads	0.08: Reflects the sensitivity of reproductive organs to radiation, with implications for hereditary effects	01	0.08
Urinary bladder, esophagus, liver, and thyroid	0.04 each: Moderately sensitive tissues, contributing to cumulative radiation risk	04	0.16
Bone surface, brain, salivary glands, and skin	0.01 each: Less sensitive tissues, but still relevant in calculating effective dose	04	0.04
Total **1.00**: Sum of all tissue weighting factors, ensuring a comprehensive assessment of radiation exposure.			
Remainder tissues *Includes adrenals, extra-thoracic region, gall bladder, heart, kidneys, lymphatic system, muscles, oral mucosa, pancreas, prostate, small intestine, spleen, thymus, and uterus/cervix*: These are grouped together under "remainder tissues" due to their lower individual weighting factors but still contribute to the overall radiation dose calculation.			

overall risk to the entire body from radiation exposure. This risk focuses on stochastic effects, which are long-term health consequences such as cancer and genetic mutations that may develop after exposure to low radiation doses. It does not directly predict deterministic effects, which are immediate tissue damage symptoms occurring at higher radiation doses.

The effective dose serves several purposes, including:

- Facilitating comparison of different diagnostic medical exposures, even across different modalities
- Guiding dosimetry-based decisions, such as the choice of radiopharmaceuticals in nuclear medicine studies
- Allowing the summation of doses from various sources, including radiopharmaceuticals and other procedures in addition to nuclear medicine
- Providing a basis for assessing radiation risks

However, the effective dose has limitations:

- It is based on sex- and age-averaged weighting factors, which may not accurately reflect individual risks, particularly for organs like the thyroid.
- It is most appropriate for assessing stochastic risk in diagnostic exposures within populations whose demographics align with the conditions used to derive the weighting factors.
- It should not be applied to situations involving radiation therapy or to individual patients; its utility is in assessing risks across populations.

10.4.5 Collective Effective Dose or Collective Dose: Assessing Population Exposure

While effective dose focuses on the risk to an individual, collective effective dose (sometimes simply called collective dose) takes a broader view. It estimates the **total** radiation exposure experienced by a **population group** from a specific radiation source.

The unit for collective effective dose is the same as effective dose—Sievert (Sv). However, it is applied to a whole population, not a single person.

Common Applications of Collective Effective Dose

- **Assessing Population Risk**: Estimating the potential for stochastic effects (cancers, genetic mutations) in a population exposed to environmental radiation sources like nuclear power plants or fallout from accidents
- **Regulatory Limits**: Setting limits on the amount of radiation a population can be exposed to from various sources
- **Cost–Benefit Analysis**: Comparing the potential health risks (estimated through collective dose) with the benefits of activities involving radiation exposure (e.g., medical imaging and industrial applications)

Calculating Collective Effective Dose

Collective effective dose (S) is calculated by summing the effective doses (E) received by all individuals in the population:

$$S = \sum E_{\mathrm{i}} \tag{10.5}$$

S: Collective effective dose (Sv)
Σ: Summation symbol
E_{i}: Effective dose received by an individual (Sv)

Collective effective dose helps us understand the overall radiation burden on a population group exposed to a specific source. It does not tell us how much radiation any one person received, but it provides a valuable tool for assessing potential health risks at the population level.

10.4.6 Dose Limit

The term "dose limit" was coined in ICRP publication 26 (1977), and earlier, the limits were considered in terms of "Maximum Permissible Dose" [3]. The dose limit is one of the three key principles of radiation protection. I have personally seen a fear of radiation among radiation workers, and many times, people have been seen escaping from their duties that involved radiation exposure, sometimes leading to conflicts among workers. As a radiological safety officer, wherever I have worked or with my YouTube channel, my sincere efforts have always been to make the people "understand the radiation and not fear unnecessarily." It is not denied that radiation is a double-edged sword, and the world has seen its darkest side in the past, but apart from that, radiation has done so much more than that to save mankind, and it is consistently doing so every day with such a great amount of diagnostic and therapeutic procedures performed every day along with many industrial uses. We are lucky to be born in this era where the world's understanding about radiation is much more than what it was 100 years ago.

The dose limits are established guidelines that specify the maximum allowable radiation doses for individuals in different exposure situations. These limits ensure that radiation exposure remains safe and minimizes the risk of harmful effects. Dose limits vary depending on the exposure situation, the individual's role, and the potential risks associated with ionizing radiation. Let us discuss these:

Different Categories Dose limits vary based on the type of individual and their role in exposure scenarios:

- *Radiation Workers*: Individuals whose occupation is to work with sources of ionizing radiation are called radiation workers and have higher dose limits than the public. However, their exposures are subject to careful monitoring and control to ensure safety.
- *Trainees in the Field of Radiation Occupation*: People aged under 16–18 years are strictly supervised as trainees for training purposes only in controlled areas [4]. However, under 16 years of age, no person is allowed for occupational exposure.
- *General Public*: The dose limits for the general public, who might be exposed to radiation from various sources in the environment or medical procedures, are set significantly lower radiation doses than radiation workers. The first recommendation on restrictions of exposures of the members of the general public came in the ICRP publication 1954, which recommended that, for prolonged exposure to a large population, the maximum permissible

dose (MPD) should be reduced by a factor of 10 below the occupational exposure. They never argued any reason, for example, "knowing the hazard" and "receiving salaries" justifies "more" radiation than the public [3]. Initial recommendations were based on possible genetic effects due to prolonged exposure; however, later, it was said that the general public includes more sensitive persons, for example, children or sick people [3].

- *Patients*: Medical procedures involving radiation, such as X-rays or computed tomography (CT) scans, are designed to keep patient doses ALARA while obtaining accurate diagnostic information.
- *Carer and Comforters*: (i) exposures of carers and comforters are limited to ensure safety and (ii) exposures due to diagnostic investigations of volunteers participating in a biomedical research program.

10.4.6.1 Dose Limit for Carers and Comforters

The IAEA's Safety Standards GSR Part 3 [4] has mentioned carers and comforters. However, there is no clear distinction between or a definition of who can be called a carer and who is a comforter. They define this as one phrase and say the Carer and Comforter the "Persons who willingly and voluntarily help (other than in their occupation) in the care, support and comfort of patients undergoing radiological procedures for medical diagnosis or medical treatment" [4].

Now consider two scenarios: first, where a nurse is standing with a patient wearing a lead apron during a radiology procedure to help the patient, and second, the child's mother is standing in the radiology procedure room to accomplish the test. In the first situation, the nurse is standing neither willingly nor voluntarily, but as her duty to help the patient and the radiology team complete the investigational procedure. So, what would she be called, carer or comforter, or is she carer and comforter both? She is a carer, and the mother would be a comforter, as without her presence, the child may not undergo the procedure because of anxiety or any other reason.

The terms "carers" and "comforters" are not formally defined, but they can be understood within the broader context of patient care and support in radiology settings. Here is a general understanding of these terms and the potential differences between them:

Carers Carers in the context of radiology investigations might refer to healthcare professionals responsible for patients' overall care and well-being before, during, and after radiological procedures. Carers can include radiologic technologists, nurses, medical assistants, and other healthcare personnel assisting patients throughout imaging. Their primary role is to ensure the safety and comfort of patients, explain the procedure, help with positioning, and ensure optimal imaging conditions.

Comforters Comforters typically refer to individuals who provide emotional and psychological support to patients undergoing medical procedures, including radiology investigations. They are often family members, friends, or volunteers who are not part of the formal healthcare team but play a vital role in helping patients feel at ease. Their primary role is to offer comfort, reassurance, and companionship to patients who may be anxious, stressed, or uncomfortable due to the medical procedure. Comforters may hold the patient's hand, encourage, engage in conversation, or offer distractions to help reduce anxiety and improve the patient's overall experience.

Their presence can positively impact a patient's emotional well-being during a potentially stressful medical procedure.

Differences

- Carers are typically healthcare professionals with specific roles and responsibilities related to the technical aspects of radiology investigations, patient safety, and healthcare delivery.
- Comforters are individuals, often from the patient's personal support network or volunteer programs, who provide emotional and

psychological support to patients but do not have formal medical responsibilities.

- Carers focus on care's technical and clinical aspects, while comforters focus on the patient's emotional and psychological needs.
- Carers work as part of the healthcare team, while comforters are external to the healthcare system, but can be invaluable in enhancing the patient's experience.

As far as "dose limit" is concerned, "the carer and comforters" are treated in one category, and the dose limit is defined by the ICRP. For individuals directly involved in providing comfort and care, excluding young children and infants, a dose constraint of 5 mSv per episode (i.e., for the duration of a specific release after therapy) is considered reasonable. This constraint should be applied with flexibility.

10.4.6.2 Dose Limits for Volunteers in Biomedical Research

Volunteers are vital in biomedical research, whether they are patients with a condition or healthy individuals. Ethical committees play a key role in approving research programs involving radiation use, such as diagnostic procedures or treatment comparisons. They need accurate data on expected radiation doses and risks based on participants' characteristics and details on who will perform the procedures. Ethical committees set dose constraints based on national or regional standards, with constraints for research with societal benefits. The ICRP provides dose constraint guidelines ranging from 0.1 to 1 mSv for minimal risk studies and up to 10 mSv for studies with significant societal benefits. Special attention is given to setting constraints for healthy volunteers repeatedly exposed to increased risks in biomedical research programs.

Different Situations of Exposure for the Dose Limit

The International Atomic Energy Agency (IAEA), in its General Safety Regulations [4], describes three scenarios of radiation exposure such as a planned exposure situation, an emergency exposure situation, and an existing exposure situation. All routine diagnostic investigations are considered under planned exposure situations. The dose limits defined by IAEA are different for all these situations. Let us understand these:

- *Planned Exposure Situation*: The planned exposure situation arises from the planned operation of a source or a planned activity resulting from an exposure due to a source [4]. In this situation, radiation exposure is intentionally initiated for a specific purpose, such as medical imaging, industrial applications, or research. The exposure is carefully planned and controlled to achieve the desired outcome while minimizing unnecessary radiation exposure to individuals. Medical diagnostic procedures, radiological treatments, and industrial radiography are examples of planned exposure situations.
- *Emergency Exposure Situation*: This is a situation of exposure that arises from an accident, a malicious act, or other unexpected event and requires prompt action to avoid or reduce adverse consequences [4]. This may result in a sudden increase in radiation exposure for individuals and can occur due to accidents, incidents, or events such as nuclear accidents or unintended exposures. During an emergency exposure situation, the primary focus is on mitigating the impact of the event, protecting individuals, and preventing further exposures. The employer is responsible for ensuring that emergency workers are not exposed to more than the planned annual dose limit for a single year, except in the case of:
  - Life-saving situations or to prevent serious injuries
  - Prevention of severe deterministic effects
  - Prevention of catastrophic conditions that can affect members of the public and the environment or
  - Minimizing large collective doses
- *Existing Exposure Situation*: An existing exposure involves ongoing or long-term exposure to ionizing radiation due to natural sources, human activities, or historical events. These situations are characterized by chronic

or prolonged exposure over time. Examples of existing exposure situations include living in areas with naturally occurring radioactive materials (e.g., radon gas exposure) or working in occupations where radiation exposure is part of the job (e.g., airline crew and nuclear industry workers).

It is important to note that radiation protection measures and guidelines differ for each exposure situation. In planned exposure situations, efforts focus on optimizing procedures, ensuring appropriate shielding, and managing doses to keep exposures ALARA. Rapid response, evacuation, and providing appropriate medical care to affected individuals are priorities in emergency exposure situations. Monitoring, dose assessment, and long-term risk management strategies are employed in existing exposure situations. These exposure situations are considered when developing radiation protection standards, guidelines, and regulations to ensure the safety of individuals and the environment in various scenarios involving ionizing radiation.

10.4.6.3 Dose Constraints and Reference Levels

Dose constraints and reference levels are utilized for optimization to ensure safety and protection. When optimizing protection, dose constraints and reference levels are applied to limit individual doses [5]. The concept of a dose constraint was first introduced in ICRP publication 60 (1991) and later explained again in publication 103 (2007) more clearly. It is an upper bound to optimization, and the dose above this is unlikely in optimized conditions for a given set of exposure, and action must be taken if it breaches. It is defined for the planned exposure situation (except in medical exposures) and provides a basic level of protection that is always lower than the prescribed dose limits. Exceeding a dose constraint does not necessarily mean non-compliance with regulatory requirements but may lead to additional follow-up actions.

Example The radiation dose limits for occupational radiation workers typically allow for an annual dose of 20 mSv averaged over 5 years, with a maximum limit of 50 mSv in a single year. In some countries like India, the single-year annual limit is 30 mSv. Additionally, during routine monitoring, the effective dose should not exceed 10 mSv within a specified quarterly monitoring period. This is an example of dose constraint where, despite not crossing the annual dose, there is a checkpoint in each monitoring period, and subsequent follow-ups are done as necessary.

The reference level is used in emergency and existing exposure situations. In the event of an emergency exposure or identification of an existing exposure, protective measures must be taken, and the doses to workers and the public should be measured or assessed. The reference level can then be a benchmark for evaluating protection options in hindsight. Depending on the protective measures' success, the doses' distribution may or may not exceed the reference level. However, any efforts should be made to reduce exposures above the reference level to a lower level, if possible [5].

The appropriate value for a constraint or reference level will vary depending on the specific situation of the exposure being evaluated. It is important to note that neither dose and risk constraints nor reference levels indicate a clear boundary between "safe" and "dangerous" conditions, nor do they signify a significant change in the associated health risks for individuals [5].

10.4.6.4 Diagnostic Reference Level

In medical diagnosis, diagnostic reference levels (DRLs) assess whether the patient dose or administered activity from a specified imaging procedure is too high or low under routine conditions. This helps determine if protection measures have been optimized or if corrective action is necessary. If such levels are deemed unusual, a local review should be initiated.

DRLs are established to help optimize the balance between obtaining high-quality diagnostic images while minimizing the radiation dose delivered to the patient. They are benchmarks to ensure that the radiation dose used in diagnostic radiology is ALARA while still producing clinically useful images. They are procedure-specific, country-specific, patient size and age-specific, and so on. Each type of exam may have its DRLs based on factors like the body part being imaged and the clinical objective.

10.4.6.5 History and Current Recommendations on Dose Limits

As mentioned above, the term "dose limit" was introduced in 1977 by the ICRP in publication 26; before that, there was a concept of "MPD." Even the terms "ALARA," that is, "As Low As Reasonably achievable," and three basic principles of radiation protection, "Justification," "Optimization," and "Application of Dose Limits," were also introduced in the same publication. However, the first advice on radiation protection was published just 1 year after the discovery of X-rays, and the importance of time, distance, and shielding was highlighted [6]. Several nations began to develop radiation protection laws in the early 1920s, but it was not until 1925 that the first International Congress of Radiology (ICR) met and discussed creating international protection standards [3].

In 1928, the International Commission on Radiation Protection was born with the name "International X-ray and Radium Protection Committee" (IXRPC), and the first recommendations were released with restrictions on the number of working hours along with recommendations on shielding and precautions to be observed by X-ray operators. These recommendations were mainly based on the deterministic effects of radiation with a certain threshold. Bo Lindell, who was once scientific secretary of ICRP during 1957–62, published "A History of Radiation Protection (1996) [1]" and estimated that occupational annual effective doses to the medical staff at the time may have averaged around 1000 mSv in ICRP (then IXRPC) the first recommendation of 1928. The Sievert unit came into existence in 1962 after recommendations from the International Commission on Radiological Units and Measurements (ICRU); however, Roentgen was then the unit for measuring radiation. The unit Roentgen was recommended by the ICRU (then the International X-Ray Unit Committee) in 1928, during the same ICR meeting where IXRPC was formed (Table 10.3).

The next ICRP recommendations were in 1934, and the exposure conditions were modi-

Table 10.3 The evolution of dose limits for occupational workers

Recommendation body and year	Dose limits	Basis and additional information
IXRPC 1928	1 Sv per year for workers	The first formal recommendation by the IXRPC, setting a relatively high limit based on the limited understanding of radiation risks at the time. This early guideline reflected the need to protect workers in emerging radiology and radium industries.
IXRPC 1934	500 mSv per year for workers	The IXRPC, now recognizing the need for stricter controls, reduced the annual dose limit by half. This change indicated growing awareness of the health risks associated with prolonged radiation exposure, although the limit was still quite high by today's standards.
ICRP 1951	150 mSv per year for workers	The ICRP further reduced the limit, reflecting improved understanding of radiation-induced health effects, particularly the long-term risks such as cancer. This marked a significant shift toward more conservative safety standards.
ICRP 1966	50 mSv per year for workers	5 mSv for members of the public
ICRP 26 (1977)	50 mSv per year for workers	1 mSv per year for members of the public
ICRP 60 (1991)	20 mSv per year for workers	1 mSv per year for members of the public
ICRP 103 (2007)	20 mSv per year for workers	1 mSv per year for members of the public

fied, corresponding to 500 mSv per year as current units. The 1938 recommendations included X-rays and gamma rays with no major obvious changes from the 1934 recommendations. After the Second World War, further recommendations came in 1951, and the corresponding annual limit for occupational effective dose was reduced to 150 mSv. The ICRP publication 9 (1966) brought substantial changes in radiation protection, further reduced the annual doses to 50 mSv, and introduced the term "dose limit" for public exposures. This was the first publication in which the philosophy of radiation protection moved from deterministic effects to stochastic effects, and the assumption of a threshold for induction of cancer was rejected [3].

The ICRP publication 26 (1977) introduced weighting factors, and publication 27 (1978) introduced the name "effective dose equivalent." The ICRP 60 (1991) brought major changes and introduced the principles of justification, optimization, and dose limits. In the same publication, the terms "effective dose" and "equivalent dose" were introduced, and the term "effective dose equivalent" was abolished. The same publication also introduced the concept of "dose constraints."

The purpose of "dose limitation" is to prevent anyone from being exposed to an unacceptable level of risk from regulated sources, whereas "dose constraint" is an individual-focused criterion applied to a single source to ensure that the most vulnerable individuals are not exposed to excessive risk from that source [3].

Publication 103 (2007) was yet another important publication from the ICRP, which was a kind of revised edition of publication 60 (1991) and emphasized the significance of optimizing radiological protection and expanded on the successful implementation of this requirement in planned exposure situations to include emergency and existing exposure situations. The dose limits were kept almost the same, with minor changes here and there. The current dose limits are mentioned in Tables 10.4, 10.5, and 10.6 for different exposure situations.

Table 10.4 Planned exposure situations

Category of exposure	ICRP 103 (2007) recommendations	Remarks
For occupational exposure of workers (above 18 years)		
Whole body dose	**20 mSv/year averaged over 5 years** (i.e., 100 mSv in 5 years), with a maximum of **50 mSv** and **30 mSv** in India in any single year.	A single year typically means a calendar year. The 5-year averaging is typically done on a rolling basis, meaning that at any given time, the previous 5 years of exposure are considered when assessing compliance with the limit [7].
Lens of eye	**20 mSv/year averaged over 5 years** (i.e., 100 mSv in 5 years), with a maximum of **50 mSv** in any single year.	The eye is particularly sensitive to radiation, and these limits are designed to prevent cataract formation and other eye injuries.
Extremities and skin (hand/feet/skin)	**500 mSv in a year**	Extremities and skin can tolerate higher doses compared to the whole body, as they have a lower risk of severe health effects from radiation exposure.
Pregnant women for the remainder of pregnancy	**1 mSv to the embryo/fetus**	This limit aims to protect the developing embryo/fetus, which is highly sensitive to radiation, particularly during the early stages of development. The dose estimation should be conducted carefully, as outlined in para 10.8 of the ICRP guidelines.
For occupational exposure of apprentices (16–18 years)		
Whole body	**6 mSv/year**	Younger workers are subject to stricter limits due to their increased susceptibility to radiation and the potential for longer lifetime exposure.
Lens of eye	**20 mSv/year**	Similar to adult workers, but applied to a younger, more vulnerable population.

(continued)

Table 10.4 (continued)

Category of exposure	ICRP 103 (2007) recommendations	Remarks
Extremities and skin (hand/feet/skin)	**150 mSv in a year**	This lower limit reflects the need for greater protection of younger individuals' extremities and skin.
Public exposure		
Whole body	**1 mSv in a year**	In certain special circumstances, a higher dose may be permitted in a single year, as long as the 5-year average does not exceed 1 mSv/year. This flexibility allows for occasional higher exposures while maintaining overall safety [8].
Lens of eye	**15 mSv in a year**	The public is generally less exposed than occupational workers, but specific organs like the eye still require protective limits due to their sensitivity.
Skin	**50 mSv in a year**	This limit is designed to protect against potential skin damage from radiation, ensuring that exposure remains within safe boundaries.

Table 10.5 Emergency exposure situations

Category of exposure	Recommendations	Remarks
For occupational exposure of workers		
Life-saving (informed volunteers)	**No dose restrictions** if the benefit to others outweighs the rescuer's life	In extreme emergency situations, where workers voluntarily engage in life-saving activities, there are no formal dose limits. This approach is based on the ethical principle that the potential benefits to others justify the risks to the rescuer. Informed consent is critical in these scenarios.
Other urgent rescue operations	**500–1000 mSv**	Effective doses below 1000 mSv should avoid serious deterministic effects, while those below 500 mSv should avoid other deterministic effects. These operations are less critical than life-saving but still require urgent action, with dose limits reflecting the need to protect the worker [9].
Other rescue operations	**≤100 mSv in a year**	These operations are less time-sensitive and involve lower risk. A dose limit of 100 mSv is set to prevent any acute effects, with a subsequent additional cancer risk of less than 1% [9]. This limit ensures the safety of workers involved in less critical rescue missions.
Public exposure		
All countermeasures combined in an overall protection strategy	**20–100 mSv/year**, depending on the situation.	This category includes measures such as foodstuff control, distribution of stable iodine, sheltering, and temporary evacuation. The dose range is flexible, allowing for appropriate response strategies based on the severity of the emergency, with emphasis on justification and optimization.

10.4.6.6 Maintaining the Dose Records

Records of occupational exposure for each worker must be kept throughout and after their working life. These records should be preserved until the worker reaches or has reached the age of 75 years and for at least 30 years after they cease working in jobs that expose them to occupational hazards. It is crucial to maintain these records to ensure the safety and well-being of the workers, both during and after their employment [2].

Table 10.6 Medical exposure situations

Category of exposure	Recommendations	Remarks
Patients	**No dose limit**	In medical situations, there are no dose limits for patients undergoing diagnostic or therapeutic procedures. Instead, the focus is on **justification** and **optimization** of the procedure. DRLs should be followed to ensure doses are kept ALARA while still providing the necessary medical benefit [5].
Volunteers for biomedical research		
Minor benefit to society	**<0.1 mSv**	In research studies where the potential benefit to society is minor, the radiation dose to volunteers should be kept below 0.1 mSv. This low dose reflects the limited benefit and aims to minimize any potential risks to the participants.
Intermediate benefit to society	**0.1–1 mSv**	For research with intermediate societal benefits, the acceptable dose range increases to 0.1–1 mSv. This range balances the moderate benefit with a slightly higher radiation dose, still ensuring that participant safety is prioritized.
Moderate benefit to society	**1–10 mSv**	In studies where the potential benefit is moderate, a dose range of 1–10 mSv is recommended. This higher dose range reflects the greater potential societal benefit and is considered acceptable as long as the risk to volunteers remains justified.
Substantial benefit to society	**>10 mSv**	For research expected to provide substantial benefits to society, doses exceeding 10 mSv may be justified. However, even in these cases, the principle of keeping radiation exposure as low as possible should still apply, with careful consideration of the risks and benefits.
Comforters and carers	**5 mSv per episode**	Comforters and carers, such as family members or friends who support patients during medical procedures, are allowed a dose limit of 5 mSv per episode. This recognizes their voluntary exposure while ensuring that their safety is not compromised, particularly when exposure is repetitive or occurs over multiple episodes.

10.5 Principles of Safe Work Practices in Diagnostic Radiology

Safe work practices in diagnostic radiology are essential to minimize the risks associated with ionizing radiation exposure for patients and healthcare workers. Implementing proper safety measures ensures that radiological procedures are performed safely and effectively. Here are some key safe work practices in diagnostic radiology:

- *ALARA Principle*: Follow the ALARA principle, which means minimizing radiation exposure doses to patients and healthcare workers while still obtaining the necessary diagnostic information.
- *Personal Protective Equipment (PPE):* Wear appropriate PPE, including lead aprons, thyroid shields, gloves, and eyewear, to reduce radiation exposure to body parts not involved in the procedure.
- *Time:* Minimize the time of radiation exposure. Ensure that efficient and accurate positioning and imaging techniques are used to reduce exposure duration for both the patient and healthcare worker.
- *Distance:* Maintain a safe distance from the radiation source. Stand behind protective barriers whenever possible during X-ray exposures.
- *Patient Positioning:* Properly position patients to obtain the required diagnostic images with the least radiation exposure. Use immobilization devices when needed.

- *Collimation:* Collimate the X-ray beam to cover only the area of interest. Avoid unnecessary radiation exposure to surrounding tissues.
- *Use of Shields:* Use lead shielding devices such as aprons, gloves, and thyroid shields to protect sensitive body areas during procedures.
- *Avoid Repeat Exposures:* Ensure that images are taken correctly the first time to prevent the need for repeat exposures, which increases radiation exposure.
- *Quality Control:* Regularly test and calibrate radiological equipment to ensure accurate dose delivery and image quality. Follow quality control procedures for equipment maintenance.
- *Radiation Monitoring:* Wear personal radiation dosimeters to monitor and record radiation exposure levels for healthcare workers. Regularly review exposure records to identify trends.
- *Communication:* Communicate with patients about the procedure, its benefits, and potential risks. Obtain informed consent for procedures involving ionizing radiation.
- *Pregnant Workers:* Pregnant workers should inform their employers about their pregnancy. Employers should take measures to limit the pregnant worker's radiation exposure during the gestational period.
- *Minimize Pediatric Exposure:* Use pediatric-specific techniques and protocols to reduce radiation exposure in pediatric patients.
- *Proper Ventilation:* Ensure proper ventilation in X-ray rooms to minimize the accumulation of airborne contaminants.
- *Education and Training:* Provide ongoing education and training to healthcare workers regarding radiation safety, including the proper use of equipment and protective measures.
- *Emergency Procedures:* Establish clear procedures for responding to radiation exposure emergencies, including contamination incidents.
- *Regulatory Compliance:* Adhere to local regulations, guidelines, and recommendations for radiation safety in diagnostic radiology

By following these safe work practices, healthcare professionals can effectively manage and minimize the risks associated with ionizing radiation exposure in diagnostic radiology environments.

10.6 Use of Barriers and Techniques for Radiation Protection in Radiology

Safe work practice necessitates good department design, different barriers, and techniques such as filtration, collimation, and patient positioning aids. The radiation protection principles are conceived during the planning and designing of the department itself. Apart from design considerations, many physical barriers, including lead aprons, shields, and the use of different aids, help to protect patients, staff, and the public from unjustified radiation. The barriers are designed to minimize the radiation dose to sensitive body parts while still obtaining diagnostically valuable images. This approach helps mitigate long-term health risks associated with cumulative radiation exposure from medical imaging procedures. Here are some primary radiation protection measures commonly used for patient protection in radiology:

10.6.1 Design and Regulations

The regulatory guidelines specify the thickness and quality of the protective materials required to achieve effective radiation shielding. The goal is to attenuate the radiation to safe levels while allowing the necessary diagnostic imaging to occur. The walls that face the X-ray source are often lined with lead or other radiation-absorbing materials. This helps prevent radiation from penetrating adjacent areas. The control panels and operator stations are shielded to minimize the operator's radiation exposure during imaging. Barriers are strategically positioned between the radiation source and individuals at risk. For example, during X-ray examinations, the X-ray tube is usually positioned behind a protective barrier, preventing radiation's direct transmission toward the operator.

10.6.2 Use of Radiation Barriers

Radiation barriers in radiology are protective structures designed to shield individuals from ionizing radiation, used in various medical imaging procedures such as X-rays and fluoroscopy. The primary purpose of radiation barriers is to reduce the exposure of individuals in the vicinity of radiological procedures to ionizing radiation. These barriers play a critical role in ensuring radiation safety for patients, healthcare workers, and anyone else who might be present in the area. Radiation barriers can come in various forms:

10.6.2.1 Lead Aprons and Shields

Lead aprons are worn by patients during X-ray examinations to shield their reproductive organs, abdomen, and other sensitive areas from radiation exposure. Gonadal shields, made of lead or other radiation-absorbing materials, are placed over the patient's pelvis during procedures involving the lower abdomen and pelvic region. Thyroid shields protect the thyroid gland from radiation exposure during X-ray procedures involving the head, neck, or upper chest. There are several varieties of lead aprons and shields designed for specific purposes:

- *Frontal Aprons*: These aprons are commonly used in radiological procedures and have thicknesses of lead equivalent of 0.25, 0.35, and 0.50 mm. They protect the torso, including the chest and abdomen, and come in different designs depending on need.
- *Thyroid Collar*: A thyroid collar is an accessory worn around the neck to shield the thyroid gland from radiation exposure. It is especially important during procedures that involve radiation directed toward the head and neck area.
- *Wraparound Aprons*: These aprons offer additional protection by wrapping around the sides, shielding the sides of the body and hips.
- *Pediatric Aprons*: Pediatric patients require radiation protection as well. Pediatric lead aprons are designed with sizes and features suitable for children, ensuring proper fit and comfort.

10.6.2.2 Lead Shields

Contact or adhesive shields are applied directly to the patient's skin overlying sensitive organs. They are used in procedures such as fluoroscopy and angiography to provide localized protection. Pediatric and neonatal shields are designed to protect infants and young children during X-ray examinations. They are tailored to their smaller size and unique anatomical considerations. Pregnancy shields protect pregnant patients and their developing fetuses from radiation exposure. These shields are typically placed over the abdomen during procedures.

- Mobile Shields: These are movable barriers made of lead or lead-equivalent materials. During procedures, they can be placed between the radiation source and personnel to provide temporary protection. Mobile shields are often used when there is a need to be close to the patient during imaging.
- Protective Eyewear: Lead glasses are designed to shield the eyes from radiation exposure. They are especially important for operators exposed to scatter radiation during procedures.
- Gonadal Shields: Gonadal shields protect the reproductive organs from radiation exposure. They are commonly used during procedures where the reproductive organs are within or near the primary X-ray beam.
- Lead Curtains and Drapes: Lead curtains and drapes can be used in radiology rooms to create additional barriers for radiation protection, especially in areas with high radiation exposure.

Regular inspection, maintenance, and quality control of lead aprons and shields are crucial to ensure their effectiveness in providing radiation protection. These measures help identify any issues or degradation in the protective properties of lead aprons and shields. The visual inspection of lead aprons and shields is important to detect any visible signs of wear, damage, or deterioration. Inspect for cracks, tears, creases, or other structural issues compromising the shielding effectiveness. Specialized lead inspection tools, such as fluoroscopes or lead detectors, can check for gaps or thinning areas in the lead lining. These tools can identify spots where the lead may have degraded, ensuring no areas of reduced shielding. Check the seams, stitching, and fasteners (such as Velcro straps) for any signs of damage and ensure that the fasteners are secure and functional to maintain the proper fit of the apron.

10.6.3 Use of Patient Positioning Aids

Proper patient positioning aids ensure accurate anatomical alignment, reducing the need for retakes and repeated exposures. These primary radiation protection devices are essential components of safe radiology practices. They help to minimize radiation exposure to critical organs and sensitive tissues, ensuring that patients receive the necessary diagnostic information while keeping their radiation dose ALARA. They come in various forms, each designed to address specific imaging needs and anatomical considerations. Here are some examples of common patient positioning aids used in radiology:

- *Immobilization Devices*: Immobilization devices are used to keep patients in a stable position during imaging. They are particularly useful for pediatric patients and those with difficulty holding still. Examples include pediatric immobilizers (used for infants and young children), head holders, and bite blocks for dental radiography.
- *Positioning Cushions and Wedges*: Positioning cushions and wedges are placed under patients to achieve proper alignment and angle during imaging. Examples include sponge cushions, body wedges, and positioning pillows for specific anatomical areas.
- *Compression Paddles*: Compression paddles are used in mammography to immobilize and flatten breast tissue. Proper compression helps improve image quality and reduces the need for retakes.
- *Alignment Guides*: Alignment guides help ensure that patients are positioned symmetrically and in proper alignment with the imaging equipment. They can be used for extremity radiography and spinal imaging.
- *Anatomical Markers*: Anatomical markers identify specific anatomical landmarks on the patient's body. They help ensure consistent positioning between images taken at different times.
- *Laser Alignment Systems*: Laser alignment systems project laser lines or dots onto the patient's body, assisting technologists in positioning the patient accurately within the imaging field.
- *Compression Bands and Straps*: During imaging, compression bands and straps secure limbs or body parts. They prevent movement and reduce the risk of motion artifacts in the images.
- *Stabilization Devices*: Stabilization devices prevent patient movement in specific imaging positions. For example, they can stabilize the head during skull X-rays.
- *Grids and Bucky Trays*: Grids and Bucky trays are used in radiography to stabilize and position the X-ray detector in alignment with the patient. They help ensure accurate and consistent image acquisition.
- *Breath-Hold Instructions*: In some cases, simple instructions are given to patients to hold their breath during imaging. This minimizes motion artifacts caused by breathing and enhances image quality.
- *Artifact Reducing Accessories*: Accessories such as lead markers, lead shields, and lead masks can reduce artifacts from dental restorations or jewelry.

These are a few examples of the many patient positioning aids used in radiology to achieve accurate and consistent patient positioning, improve image quality, and optimize radiation protection. The choice of positioning aid depends on the type of imaging procedure, the patient's condition, and the anatomical area being imaged.

10.6.4 Use of Filtration

Filtration refers to removing low-energy, less penetrating X-rays from the X-ray beam before it reaches the patient. This has the effect of reducing patient dose while still maintaining image quality. It is achieved by inserting a filter made of a material like aluminum into the X-ray beam. This filter selectively absorbs the lower-energy X-rays, which contribute less to image formation but can contribute significantly to patient dose. It helps to "harden" the X-ray beam by removing the softer, less penetrating X-rays while allowing the higher-energy X-rays to penetrate deeper and contribute to the diagnostic image. In addition to reducing patient dose, effective filtration helps improve image quality by reducing scatter radiation and increasing the image's contrast.

10.6.5 Use of Collimation

Collimation involves restricting the X-ray beam to only cover the specific area of interest of the patient. It is achieved by adjusting the size and shape of the X-ray field using lead shutters or other mechanisms on the X-ray tube housing. By limiting the X-ray field to the imaged anatomical region, collimation helps minimize unnecessary radiation exposure to surrounding tissues and organs. It prevents unnecessary exposure of healthy tissues and organs not part of the diagnostic region. This reduces the overall radiation dose to the patient and minimizes the potential risk of harmful effects from radiation. By focusing the X-ray beam solely on the area of interest, collimation contributes to better image clarity and resolution. Reduced scatter leads to sharper images with improved contrast and detail.

10.6.6 Use of Intensifying Screen

Intensifying screens are combined with X-ray film to amplify the amount of visible light produced from the X-ray exposure. This allows lower X-ray doses to achieve the same image exposure level, thereby reducing the radiation dose delivered to the patient. In modern digital radiography and computed radiography (CR) systems, digital detectors have largely replaced intensifying screens, offering benefits such as immediate image capture and the potential for further dose reduction through post-processing adjustments.

10.6.7 Regular Staff Training and Equipment Quality Control

Regular checks and quality control measures are conducted to ensure the effectiveness of radiation barriers. This might involve radiation measurements to verify that the shielding provides the intended protection.

Healthcare workers are trained to use radiation barriers correctly and effectively. This includes understanding the appropriate use of lead aprons, positioning mobile shields, and other safety practices; training should be refreshed annually to ensure compliance with current standards.

10.7 Regulatory Bodies

Several regulatory bodies and organizations are responsible for establishing and enforcing radiation protection standards and guidelines to ensure the safe and responsible use of ionizing radiation in various fields. These bodies set standards for radiation safety, dose limits, equipment specifications, and practices to protect individuals, workers, patients, and the environment. Some of the notable regulatory bodies for radiation protection include the following.

10.7.1 International Commission on Radiological Protection

The ICRP is an independent international organization that provides recommendations and guidance on radiation protection to protect people and the environment from the harmful effects of ionizing radiation. Established in 1928, the ICRP is recognized as a leading authority in radiation protection and plays a crucial role in global radiation safety standards and practices. It consists of a group of international experts from various fields related to radiation protection, including radiology, nuclear medicine, epidemiology, physics, and other scientific disciplines. These experts contribute their knowledge and experience to develop evidence-based recommendations, principles, and guidelines for radiation protection. These recommendations are widely used by national regulatory authorities, governments, industries, healthcare organizations, and other stakeholders to develop radiation protection regulations and practices.

10.7.2 IAEA

The IAEA, established on July 29, 1957, is a United Nations agency promoting the peaceful use of nuclear energy and technology. It develops safety standards, guidelines, and best practices for radiation protection, nuclear safety, and security. These standards provide a framework for member states to establish and maintain safe practices in various ionizing radiation applications. It also offers technical assistance, training programs, and workshops to enhance the capabilities of professionals working with ionizing radiation.

10.7.3 World Health Organization (WHO)

The WHO is a specialized agency of the United Nations that focuses on international public health issues. While the WHO's primary mandate is broader than radiation protection, it plays a significant role in addressing radiation-related health concerns and providing guidance on radiation protection.

While the IAEA and the WHO play roles in radiation protection, their primary mandates and focus areas are distinct. However, their work has some overlapping aspects due to the interconnectedness of public health and radiation safety. The primary mandate of the WHO is to address global health issues and promote public health. It focuses on various health concerns, including communicable diseases, non-communicable diseases, health systems, and environmental health.

10.7.4 National Regulatory Authorities

Many countries typically have their national regulatory authority responsible for overseeing radiation protection and safety within their borders. Examples include the Atomic Energy Regulatory Board in India. The Nuclear Regulatory Commission (NRC) in the United States, the Health and Safety Executive in the United Kingdom, the Autorité de Sûreté Nucléaire in France, and so on. The European Commission sets radiation protection standards and guidelines for European Union member states.

10.7.5 Food and Agriculture Organization (FAO)

FAO, a specialized agency of the United Nations, guides radiation protection in food safety, including minimizing contamination in agricultural products after nuclear accidents.

10.7.6 United Nations Scientific Committee on the Effects of Atomic Radiation (UNSCEAR)

UNSCEAR assesses and reports the levels and effects of ionizing radiation exposure, both natural and man-made, on human health and the environment.

10.7.7 Health and Medical Organizations

Various medical and health organizations, such as the American College of Radiology and the European Society of Radiology, provide guidelines for radiation protection in medical imaging and procedures.

10.7.8 Industry-Specific Authorities

Different industries using ionizing radiation have specific regulatory bodies overseeing their radiation protection practices. For example, the U.S. NRC oversees nuclear power plants, and the International Maritime Organization deals with radiation protection in maritime transport of radioactive materials.

These regulatory bodies collaborate globally to develop standards, guidelines, and recommendations that contribute to consistent and effective radiation protection practices worldwide. Their efforts aim to ensure that radiation-related activities are carried out safely while minimizing potential risks to human health and the environment.

10.8 Biological Effects of Radiation

Radiation can have biological effects on living organisms due to its ability to ionize atoms and molecules within cells. These effects can vary depending on factors such as the type of radiation, the dose received, the duration of exposure, and the sensitivity of the tissues involved. Studies suggest that most cancers begin with damage to individual cells, resulting in the deregulation of cell growth and a loss of control over cell proliferation [10]. While these changes may occur, they do not lead to malignancy until chemicals or hormones activate them in the surrounding environment. Radiation exposure can contribute to the mutation process that leads to cancer, but it is only one step among many. Many cancers are believed to originate from genetic mutations or damage to individual cells, disrupting normal cell growth and regulation. The process by which normal cells transform into cancer cells is known as carcinogenesis. A simplified overview of how this process works:

- *Initiation*: Carcinogenesis often begins with a genetic mutation or damage to the DNA within a single cell. Various factors, including exposure to carcinogens such as radiation, chemicals, certain viruses, or genetic predisposition, can cause this damage.
- *Promotion*: After the initial genetic damage, certain factors can promote the growth of the mutated cell. These factors might include chronic inflammation, hormonal imbalances, or ongoing exposure to carcinogens. The promotion stage encourages the mutated cell to divide and proliferate more rapidly than normal cells.
- *Progression*: Additional genetic changes accumulate in the rapidly dividing cells during progression. These changes can confer advantages to the cells, allowing them to evade the body's natural mechanisms for controlling cell growth and repair. The cells become more aggressive, and their ability to invade nearby tissues and spread to other body parts (metastasis) increases.
- *Metastasis*: If cancer cells successfully invade nearby tissues and enter the bloodstream or lymphatic system, they can spread to other parts of the body. This is how cancer can establish secondary tumors in distant locations from the original site.
- *Loss of Cellular Control*: One hallmark of cancer is the loss of cellular control mechanisms. Normal cells have built-in checks and balances that regulate their growth, repair, and death. Cancer cells often bypass or disrupt these controls, leading to uncontrolled growth and proliferation.
- *Genomic Instability*: Cancer cells frequently exhibit genomic instability, meaning that they have a high rate of genetic mutations and chromosomal abnormalities. This contributes to the heterogeneity of cancer and its ability to adapt and survive in different environments.

It is important to note that not all genetic mutations or cellular damage lead to cancer. The body has mechanisms to repair DNA damage and eliminate cells with irreparable mutations. However, in cases where these repair mechanisms fail or are overwhelmed, cancerous transformation can occur.

Understanding the molecular and cellular processes underlying carcinogenesis is essential for developing effective strategies for cancer prevention, early detection, and treatment. While radiation exposure can potentially contribute to genetic mutations that initiate cancer, modern medical practices prioritize minimizing radiation exposure while maximizing the benefits of diagnostic and therapeutic procedures.

The biological effects of radiation can be categorized into two main types: deterministic effects and stochastic effects.

10.8.1 Deterministic Effects

Deterministic effects are biological effects of radiation exposure with a threshold dose below which they do not occur. These effects become more severe as the radiation dose increases above the threshold. Unlike stochastic effects, which are probabilistic and have no dose threshold, deterministic effects are directly related to the dose received. Here are some examples of deterministic effects:

- *Acute Radiation Syndrome (ARS):* ARS occurs after exposure to high doses of radiation over a short period, typically within hours to days. Symptoms include nausea, vomiting, diarrhea, fever, fatigue, and decreased blood cell counts. The severity of ARS is dose-dependent, and exposure levels well above diagnostic radiology doses are required to trigger ARS. The threshold dose is above 1 Gy. ARS can occur at doses above 1 Gy, with symptoms becoming more severe as the dose increases. However, severe ARS symptoms typically occur at 3 Gy or higher doses.
- *Skin Erythema (Redness) and Burns*: At higher doses of radiation, skin can experience erythema (reddening) and, in extreme cases, burns. The severity of these effects increases with the radiation dose. This effect is commonly observed when high doses are used to treat tumors in radiation therapy settings. The threshold dose is around 2 Gy (gray) or higher. The reddening of the skin can occur at doses above 2 Gy, and burns can occur at higher doses.
- *Cataract Formation:* Prolonged exposure to relatively high doses of radiation, such as those received by individuals working with ionizing radiation without proper protection, can lead to the formation of cataracts in the lens of the eye. The threshold dose varies, but it is around 2–5 Gy Gy, depending on exposure duration. The threshold dose for cataract formation can vary depending on factors like the type of radiation and the duration of exposure. In some cases, the threshold may be as low as 1.5–2 Gy, while other studies suggest cataracts may not develop until doses exceed 5 Gy [11].
- *Hematopoietic (Blood Cell) Syndrome:* At very high doses, radiation can damage bone marrow, where blood cells are produced. This can lead to decreased blood cell counts, including red blood cells, white blood cells, and platelets, resulting in anemia, susceptibility to infections, and bleeding disorders. The threshold dose is around 2–5 Gy. Symptoms become more severe as the dose increases. At doses around 2–5 Gy, there can be a noticeable decrease in blood cell counts.
- *Gastrointestinal Syndrome:* Extremely high doses of radiation can damage the lining of the gastrointestinal tract, leading to severe nausea, vomiting, and diarrhea. This can result in fluid loss, electrolyte imbalance, and potentially fatal outcomes. The threshold dose is around 6–30 Gy. Symptoms become severe at doses above 6 Gy and can be fatal at around 30 Gy or higher.

It is important to emphasize that deterministic effects only occur above a certain threshold dose. Below this threshold, these effects do not manifest, and the body's natural repair mechanisms can usually handle radiation-induced damage. Radiation protection aims to ensure that radiation doses are kept well below the levels where deterministic effects could occur. In medical practices, such as diagnostic imaging, radiation doses are carefully controlled to prevent deterministic effects by following the principle of ALARA to optimize image quality while minimizing the risk of harmful effects.

10.8.2 Stochastic Effects

Stochastic or probabilistic effects are biological effects of radiation exposure that occur randomly and have no threshold dose. Unlike deterministic effects, which become more severe as the radiation dose increases, stochastic effects are characterized by their probability of occurrence increasing with higher doses. In other words, there is no minimum dose below which these effects do not occur; they can occur even at very low doses, but their likelihood is proportional to the dose received. It can be characterized by the following:

- *No Threshold Dose*: Unlike deterministic effects, which have a threshold dose below which they do not occur, stochastic effects have no dose threshold. Even the smallest dose of radiation carries some probability of causing a stochastic effect.
- *Probabilistic Nature*: Stochastic effects occur randomly, and their occurrence is governed by probability. They cannot be predicted with certainty for an individual, but their likelihood increases with higher doses of radiation.
- *Dose-Response Relationship*: The probability of a stochastic effect occurring increases with the radiation dose received. This means that higher doses are associated with a higher likelihood of an effect, but there is no dose at which the effect becomes certain.
- *Delayed Onset*: Stochastic effects may have a latency period between the time of radiation exposure and the appearance of the effect. This delay can make it challenging to attribute an effect to a specific exposure directly.

Examples of stochastic effects are as follows:

- *Cancer:* Stochastic effects include an increased risk of developing cancer due to radiation exposure. Ionizing radiation can damage DNA within cells, potentially leading to genetic mutations. These mutations can accumulate over time and increase the likelihood of cancer development. The risk of cancer from radiation exposure is considered a stochastic effect because it does not have a dose threshold; any dose of radiation carries some risk of inducing cancer, no matter how small.
- *Hereditary Effects*: Radiation exposure can also increase the risk of hereditary effects, where genetic mutations are passed down to future generations through reproductive cells (sperm and eggs). The risk of hereditary effects is also considered a stochastic effect, as there is no dose threshold below which these effects do not occur. However, the magnitude of the risk is generally much smaller compared to the risk of cancer.
- *Genetic Effects*: Stochastic genetic effects result from changes in the DNA of germ cells (reproductive cells, such as eggs and sperm) due to radiation exposure. These changes, known as mutations, can be passed on to future generations if they occur in the reproductive cells. However, it is important to note that the likelihood of genetic effects due to radiation exposure is generally much smaller than cancer risk.

"Genetic effects" and "hereditary effects" are related concepts, but they refer to slightly different outcomes of radiation exposure to genetic material, as discussed above. Hereditary effects are a subset of genetic effects and are of particular concern because they can impact the health of future generations. All hereditary effects are genetic, but not all are necessarily hereditary. Efforts to minimize radiation exposure, especially in reproductive cells, aim to reduce the potential for hereditary effects and their associated risks. Other genetic effects are Somatic mutations, that is, changes in the DNA of somatic cells, cancer, chromosomal aberrations, cell death and apoptosis, and genomic instability.

To mitigate stochastic effects, radiation protection principles such as the ALARA principle are followed to minimize radiation exposure. For medical and non-medical applications, efforts are made to limit radiation doses to the lowest achievable levels while achieving the intended diagnostic or therapeutic outcomes.

10.9 Female Patients, Female Radiation Workers, and the Effects of Radiation on the Fetus

Special care must be taken with females of childbearing age when dealing in the radiology department, as radiation exposure during pregnancy can pose risks to the developing fetus. When discussing the potential risks to a fetus, it is important to discuss female patients and female radiation workers separately. Though the effect of radiation on the fetus is considered to be the same in both cases, still, in the case of female radiation workers, the questions would be more and can be:

- Should I continue to work as a radiation worker when I am pregnant or planning to be pregnant?
- Do I need to inform the employer? Is it necessary, and if yes, when should I?
- Should my working conditions be modified once I am pregnant, and is it my right?
- Will I be removed from my job, or will there be any discrimination if I notify my pregnancy?
- How much is the risk to my baby if I continue my job?
- How do I measure the doses to my fetus?

As radiation workers, we are supposed to protect our patients from unnecessary radiation burden, and this liability increases when the patient is female of childbearing age as they may be carrying an unborn child. The fetus and the female patient will be treated as separate entities, and radiation safety precautions are to be taken accordingly. Along with safety, the documentation of the proceedings is equally important to avoid any legal issues in the future.

We have four key points in our discussion: first, conducting different diagnostic procedures during pregnancy; second, the effect of radiation on the fetus during different phases of pregnancy; third, handling and record keeping in case of female patients of childbearing age; and fourth, as female radiation workers, the answer to the abovementioned questions.

When we go further in our discussion, the terms dose, Gray, and Sievert will be used. Though they have been explained in detail in Chap. 1, just for refreshing, the absorbed doses are termed as doses in further discussions. Gray and Sieverts can be used interchangeably as both are the same in the case of X-rays, gamma rays, and electrons, and these are only used in radiology or diagnostic nuclear medicine. Most of the contents discussed below have been adapted from ICRP publication 84 [12].

10.9.1 Conducting Different Diagnostic Procedures During Pregnancy

Properly conducted diagnostic procedures during pregnancy generally do not significantly raise risk beyond the natural occurrence. Yet, higher doses in therapeutic procedures can harm the fetus. Risks are highest during early development, less in the second trimester, and lowest in the third. The fetus is considered a member of the public, and doses to the fetus are not justified until it is a direct beneficiary. However, in situations where the diagnostic procedures are unavoidable to the woman who is carrying conceptus, for example, in case of a road traffic accident or any other situation requiring urgent intervention and the risk to the mother is more than the risk to the fetus, the procedure must be carried out.

Any doses less than 100 mGy are considered safer for fetuses, and malformations due to radiation are unlikely. In case of higher doses than 100 mGy, and pregnancy is between the 3rd and the 15th week of gestation, the risk of malformation increases and there may be a decrease in intelligence quotient (IQ) and possible retardation. However, most diagnostic procedures do not significantly increase the risk of fetal death, deformity, or impaired mental development. The fetal dose can approach or exceed 50 mGy during barium enema if the fluoroscopy time crosses 7 minutes. Otherwise, with good technique, the doses during barium enema are 3–7 mGy. If performed properly, the fetal dose of 100 mGy does not reach with 3 pelvic CR scans or with 20 conventional diagnostic X-rays of the abdomen or pelvis. At doses 100–200 mGy, the risk of malformations is low, but the risk increases with increasing dose.

If the X-ray equipment is adequately insulated and X-ray beam collimation is utilized, clinically required radiography or fluoroscopy of distant from the fetus locations, such as the chest, skull, or limbs (other than the hip), can be performed safely at any time throughout pregnancy without any modification or tailoring of the protocol. If the conceptus is in the primary beam of radiation such as high-dose abdominal or pelvic CT or fluoroscopy, the fetal dose estimation is to be carried out, and the related risk is to be informed to the concerned individuals for their informed choice. During abdominal CT scans, the typical doses to the fetus can be 10–40 mGy. However, the CT has the advantage of tight collimation, and scanning the precise area of interest rather than the entire abdomen and pelvis will help reduce fetal dose. Table 10.7 gives an outline of approximate fetal doses from common diagnostic procedures.

When fetal radiation exposure cannot be completely avoided, efforts should be focused on minimizing the absorbed dose to the fetus. However, any adjustments made should not compromise the diagnostic effectiveness of the radiological examination. Techniques such as narrowing the beam collimation to the specific area of interest, raising the kilovolt peak (kVp), eliminating anti-scatter grids, and reducing the number of radiographs taken are commonly employed to tailor the examinations and decrease fetal exposure. These methods are frequently employed to customize procedures and mitigate radiation exposure to the fetus.

Table 10.7 Approximate fetal doses from common diagnostic procedures in the United Kingdom

Examination	Mean (mGy)	Maximum (mGy)
Conventional X-ray examinations		
Abdomen	1.4	4.2
Chest	<0.01	<0.01
Intravenous urogram	1.7	10
Lumbar spine	1.7	10
Pelvis	1.1	4
Skull	<0.01	<0.01
Thoracic spine	<0.01	<0.01
Fluoroscopic examinations		
Barium meal (UGI)	1.1	5.8
Barium enema	6.8	24
CT		
Abdomen	8.0	49
Chest	0.06	0.96
Head	<0.005	<0.005
Lumbar spine	2.4	8.6
Pelvis	25	79
Nuclear medicine		
^{99m}Tc bone scan	3.3	4.6
^{99m}Tc lung perfusion	0.2	0.4
^{99m}Tc lung ventilation	0.3	1.2
^{99m}Tc renal scan (DTPA)	1.5	4.0
^{99m}Tc thyroid scan (pertechnetate)	0.7	1.6
^{99m}Tc dynamic cardiac scan (RBC)	3.4	3.7
^{201}Tl myocardial perfusion	3.7	4.0
^{131}I thyroid metastases	–	22.0

Reference: Sharp et al. [13]

10.9.2 Effects of Radiation on the Fetus During Different Phases of Pregnancy

The effect of radiation on the fetus mainly depends on the conceptus age or the gestation period (Table 10.8). The gestation period can be divided into three phases:

Table 10.8 Probability of bearing healthy children as a function of radiation dose

Absorbed dose to conceptus (mGy)	Probability of no malformation (%)	Probability of no cancer development by age 19 (%)	Additional information
0	97.0	99.7	Represents natural background radiation exposure
0.5	97.0	99.7	Minimal dose increase, no significant change in probability
1	97.0	99.7	Common threshold for diagnostic imaging, negligible risk increase
2.5	97.0	99.7	Within safe limits for diagnostic purposes
5	97.0	99.7	Still considered safe with minimal impact on health outcomes
10	97.0	99.6	Slightly lower probability of avoiding cancer development
50	97.0	99.4	Noticeable reduction in the probability of avoiding cancer.
100	Close to 97.0	99.1	Higher radiation exposure, though significant effects are still uncommon

Reference ICRP 84 [14]

1. The pre-implantation period from conception until implantation, that is, the journey of the fertilized egg from the fallopian tube to the uterus and its eventual attachment to the uterine lining. It begins at the moment of fertilization, when a sperm cell penetrates an egg, forming a fertilized egg or zygote. This zygote then undergoes several divisions as it travels through the fallopian tube toward the uterus.
2. The phase of major organ formation spanning roughly from the 3rd to the 8th week after conception.
3. The fetal development phase extends from the 9th week until birth. This later phase encompasses the crucial central nervous system development period, occurring between the 8th and 25th weeks.

In the first 2 weeks, that is, phase I of pregnancy, malformations or fetal death is unlikely, even though only the development of the central nervous system and the heart begins during this period. Malformations may occur, especially in the organs under development at the time of exposure, during the remaining period of major organogenesis, which is typically understood to begin from the third week following conception.

Ionizing radiation can cause a variety of effects once it crosses a threshold. Less than 100 mGy of radiation is considered safer for fetuses, and malformations due to radiation are unlikely. The threshold, that is, 100–200 mGy or higher, can lead to various outcomes, including lethality, central nervous system issues, cataracts, growth problems, and behavioral disorders. Radiation-related disorders are rarely seen in humans without associated neuropathology since the fetal neural system is extremely sensitive and goes through a lengthy development phase. This illness is recognizable but can be brought on by other dangerous substances.

The clinical effects of radiation result from (1) cell killing or (2) unrepaired/mis-repaired DNA damage. Unrepaired/mis-repaired DNA damage leads to conditions such as leukemia, cancer, and hereditary effects. The likelihood of such effects increases with dose. CNS sensitivity peaks at 8–15 weeks post-conception; doses exceeding 100 mGy can reduce IQ. The situation is less clear-cut in the intermediate dose range of 100–500 mGy. However, these situations do not occur very frequently. At 1000 mGy, the likelihood of significant IQ reduction rises to about 40%, exceeding the 3% spontaneous rate. Effects diminish after 25 weeks of gestation.

10.9.3 Safety and Handling of Female Patients of Childbearing Age

While handling female patients of childbearing age, all such patients should be considered pregnant until it is proven that she is not pregnant or has a history of hysterectomy or tubal ligation. In routine practice, every woman of reproductive age should be asked about her menstrual history. However, in many cases, menstrual history may not give accurate information about her pregnancy. For example, the woman can get pregnant on the 14th day following the last menstrual period and come to you on the 25th. We assume that she would not be pregnant if the last period was within a month. However, in reality, she can be pregnant. The urine pregnancy tests or blood serum (human chorionic gonadotropin test) give reliable results 6–12 days post-conception, typically around the 20th–26th day of the menstrual cycle. However, this approach is not commonly employed for low-dose diagnostic tests but can be opted for if there is a chance of high radiation dose to the pelvis.

To reduce the occurrence of unintended radiation exposures to the embryo and fetus, it is recommended to display advisory notices at various locations within diagnostic radiology departments, with a particular focus on the reception area. Additionally, these notices should be placed in areas where diagnostic X-ray equipment is used. These notices should be in bilingual format with one language as local (Fig. 10.1).

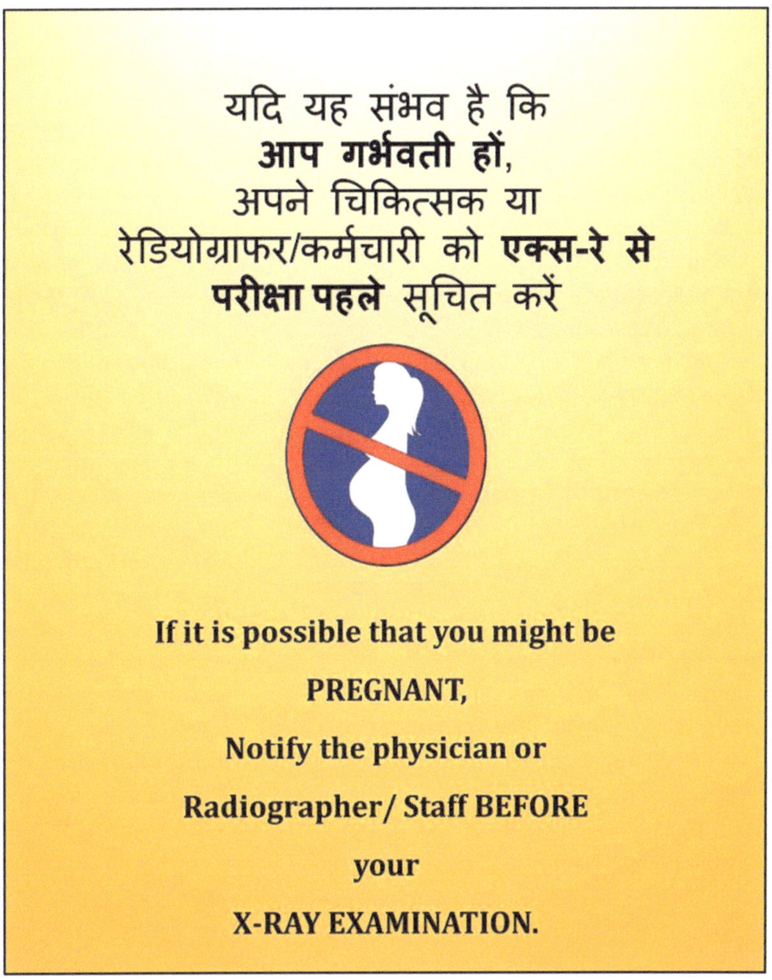

Fig. 10.1 Bilingual caution notice for pregnancy

Informed Consent

In medicine, informed consent often dictates that individuals must voluntarily consent to non-emergency medical procedures after being fully informed of any potential hazards to their health or way of life. The pregnant patient or worker has a right to be informed about the scope and nature of any radiation effects that could develop during pregnancy. Usually, the only information required for low-dosage procedures, such as a chest X-ray, is a verbal assurance that the danger is extremely low. When fetal dosages are 1 mGy and above, a more thorough explanation would typically be needed. The consent forms are to be designed to not only include potential radiation risks but also cover alternative treatment options, including non-radiological options and the harm from not having the medical procedure.

If the radiological procedure is carried out knowing that the patient is carrying conceptus, the fetal dose estimation will be carried out and documented. This should provide information on the technical factors such as details of beam collimation to the specific area of interest, kVp, milliampere-seconds, use of anti-scatter grids, number of radiographs, fluoroscopy time, and so on. A qualified medical physicist should perform such calculations, and the mother should be informed of potential dangers. These records are typically to be preserved until the child becomes an adult or as per local regulations.

10.9.4 Pregnant Female Radiation Worker

The dose limits for occupational exposure are the same for men and women until the pregnancy is declared. If the woman is or may be pregnant, additional measures must be taken to protect the unborn child and keep the radiation doses less than 1 mSv as with the general public. As soon as a woman learns about her pregnancy, she should inform the employer about it; though it is not mandatory, informing about the pregnancy can always be beneficial [4]. Once the employer is informed, they may consider modifying working conditions so that conceptus should not exceed the dose limit of 1 mGy during the remainder of pregnancy. In normal working conditions, the dose to the fetus does not exceed 1 mGy, even when working conditions are not modified. For precautionary measures, the employer should review the working conditions and restrict where there is a high accidental probability of doses or chances of high intake of radiopharmaceuticals.

The responsibility of the unborn child's safety lies on both the employer and the pregnant worker, and the first responsibility is the woman herself. However, it is important to note that, while modifying working conditions, there should not be any unnecessary discrimination against pregnant workers. Sometimes, pregnant workers may request a change to a radiation-free work environment to avoid minimal additional risks. The employer might accommodate such requests to pre-empt potential complications if the employee gives birth to a child with an unforeseen congenital condition (which statistically happens around 2–4% of 100 births). The change in working conditions is not required to be mandatory from a radiation safety perspective, but it can depend on company size to accommodate such requests. Approximate risks during pregnancy in a population that has not been exposed to radiation include a rate of spontaneous abortion of 10–20%, a rate of major malformations of 2–4%, a rate of intrauterine growth retardation of 4% (mostly caused by hypertension), and a rate of genetic diseases of 5–10%.

If a change is considered, pregnant workers may be transferred from fluoroscopy to CT scanning or an area with less scattered radiation. In nuclear medicine departments, pregnant workers might spend less time in the radiopharmacy or their involvement with radioiodine solutions. In the context of radiotherapy using sealed sources, pregnant technicians could be excluded from participating in manual brachytherapy procedures. However, there is ethical involvement in all such situations since the co-worker has to incur additional radiation exposure.

Let us consider where a worker desires to persist in her current role or if the employer relies on her only to ensure patient care. This is completely acceptable from the radiation protection perspective as long as the estimated fetal dose remains within the advised limit of 1 mGy after the pregnancy is reported. However, it is prudent to assess the work environment to ensure the occurrence of high-dose accidents. In all such cases, there should be careful monitoring of radiation doses to the fetus.

To monitor the radiation dose to the fetus, the pregnant worker is to wear an additional radiation monitor at the abdomen level; a pocket dosimeter or an additional thermo-luminescent dosimeter (TLD) can suffice for this need. While estimating the dose to the fetus, a few facts to consider are as follows:

- The fetal dose estimation from a personal dosimeter worn by diagnostic radiology staff could be overestimated by a factor of around 10 or even more.
- When the dosimeter is worn outside a lead apron, the recorded dose might be approximately 100 times greater than the actual fetal dose.
- Individuals in nuclear medicine and radiation therapy typically do not wear lead aprons and encounter radiation of higher photon energies. Despite this, fetal doses will not cross 25% of the measurement indicated by the personal dosimeter.

It is important to consider additional factors when assessing the activities of pregnant workers. Within a medical environment, tasks such as lifting patients and assuming positions that involve stooping or bending below knee level are common. Various national organizations have set forth guidelines unrelated to radiation, addressing these activities at different pregnancy stages and keeping them in mind.

10.10 Radiation Area and Its Classification

In radiology, different areas have different levels of severity when we talk about radiation; therefore, its access is regulated. The different areas are controlled, supervised, and unsupervised, with different access levels and radiation safety protocols within a facility. These areas are designed to ensure the safety of patients, healthcare workers, and the general public. Here is an overview of each type of area:

10.10.1 Controlled Area

A controlled area is where radiation levels can be higher due to the presence of radiation sources or equipment. Access to controlled areas is restricted and controlled through physical barriers, access controls, and signage. Personnel working in controlled areas must adhere to appropriate radiation safety protocols. Examples of controlled areas are CT scan rooms, interventional radiology suites, C-arm fluoroscopy suites, nuclear medicine, radiopharmacy or hot labs, injection rooms, radioactive source storage rooms, and radioactive waste storage rooms fall under this classification.

10.10.2 Supervised Area

A supervised area is where radiation levels are relatively lower than the controlled areas but still require oversight due to the presence of radiation sources or equipment nearby. Access to supervised areas might be restricted to authorized personnel, but the level of access control might be less stringent than in controlled areas. Personnel working in supervised areas still need to follow radiation safety guidelines. Examples of supervised areas include radiography rooms, general fluoroscopy suites, corridors, and areas around CT machines.

10.10.3 Unsupervised Area

An unsupervised area is where radiation levels are low and do not require constant oversight or specific radiation safety protocols. Access to unsupervised areas is typically less restricted, and personnel may not need to wear lead aprons or dosimeters. Common areas, waiting rooms, reception, and administrative offices are unsupervised areas where the general public or non-radiation workers might spend time.

Regulatory guidelines and institutional policies determine the classification of areas as controlled, supervised, or unsupervised. These classifications ensure that appropriate safety measures are in place to protect individuals from unnecessary radiation exposure. It is important for healthcare personnel to be aware of the classification of different areas and to follow the corresponding radiation safety practices to maintain a safe environment for both staff and patients.

10.11 Personal Monitoring Devices

Personal monitoring devices are crucial tools in radiology and other fields involving ionizing radiation to ensure the safety of healthcare workers and individuals who may be exposed to radiation. These devices are worn by personnel to measure their radiation exposure levels and help maintain radiation doses within safe limits. Several types of personal monitoring devices are used; examples are TLDs, optically stimulated luminescence dosimeters (OSLDs), pocket ionization chambers, digital pocket dosimeters, film badges, and electronic personal dosimeters.

(The following text is extracted from "Radiation Safety Guide for Nuclear Medicine Professionals (2022)" by Pankaj Tandon, Dibya Prakash, Subhash Chand Kheruka, and Nagesh N Bhatt. Reprinted with permission, with little modifications.)

10.11.1 Thermo-Luminescent Dosimeters

TLDs are widely used across many countries to monitor radiation exposure among radiation workers. These passive detectors record radiation doses and provide readings when stimulated by heat. They are composed of insulating materials doped with specific impurities. When exposed to radiation, the deposited energy becomes trapped at defect sites within the material. Upon heating, this trapped energy is released in the form of visible light, which is then converted into electrical signals and amplified using photomultiplier tubes. The intensity of the emitted light directly correlates with the amount of radiation absorbed.

According to the UNSCEAR 2021 Report, approximately 11.4 million workers worldwide were monitored for radiation exposure between 2010 and 2014, with the medical sector accounting for nearly 80% of the total [15]. Different countries employ various TLD materials in their personal monitoring programs, depending on factors such as availability and sensitivity.

Several materials have been explored for use in TLDs, including calcium sulfate dysprosium-activated ($CaSO_4$:Dy), lithium fluoride (LiF), lithium borate manganese-activated ($Li_2B_4O_7$:Mn), calcium fluoride dysprosium-activated (CaF_2:Dy), calcium sulfate dysprosium and manganese-activated ($CaSO_4$:Dy, Mn), calcium fluoride manganese-activated (CaF_2:Mn), and lithium fluoride doped with magnesium, copper, and phosphorus (LiF: Mg, Cu, P).

- India, Australia, and Brazil primarily use $CaSO_4$:Dy TLDs due to their superior sensitivity and local availability.
- Many other regions worldwide utilize LiF-based TLDs.
- The United States and several European countries rely on LiF: Mg, Ti (commercially called TLD-100) and LiF: Mg, Cu, P (TLD-100H, TLD-600H, TLD-700H).
- Japan predominantly employs $Li_2B_4O_7$:Cu and $CaSO_4$:Tm for radiation monitoring.
- China also adopts LiF: Mg, Cu, P (GR-200) for its monitoring programs.
- Russia primarily uses LiF: Mg, Ti (DTG-4).
- Certain parts of the United States have integrated optically stimulated luminescence dosimeters into their monitoring systems.

A detailed comparison of the properties of various TLD materials used globally is provided in Table 10.9.

10.11.1.1 TLD-100, TLD-600, and TLD-700 Dosimeters

TLD-100, developed by Thermo Fisher Scientific (formerly Harshaw Chemical Company), contains lithium in its natural isotopic composition,

Table 10.9 Properties of some thermos-luminescent materials

TLD type	Effective atomic number Z_{eff}	TL main peak (°C)	Emission maximum (nm)	Relative sensitivity[a]	Fading at 25 °C, when stored in the dark	Useful dose range
LiF: Mg, Ti	8.14	200	400	1	5%/year	20 μGy–10 Gy
LiF: Mg, Cu, P	8.14	210	368	40	5%/year	0.2 μGy–10 Gy
LiF: Mg, Cu, Si	8.14	240	384	55	Negligible	1 μGy–20 Gy
$Li_2B_4O_7$:Mn	7.3	220	605	0.40	4% monthly	0.1 mGy–3 Gy
$Li_2B_4O_7$:Cu	7.3	205	368	8	10%/2 months	10 μGy–10^3 Gy
MgB_4O_7:Dy/Tm	8.4	190	490	67	4%/month	5 μGy–50 Gy
BeO	7.1	190	330	≈1.00	8%/2 month	0.1 mGy–0.5 Gy
Mg_2SiO_4:Tb	11	200	380–400	40–53	Very slight	10 μGy–1 Gy
$CaSO_4$:Dy	15.3	220	480–570	30–40	1%/2 monthly	2 μGy–10 Gy
$CaSO_4$:Tm	15.3	220	452	30–40	1–2%/2 months	2 μGy–10 Gy
CaF_2:Mn	16.3	260	500	5	16%/2 weeks	10 μGy–10 Gy
CaF_2 (Natural)	16.3	260	380	23	Insignificant	10 μGy–50 Gy
CaF_2:Dy	16.3	215	480–570	15	8%/2 months	10 μGy–10 Gy
Al_2O_3:C	10.2	190	420	60	5%/year	0.1 μGy–10 Gy

Table originally published in Bhatt and Kulkarni [16]. Reprinted with the kind permission of Trans Tech Publications
[a]As compared to LiF: Mg, Ti

with 7.5% of ^{6}Li and 92.5% of ^{7}Li. This dosimeter is sensitive not only to photons and electrons but also to neutrons, particularly thermal neutrons [17].

- TLD-600 is highly sensitive to both thermal neutrons and gamma radiation due to its high ^{6}Li content (95.62%).
- TLD-700, in contrast, is primarily sensitive to gamma radiation, as it is enriched with ^{7}Li (99.99%) [18].

Since ^{6}Li has a much higher neutron cross-section than ^{7}Li, TLD-600 exhibits greater neutron sensitivity compared to TLD-700 [18]. Although TLD-100 is widely used in radiation clinics, it tends to over-respond at higher energies, limiting its effectiveness in certain applications [17]. The fundamental detection mechanism remains consistent across different types of TLDs.

10.11.1.2 $CaSO_4$:Dy Thermo-Luminescent Dosimeters

A simple and effective method for producing $CaSO_4$:Dy phosphor for TLD applications was first described by Yamashita et al. in 1968 [18]. The phosphor is synthesized by dissolving high-purity calcium sulfate ($CaSO_4$) and dysprosium oxide (Dy_2O_3) in concentrated sulfuric acid (H_2SO_4). The mixture is then crystallized through distillation under reduced pressure, followed by annealing and quenching to enhance its sensitivity.

Since the crystalline $CaSO_4$:Dy material cannot be directly formed into pellets, it is blended with Teflon to create a homogeneous composite. The final composition consists of $CaSO_4$:Dy phosphor powder (grain size <75 μm) and Teflon resin in a 1:3 weight ratio, which is then processed into discs (280 mg each, 0.8 mm thick, and 1.35 cm in diameter). These discs are initially cold-pressed and subsequently subjected to a 400 °C heat treatment for 1 hour, ensuring mechanical strength and flexibility.

In India, commercial production of $CaSO_4$:Dy TLDs is carried out by Renentech Laboratories Pvt. Ltd., Mumbai, with a batch production capacity of 600 g [16].

Bhabha Atomic Research Centre (BARC) TLD Design

TLDs developed by the BARC incorporate a well-defined three-zone structure:

- Top Section: A circular metal filter (13 mm diameter on the front cover, 12 mm on the back cover) consisting of 1 mm aluminum and 1 mm copper layers, with the copper filter positioned closer to the TLD disc
- Middle Section: A rectangular plastic filter (30 mm × 20 mm) on the front cover, paired with a circular filter (25 mm diameter) on the back cover
- Bottom Section: An open-window region (15 mm diameter on the front cover, 13 mm on the back cover), allowing exposure to radiation

These TLDs are capable of detecting beta, gamma, and X-ray radiation, covering a dose range from 0.1 mSv to 10 Sv [16]. They are known for their high sensitivity, low fading properties, and domestic production advantages. Additionally, the readout time for these TLDs is 100 seconds per badge, making them efficient for radiation monitoring (Figs. 10.2, 10.3, 10.4, and 10.5).

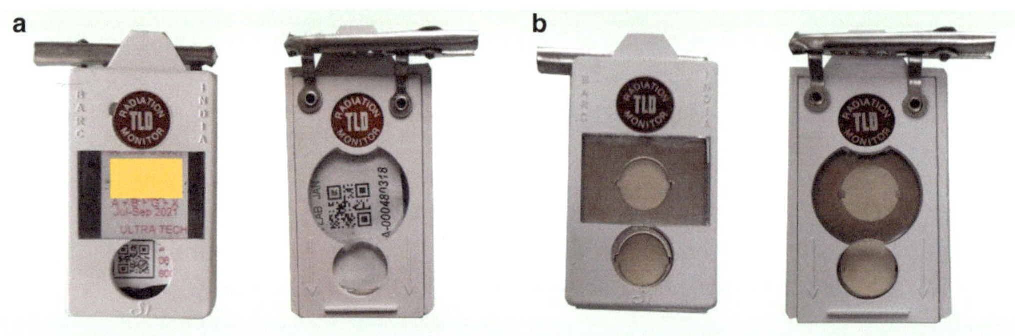

Fig. 10.2 (**a**) Front and back views of TLDs. (**b**) Demonstration of how the dosimeter interacts with radiation when placed inside the TLD cover. This image is for illustrative purposes only; removing the TLD from its protective plastic cover is not recommended. (Copyright Springer Nature [19]. Reprinted with permission)

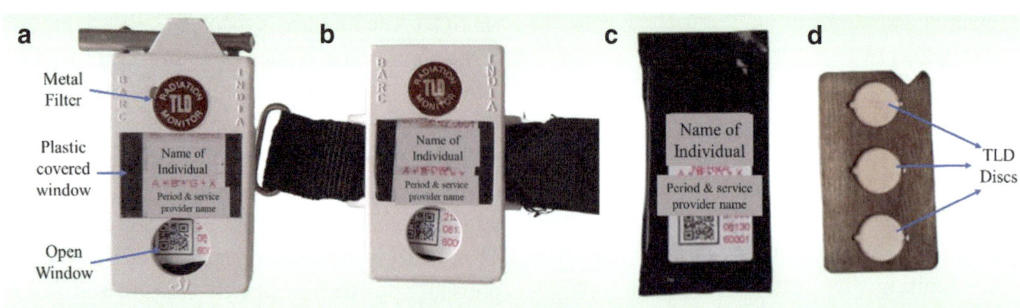

Fig. 10.3 Different types of TLDs: (**a**) Chest TLD featuring three windows. (**b**) Wrist TLD, designed for monitoring radiation exposure to the hands and forearms. (**c**) TLDs in their protective plastic covers, labeled with individual names as received from the vendor. (**d**) TLD discs mounted on a 1-mm aluminum plate for secure placement. (Copyright Springer Nature [19]. Reprinted with permission)

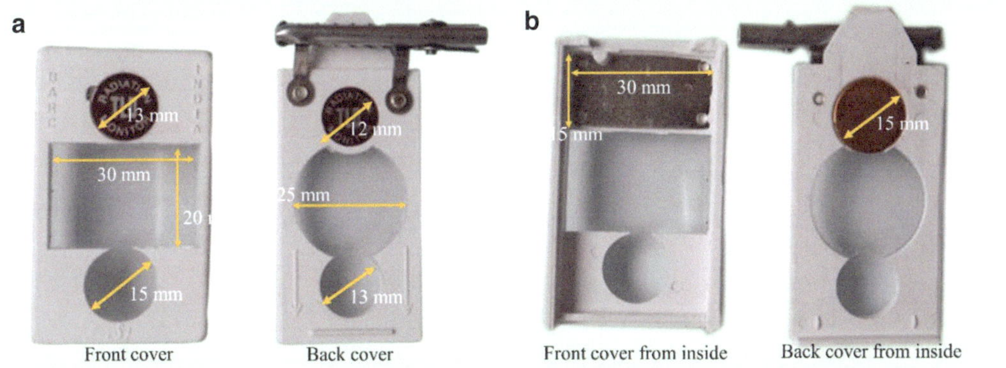

Fig. 10.4 Dimensions of TLD covers from different perspectives: (**a**) External view of the TLD cover. (**b**) Internal view showing the structural details. (Copyright Springer Nature [19]. Reprinted with permission)

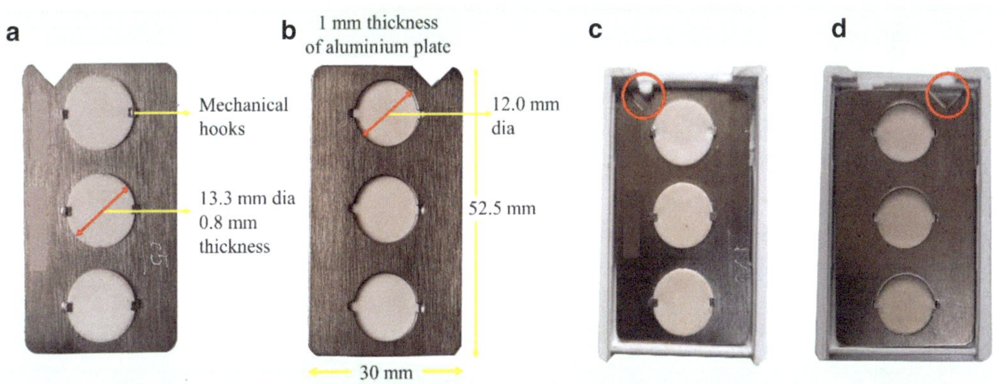

Fig. 10.5 (**a**, **b**) Thermo-luminescent pellets mounted on an aluminum plate, secured with mechanical clips of varying dimensions. (**c**) Correctly positioned TLD inside its cover, aligned with the V-notch in the plastic casing. (**d**) Incorrectly placed TLD, showing a complete misalignment within the cover. (Copyright Springer Nature [19]. Reprinted with permission)

Mechanism of Detection

Scintillation detectors function by emitting light photons when exposed to radiation, a process known as prompt luminescence. Radiation interacts with the detector material, generating electrons and holes, which then recombine at activator sites, releasing detectable light photons.

Although thermo-luminescent materials also generate electrons and holes upon radiation exposure, these charges become trapped within the energy gap between the valence and conduction bands at designated luminescence and trapping centers (TCs). When subjected to thermal or optical stimulation, the trapped electrons are released, producing light photons in proportion to the absorbed radiation dose. This characteristic enables dose integration over a specific time interval (Fig. 10.6).

TLDs are specifically engineered with materials that contain a high density of TCs and luminescence centers (LCs), with energy levels within the bandgap. Upon radiation exposure, the material does not produce an immediate signal but instead stores the energy by accumulating trapped charges, directly proportional to the incident radiation dose. Since TLDs operate without an

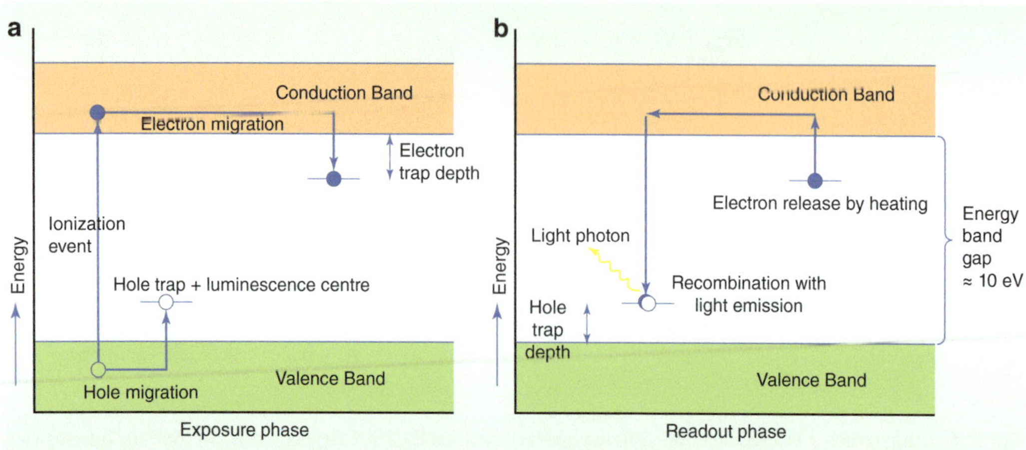

Fig. 10.6 TLDs energy band. (Copyright Springer Nature [19]. Reprinted with permission)

external voltage, the movement of electrons within the conduction band occurs randomly. Some of these electrons become captured at different TCs, where they remain until released by thermal or optical stimulation. Once freed, these electrons generate photons at LCs, producing a measurable signal during the readout phase.

The readout process for TLDs typically occurs within a temperature range of 175–250 °C, as seen in $CaSO_4$:Dy Teflon Discs, which exhibit a peak luminescence around 240 °C. Specialized TL readers, which are commercially available, facilitate this process. For complete signal erasure, a higher-temperature readout at 300–400 °C (thermal oven) or post-readout annealing is performed, effectively resetting the TLD by depleting all TCs and LCs. This allows the recycling and repeated use of the same TLD material multiple times without significant sensitivity degradation [20].

10.11.1.3 Advantages of $CaSO_4$:Dy TLDs

- **High Sensitivity and Linearity**:

  $CaSO_4$:Dy TLDs demonstrate exceptional sensitivity and linearity when exposed to various types of ionizing radiation, including X-rays, gamma rays, and beta particles. This characteristic allows them to measure radiation doses accurately across different exposure levels. Their linear dose-response simplifies radiation dose calculations and assessments, making them effective in diverse radiation environments.
- **Energy Independence**:

  These TLDs maintain a consistent response across a broad range of radiation energies, making them suitable for monitoring various radiation sources. While slight variations in response may occur depending on radiation energy, they remain within an acceptable tolerance range, ensuring reliable dosimetry for most practical applications.
- **Efficient Readout Process**:

  The trapped electrons within $CaSO_4$:Dy TLDs can be efficiently read using automated TLD readers, which apply controlled heating to release the stored energy as light photons. The emitted light is then measured to determine radiation exposure levels with high accuracy.
- **Reusability and Cost-Effectiveness**:

  After measurement, $CaSO_4$:Dy TLDs can be annealed (heated at high temperatures) to reset the trapped electrons, allowing them to be reused multiple times. This capability makes them an economical choice for long-term radiation monitoring.
- **Long-Term Stability**:

  These dosimeters offer excellent signal stability over time, a crucial factor for maintaining accuracy in prolonged radiation monitoring programs. Their low fading rate ensures reliable measurements even after extended exposure periods.

- **Quality Assurance in Radiation Dosimetry**:
  $CaSO_4$:Dy TLDs play a critical role in radiation therapy and medical imaging quality assurance. They are commonly used to verify treatment plans, confirm dose delivery accuracy, and assess the functionality of radiation equipment.
- **Environmental Resilience**:
  Unlike some other dosimeters, $CaSO_4$:Dy TLDs are less affected by environmental factors such as temperature fluctuations and humidity. This enhances their reliability in varied working conditions, making them ideal for both clinical and industrial radiation monitoring.
- **Dose Distribution Mapping**:
  In medical applications, these TLDs are used for dose distribution mapping, which helps optimize radiation treatment planning and patient safety by ensuring accurate dose delivery during medical procedures.
- **Regulatory Approval and Industry Recognition**:
  $CaSO_4$:Dy TLDs are widely accepted by regulatory authorities and standards organizations for radiation monitoring and personnel dose assessment. Their recognition ensures compliance with radiation safety guidelines in healthcare, research, and nuclear industries.
- **Personal Radiation Dosimetry**:
  These TLDs are extensively used for individual radiation exposure monitoring, particularly among healthcare professionals, radiation workers, and individuals exposed to ionizing radiation in various occupational settings.

While $CaSO_4$:Dy TLDs offer numerous advantages, achieving precise and reliable dose measurements requires proper calibration, careful handling, and adherence to standardized readout procedures. Regular maintenance and quality control checks are essential for ensuring consistent performance in radiation monitoring.

10.11.1.4 Disadvantages of $CaSO_4$:Dy TLDs

- **Limited β-Dosimetry Performance**:
  $CaSO_4$:Dy TLDs have a significant drawback in beta (β) radiation dosimetry. Their thick dosimeter disc leads to a very low thermoluminescent (TL) response for β-rays with a maximum energy (Emax) below 0.8 MeV, making them less effective for lower-energy beta radiation measurements.
- **Inability to Detect Neutrons**:
  These TLDs cannot measure neutron radiation, limiting their applicability in mixed radiation fields where neutron dosimetry is required, such as nuclear reactor environments and radiation protection monitoring.
- **Fade Effect (Signal Loss Over Time)**:
  Like many other TL materials, $CaSO_4$:Dy TLDs are susceptible to the fade effect, where the stored energy gradually dissipates over time after exposure. If there is a delay in the readout process, this signal loss can lead to slight inaccuracies in dose measurement. Proper storage conditions and timely readout are necessary to minimize this issue.
- **Dose Rate Dependence**:
  $CaSO_4$:Dy TLDs exhibit a certain degree of dependence on the radiation dose rate, meaning their response can vary based on how quickly the radiation is delivered. This characteristic may affect measurement accuracy in high-dose-rate conditions, such as during certain radiation therapy procedures or industrial radiation exposure scenarios.

Despite these limitations, proper calibration, readout timing, and dose rate corrections can help mitigate some of these drawbacks, ensuring accurate and reliable radiation dosimetry.

10.11.1.5 Optically Stimulated Luminescence Dosimeters

OSLDs function similarly to TLDs but use a different mechanism to release stored energy. Instead of heat stimulation, OSLDs utilize light exposure to release luminescence, which is proportional to the radiation dose absorbed.

Mechanism of Operation

- OSLDs are stimulated using light rather than heat.
- The light source can operate in continuous-wave mode (constant intensity) or pulsed mode (varying intensity).
- A laser, light-emitting diode, or broadband lamp is used to stimulate the luminescent material.
- The intensity of the emitted light corresponds to the radiation dose received.

Materials Used in OSLDs

- Common OSLD materials include aluminum oxide carbon-activated (Al_2O_3:C) and beryllium oxide (BeO).
- The material choice depends on:
  - Luminescence efficiency
  - Sensitivity and stability
  - Application requirements
  - Cost, toxicity, and ease of fabrication

Advantages of OSLDs Over TLDs

- Immediate Readout: OSLDs provide near-instantaneous dose readings after exposure, while TLDs require post-exposure processing.
- Reusability: OSLDs can be read multiple times, reducing costs compared to single-use TLDs.
- Dose History Storage: OSLDs retain dose history, allowing users to access past exposure data easily.
- Linear Dose Response: OSLDs exhibit a linear response to radiation doses across a wide range.
- Energy Independence: OSLDs have a relatively uniform response to different types of radiation.
- Efficient Readout: Automated OSLD readers ensure fast and consistent dose measurements.
- Compact and Lightweight: OSLDs are small, easy to handle, and comfortable for personal dosimetry.

Advantages of TLDs Over OSLDs

- Long-Term Stability: TLDs exhibit excellent dose retention, making them reliable for long-term monitoring.
- Dose Rate Independence: TLDs typically show less dependency on dose rate variations compared to OSLDs.
- Robustness: TLDs are more durable and can withstand harsh environmental conditions better.
- Versatile Applications: TLDs have established calibration protocols for different radiation sources and energies.
- Proven Reliability: With a long history of successful use, TLDs are widely accepted in radiation protection and medical applications.
- Cost-Effectiveness: TLDs can be more economical, especially in single-use scenarios.

Choosing Between OSLDs and TLDs

Both OSLDs and TLDs offer unique benefits and have specific limitations. The selection of the appropriate dosimeter depends on:

- Application type (e.g., medical, industrial, and environmental monitoring)
- Desired features (e.g., immediate readout, reusability, and long-term stability)
- Radiation environment (e.g., dose rate variations and exposure conditions)
- Regulatory compliance
- Available technology and cost considerations

Proper selection ensures accurate radiation monitoring and safety assurance for the intended application.

(The following text is extracted from "Radiation Safety Guide for Nuclear Medicine Professionals (2022)" by Pankaj Tandon, Dibya Prakash, Subhash Chand Kheruka, and Nagesh N Bhatt. Reprinted with permission, with little modifications.)

10.11.2 Pocket Ionization Chambers

Pocket ionization chambers are small, handheld devices that directly measure ionization produced by ionizing radiation in air. They provide real-time dose rate measurements, making them useful for personal radiation monitoring, particularly in environments with variable radiation levels. These devices operate based on the principle of charge integration:

- The chamber contains a small gas-filled ionization chamber that is pre-charged before use.
- When exposed to radiation, ionization occurs within the chamber, causing a drop in voltage.
- The voltage drop is directly proportional to the amount of radiation detected.
- A scale calibrated in radiation dose units converts this voltage change into a readable dose measurement.

The voltage difference across the capacitor in the ionization chamber is given by

$$\Delta V = \frac{\Delta Q}{C} \tag{10.6}$$

where:

- ΔV = Voltage difference
- ΔQ = Collected charge due to radiation exposure
- C = Capacitance of the chamber

The device contains an integrated quartz fiber electroscope, which allows for visual dose readings when observed against light. When the device is fully charged, the initial reading remains at zero. As radiation interacts with the chamber, the charge gradually decreases, and the electroscope displays the corresponding dose.

Key Features and Limitations

- **Real-Time Monitoring**: Provides instantaneous dose readings.
- **High Accuracy**: When operated within its specified range, accuracy is maintained within a few percent.
- **Compact and Portable**: Lightweight design makes it ideal for personal dosimetry.
- **Direct Reading Capability**: Users can check their radiation exposure without requiring external processing.
- **Leakage Current Limitation**: Over time, a small leakage current flows across the insulator surface, limiting the ultimate sensitivity of the device.
- **Charge Stability**: The initial charge may degrade over prolonged storage, requiring periodic recalibration.

Applications

- **Personal radiation dosimetry** for healthcare professionals, nuclear industry workers, and emergency responders
- **Radiation surveying** in nuclear facilities, laboratories, and accident sites
- **Short-term exposure monitoring** in high-radiation environments (Fig. 10.7)

10.11.3 Digital Pocket Dosimeter

Digital pocket dosimeters are compact, portable devices designed to provide real-time radiation dose readings in a digital format. These dosimeters are both lightweight and user-friendly, offering immediate feedback on radiation exposure levels, making them ideal for personal radiation monitoring.

Working Principle

Digital pocket dosimeters are based on semiconductor detection technology, specifically utilizing a PN-junction silicon (Si) semiconductor detector. These devices are typically designed to detect X-rays and gamma radiation with energies greater than 40 keV. They are available in different models from different manufacturers with little variations in their manufacturing and capabilities (one model is shown in Fig. 10.8). In the presence of ionizing radiation, the dosimeter operates as follows:

1. **Silicon Rectifier Diode**: A reverse-biased silicon rectifier diode is the core of the detec-

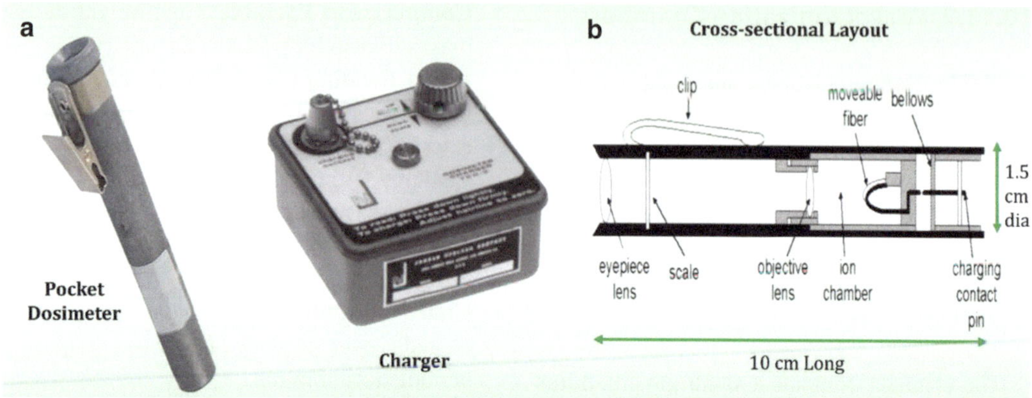

Fig. 10.7 Analog pocket dosimeter. (**a**) External view of the analog pocket dosimeter (left) and its charger (right) used for measuring accumulated radiation dose. (**b**) Cross-sectional layout of the pocket dosimeter showing internal components, including the clip, eyepiece lens, scale, objective lens, ion chamber, movable fiber, bellows, and charging contact pin (Copyright Springer Nature [19]. Reprinted with permission)

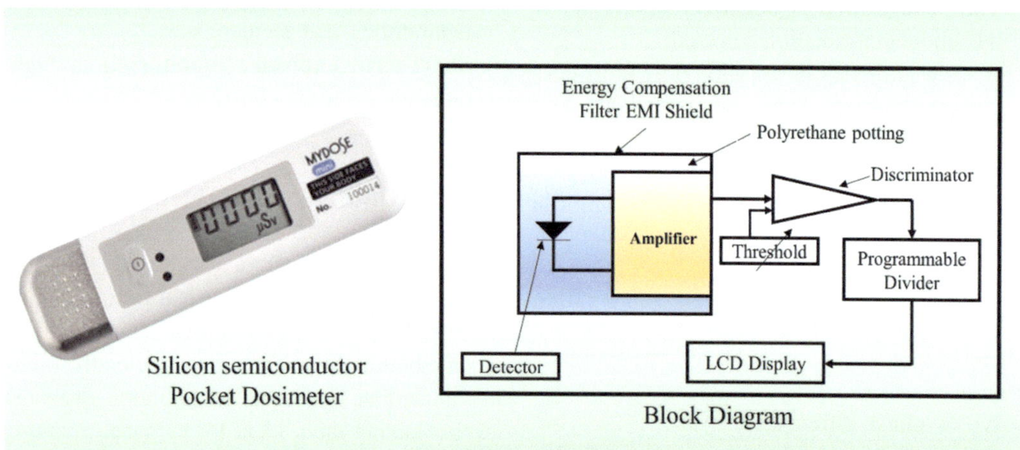

Fig. 10.8 Digital pocket dosimeter. (Copyright Springer Nature [19]. Reprinted with permission)

tion system, functioning at approximately 4 V.

2. **Charge Amplification**: Radiation interacting with the silicon detector generates pulses, which are then amplified by a charge-sensitive amplifier. The amplification process is powered by a low-power complementary metal–oxide–semiconductor integrated circuit.

Energy Compensation and Noise Filtering

To ensure accurate readings, the dosimeter incorporates an energy compensation filter, which serves two functions:

- **Electromagnetic shielding** to protect the sensitive components from interference
- **Noise suppression**, enabling the dosimeter to filter out irrelevant noise by using a **threshold voltage discriminator**

Once the signal is processed, the output pulses from the discriminator are sent to a programmable divider circuit, which is specifically calibrated so that the dosimeter displays one count for each 1 µSv of exposure to ^{137}Cs gamma radiation. This precise calibration allows for reliable dose readings over time. The accumulated counts are then displayed on a digit-counter liquid crystal display (LCD) module for easy interpretation.

The device is powered by coin-type lithium batteries, with some models featuring a "Battery Low" indicator to alert the user when power is running low. For durability, the entire system is encased in an anti-vibration polyurethane housing, ensuring protection from physical damage and ensuring consistent performance in various conditions.

10.11.4 Film Badges

Film badges are radiation monitoring devices that use photographic film to measure exposure levels. When exposed to radiation, the film undergoes darkening (optical density), with the degree of darkening corresponding to the radiation dose received. After exposure, the film is processed and analyzed, allowing for an estimate of the total radiation dose.

Although film badges have become less common due to advancements in digital dosimetry and more precise real-time monitoring devices, they are still used in certain applications where cost-effectiveness and long-term dose recording are priorities.

10.11.5 Extremity Monitors

Extremity monitors are specialized radiation dosimeters designed to measure localized radiation exposure to specific body parts, such as the hands, fingers, and wrists. Common types include ring dosimeters and wrist dosimeters, which are worn by individuals who work in environments where extremities are at higher risk of radiation exposure.

These monitoring devices play a crucial role in radiation safety, particularly in radiology, nuclear medicine, and radiation therapy. By continuously tracking radiation doses to extremities, they help ensure that exposure levels remain within regulated safety limits, allowing healthcare facilities to effectively manage occupational radiation risks for their staff.

10.12 Radiation Emergencies

Radiological emergencies in radiology refer to unexpected events or situations that pose a risk of radiation exposure to patients, radiology staff, or the public. These emergencies can result from equipment malfunction, human error, natural disasters, or other unforeseen circumstances. Handling radiological emergencies effectively is crucial to minimize radiation exposure and ensure the safety of all individuals involved. Here are some common radiological emergencies in radiology:

- **Equipment Malfunction**: Malfunctions in radiological equipment, such as X-ray machines or CT scanners, can lead to unintended radiation exposure to the patients and staff. These emergencies can vary in severity, but they all require prompt and appropriate responses to ensure safety. Emergency protocols should be in place to shut down malfunctioning equipment and prevent further exposure.
- The following actions should be taken in case of equipment malfunction:
  - *Immediate Response*: Operators should be trained to recognize equipment malfunctions and respond promptly by shutting down the equipment and taking appropriate safety measures.
  - *Notification*: The facility's radiation safety officer (RSO) or responsible authority should be notified immediately.
  - *Patient Assessment*: In cases involving patient exposure, affected patients should be assessed for potential health impacts, and medical care should be provided as needed.
  - *Investigation and Repair*: A thorough investigation of the equipment malfunction should be conducted, and qualified technicians should make the necessary repairs.
  - *Reporting and Documentation*: All equipment malfunctions and related incidents should be documented and reported to the appropriate regulatory authorities.

Preventive maintenance, regular equipment inspections, and ongoing staff training are essential to minimize the risk of equipment malfunctions in radiology departments and ensure a swift and effective response in emergencies.

- **Accidental Exposure**: Accidental radiation exposure may occur due to operator error, incorrect settings, equipment misalignment, malfunctions, or miscommunications. Protocols for minimizing exposure and reporting incidents are essential.

In any accidental exposure situation, the first step is to immediately cease the radiation source, such as turning off the X-ray machine or CT scanner and ensuring the safety of patients and healthcare workers. Evacuate the area if necessary to minimize further exposure.

The RSO or supervisor should be notified immediately to assess the situation and provide guidance. If patients are involved, medical personnel should be alerted to assess and address any potential health effects.

Root Cause Analysis Conduct a thorough investigation to determine the cause of the accidental exposure. This may involve assessing equipment performance, operator actions, and communication breakdowns.

Documentation and Reporting All details of the accidental exposure incident should be documented, including exposure levels, circumstances, and actions taken. The accidental radiation exposures must be reported to the relevant regulatory authorities.

Corrective Actions and Prevention

- Verify and rectify any equipment issues that contributed to the exposure.
- Implement regular maintenance and inspection procedures.
- Enhance staff training programs to prevent similar incidents and improve communication protocols.
- Review and update radiological procedures to incorporate lessons learned from the incident.
- Continue monitoring and providing necessary medical care to affected patients.
- In the case of healthcare workers who were accidentally exposed should receive appropriate medical follow-up and monitoring.

Establishing a culture of safety within radiology departments is crucial, emphasizing prevention, training, and effective response protocols to minimize the risk of accidental radiation exposure incidents.

- **Terrorism or Sabotage**: Radiology facilities and equipment can be potential targets for terrorism or sabotage. Security measures and response plans are essential to address such threats.

10.12.1 General Preparedness for Radiological Emergencies

In radiology, preparedness for radiological emergencies involves several key elements, including:

- Emergency Response Plans: Facilities should have comprehensive emergency response plans that outline procedures for different types of emergencies.
- Training and Drills: Staff should receive regular training and participate in drills to ensure they understand emergency procedures and can respond effectively.
- Radiation Monitoring: Monitoring equipment and personnel dosimeters should be used to track radiation exposure during emergencies.
- Communication: Effective communication is essential for coordinating responses and notifying appropriate authorities and the public when necessary.
- RSOs: Appointing a qualified RSO is critical for ensuring proper radiation safety measures and emergency response.

Radiological emergencies are rare but can have serious consequences if not managed properly. A proactive approach to safety, including planning, training, and ongoing monitoring, is essential in radiology to prevent and respond to such emergencies effectively.

Exercise

Multiple Choice Questions (MCQs)

1. Who is considered the first "Radiation protection officer" for his work in protecting mine workers from radon exposure?
   A. Marie Curie
   B. Wilhelm Roentgen
   C. Georg Bauer (Agricola)
   D. Henri Becquerel
2. What type of radiation is capable of removing tightly bound electrons from atoms, creating ions?
   A. Non-ionizing radiation
   B. Visible light
   C. Ionizing radiation
   D. Infrared radiation
3. What principle is encapsulated by the acronym ALARA in radiation protection?
   A. As Low As Radiation Achieved
   B. As Long As Reasonable Action
   C. As Low As Reasonably Achievable
   D. As Long As Radiation Accumulated
4. What is the primary goal of dose limitation in radiation protection?
   A. To ensure maximum radiation exposure
   B. To balance economic benefits with radiation exposure
   C. To prevent harmful health effects
   D. To allow unrestricted use of radiation
5. For how long should records of occupational radiation exposure be maintained after a worker's employment ends?
   A. 10 years
   B. 20 years
   C. 30 years
   D. 50 years
6. Which principle emphasizes reducing the duration of exposure to ionizing radiation?
   A. Distance
   B. Shielding
   C. Time
   D. Dose limitation
7. According to the inverse square law, if the distance between a radiation source and an individual is doubled, the radiation intensity will:
   A. Double
   B. Halve
   C. Reduce to one-fourth
   D. Remain the same
8. What is the SI unit for absorbed dose?
   A. Rad
   B. Sievert
   C. Gray
   D. Roentgen
9. What is the primary purpose of the radiation weighting factor (wR) in calculating the equivalent dose?
   A. To account for different radiation types
   B. To measure absorbed dose
   C. To determine shielding thickness
   D. To calculate distance from the source
10. What does the term "collective effective dose" refer to?
    A. The dose received by a single individual
    B. The total radiation dose experienced by a population
    C. The radiation dose measured over a specific time
    D. The effective dose for a medical procedure
11. What term did the ICRP introduce in 1977 related to radiation protection?
    A. Maximum permissible dose
    B. Radiation safety level
    C. Dose limit
    D. Radiological safety measure
12. What is the primary role of a comforter during radiological procedures?
    A. Assisting with technical aspects of imaging
    B. Providing emotional and psychological support

C. Operating imaging equipment
D. Supervising medical trainees

13. Which situation does NOT typically involve a planned exposure situation?
    A. Medical diagnostic procedures
    B. Industrial radiography
    C. Nuclear accidents
    D. Research activities
14. What is the maximum allowable dose for the general public per year according to ICRP publication 103 (2007)?
    A. 5 mSv
    B. 10 mSv
    C. 1 mSv
    D. 50 mSv
15. In what year did the ICRP reduce the annual dose limit for occupational workers to 20 mSv per year?
    A. 1977
    B. 1991
    C. 2007
    D. 2011
16. What does the ALARA principle stand for?
    A. As Little As Radiation Achievable
    B. As Low As Reasonably Achievable
    C. As Long As Reasonable Achievable
    D. As Large As Radiation Acceptable
17. Which of the following is NOT mentioned as PPE in diagnostic radiology?
    A. Lead aprons
    B. Thyroid shields
    C. Goggles
    D. Helmets
18. What is the purpose of collimation in diagnostic radiology?
    A. Increase patient exposure to radiation
    B. Focus the X-ray beam only on the area of interest
    C. Measure the radiation exposure level
    D. Amplify the X-ray beam intensity
19. What are lead aprons used for in radiology?
    A. To reduce noise during procedures
    B. To protect the patient and staff from ionizing radiation
    C. To assist in patient positioning
    D. To measure radiation doses
20. Which device is used in mammography to immobilize and flatten breast tissue?
    A. Immobilization device
    B. Compression paddle
    C. Lead shield
    D. Thyroid collar
21. Which of the following organizations is responsible for providing recommendations and guidance on radiation protection and was established in 1928?
    A. IAEA
    B. ICRP
    C. WHO
    D. UNSCEAR
22. What is the primary mandate of the WHO in relation to radiation protection?
    A. To develop safety standards and guidelines for radiation protection
    B. To focus on international public health issues
    C. To provide technical assistance and training programs
    D. To assess and report on the effects of ionizing radiation
23. The International Atomic Energy Agency (IAEA) was established on which date?
    A. July 29, 1957
    B. January 1, 1948
    C. October 15, 1960
    D. March 3, 1972
24. What type of radiation effects are characterized by a threshold dose below which they do not occur?
    A. Stochastic effects
    B. Deterministic effects
    C. Acute effects
    D. Chronic effects
25. Which of the following is an example of a deterministic effect of radiation exposure?
    A. Cancer
    B. Genetic mutations
    C. Cataract formation
    D. Hereditary effects
26. Which of the following statements is true regarding radiation exposure during pregnancy?
    A. Radiation exposure during the first 2 weeks of pregnancy always results in malformations.
    B. Risks from radiation exposure to the fetus are highest during early development.

C. Diagnostic procedures involving high doses of radiation are always safe for the fetus.
D. Radiation exposure during the third trimester has the highest risk of causing birth defects.

27. What should be done if a female radiation worker becomes pregnant?
A. She must immediately stop working in any radiation area.
B. She is not required to inform her employer about her pregnancy.
C. Her employer may need to modify her working conditions to reduce radiation exposure to the fetus.
D. She should work under the same conditions without any changes.

28. Which of the following is NOT considered a controlled area in radiology?
A. CT scan rooms
B. Radioactive waste storage rooms
C. General fluoroscopy suites
D. Reception areas

29. During which phase of pregnancy is the fetus considered most sensitive to radiation?
A. Pre-implantation period
B. Major organ formation
C. Fetal development phase
D. Third trimester

30. What is the recommended dose limit for fetal exposure to radiation during pregnancy?
A. 100 mGy
B. 10 mGy
C. 1 mSv
D. 1 mGy

31. What is the primary material used in the commercial TLD-100 dosimeters in the United States?
A. Calcium sulfate dysprosium activated (CaSO4)
B. Lithium fluoride (LiF: Mg, Ti)
C. Lithium bromate manganese activated (Li2B4O7)
D. Calcium fluoride dysprosium activated (CaF2)

32. Which of the following TLDs has the highest relative sensitivity?
A. LiF: Mg, Ti
B. LiF: Mg, Cu, P
C. Li2B4O7
D. CaF2

33. What is a major advantage of CaSO4 TLDs?
A. High sensitivity to beta rays
B. Energy-dependent response
C. Reusability
D. Sensitivity to neutrons

34. Which material is commonly used in OSLDs?
A. Calcium fluoride
B. Aluminum oxide carbon activated (Al2O3)
C. Lithium fluoride
D. Beryllium Oxide (BeO)

35. What does a digital pocket dosimeter primarily use for radiation detection?
A. Gas-filled ionization chamber
B. Thermo-luminescent material
C. PN-junction silicon (Si) semiconductor
D. Photographic film

36. Which of the following is NOT a type of personal monitoring device mentioned in the text?
A. TLDs
B. Digital pocket dosimeters
C. Gas chromatographs
D. Film badges

37. What is the primary mechanism by which TLDs detect radiation?
A. Emission of sound waves
B. Light emission upon heating
C. Chemical reaction with radiation
D. Electrical charge accumulation

38. Which TLD material is used in the United States and many parts of Europe?
A. Lithium fluoride (LiF) with magnesium and titanium (LiF: Mg, Ti)
B. Calcium sulfate dysprosium activated (CaSO4)
C. Lithium bromate manganese activated (Li2B4O7)
D. Beryllium oxide (BeO)

39. What does the “fade effect” refer to in TLDs?
A. Increase in sensitivity over time
B. Loss of stored energy over time
C. Immediate response to radiation
D. Enhanced accuracy with higher doses

40. Which of the following is an advantage of OSLDs over TLDs?
    A. Higher dose rate dependence
    B. Immediate or near real-time dose readings
    C. Less reusability
    D. More complex readout process

Short Questions

1. What is the difference between radiation protection and radiation safety?
2. Explain the importance of dose monitoring and record keeping in radiation protection.
3. Explain the principle of "shielding" in radiation protection.
4. What is the importance of dose rate in determining the biological effects of radiation?
5. What is the difference between "carers" and "comforters" in the context of radiology investigations?
6. Explain the concept of dose constraints and its significance in radiation protection.
7. Describe the importance of proper ventilation in X-ray rooms.
8. What are the different types of lead shields used for patient protection in diagnostic radiology?
9. Describe the role of the UNSCEAR in radiation protection.
10. Explain the difference between deterministic and stochastic effects of radiation.
11. Explain the key considerations when conducting diagnostic procedures during pregnancy.
12. How should female patients of childbearing age be handled to minimize unintended radiation exposure?
13. Describe the process of how TLDs detect radiation.
14. Explain the main differences between OSLDs and TLDs.
15. Explain the preparation method of CaSO4.
16. TLDs as described in the text.
17. Describe the process and advantages of using digital pocket dosimeters for radiation measurement.

Long Questions

1. Discuss the three key principles of radiation protection: Justification, Optimization, and Dose Limitation. How do these principles work together to ensure safe and effective use of ionizing radiation?
2. Discuss the concepts of radiation absorbed dose, equivalent dose, and effective dose. How do these measurements differ, and what are their roles in radiation protection?
3. Discuss the evolution of dose limits from the IXRPC recommendations of 1928 to the current ICRP guidelines. Include key changes and the rationale behind these changes.
4. Discuss the role of patient positioning aids in minimizing radiation exposure and improving image quality in radiology. Include examples of common aids and their specific applications.
5. Discuss the process of carcinogenesis and how radiation exposure can contribute to this process. Include the stages of carcinogenesis and describe how radiation fits into this process.
6. Discuss the responsibilities of both the employer and the pregnant radiation worker in ensuring the safety of the fetus from radiation exposure. How should working conditions be adjusted, and what measures should be taken to monitor and manage radiation doses?
7. Discuss the advantages and disadvantages of using CaSO4 TLDs in radiation monitoring. Include considerations of sensitivity, energy independence, and limitations in your response.
8. Discuss the role and importance of personal monitoring devices in ensuring radiation safety for healthcare workers, highlighting their different types and the advantages and disadvantages associated with each type. How do they contribute to maintaining radiation doses within safe limits?

Answers for MCQs

1. C. Georg Bauer (Agricola)
2. C. Ionizing radiation
3. C. As Low As Reasonably Achievable
4. C. To prevent harmful health effects
5. C. 30 years
6. C. Time
7. C. Reduce to one-fourth
8. C. Gray
9. A. To account for different radiation types
10. B. The total radiation dose experienced by a population
11. C. Dose limit
12. B. Providing emotional and psychological support
13. C. Nuclear accidents
14. C. 1 mSv
15. B. 1991
16. B. As Low As Reasonably Achievable
17. D. Helmets
18. B. Focus the X-ray beam only on the area of interest
19. B. To protect the patient and staff from ionizing radiation
20. B. Compression paddle
21. B. ICRP
22. B. To focus on international public health issues
23. A. July 29, 1957
24. B. Deterministic effects
25. C. Cataract formation
26. B. Risks from radiation exposure to the fetus are highest during early development.
27. C. Her employer may need to modify her working conditions to reduce radiation exposure to the fetus.
28. D. Reception areas
29. B. Major organ formation
30. D. 1 mGy
31. B. Lithium fluoride (LiF: Mg, Ti)
32. B. LiF: Mg, Cu, P
33. C. Reusability
34. B. Aluminum oxide carbon activated (Al2O3)
35. C. PN-junction Silicon (Si) semiconductor
36. C. Gas chromatographs
37. B. Light emission upon heating
38. A. Lithium fluoride (LiF) with magnesium and titanium (LiF: Mg, Ti)
39. B. Loss of stored energy over time
40. B. Immediate or near-real-time dose readings

References

1. Lindell B. A history of radiation protection. Radiat Prot Dosim. 1996;68(1):83–95. https://doi.org/10.1093/oxfordjournals.rpd.a031856.
2. IAEA Safety Standards for protecting people and the environment General Safety Guide No. GSG-7 Occupational Radiation Protection Jointly sponsored by. 2018. [Online]. Available: http://www-ns.iaea.org/standards/.
3. Clarke RH, Valentin J. The history of ICRP and the evolution of its policies. Ann ICRP. 2009;39(1):75–110. https://doi.org/10.1016/j.icrp.2009.07.009.
4. IAEA Safety Standards for protecting people and the environment GSR Part 3. 2014. [Online]. Available: http://ec.europa.eu/dgs/communication/services/visual_identity/index_en.htm.
5. ICRP. Publication 103 (2007): Annals of the ICRP Published on behalf of the International Commission on Radiological Protection. 2007.
6. Fuchs WC. Effect of the Röntgen rays on the skin. Western Electrician. 1896:291.
7. International Commission on Radiological Protection and Jack. Valentin. Analysis of the criteria used by the International Commission on Radiological Protection to justify the setting of numerical protection level values. New York: Elsevier; 2007.
8. IAEA Safety Standards for protecting people and the environment Specific Safety Guide No. SSG-46 Radiation Protection and Safety in Medical Uses of Ionizing Radiation. 2014. [Online]. Available: http://www-ns.iaea.org/standards/.
9. Alexakhin PR, et al. ICRP Publication 96 – Annals of the ICRP Published on behalf of the International Commission on Radiological Protection. 2005. [Online]. Available: http://www.elsevier.com/locate/jnlabr/jaicrp.
10. Tandon P, Prakash D, Kheruka SC, Bhat NN. Radiation protection standards in relation to ICRP recommendations. In: Radiation safety guide for nuclear medicine professionals. Singapore: Springer Nature Singapore; 2022. p. 37–47. https://doi.org/10.1007/978-981-19-4518-2_4.
11. Rao S. Biological bases for the revision of dose limits to the eye lens. J Med Phys. 2016;41(4):211. https://doi.org/10.4103/0971-6203.195183.
12. Valentin J. Annals of the ICRP pregnancy and medical radiation. 2000. p. 43–62.

13. Sharp C, Shrimpton JA, Bury RF. Diagnostic medical exposures: Advice on exposure to ionising radiation during pregnancy. Didcot (UK): National Radiological Protection Board; 1998.
14. Valentin J, editor. Pregnancy and medical radiation. Ann ICRP. 2000;30(1):1–43. Oxford (UK): Elsevier Science Ltd; 2000.
15. Report of the United Nations Scientific Committee on the Effects of Atomic Radiation Sixty-seventh and sixty-eighth sessions (2–6 November). General Assembly Official Records Seventy-sixth Session Supplement No. 46. 2021. Accessed 16 Aug 2023. [Online]. Available: https://www.unscear.org/docs/GAreports/2021/2021_GA_A-76-46_E.pdf.
16. Bhatt BC, Kulkarni MS. Thermoluminescent phosphors for radiation dosimetry. Defect Diffus Forum. 2014;347:179–227. https://doi.org/10.4028/www.scientific.net/DDF.347.179.
17. Kry SF, Price M, Followill D, Mourtada F, Salehpour M. The use of LiF (TLD-100) as an out-to-field dosimeter. J Appl Clin Med Phys. 2007;8(4):169–75. https://doi.org/10.1120/jacmp.v8i4.2679.
18. Cavalieri TA, Castro VA, Siqueira PTD. Differences in TLD-600 and TLD-700 glow curves derived from distinct mixed gamma/neutron field irradiations. Radiat Prot Dosimetry. 2013;154(1-4):24–29. Oxford University Press, Oxford, UK.
19. Tandon P, Prakash D, Kheruka SC, Bhat NN. Working mechanism of radiation detectors used in nuclear medicine. In: Radiation safety guide for nuclear medicine professionals. Singapore: Springer Nature Singapore; 2022. p. 153–75. https://doi.org/10.1007/978-981-19-4518-2_15.
20. Knoll G. Miscellaneous detector type. In: Radiation detection and measurement. New York: John Wiley; 2010.

11 General Safety and Pediatric Care in Radiological Procedures

Learning Objectives

General Safety and Pediatric Care in Radiological Procedures	A Peek into the Approach Involved in Pediatric Patient Preparation
Introduction: Legislation, Justification, and Optimization	Immobilization Tools in Pediatric Imaging
Principles of Pediatric Imaging	Radiographic Technical Considerations for Supplementing Immobilization Techniques
Safety Precautions in Pediatric Ionizing Radiation Imaging Based on the Imaging Modality	Approaching Children with Special Needs
Radiation Safety Precautions During X-Ray/Fluoroscopy Procedures for Pediatric Imaging	Imaging Room Design Specifications for Pediatric Radiography
Radiation Safety Precautions During Computed Tomography Pediatric Imaging	Pediatric Imaging Device Equipment Specifications for Industry Manufacturers
FDA's Responsibilities in X-Ray Safety	Dose Considerations and Radiation Protection in Pediatric Imaging
Guidelines for Imaging Technologists and Healthcare Professionals	Diagnostic Reference Ranges in Pediatric Radiography
Guidelines for Pediatric Population Patients, Parents, and Caregivers	Image Quality and Dosimetry in Pediatric Radiography
Impact of Psychological Factors and Child Development in Pediatric Radiography	Routine Pediatric Radiological Examinations and Referral Criteria
Child Versus Adult Anatomical Differences	AI and Pediatric Radiography

11.1 Introduction: Legislation, Justification, and Optimization

The primary goal of any radiology and imaging department is to achieve the optimum diagnostic image quality while minimizing the patient's radiation dose. This goal becomes more sensitive and important when it comes to pediatric radiographic procedures. Depending on the radiation dose of the radiological procedure, the pediatric age group is at a two to three times higher risk of developing late effects of radiation, either late somatic or late deterministic effects [1–4].

Quality and safety guidelines for pediatric imaging procedures have been established globally by all communities and bodies governing medical imaging, radiology, and radiography legislation. The primary focus is on the safety and radiation dose to the pediatric age group during diagnostic imaging procedures. Several recommendations and guidelines for pediatric imaging quality and dose are available online. These guidelines concentrate on image quality,

D. Prakash, R. P. Kotian, *Fundamentals of X-ray Imaging*,
https://doi.org/10.1007/978-981-96-7328-5_11

gold-standard pediatric imaging methods, and technical parameters such as kVp, mAs, grid, and so on.

The current trend in pediatric radiological imaging is heavily reliant on the use of national and international reference dose ranges published by radiation regulatory bodies for all common pediatric radiological procedures that use ionizing radiation. These reference dose data are based on the survey's rounded third-quartile values and are reviewed every 3–5 years. The main disadvantage of these reference ranges is that the children vary in size and shape, resulting in less significant data reporting. As a result, regulatory bodies around the world have standardized doses for five to seven standard sizes. The need for local, national, and international diagnostic reference ranges in the pediatric population is high in today's medical imaging era [5–12].

There has been a lot of debate lately when it comes to the justification of practice in terms of radiation dose in pediatric radiography. It is the collective responsibility of the treating physician, radiologist, and imaging technologist to ensure that the type of radiological procedure is suitable based on the risk versus benefit analogy to the patient. The use of non-ionizing radiation, that is, ultrasonography and magnetic resonance imaging (MRI) for the initial diagnosis, may totally eliminate the need for a radiological procedure employing ionizing X-rays. The International Commission on Radiological Protection has laid down guidelines regarding the justification of radiological procedures based on the following criteria:

- Benefit versus risk (The use of radiological procedures should produce more benefit towards the treatment of the patient than harm.)
- The use of the radiological procedure, only when required for a specific disease and age group, contributes toward the early accurate diagnosis and quick treatment opportunity.
- The use of non-ionizing modalities in children requiring follow-up radiological procedures.
- Referral guidelines on the need for justification regarding appropriate imaging pathways in pediatric imaging. This is further achieved after answering a set of frequent clinical questions of the patient to be imaged.

Hence, to conclude this section on the justification of practice in pediatric radiological procedures, it is not very important to compare the referral criteria and investigations in both case scenarios when a procedure is needed and vice versa [13–15].

After a pediatric radiological procedure has been justified, the final step that must be prioritized is technique optimization. Medical imaging technologists/professionals and radiologists have the necessary expertise and knowledge to assist and guide referring physicians. Individual advice may not be possible during a typical busy working day, so set guidelines are followed by both the referring physician and the imaging technologist. Finally, legislation guidelines, practice justification, and technique optimization serve as the foundation for pediatric radiological procedures [16].

11.2 Principles of Pediatric Imaging

Pediatric imaging principles involve techniques and practices that are modified to meet the particular requirements of children. These principles are as follows:

1. **Radiation Safety:** Because developing cells are more sensitive to damage, children are more vulnerable to the harmful effects of ionizing radiation than adults. As a result, pediatric imaging should use the lowest possible dose of radiation to provide diagnostic information.
2. **Pediatric-Friendly Environment:** Children may experience anxiety and fear when undergoing medical imaging, so it is critical to create a child-friendly environment that allows them to feel at ease and relaxed. Distraction techniques, providing a soothing environment, and using child-sized equipment are all examples of this.

3. **Age group-based Imaging Techniques:** Because children's anatomical and physiological characteristics differ from those of adults, imaging techniques should be tailored to their age and developmental stage. For infants and young children, for example, ultrasound or MRI may be preferred over computed tomography (CT) because it does not use ionizing radiation and is less invasive.
4. **Multidisciplinary Hybrid Team:** Pediatric imaging necessitates the collaboration of pediatric radiologists, pediatricians, surgeons, and other healthcare professionals. This multidisciplinary approach ensures that imaging is used to provide accurate diagnoses, develop appropriate treatment plans, and track the progress of the child over time.
5. **Parental Role:** Parents are vital partners in their child's care and should be involved in the imaging process. This includes informing the child's medical history to the radiologist, explaining the imaging procedure to the child, and providing emotional support during the procedure.

Working with pediatric patients requires exceptional skills and the threshold experience required by statutory bodies in their respective countries to gain the patient's confidence, trust, and, most importantly, their support and cooperation. The most prestigious tertiary care facilities around the world have a dedicated pediatric core radiology team of professionals to deal with children's imaging needs and provide necessary guidance. This approach will result in a continuous understanding of the child's needs, pathology imaging, psychological support, overall development, and smooth operation of the entire pediatric imaging process in the radiology department. This qualified core team should be well-equipped with cutting-edge technology and equipment that uses artificial intelligence (AI) to reduce radiation dose while also being child-friendly.

Before performing pediatric radiology imaging, all X-ray radiological technologists must follow the ionizing radiation regulations of as low as reasonably achievable (ALARA) principles, justification, optimization, and radiation protection [17–19]. Overall, pediatric imaging principles prioritize the child's safety and comfort while providing accurate diagnostic information to guide the child's care.

11.3 Safety Precautions in Pediatric Ionizing Radiation Imaging Based on the Imaging Modality

When it comes to imaging children with ionizing radiation, predictions and research questions remain unanswered. Due to a lack of research data in pediatrics, it is still difficult to determine how safe each imaging modality is! The most recent scientific evidence sheds light on the small but definite risk of radiation dose in children from CT, fluoroscopy, and X-ray imaging. The use of fluoroscopic imaging should be decided based on benefit versus risk to the child, and the intermittent technique is the key to low-dose imaging. Although there have been few reports of MRI and ultrasound imaging causing harm, it is best practice to begin a radiological examination with pediatric patients using non-ionizing radiation. The most recent trend in pediatric imaging focuses on starting with an ultrasound or MRI scan, then using X-ray, fluoroscopy, and CT to determine the benefit versus risk analogy [20].

11.3.1 Radiation Safety Precautions During X-Ray/Fluoroscopy Procedures for Pediatric Imaging

When compared to traditional old X-ray units, the most recent X-ray imaging system employing cutting-edge advanced selenium digital detectors in conjunction with AI has significantly reduced the radiation dose. However, the Food and Drug Administration (FDA) and the Federal Food, Drug, and Cosmetic Act have established guidelines for the age, shape, and size of pediatric patients, which will be useful in determining the actual radiation dose required to produce an optimum image quality. The radiation risk of X-rays in pediatric imaging is relatively low in comparison to the greater benefits they provide. All pediatric X-ray examinations should follow the following procedures:

- Pediatric patients are highly radiosensitive compared to adults, and the cancer risk in later life is high (i.e., stochastic effects of radiation).
- Utilization of specially designed protocols, manual or automatic exposure controls (AEC), and X-ray units with digital radiography (DR) for pediatric imaging.
- The life expectancy of a pediatric patient is much higher compared to an adult patient. Hence, ALARA principles should be followed to avoid the unnecessary risk of cancer.
- X-ray exams should be properly justified by the treating physician in terms of their clinical question and treatment regime [21].

11.3.2 Radiation Safety Precautions During CT Pediatric Imaging

CT scanning is a popular imaging modality in pediatric radiology, but it exposes patients to ionizing radiation. To reduce radiation dose to pediatric patients, it is critical to use appropriate radiation safety precautions during CT imaging [22]. Here are some crucial radiation safety precautions:

1. **ALARA Principle:** This principle emphasizes the importance of keeping the radiation dose as low as reasonably achievable while still obtaining the necessary diagnostic information. This means that the CT scan should be justified based on the medical condition, and alternative imaging modalities, if possible, should be considered [23].
2. **Low-Dose Pediatric Protocols:** Pediatric imaging protocols should be optimized to reduce radiation dose. Pediatric CT protocols typically use lower radiation doses than adult protocols, with parameters adjusted based on the child's age, weight, and size. To optimize exposure settings and assess the need for CT in an individual patient, educate the entire pediatric imaging team through journal publications and conferences within and outside of the radiology specialties [24].
3. **Shielding:** To protect sensitive organs from radiation exposure during a CT scan, such as the thyroid gland and gonads, lead shields or aprons can be used.
4. **Dose Modulation and Optimization Techniques:** For example, automatic tube current modulation can be used to adjust the radiation dose based on the patient's size and anatomy. This reduces the radiation dose to body parts that are not useful for diagnostic purposes [25, 26].
5. **Quality Assurance:** CT equipment should be regularly maintained and calibrated to ensure that image quality is optimized and radiation dose is kept to a minimum.
6. **Patient Education:** Parents and caregivers should be informed about the risks and benefits of CT imaging, as well as the radiation dose involved. They should also be taught how to position the child correctly during the CT scan to minimize motion artifacts and the need for repeat imaging.
7. **Research:** It is also instrumental to conduct additional research to determine the relationship between CT quality and dose, to personalize CT scanning for individual children, and to clarify the link between CT radiation and cancer risk.

In summary, radiation safety precautions for pediatric CT imaging include the use of optimized protocols, shielding, dose modulation techniques, image quality assurance, and patient education. To reduce the radiation dose to pediatric patients, the ALARA principle should always be followed.

11.3.3 FDA's Responsibilities in X-Ray Safety

The FDA works with imaging societies, associations, and governing bodies around the world to develop a database to reduce radiation doses to children from X-ray exposure by enforcing the following:

- Empowering X-ray/CT manufacturers to focus on and design units specifically for pediatric patients. Special protocols for different patient sizes and shapes must be incorporated into the X-ray/CT unit.
- Providing a special user manual guide on pediatric radiation safety and imaging for technologists operating pediatric X-ray/CT units.
- Fostering and establishing relationships between manufacturers and healthcare professionals to improve device design and user instructions.
- Increasing public awareness of the importance of radiation protection principles in hospital quality assurance, as well as personnel training and certification requirements.

11.3.4 Guidelines for Imaging Technologists and Healthcare Professionals

The FDA advises healthcare professionals and hospital administrators to take extra precautions in reducing radiation exposure to the pediatric population by taking the following steps:

- Discuss the purpose of the examination, explaining the benefits versus risks to the parent for a clear understanding.
- Reduce the number of unwanted referrals by proper communication to answer the clinical question and employ non-ionizing radiation techniques for imaging.
- For a dedicated pediatric center, purchasing specially designed units for pediatric imaging is advised.
- It is recommended to use pediatric protocols only and refer to diagnostic reference levels for pediatric patients.
- It is also very instrumental to report adverse radiation incidents to the FDA.

11.3.5 Guidelines for Pediatric Population Patients, Parents, and Caregivers

- Maintain a record of your children's X-ray imaging to aid in your discussion with the referring physician when a new X-ray is recommended.
- Inquire with the referring physician about the advantages and disadvantages of imaging procedures and available alternatives.
- Ask the imaging department about the adverse harmful effects of X-ray and any specific patient preparation needed (e.g., contrast agent, sedation, and bowel preparation).
- Report adverse radiation effects to the FDA [27, 28].

11.4 Impact of Psychological Factors and Child Development in Pediatric Radiography

Neonates in the age group of older children are among the pediatric patients who visit the radiology department, and each group of patients may react differently in the imaging department. In the presence of their parents, such young children may be unable to comprehend an explanation provided by the imaging technologist. The greatest challenge for an imaging technologist is to add to the perception of time and disorientation in imaging such as in children. Young children are in pain, fear, and anxiety, making cooperation and completing the imaging examination difficult. A trained imaging technologist's expertise is tested by how they handle a pediatric patient with the wise assistance of their parents in a kind and sympathetic manner. Regardless of how kind the technologist is to the patient, the ultimate compassion provided by the child's parents is unrivalled. As a result, the parent's role in pediatric imaging is critical. The pediatric patient's appointment should begin with clear instructions to their parents to bring their child's favorite toys, accessories, or any specific items that would make them happy and comfortable during the imaging procedure. Following this, important user-friendly handouts explaining the imaging procedures to be performed, along with their do's and don'ts, should be provided. Second, all necessary information for the imaging procedure should indeed be given to the child only in the presence of their parents. Having said that, it is critical to be soft, and clear, and use short, simple sentences when explaining important steps of the imaging procedure to the patient and parent. The time required for a specific imaging procedure will be determined by the modality used, the use of contrast agents, and the pediatric patient's overall cooperation. Third, because the parents of these pediatric patients are usually stressed and worried, it is critical to calm them down before beginning the actual pediatric radiography process. Things do not always go as planned, and parents become disoriented, upset, and angry during the procedure for a variety of reasons. It is best to take them to your department staff cabin room and handle them professionally. Involving the radiology manager and possibly the Head of Radiology in the discussion of the next steps for pediatric imaging can help to avoid major issues.

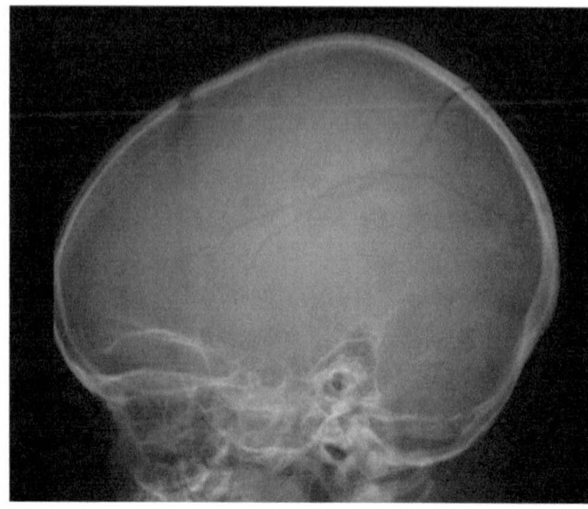

Fig. 11.1 Child lateral skull view

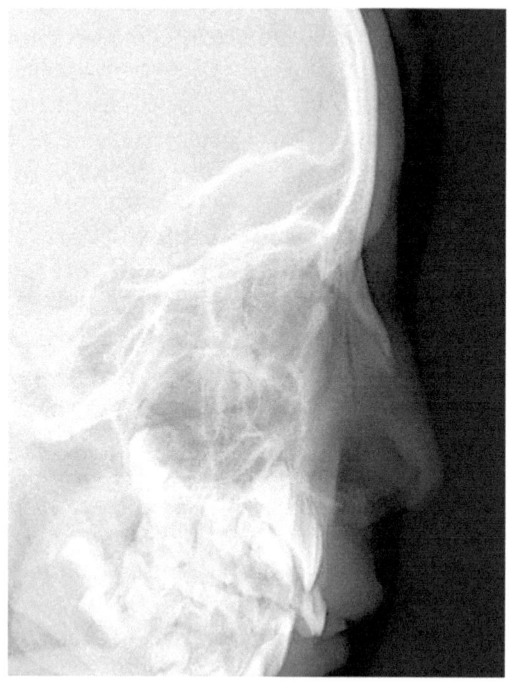

Fig. 11.2 Child nasal bone lateral view

11.5 Child Versus Adult Anatomical Differences

There are noteworthy differences between adult and children's bodies, which makes it imperative to utilize safety precautions while performing pediatric radiography. The overall body size of children is not only smaller, but their internal body makeup is also very different. The following points should be taken into consideration before performing pediatric radiography:

- Thin skull vaults and vascular demarcations are not seen before the age of one in babies, as depicted in Fig. 11.1.
- Nasal bone ossification is only seen after 3 years of age in children, as depicted in Fig. 11.2.
- Paranasal air sinuses pneumatization is only seen after 6 years of age in children, as depicted in Fig. 11.3.
- Scaphoid bone ossification is seen after 6 years of age in children.
- When compared to adult chest X-ray imaging on anterior–posterior (AP) projections, heart enlargement is minimal in children due to the smaller depth of the thoracic cavity, as depicted in Fig. 11.4.

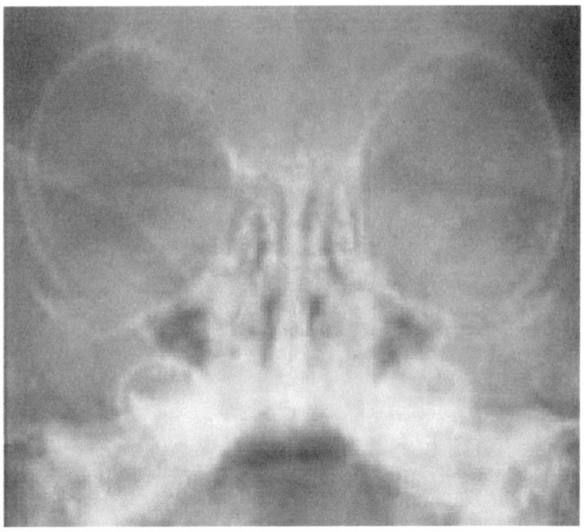

Fig. 11.3 Child Paranasal sinus (PNS) water's view

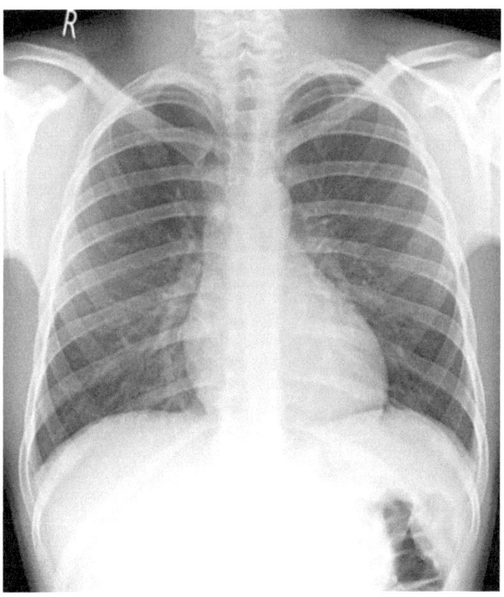

Fig. 11.4 Child AP chest view

- Thymus is an important area to investigate for pediatric imaging as it can mimic pathology in the form of a mediastinal shadow.
- Ossification centers are not well developed in pediatric patients and should be dealt with in the most recent reference articles published online.
- The faster heart and respiratory rates in children should be taken into consideration before planning radiographic procedures.
- The most radiosensitive organ to ionizing radiation is the bone marrow, which is abundantly available in all bones of the child.

These anatomical differences should be considered when optimizing techniques and planning specific radiographic views in pediatric radiography [29].

11.6 A Peek into the Approach Involved in Pediatric Patient Preparation

The main goal of preparing a pediatric patient before the procedure is to reduce stress and anxiety and improve the child's overall cooperation. The imaging technologist should always make a friendly but professional introduction to the child and his parent. At the beginning of the imaging procedure, it is also critical to confirm the referring physician's order and reconfirm the pediatric patient's vital details. It is also recommended that the imaging technologist accompany the child and parent to the well-prepared X-ray/CT/fluoroscopic room, which is equipped with all necessary equipment such as X-ray tubes, imaging consoles, table height adjustments, and other immobilization devices. According to radiation safety guidelines, a single or both parents can be used to assist in the required pediatric imaging procedure, depending on the child's level of cooperation. Throughout the imaging procedure, the imaging technologist should constantly cheer and appreciate the child, and keep small trinkets, gifts, or something special as a token of appreciation. However, it is also important to be truthful in answering all questions about the pediatric imaging procedure [30, 31].

According to ethical guidelines, the imaging technologist should never reveal the procedure's results or diagnosis. The referring physician has the sole authority to share, discuss, and plan treatment for the pediatric patient. Children admitted to the radiology department as inpatients should always be escorted by a nurse, with all IV contrast lines, intravenous (IV) fluids, drainage tubes, and oxygen supply arrangements in place before the imaging procedure begins. Protocols for contagious diseases such as COVID 19 should be well maintained and strictly followed for all pediatric procedures. Furthermore, avoid placing such vulnerable pediatric patients near general patient traffic and plan the procedure accordingly. The use of masks, aprons, gloves, and antiseptic handwashing practices should be followed by all radiology department personnel. It is also recommended that the radiology department disinfect the room after each pediatric population imaging procedure. Outpatient pediatric patients, on the other hand, do not require any special preparations when compared to vulnerable pediatric inpatients. An imaging technologist must use special care and expertise when manipulating a prone invertogram radiograph for assessment of the anus within 24 hours of birth, where the patient is radiographed and held still for 15 minutes before the exposure.

11.6.1 Immobilization Tools in Pediatric Imaging

Pediatric immobilization is a technique used in radiography and other types of imaging to keep children still during examinations. The primary goal of using immobilization tools is to reduce the need for unnecessary repeat examinations due to motion artifacts and thus to reduce the overall radiation dose to the child, who is affected more than ten times that of adults. The hallmark of a successful pediatric imaging procedure is the wise application of these available tools and immobilization accessories. These tools should be simple to use and adaptable to a wide range of sizes. These instruments should be tailored to the anatomical region and the corresponding pediatric imaging technique. These immobilization tools cause artifacts in radiographic images and should be used with caution. The decision to use various immobilization techniques and devices is crafted either through individual department's protocols or at the imaging technologist's discretion. Because the age and maturity of the child may influence the technique used, studies have revealed a potential need for specific immobilization guidelines to assist the imaging technologist [12, 16, 32–35]. The following immobilization techniques and immobilization devices should be used collectively to avoid repeat examinations in pediatric imaging.

Immobilization Techniques

- Colorful toys and distracting objects
- Colorful room ambience and lighting
- Verbal friendly techniques
- Use of music and electronic gadgets
- Physical help from the parent
- Feed and sleep technique
- Monitored sedation technique

Immobilization Devices

- The Pigg-O-Stat—a specialized device used for pediatric chest radiography for child immobilization for over 40 years
- Swaddling devices
- Soft sticky tapes
- Velcro straps
- Lightweight colorful sandbags
- Soft sheets
- Radiolucent neon sponge blocks
- Colorful stockings
- Soft non-allergenic compression and ace bandages

Note All the abovementioned items should be cleaned with bleach/antiseptic solutions after each procedure or should be disposable.

Due to the child's lack of cooperation, the immobilization techniques and devices mentioned above may fail to perform the pediatric imaging procedure in some cases. In these cases, restraint techniques involving manual physical force can be used only with the consent of the child (which is not always possible) or the parent. Restraint techniques, in both scenarios, cause unwanted anxiety and post-traumatic stress for future imaging studies.

11.6.2 Radiographic Technical Considerations for Supplementing Immobilization Techniques

- Utilization of high tube mA techniques to reduce the exposure time
- The shortest exposure time reduces image blurring due to child motion
- Using the right immobilization technique and device for a particular procedure
- Good communication skills with effective management techniques
- Use of AI coupled with automatic exposure control to reduce the overall radiation dose of the procedure

11.6.3 Approaching Children with Special Needs

The importance of approaching a child with special needs and people of determination doubles the imaging technologist's responsibility in terms of ethical care and support practice. It is also critical to conduct an in-depth analysis of the child's handicapped status based on location and extent. It is not recommended to make assumptions about the child's disability before the start of the imaging procedure. In the presence of their parents, the technologist should spend some quality time with children of all abilities, explaining the details of the technique. The simple presence of the child's parent adds a lot of value and eases the overall process of the pediatric imaging procedure. The support in lifting, shifting, transferring, rotating, and introduction of contrast medium can be easily performed if the child's parent is helpful and cooperative.

11.7 Imaging Room Design Specifications and Devices Used to Distract Pediatric Radiography Patients

Waiting Area

The pediatric patient's first impression as they enter the radiology reception area with their parent is critical to the overall success of the imaging procedure. The receptionists should engage with the pediatric patients as soon as possible because these customers are always anxious and concerned about their child's health status. This approach will relax the patient and their parent and make them feel at ease in the radiology department. To effectively manage pediatric patients, reception staff should have extensive experience with child psychological needs as well as a friendly demeanor. The department's waiting area should be colorful and well-stocked with toys, gaming devices, crayons, color-paint books, and child-friendly materials for all ages. The appointment of a playing therapist at the reception desk may be beneficial when dealing with patients undergoing complex procedures.

X-Ray Imaging Room

The imaging room should always be prepared with proper sanitation treatment before the start of the pediatric patient examination. It is not advisable to keep the patient waiting due to room preparation because this adds to the child's and parents' anxiety. The imaging room should be well-lit, colorful, and appealing, in addition to placing child-friendly paintings, charts, and stickers on the wall painted with bright colors. Soft toys and other tools should be used to divert the child's attention away from the fear of the imaging procedure. Light music has been shown to improve the overall success rate of pediatric radiographic examinations. Contrast media, injection syringes, and other frightening imaging equipment should be kept hidden until imaging is needed.

11.8 Pediatric Imaging Device Equipment Specifications for Industry Manufacturers

The FDA and all international regulatory bodies have established guidelines for all X-ray manufacturing companies, which are available online, to encourage pediatric patients' radiation safety to be prioritized when designing X-ray Imaging units. The following are the most important criteria to consider:

- Pre-set radiation dose optimization features such as automatic exposure control using AI to ensure that the X-ray system operates at the lowest radiation dose for pediatric patients while providing images of the highest quality adequate for clinical diagnosis and treatment.
- Management of user-friendly instructions and operating systems to assist imaging technologists in modulating, operating, and performing setting changes for pediatric patients of various sizes across all healthcare hospitals and units.
- Market and promote the guidelines for using X-ray imaging safely during pediatric radiography. The FDA recommends that old X-ray units sold globally be upgraded with the necessary software and hardware to keep radiation doses in pediatric radiographic procedures to a minimum. All existing customers and healthcare providers should be given the necessary assistance to ensure the safety of using older X-ray units on pediatric patients.
- Dose pop-ups and automatic alarms for all pediatric imaging procedures employing X-rays.
- Reach out to medical imaging societies and communities around the world for feedback on pediatric safety and imaging.

11.9 Dose Considerations and Radiation Protection in Pediatric Imaging

Pediatric radiation dose is an important consideration in pediatric medical imaging. Children are more vulnerable to the harmful effects of radiation than adults, and ionizing radiation exposure can increase their likelihood of getting cancer later in life [36, 37]. Radiologists and radiologic technologists use a variety of specialized techniques to reduce radiation dose in pediatric imaging, including:

1. **Modulating Radiation Parameters:** Radiation dose can be reduced by optimizing radiation dose parameters such as tube voltage and current, exposure time, and image processing.
2. **Precise Planning of the Imaging Area:** Imaging only the area of interest and limiting the field of view can significantly decrease the radiation dose in many cases.
3. **Protective Shielding:** Radiation exposure to surrounding tissues can be reduced by using lead aprons, thyroid shields, gonadal shields, and other shielding materials.
4. **Use of Non-Ionizing Imaging Modalities:** Based on specific indication cases, non-ionizing radiation imaging modalities such as ultrasound or MRI can be used instead of X-rays or CT scans.
5. **Utilizing Low-Dose Protocol with Tracking and Monitoring Systems:** Imaging departments use sophisticated dose tracking and monitoring systems to keep track of the radiation dose delivered to a patient and adjust imaging protocols as needed.

In addition to these techniques, imaging professionals should closely examine the justification for the imaging exam, guaranteeing that the benefit outweighs the potential risk from radiation exposure. Overall, minimizing pediatric radiation dose is an important aspect of pediatric radiology because it ensures the child's safety and lowers their risk of developing cancer later in life.

11.9.1 Diagnostic Reference Ranges in Pediatric Radiography

In pediatric radiography, diagnostic reference ranges refer to the range of values considered normal for a specific diagnostic test or procedure in children of a certain age group. These reference ranges are critical for interpreting imaging test results and making a diagnosis. Diagnostic reference ranges in pediatric radiography are typically based on the child's age, weight, height, and the specific test being performed. For example, the reference range for a newborn's chest X-ray will differ from that for a chest X-ray in a 10-year-old. The American College of Radiology

(ACR) has issued guidelines for the proper use of diagnostic imaging in pediatric patients, including reference ranges for various diagnostic tests. The ACR also offers a free online tool called the ACR Appropriateness Criteria, which advises on the best imaging studies for specific clinical scenarios in pediatric patients. When interpreting the results of a radiographic study, imaging technologists, radiologists, and other healthcare providers must consider the child's clinical presentation, medical history, and other diagnostic test results in addition to reference ranges.

It is critical to remember that pediatric patients are not simply small adults; their diagnostic reference ranges may differ significantly from adults. As a result, it is critical in pediatric radiography to use age-specific reference ranges to ensure accurate interpretation and diagnosis [38–42].

11.9.2 Image Quality and Dosimetry in Pediatric Radiography

When it comes to pediatric radiography, image quality and dosimetry are two critical factors that need to be carefully examined.

Image Quality The quality of the radiographic image is critical to ensuring that it contains the information required for a proper diagnosis. Because of the child's smaller size and the need to reduce radiation exposure as much as possible, pediatric radiography requires special attention to image quality. To improve image quality while reducing radiation exposure, radiologic technologists have used appropriate techniques and equipment, such as high-speed film, high-frequency generators, and appropriate grids in the past. Most recently, computed radiography and DR employing automatic exposure controls have significantly reduced pediatric patient radiation doses.

Dosimetry Dosimetry is the measurement of radiation dose, and it is critical in pediatric radiography to monitor radiation exposure levels. Children are more sensitive to radiation than adults, and long-term risks from ionizing radiation include an increased risk of cancer. As a result, radiologic technologists must use the lowest possible radiation dose to obtain diagnostic-quality images. Radiation dose to children can be reduced by using techniques such as collimation, shielding, and exposure factor adjustment.

It is also important to remember that different exposure parameters may be required for children depending on their size and developmental stage. As a result, radiologic imaging technologists must carefully assess each child and adjust the exposure parameters to ensure the lowest possible radiation dose while obtaining optimum-quality diagnostic images [43].

Finally, when performing pediatric radiography, it is critical to carefully consider image quality and dosimetry. Using appropriate techniques and equipment, monitoring radiation exposure levels, and adjusting exposure parameters based on the child's size and developmental stage can help reduce the risks of ionizing radiation exposure while obtaining accurate diagnostic images [3, 31].

11.10 Routine Pediatric Radiological Examinations, Recommended Projections, and Referral Criteria

The most common pediatric radiological procedures are listed below:

Recommended Projections:
Posterior–Anterior View and AP View

- Chest—neonatal, post-neonatal, infant, and elderly children
- Skull and paranasal air sinuses
- Abdomen series
- Pelvis and hips (limb length assessment X-rays)
- Spine (scoliosis and kyphosis)
- Bone age and extremities (feet, elbow, hands, and knees)
- Skeletal survey for various specific indications
- Dental radiography
- Fluoroscopic procedures (IVU and barium studies)

- CT brain, spine, and abdomen—complex abnormalities not assessed using routine radiography

The most common indications for pediatric radiological procedures are listed below:

Some Pathologies Would Require the Chest and Abdomen to be Radiographed on a Single Image

- Lung pathologies: thoracic cage pathology, respiratory difficulties, pleural effusion, pneumothorax, and chronic lung diseases
- Heart cyanosis and heart murmur
- Esophageal atresia
- Infection
- Aspiration (meconium)
- Confirming the position of catheters/tubes
- After any post-operative procedure
- Skeletal survey syndrome
- Suspected antenatal abnormality
- Abdomen pathology—diaphragmatic hernia

11.11 Recent Advancements in Pediatric Radiography Imaging Techniques

Pediatric radiography imaging techniques have advanced significantly in recent years as a result of technological advancements and field research. Here are a few examples of recent advances in pediatric radiography imaging techniques:

1. **DR:** In many cases, DR has supplanted film-based radiography. Superior image quality, faster image acquisition, and lower radiation doses are all advantages of DR systems. In pediatric imaging, where low radiation doses are critical, DR is especially useful.
2. **Cone Beam CT (CBCT):** CBCT is a type of CT imaging that produces 3D images of the body by using a cone-shaped X-ray beam and a detector. In comparison to traditional CT scans, CBCT provides high-resolution images with lower radiation doses. In pediatric imaging, CBCT is useful for evaluating complex fractures, dental and facial abnormalities, and other musculoskeletal conditions.
3. **MRI:** MRI is a non-invasive imaging technique that produces detailed images of the body by using magnetic fields and radio waves. Because it does not use ionizing radiation, MRI is especially useful in pediatric imaging. This makes it safer for children. Recent advances in MRI technology have improved image quality and reduced scan times, making the procedure more bearable for children.
4. **Ultrasound:** Ultrasound imaging creates images of the body by using high-frequency sound waves. Because ultrasound is non-invasive and does not use ionizing radiation, it is suitable for use in children. Recent advances in ultrasound technology, such as 3D and 4D imaging, have improved diagnostic accuracy and made complex structures easier to visualize.
5. **Image Processing Techniques:** Image processing advances have improved image quality, reduced image noise, and allowed for the creation of 3D and 4D images. Image processing techniques such as computer-aided detection and machine learning algorithms are being used to improve diagnostic accuracy and decrease the need for repeat imaging.

Finally, recent advances in pediatric radiography imaging techniques have resulted in improved image quality, lower radiation exposure, and increased diagnostic accuracy. These advancements in pediatric imaging have made it safer and more tolerable for children, which is critical for ensuring that children receive the best possible care.

11.11.1 AI and Pediatric Radiography

AI has the potential to transform pediatric radiography by improving diagnostic accuracy, reducing errors, and increasing efficiency. Here are some examples of how AI is being used in pediatric radiography:

1. **Image Analysis:** Medical images can be analyzed by AI algorithms to detect and quantify abnormalities that are difficult to detect with the naked eye. AI algorithms can assist imaging technologists and radiologists in identifying and classifying abnormalities in pediatric radiography, such as bone fractures, lung nodules, and brain tumors.
2. **Workflow Optimization:** AI can also aid in the optimization of pediatric radiography workflow by automating routine tasks and reducing the time required for image analysis. AI algorithms can triage images, prioritize urgent cases, and alert radiologists to abnormalities that require immediate attention.
3. **Radiation Dose Reduction:** By optimizing imaging protocols and reducing the number of unnecessary scans, AI can help reduce radiation exposure in pediatric radiography. Based on patient characteristics and clinical indications, AI algorithms can predict the required radiation dose for each imaging study, ensuring that the dose is tailored to the child's needs.
4. **Predictive Modeling:** AI can be used to create predictive models that identify children who are at risk of developing certain diseases. These models can aid in the direction of screening and monitoring programs, allowing for earlier detection and treatment.
5. **Education and Training:** AI can be used to create educational and training tools for imaging technologists, radiologists, and other healthcare professionals. AI algorithms can provide feedback on image interpretation, assist in the identification of areas for improvement, and provide ongoing training and support.

To summarize, AI has the potential to transform pediatric radiography by improving diagnostic accuracy, reducing errors, and increasing efficiency [44–50]. However, it is critical to ensure that these technologies are used safely and ethically and that they supplement rather than replace image technologists, radiologists, and other healthcare professional's expertise.

Learning Outcomes/Summary

Pediatric patient care entails providing specialized care to children during medical imaging procedures in radiology. The goal is to minimize the child's discomfort and anxiety while ensuring accurate diagnostic results.

The following are some important aspects of pediatric patient care in radiology:

1. Effective communication with the child and their parents is essential for reducing fear and anxiety. Radiology staff should explain the procedure to the child and parents in age-appropriate language, answer questions, and reassure them.
2. Patient Positioning: Because children may have difficulty remaining still during imaging procedures, it is critical to position them correctly to ensure the best diagnostic results possible. Specialized equipment and techniques discussed earlier in this chapter may be used to immobilize the child in a comfortable and safe position.
3. Radiation Protection: Children are more sensitive to radiation than adults, so special precautions must be taken to reduce radiation exposure. Radiology personnel should use the lowest radiation dose possible while still providing accurate diagnostic results.
4. Sedation and Anesthesia: Sedation or anesthesia may be required to keep the child still during some imaging procedures. Radiology staff should have specialized training and experience in pediatric sedation and anesthesia to ensure safety and comfort.
5. Follow-Up Care: Following the imaging procedure, radiology staff should provide appropriate follow-up care and inform the child's healthcare team of the results. They should also address any concerns or questions raised by the child or parents.

Overall, high-quality pediatric patient care in radiology necessitates specialized training, expertise, and a compassionate approach that considers the unique needs of children and their families.

Exercise

Multiple Choice Questions (MCQs)

1. What is the primary goal of a radiology and imaging department?
   A. Maximizing patient throughput
   B. Minimizing equipment costs
   C. Achieving optimum diagnostic image quality with minimal radiation dose
   D. Reducing wait times for appointments
2. According to the text, pediatric patients are at a higher risk of developing which of the following due to radiation exposure?
   A. Early onset diabetes
   B. Late somatic or late deterministic effects
   C. Immediate radiation burns
   D. Short-term memory loss
3. What principle should be followed to avoid unnecessary radiation risk in pediatric X-ray exams?
   A. Maximum intensity projection
   B. ALARA (As Low As Reasonably Achievable)
   C. Maximum radiation principle
   D. Minimum dose strategy
4. What is the benefit of using the most recent X-ray imaging systems with advanced selenium digital detectors?
   A. They are cheaper to operate
   B. They significantly reduce radiation dose
   C. They produce faster results
   D. They are easier to maintain
5. What is a key feature of pediatric-friendly environments in imaging?
   A. Use of larger equipment
   B. Use of distraction techniques
   C. Quick imaging sessions
   D. Strict enforcement of quiet zones
6. What does the FDA encourage X-ray/CT manufacturers to design specifically for pediatric patients?
   A. Faster imaging units
   B. Larger units
   C. Units with special protocols for different patient sizes and shapes
   D. More expensive equipment
7. According to the guidelines for imaging technologists, what should be reduced to minimize radiation exposure in pediatric patients?
   A. Number of referrals
   B. Cost of imaging procedures
   C. Duration of imaging sessions
   D. Number of imaging modalities used
8. Which of the following is an important consideration in pediatric radiography due to anatomical differences from adults?
   A. Thicker skull vaults in children
   B. Rapid ossification of bones
   C. Faster heart and respiratory rates
   D. Less sensitivity to radiation
9. What role do parents play in pediatric imaging, according to the text?
   A. They provide technical assistance
   B. They give consent and emotional support
   C. They perform the imaging
   D. They interpret the results
10. Why is the thymus an important area to investigate in pediatric imaging?
   A. It is always indicative of disease
   B. It can mimic mediastinal pathology
   C. It is a common site of injury
   D. It is not visible in children
11. What is the primary goal of preparing a pediatric patient before an imaging procedure?
   A. To speed up the procedure
   B. To reduce stress and anxiety
   C. To increase the radiation dose
   D. To inform them of the results
12. Which immobilization device has been used for over 40 years in pediatric chest radiography?
   A. Swaddling devices
   B. The Pigg-O-Stat
   C. Soft sticky tapes
   D. Velcro straps
13. What is recommended for imaging rooms to help relax pediatric patients?
   A. Bright lights and loud music
   B. Child-friendly paintings and toys
   C. Dark and quiet environments
   D. Keeping all equipment visible

14. What should be done to the imaging equipment after each pediatric procedure?
    A. Leave it as is
    B. Dispose of it
    C. Clean with bleach/antiseptic solutions
    D. Store it in a different room
15. What is a critical aspect of pediatric radiology in terms of radiation dose?
    A. Increasing radiation exposure
    B. Reducing radiation dose
    C. Ignoring radiation safety
    D. Using only adult reference ranges
16. What imaging technique has replaced film-based radiography due to superior image quality and lower radiation doses?
    A. CBCT
    B. MRI
    C. DR
    D. Ultrasound
17. What is a common indication for pediatric chest and abdomen radiography?
    A. Brain tumor
    B. Diaphragmatic hernia
    C. Bone fracture
    D. Dental abnormalities
18. Which recent advancement in imaging does not use ionizing radiation, making it safer for children?
    A. CT
    B. DR
    C. MRI
    D. Fluoroscopy
19. What role does AI play in pediatric radiography?
    A. Replaces radiologists entirely
    B. Increases radiation doses
    C. Automates routine tasks and improves diagnostic accuracy
    D. Eliminates the need for imaging
20. What is essential in ensuring high-quality pediatric patient care in radiology?
    A. Ignoring the child's discomfort
    B. Using the highest radiation dose
    C. Specialized training and compassionate approach
    D. Performing procedures without consent

Short Questions

1. Explain the importance of a multidisciplinary hybrid team in pediatric imaging.
2. Describe the significance of the ALARA principle in pediatric CT imaging.
3. Describe the responsibilities of the FDA in ensuring X-ray safety for pediatric patients.
4. How do psychological factors impact pediatric patients during radiography?
5. Discuss the ethical guidelines for imaging technologists regarding the disclosure of procedure results.
6. Describe the importance of diagnostic reference ranges in pediatric radiography.
7. Describe the benefits of using CBCT in pediatric imaging.
8. What are the key considerations for radiation protection in pediatric radiography?

Long Question

1. Discuss the various radiation safety precautions that should be taken during pediatric imaging procedures involving ionizing radiation, with a focus on the differences between X-ray/fluoroscopy and CT scans.
2. Discuss the anatomical differences between children and adults that must be considered when planning and optimizing pediatric radiographic techniques.
3. Explain the considerations and techniques involved in minimizing radiation exposure in pediatric imaging, including the use of non-ionizing imaging modalities.
4. Discuss the impact of recent advancements, including DR, MRI, and AI, on the quality and safety of pediatric imaging.

Answers for MCQs

1. C. Achieving optimum diagnostic image quality with minimal radiation dose
2. B. Late somatic or late deterministic effects

3. B. ALARA (As Low As Reasonably Achievable)
4. B. They significantly reduce radiation dose
5. B. Use of distraction techniques
6. C. Units with special protocols for different patient sizes and shapes
7. A. Number of referrals
8. C. Faster heart and respiratory rates
9. B. They give consent and emotional support
10. B. It can mimic mediastinal pathology
11. B. To reduce stress and anxiety
12. B. The Pigg-O-Stat
13. B. Child-friendly paintings and toys
14. C. Clean with bleach/antiseptic solutions
15. B. Reducing radiation dose
16. C. DR
17. B. Diaphragmatic hernia
18. C. MRI
19. C. Automates routine tasks and improves diagnostic accuracy
20. C. Specialized training and compassionate approach

References

1. Rahu M. Health effects of the Chernobyl accident: fears, rumours and the truth. Eur J Cancer. 2003;39(3):295.
2. Thomas D, Darby S, Fagnani F, Hubert P, Vaeth M, Weiss K. Definition and estimation of lifetime detriment from radiation exposures: principles and methods. Health Phys. 1992;63(3):259.
3. Regulla DF, Eder H. Patient exposure in medical X-ray imaging in Europe. Radiat Prot Dosim. 2005;114(1–3):11.
4. Charles M. UNSCEAR report 2000: sources and effects of ionizing radiation. United Nations Scientific Comittee on the Effects of Atomic Radiation. J Radiol Prot. 2001;21(1):83.
5. Rawashdeh M, Saade C, Zaitoun M, Abdelrahman M, Brennan P, Alewaidat H, et al. Establishment of diagnostic reference levels in cardiac computed tomography. J Appl Clin Med Phys. 2019;20(10):181.
6. MacDougall RD, Kleinman PL, Callahan MJ. Size-based protocol optimization using automatic tube current modulation and automatic kV selection in computed tomography. J Appl Clin Med Phys. 2016;17(1):328.
7. Goske MJ, Strauss KJ, Coombs LP, Mandel KE, Towbin AJ, Larson DB, et al. Diagnostic reference ranges for pediatric abdominal CT. Radiology. 2013;268(1):208.
8. Strauss KJ, Goske MJ, Towbin AJ, Sengupta D, Callahan MJ, Darge K, et al. Pediatric chest CT diagnostic reference ranges: development and application. Radiology. 2017;284(1):219.
9. Jose A, Saravana Kumar A, Govindarajan KN, Manimaran P. Assessment of regional pediatric diagnostic reference levels for panoramic radiography using dose area product. J Med Phys. 2020;45(3):182.
10. Martin CJ. Optimisation in general radiography. Biomed Imaging Intervention J. 2007;3:e18.
11. Lynch T, Bialy L, Kellner JD, Osmond MH, Klassen TP, Durec T, et al. A systematic review on the diagnosis of pediatric bacterial pneumonia: when gold is bronze. PLoS One. 2010;5(8):e11989.
12. Porto L, Lunelli N, Paschuk S, Oliveira A, Ferreira JL, Schelin H, et al. Evaluation of entrance surface air kerma in pediatric chest radiography. Radiat Phys Chem. 2014;104:252.
13. Sanchez R, Khong PL, Ringertz H. Radiologic protection in pediatric radiology: ICRP recommendations. Pediatr Radiol. 2013;43:920.
14. ICRP, Khong PL, Ringertz H, Donoghue V, Frush D, Rehani M, et al. ICRP Publication 121: radiological protection in paediatric diagnostic and interventional radiology. Ann ICRP. 2013;42(2):1.
15. Corrigendum to ICRP Publication 121: radiological protection in paediatric diagnostic and interventional radiology. Ann ICRP. 2013;42(2):1–63. https://doi.org/10.1016/j.icrp.2012.10.001. Ann ICRP. 2021.
16. Portelli JL. Benefit-risk communication in paediatric radiology. Pediatr Radiol. 2019;49.
17. Strauss KJ, Kaste SC. ALARA in pediatric interventional and fluoroscopic imaging: striving to keep radiation doses as low as possible during fluoroscopy of pediatric patients-a white paper executive summary. J Am Coll Radiol. 2006;3(9):686.
18. Sodhi KS, Krishna S, Saxena AK, Sinha A, Khandelwal N, Lee EY. Clinical application of "Justification" and "Optimization" principle of ALARA in pediatric CT imaging: 'how many children can be protected from unnecessary radiation?'. Eur J Radiol. 2015;84(9):1752.
19. Portelli JL, McNulty JP, Bezzina P, Rainford L. Paediatric imaging radiation dose awareness and use of referral guidelines amongst radiology practitioners and radiographers. Insights Imaging. 2016;7(1):145.
20. John SD, Moore QT, Herrmann T, Don S, Powers K, Smith SN, et al. The image gently pediatric digital radiography safety checklist: tools for improving pediatric radiography. J Am Coll Radiol. 2013;10(10):781.
21. National Cancer Institute. Radiation risks and pediatric computed tomography (CT): a guide for health care providers. National Cancer Institute; 2012.
22. Brody AS, Frush DP, Huda W, Brent RL, DiPietro MA, Applegate KE, et al. Radiation risk to children from computed tomography. Pediatrics. 2007;120(3):677.

23. Marin JR, Wang L, Winger DG, Mannix RC. Variation in computed tomography imaging for pediatric injury-related emergency visits. J Pediatr. 2015;167(4):897.
24. Frush DJ, Commander CW, Hartman TS, Cecil AK, Handly BD, Park DB, et al. Utilization of computed tomography imaging in the pediatric emergency department. Pediatr Radiol. 2020;50(4):470.
25. Nardo L, Schmall JP, Werner TJ, Malogolowkin M, Badawi RD, Alavi A. Potential roles of total-body PET/computed tomography in pediatric imaging. PET Clin. 2020;15:271.
26. Young C, Owens CM. Pediatric computed tomography imaging guideline. Acta Radiol. 2013;54:998.
27. National Cancer Institute. Radiation risks and pediatric computed tomography (CT): a guide for health care providers. National Cancer Institute; 2018.
28. Blackmore CC, Medina LS. Evidence-based radiology and the ACR Appropriateness Criteria®. J Am Coll Radiol. 2006;3(7):505.
29. Chang SE, Erickson KI, Ambrose NG, Hasegawa-Johnson MA, Ludlow CL. Brain anatomy differences in childhood stuttering. Neuroimage. 2008;39(3):1333.
30. Delis H, Homolka P, Chapple CL, Costa PR, Attalla E, Lubis LE, et al. Developing and implementing a multi-modality imaging optimization study in paediatric radiology: experience and recommendations from an IAEA coordinated research project. Phys Med. 2021;82:255.
31. Pratama IBGP, Mulia IR. Diagnostic reference level (DRL) analysis of CT scan modality for head procedure on pediatric patient. In: AIP conference proceedings; 2021.
32. Raissaki MT. Pediatric radiation protection. Eur Radiol Suppl. 2004;14:74.
33. Minigh J. Pediatric radiation protection. Radiol Technol. 2005;76:365.
34. Stephenson SK. Radiation protection in pediatric radiology. Int J Radiat Biol. 1982;42(4).
35. Furlow B. Radiation protection in pediatric imaging. Radiol Technol. 2011;82:421.
36. Vassileva J, Rehani MM, Applegate K, Ahmed NA, Al-Dhuhli H, Al-Naemi HM, et al. IAEA survey of paediatric computed tomography practice in 40 countries in Asia, Europe, Latin America and Africa: procedures and protocols. Eur Radiol. 2013;23(3):623.
37. Poli GL, Coca M, Torres L, Fahey F, Lassmann M, Chapple CL, et al. Developing and implementing an imaging optimization study in pediatric nuclear medicine: experience and recommendations from an IAEA-coordinated research project. J Nucl Med. 2021;62(4):570.
38. Lackay O, Horn-Lodewyk J, Muller H. A practical guide for paediatric diagnostic reference levels (PiDRLs). J Med Imaging Radiat Sci. 2022;53(1):123.
39. Tschauner S, Marterer R, Gübitz M, Kalmar PI, Talakic E, Weissensteiner S, et al. European guidelines for AP/PA chest X-rays: routinely satisfiable in a paediatric radiology division? Eur Radiol. 2016;26(2):495.
40. Schegerer A, Loose R, Heuser LJ, Brix G. Diagnostic reference levels for diagnostic and interventional X-ray procedures in Germany: update and handling. RoFo Fortschritte auf dem Gebiet der Rontgenstrahlen und der Bildgeb Verfahren. 2019;191(8):739.
41. Goske MJ. Diagnostic reference ranges and the American College of Radiology Dose Index Registry: the pediatric experience. Pediatr Radiol. 2014;44:506.
42. Goske MJ, Strauss KJ, Coombs LP, Mandel KE, Towbin AJ, Larson DB, et al. Diagnostic reference ranges for paediatric CT. Radiology. 2013;268(1):208.
43. Paulo G, Vaño E, Rodrigues A. Diagnostic reference levels in plain radiography for paediatric imaging: a Portuguese study. Radiography. 2016;22(1):e34.
44. Wang F, Gu X, Chen S, Liu Y, Shen Q, Pan H, et al. Artificial intelligence system can achieve comparable results to experts for bone age assessment of Chinese children with abnormal growth and development. PeerJ. 2020;8:e8854.
45. Yi PH, Kim TK, Wei J, Shin J, Hui FK, Sair HI, et al. Automated semantic labeling of pediatric musculoskeletal radiographs using deep learning. Pediatr Radiol. 2019;49(8):1066.
46. Behzadi-khormouji H, Rostami H, Salehi S, Derakhshande-Rishehri T, Masoumi M, Salemi S, et al. Deep learning, reusable and problem-based architectures for detection of consolidation on chest X-ray images. Comput Methods Prog Biomed. 2020;185:105162.
47. Meda KC, Milla SS, Rostad BS. Artificial intelligence research within reach: an object detection model to identify rickets on pediatric wrist radiographs. Pediatr Radiol. 2021;51(5):782.
48. Mahomed N, van Ginneken B, Philipsen RHHM, Melendez J, Moore DP, Moodley H, et al. Computer-aided diagnosis for World Health Organization-defined chest radiograph primary-endpoint pneumonia in children. Pediatr Radiol. 2020;50(4):482.
49. Choi JW, Cho YJ, Ha JY, Lee YY, Koh SY, Seo JY, et al. Deep learning-assisted diagnosis of pediatric skull fractures on plain radiographs. Korean J Radiol. 2022;23(3):343.
50. Schalekamp S, Klein WM, van Leeuwen KG. Current and emerging artificial intelligence applications in chest imaging: a pediatric perspective. Pediatr Radiol. 2022;52:2120.

12 Role of Nursing Care in Radiological Procedures

Learning Objectives

D. Prakash, R. P. Kotian, *Fundamentals of X-ray Imaging*,
https://doi.org/10.1007/978-981-96-7328-5_12

12.1 Introduction

Radiology is a rapidly growing field due to advancements in technology and imaging. With the help of radiological techniques, percutaneous minimally invasive procedures are reducing patient pain, recovery time, and hospital stays while increasing outcomes. In cases where surgery is not appropriate, radiofrequency ablation offers an alternative therapy for patients with liver cancer. Image-guided biopsies have largely replaced exploratory laparotomies, which are traditionally costly surgical procedures.

A growing radiology department will certainly require skilled radiology nurses in order to achieve the best possible outcomes for patients. Additionally, nursing students rarely participate in radiology rotations, and nurses have limited exposure to radiology. In consequence, radiology nursing has become one of the least known specialties and has a less defined career path [1].

The radiology nurse's position requires extensive knowledge, skill, and independence because radiology nurses serve patients with varying needs and limited information. A radiology nurse often initiates or checks peripheral intravenous lines, examines infusion ports, administers medications, monitors vital signs, suctions patients, implants Foley catheters, and assists patients with their personal needs. As well as notifying the radiology technologist or radiologist of unexpected patient needs, the radiology nurse performs specialist nursing tasks, such as administering intravenous sedation or analgesia during particular procedures and closely monitoring patients. Nursing care is required for patients transferring from intensive care units (ICUs), for those in emergency circumstances, for children, and for those who require sedation in radiology departments [2].

A radiology nurse's other responsibility is teaching patients, their families, students, and other nurses about patient care. They train the radiology staff on new nursing rules and national standards as soon as they are implemented. In addition to collecting data, keeping records, and reporting results, radiology nurses dedicate significant time and effort to quality improvement and infection control programs [3].

Radiology nurses are organized individuals who coordinate ecological and system assets to provide excellent treatment. To provide optimal and safe care, they combine knowledge and abilities from other nursing specializations. Like nurses in operating rooms, they are experts at positioning, comforting, and preventing falls in patients. They conduct rapid assessments, coordinate patient flow, and coordinate patient care, just as ambulatory and emergency department (ED) nurses do. As ICU nurses manage complex care (e.g., hemodynamic monitoring and vasoactive drip titration), they also manage complex care for patients. Nurses in radiology are skilled at delivering minimal to moderate pain management and sedation to patients. The care they provide is governed by federal and state laws and regulations. They are also guided by professional organizations such as the American College of Radiology and the Association for Radiologic and Imaging Nursing [4–6].

The radiology nurse is an integral part of the triad of radiologists, technologists, and nurses in radiology. Patients are at the center of the trio's commitment to compassion, support, and therapeutic environments. In preparation for and after the radiological procedure, they explain what patients can expect. Nurses in radiology are sensitive to the cultural needs of their patients and families and provide culturally competent care.

12.2 Role of Nursing Care in Radiological Procedures: What It Takes to Specialize in This Area

Nursing radiology, also known as radiologic nursing, is an important aspect of medical imaging since it provides patient care and assistance during the radiological procedure. Here are some important features of the role:

1. **Patient Preparation:** An essential part of nursing in radiology is preparing patients for a range of imaging procedures, such as X-rays,

computed tomography (CT) scans, magnetic resonance imaging (MRI), ultrasounds, and nuclear medicine examinations. This preparation may include explaining the procedure to the patient, gathering pertinent medical information, and ensuring that the patient knows any pre-operation instructions, such as fasting or drug protocols.

2. **Safety and Comfort:** Radiology nurses are responsible for assuring patient safety and comfort during imaging treatments. They may help patients position themselves correctly for imaging, give comfort measures such as blankets or pillows, and address any questions or concerns the patient may have regarding the procedure.
3. **Administration of Contrast Agents:** Contrast agents may be used in certain imaging procedures, such as CT scans and MRIs, to make specific structures or abnormalities more visible. Nursing radiologists are primarily in charge of giving these contrast agents, monitoring the patient for adverse responses, and implementing appropriate measures as needed.
4. **Monitoring Vital Signs:** Throughout the imaging procedure, nurses check the patient's vital signs to guarantee their safety and well-being. This includes monitoring heart rate, blood pressure, breathing rate, and oxygen saturation, especially during procedures that may be uncomfortable or require contrast agents.
5. **Patient Education and Support:** Teaching patients about the imaging procedure, including what to anticipate during the process and any potential dangers or side effects, is a key component of nursing radiology. Additionally, nurses offer assistance to patients and their families by answering any queries or worries they may have and reassuring them throughout the imaging procedure.
6. **Collaboration With Radiology Team:** Radiologic technologists, radiologists, and other medical professionals involved in imaging work closely with radiology nurses. They work together to make sure imaging operations are carried out properly and successfully, and they let the other members of the team know about any pertinent patient information or concerns.
7. **Post-Procedure Care:** Nursing radiology continues to care for patients while they recuperate from the imaging process. This could involve keeping an eye out for any delayed reactions to contrast materials, helping patients move around after the procedure, and making sure that they get any instructions or follow-up care that they require.

The importance of nurses to the healthcare system and the hospital system has been substantiated by abundant research over the past few decades. It has been demonstrated that nursing improves the quality and availability of healthcare in several studies and assessments.

Radiology nurses are currently involved in diagnostic imaging and interventional treatment. In addition to providing comfort and safety, they also assess and educate patients, monitor vital signs, and administer medication. Nurses have the most extensive patient interaction of any healthcare practitioner; thus, they have a significant opportunity to affect patient outcomes in radiological settings. A radiology nurse's position involves extensive knowledge, skill, and independence because they care for a diverse spectrum of patients with variable requirements and limited information.

Radiology nurses are responsible for establishing IV access, dispensing prescriptions, monitoring vital signs, aiding patients, and performing specialist nursing responsibilities such as administering contrast media. Also, they spend considerable time collecting data, maintaining records, and improving quality. Radiology nurses provide high-quality treatment to a varied patient population while also serving as educators and advocates within the radiology department. In the upcoming sections of this chapter, we shall go over the tasks and duties performed by nurses in the radiology department during different varieties of examinations [7–9].

Generally, nursing radiology plays a critical role in the safe and effective delivery of medical imaging services, focusing on patient care, safety, and comfort throughout the imaging process.

12.3 Nursing Perspective: Patient Care and Assessment in Various Radiological Procedures

In radiology, imaging technology such as X-rays, CT scans, ultrasounds, and MRI scans are used to diagnose and treat medical conditions. Patient care and assessment in these procedures are critical to ensuring accurate imaging results and patient safety. Here are some important aspects to consider for radiology nursing staff:

1. **Patient Preparation:** Before a radiological procedure, patients may need to fast, drink contrast material, or take certain drugs. It is critical for nursing personnel to provide the patient with precise instructions and answer any concerns they may have.
2. **Before starting the process**, radiology nurses should review the patient's medical history, allergies, and current health status. This information assists in identifying the best imaging approach and guaranteeing the patient's safety.
3. **Effective Communication:** Explain each phase of the procedure and address any concerns or questions the patient may have. This helps to minimize anxiety and enhances the entire patient experience.
4. **Positioning:** Proper patient positioning ensures clear and accurate imaging results. Healthcare personnel should make sure that the patient is comfortable and in the proper position for the treatment.
5. **Monitoring:** Radiology nurses should monitor patients' vital signs during radiological procedures to prevent problems or bad reactions. In the event of an abnormality, prompt intervention may be required.
6. **Following radiological procedures**, nurses should follow patients for any acute adverse effects or problems. Patients should be given post-procedure care instructions, such as drinking water and relaxing [10–12].

Patient care and assessment during radiological operations are critical to guaranteeing the patient's safety and well-being. Radiology nurses should deliver quality care and reliable imaging results by adhering to established protocols and communication techniques.

12.4 Impact of Nursing Radiology Professionals

12.4.1 What Is the Main Role of a Radiology Nurse?

Nurses who work in radiology work in a variety of environments, including universities, community hospitals, and outpatient imaging centers. Radiology has many different subspecialties, including ultrasound, MRI, CT, interventional radiology (IR), neuro-IR, and radiology-oncology. Nurses value autonomy and diversity of responsibilities as part of a small team of experienced professionals. Here are some listed nursing tasks performed at radiology:

- Answering any questions patients may have about their upcoming X-ray procedures
- Identifying any allergies or health issues before the procedure
- Monitoring and assessing the body temperature and blood pressure of radiology patients
- Administering any needed medications, light anesthesia, or sedation
- Performing intravenous injections as needed
- Ensure that the patient recovers from the procedure and is safely discharged.

Radiology nurses treat patients of all ages and levels of acuity with their diverse skill sets. An MRI patient can receive glucagon, respond to an emergency contrast media response, and then undergo a high-risk interventional surgery by transfusing blood into a bleeding patient in one visit. It is important for nurses to be flexible and comfortable with changing routines in this environment [13, 14].

12.4.2 What Are the Radiology Nursing Safety Concerns?

Radiology can be a high-risk specialty, with patients suffering from stable to severe illnesses. There are many factors that can cause patients to get sick quickly, including falls, pressure injuries, radiation overexposure, and infections. Physio-psycho-social changes are meticulously monitored and managed by radiation nurses. Despite the fact that radiology nurses only care for patients for a brief time, they are strong advocates for patient safety. The patient typically receives nursing care before entering the department of radiology. Inpatients and outpatients may be treated together or exclusively as outpatients, depending on the context. Radiology nurses call outpatients a few days before the procedure and establish rapport. Screening is conducted during the call (such as checking for allergies and reviewing current medications), as well as instructions (about Nil Per oral (NPO) requirements and what to expect the day of the procedure). In order to meet patients' needs, radiology nurses communicate regularly with radiologists and other care team members [15].

12.4.3 Before the Procedure

Radiology nurses complete pre-procedure checklists and evaluate assessment data. When necessary, he or she consults with a pharmacist to ensure that medication is used safely.

12.4.4 During the Procedure

Radiology nurses closely monitor patients, provide comfort, and administer medications as prescribed.

12.4.5 Following the Procedure

The patient will be moved to a para-anesthesia care unit (PACU), inpatient unit, or intra-departmental recovery area. Upon release, the radiology nurse contacts the patient to assess any post-procedure issues and reinforce all training. Pre-screenings and other care needs are communicated primarily between radiology nurses and the patient's bedside nurses in the periprocedural process, which is the same for outpatients. Radiology nurses confirm with bedside nurses that pre-procedural checklists and orders have been completed before transferring to radiology.

Radiology nurses are also expected to respond to emergencies and adverse events as part of their quality and safety monitoring and performance improvement duties.

12.4.6 Nursing Efficiency

Radiology nurses coordinate care. In addition to coordinating radiology care, they assist inpatient units, pharmacies, PACUs, anesthesia, and infection prevention. To provide the best possible treatment for patients, they urge team members to collaborate and contribute. Additionally, they reduce waiting time and prevent unnecessary delays by improving throughput.

Nurses in radiology are often faced with operational flow issues such as double-ups, no-shows, and walk-in patients. In addition to providing direct patient care, radiology nurses also handle non-direct care tasks, such as problem solving, phone calls, setup, and clean-up. Patient contacts are usually not measured in terms of productivity because they are episodic. Nurses are responsible for continuously triaging and prioritizing patient care, taking into account urgent or emergent cases as well as changes in patient status [16, 17].

12.4.7 How Do Radiology Nurses Create an Impact on Patient Care?

Radiology nurses play a pivotal role in patient care since they provide specialized care to patients undergoing radiological procedures. They contribute to the safety and well-being of patients before, during, and after imaging procedures. Radiology nurses contribute to patient care in a variety of ways, including:

1. **Patient Education:** Radiology nurses advise patients on what kind of procedure they will have, what to anticipate, and how to get ready. They assist in reducing patients' fear and encourage collaboration and understanding by educating them.
2. **Patient Monitoring:** To guarantee patients' comfort and safety throughout imaging examinations, radiology nurses keep a constant eye on their well-being. Vital signs are evaluated, complications or negative reactions are monitored, and necessary action is taken.
3. **Delivering Medicine and IV Fluids:** To keep patients comfortable and guarantee the accuracy of the test results, radiology nurses may give medication or IV fluids as needed during imaging procedures.
4. **Offering Emotional Support:** Radiology nurses frequently assist patients who are apprehensive or uneasy about having imaging tests done. To put patients at ease, they offer emotional support, assurance, and encouragement.
5. **Acting as an Advocate for Patients:** Radiology nurses represent patients' interests by making sure that their wants and worries are met and that they get the best treatment available.

All things considered, radiology nurses are essential to guaranteeing the security, comfort, and well-being of patients having radiological treatments. Their knowledge and specialized treatment improve the patient experience as a whole and lead to successful results.

12.4.8 What Education and Training Do Radiology Nursing Staff Require?

Registered nurses (RNs) perform general nursing duties in a hospital setting. However, to specialize in another field (like radiology), further studies are necessary. Nurses who are interested in a more specialized career can benefit from postgraduate Nurse Practitioner (NP) to Registered Nurse (RN) programs. To specialize as a radiology nurse, it is necessary to follow a study program that teaches the necessary technical skills to assist with radiology procedures.

Radiology nurses begin their careers with an associate's degree in nursing and an RN licensure. Due to the complexity and variety of acuity of their patients, nurses are typically required to possess basic and advanced cardiac life support certifications.

The majority of radiology nurses come from the ICU, ED, or post-acute care unit. Even seasoned nurses who are professionals in their former specialization can find the environment difficult to adjust to at first in radiology. The learning curve is influenced by several factors, including multiple modalities, procedures, a mix of skills, and autonomy. However, once nurses have adjusted, they rarely wish to quit this specialization [17, 18].

12.4.9 Dealing with Acute Situations: Nursing Angle

In a variety of healthcare settings, acute circumstances may emerge. Nursing personnel are prepared to address these scenarios. In an emergency, nurses need to maintain composure, make prompt decisions, and put the patient's needs first. Acute conditions that nurses frequently deal with include severe allergic responses, respiratory distress, cardiac arrest, and traumatic traumas. In these circumstances, nurses have to move quickly to stabilize the patient, administer interventions that could save their lives, and efficiently communicate with members of the healthcare team. In addition, radiology nurses need to be ready to support patients and their families emotionally, successfully manage pain, and speak up for patients' rights to the right care. They also need to be able to spot indicators that a patient's condition is getting worse or deteriorating and know when to increase care. Nurses need to collaborate with other healthcare workers, stay calm under pressure, and maintain current training and certifications in order to handle acute circumstances effectively. In emergency situations, nurses may assist in guaranteeing the best possible results for their patients by being proactive and well-prepared [19].

12.5 Infection Control and Sterilization Techniques

Infection control is the process of developing policies and procedures to manage and minimize the transmission of illnesses within hospitals and other healthcare settings, with the primary goal of lowering infection rates. The basic purpose of an infection control program is to prevent and contain the spread of infections. Depending on the microorganism in question, specific precautions must be taken. Examples of indications for transmission-based precautions are as follows:

- **Standard Precautions:** These practices apply to all patient care situations, including hand hygiene, personal protective equipment (PPE) use, patient placement, equipment cleaning and disinfection, laundry management, injection safety, and sharp object disposal.
- **Contact Precautions:** Used for patients with suspected or confirmed infections that can spread through contact. In addition to basic precautions, measures such as restricting patient movement, using disposable patient care equipment, and carrying out rigorous cleaning and disinfection procedures are essential. Patients with acute infectious diarrhea (e.g., *Clostridium difficile*), vesicular rash, respiratory tract infections caused by multidrug-resistant organisms, or exposed abscesses or draining wounds should adopt contact precautions.
- **Droplet Precautions:** Applied to individuals with suspected or actual infections that can be spread by respiratory droplets. This includes applying a mask to the patient and using basic precautions, as well as limiting patient movement. Patients with respiratory tract infections in infants and young children, petechial or ecchymotic rashes with fever, or meningitis are subjected to droplet precautions.
- **Airborne Precautions:** Used for patients with confirmed or suspected airborne illnesses. These patients must be segregated in an airborne infection isolation room and given all of the previously indicated safeguards. Tuberculosis, measles, chickenpox, and disseminated herpes zoster are some infections that require airborne protection. Patients with suspected diseases, such as vesicular rashes, cough/fever with lung infiltration, or maculopapular rashes with cough/coryza/fever, require airborne protection.

Several indications may necessitate a mix of precautions to achieve efficient infection management. For example, individuals suspected of having *Clostridium difficile* must take both contact and standard precautions, whereas those with tuberculosis must take airborne, contact, and standard precautions. Healthcare facilities must have the resources to follow standard safeguards for all patients. Hand hygiene is critical to reducing illness transmission, which can be accomplished by washing your hands with soap and warm water or by using alcohol-based hand sanitizers. Standard precautions include changing gloves for each patient and disposing of them after each interaction. Infection control equipment also comprises housekeeping tools for routine sanitation and disinfection of medical equipment, surfaces, and flooring.

12.5.1 The Below-Mentioned Measures Should Be Implemented in Healthcare Facilities to Ensure an Effective Infection Control Program, and the Radiology Nursing Staff Should Take a Lead Role

- Surveillance involves tracking infection rates and trends in high-risk settings such as ICUs and surgery units.
- Isolation involves separating contaminated individuals to prevent the spread of microbes to others.
- Identifying and managing epidemics using surveillance systems. To prevent the spread of illness, infected patients should be isolated when needed, and appropriate contact precautions should be implemented.
- Education: Seminars and workshops help healthcare providers understand how to avoid infectious disease transmission.

- Employee Health: Working closely with employee health services to ensure staff well-being and infection prevention. This includes limiting exposure to blood-borne and other infectious diseases. New personnel should typically be screened to ensure that they are immunized and resistant to common communicable diseases. Encourage annual influenza vaccinations, as well as implement proactive campaigns and policies to engage personnel in infection prevention.
- Sterilizing and cleaning medical and surgical tools are critical for preventing the spread of infectious pathogens to patients. Healthcare rules should specify whether cleaning, disinfection, or sterilization is required for specific products based on their intended purpose.

Sterilization is the process of destroying all microorganisms in healthcare settings through physical or chemical means. In healthcare settings, steam under pressure, dry heat, hydrogen peroxide gas, and liquid chemicals are commonly used to sterilize. Disinfection is a method that removes a major portion or all of pathogenic germs from inanimate items, excluding bacterial spores. In hospital settings, liquid chemicals or wet pasteurization are frequently utilized for disinfection. The disinfection process can, however, be negatively impacted by a number of factors. It is important to consider several factors when performing disinfection and sterilization, such as the cleanliness of the object before disinfection, the proportion of organic and inorganic materials, the kind and magnitude of contamination by microorganisms, concentrations and lengths of exposure, physical characteristics (such as crevices, hinges, and lumens), biofilms, temperatures and pH levels during disinfection, and humidity levels.

Depending on how an item will be used, a different level of disinfection or sterilization is required: surgical instruments placed on sterile tissue, endoscopes placed on mucous membranes, and stethoscopes placed on intact skin all require different levels of sterilization, high-level disinfection, and low-level disinfection. To do high-level disinfection and sterilization, it is necessary to clean the area first. It is important for users to weigh the benefits and drawbacks of several methods of disinfection or sterilization before choosing one. Healthcare facilities can reduce the risk of infection by following these guidelines, improving disinfection and sterilization methods [20–22].

Sterilization techniques and the commonly used applications

Technique	Example	Target microorganism	Application
High temperature	Steam, dry heat	All forms of microbes (vegetative and spore)	Heat-tolerant surgical instruments Semicritical patient care items
Low temperature	Ethylene oxide gas, hydrogen peroxide, ozone gas, plasma gaseous chlorine dioxide	Gram-positive and -negative bacteria, mycobacteria, lipid-enveloped viruses	Heat-sensitive critical items. Semiradial patient care items
Liquid chemicals	Chemical sterilant	Prions (resistant to any form of sterilization)	Heat-sensitive critical items Semicritical patient care items (that can be immersed)

Disinfection techniques and the commonly used applications

Technique	Example	Target microorganism	Application
Heat	Pasteurization	All vegetative forms of microorganisms	Respiratory therapy equipment
Chemicals	Chemical sterilant	Gram-positive and -negative bacteria, mycobacteria, lipid-enveloped viruses	GI endoscopes, bronchoscopes
Intermediate level disinfectant	Chlorine-based products, phenolics	Gram-positive and -negative bacteria, enveloped and non-enveloped viruses, mycobacteria	Soiled noncritical items Surfaces contaminated with blood Devices contaminated with body fluids
Low-level disinfectant	Chlorine-based products, phenolics, quaternary ammonium compounds, 70–90% alcohol	Vegetative forms of bacteria, lipophilic viruses, and some fungi	Noncritical patient care items

12.6 Nursing Care and Role in Emergency Medications in Case of Contrast Reaction: Nursing Responsibilities for CT Scan

Nursing care is critical during CT treatments to ensure patient safety, comfort, and the best possible imaging results. Here are several important components of nursing care during CT treatments.

1. **Pre-Procedure Preparation:**
   - Determine whether the patient has allergies or any contraindications to contrast media, as well as his or her medical history.
   - Provide the patient with information about the procedure, including its purpose, potential risks, and what to expect during the procedure.
   - Ensure that the patient is appropriately dressed and remove any metallic objects or clothing that may interfere with imaging.
2. **Patient Positioning:**
   - Assist the patient in assuming the required position for the CT scan, which may involve lying flat on the CT table.
   - Provide support and padding to ensure the patient's comfort and maintain proper alignment.
3. **Administration of Contrast Media:**
   - If contrast-enhanced CT is planned, verify the patient's renal function and assess for allergies to iodinated contrast media.
   - Start an intravenous (IV) line for contrast administration, following hospital protocols for IV access and contrast injection.
   - Monitor for signs of contrast reactions, such as itching, flushing, or difficulty breathing, and be prepared to intervene promptly if needed.
4. **Communication and Reassurance:**
   - Explain each step to the patient and provide reassurance as necessary during the procedure.
   - Teach the patient how important it is to remain still during the scan so that clear images can be obtained.
   - Answer questions or concerns the patient may have, and provide support throughout the process.
5. **Monitoring:**
   - The heart rate, blood pressure, breathing rate, and oxygen saturation should all be monitored before, during, and after the CT scan.
   - Stay vigilant for any signs of distress or adverse reactions, such as contrast-induced nephropathy or anaphylaxis, and intervene promptly as necessary.

6. **Post-Procedure Care:**
   - After the CT scan, assist the patient in getting up from the table and provide any necessary support for ambulation.
   - Monitor the patient for any delayed reactions or complications following contrast administration.
   - Document the procedure, including any contrast used, patient responses, and any adverse events, in the medical record.

Overall, nursing care during CT procedures involves thorough assessment, preparation, support, monitoring, and communication to ensure the safety and well-being of the patient throughout the imaging process. When it comes to CT scans, it is essential to collaborate with other members of the healthcare team, including radiologists and technologists.

In the event of a contrast reaction, nurses are essential in administering emergency treatment. Prompt management is crucial to prevent further complications, as contrast reactions can range in severity from mild to severe. First and foremost, nurses need to be aware of the warning signs and symptoms of contrast reactions, which can include fever, hives, itching, breathing difficulties, and variations in heart rate and blood pressure. Emergency drugs such as bronchodilators, corticosteroids, and antihistamines that may be used to treat these responses should also be known to radiology nurses. Nurses should evaluate the patient's vital signs and symptoms as soon as possible and alert the healthcare practitioner right away if a contrast response occurs.

In addition to monitoring the patient's response to therapy, recording the events leading up to, during, and following the reaction, the nurse may be in charge of giving emergency drugs as directed by the physician. Furthermore, during this trying time, nurses ought to comfort and reassure the patient and their family. It is critical for nurses to collaborate well with the medical staff and make sure that patients receive the right treatment when they need it. All things considered, nurses are essential in managing contrast responses and must be ready to act swiftly and decisively to guarantee the patient's best course of care [23].

12.6.1 Nursing Care During Computed Tomographic Procedures Using Contrast Media: Prevention, Detection, and Treatment of Effects Caused by Iodinated Contrast

The nursing team involved in CT services has an essential role in preventing, detecting, and treating the harmful consequences of iodinated contrast use. Nursing in radiology investigates the presence of risk factors for these reactions, establishes venous access, and administers contrast agents. Furthermore, radiology nurses recognize indicators of systemic or local adverse reactions and provide the appropriate treatment for each instance. As a result, monitoring adverse events resulting from CT is a tool for assessing care delivery in radiology as well as an important indicator of care quality.

Contrast media extravasation is an unexpected effect of intravenous contrast media injection that happens in individuals undergoing CT. Its effects vary from mild to severe. It may cause excessive muscular pressure, leading to cell death and ischemia in the affected area. Nurses play a key role in assessing, preventing, and providing nursing care when contrast media extravasation occurs. As a result, when this adverse event occurs, nurses must have the information, skills, experience, and ability to ensure patient safety and reduce the degree of complications.

The responsibilities of a radiology nurse include taking the history, obtaining informed consent, preparing them, providing education, and monitoring the process. Professional nurses should understand the nursing practices and principles that underlie CT in order to ensure its safety and accuracy [24–26]. An individual undergoing CT will require the following nursing interventions and considerations:

12.6.2 Nursing Intervention Before the Procedure

The nursing interventions before CT are as follows:

- Obtain a signed informed consent form.
- Check for allergies: Before using contrast media, ensure that you have no past allergies to iodinated dyes or shellfish.
- Inquire about the patient's health history, including recent illnesses, medical conditions, and current medications. The use of oral or intravenous contrast material is determined by the type of CT scan.
- Check the patient's NPO status and advise them not to eat or drink, especially for contrast-enhanced studies.
- Instruct patients to dress comfortably and loosely for the exam.
- Informing the patient about the contrast media: Instruct the patient that they will feel a slight flush after the needle is punctured, and a minor pain will occur after an intravenous contrast medium is injected.
- When the patient is being examined, ask him or her to remain quiet and report any symptoms, including itching, difficulty breathing or swallowing, nausea, vomiting, dizziness, or headaches.
- Explain the duration of the procedure, which may range from 5 to 20 min depending on the type of scan and the patient's ability to relax.

12.6.3 Nursing Intervention After the Procedure

Post-procedure nursing interventions that the radiology nurse should be aware of after a CT scan include:

- Resume normal diet and activities, unless told differently.
- Advise patients to consume additional fluids (if given a contrast). This increases dye excretion.
- Nurses should inform medical teams of the risk factor.
- Observe the patients receiving intravenous contrast depending on the procedure and their clinical condition.
- After administering contrast media, leave the intravenous cannula in place and observe the patient for at least 15 min.
- Patients with a higher risk of anaphylaxis should have a 30-min interval.

12.6.4 Nursing: Intravenous Contrast Checklist

- Ensure that the patient has an appropriate gauge intravenous cannula for the injection rate of the contrast media:
- 22 g or larger for injections 3 mL/second
- 20 g or larger for injections 5 mL/second
- 18 g or larger for injections 6–7 mL/second
- Ensure that large veins are used, preferably Cubital Fossa, backs of hands should be avoided.
- Ensure that all cannulas are flushed and patent prior to injection.

12.6.5 Storage, Preparation, and Documentation of Contrast Media

Iodinated contrast media should be stored at room temperature, away from direct sunlight. Before using, iodinated contrast medium should be stored at 30–37 °C. Injection pressure and viscosity of the media are reduced as a result. The iodinated contrast media is dated using a date inserted in the warmer. Over 30-day-old iodinated contrast media should be discarded.

Aseptic preparation of iodinated contrast medium is important. Upon opening an iodinated contrast material, it must be thrown away within 24 h. Each contrast bottle's batch number and expiration date should be recorded in the patient's clinical record and any relevant clinical information system. In the patient's notes, the prescription chart/contrast order form, and the clinical area's relevant information system, the contrast and volume utilized should be noted.

12.7 Nursing Care in Bedside Radiography

Providing care to patients who require mobile radiography is a crucial role for radiology nurses. Whenever a patient cannot be transported to the radiology department due to their medical condition, mobile radiography is requested. It is important that nurses, doctors, and radiographers who participate in mobile radiography are aware of this subject. Modern practice is characterized by the evaluation and referral of patients for limited radiological studies by nurse consultants and advanced practitioners [27].

Imaging patients outside of a radiology department is done with mobile X-ray equipment. Originally designed so that they could be disassembled and assembled at the patient's bedside, portable X-rays are commonly referred to as portable imaging studies. The power output of portable X-ray systems was limited, the radiation doses were excessive, and the quality of the images was poor. Due to these reasons, portable X-ray machines are no longer used in medicine. Despite this, mobile radiography is often referred to as "portable X-rays" among health professionals [28].

Most hospitals have mobile X-ray systems available for patients whose care could be compromised by moving to the radiology department. Thus, mobile radiography should only be used by patients who cannot be transferred to a radiology department without risking their health. There are a number of places where these patients can be treated, including ICUs, coronary care units, cardiac surgery units, and resuscitation units in EDs (recovery rooms).

In hospital wards or other hospital settings, mobile radiography may also be used on unstable patients, but it should be limited due to radiation protection guidelines. While normal wards are not designed this way, special care units typically have lead walls or concrete walls to shield ionizing radiation. Mobile X-ray devices are commonly used in hospitals to perform chest X-rays. It is possible to perform other radiological exams with a portable X-ray unit, but there are limitations, such as low-quality images and radiation shielding. Most portable X-ray machines are used to examine tracheostomies, nasogastric tubes, central lines, central venous catheters, and trauma injuries in patients who require special care [29, 30].

Mobile radiography involves three types of health professionals: advocating doctors, radiographers, and nurses. It is important to discuss the patient's requirements with the referring doctor before requesting a portable X-ray from the radiology department. During an imaging examination, the radiographer communicates with the nurse(s) and positions and immobilizes the patient. In order to undertake this position, radiographers are trained, and educational materials are provided from their perspective. It is, however, imperative to provide educational literature on this topic for radiology nurses and to recognize the subspecialty of nursing in radiology [31].

12.7.1 A Workflow Relationship: Between Referring Medical Doctor, Medical Imaging Technologist, and Radiology Nurse

The referring doctor, the radiographer, and the nurse involved in mobile radiography must work together to obtain high-quality diagnostic images. X-ray requests for mobile X-rays should be submitted electronically via the radiology information system. When an urgent situation necessitates an X-ray, radiology departments should be notified by phone, bleep systems, or by mail. When a radiographer arrives on a ward or unit, he or she should establish rapport with the nurses and inquire about the patient's condition. The radiographer should consult with the nurse before moving or disturbing the patient. The nurse is aware of the patient's condition and needs in this case. Elevating the patient is necessary for nurses and support personnel to place the X-ray plate or detector and communicate with the patient.

When the X-rays are available on the PACS system or in hard copies after the imaging examination, nurses and referring doctors should be informed. Radiographers need a written request before performing digital radiography and processing CR plates for analog imaging. A lack of understanding of the processing may lead physicians to request an imaging examination before they submit a written request.

12.7.2 Control During Mobile Radiography

Infection control is crucial to the management of all patients, especially those in special care units. It is the nurses' responsibility to communicate any infection control measures to the radiographers and to ensure that all control measures are implemented to prevent contamination during mobile radiography. Infections can spread from transportable X-ray equipment, Computed Radiography (CR) plates, or digital detectors, as well as lead aprons. Therefore, the nurse is responsible for ensuring that all workers who interact with the patient follow the local infection control protocol.

Dedicated mobile X-ray machines should be kept on site in special care units. Alternatively, mobile X-ray equipment should be cleaned with antiseptic solution before moving to an infection-control area. The World Health Organization recommends that each staff member follow the "Five seconds of hand hygiene." A nurse or radiographer is reminded to practice hand hygiene when interacting with patients, performing cleaning/aseptic procedures, being exposed to body fluids or risks, touching a patient, and touching the surroundings of the patient as part of this infection control measure.

In order to prevent contamination from body fluids, the CR plate or digital detector should be covered with a suitable cover, such as plastic. Working with patients with highly contagious infections, such as COVID-19 and methicillin-resistant *Staphylococcus aureus*, requires PPE. After the imaging test, the PPE should be properly removed and disposed of. Lead aprons and mobile X-ray equipment should also be disinfected [32, 33].

12.8 Nursing Care, Preparation, and Examinations in Gastrointestinal Studies

When it comes to gastrointestinal (GIT) procedures within radiology, nursing care is pivotal in ensuring patient comfort, safety, and success of the procedure. Below are key considerations for nursing care during GIT procedures in a radiology setting:

1. **Pre-Procedure Preparation:**
   - Review the medical history, including allergies, previous surgeries, and current medications.
   - Verify the procedure to be performed and ensure that informed consent is obtained.
   - Educate the patient about the procedure, including preparation instructions (such as fasting or bowel cleansing), its purpose, potential risks, and what to expect during and after the procedure.
2. **Patient Positioning and Comfort:**
   - Assist the patient in assuming the required position for the procedure, whether it involves lying on an imaging table, sitting, or standing.
   - Provide support and positioning aids to ensure the patient's comfort throughout the procedure.
3. **Administration of Medications and Contrast Media:**
   - Administer medications as prescribed, such as sedatives or analgesics, to help alleviate anxiety and discomfort during the procedure.
   - Prepare and administer any contrast media required for the imaging study, following hospital protocols and verifying the patient's renal function and allergies.
4. **Monitoring and Assessment:**
   - Monitor the patient's vital signs before, during, and after the procedure.
   - In case of allergic reactions or contrast-induced nephropathy, assess the patient and intervene immediately if the symptoms persist.

5. **Collaboration With the Radiology Team:**
   - To ensure the smooth execution of the procedure, work closely with radiologists, radiologic technologists, and other healthcare providers.
   - Assist the radiologist as needed during image acquisition, such as by providing positioning assistance or helping with patient immobilization.
6. **Patient Education and Post-Procedure Care:**
   - Inform the patient of any dietary or activity restrictions and side effects to watch for after the procedure.
   - Assess the patient for immediate post-procedure complications, such as bleeding, perforation, or allergic reactions, and initiate appropriate interventions as required.
   - Document the procedure, including medications administered, patient responses, and any adverse events, in the medical record.

Throughout the GIT procedure, effective communication with the patient, collaboration with the radiology team, and vigilant monitoring are essential components of nursing care to ensure a safe and successful outcome for the patient.

GIT examinations include a variety of diagnostic methods designed to visualize the digestive tract and identify different disorders, including ulcers, tumors, and inflammatory bowel disease. As an essential element of the healthcare team, the radiology nurse has a critical responsibility in assuring patient comfort, safety, and adherence to the examination procedure. This position requires providing thorough nursing care, precise preparation, and careful monitoring during the examination process [34].

#GIT Examination Types

A. **Upper GIT Series (UGI):** This involves using contrast media that is given orally or through a nasogastric tube to visualize the stomach, duodenum, and esophagus.

B. **Barium Swallow (Esophageal):** This procedure looks for abnormalities in the esophagus, like tumors or strictures.

C. **Small Bowel Series:** Screens for malabsorption disorders and Crohn's disease in the small intestine.

D. **Barium Enema (Lower GI Series):** Screens for tumors, inflammatory diseases, and polyps in the colon and rectum.

E. **Colonoscopy and Sigmoidoscopy:** A flexible scope is used to directly visualize the colon and rectum to detect colorectal cancer, polyps, or inflammatory bowel disease.

12.8.1 Nursing Care and Preparation: Before the Examination

- **Patient Education:** Radiology nurses explain to patients the purpose and duration of their procedure, as well as potential discomfort.
- **Preparation Instructions:** Provides clear instructions regarding dietary restrictions, bowel preparation (such as laxatives or enemas), and medication adjustments as per the physician's orders.
- **Assessment and Consent:** Performs a thorough medical history assessment, checks for allergies, and determines the patient's current medication. Obtains informed consent for the procedure.

12.8.2 Nursing Care and Preparation: During the Examination

- **Patient Positioning:** Assists the patient into the required positions for optimal imaging, ensuring comfort and safety.
- **Administration of Contrast Media:** Collaborates with the radiologist in administering oral or rectal contrast agents, monitoring for any adverse reactions such as allergic responses or aspiration.
- **Patient Monitoring:** Monitors vital signs, patient comfort, and response throughout the procedure, promptly addressing any concerns or complications.

12.8.3 Nursing Care and Preparation: After the Examination

- **Post-Procedure Care:** Provides post-procedural care, including monitoring for delayed reactions to contrast media, ensuring adequate hydration, and assisting with post-procedure ambulation.
- **Patient Education:** Offers guidance on resuming normal activities, dietary considerations, and any follow-up appointments or tests as recommended by the healthcare provider.

The radiology nurse serves as a patient advocate, educator, and coordinator throughout the GIT examination process. They should collaborate closely with the interdisciplinary team, including radiologists, gastroenterologists, and imaging technologists, to ensure the seamless delivery of care and the attainment of optimal imaging outcomes while prioritizing patient safety and comfort [35–38].

12.9 Nursing Care During Radiological Special Procedures Using Fluoroscopy

Fluoroscopy, a radiological technique, is crucial for the diagnosis and treatment of various conditions, such as vascular disorders, GIT abnormalities, and IR procedures. The radiology nurse has a vital responsibility in ensuring the safety and comfort of patients, as well as facilitating effective collaboration among the multidisciplinary team. Radiological special procedures that utilize fluoroscopy include angiography, which shows blood vessels in order to identify diseases such as vascular malformations, aneurysms, and blockages in the arteries.

During radiological special procedures utilizing fluoroscopy, nursing care is crucial to ensure patient safety, comfort, and effective procedural outcomes. Here is a detailed outline of nursing responsibilities throughout the process:

1. **Pre-Procedure Preparation:**
   - Ensure that the patient understands the procedure to be performed.
   - Confirm informed consent and answer any questions the patient may have.
   - Assess the patient's medical history, current medications, any past adverse reactions to anesthesia, or contrast media.
   - Provide clear instructions on fasting, medication adjustments, and any necessary bowel preparation for the procedure.
   - Ensure that appropriate pre-procedural tests, such as laboratory work or imaging studies, have been completed.
2. **Patient Assessment and Monitoring:**
   - Assess the patient's vital signs such as blood pressure, heart rate, and respiratory rate before, during, and after the procedure.
   - Monitor the patient's level of consciousness, pain, and overall comfort throughout the procedure.
   - Continuously monitor for signs of complications, such as allergic reactions to contrast media, respiratory distress, or hemodynamic instability.
3. **Administration of Medications and Contrast Media:**
   - Administer pre-procedural medications as prescribed, such as sedatives or anxiolytics, to reduce anxiety and promote relaxation.
   - Prepare and administer contrast media as directed by the radiologist, ensuring accurate dosage calculation and appropriate timing of administration.
   - Ensure that the patient is not experiencing any adverse reactions to medications or contrast media, such as allergic reactions, and intervene as quickly as possible if necessary.
4. **Radiation Safety:**
   - Ensure that the patient and all personnel in the fluoroscopy suite are appropriately shielded from radiation using lead aprons, thyroid shield, and lead glass.
   - Follow radiation safety protocols, including minimizing fluoroscopy time and keep-

ing the radiation source as far from the patient as possible while maintaining image quality.
   - Use fluoroscopy pulse modes or low-dose protocols whenever feasible to reduce radiation exposure to both patients and staff.
5. **Communication and Collaboration:**
   - Communicate openly throughout the procedure with the radiologist, radiologic technologist, and other members of the healthcare team.
   - Collaborate closely with the radiologist to ensure optimal imaging quality and accurate interpretation of fluoroscopic images.
   - Provide clear and concise instructions to the patient during the procedure, explaining each step and offering reassurance as needed.
6. **Post-Procedure Care:**
   - Monitor the patient closely in the immediate post-procedural period for any signs of complications, such as bleeding, hematoma formation, or respiratory distress.
   - The nurse should inform the patient about any restrictions on activities, any dietary considerations, and any potential complications that should be addressed immediately after surgery.
   - Document the procedure, including medication administration, patient responses, any adverse events, and post-procedural care provided, in the patient's medical record.

By adhering to these guidelines and providing attentive nursing care, healthcare providers can contribute to the safe and successful completion of radiological special procedures using fluoroscopy while promoting positive patient outcomes and experiences. Below are the different types of radiological procedures performed under fluoroscopy:

A. **GIT Fluoroscopy:** This diagnostic technique examines the anatomy and function of the digestive tract, encompassing barium enemas, esophagrams, and swallowing studies.
B. **Procedures in IR:** These encompass a broad spectrum of minimally invasive treatments, including biopsies, catheter-based interventions, and central line implantations.
C. **Fluoroscopically-Guided Pain Management:** This type of pain management uses fluoroscopic guidance to administer therapeutic injections or nerve blocks.

Nursing Care During Radiological Special Procedures:

12.9.1 Nursing Care: Pre-procedure Preparation

Patient Assessment: The radiology nurse performs an accurate assessment to detect any contraindications, allergies, or possible risks linked to the procedure.

Patient Education: Offers comprehensive information regarding the procedure, including its purposes, possible risks, and expected outcomes. Addresses all questions or concerns that the patient may have.

Obtain Consent: Following a thorough explanation of the procedure and its associated risks to the patient or their legal representative, ensure that they provide their informed consent.

12.9.2 Nursing Care and Preparation: During the Procedure

Patient Positioning: Assists in positioning the patient on the fluoroscopy table, ensuring correct alignment for accurate imaging and procedural access.

Radiation Safety: Implements radiation safety protocols to protect both patients and healthcare workers, such as utilizing lead aprons, thyroid shields, and radiation monitoring devices.

Medication Administration: Administers prescribed medications, such as sedatives or analgesics, to enhance patient comfort and cooperation during the procedure.

Collaboration: Participating in close cooperation with the radiologist and imaging technologist team members to assist in the preparation of equipment, administration of contrast agents, and guidance during procedures using fluoroscopy.

12.9.3 Nursing Care and Preparation: Aftercare

Monitoring: The radiology nurse monitors the patient's vital signs, neurological condition, and intervention site for any possible signs of complications, such as hemorrhaging or allergic responses.

Patient Comfort: Provides comfort measures, reassurance, and emotional support to the patient post-procedure.

Discharge Instructions: Provides instructions for post-hospitalization care, including limitations on physical activity, proper wound treatment, and effective medication administration. Addresses any potential issues or symptoms that may arise after the procedure.

Radiology nurses serve as a vital link between the patient, the healthcare team, and the procedural environment during radiological procedures involving fluoroscopy. They promote patient safety, facilitate efficient communication, and ensure compliance with nursing care and procedural protocols [39–41].

12.10 Nursing Care During Mammography

In medical imaging, mammography is used to detect and diagnose breast disorders, such as breast cancer. Mammography consists of two different types: analog (film-screen) and digital. Certain conditions may also require sophisticated or specialized mammography techniques. There are several types and advancements in mammography.

1. **Conventional (Film-Screen) Mammography**

   The traditional mammography procedure captured and recorded images using X-ray film and a cassette. Advantages include being cost-effective, widely available, and in use for many years after its invention. Disadvantages include lower image contrast than digital mammography, longer processing periods, and the requirement for chemical processing.
2. **Full-Field Digital Mammography** (FFDM), or digital mammography, works similarly to screen-film mammography (SFM). Digital signals are used in FFDM instead of traditional X-ray films, as in SFM. A computer monitor or special films are used to view images of the breast. The advantages of this technology include improving image quality, enhancing images for better viewing, storing and retrieving digital data more quickly, and using artificial intelligence to reduce radiation doses. The disadvantages include a higher starting cost than analog mammography.
3. **3D mammography (Digital Breast Tomosynthesis):**

   This imaging technique obtains several X-ray images of the breast from various angles to reconstruct three-dimensional images. Advantages include improved identification of breast cancer, particularly in dense breast tissue, and fewer false positives. Disadvantages include higher radiation exposure than regular 2D mammography.
4. **Contrast-Enhanced Mammography:**

   A contrast agent is injected prior to mammography to improve the visibility of blood vessels and breast abnormalities. The advantages are improved lesion detection, particularly in women with dense breast tissue. The cons are limited availability and increasing cost.
5. **Positron Emission Mammography (PEM):**

   A radioactive tracer is injected, and a PET scanner is used to image the breasts. The advantages include high-resolution imaging and early diagnosis of tiny lesions. The disadvantages include limited availability, increased cost, and increased radiation.

6. **Computer-Assisted Detection System**

   The technology scans mammography images for abnormal areas, such as density, abnormal size, or calcifications, which may suggest cancer. A radiologist will further examine abnormal spots after "marking" them. Patients' specific circumstances, breast density, and healthcare providers' preferences all play a role in the choice of mammography technique. Technological advancements continue to change mammography, which is being studied in order to increase early detection and limit radiation exposure.

12.10.1 Mammography Indications

- The mammogram can also be used to find out if a patient is suffering from breast pain, nipple retraction, or discharge.
- Examine palpable and unpalpable lumps in the breast.
- Check for malignant tumors.
- Monitor the effectiveness of radiation therapy.
- Evaluate the opposite breast post-mastectomy.

12.10.2 Contraindications

- Women who are pregnant should not undergo radiation procedures unless the benefits far outweigh the risks.
- Patients younger than 25 years or with dense breast tissue.

12.10.3 Compounding Factors

Several factors can affect the study outcome, including the use of antiperspirants (deodorants), talcum powder, lotions, or creams underarms and breasts, the failure to remove metallic objects and clothing, previous breast surgery, active lactation, glandular breasts (common in women under 30 years), and placement of implants. Before mammography procedures, nursing staff play a pivotal role in educating the patients [42].

12.10.4 Nursing Responsibility During Mammography

Prior to mammography, the following nursing interventions are needed:

- Explain what will happen after the technique. The patient should be informed where and who will perform the test. It may be necessary to ask the patient to wait while the films are examined to ensure they are readable, despite the fact that the test only takes around 15 min. It is important to let her know that false positives are common.
- Encourage patients to express their fears and concerns about the surgery. Answer any questions the patient may have and clarify any misconceptions they may have about the operation.
- Eliminate the interfering elements. Do not allow the patient to use deodorant or powder under his or her arms before the examination.
- Assign a senior technician to a patient with breast implants. Instruct the patient to notify the staff if he or she has breast implants so that a technologist familiar with imaging implants can be available.

Prepare the patient. Just before the test, the patient should be given a gown that opens in the front and instructed to remove all jewelry and clothing above the waist.

12.10.5 Nursing Responsibility During Mammography: During the Procedure

During mammography, the nurse intervenes with the imaging technologist as follows:

- Assist in positioning the patient. An X-ray machine should be adjusted to the breast level when the patient is standing or sitting. Make

sure that the patient's arms are out of the imaging area.
- Inform the patient that some discomfort may be experienced because of breast compression, which may cause pain/discomfort.
- Ensure that the patient follows directions and cooperates completely. Instruct the patient to remain still throughout the procedure, as movement can produce unreliable results. Ask the patient to hold her breath during X-rays.

12.10.6 Nursing Responsibility During Mammography

Nurses should document the following nursing interventions after a procedure:

- Provide information about the availability of results.
- Provide a copy of the report to the patient, which will be discussed with the requesting physician.
- Confirm the physician's information.
- In the event of an abnormality, assist the patient in arranging additional testing, therapy, or referral to another healthcare provider [42–51].

12.10.7 Mammography: Normal and Abnormal Results

Normal findings in mammography will show:

- Normal breast tissue, with an absence of cysts, tumors, or calcification

Abnormalities in mammography will reveal:

- Abscesses or cysts
- Tumors
- Calcifications
- Hematoma resulting from trauma
- Mastitis
- Soft tissue masses
- Vascular calcification

12.11 Nursing Care During Biopsies and Fine-Needle Aspiration Studies: Fine-Needle Aspiration Cytology: The Nurse's Role

Fine Needle Aspiration Cytology (FNAC) is the aspiration of tissue cells from a tumor or visible lesion for diagnostic analysis. It is a straightforward, accurate, quick, and inexpensive treatment that provides an alternate diagnostic modality to surgery. The success of an FNAC procedure is heavily reliant on the team of clinicians who perform it. Nurses are an important and integral part of these teams.

FNAC uses a fine-bore needle (gauge 21–25), either individually or with a syringe. In the aforementioned scenario, a syringe holder is commonly used for stabilizing the syringe. The needle is inserted into the desired lesion, and many passes are made in different directions to optimize sampling. If a syringe is used, suction can be used to increase the cellular extraction. The entire procedure, including the preliminary review of the material, usually takes no more than 30 min. The patient experiences discomfort comparable to a venipuncture, especially with a superficial FNAC. Imaging modalities such as fluoroscopy, ultrasound, CT, and endoscopic procedures can detect small, deep, mobile lesions that would otherwise be difficult to detect or palpate. Because of the availability of various modalities, there are relatively few organs or bodily areas that an aspiration needle cannot easily access.

Biopsies are medical procedures that involve removing a small sample of tissue or cells from a patient's body and examining it under a microscope. In addition to diagnosing or evaluating cancer, infections, inflammatory disorders, and other abnormalities, biopsy is used to evaluate a variety of medical conditions [52]. Biopsies are classified into numerous varieties, and the procedure used is determined by the suspected ailment and the location of the abnormal tissue. Some frequent types of biopsies are as follows:

1. **Needle Biopsy:** Tissue or fluid can be retrieved with a thin, hollow needle. Fine-needle aspiration (FNA), core needle biopsy,

and vacuum-assisted biopsy are three types of needle biopsies.
2. **Surgical Biopsy:** A surgeon performs this type of biopsy by removing a larger amount of tissue during a minor surgical procedure. Surgical biopsies are commonly used when a larger sample is required or the tissue is located deep within the body.
3. **Endoscopic Biopsy:** The biopsy instrument is directed to the desired location with the help of an endoscope, a thin, flexible tube with a camera and light. This form of biopsy is commonly used to examine the GIT tract, respiratory system, or other internal organs.
4. **Skin Biopsy:** This entails removing a small portion of skin for examination. Skin biopsies are commonly used to identify skin problems, including dermatitis or skin cancer.

Following the biopsy, the obtained tissue is submitted to a pathology laboratory and examined by a pathologist. The biopsy results help define the nature of the tissue, whether malignant or non-cancerous, and provide critical information for developing a suitable treatment plan. There are a few risks or problems associated with biopsy operations.

12.11.1 Nurse's Role in FNAC and Biopsy

In FNAC, the radiology nurse assumes the lead role. The nurse is involved in the care of such patients throughout the entire process, from initial contact to discharge. Initially, the nurse's responsibilities included patient education, screening (for coagulation disorders), and informed consent. First, the nurse explains the procedure and addresses any questions the patient may have. FNAC of the liver or lung requires coagulation tests, like prothrombin time and active partial thromboplastin time, to be performed before surgery. Furthermore, the nurse inquires about any medications that may influence platelet function or coagulation, such as aspirin, warfarin, or clopidogrel. The presence of such medications is not always a contraindication to superficial FNAC, since this type of technique can be conducted without considerable risk of bleeding, even in patients taking anticoagulants. A complete list of the patient's medications is gathered by the radiology nurse.

Once these difficulties have been resolved, the nurse, together with the cytopathologist/imaging technologist or other engaged physician, asks the patient to sign a consent form. Following the interview, the nurse records clinical data in the patient's chart and prepares and manages the supplies that the team will require. In the case of radiographically guided FNAC, the nurse normally performs these activities, while the CT or ultrasound technologist locates the biopsy site. Once the procedure begins, the nurse should be in control of monitoring the patient. If conscious sedation is required, the nurse provides the proper medicines and supervises the patient in accordance with the hospital's standard of care protocols. Vital sign monitoring is required when a patient is sedated, but it is usually unnecessary in the majority of superficial FNAC procedures. Even without sedation, most patients are digitally monitored for blood pressure, electrocardiographic tracing, and oxygen saturation. The nurse also provides emotional support to the patient as needed when using the aspiration needle. The function of the nurse in specimen triage is to route the specimen and request any tests that the specialized provider deems essential.

The nurse next applies antibiotic ointment and an adhesive bandage to the puncture site while continuing to check for bleeding or swelling. If the FNAC technique involves a major organ or anesthesia is required, the patient must rest for at least 30 min. Similarly, the nurse is responsible for monitoring the patient's vital signs until release. Nurses give discharge instructions and answer any questions when patients are ready to go home. Nursing care during biopsies and FNA exams is essential for patient comfort, safety, and effective therapy. Here are some critical considerations for nursing care throughout these procedures [53–55].

12.11.2 Nursing Role: Before the Procedure

1. **Patient Education:**
   - Explain the purpose, procedure, and potential risks to the patient.
   - Provide information about necessary preparations, such as fasting or discontinuing specific drugs.
2. **Informed Consent**:
   - Ensure that the patient understands the entire procedure and provides informed consent.
3. **Pre-Procedure Assessment:**
   - Assess the patient's current medications and medical history.
   - Check vital signs to ensure that the patient is stable.
4. **Preparation of the Patient:**
   - Position the patient comfortably and emphasize the significance of remaining still throughout the treatment.
   - Use adequate drapery to protect privacy.

12.11.3 Nursing Role: During the Procedure

1. **Assistance to the Physician:**
   - Assist the physician or healthcare practitioner in situating the patient and locating the target location for biopsy or FNA.
2. **Monitoring:**
   - Monitor vital indicators throughout the treatment.
   - Observe the patient for any signs of discomfort or distress.
3. **Patient Comfort:**
   - Use local anesthetic as advised by your healthcare professional to alleviate pain and discomfort.
   - Offer emotional support and reassurance during the process.
4. **Infection Control:**
   - Use stringent aseptic methods to decrease the risk of infection.
   - Ensure that healthcare providers use sterile equipment and use proper protective gear.
5. **Documentation:**
   - Document the procedure, including patient replies, vital signs, and potential consequences.
   - Record biopsy details, including kind, location, and sample collection.

12.11.4 Nursing Role: After the Procedure

1. **Monitoring and Observation**
   - Monitor the patient for acute post-procedure problems, such as bleeding or infection.
   - Continue to monitor vital signs and record any changes.
2. **Pain Management:**
   - Provide pain relief as suggested by the healthcare provider.
3. **Patient Education:**
   - Provide post-procedure care instructions, including restrictions on activities and medications.
   - Inform patients about possible side effects and when to seek medical assistance.
4. **Follow-Up:**
   - Schedule any required follow-up visits for the patient.
   - Ensure that the patient understands the need to report any odd symptoms or complications.
5. **Emotional Support:**
   - Provide emotional support and address the patient's problems and anxieties.

Effective communication, attention to minutiae, and an emphasis on patients are critical aspects of nursing care during biopsies and FNA examinations. Always follow institutional protocols and work collaboratively with the healthcare team to deliver complete treatment [56–58].

12.12 Nursing Responsibilities for Chest X-Ray Examinations

The following nursing interventions and nursing care considerations are given to the patient:

12.12.1 Nursing Interventions: Before Chest X-Ray

- Make sure that all metal components are removed. Jewelry, pins, buttons, and other items might make viewing the chest difficult.
- No preparation is needed. It is not necessary to fast or restrict medication unless prescribed by a physician.
- Ensure that the patient is not pregnant or suspected of being pregnant. It is usually not recommended to take X-rays during pregnancy unless the benefits outweigh the risks.
- Assess the patient's breath-holding capacity. An X-ray can be more clearly seen if one holds their breath after inhaling.
- Provide proper clothing. In order to undergo an X-ray procedure, patients should remove all clothing up to their waists and wear an X-ray gown.
- The patient should be instructed to comply during the X-ray. Any movement would reduce the quality of the image, so the patient should remain calm [59–61].

12.12.2 Nursing Interventions: After Chest X-Ray

- No special care is required.
- Ensure patient comfort. The patient should be adjusted correctly if the chest x-ray is done at the bedside.

12.12.3 Normal Findings in a Chest X-Ray

- Normal lung fields, heart size, mediastinum, thoracic vertebra, ribs, and diaphragm

12.12.3.1 Abnormal Results in a Chest X-Ray

Chest X-rays can reveal the following abnormalities

- Atelectasis
- Bronchitis
- Cardiomegaly
- Hyperinflated lungs with flattened diaphragm
- Images of radiopaque objects lodged in the pulmonary system
- Lung infiltrates that are irregular and patchy
- Lung tumors
- An improperly positioned tube or wire
- Bones that are misaligned or broken
- Pericardial effusion
- Pericarditis
- Pleural effusion
- Pneumothorax
- Pulmonary bases, infiltrates, fibrosis
- Scoliosis
- Swollen lymph nodes
- Tuberculosis
- Widened mediastinum

12.13 Summary

- Radiology nursing is a lesser-known specialization that may not be the most intuitive career choice for nurses.
- A number of contexts are affected by them, including university medical facilities, community hospitals, and independent radiology clinics.
- Nurses play a crucial part in radiology procedures, from preparation to follow-up.

Exercise

Multiple Choice Questions (MCQs)

1. What is a major advantage of percutaneous minimally invasive procedures in radiology?
   A. Increased pain
   B. Longer hospital stays
   C. Reduced recovery time
   D. Higher cost

2. What role does a radiology nurse play during imaging procedures?
   A. Conducting surgery
   B. Administering contrast agents
   C. Operating imaging equipment
   D. Diagnosing medical conditions
3. Which organization guides the practice of radiology nurses?
   A. American Medical Association
   B. American College of Radiology
   C. World Health Organization
   D. Centers for Disease Control and Prevention
4. What is the primary responsibility of radiology nurses regarding patient safety during imaging procedures?
   A. Designing imaging equipment
   B. Monitoring vital signs
   C. Writing prescriptions
   D. Performing laboratory tests
5. What is an essential part of patient preparation for radiological procedures?
   A. Ignoring patient concerns
   B. Administering surgery
   C. Providing precise instructions
   D. Skipping medical history review
6. What is one of the primary roles of radiology nurses before a procedure?
   A. Designing imaging equipment
   B. Performing surgery
   C. Completing pre-procedure checklists
   D. Writing prescriptions
7. How do radiology nurses contribute to patient safety during imaging procedures?
   A. Operating the imaging machines
   B. Administering heavy sedation
   C. Monitoring vital signs
   D. Performing diagnostic tests
8. Which of the following is a key responsibility of radiology nurses in relation to patient care?
   A. Interpreting imaging results
   B. Offering emotional support to patients
   C. Conducting radiological research
   D. Managing hospital administration
9. What do radiology nurses do during the procedure?
   A. Operate CT scanners
   B. Perform the actual imaging
   C. Administer medications and provide comfort
   D. Diagnose medical conditions
10. How do radiology nurses help in ensuring patient comfort?
    A. By setting up imaging equipment
    B. By explaining the procedure and offering reassurance
    C. By conducting post-procedure surgeries
    D. By minimizing their contact with patients
11. What is a typical starting qualification for a radiology nurse?
    A. Master's degree in nursing
    B. Associate's degree in nursing
    C. PhD in radiology
    D. Certificate in emergency care
12. What types of situations do radiology nurses need to handle in their role?
    A. Administrative issues
    B. Routine check-ups
    C. Acute situations such as allergic reactions and cardiac arrest
    D. Surgical procedures
13. What is a key component of infection control in healthcare settings?
    A. Limiting patient access to radiology
    B. Regular staff meetings
    C. Hand hygiene and proper use of PPE
    D. Daily health check-ups for all staff
14. Which of the following is a technique used for sterilization in health care?
    A. Wet pasteurization
    B. Ethylene oxide gas
    C. 70–90% alcohol
    D. Chlorine-based products
15. In the event of a contrast reaction during a CT scan, what is one of the nurse's responsibilities?
    A. Operating the CT machine
    B. Informing the patient's family about the procedure
    C. Administering emergency medications as needed
    D. Analyzing CT scan results
16. Before a CT scan, why is it important to check a patient's NPO status?
    A. To prevent discomfort from lying down
    B. To avoid contrast media-related complications

C. To reduce the risk of aspiration
D. To ensure patient hydration

17. How long should patients with a higher risk of anaphylaxis be observed after receiving intravenous contrast?
A. 10 min
B. 15 min
C. 20 min
D. 30 min

18. What gauge intravenous cannula should be used for injections at a rate of 5 mL/second?
A. 22 g
B. 20 g
C. 18 g
D. 16 g

19. Which of the following is NOT a typical responsibility of radiology nurses during mobile radiography?
A. Patient positioning
B. Administering sedation
C. Infection control measures
D. Operating the X-ray machine

20. During a GIT procedure, what is the purpose of administering contrast media?
A. To sedate the patient
B. To visualize the digestive tract
C. To relieve discomfort
D. To increase hydration

21. What is the primary role of a radiology nurse during a fluoroscopic procedure?
A. Administering radiation
B. Performing the procedure
C. Ensuring patient safety and comfort
D. Writing the radiology report

22. Which of the following is NOT a type of radiological procedure performed under fluoroscopy?
A. Angiography
B. PEM
C. GIT fluoroscopy
D. IR

23. During mammography, what should patients be instructed to avoid to ensure accurate results?
A. Eating before the test
B. Using deodorants or powders
C. Drinking water
D. Exercising

24. What is the nurse's responsibility in the case of a patient with breast implants during mammography?
A. Remove the implants
B. Assign a junior technician
C. Ensure that a technologist familiar with imaging implants is available
D. Administer additional contrast

25. Which of the following is NOT a type of biopsy?
A. Endoscopic biopsy
B. Needle biopsy
C. FNAC biopsy
D. Radiographic biopsy

26. What is the primary purpose of providing patient education before a biopsy or FNA?
A. To obtain informed consent
B. To explain potential risks and procedures
C. To ensure patient comfort
D. To prepare the equipment

27. During a biopsy procedure, what is a critical aspect of the nurse's role in infection control?
A. Monitoring the patient's vital signs
B. Providing emotional support
C. Using stringent aseptic methods
D. Documenting the procedure

28. What should be done before a chest X-ray to ensure clear imaging?
A. Patient fasting
B. Removal of all metal components
C. Use of local anesthetics
D. Providing sedation

29. What should a nurse do if a patient is suspected to be pregnant before a chest X-ray?
A. Proceed with the X-ray without changes
B. Cancel the X-ray
C. Assess the need for the X-ray and consider alternatives
D. Provide pain relief

30. Which of the following is NOT typically found in an abnormal chest X-ray?
A. Normal lung fields
B. Pleural effusion
C. Pneumothorax
D. Cardiomegaly

Short Questions

1. Describe the responsibilities of radiology nurses in post-procedure care.
2. What skills and knowledge are crucial for a radiology nurse to provide high-quality patient care?
3. What are the responsibilities of radiology nurses after a radiological procedure?
4. How do radiology nurses act as advocates for patients during imaging procedures?
5. What are the key elements of nursing care during CT procedures?
6. Describe the role of radiology nurses in infection control and sterilization.
7. What are the key components of nursing care during GIT procedures?
8. Describe the infection control measures that should be implemented during mobile radiography.
9. Describe the purpose of administering contrast media during radiological procedures.
10. What precautions should a radiology nurse take to ensure radiation safety during fluoroscopic procedures?
11. What are the essential components of pre-procedure assessment by a nurse before a biopsy?
12. Describe the nursing interventions required for patient monitoring and observation after a biopsy procedure.

Long Questions

1. Discuss the various roles and responsibilities of radiology nurses, highlighting their importance in ensuring patient safety and effective delivery of medical imaging services.
2. Discuss the various ways in which radiology nurses impact patient care, particularly focusing on their roles before, during, and after imaging procedures.
3. Discuss the comprehensive responsibilities of radiology nurses, including their role in acute situations, infection control, and during CT procedures with contrast media. Highlight the importance of their contributions to patient safety and care.
4. Discuss the role of radiology nurses in the workflow relationship between referring doctors, medical imaging technologists, and other healthcare providers during mobile radiography. Include details on patient communication, infection control, and collaboration within the interdisciplinary team.
5. Discuss the nursing responsibilities before, during, and after mammography, highlighting the importance of patient education and safety protocols.
6. Discuss the nursing responsibilities before, during, and after a chest X-ray examination, emphasizing patient safety and communication.

Answers for MCQ

1. C. Reduced recovery time
2. B. Administering contrast agents
3. B. American College of Radiology
4. B. Monitoring vital signs
5. C. Providing precise instructions
6. C. Completing pre-procedure checklists
7. C. Monitoring vital signs
8. B. Offering emotional support to patients
9. C. Administer medications and provide comfort
10. B. By explaining the procedure and offering reassurance
11. B. Associate's degree in nursing
12. C. Acute situations such as allergic reactions and cardiac arrest
13. C. Hand hygiene and proper use of PPE
14. B. Ethylene oxide gas
15. C. Administering emergency medications as needed
16. C. To reduce the risk of aspiration
17. D. 30 min
18. B. 20 g
19. D. Operating the X-ray machine
20. B. To visualize the digestive tract
21. C. Ensuring patient safety and comfort
22. B. PEM
23. B. Using deodorants or powders

24. C. Ensure a technologist familiar with imaging implants is available
25. D. Radiographic biopsy
26. B. To explain potential risks and procedures
27. C. Using stringent aseptic methods
28. B. Removal of all metal components
29. C. Assess the need for the X-ray and consider alternatives
30. A. Normal lung fields

References

1. Blevins SJ. The role of the radiology nurse. Radiol Manage. 1994;16(4):46–8.
2. Cadet MJ. What is the role of the quality improvement radiology nurse? J Radiol Nurs. 2021;40(4):339–44.
3. Jones AK, Ramirez JA. The role of the radiology nurse in managing radiation dose during fluoroscopically guided interventional procedures. J Radiol Nurs. 2022;41:201.
4. Dickinson J. The essentials of expert witnessing for the radiology nurse. J Radiol Nurs. 2015;34(1):8.
5. Othman K, Arabi M. Radiology nursing Saudi career development program: single center experience. J Radiol Nurs. 2023;42(1):136.
6. Hardy M, Barrett C. Interpretation of trauma radiographs by radiographers and nurses in the UK: a comparative study. Br J Radiol. 2004;77(920):657.
7. Collette CL. Understanding patients' needs is the foundation of perioperative nursing. AORN J. 2000;71(3):629.
8. Archibong U, Dunn A, Hepworth D, Kenworthy D, Milner SC. Filling the gap: a research-based radiological awareness programme for nurses. Clin Eff Nurs. 2001;5(4):152.
9. Askari-Majdabadi H, Valinejadi A, Mohammadpour A, Bouraghi H, Abbasy Z, Alaei S. Use of health information technology in patients care management: a mixed methods study in Iran. Acta Inform Med. 2019;27(5):311.
10. Benabbas R, Hanna M, Shah J, Sinert R. Diagnostic accuracy of history, physical examination, laboratory tests, and point-of-care ultrasound for pediatric acute appendicitis in the emergency department: a systematic review and meta-analysis. Acad Emerg Med. 2017;24(5):523–51.
11. Jaspan O, Wysocka A, Sanchez C, Schweitzer AD. Improving the relationship between confidence and competence: implications for diagnostic radiology training from the psychology and medical literature. Acad Radiol. 2022;29:428.
12. Rockall AG, Justich C, Helbich T, Vilgrain V. Patient communication in radiology: moving up the agenda. Eur J Radiol. 2022;155:155.
13. Bwanga O, Chanda E, Mwale A, Maliti BK. Radiology nursing: a little-known speciality in Zambia. South Asian Res J Nurs Healthc. 2020;2(4):56.
14. Aita V, Dodendorf DM, Lebsack JA, Tallia AF, Crabtree BF. Patient care staffing patterns and roles in community-based family practices. J Fam Pract. 2001;50(10):889.
15. Jalal S, Parker W, Ferguson D, Nicolaou S. Exploring the role of artificial intelligence in an emergency and trauma radiology department. Can Assoc Radiol J. 2021;72:167.
16. Andersson BT, Fridlund B, Elgán C, Axelsson ÅB. Radiographers' areas of professional competence related to good nursing care. Scand J Caring Sci. 2008;22(3):401–9.
17. Duszak R, Walls DG, Wang JM, Hemingway J, Hughes DR, Small WC, et al. Expanding roles of nurse practitioners and physician assistants as providers of nonvascular invasive radiology procedures. J Am Coll Radiol. 2015;12(3):284.
18. Kuhlman M, Meyer M, Krupinski EA. Direct reporting of results to patients. The future of radiology? Acad Radiol. 2012;19(6):646.
19. Holbrook K, Greene R. Patient care in radiography by Ruth Ann Ehrlich and Ellen Doble McCloskey St. Louis. Magn Reson Imaging. 1994;12(8):311.
20. Mohapatra S. Sterilization and disinfection. In: Essentials of neuroanesthesia. Academic Press; 2017.
21. Taneja N, Emmanuel R, Chari PS, Sharma M. A prospective study of hospital-acquired infections in burn patients at a tertiary care referral Centre in North India. Burns. 2004;30(7):665.
22. Stützle H, Puhlmann M, Kessler S, Schweiberer L. Sterilization of partially demineralized bone matrix: the effects of different sterilization techniques on osteogenetic properties. J Surg Res. 1995;59(5):614.
23. Coupal TM, Buckley AR, Bhalla S, Li JL, Ho SGF, Holmes A, et al. Management of acute contrast reactions—understanding radiologists' preparedness and the efficacy of simulation-based training in Canada. Can Assoc Radiol J. 2018;69(4):349.
24. Kim MH, Park CH, Kim DI, Kim KM, Kim HK, Lim KH, et al. Surveillance of contrast-media-induced hypersensitivity reactions using signals from an electronic medical recording system. Ann Allergy Asthma Immunol. 2012;108(3):167.
25. Moyo M. Radiology nursing: a growing specialty, vol. 14. Am Nurse Today; 2019. p. 73–5.
26. Shin J, Yun S, Jin S, Noh GO. Developing an evidence-based nursing protocol using early epinephrine administration for anaphylaxis caused by computed tomography contrast agents. J Radiol Nurs. 2021;40(4):357.
27. Khalid Alshamrani KA. Radiation safety while providing bedside care during portable radiog-raphy procedures: knowledge and awareness of respiratory therapists and ICU nurses. J King Abdulaziz Univ Eng Sci. 2022;32(1):25.
28. Leong CS, Cascade PN, Kazerooni EA, Bolling SF, Deeb GM. Bedside chest radiography as part of a

postcardiac surgery critical care pathway: a means of decreasing utilization without adverse clinical impact. Crit Care Med. 2000;28(2):383.
29. Audin CR, Aran S, Muse VV, Abbott GF, Ackman JB, Sharma A, et al. Bedside chest radiographs in the intensive care setting: wireless direct radiography compared to computed radiography. Curr Probl Diagn Radiol. 2018;47(6):397.
30. Peris A, Tutino L, Zagli G, Batacchi S, Cianchi G, Spina R, et al. The use of point-of-care bedside lung ultrasound significantly reduces the number of radiographs and computed tomography scans in critically ill patients. Anesth Analg. 2010;111(3):687.
31. Alrajab S, Youssef AM, Akkus NI, Caldito G. Pleural ultrasonography versus chest radiography for the diagnosis of pneumothorax: review of the literature and meta-analysis. Crit Care. 2013;17(5):R208.
32. Chiang HW, Liu YL, Chen TR, Chen CL, Chiang HJ, Chao SY. Scattered radiation doses absorbed by technicians at different distances from X-ray exposure: experiments on prosthesis. Biomed Mater Eng. 2015;26:26.
33. Azimi H, Teimouri ZM, Mousavi S, Leyli hsan KN, Jafaraghaee F. Individual protection adopted by ICU nurses against radiation and its related factors. J Holist Nurs Midwifery. 2018;28(1):18–25.
34. Acauan LV, Seda JM, Silva SC, Paes GO, Trotte LA, Stipp MA. The performance of the nursing team in outpatient radiology and diagnostic imaging services. Rev Gauch Enferm. 2022;43:43.
35. Vealé BL, Wagner JB. Changes in shielding practice for radiographers—implications for radiologic and imaging nursing. J Radiol Nurs. 2021;40(4):353–6.
36. Laukhuf G, Myrthil M, Cramer SJ. Joint Association for Radiologic and Imaging Nursing, radiologic nursing certification board, and radiologic nursing certification task force position paper: the value of certification in radiologic nursing. J Radiol Nurs. 2015;34:157.
37. Menon Murali K. Technician who got stuck to MRI machine in Mumbai hospital gets Rs 1 cr [Internet]. 2017 [cited 2018 Nov 26]. Available from: https://bangaloremirror.indiatimes.com/news/india/technician-who-got-stuck-to-mri-machine-in-mumbai-hospital-gets-rs-1-cr/articleshow/56976834.cms.
38. Anderson TJ, Erdmann AL, Backes MTS. Nursing care management in radiation protection in interventional radiology. Rev Gauch Enferm. 2022;43:43.
39. Neumann DA, DeLegge MH. Gastric versus small-bowel tube feeding in the intensive care unit: a prospective comparison of efficacy. Crit Care Med. 2002;30(7):1436.
40. Queiroz CG, Duarte FH, Sarmento SD, Dantas JK, Dantas DV, Dantas RA. Gastrointestinal tube insertion techniques in critical patients: scoping review. Texto e Contexto Enfermagem. 2021;30:e20210017.
41. Wang Y, Zhang J, Ma X, Bi C, Gao H. Swallowing function and neuropsychological status in patients with dysphagia after stroke: literature review and nursing intervention. Int J Clin Exp Med. 2023;16(1):1–7.
42. Fernández-Feito A, Lana A, Cabello-Gutiérrez L, Franco-Correia S, Baldonedo-Cernuda R, Mosteiro-Díaz P. Face-to-face information and emotional support from trained nurses reduce pain during screening mammography: results from a randomized controlled trial. Pain Manag Nurs. 2015;16(6):862–70.
43. Sinclair P, Kable A, Levett-Jones T. The effectiveness of internet-based e-learning on clinician behavior and patient outcomes: a systematic review protocol. Int J Nurs Stud. JBI database of systematic reviews and implementation reports. 2015;13:52.
44. DeLano N, Lane S, De Mayo M. Implementing a breast screening assessment tool in the inpatient setting ...Academy of Oncology Nurse & Patient Navigators, November 17–20, 2016, Las Vegas, Nevada J Oncol Navig Surviv 2016;7(9).
45. Venkataraman S. Breast imaging for cancer screening: mammography and ultrasonography. Uptodate; 2015.
46. Jerome-D'Emilia B, Suplee PD, Akincigil A. Validation of the Spanish version of the mammography-specific self-efficacy scale. Oncol Nurs Forum. 2015;42(3):E279.
47. Larsson LG, Andersson I, Bjurstam N, Fagerberg G, Frisell J, Tabár L, et al. Updated overview of the Swedish randomized trials on breast cancer screening with mammography: age group 40–49 at randomization. J Natl Cancer Inst Monogr. 1997;22:57.
48. Larsson LG, Nyström L, Wall S, Rutqvist L, Andersson I, Bjurstam N, et al. The Swedish randomised mammography screening trials: analysis of their effect on the breast cancer related excess mortality. J Med Screen. 1996;3(3):129.
49. Nyström L, Wall S, Rutqvist LE, Lindgren A, Lindqvist M, Rydén S, et al. Breast cancer screening with mammography: overview of Swedish randomised trials. Lancet. 1993;341(8851):973.
50. Nystrom L, Rutqvist LE, Wall S, Lindgren A, Lindqvist M, Ryden S, et al. Breast cancer screening with mammography.: overview of Swedish randomised trials [see comments] [published erratum appears in Lancet 1993 Nov 27;342(8883):1372]. Lancet. 1993;341(8851):973.
51. Nyström L, Andersson I, Bjurstam N, Frisell J, Nordenskjöld B, Rutqvist LE. Long-term effects of mammography screening: updated overview of the Swedish randomised trials. Lancet. 2002;359(9310):909.
52. Sugimoto Y, Ito Y, Shimokawa T, Shiozaki Y, Mazaki T. Percutaneous screw fixation for traumatic spondylolisthesis of the axis using iso-c3d fluoroscopy-assisted navigation (case report). Minim Invasive Neurosurg. 2010;53(2):83.
53. Lin MG, Wei FL, Yi XY, Yu L. The nursing care for patients receiving percutaneous fluoroscopy-guided gastrostomy for treatment of dysphagia caused by head and neck cancer. J Interv Radiol. 2014;23(7):637–9.

54. Lin M, Wei F, Yi X, Yu L. The nursing care for patients receiving percutaneous fluoroscopy-guided gastrostomy for treatment of dysphagia caused by head and neck cancer. J Interv Radiol. 2014;23(7):637–9.
55. Askey J, Clements W. A single-center experience of fluoroscopic-guided peripherally inserted central catheter insertion by nursing staff: rationale and clinical outcomes. J Radiol Nurs. 2019;38(3):155.
56. Kwok CS, Naneishvili T, Curry S, Aston C, Beeston M, Chell S, et al. Description and development of a nurse-led cardiac assessment team. Futur Healthc J. 2020;7(1):78.
57. Hooper KP, Anstey MH, Litton E. Safety and efficacy of routine diagnostic test reduction interventions in patients admitted to the intensive care unit: a systematic review and meta-analysis. Anaesth Intensive Care. 2021;49:23.
58. Mohammadpour A, Mohammadian B, Basiri Moghadam M, Nematollahi MR. The effects of topical heat therapy on chest pain in patients with acute coronary syndrome: a randomised double-blind placebo-controlled clinical trial. J Clin Nurs. 2014;23(23–24):3460–7.
59. Ganapathy A, Adhikari NKJ, Spiegelman J, Scales DC. Routine chest x-rays in intensive care units: a systematic review and meta-analysis. Crit Care. 2012;16(2):R68.
60. Johnson M, Goodacre S, Tod A, Read S. Patients' opinions of acute chest pain care: a qualitative evaluation of chest pain units. J Adv Nurs. 2009;65(1):120.
61. Siebens K, Moons P, De Geest S, Miljoen H, Drew BJ, Vrints C. The role of nurses in a chest pain unit. Eur J Cardiovasc Nurs. 2007;6(4):265.